WITHDRAWN

LIVERPOOL JMU LIBRARY

3 1111 01467 2990

SIDE EFFECTS OF DRUGS ANNUAL

VOLUME 37

Side Effects of Drugs Annual

Volume 37

Honorary Editor

Prof. M.N.G. Dukes, Oslo, Norway

SIDE EFFECTS OF DRUGS ANNUAL

VOLUME 37

A worldwide yearly survey of new data
in adverse drug reactions

Editor

SIDHARTHA D. RAY, PhD., FACN
Manchester University College of Pharmacy, USA

Associate Editors

JOSHUA P. GRAY, PhD.
United States Coast Guard Academy, USA

MARY E. KIERSMA, PharmD, PhD.
Accreditation Council for Pharmacy Education (ACPE), USA

ELSEVIER AMSTERDAM • BOSTON • HEIDELBERG • LONDON • NEW YORK • OXFORD
PARIS • SAN DIEGO • SAN FRANCISCO • SINGAPORE • SYDNEY • TOKYO

Elsevier
Radarweg 29, PO Box 211, 1000 AE Amsterdam, Netherlands
The Boulevard, Langford Lane, Kidlington, Oxford OX5 1GB, UK
225 Wyman Street, Waltham, MA 02451, USA

First edition 2015

Copyright © 2015 Elsevier B.V. All rights reserved

No part of this publication may be reproduced or transmitted in any form or by any means, electronic or mechanical, including photocopying, recording, or any information storage and retrieval system, without permission in writing from the publisher. Details on how to seek permission, further information about the Publisher's permissions policies and our arrangements with organizations such as the Copyright Clearance Center and the Copyright Licensing Agency, can be found at our website: www.elsevier.com/permissions.

This book and the individual contributions contained in it are protected under copyright by the Publisher (other than as may be noted herein).

Notices
Knowledge and best practice in this field are constantly changing. As new research and experience broaden our understanding, changes in research methods, professional practices, or medical treatment may become necessary.

Practitioners and researchers must always rely on their own experience and knowledge in evaluating and using any information, methods, compounds, or experiments described herein. In using such information or methods they should be mindful of their own safety and the safety of others, including parties for whom they have a professional responsibility.

To the fullest extent of the law, neither the Publisher nor the authors, contributors, or editors, assume any liability for any injury and/or damage to persons or property as a matter of products liability, negligence or otherwise, or from any use or operation of any methods, products, instructions, or ideas contained in the material herein.

ISBN: 978-0-444-63525-9
ISSN: 0378-6080

For information on all Elsevier publications
visit our website at http://store.elsevier.com/

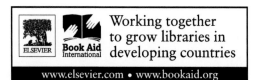

Working together
to grow libraries in
developing countries

www.elsevier.com • www.bookaid.org

Contributors

Nazeer Ahmed Department of Pharmacy, Johns Hopkins Bayview Medical Center, Baltimore, MD, USA

A. Ali Campbell University College of Pharmacy and Health Sciences, Buies Creek, NC, USA

G. Baker University of Alberta, Edmonton, AB, Canada

Robert D. Beckett Drug Information Center, Manchester University College of Pharmacy, Fort Wayne, IN, USA

Nicholas T. Bello Department of Animal Sciences, School of Environmental and Biological Sciences, Rutgers, The State University of New Jersey, New Brunswick, NJ, USA

Adrienne T. Black 3E Company, Carlsbad, CA, and Institute of Public Health, New York Medical College, Valhalla, NY, USA

Kristien Boelaert Centre for Endocrinology, Diabetes and Metabolism, University of Birmingham, Birmingham, United Kingdom

Alison Brophy Clinical Assistant Professor, Rutgers, the State University of New Jersey, Piscataway, and Critical Care Clinical Pharmacist, Saint Barnabas Medical Center, Livingston, NJ, USA

Santos Castañeda Department of Rheumatology, IIS-IPrincesa, Hospital Universitario de La Princesa, Madrid, Spain

Peter R. Chai Division of Medical Toxicology, Department of Emergency Medicine, University of Massachusetts Medical School, Worcester, MA, USA

K. Chan The National Institute of Complementary Medicine, University of Western Sydney, Penrith, NSW, Australia

Saira B. Chaudhry Ernest Mario School of Pharmacy, Rutgers University, The State University of New Jersey, Piscataway, New Jersey and Jersey Shore University Medical Center, Neptune, New Jersey

Vasileios Chortis Centre for Endocrinology, Diabetes and Metabolism, University of Birmingham, Birmingham, United Kingdom

P. Chue University of Alberta, Edmonton, AB, Canada

Stephen Curran Fieldhead Hospital, South West Yorkshire Partnership NHS Foundation Trust, Wakefield, United Kingdom

K.M. Damer Butler University College of Pharmacy and Health Sciences, Indianapolis, IN, USA

Gwyneth A. Davies Swansea University Medical School, Swansea, United Kingdom

Rahul Deshmukh Department of Pharmaceutical Sciences, Rosalind Franklin University of Medicine and Science, College of Pharmacy, North Chicago, IL, USA

A. Dethloff Saint Joseph Regional Medical Center, Mishawaka, IN, USA

Sujana Dontukurthy Department of Anesthesiology, New York Methodist Hospital, Brooklyn, NY, USA

Alisa K. Escaño Department of Pharmacotherapy & Outcomes Science, Virginia Commonwealth University School of Pharmacy, Falls Church, VA, USA

K. Evoy Saint Joseph Regional Medical Center, Mishawaka, IN, USA

Jingyang Fan SIUE School of Pharmacy, Edwardsville, IL, USA

Swaran J.S. Flora Drug Discovery and Regulatory Toxicology Division, Defence Research and Development Establishment, Gwalior, India

Lynn Frendak Department of Pharmacy, Johns Hopkins Bayview Medical Center, Baltimore, MD, USA

Rebecca Gale Anaesthesia and Critical Care, Royal Liverpool Hospital, Liverpool, United Kingdom

Jason C. Gallagher Temple University, Philadelphia, PA, USA

Jayan George Swansea University Medical School, Swansea, United Kingdom

Tatsuya Gomi Department of Radiology, Ohashi Medical Center, Toho University, Tokyo, Japan

Joshua P. Gray Department of Science, United States Coast Guard Academy, New London, CT, USA

Matthew K. Griswold Division of Medical Toxicology, Department of Emergency Medicine, University of Massachusetts Medical School, Worcester, MA, USA

Alison Hall Anaesthesia and Critical Care, Royal Liverpool Hospital, Liverpool, United Kingdom

Makoto Hasegawa Department of Radiology, Ohashi Medical Center, Toho University, Tokyo, Japan

J. Helmen Saint Joseph Regional Medical Center, Mishawaka, IN, USA

Gary L. Hite Department of Pharmaceutical Sciences, Manchester University College of Pharmacy, Fort Wayne, IN, USA

Lokesh K. Jha Sanford Center for Digestive Disease, Sanford Health, Sioux Falls, SD, USA

C.M. Jung Butler University College of Pharmacy and Health Sciences, and Eskenazi Health, Indianapolis, IN, USA

Allison Kalstein Department of Anesthesiology, New York Methodist Hospital, Brooklyn, NY, USA

Abigail Kay Department of Psychiatry and Human Behavior-Division of Substance Abuse, Thomas Jefferson University Hospital, Philadelphia, PA, USA

Sipan Keshishyan Department of Pharmaceutical Sciences, Manchester University College of Pharmacy, Fort Wayne, IN, USA

M.K. Kharel School of Pharmacy and Health Professions, University of Maryland Eastern Shore, Princess Anne, MD, USA

Catherine Kiruthi Department of Pharmacy, Johns Hopkins Bayview Medical Center, Baltimore, MD, USA

Justin D. Kreuter Department of Laboratory Medicine and Pathology, Mayo Clinic, Rochester, MN, USA

Dirk W. Lachenmeier Chemisches und Veterinäruntersuchungsamt (CVUA) Karlsruhe, Karlsruhe, Germany

Ashakumary Lakshmikuttyamma Department of Pharmaceutical Sciences, Jefferson College of Pharmacy, Thomas Jefferson University Hospital, Philadelphia, PA, USA

Lucia Rivera Lara Departments of Neurology, Anesthesiology, and Critical Care Medicine, Johns Hopkins Medicine, Baltimore, MD, USA

R. Latini Department of Cardiovascular Research, IRCCS-Istituto di Ricerche Farmacologiche Mario Negri, Milan, Italy

L. Lim Purdue University, West Lafayette, IN, USA

Z.X. Lin School of Chinese Medicine, Faculty of Medicine, The Chinese University of Hong Kong, Shatin, N.T., Hong Kong SAR, PR China

Mei T. Liu Ernest Mario School of Pharmacy at Rutgers, The State University of New Jersey, Piscataway, NJ, USA

Alicia G. Lydecker Division of Medical Toxicology, Department of Emergency Medicine, University of Massachusetts Medical School, Worcester, MA, USA

C.M. Maffeo Butler University College of Pharmacy and Health Sciences, Indianapolis, IN, USA

Arduino A. Mangoni Department of Clinical Pharmacology, School of Medicine, Flinders University and Flinders Medical Centre, Bedford Park, SA, Australia

Megan E. Maroney Ernest Mario School of Pharmacy at Rutgers, The State University of New Jersey, Piscataway, NJ, USA

Ashley Martinelli Department of Pharmacy, Johns Hopkins Bayview Medical Center, Baltimore, MD, USA

Cassandra Maynard SIUE School of Pharmacy, Edwardsville, IL, USA

Dayna S. McManus Department of Pharmacy Services, Inova Farifax Hospital, Falls Church, VA, USA

Calvin J. Meaney Department of Pharmacy Practice, School of Pharmacy and Pharmaceutical Sciences, State University of New York at Buffalo, Buffalo, NY, USA

Tahir Mehmood Department of Laboratory Medicine and Pathology, Mayo Clinic, Rochester, MN, USA

Marta Martín Millán Department of Internal Medicine, IFIMAV, Hospital Universitario Marqués de Valdecilla, Santander, Cantabria, Spain

Philip B. Mitchell School of Psychiatry, University of New South Wales, and Black Dog Institute, Sydney, NSW, Australia

Vicky V. Mody Associate Professor of Pharmaceutical Sciences, PCOM School of Pharmacy, Suwanee, GA, USA

Sandeep Mukherjee Creighton University Medical Center, Omaha, NE, USA

Shabir Musa Fieldhead Hospital, South West Yorkshire Partnership NHS Foundation Trust, Wakefield, United Kingdom

Toshio Nakaki Department of Pharmacology, Teikyo University School of Medicine, Tokyo, Japan

Anjan Nan Department of Pharmaceutical Sciences, University of Maryland Eastern Shore School of Pharmacy, Princess Anne, MD, USA

D. Nguyen Baylor College of Medicine, Houston, TX, USA

A. Nobili Department of Neuroscience, IRCCS-Istituto di Ricerche Farmacologiche Mario Negri, Milan, Italy

John D. Noti Allergy and Clinical Immunology Branch, Health Effects Laboratory Division, National Institute for Occupational Safety and Health, Centers for Disease Control and Prevention, Morgantown, WV, USA

Igho J. Onakpoya Nuffield Department of Primary Care Health Sciences, Oxford, United Kingdom

Yekaterina Opsha Rutgers, the State University of New Jersey, Piscataway, and Saint Barnabas Medical Center, Livingston, NJ, USA

Sreekumar Othumpangat Allergy and Clinical Immunology Branch, Health Effects Laboratory Division, National Institute for Occupational Safety and Health, Centers for Disease Control and Prevention, Morgantown, WV, USA

Vidhu Pachauri Drug Discovery and Regulatory Toxicology Division, Defence Research and Development Establishment, Gwalior, India

L. Pasina Department of Neuroscience, IRCCS-Istituto di Ricerche Farmacologiche Mario Negri, Milan, Italy

Michelle M. Peahota Infectious Diseases, Thomas Jefferson University Hospital, Philadelphia, PA, USA

Alyssa N. Petry Department of Pharmaceutical Sciences, Manchester University College of Pharmacy, Fort Wayne, IN, USA

Alan Polnariev VA Healthcare System, East Orange, NJ, and College of Pharmacy, University of Florida, Gainesville, FL, USA

H. Raber Saint Joseph Regional Medical Center, Mishawaka, IN, USA

Sidhartha D. Ray Department of Pharmaceutical Sciences, Manchester University College of Pharmacy, Fort Wayne, IN, USA

David Reeves Department of Pharmacy Practice, College of Pharmacy and Health Sciences, Butler University, Indianapolis, IN, USA

Lucia Rose Infectious Diseases, Cooper University Hospital, One Cooper Plaza, Camden, NJ, USA

Amir Sajjadi St Mary's House, St Mary's Road, Leeds and York Partnerships-NHS Foundation Trust, Leeds, West Yorkshire, United Kingdom

Karin Sandoval Department of Pharmaceutical Sciences, School of Pharmacy, Southern Illinois University Edwardsville, Edwardsville, IL, USA

Vikas Sehdev Division of Pharmaceutical Sciences, Arnold & Marie Schwartz College of Pharmacy and Health Sciences, Long Island University, Brooklyn, NY, USA

Mona U. Shah Department of Pharmacy, Inova Fairfax Hospital, Falls Church, VA, USA

Samit Shah Department of Biopharmaceutical Sciences, KGI School of Pharmacy, Claremont, CA, USA

E. Sheridan Saint Joseph Regional Medical Center, Mishawaka, IN, USA

Ajay N. Singh Department of Pharmaceutical Sciences, South University School of Pharmacy, Appalachian College of Pharmacy, Oakwood, VA, USA

Thomas R. Smith Manchester University College of Pharmacy, Fort Wayne, IN, USA

Jonathan Smithson School of Psychiatry, University of New South Wales, and Black Dog Institute, Sydney, NSW, Australia

Brian Spoelhof Department of Pharmacy, Johns Hopkins Bayview Medical Center, Baltimore, MD, USA

Shehnoor Tarique Swansea University Medical School, Swansea, United Kingdom

Michelle J. Taylor Department of Laboratory Medicine and Pathology, Mayo Clinic, Rochester, MN, USA

F.R. Tejada School of Pharmacy and Health Professions, University of Maryland Eastern Shore, Princess Anne, MD, USA

Scott Thurston Department of Pharmaceutical Sciences, Manchester University College of Pharmacy, Fort Wayne, IN, USA

A.R. Walk School of Pharmacy and Health Professions, University of Maryland Eastern Shore, Princess Anne, MD, USA

Andrea L. Wilhite Manchester University College of Pharmacy, Fort Wayne, IN, USA

Ken Witt Department of Pharmaceutical Sciences, School of Pharmacy, Southern Illinois University Edwardsville, Edwardsville, IL, USA

Joel Yarmush Department of Anesthesiology, New York Methodist Hospital, Brooklyn, NY, USA

H.W. Zhang School of Chinese Medicine, Faculty of Medicine, The Chinese University of Hong Kong, Shatin, N.T., Hong Kong SAR, PR China

Contents

Preface

Side Effects of Drugs: Annual (*SEDA*) is a yearly publication focused on existing, new and evolving side effects of drugs encountered by a broad range of healthcare professionals including physicians, pharmacists, nurse practitioners and advisors of poison control centres. This 37th edition of *SEDA* includes analyses of the side effects of drugs using both clinical trials and case-based principles which include encounters identified during bedside clinical practice over the 18 months since the previous edition. *SEDA* seeks to summarize the entire body of relevant medical literature into a single volume with dual goals of being comprehensive and of identifying emerging trends and themes in medicine as related to side effects and adverse drug effects (ADEs).

With a broad range of topics authored by practising clinicians and scientists, *SEDA* is a comprehensive and reliable reference to be used in clinical practice. The majority of the chapters include relevant case studies that are not only peer-reviewed but also have a forward-looking, learning-based focus suitable for practitioners as well as students in training. The nationally and internationally known contributors believe this educational resource can be used to stimulate an active learning environment in a variety of settings. Each chapter in this volume has been reviewed by the editors, experienced clinical educators, actively practising clinicians and scientists to ensure the accuracy and timeliness of the information. The overall objective is to provide a framework for further understanding the intellectual approaches in analysing the implications of the case studies and their appropriateness when dispensing medications, as well as interpreting adverse drug reactions (ADRs), toxicity and outcomes resulting from medication errors.

This issue of *SEDA* is the first to include concepts from pharmacogenomics/pharmacogenetics and personalized medicine. Due to the advances in science, the genetic profiles of patients must be considered in the aetiology of side effects, especially for medications provided to very large populations. This marks the first phase of genome-based personalized medicine, in which side effects of common medications are linked to polymorphisms in one or more genes. A focus on personalized medicine should lead to major advances for patient care and awareness among clinicians to deliver the most effective medication for the patient. This modality should considerably improve 'appropriate medication use' and enable the clinicians to predetermine 'the good versus the bad responders', and help reduce ADRs. Overall, clinicians will have a better control on 'predictability and preventability' of ADEs induced by certain medications. Over time, it is anticipated that pharmacogenetics and personalized medicine will become an integral part of the practice sciences. *SEDA* will continue to highlight the genetic basis of side effects in future editions.

The collective wisdom, expertise and experience of the editors, authors and reviewers were vital in the creation of a volume of this breadth. Reviewing the appropriateness, timeliness and organization of this edition consumed an enormous amount of energy by the authors, reviewers and the editorial team, which we hope will facilitate the flow of information both inter-professionally among health practitioners, professionals in training and students, and will ultimately improve patient care. Scanning for accuracy, rebuilding and reorganizing information between each edition is not an easy task; therefore, the editors have the difficult task of accepting or rejecting information. The editorial team will consider this undertaking worthwhile if this publication helps to provide better patient care; fulfils the needs of the healthcare professionals in sorting out side effects of medications, medication errors or adverse events; and stimulates interest among those working and studying medicine, pharmacy, nursing, physical therapy and chiropractic medicine, and those working in the basic therapeutic arms of pharmacology, toxicology, medicinal chemistry and pathophysiology.

Editors of this volume gratefully acknowledge the leadership provided by the former editor Prof. J. K. Aronson, all the contributors and reviewers, and will continue to maintain the legacy of this publication by building on their hard work. The editors would also like to extend special thanks for the excellent support and assistance provided by Ms. Zoe Kruz (Publisher, serials and series) and Ms. Sarah Lay (Senior Editorial Project Manager) during the compilation of this work.

Sidhartha D. Ray
Editor
Joshua P. Gray
Associate Editor
Mary E. Kiersma
Associate Editor

Special Reviews in SEDA 37

Table of Essays, Annuals 1–36

Abbreviations

The following abbreviations are used throughout the SEDA series.

2,4-DMA	2,4-Dimethoxyamfetamine
3,4-DMA	3,4-Dimethoxyamfetamine
3TC	Lamivudine (dideoxythiacytidine)
ADHD	Attention deficit hyperactivity disorder
ADP	Adenosine diphosphate
ANA	Antinuclear antibody
ANCA	Antineutrophil cytoplasmic antibody
aP	Acellular pertussis
APACHE	Acute physiology and chronic health evaluation (score)
aPTT	Activated partial thromboplastin time
ASA	American Society of Anesthesiologists
ASCA	*Anti-Saccharomyces cerevisiae* antibody
AUC	The area under the concentration versus time curve from zero to infinity
$AUC_{0\to x}$	The area under the concentration versus time curve from zero to time x
$AUC_{0\to t}$	The area under the concentration versus time curve from zero to the time of the last sample
AUC_τ	The area under the concentration versus time curve during a dosage interval
AVA	Anthrax vaccine adsorbed
AZT	Zidovudine (azidothymidine)
BCG	Bacillus Calmette Guérin
bd	Twice a day (bis in die)
BIS	Bispectral index
BMI	Body mass index
CAPD	Continuous ambulatory peritoneal dialysis
CD [4, 8, etc]	Cluster of differentiation (describing various glycoproteins that are expressed on the surfaces of T cells, B cells and other cells, with varying functions)
CI	Confidence interval
C_{max}	Maximum (peak) concentration after a dose
$C_{ss.max}$	Maximum (peak) concentration after a dose at steady state
$C_{ss.min}$	Minimum (trough) concentration after a dose at steady state
COX-1 and COX-2	Cyclo-oxygenase enzyme isoforms 1 and 2
CT	Computed tomography
CYP (e.g. CYP2D6, CYP3A4)	Cytochrome P450 isoenzymes
D4T	Stavudine (didehydrodideoxythmidine)
DDC	Zalcitabine (dideoxycytidine)
DDI	Didanosine (dideoxyinosine)
DMA	Dimethoxyamfetamine; *see also* 2,4-DMA, 3,4-DMA
DMMDA	2,5-Dimethoxy-3,4-methylenedioxyamfetamine
DMMDA-2	2,3-Dimethoxy-4,5-methylenedioxyamfetamine
DTaP	Diphtheria + tetanus toxoids + acellular pertussis
DTaP-Hib-IPV-HB	Diphtheria + tetanus toxoids + acellular pertussis + IPV + Hib + hepatitis B (hexavalent vaccine)
DT-IPV	Diphtheria + tetanus toxoids + inactivated polio vaccine
DTP	Diphtheria + tetanus toxoids + pertussis vaccine
DTwP	Diphtheria + tetanus toxoids + whole cell pertussis
eGFR	Estimated glomerular filtration rate
ESR	Erythrocyte sedimentation rate
FDA	(US) Food and Drug Administration
FEV_1	Forced expiratory volume in 1 s
FTC	Emtricitabine
FVC	Forced vital capacity
G6PD	Glucose-6-phosphate dehydrogenase
GSH	Glutathione
GST	Glutathione S-transferase
HAV	Hepatitis A virus
HbA_{1c}	Hemoglobin A_{1c}
HbOC	Conjugated Hib vaccine (Hib capsular antigen polyribosylphosphate covalently linked to the nontoxic diphtheria toxin variant CRM197)
HBV	Hepatitis B virus

HDL, LDL, VLDL	High-density lipoprotein, low-density lipoprotein, and very low density lipoprotein (cholesterol)
Hib	*Haemophilus influenzae* type b
HIV	Human immunodeficiency virus
hplc	High-performance liquid chromatography
HPV	Human papilloma virus
HR	Hazard ratio
HZV	Herpes zoster virus vaccine
ICER	Incremental cost-effectiveness ratio
Ig (IgA, IgE, IgM)	Immunoglobulin (A, E, M)
IGF	Insulin-like growth factor
INN	International Nonproprietary Name (rINN = recommended; pINN = provisional)
INR	International normalized ratio
IPV	Inactivated polio vaccine
IQ [range], IQR	Interquartile [range]
JE	Japanese encephalitis vaccine
LABA	Long-acting beta-adrenoceptor agonist
MAC	Minimum alveolar concentration
MCV4	4-valent (Serogroups A, C, W, Y) meningococcal Conjugate vaccine
MDA	3,4-Methylenedioxyamfetamine
MDI	Metered-dose inhaler
MDMA	3,4-Methylenedioxymetamfetamine
MenB	Monovalent serogroup B meningoccocal vaccine
MenC	Monovalent serogroup C meningoccocal conjugate vaccine
MIC	Minimum inhibitory concentration
MIM	Mendelian Inheritance in Man (see http://www.ncbi.nlm.nih.gov/omim/607686)
MMDA	3-Methoxy-4,5-methylenedioxyamfetamine
MMDA-2	2-Methoxy-4,5-methylendioxyamfetamine
MMDA-3a	2-Methoxy-3,4-methylenedioxyamfetamine
MMR	Measles + mumps + rubella
MMRV	Measles + mumps + rubella + varicella
MPSV4	4-Valent (serogroups A, C, W, Y) meningococcal polysaccharide vaccine
MR	Measles + rubella vaccine
MRI	Magnetic resonance imaging
NMS	Neuroleptic malignant syndrome
NNRTI	Non-nucleoside analogue reverse transcriptase inhibitor
NNT, NNT_B, NNT_H	Number needed to treat (for benefit, for harm)
NRTI	Nucleoside analogue reverse transcriptase inhibitor
NSAIDs	Nonsteroidal anti-inflammatory drugs
od	Once a day (omne die)
OMIM	Online Mendelian Inheritance in Man (see http://www.ncbi.nlm.nih.gov/omim/607686)
OPV	Oral polio vaccine
OR	Odds ratio
OROS	Osmotic-release oral system
PCR	Polymerase chain reaction
PMA	Paramethoxyamfetamine
PMMA	Paramethoxymetamfetamine
PPAR	Peroxisome proliferator-activated receptor
ppb	Parts per billion
PPD	Purified protein derivative
ppm	Parts per million
PRP-CRM	*See* HbOC
PRP-D-Hib	Conjugated Hib vaccine(Hib capsular antigen polyribosylphosphate covalently Linked to a mutant polypeptide of diphtheria toxin)
PT	Prothrombin time
PTT	Partial thromboplastin time
QALY	Quality-adjusted life year
qds	Four times a day (quater die summendum)
ROC curve	Receiver-operator characteristic curve
RR	Risk ratio or relative risk
RT-PCR	Reverse transcriptase polymerase chain reaction
SABA	Short-acting beta-adrenoceptor agonist
SMR	Standardized mortality rate
SNP	Single nucleotide polymorphism
SNRI	Serotonin and noradrenaline reuptake inhibitor
SSRI	Selective serotonin reuptake inhibitor

SV40	Simian virus 40
Td	Diphtheria + tetanus toxoids (adult formulation)
Tdap:	Tetanus toxoid + reduced diphtheria toxoid + acellular pertussis
tds	Three times a day (ter die summendum)
TeMA	2,3,4,5-Tetramethoxyamfetamine
TMA	3,4,5-Trimethoxyamfetamine
TMA-2	2,4,5-Trimethoxyamfetamine
t_{max}	The time at which C_{max} is reached
TMC125	Etravirine
TMC 278	Rilpivirine
V_{max}	Maximum velocity (of a reaction)
wP	Whole cell pertussis
VZV	*Varicella zoster* vaccine
YF	Yellow fever
YFV	Yellow fever virus

ADRs, ADEs and SEDs: A Bird's Eye View

*Sidhartha D. Ray**,1*, *Robert D. Beckett†*, *David F. Kisor**, *Joshua P. Gray‡*, *Mary E. Kiersma§*

*Department of Pharmaceutical Sciences, Manchester University College of Pharmacy, Fort Wayne, IN, USA
†Director of the Drug Information Center, Manchester University College of Pharmacy, Fort Wayne, IN, USA
‡Departments of Chemistry and Science, United States Coast Guard Academy, New London, CT, USA
§Accreditation Council for Pharmacy Education (ACPE), Chicago, IL, USA
1Corresponding author: Email: sdray@manchester.edu

I INTRODUCTION

Adverse drug events (ADEs), drug-induced toxicity and side effects are a significant concern. ADEs are known to pose a significant morbidity, mortality, and cost burden to society; however, there is a lack of strong evidence to determine their precise impact. The landmark Institute of Medicine (IOM) report *To Err is Human* implicated adverse drug events in 7000 annual deaths at an estimated cost of $2 billion [1]. However, the US Department of Health and Human Services estimates 770 000 people are injured or die each year in hospitals from ADEs, which costs up to $5.6 million each year per hospital excluding the other accessory costs (e.g., hospital admissions due to ADEs, malpractice and litigation costs, or the costs of injuries). Nationally, hospitals spend $1.56–5.6 billion each year to treat patients who suffer ADEs during hospitalization [2]. A second landmark study suggests that approximately 28% of ADEs are preventable through optimization of medication safety and distribution systems, provision and dissemination of timely patient and medication information, and staffing assignments [3]. Subsequent recent investigations suggest these numbers might be conservative estimates of the morbidity and mortality impact of ADEs [4].

A Analysis of ADEs, ADRs, Side Effects and Toxicity

A recent report suggested that ADEs and/or side effects of drugs occur in approximately 30% of hospitalized patients [5]. The American Society of Health-System Pharmacists (ASHP) defines medication misadventures as unexpected, undesirable iatrogenic hazards or events where a medication was implicated [1]. These events can be broadly divided into two categories: (i) medication errors (i.e., preventable events that may cause or contain inappropriate use), and (ii) adverse drug events (i.e., any injury, whether minor or significant, caused by a medication or lack thereof). Another significant ADE-generating category that can be added to the list is lack of incorporation of pre-existing condition(s) or pharmacogenomics factors. This work focuses on adverse drug events; however, it should be noted that adverse drug events may or may not occur secondary to a medication error.

The lack of more up to date epidemiological data regarding the impact of ADEs is largely due to challenges with low adverse drug event reporting. ASHP recommends that health systems implement adverse drug reaction (ADR) monitoring programs in order to (i) mitigate ADR risks for specific patients and expedite reporting to clinicians involved in care of patients who do experience ADRs and (ii) gather pharmacovigilance information that can be reported to pharmaceutical companies and regulatory bodies [6]. Factors that may increase the risk for ADEs include polypharmacy, multiple concomitant disease states, pediatric or geriatric status, female sex, genetic variance, and drug factors, such as class and route of administration. The Institute for Safe Medication Practices (ISMP) defines high-alert medications as those with high risk for harmful events, especially when used in error [6]. Examples include antithrombotic agents, cancer chemotherapy, insulin, opioids, and neuromuscular blockers.

B Terminology

ADEs may be further classified based on expected severity into adverse drug reactions (ADRs) or adverse effects (also known as side effects). ASHP defines ADRs as an "unexpected, unintended, undesired, or excessive response to a drug" resulting in death, disability, or harm [5]. The World Health Organization (WHO) has traditionally defined an ADR as a "response to a drug that is noxious and unintended and occurs at doses normally used"; however, another proposed definition, intended to highlight the seriousness of ADRs is "an appreciably harmful or unpleasant reaction, resulting from an intervention related to the use of a medicinal product, which predicts hazard from future administration and warrants prevention or specific treatment, or alteration of the dosage regimen, or withdrawal of the product" [7]. Under all definitions, ADRs are distinguished from side effects in that they generally necessitate some type of modification to the patient's therapeutic regimen. Such modifications could include discontinuing treatment, changing medications, significantly altering the dose, elevating or prolonging care received by the patient, or changing diagnosis or prognosis. ADRs include drug allergies, immunologic hypersensitivities, and idiosyncratic reactions. In contrast, side effects, or adverse effects, are defined as "expected, well-known reaction resulting in little or no change in patient management" [5]. Side effects occur at predictable frequency and are often dose-related, whereas ADRs are less foreseeable [7,8].

Two additional types of adverse drug events are drug-induced diseases and toxicity. Drug-induced diseases are defined as an "unintended effect of a drug that results in mortality or morbidity with symptoms sufficient to prompt a patient to seek medical attention, require

hospitalization, or both" [9]. In other words, a drug-induced disease has elements of an ADR (i.e., significant severity, elevated levels of patient care) and adverse effects (i.e., predictability, consistent symptoms). Toxicity is a less precisely defined term referring to the ability of a substance "to cause injury to living organisms as a result of physicochemical interaction" [10]. This term is applied to both medication and non-medication types of substances, while "ADRs," "side effects," and "drug-induced diseases" typically only refer to medications. When applied to medication use, toxicity typically refers to use at higher than normal dosing or accumulated supratherapeutic exposure over time, while ADRs, side effects, and drug-induced diseases are associated with normal therapeutic use.

Although the title of this book is "Side Effects of Drugs," this work provides emerging information for all adverse drug events including ADRs, side effects, drug-induced diseases, toxicity, and other situations less clearly classifiable into a particular category, such as effects subsequent to drug interactions with other drugs, foods, and cosmetics. Pharmacogenetic considerations have been incorporated in several chapters as appropriate and subject to availability of literature.

C EIDOS

Adverse drug reactions are described in SEDA using two complementary systems, EIDOS and DOTS [13,14, 15]. These two systems are illustrated in Figures 1 and 2

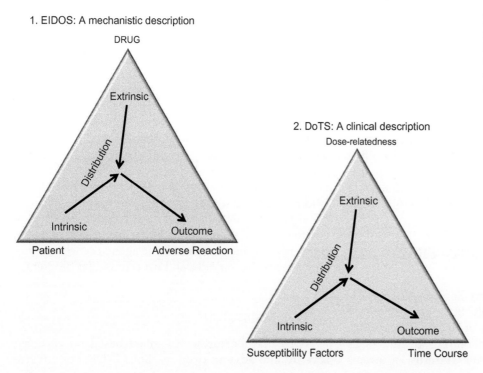

1. EIDOS: A mechanistic description

2. DoTS: A clinical description

FIGURE 1 Describing adverse drug reactions—two complementary systems. Note that the triad of drug–patient–adverse reaction appears outside the triangle in EIDOS and inside the triangle in DoTS, leading to Figure 2.

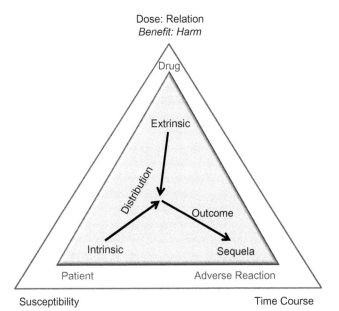

Dose: Relation
Benefit: Harm

FIGURE 2 How the EIDOS and DoTS systems relate to each other. Here the two triangles in Figure 1 are superimposed, to show the relation between the two systems. An adverse reaction occurs when a drug is given to a patient. Adverse reactions can be classified mechanistically (EIDOS) by noting that when the Extrinsic (drug) species and an Intrinsic (patient) species, are co-Distributed, a pharmacological or other effect (the Outcome) results in the adverse reaction (the Sequela). The adverse reaction can be further classified (DoTS) by considering its three main features—its Dose-relatedness, its Time-course, and individual Susceptibility.

and general templates for describing reactions in this way are shown in Figures 3–5. Examples of their use have been discussed elsewhere [16–20].

The EIDOS mechanistic description of adverse drug reactions [15] has five elements:

- the *Extrinsic* species that initiates the reaction (Table 1);
- the *Intrinsic* species that it affects;
- the *Distribution* of these species in the body;
- the (physiological or pathological) *Outcome* (Table 2), which is the adverse effect;
- the *Sequela*, which is the adverse reaction.

Extrinsic species This can be the parent compound, an excipient, a contaminant or adulterant, a degradation product, or a derivative of any of these (e.g. a metabolite) (for examples see Table 1).

Intrinsic species This is usually the endogenous molecule with which the extrinsic species interacts; this can be a nucleic acid, an enzyme, a receptor, an ion channel or transporter, or some other protein.

Distribution A drug will not produce an adverse effect if it is not distributed to the same site as the target species that mediates the adverse effect. Thus, the pharmacokinetics of the extrinsic species can affect the occurrence of adverse reactions.

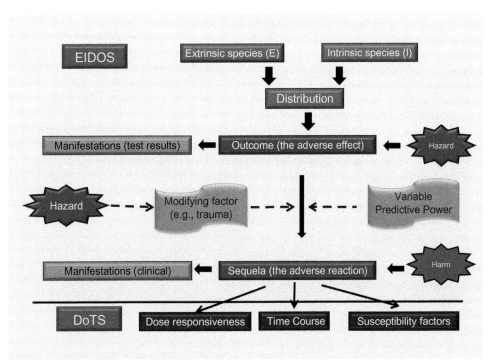

FIGURE 3 A general form of the EIDOS and DoTS template for describing an adverse effect or an adverse reaction.

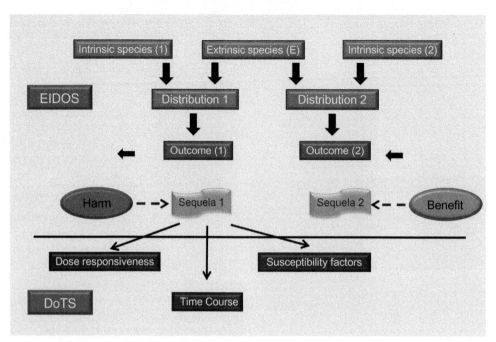

FIGURE 4 A general form of the EIDOS and DoTS template for describing two mechanisms of an adverse reaction or (illustrated here) the balance of benefit to harm, each mediated by a different mechanism.

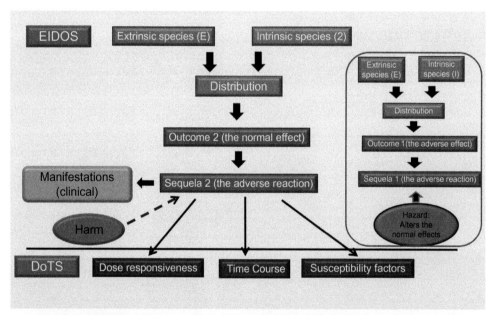

FIGURE 5 A general form of the EIDOS and DoTS template for describing an adverse drug interaction.

Outcome Interactions between extrinsic and intrinsic species in the production of an adverse effect can result in physiological or pathological changes (for examples see Table 2). Physiological changes can involve either increased actions (e.g. clotting due to tranexamic acid) or decreased actions (e.g. bradycardia due to beta-adrenoceptor antagonists). Pathological changes can involve cellular adaptations (atrophy, hypertrophy, hyperplasia, metaplasia and neoplasia), altered cell function (e.g. mast cell degranulation in IgE-mediated anaphylactic reactions) or cell damage (e.g. cell lysis, necrosis or apoptosis).

Sequela The sequela of the changes induced by a drug describes the clinically recognizable adverse drug

TABLE 1 The EIDOS Mechanistic Description of Adverse Drug Effects and Reactions

Feature	Varieties	Examples
E. Extrinsic species	1. The parent compound	Insulin
	2. An excipient	Polyoxyl 35 castor oil
	3. A contaminant	1,1-ethylidenebis [l-tryptophan]
	4. An adulterant	Lead in herbal medicines
	5. A degradation product formed before the drug enters the body	Outdated tetracycline
	6. A derivative of any of these (e.g. a metabolite)	Acrolein (from cyclophosphamide)
I. The intrinsic species and the nature of its interaction with the extrinsic species		
(a) Molecular	1. Nucleic acids	
	(a) DNA	Melphalan
	(b) RNA	Mitoxantrone
	2. Enzymes	
	(a) Reversible effect	Edrophonium
	(b) Irreversible effect	Malathion
	3. Receptors	
	(a) Reversible effect	Prazosin
	(b) Irreversible effect	Phenoxybenzamine
	4. Ion channels/transporters	Calcium channel blockers; digoxin and Na^+–K^+–ATPase
	5. Other proteins	
	(a) Immunological proteins	Penicilloyl residue hapten
	(b) Tissue proteins	N-acetyl-p-benzoquinone-imine (paracetamol [acetaminophen])
(b) Extracellular	1. Water	Dextrose 5%
	2. Hydrogen ions (pH)	Sodium bicarbonate
	3. Other ions	Sodium ticarcillin
(c) Physical or physicochemical	1. Direct tissue damage	Intrathecal vincristine
	2. Altered physicochemical nature of the extrinsic species	Sulindac precipitation
D. Distribution	1. Where in the body the extrinsic and intrinsic species occur (affected by pharmacokinetics)	Antihistamines cause drowsiness only if they affect histamine H_1 receptors in the brain
O. Outcome (physiological or pathological change)	The adverse effect (see Table 2)	
S. Sequela	The adverse reaction (use the Dose, Time, Susceptibility [DoTS] descriptive system)	

reaction, of which there may be more than one. Sequelae can be classified using the DoTS system.

D DOTS

In the DoTS system (SEDA-28, xxvii–xxxiii; 1,2) adverse drug reactions are described according to the *Dose* at which they usually occur, the *Time-course* over which they occur, and the *Susceptibility factors* that make them more likely, as follows:

- *Relation to dose*
  - Toxic reactions (reactions that occur at supratherapeutic doses)
  - Collateral reactions (reactions that occur at standard therapeutic doses)

TABLE 2 Examples of Physiological and Pathological Changes in Adverse Drug Effects (Some Categories can be Broken Down Further)

Type of change	Examples
1. Physiological changes	
(a) Increased actions	Hypertension (monoamine oxidase inhibitors); clotting (tranexamic acid)
(b) Decreased actions	Bradycardia (beta-adrenoceptor antagonists); QT interval prolongation (antiarrhythmic drugs)
2. Cellular adaptations	
(a) Atrophy	Lipoatrophy (subcutaneous insulin); glucocorticosteroid-induced myopathy
(b) Hypertrophy	Gynecomastia (spironolactone)
(c) Hyperplasia	Pulmonary fibrosis (busulfan); retroperitoneal fibrosis (methysergide)
(d) Metaplasia	Lacrimal canalicular squamous metaplasia (fluorouracil)
(e) Neoplasia	
– Benign	Hepatoma (anabolic steroids)
– Malignant	
– Hormonal	Vaginal adenocarcinoma (diethylstilbestrol)
– Genotoxic	Transitional cell carcinoma of bladder (cyclophosphamide)
– Immune suppression	Lymphoproliferative tumors (ciclosporin)
3. Altered cell function	IgE-mediated mast cell degranulation (class I immunological reactions)
4. Cell damage	
(a) Acute reversible damage	
– Chemical damage	Periodontitis (local application of methylene dioxymetamfetamine [MDMA, 'ecstasy'])
– Immunological reactions	Class III immunological reactions
(b) Irreversible injury	
– Cell lysis	Class II immunological reactions
– Necrosis	Class IV immunological reactions; hepatotoxicity (paracetamol, after apoptosis)
– Apoptosis	Liver damage (troglitazone)
5. Intracellular accumulations	
(a) Calcification	Milk-alkali syndrome
(b) Drug deposition	Crystal-storing histiocytosis (clofazimine) Skin pigmentation (amiodarone)

- ○ Hypersusceptibility reactions (reactions that occur at subtherapeutic doses in susceptible individuals)
- *Time course*
  - ○ Time-independent reactions (reactions that occur at any time during a course of therapy)
  - ○ Time-dependent reactions
    - Immediate or rapid reactions (reactions that occur only when drug administration is too rapid)
    - First-dose reactions (reactions that occur after the first dose of a course of treatment and not necessarily thereafter)
    - Early tolerant and early persistent reactions (reactions that occur early in treatment then either abate with continuing treatment, owing to tolerance, or persist)
    - Intermediate reactions (reactions that occur after some delay but with less risk during longer term therapy, owing to the 'healthy survivor' effect)
    - Late reactions (reactions the risk of which increases with continued or repeated exposure)
    - Withdrawal reactions (reactions that occur when, after prolonged treatment, a drug is withdrawn or its effective dose is reduced)
    - Delayed reactions (reactions that occur at some time after exposure, even if the drug is withdrawn before the reaction appears)
- *Susceptibility factors*
  Genetic
  Age
  Sex
  Physiological variation (e.g. weight, pregnancy)
  Exogenous factors (for example the effects of other drugs, devices, surgical procedures, food, smoking)
  Diseases

E WHO Classification

Although not systematically used in Side Effects of Drugs Annual, the WHO classification, used at the Uppsala Monitoring Center, is a useful schematic to consider in assessing ADRs and adverse effects. Possible classifications include:

- Type A (dose-related, "augmented"), more common events that tend to be related to the pharmacology of the drug, have a mechanistic basis, and result in lower mortality;
- Type B (non-dose-related, "bizarre"), less common, unpredictable events that are not related to the pharmacology of the drug;
- Type C (dose-related and time-related, "chronic"), events that are related to cumulative dose received over time;
- Type D (time-related, "delayed"), events that are usually dose-related but do not become apparent until significant time has elapsed since exposure to the drug;
- Type E (withdrawal, "end of use"), events that occur soon after the use of the drug;

- Type F (unexpected lack of efficacy, "failure"), common, dose-related events where the drug effectiveness is lacking, often due to drug interactions.

REFERENCES ON ADVERSE DRUG REACTIONS

[1] Kohn, LT, Corrigan JM, Donaldson MS, editors. *To Err is Human: Building a Safer Health System.* Washington, DC National Academy Press; 1999: 1-8.

[2] US Department of Health & Human Services Report: http://archive.ahrq.gov/research/findings/factsheets/errors-safety/aderia/ade.html.

[3] Leape LL, Bates DW, Cullen DJ, et al. Systems analysis of adverse drug events. JAMA. 1995; 274 (1):35-43.

[4] James JT. A new, evidence-based estimate of patient harms associated with hospital care. J Patient Saf. 2013; 9(3):122-128.

[5] Wang G, Jung K, Winnenburg R, Shah NH. A method for systematic discovery of adverse drug events from clinical notes. J Am Med Inform Assoc. 2015 Jul 31. pii: ocv102. doi: 10.1093/jamia/ocv102.

[6] American Society of Health-Systems Pharmacists. Positions. Medication Misadventures. http://www.ashp.org/DocLibrary/BestPractices/MedMisPositions.aspx.

[7] American Society of Health-Systems Pharmacists. Guidelines. ASHP Guidelines on adverse drug reaction monitoring and reporting. http://www.ashp.org/DocLibrary/BestPractices/MedMisGdlADR.aspx.

[8] Institute for Safe Medication Practices. ISMP list of high-alert medications in acute care settings. http://www.ismp.org/Tools/institutionalhighAlert.asp.

[9] Edwards IR, Aronson JK. Adverse drug reactions: Definitions, diagnosis, and management. Lancet. 2000; 356:1255-59.

[10] Cochrane ZR, Hein D, Gregory PJ. Medication misadventures I: adverse drug reactions. In: Malone PM, Kier KL, Stanovich JE, Malone MJ, editors. Drug Information: A Guide for Pharmacists, 5th edition. New York, NY: McGraw-Hill; 2013.

[11] Tisdale JE, Miller DA, editors. Drug-Induced Diseases: Prevention, Detection, and Management. 2nd edition. Bethesda, MD: American Society of Health-System Pharmacists; 2010.

[12] Wexler P, Abdollahi M, Peyster AD, et al., editors. Encyclopedia of Toxicology. 3rd edition. Burlington, MA: Academic Press, Elsevier; 2014.

[13] Aronson JK, Ferner RE. Joining the DoTS. New approach to classifying adverse drug reactions. BMJ. 2003; 327:1222–1225.

[14] Aronson JK, Ferner RE. Clarification of terminology in drug safety. Drug Saf. 2005; 28(10):851–870.

[15] Ferner RE, Aronson JK. EIDOS: a mechanistic classification of adverse drug effects. Drug Saf. 2010; 33(1):13–23.

[16] Callréus T. Use of the dose, time, susceptibility (DoTS) classification scheme for adverse drug reactions in pharmacovigilance planning. Drug Saf. 2006; 29(7):557–566.

[17] Aronson JK, Price D, Ferner R.E. A strategy for regulatory action when new adverse effects of a licensed product emerge. Drug Saf. 2009; 32(2):91–98.

[18] Calderón-Ospina C, Bustamante-Rojas C. The DoTS classification is a useful way to classify adverse drug reactions: a preliminary study in hospitalized patients. Int J Pharm Pract. 2010; 18(4):230–235.

[19] Ferner RE, Aronson JK. Preventability of drug-related harms. Part 1: A systematic review. Drug Saf. 2010; 33(11):985–994.

[20] Aronson JK, Ferner RE. Preventability of drug-related harms. Part 2: Proposed criteria, based on frameworks that classify adverse drug reactions. Drug Saf. 2010; 33(11):995–1002.

II PHARMACOGENOMICS CONSIDERATIONS

A Introduction

Advances in medical genomics have generated considerable beneficiaries for precision (personalized) medicine through the identification of genetic variants that alter drug response relative to drug efficacy or leading to either an exacerbation or minimization of adverse drug reactions (ADRs). The cost and turn-around-time of genetic tests have slowed rapid uptake of the clinical application of pharmacogenetics. However, this is improving as the rate of uptake is increasing. It is anticipated that clinicians' attitudes toward multiplex genomic testing may be vital to the success of translational programs. Exploratory studies to investigate the action of drugs require ethnic considerations be kept as an integral parameter in publicly funded programs in several countries. It has been suggested that pharmacogenetic profiles of patients be analyzed when administering and tailoring drug therapy.

The past decade has witnessed an explosion in the development, implementation and availability of genetic testing strategies that can envisage hereditary variations to drug responses in living systems. Compelling statistics on ADRs remain a primary component for driving such testing. In the United States, ADRs occur in nearly 10% of patients taking prescription medications in the ambulatory setting and cause an estimated 100 000 deaths annually in hospitalized patients [1,2]. Although many nongenetic factors, such as age, organ function, concomitant therapy, drug interactions, and pathophysiology of the disease influence the effects of medications, it has been projected that genetics can account for 20–95% of variability in drug disposition and effects [3]. More than one-fourth of primary care patients are taking a medication that commonly causes ADRs and are under the control of genetically variable factors [4,5]. The United States Food and Drug Administration has made considerable efforts in informing prescribers about the potential for ADRs and improving labeling of drugs that are subject to variable patient response because of certain genetic variations [6]. Information pertaining to pharmacogenomics considerations is indicated on the labels of over 130 drugs, and it has been estimated that 25% of medications used in the outpatient setting have pharmacogenomic information in the package labeling [7,8].

B The Context of Pharmacogenomics

The interaction between a drug and a gene product (e.g., functional protein) affecting an individual's response to the drug, i.e., pharmacogenetics (PGt), represents a clear application of the EIDOS mechanism description of an adverse drug reaction when the drug–gene interaction produces a collateral reaction as described using the DoTS system [9].

The gene products of interest relative to drug–gene interactions include receptors, signaling proteins, target enzymes, drug transporters and drug-metabolizing enzymes [10]. Gene variants, a consequence of single nucleotide polymorphisms (SNPs) or insertions or deletions (indels) among other DNA alterations or duplications can result in outcomes with deleterious effects resulting in sequela. Here, ranging from an exaggerated clinical response (e.g. bleeding as can be seen with warfarin in an individual with decreased production of the target enzyme vitamin K epoxide reductase subunit 1 (VKORC1) in an individual with an A/A VKORC1 genotype) to death, in an individual with multiple copies of CYP2D6 who dies due to morphine overdose following the administration of codeine [11,12]. Another example of a drug–gene interaction resulting in an adverse effect and observed sequela involves decreased activity of the organic anion transporter protein 1B1 (OATP1B1), a product of the solute carrier transporter gene SLCO1B1, in an individual with a C/T or C/C genotype who experiences myopathy following administration of simvastatin in the treatment of hypercholesterolemia [13]. The above mentioned drug–gene interactions result in collateral reactions as the above mentioned outcomes and sequela are seen at standard therapeutic doses.

Perhaps the most studied drug–gene interactions are related to the activity of drug-metabolizing gene products, e.g. cytochrome P450 enzymes (CYPs), thiopurine methyl transferase (TPMT), and dihydropyrimidine dehydrogenase (DPD). Here, gene variants, most often a consequence of a SNP or a combination of SNPs (haplotype), result in decreased drug metabolism altering the pharmacokinetic parameter clearance, which influences the required maintenance dose of a given drug. Table 3 presents examples of gene variants and

TABLE 3 Drug (Extrinsic)–Gene (Intrinsic) Interactions and Example Outcomes and Sequela

Drug–gene(s) interaction	Example Gene variant[a]/metabolizer phenotype[b]	Effect on drug metabolism/ clearance (CL)	Other pharmacokinetic consequences[c,d]	Example Outcome	Example sequela
Amitriptyline–CYP2D6/CYP2C19	CYP2D6*4/*4, CYP2C19*2/*2; PM, PM	Significantly decrease	Increased drug exposure: higher AUC and longer $t_{1/2}$	Central nervous system stimulation	Agitation
Mercaptopurine–TPMT	TPMT*1/*3C; IM	Somewhat decrease	Increased drug exposure: higher AUC and longer $t_{1/2}$	Immunosuppression	Infection
Citalopram–CYP2C19	CYP2C19*2/*2; PM	Significantly decrease	Increased drug exposure: higher AUC and longer $t_{1/2}$	Prolonged QT interval	Torsades-de-pointes
Codeine–CYP2D6	CYP2D6*2xN; UM	Significantly increase	Increased metabolite exposure	CNS depression	Respiratory arrest/death
Warfarin–CYP2C9	CYP2C9*3/*3; PM	Significantly decrease	Increased drug exposure: higher AUC and longer $t_{1/2}$	Decreased formation of vitamin K-dependent clotting factors	Bleeding

[a] "Star" nomenclature [13].
[b] Metabolizer phenotype: PM = poor metabolizer, IM = intermediate metabolizer, UM = ultrarapid metabolizer.
[c] AUC = area under the plasma drug concentration versus time curve.
[d] $t_{1/2}$ = half-life.

the effects on the pharmacokinetics resulting in outcomes with noted sequela.

The intrinsic genetic influence on the drug–receptor or drug–target enzyme interaction, drug transporter, and/or drug-metabolizing enzyme can influence an individual's response to the administration of standard doses of a given drug. Here, the collateral reactions can result in outcomes with significant sequela. As technology allows, preemptive genetic testing of patients will allow for appropriate drug/drug dose selection as to decrease/avoid the risk of adverse drug reactions.

REFERENCES PHARMACOGENOMICS CONSIDERATIONS

[1] Taché SV, Sönnichsen A, Ashcroft DM. Prevalence of adverse drug events in ambulatory care: a systematic review. Ann Pharmacother. 2011; 45(7–8):977–989.

[2] Lazarou J, Pomeranz B, Corey PN. Incidence of adverse drug reactions in hospitalized patients: a meta-analysis of prospective studies. JAMA. 1998; 279(15):1200–1205.

[3] Evans WE., McLeod HL. Pharmacogenomics: Drug Disposition, Drug Targets, and Side Effects. N Engl J Med 2003; 348:538-549.

[4] Grice GR, Seaton TL, Woodland AM, McLeod HL. Defining the opportunity for pharmacogenetic intervention in primary care. Pharmacogenomics. 2006; 7(1):61–65.

[5] Kisor DF, Munro C, Loudermilk E. Pharmacogenomics and the most commonly prescribed drugs of 2011. Pharm Times. 2012; 78(12):85–96.

[6] US Food and Drug Administration. Table of pharmacogenomic biomarkers in drug labeling. Available from: http://www.fda.gov/drugs/scienceresearch/researchareas/pharmacogenetics/ucm083378.htm. Accessed September 1, 2015.

[7] Frueh FW, Amur S, Mummaneni P, et al. Pharmacogenomic biomarker information in drug labels approved by the United States food and drug administration: prevalence of related drug use. Pharmacotherapy. 2008; 28(8):992–998.

[8] Johansen Taber KA, Dickinson BD. Pharmacogenomic knowledge gaps and educational resource needs among physicians in selected specialties. Pharmgenomics Pers. Med. 2014 Jul 10; 7:145-62. doi: 10.2147/PGPM.S63715. eCollection 2014.

[9] Aronson JK, Ferner RE. Joining the DoTS. New approach to classifying adverse drug reactions. BMJ. 2003; 327:1222–5.

[10] Ma Q, Lu AYH. Pharmacogenetics, pharmacogenomics, and individualized medicine. Pharmacol Rev. 2011; 63(2):437-459.

[11] Johnson JA, Gong L, Whirl-Carrillo M, et al. Clinical Pharmacogenetics Implementation Consortium guidelines for CYP2C9 and VKORC1 genotypes and warfarin dosing. Clin Pharmacol Ther. 2011; 90(4):625–629.

[12] Crews KR, Gaedigk A, Dunnenberger HM, et al. Clinical Pharmacogenetics Implementation Consortium (CPIC) guidelines for codeine therapy in the context of cytochrome P450 2D6 (CYP2D6) genotype: supplementary data. Clin Pharmacol Ther. 2012; 91(2):321–326.

[13] Ramsey LB, Johnson SG, Caudle KE, et al. The Clinical Pharmacogenetics Implementation Consortium Guideline for SLCO1B1 and Simvastatin-Induced Myopathy: 2014 Update. Clin Pharmacol Ther. Online publication. doi:10.1038/clpt.2014.125.

[14] Robarge JD, Li L, Desta Z, Nguyen A, Flockhart DA. The star-allele nomenclature: retooling for translational genomics. Clin Pharmacol Ther. 2007; 82(3):244-8.

III IMMUNOLOGICAL REACTIONS

The immunological reactions are diverse and varied but considered specific. Nearly five decades ago, Karl Landsteiner's ground-breaking work "The Specificity of Serological Reactions" set the standard in experimental immunology. Several new discoveries in immunology in the 20th century, such as 'CD' receptors (cluster of differentiation), recognition of 'self' versus 'non-self', a large family of cytokines and antigenic specificity, became instrumental in describing immunological reactions. The most widely accepted classification divides immunological reactions (drug allergies or otherwise) into four pathophysiological types, namely anaphylaxis (immediate type or Type I hypersensitivity), antibody-mediated cytotoxic reactions (cytotoxic type or Type II hypersensitivity), immune complex-mediated reactions (toxic-complex syndrome or Type III hypersensitivity), and cell-mediated immunity (delayed-type hypersensitivity or Type IV hypersensitivity). Although Gell and Coomb's classification was proposed more than 30 years ago, it is still widely used [1–3].

A Type I Reactions (IgE-Mediated Anaphylaxis; Immediate Hypersensitivity)

In Type I reactions, the drug or its metabolite interacts with IgE molecules bound to specific type of cells (mast cells and basophils). This triggers a process that leads to the release of pharmacological mediators (histamine, 5-hydroxytryptamine, kinins, and arachidonic acid derivatives), which cause the allergic response. Mounting of such a reaction depends exclusively upon exposure to the same assaulting agent (antigen, allergen or metabolite) for the second time and the severity depends on the level of exposure. The clinical effects [2] are due to smooth muscle contraction, vasodilatation, and increased capillary permeability. The symptoms include faintness, lightheadedness, pruritus, nausea, vomiting, abdominal pain, and a feeling of impending doom (angor animi). The signs include urticaria, conjunctivitis, rhinitis, laryngeal edema, bronchial asthma and pulmonary edema, angioedema, and anaphylactic shock; takotsubo cardiomyopathy can occur, as can Kounis syndrome (an acute coronary episode associated with an allergic reaction). Not all Type I reactions are IgE-dependent; however, adverse reactions that are mediated by direct histamine release have conventionally been called anaphylactoid reactions, but are better classified as non-IgE-mediated anaphylactic reactions. Cytokines, such as IL-4, IL-5, IL-6 and IL-13, either mediate or influence this class of hypersensitivity reaction. Representative agents that are known to induce such reactions include: Gelatin, Gentamicin, Kanamycin, Neomycin, Penicillins, Polymyxin B, Streptomycin and Thiomersal [1–3].

B Type II Reactions (Cytotoxic Reactions)

Type II reactions involve circulating immunoglobulins G or M (or rarely IgA) binding with cell-surface antigens (membrane constituent or protein) and interacting with an antigen formed by a hapten (drug or metabolite) and subsequently fixing complement. Complement is then activated leading to cytolysis. Type II reactions often involve antibody-mediated cytotoxicity directed to the membranes of erythrocytes, leukocytes, platelets, and probably hematopoietic precursor cells in the bone marrow. Drugs that are typically involved are methyldopa (hemolytic anemia), aminopyrine (leukopenia), and heparin (thrombocytopenia) with mostly hematological consequences, including thrombocytopenia, neutropenia, and hemolytic anemia [1–3].

C Type III Reactions (Immune Complex Reactions)

In Type III reactions, formation of an immune complex and its deposition on tissue surface serve as primary initiators. Occasionally, immune complexes bind to endothelial cells and lead to immune complex deposition with subsequent complement activation in the linings of blood vessels. Circumstances that govern immune formation or immune complex disease remain unclear to date, and it usually occurs without symptoms. The clinical symptoms of a Type III reaction include serum sickness (e.g., β-lactams), drug-induced lupus erythematosus (e.g., quinidine), and vasculitis (e.g., minocycline). Type III reactions can result in acute interstitial nephritis or serum sickness (fever, arthritis, enlarged lymph nodes, urticaria, and maculopapular rashes) [1–3].

D Type IV Reactions (Cell-Mediated or Delayed Hypersensitivity Reactions)

Type IV reactions are initiated when hapten–protein antigenic complex-mediated sensitized T lymphocytes meet the assaulting immunogen for the second time; usually this leads to severe inflammation. Type IV reactions are exemplified by contact dermatitis. Pseudoallergic reactions resemble allergic reactions clinically but are not immunologically mediated. Examples include asthma and rashes caused by aspirin and maculopapular erythematous rashes due to ampicillin or amoxicillin in the absence of penicillin hypersensitivity. A few other entities that can initiate this reaction are: sulfonamides, anticonvulsants (phenytoin, carbamazepine, and phenobarbital), NSAIDs (aspirin, naproxen, nabumetone, and ketoprofen), antiretroviral agents and cephalosporins [1–4].

E Other types of reactions

Several types of adverse drug reactions do not easily fit into Gell and Coomb's classification scheme. These include most cutaneous hypersensitivity reactions (such as toxic epidermal necrolysis), 'immune-allergic' hepatitis and hypersensitivity pneumonitis. Another difficulty is that allergic drug reactions can occur via more than one mechanism; picryl chloride in mice induces both Type I and Type IV responses. Although other classification schemes have been proposed, Gell and Coomb's system remains the most widely utilized scheme [4–7].

REFERENCES

[1] Coombs RRA, Gell PGH. Classification of allergic reactions responsible for clinical hypersensitivity and disease. In: Gell PGH, Coombs RRA, Lachmann PJ, editors. Clinical Aspects of Immunology. London: Blackwell Scientific Publications; 1975. p. 761–81.

[2] Schnyder B, Pichler W. Mechanisms of Drug-Induced Allergy. Mayo Clin Proc. Mar 2009; 84(3): 268–272.

[3] Boyman O, Comte D, Spertini F. Adverse reactions to biologic agents and their medical management. Nat Rev Rheumatol., 2014 Aug 12. doi: 10.1038/nrrheum.2014.123. [Epub ahead of print].

[4] Brown SGA. Clinical features and severity grading of anaphylaxis. J Allergy Clin Immunol 2004; 114(2): 371–6.

[5] Johansson SGO, Hourihane JO, Bousquet J, Bruijnzeel-Koomen C, Dreborg S, Haahtela T, Kowalski ML, Mygind N, Ring J, van Cauwenberge P, van Hage- Hamsten M, Wüthrich B. A revised nomenclature for allergy. An EAACI position statement from the EAACI nomenclature task force. Allergy 2001; 56(9): 813–24.

[6] Uzzaman A, Cho SH. Chapter 28: Classification of hypersensitivity reactions. Allergy Asthma Proc. 2012 May-Jun; 33 Suppl 1:S96-9.

[7] Descotes J, Choquet-Kastylevsky G. Toxicology, 2001; 158(1-2):43-9. Gell and Coombs's classification: is it still valid?

IV ANALYSIS OF TOXICOLOGICAL REACTIONS

A Potentiation Reactions

This type of reaction occurs only when one non-toxic chemical interacts with another non-toxic chemical, or one non-toxic chemical interacts with another toxic chemical at low doses (subtoxic, acutely toxic). An alternate interpretation could be when two drugs are taken together, one of them intensifies the action of the other. In such scenarios, if the final outcome is high toxicity, then the final outcome is called a potentiation (increasing the toxic effect of 'Y' by 'X'). Theoretically, it can be expressed as: $x + y = M$ $(1 + 0 = 4)$.

Examples: (i) When chronic or regular alcohol drinkers consume therapeutic doses of acetaminophen, it can lead to alcohol-potentiated acetaminophen-induced hepatoxicity (cause: ethanol-induced massive CYP2E1 induction in the liver); (ii) Avoid iron supplements in patients on doxorubicin therapy to prevent possible potentiation of doxorubicin-induced cardiotoxicity (cause: hydroxyl radical formation and redox cycling of doxorubicin); (iii) Phenergan®, an antihistamine, when given with a painkilling narcotic such as meperidine (Demerol®) can intensify its effect; therefore, reducing the dose of the narcotic is advised; (iv) Ethanol potentiation of CCl_4-induced hepatotoxicity; (v) Use of phenytoin and calcium-channel blockers combination should be used with caution.

B Synergistic Effect

Synergism is somewhat similar to potentiation. When two drugs are taken together that are similar in action, such as barbiturates and alcohol, which are both depressants, an effect exaggerated out of proportion to that of each drug taken separately at the given dose may occur (mathematically: $1 + 1 = 4$). Normally, taken alone, neither substance would cause serious harm, but if taken together, the combination could cause coma or death. Another established example: when smokers get exposed to asbestos.

C Additive Effect

Additive effect is defined as a consequence which follows exposure to two or more physicochemical agents which act jointly but do not interact, or commonly, the total effect is the simple sum of the effects of separate exposure to the agents under the same conditions. This could be represented by $1 + 1 = 2$: (i) one example would be barbiturate and a tranquilizer when given together before surgery to relax the patient; (ii) a second example would be the toxic effect on bone marrow that follows after AZT + Ganciclovir or AZT + Clotrimazole administration.

D Antagonistic Effects

Antagonistic effects occur when two drugs/chemicals are administered simultaneously or one followed by the other, and the net effect of the final outcome of the reaction is negligible or zero. This could be expressed by $1 + 1 = 0$. An example might be the use of a tranquilizer to stop the action of LSD.

Examples: (i) When ethanol is administered to methanol-poisoned patient; (ii) NSAIDs administered to diuretics (hydrochlorothiazide/Furosemide): Reduce diuretics effectiveness; (iii) Certain β-blockers (INDERAL®) taken to control high blood pressure and heart disease counteract β-adrenergic stimulants, such as Albuterol®.

REFERENCES

[1] Ray SD, Mehendale HM. Potentiation of CCl4 and CHCl3 hepatotoxicity and lethality by various alcohols. Fundam Appl Toxicol. 1990; 15(3):429-40.

[2] Gammella, E., Maccarinelli, F., Buratti, P., et al. The role of iron in anthracycline cardiotoxicity. Front Pharmacol. 2014; 5:25. doi: 10.3389/ fphar.2014.00025. eCollection 2014.

[3] NLM's Toxlearn tutorials: http://toxlearn.nlm.nih. gov/Module1.htm.

[4] NLM's Toxtutor (visit interactions): http://sis.nlm. nih.gov/enviro/toxtutor/Tox1/a42.htm.

V GRADES OF ADVERSE DRUG REACTIONS

Drugs and chemicals may exhibit adverse drug reactions (ADR, or adverse drug effect) that may include unwanted (side effects), uncomfortable (system dysfunction), or dangerous effects (toxic). ADRs are a form of manifestation of toxicity, which may occur after overexposure or high-level exposure or, in some circumstances, after exposure to therapeutic doses but often with an underlying cause (pre-existing condition). In contrast, 'Side effect' is an imprecise term often used to refer to a drug's unintended effects that occur within the therapeutic range [1]. Risk–benefit analysis provides a window into the decision-making process prior to prescribing a medication. Patient characteristics such as age, gender, ethnic background, pre-existing conditions, nutritional status, genetic pre-disposition or geographic factors, as well as drug factors (e.g., type of drug, administration route, treatment duration, dosage, and bioavailability) may profoundly influence ADR outcomes. Drug-induced adverse events can be categorized as unexpected, serious or life-threatening.

Adverse drug reactions are graded according to intensity, using a scheme that was originally introduced by the US National Cancer Institute to describe the intensity of reactions to drugs used in cancer chemotherapy [2]. This scheme is now widely used to grade the intensity of other types of adverse reactions, although it does not always apply so clearly to them. The scheme assigns grades as follows:

- Grade 1 ≡ mild;
- Grade 2 ≡ moderate;
- Grade 3 ≡ severe;
- Grade 4 ≡ life-threatening or disabling;
- Grade 5 ≡ death.

Then, instead of providing general definitions of the terms "mild", "moderate", "severe", and "life-threatening or disabling", the system describes what they mean operationally in terms of each adverse reaction, in each case the intensity being described in narrative terms. For example, hemolysis is graded as follows:

- Grade 1: Laboratory evidence of hemolysis only (e.g. direct antiglobulin test; presence of schistocytes).
- Grade 2: Evidence of red cell destruction and ≥2 g/dl decrease in hemoglobin, no transfusion.
- Grade 3: Transfusion or medical intervention (for example, steroids) indicated.
- Grade 4: Catastrophic consequences (for example, renal failure, hypotension, bronchospasm, emergency splenectomy).
- Grade 5: Death.

Not all adverse reactions are assigned all grades. For example, serum sickness is classified as being of grade 3 or grade 5 only; i.e. it is always either severe or fatal.

The system is less good at classifying subjective reactions. For example, fatigue is graded as follows:

- Grade 1: Mild fatigue over baseline.
- Grade 2: Moderate or causing difficulty performing some activities of daily living.
- Grade 3: Severe fatigue interfering with activities of daily living.
- Grade 4: Disabling.

Attribution categories can be defined as follows:

- **(i)** Definite: The adverse event is clearly related to the investigational agent(s).
- **(ii)** Probable: The adverse event is likely related to the investigational agent(s).
- **(iii)** Possible: The adverse event may be related to the investigational agent(s).
- **(iv)** Unlikely: The adverse event is doubtfully related to the investigational agent(s).
- **(v)** Unrelated: The adverse event is clearly NOT related to the investigational agent(s).

REFERENCES

[1] Merck Manuals: http://www.merckmanuals.com/professional/clinical_pharmacology/adverse_drug_reactions/adverse_drug_reactions.html.

[2] National Cancer Institute. Common Terminology Criteria for Adverse Events v3.0 (CTCAE). 9 August, 2006. http://ctep.cancer.gov/protocolDevelopment/electronic_applications/docs/ctcaev3.pdf.

VI FDA PREGNANCY CATEGORIES/ CLASSIFICATION OF TERATOGENICITY

The FDA has established five categories to indicate the potential of a drug to cause birth defects if used during pregnancy. The categories are determined by the reliability of documentation and the risk-to-benefit ratio. They do not take into account any risks from pharmaceutical agents or their metabolites in breast milk. The pregnancy categories are:

Category A: Adequate and well-controlled studies have failed to demonstrate a risk to the fetus in the first trimester of pregnancy (and there is no evidence of risk in later trimesters).

Example drugs or substances: levothyroxine, folic acid, magnesium sulfate, liothyronine.

Category B: Animal reproduction studies have failed to demonstrate a risk to the fetus and there are no adequate and well-controlled studies in pregnant women.

Example drugs: metformin, hydrochlorothiazide, cyclobenzaprine, amoxicillin, pantoprazole.

Category C: Animal reproduction studies have shown an adverse effect on the fetus and there are no adequate and well-controlled studies in humans, but potential benefits may warrant use of the drug in pregnant women despite potential risks.

Example drugs: tramadol, gabapentin, amlodipine, trazodone, prednisone.

Category D: There is positive evidence of human fetal risk based on adverse reaction data from investigational or marketing experience or studies in humans, but potential benefits may warrant use of the drug in pregnant women despite potential risks.

Example drugs: lisinopril, alprazolam, losartan, clonazepam, lorazepam.

Category X: Studies in animals or humans have demonstrated fetal abnormalities and/or there is positive evidence of human fetal risk based on adverse reaction data from investigational or marketing experience, and the risks involved in use of the drug in pregnant women clearly outweigh potential benefits.

Example drugs: atorvastatin, simvastatin, warfarin, methotrexate, finasteride.

Category N: FDA has not classified the drug.

Example drugs: aspirin, oxycodone, hydroxyzine, acetaminophen, diazepam.

The most recent (Dec 3, 2014) USFDA rulings on changes to pregnancy and lactation labeling information for prescription drug and biological products can be found at: http://www.fda.gov/NewsEvents/Newsroom/PressAnnouncements/ucm425317.htm

REFERENCES

[1] Doering PL, Boothby LA, Cheok M. Review of pregnancy labeling of prescription drugs: is the current system adequate to inform of risks? Am J Obstet Gynecol 2002; 187(2): 333–9.

[2] Ramoz LL, Patel-Shori NM. Recent changes in pregnancy and lactation labeling: retirement of risk categories. Pharmacotherapy, 2014; 34(4):389-95. doi: 10.1002/phar.

[3] Drugs.com: http://www.drugs.com/pregnancy-categories.html.

CONCLUSION

Adverse drug events, including ADRs, side effects, drug-induced diseases, toxicity, pharmacogenetics and immunologic reactions, represent a significant burden to patients, health care systems, and society. It is the goal of *Side Effects of Drugs Annual* to summarize and evaluate important new evidence-based information in order to guide clinicians in the prevention, monitoring, and assessment of adverse drug events in their patients. The work provides not only a summary of this essential new data, but suggestions for how it may be interpreted and implications for practice.

1

Central Nervous System Stimulants and Drugs That Suppress Appetite

Nicholas T. Bello[1]

Department of Animal Sciences, School of Environmental and Biological Sciences, Rutgers, The State University of New Jersey, New Brunswick, NJ, USA

[1]Corresponding author: ntbello@aesop.rutgers.edu

Amphetamine and Amphetamine Derivates [SEDA-15, 180; SEDA-32, 1; SEDA-33, 1; SEDA-34, 1; SEDA-35, 1; SEDA-36, 1]

Key to abbreviations of amphetamines:

MDA: 3,4-methylenedioxyamphetamine
MDMA: 3,4-methylenedioxymetamphetamine

Studies

A three-period (7 days/period) randomized crossover study ($n=18$) was published comparing lisdexamfetamine dimesylate (50 mg/kg), mixed amphetamines salt-immediate release (20 mg/day), and placebo on daily cognition patterns. A total of 12, 9, and 8 subjects, respectively, reported treatment-emergent adverse events (TEAE). Most common reported TEAEs with lisdexamfetamine dimesylate were dry mouth (33.3%) and decreased appetite (23.5%). Dry mouth (23.5%) was reported with mixed amphetamines salt-immediate release, and headache (17.6%) was reported with placebo [1c].

An examination of all case reports submitted to the FDA Adverse Event Reporting System (FAERS) for approved use in children (1–18 years old) revealed 1511 cases were submitted for lisdexamfetamine. Of those cases 138 were classified as an adverse event with a serious outcome (AESO) with insomnia (18%), agitation (16%), and aggression (15.9%) being the most common in all age groups. In the 12- to 18-year-old age group, which is the more likely age group to abuse stimulants, off-label use (42.4%) was the most commonly AESO with lisdexamfetamine. In comparison, methylphenidate had a total of 4055 cases reported with 542 being classified

as an AESO. For all age groups, sudden death (7.2%), aggression (7%) and agitation (6.6%) were reported with methylphenidate. In the 12- to 18-year-old age group, suicide attempt (9.5%) was the most commonly AESO with methylphenidate [2M].

In study examining Veterans Affairs administration data for a 5-year period to evaluate the use of health services by patients ($n=718$) with methamphetamine use disorder (MUD) compared with patients ($n=744$) with alcohol use disorder. Patients with MUD were more likely to have an inpatient hospitalization [Odds Ratio (OR) 1.8; 95% CI: 1.4–2.3], discharge from hospitalization against medical advice (OR 2.6; 95% CI: 1.9–3.7), and have more missed appointments of the 5-year period ($P<0.001$) [3C].

A cross-sectional study of methamphetamine-dependent subjects ($n=100$) revealed 36% met the criteria for a current psychiatric disorder. Subjects were predominately male (72%) and 80% consumed 1 g of methamphetamine per week. Median duration of methamphetamine use was 7 years. Most commonly diagnosed psychiatric illnesses were mood disorders (16%), psychotic disorders (13%), and anxiety disorders (7%). Methamphetamine-induced psychiatric disorders accounted for 4% of the mood disorders and 4% of psychotic disorders in the total population [4c].

Data collected during a 2-year period from the Iran Psychiatric Hospital in Tehran revealed 111 patients with methamphetamine-induced psychosis. The most common psychotic symptoms were persecutory delusions (82%), auditory hallucinations (44.1%) and grandiosity delusions (26.1%). The mean duration of psychotic episode was 17.37 days [5c].

© 2015 Elsevier B.V. All rights reserved.

Cases

- A 31-year-old male with a high fever, dyspnea, and a productive cough was hospitalized after a few hours of smoking amphetamine. He was a chronic user of amphetamine (>1 year). He was diagnosed with acute eosinophilic pneumonia (AEP), which was successfully treated with corticosteroids and discharged 19 days later [6A].
- A 27-year-old female presented with a 2-week history of non-productive cough, dyspnea, subjective fever, and arthralgias. Based on the clinical impression of sepsis secondary to atypical pneumonia, patient was discharged from the hospital after a 12-day course of antibiotics. Two days after discharge she returned the hospital with seizure activity. Patient admitted to extensive methamphetamine use. Further testing revealed a vasculitis without confirmatory histological markers of true vasculitis. Hence, the patient was diagnosis of methamphetamine-induced pseudovasculitis. Avoidance of methamphetamine by the patient resolved the condition [7A].

Ecstasy (3,4-Methylenedioxy-N-Methylamphetamine; MDMA)

Studies

An investigational study to determine the peripheral mononuclear cells serotonin transporter (5-HTT) gene expression changes associated with the subjective psychology assessment following MDMA intake was performed in recreational MDMA users ($n = 18$). The serotonin transporter is responsible for removing extracellular serotonin, hence is involved in serotonin signaling. Serotonin mechanisms have been implicated in the subjective response, as well as the adverse effects, of MDMA [8H]. Each subjects received MDMA (75 mg) and placebo in randomized double-blind crossover design. Dosing was separated by 7 days. There was a positive correlation between 5-HTT gene expression after MDMA intake and fatigue ($r = 0.585$; $P < 0.05$) as well as confusion ($r = 0.597$; $P < 0.05$). With respect to genotypes of 5-HTT linked polymorphism region, there was a trend for larger gene expression changes in the l/l compared with */s carriers [9c].

Cases

- A 20-year-old man was hospitalized who presented with aggressive behavior, respiratory depression, and a brief episode of apnea. He was diagnosed with diffuse alveolar hemorrhage upon X-ray examination, which resolved after 48 hours without respiratory complications. Patient had taken ecstasy at a party and tested positive for MDMA at the time of hospital admission [10A].

- A 19-month-old male child was admitted to the hospital presenting with staring (wild glance), bruxism, and erratic arm movements. No heart, lung, abdomen abnormalities were noted upon examination. MDMA and MDA were detected in the urine. Three days after admission, the child was discharged without maintenance treatment [11A].
- A 20-month-old female child was admitted to hospital for convulsions. Clinical examination demonstrated mydriasis, tachycardia, and rotation of lower limbs, rigidity, and hyperthermia. EEG and imaging were normal. Urine was initially (immunoassay) positive for amphetamines, methamphetamines and benzodiazepines. Further urine testing (GC–MS) revealed the presence of MDMA, MDA, and diazepam, and a trace of cocaine. Child's condition normalized over time [11A].
- A 19-year-old male presented with acute dyspnea. Mediastinal emphysema and epidural pneumatosis of the thoracic spine were revealed by total body CT scan. Patient consumed oral ecstasy and engaged in intense dancing prior to hospital admission [12A].
- A 27-year-old woman was hospitalized for edema of the lower limbs, ascites, and abnormal liver function tests. She had a 9-month history of orally ingesting ecstasy and administering intra-nasal cocaine two to four times a week. Histological assessment of the liver showed bridging fibrosis, stromal collapse, and proliferation of the cholangioles. Patient was hospitalized for 3 weeks, and stopped using ecstasy and cocaine. After an 8-year period of ecstasy and cocaine abstinence, her clinical examination, liver function tests, and liver elasticity were normal [13A].

Methylphenidate [SEDA-15, 2307; SEDA-32, 10; SEDA-33, 7; SEDA-34, 5; SEDA-35, 1; SEDA-36, 1]

Studies

A pharmacokinetics and safety study to evaluate multilayered extended-release bead methylphenidate (MPH-MLR) capsule (80 mg/daily), MPH-MLR sprinkle (80 mg/daily; 37% immediate release), or immediate release MPH capsule (25 mg/three times daily) used adult healthy subjects ($n = 26$) in a crossover design. Fourteen subjects (53.8%) experienced one or more mild or moderate TEAE. There were no differences between the number of subjects that reported a TEAE with capsule ($n = 8$) or sprinkle ($n = 8$). Nine subjects reported TEAEs with immediate release MPH capsule. Most commonly reported TEAEs were headache, dizziness, dry mouth, nausea, and anxiety [14c]. In a double-blind crossover study in children (6–12 years old; $n = 26$) diagnosed with attention deficit hyperactive disorder (ADHD), the effectiveness of the MPH-MLR capsule was evaluated in classroom situation. After a 2- to 4-week dose optimization phase (15–40 mg/daily), there was a 2-week cross-over evaluation phase (1 week placebo or 1 week MPH-MLR or vice versa), and 30-day safety follow-up phase. During the dose optimization (open-label) phase, the most common TEAEs were insomnia (30.8%), decreased appetite (23.1%), headache (23.1%), irritability (19.2%), pyrexia (15.4%) cough (15.4%), otitis media (11.5%), abdominal pain (11.5%), vomiting (11.5%), nasal congestion (11.5%), and rhinorrhea (11.5%). The most common TEAEs with MPH-MLR during the evaluation phase were headache (14.3%), abdominal pain (9.5%), and pyrexia (9.5%), whereas abdominal pain (4.5%), rhinitis (4.5%), insomnia (4.5%) and irritability (4.5%) were reported with placebo [15c].

Adult ADHD patients in a dose optimization study of a modified release long acting MPH (MPH-LA) were randomized to receive 40 mg ($n = 181$), 60 mg ($n = 182$), 80 mg ($n = 181$) or placebo ($n = 181$) daily for 5-week open-label study. The percentage of patients experiencing TEAE was 65.2%; the most common were headache (13.4%), decreased appetite (10.7%), dry mouth (8.6%), and nasopharyngitis (7.4%). Serious TEAEs were concussion (0.2%), rib fracture (0.2%), and panic attack (0.2%). The percentage of TEAE leading to discontinuation was 3.8%. Additional alterations were noted in electrocardiogram assessments revealing MPH-LA resulted in QTcB (13.2%) and QT (5.2%) increases from baseline >30 ms [16C].

A prospective study in children diagnosed with ADHD ($n = 77$) was performed to assess the influence of polymorphisms of the *carboxylesterase 1A1* (*CES1 A1*) gene on the effectiveness of 6-week MPH treatment course. Methylphenidate is metabolized by the liver carboxylesterase 1A1 and has a potential role in the variable MPH response in ADHD subjects. Seven polymorphisms of the *CES1 A1* gene were identified in the subject population. Children receiving the immediate release MPH, the *rs2244613* polymorphism was a significant predictor of the subjective rating of sadness ($P = 0.032$). That is, children with ADHD receiving immediate release MPH that were homozygous for the A allele ($n = 29$) were significantly more likely to experience the side effect of sadness than children heterozygous or with no copies of the A allele ($n = 12$). A significant association of a diagnosis of ADHD and the haplotype of A allele of the *rs2244613* and G allele of the *rs2002577* polymorphisms of the *CES1* genes was found. These *CES1* markers were also in linkage disequilibrium with two markers (*rs5569 and rs2242447*) of the norepinephrine transporter (NET) gene (*SLC6A2*) [17c].

In another association study in children and adolescents with ADHD ($n = 139$), the *SLC6A2* gene marker, *rs192303*, was identified with a reduction of ADHD symptoms in patients using the osmotic-controlled oral delivery system methylphenidate (OROS MPH) [18c].

In a 4-week trial of OROS-MPH of MPH-naive children and adolescents with ADHD ($n = 134$) there was a strong association (OR 5.72, $P = 0.008$) with *ABCB1* polymorphisms (c.2677G > A/T; p.Ala893Thr/Ser, *rs2032582*) and adverse drug reactions (ADRs). While the association was not stratified based on individual ADRs, the most common TEAEs were poor appetite (56.7%), sleep disturbances (41.8%), talking little with others (22.4%), and irritability (20.9%) [19c]. The *ABCB1* gene is expressed in the epithelium of the choroid plexus and luminal surface of the brain. *ABCB1* encodes a drug transporter that is a membrane transporter belonging to the adenosine triphosphate (ATP)-bind cassette family. In HEK293T cells, the ATPase activity was only 15% in the c.2677T allele of that c.2677A and c.2677G expressing cells. This preliminary finding suggests a functional consequence of an impaired clearance of MPH in children and adolescents with TT genotype at the c.2677 locus [19c].

Cases

- A 20-year-old male of normal height and weight complained of "delayed puberty." He reported high-pitched voice, lack of libido, low energy levels, chronic fatigue, and poor erectile function. His past medical history revealed he was prescribed methylphenidate for approximately 17 years. He had stopped using methylphenidate a few years ago. Patient began testosterone supplementation and reported marked improvement after 4 months [20A]. Although the mechanism was unknown, Ramasay and colleagues speculate chronic methylphenidate played a role in the impaired full development of secondary sexual characteristic in this patient based on preclinical studies [20A,21E].

- Increased a daily dosing of methylphenidate from 60 to 80 mg daily (with supplemental 10 mg dosing as needed) was suspected as a causative agent in cardiovascular abnormalities (i.e., tachycardia and radiating chest pain) in a 41-year-old Norwegian male with ADHD. Patient was given standard care for cardiovascular symptoms, acetylsalicylic acid (75 mg daily), tricagrelor (90 mg twice daily), and atorvastatin (10 mg daily). Methylphenidate dose was also reduced to 30 mg twice daily. Patient was discharged from the hospital [22A].

- A 26-year-old male was admitted to the emergency room for dyspnea. During examination he suddenly expressed suicidal ideation and was admitted to psychiatry department where he displayed somnolence, disorganized and accelerated thinking, and marked psychomotor agitation. Approximately 8 hours after admission, patient serum levels of methylphenidate were subnormal (3 µg/l; reference range 8–30 µg/l), whereas the inactive metabolic of methylphenidate, ritalinic acid, was elevated (821 µg/l; reference range 80–300 µg/l). Patient was reportedly taking methylphenidate (160 mg daily) prior to admission. No other medications or pathology were noted. Patient refused treatment and left the hospital by his own request after 3 days [23A].

- Sudden hearing loss occurred in 8-year-old female with ADHD being treated with methylphenidate (5 mg twice daily). Sensorineural hearing loss began 4 days after beginning methylphenidate treatment and was progressive and irreversible at 2 months with a course of standard therapy (e.g. oral corticosteroid, hyperbaric oxygen sessions, and additional therapies). The mechanism of sensorineural hearing loss by methylphenidate is unknown [24A].

- Two patients (61-year-old right-handed female; 54-year-old right-handed male) that suffered ischemic stroke of the left middle cerebral artery (MCA) developed dyskinesia after treatment with methylphenidate. The female patient developed involuntary, flexion, and extension movements of the right arm, which was hemiplegic. Onset of dyskinetic signs developed 2 days following increasing the dosage from 5 to 10 mg (three times daily). Dyskinetic movements resolved 48 hours following cessation of methylphenidate. In the male patient onset of dyskinesia developed 24 hours after 10 mg (three times daily). Patient displayed tongue protrusion, smacking movements of the lips, abnormal posturing of neck and left hand. Signs resolved within 72 hours after cessation of methylphenidate [25A]. Sudden onset of dyskinesia is likely a result of overstimulation of dopamine receptors by increasing extracellular dopamine levels by methylphenidate inhibiting transmitter reuptake [25A].

- A 23-month-old male was brought to the emergency after accidentally ingesting an unknown quantity of methylphenidate. His pupils were dilated and had repetitive tongue thrusting to the left, left laterocollis, and grimace of the left face. The boy was responsive and had a normal neurological examination. Diphenhydramine was given twice over a 15-hour period and he remained in the hospital overnight for observation. A follow-up examination after 14 months revealed normal growth and development and no evidence of dyskinesia [26A].

METHYLXANTHINES

Caffeine [SEDA-15, 588; SEDA-32, 14; SEDA-33, 11; SEDA-34, 6; SEDA-36, 1]

Studies

A meta-analysis found an association between high maternal caffeine intake (>350 mg/day) during pregnancy and low birth weight that included 9 prospective studies (90 747 participants and 6303 cases). Low birth weight was defined as less than 2500 g, which included small for gestational age (SGA) and intrauterine growth restriction (IUGR). The relative risk for low birth weight stratified for caffeine ingestion was as follows: low caffeine intake (50–149 mg/day) (RR 1.13; 95% CI: 1.06–1.21), for moderate caffeine intake (150–349 mg/day) (RR 1.38; 95% CI: 1.18–1.62) and for high caffeine intake (>350 mg/kg) (RR 1.60; 95% CI: 1.24–2.08). In the same meta-analysis, an additional 6 prospective studies were used to assess birth weight as a continuous variable and using no or very low maternal caffeine as a comparison group. It was determine that birth weight was 9 g lower in the low caffeine group, 33 g lower in the moderate caffeine group, and 69 g lower in the high caffeine group [27M]. The exact mechanism for the association between high caffeine intake and low birth weight remains unknown.

A randomized placebo control crossover study in athletes ($n = 90$) demonstrated that caffeinated beverages or "energy drinks" increased sport performance, but had higher percentage of reported adverse effects. Subjects were exposed to two training session separated by 1 week and randomly received a caffeinated (3 mg/kg) or non-caffeinated (placebo) beverage at each session. Subjective reports of insomnia (31.2% caffeine vs. 10.4% placebo) and nervousness (13.2% caffeine vs. 0% placebo) were significantly higher in the sessions following ingestion of caffeinated beverages [28c].

Cases

- A 42-year-old man with a history of schizoaffective disorder and caffeine overdose was admitted to the emergency room after ingesting 24 g of caffeine. Patient was attempting suicide and was found 4 days after ingestion. Four days prior to admission he reported uncontrollable vomiting, diarrhea, and loss of consciousness. He denied polysubstance abuse and was noncompliant with his prescribed medications (lithium and olanzapine). Laboratory tested were consistent with acute renal failure and rhabdomyolysis (creatinine 10.2 mg/dl). Patient received daily hemodialysis for 9 days and was transferred to the inpatient psychiatric unit [29A].

- Two cases of fatal caffeine overdose as a result of ingestion of caffeine powder were reported. One case involved an 18-year-old male that was using caffeine powder as a pre-workout supplement. Cause of death was cardiac arrest and a seizure from caffeine ingestion (blood caffeine was >70 mg/l). Another similar case involved a 39-year-old male that was a "physical fitness buff." An opened bag of caffeine was found in his vehicle and he was found deceased on his doorstep (blood caffeine was 350 mg/l) [30r].

Selective Norepinephrine Reuptake Inhibitors
Atomoxetine [SEDA-33, 6; SEDA-34, 4; SEDA-36, 1]

Studies

A meta-analysis including 25 double-blinded randomized controlled trials ($n = 3923$, 56 treatment arms) was used to assess the efficacy and safety in children and adolescents with ADHD. The mean duration of treatment was 8.6 weeks (4–18 weeks). The discontinuation rate due to TEAE was higher with atomoxetine than placebo (RR 1.89; 95% CI: 1.08–3.31; $P = 0.03$). Atomoxetine had higher rates more than 1 TEAE (70.4% versus 56.1% for placebo) and more than 1 psychiatric-TEAE (21.5% versus 7.4% for placebo). Gastrointestinal TEAEs (22.1% versus 12.4% for placebo), CNS symptoms such as hostility, irritability, aggression, anger, belligerence, and disruptive behavior (21.8% versus 15.2% for placebo), anorexia (19.2% versus 5.2% for placebo) and fatigue (11.7% versus 4.6% for placebo) were significantly ($P < 0.001$ for all) higher in atomoxetine compared with placebo-treated subjects. Subjects treated with atomoxetine lost 3.9% greater baseline body weight than placebo-treated subjects. In studies that reported cardiovascular outcomes, atomoxetine resulted in an increase in diastolic and systolic blood pressure. For heart rate there was a weighted mean difference of 6 bpm for atomoxetine-treated individuals. There were also more atomoxetine-treated patients with an >25 beats/min to >100 beats/min (6.9% versus 1.3% for placebo $P = 0.04$) elevation than placebo. Electrocardiogram data also revealed atomoxetine shortened QTc compared with placebo ($P < 0.0001$) [31M].

A head-to-head double-blinded randomized active-controlled trial compared lisdexamfetamine dimesylate (30–70 mg/daily) with atomoxetine (10–100 mg/daily) in children and adolescents with ADHD ($n = 267$) for 9 weeks. The percentage of subjects reporting TEAEs were similar for lisdexamfetamine (71.9%) and atomoxetine (70.9%) as were reports of TEAE that led to discontinuation (6.3% for lisdexamfetamine; 7.5% for atomoxetine). For lisdexamfetamine the most common TEAEs were decreased appetite (25.8%), decreased weight (21.9%), headache (13.3%), nausea (12.5%), and insomnia (11.7%). For atomoxetine the most common TEAEs were headache (16.4%), nausea (15.7%), somnolence (11.9%), decreased appetite (10.4%), and fatigue (10.4%). Lisdexamfetamine and atomoxetine were both associated with elevated cardiovascular measurements. Mean change from baseline for systolic blood pressure was +0.7 mm Hg for lisdexamfetamine and +0.6 mm Hg for atomoxetine; diastolic blood pressure elevation was +0.1 mm Hg for lisdexamfetamine and +1.3 mm Hg for atomoxetine. Elevation in pulse rate was +3.6 bpm for lisdexamfetamine and +3.7 bpm for atomoxetine [32C].

A head-to-head open-label randomized trial compared immediate-release methylphenidate (0.2–1 mg/kg/daily) with atomoxetine (0.5–1.2 mg/kg/daily) in children and adolescents with ADHD ($n = 69$) for 8 weeks. The percentage of subjects reporting TEAEs was 55% for methylphenidate and 56% for atomoxetine. For methylphenidate the most common TEAEs were decreased appetite (43.8%), headache (12.5%), pain abdomen (9.4%), irritability (6.3%) and fatigue (6.3%). The most common TEAEs were decreased appetite (33.3%), irritability (19.4%), drowsiness (16.7%), headache (5.6%), and urinary incontinence (5.6%) for atomoxetine. The atomoxetine-treated group demonstrated an increase in heart rate (mean difference from baseline +7 bpm; $P = 0.021$) [33]. In patients ($n = 27$) with postural tachycardia syndrome (POTS), acute doses (40 mg) of atomoxetine also demonstrated an increase in standing heart rate (+6 to 15 bpm) compared with placebo [34C].

Cases

- A 7-year-old male with ADHD-related symptoms and oppositional defiant disorder (ODD) previously received extended-release methylphenidate (up to 36 mg/day) and reported dry mouth, moderate weakness, and moderate introverted behavior. Patient was switched to atomoxetine (18 mg/daily) and was gradually increased to 40 mg/day over a course of approximately 2 months. However, 1 week after starting the 35 mg/day dose, repetitive bouts of nocturnal bruxism (3–5 min) were noted. The bruxism also started to emerge during the waking hours. When the child received the 40 mg/day dose the bruxism frequency and severity worsened. The bruxism subsided within a week after reduction of atomoxetine to 25 mg/day. The mechanism of atomoxetine-induced bruxism is unknown [35A].

- A 7-year-old male with ADHD developed a noticeable change in posture 3 weeks after starting atomoxetine (10 mg/day). The child had a forward bending (60 degrees from the vertical plane) of his trunk, which made him incapable of sitting in his chair during class. Hematological and neurologic examinations were normal. Atomoxetine was discontinued and child was placed on diazepam (5 mg oral). After 1 month his posture improved and his back straighten to a 45 degree bend. ADHD symptoms were controlled with methylphenidate (10 mg). After 2 years his back had approximately 15 degree bend. The mechanism of atomoxetine-induced camptocormia is unknown [36A].

- A 12-year-old female with ADHD received extended release amphetamine salts (10 mg/day) for 1.5 years. Her low weight gain and "feeling numb" on amphetamine salts, prompted her physician to reduce her dose to 5 mg and "add-on" atomoxetine

(10 mg/day). After 10 days her atomoxetine dose was increased to 25 mg/day. After 2 days, the girl complained of severe anxiety, restlessness, and agitation. Symptoms resolved 4 days after discontinuation of amphetamine salts and atomoxetine. Atomoxetine was the suspected agent for the drug-induced akathisia, because the patient was previously on a higher dose of the amphetamine salts without incident [37A].

- A 11-year-old male with ADHD treated for 2 years with atomoxetine lost consciousness and was unresponsive. Upon arrival at the emergency room he was drowsy and confused. In the preceding month the child's atomoxetine dose was increased from 0.7 to 1.2 mg/kg/day. Hematological testing show brain natriuretic peptide (BNP) was elevated (19.7 mg/dl, reference range <18.4 mg/dl). Chest X-ray revealed an enlarged heart. Electrocardiogram demonstrated bradycardia (56 bpm) and prolonged QTc interval (500 ms); after 9 hours the QTc interval was still prolonged in length (829 ms) and bradycardia slightly improved (61 bpm). Atomoxetine was discontinued and the child received a beta blocker (bisoprolol 0.01 mg/kg/day) and lidocaine. The next day, however, his bradycardia worsened (31 bpm) and he was implanted with a temporary pacemaker. He was monitored in the hospital for 4 weeks. After atomoxetine was discontinued for 5 months, the child had normal cardiac function and cardiac stress test. Normal QTc (395 ms) was noted and the child was asymptomatic at 1-year follow-up. No major mutations of the long QT syndrome (LQTS) genes were found [38A]. Peripheral adrenergic mechanisms (blood born catecholamines or peripheral nerve terminals) were implicated in the atomoxetine effect on the cardiovascular impairments [39A].
- A 10-year-old female with ADHD developed coldness and ecchymosis in her hands and feet that emerged shortly (1–2 hours) after her daily atomoxetine (18 mg/day). Atomoxetine doses were maintained at 10 mg/day and symptoms of Raynaud's phenomenon resolved [40A].
- A 6-year-old male with ADHD and a chronic motor tic disorder was receiving atomoxetine (25 mg/day) and aripiprazole (10 mg/day). At 7 years old, his dose of atomoxetine was increased to 40 mg/day. After 3 weeks, the boy developed auditory hallucinations. The hallucinations involved a male voice calling the boy's name. He was responsive to the auditory hallucinations. The boy also displayed accompanying behaviors of elevated and irritable mood, insomnia, excessive talking, and argumentative behaviors with peers. Consequently, atomoxetine was reduced to 25 mg/day and the auditory hallucinations and accompanying manic behaviors subsided within

2 weeks. At 8 years old, the boy was placed on alternating schedule of atomoxetine 25 or 40 mg every other day. The dose was accidentally increased by the parents to 40 mg and manic behaviors emerged without auditory hallucinations [41A].
- The combination of atomoxetine (40 mg/day) and aripiprazole (5 mg/day) caused recurrent penile erections (i.e., 10 times a day, lasting a few minutes, sometimes painful) in an 11-year-old male with ADHD and chronic tics. The occurrence of excessive erections ceased 8 days after discontinuation of atomoxetine. Aripiprazole was continued for 2 years without incident of recurrent penile erections [42r].

VIGILANCE PROMOTING DRUGS

Modafinil and Armodafinil [SEDA-15, 2369; SEDA-32, 6; SEDA-33, 11; SEDA-34, 6; SEDA-36, 1]

Studies

In a randomized placebo-controlled crossover study in adult male subjects ($n=32$) with mild to moderate obstructive sleep apnea (OSA), the safety and daytime wakeful effectiveness of modafinil was assessed. Subjects were included if they were not currently (within the last 3 months) using any other treatment for the OSA, such as continuous positive airway pressure or mandibular advance splint. Each subject randomly received modafinil (200 mg/daily) or placebo for 2 weeks with a 2-week washout before treatment crossover. TEAEs were reported in more subjects during the modafinil treatment (RR 2.7; 95% CI: 1.4–5.3; $P=0.003$) [43c]. The TEAEs with modafinil were mild and included trouble sleeping ($n=5$), mood changes ($n=4$), nausea ($n=2$), tight cough ($n=1$), and palpitations ($n=1$) [43c]. The safety of modafinil (200 mg/daily) was also compared with placebo in double-blinded study in Japanese patients with OSA for 4 weeks. Patients ($n=114$) in this study, however, were concurrently being treated with a positive airway pressure device. The percentage of subjects reporting TEAEs was not significantly different between modafinil (36.5%) and placebo (22.6%) groups. The most frequent TEAEs in the modafinil group were headache (11.5%), insomnia (3.8%), and palpitation (3.5%). The onset of the highest frequency of TEAEs was 7 days after initiation of treatment (either in the modafinil or placebo group) [44c].

In a randomized placebo-controlled crossover study, modafinil (100 mg/daily) resulted in an acute (4-hour post-administration) increase in seated (+5 mm Hg; $P=0.002$) and standing (+3 mm Hg; $P=0.002$) systolic blood pressure in patients with POTS ($n=54$). The clinical significance of this increase in systolic blood pressure is unknown; however, modafinil did not increase the heart rate or standing orthostatic symptoms [45c]. In a double-blinded placebo-controlled study, modafinil (200 or 400 mg/daily) was compared with pitolisant (100, 200, or 400 mg/daily) for safety and efficacy in subjects with narcolepsy ($n=94$) for 8 weeks. Pitolisant is a centrally acting selective histamine (H3) receptor inverse agonist to promote wakefulness. The percentage of subjects reporting TEAEs for pitolisant was 70%, 78% for modafinil, and 33% for placebo. Serious TEAEs were reported for pitolistant, which include abdominal pain or discomfort (3%). More serious TEAEs were reported with modafinil, including abdominal pain or discomfort (3%), abnormal behavior (3%), amphetamine-like withdrawal (3%), inner ear disorders (3%), and lymphadenopathy (3%). The most common TEAEs for pitolisant were headache (35%), insomnia (10%), nausea (6%), and abdominal discomfort or pain (6%). The most common TEAEs for modafinil were headache (18%), abdominal discomfort or pain (18%), diarrhea (12%), dizziness (12%), amphetamine-like withdrawal (10%), anxiety (6%), and irritability (6%) [46C].

Armodafinil (R-enantiomer of modafinil; 50, 150 or 250 mg/daily) was examined for efficacy and safety in promoting wakefulness in mild or moderate closed traumatic brain injured (TBI) subjects ($n=117$). The first phase of the study was 12-week randomized placebo-controlled double-blinded followed by a second phase 12-month open-label trial (150 or 250 mg/daily). During the double-blinded phase the percentage of subjects reporting TEAE were similar between armodafinil (53%) and placebo (48%). For armodafinil, headache (17%), nausea (10%) and anxiety (8%) were the most common TEAEs. During the open-labeled phase, 62% of subjects reported at least 1TEAE. One serious TEAE of moderate psychotic disorder occurred, which resolved after armodafinil was discontinued. The most common TEAEs, which were mild or moderate, were headache (15%), upper respiratory infection (9%), insomnia (6%), and nausea (6%) [47c].

The efficacy and safety of armodafinil (150 or 200 mg/daily) in adults ($n=433$) with major depressive episodes associated with bipolar I disorder was assessed by randomized placebo-controlled double-blinded study for 8 weeks. Serious TEAEs occurred in 2% (150 mg/daily) and 6% (200 mg/daily) of armodafinil subject groups. In the 150 mg group, the serious TEAEs were psychotic disorder ($n=2$), irritability ($n=1$), suicidal ideation ($n=1$), aggression ($n=1$), and depressive syndrome ($n=1$). In the 200 mg group, the serious TEAEs included acute hepatitis ($n=1$) and acute liver failure leading to death ($n=1$). For the 150 mg group, one patient developed a drug eruption and pruritic rash, and a patient that developed a contact dermatitis in the placebo group. Subjects experiencing at least 1 TEAE for placebo were 46%,

150 mg were 48%, and 200 mg were 72%. For the 150 mg group, the most common TEAEs were headache (10%), diarrhea (9%), and nausea (6%). For the 200 mg group, the most common TEAEs were headache (22%), insomnia (13%), nausea (9%), and diarrhea (6%) [48C].

Cases

- A 17-year-old male patient diagnosed with obsessive-compulsive disorder (OCD), chronic tic disorder, and primary derealization syndrome was receiving fluoxetine (40 mg/daily) and haloperidol (2 mg/day). The patient complained of excessive daytime sedation and was prescribed modafinil (200 mg/day). Since an exacerbation of tics was noted, the modafinil dose was reduced (150 mg/day) and 80% improvement in tics was noted after 2 months [49A]. The mechanism of tic exacerbation by modafinil is unknown.

- A 21-year-old male patient was using modafinil intermittently (200 mg/day up to 1600 mg/day) for about 2 years without a prescription to improve scholastic performance and prepare for college entrance exams. After about a month break he began using modafinil again and was using 1600 mg/day within a week. After 5 or 6 days he developed delusions for about 1 week and reduced his modafinil daily doses (800 mg). He was referred to psychiatric unit and began risperidone (4 mg/day; later switched to quetiapine 50 mg/day) and fluoxetine (20 mg/day). After 3 weeks of stopping of modafinil, the patient was asymptomatic upon psychiatric examination, suggestive of modafinil-induced psychosis [50A].

- Armodafinil (150 mg/day) resulted in manic symptoms in a 19-year-old female diagnosed with paranoid schizophrenia. She did not present with mania prior to initiation of armodafinil treatment which was administered for excessive daytime sleepiness. She was co-currently being treated with trihexyphenidyl (4 mg/day) and aripiprazole (30 mg/day). One year after the first episode of armodafinil-induced manic episodes, armodafinil was introduced at a lower dose (50 mg/day) without recurrence of mania [51A].

Drugs That Suppress Appetite [SEDA-30, 7; SEDA-32, 16; SEDA-33, 13; SEDA-34, 8; SEDA-36, 1]

Lorcaserin

In 2012, the US Food and Drug Agency (FDA) approved a novel centrally acting selective serotonin (5-hydroxytryptamine, 5HT) 2C receptor agonist named lorcaserin (Belviq®, Arena Pharmaceuticals, San Diego, CA). Lorcaserin (10 mg; twice daily) is a medication for weight loss in obese (BMI > 30 kg/m²) or overweight

(BMI > 27 kg/m^2) individuals with a related comorbidity (e.g., type II diabetes mellitus, hypertension, or dyslipidemia) [52S]. Even though lorcaserin has approximately 10- to 50-fold higher affinity for the feeding-related 5HT2C receptor than any other 5HT receptor [53H], lorcaserin doses that exceeded recommended doses for weight loss were reported to promote feelings of euphoria, disassociation, or hallucinations (0.1% placebo-subtracted rate of occurrence) [52S]. Lorcaserin also has the potential to induce life-threatening serotonin syndrome, when taken with other serotonergic medications [54H]. The US Drug Enforcement Administration (DEA) has labeled lorcaserin as a controlled substance (schedule IV).

Studies

In two Phase III placebo-controlled, double-blind, randomized trial the efficacy and safety of lorcaserin (10 mg; twice daily) was evaluated in obese individuals ($n = 7190$). The duration of the studies was 52 weeks. The percentage of subjects experiencing TEAEs in the lorcaserin (82.8%) and placebo (75.5%) groups were similar. In the lorcaserin group, the most commonly reported TEAEs were headache (16.8%), upper respiratory infections (13.7%), nasopharyngitis (13%), dizziness (8.5%), nausea (8.3%), sinusitis (7.4%), and fatigue (7.2%). Headache was the only TEAE associated with a discontinuation rate greater than 1% (1.3% in lorcaserin versus 0.8% in placebo groups) [55C].

Naltrexone Sustained-Release/Bupropion Sustained-Release

In 2014, the USFDA approved a combination formulation of a fixed dose of naltrexone sustained-release (32 mg) and bupropion sustained-release (360 mg) two tablets (twice daily) (Contrave®; Orexigen, La Jolla, CA) for weight loss in obese (BMI > 30 kg/m^2) or overweight (BMI > 27 kg/m^2) individuals with a related comorbidity (e.g., type II diabetes mellitus, hypertension, or dyslipidemia). Naltrexone sustained-release/bupropion sustained-release has black box warning for suicide ideation and behaviors [56S], however does not have an abuse potential and is not a scheduled controlled substance [56S,57H].

Studies

A randomized placebo-controlled Phase II study in obese subjects ($n = 107$) was designed to determine the safety and efficacy of naltrexone immediate-release (16, 32, or 48 mg/day) and bupropion sustained-release (400 mg/day) alone or in combination during a 24-week time frame. Most commonly reported TEAEs with naltrexone/bupropion combined therapy were nausea (28–41% versus placebo 3.5%), headache (6.3–14.3% versus placebo 7.1%), dizziness (9.5–12.5% versus placebo 0%), and vomiting (6.3–11.5% versus placebo 1.2%). Nausea was

dose-related to naltrexone. Both nausea and dizziness were the only TEAEs that resulted in greater than a 5% discontinuation rate and reported more frequently with combined therapy [58C]. In a fixed dose formulation naltrexone sustained-release (32 mg)/bupropion sustained-release (360 mg) was compared to placebo in a double-blinded randomized trial for 56 weeks in obese subjects with type II diabetes mellitus ($n = 505$). Doses of naltrexone sustained-release/bupropion sustained-release were gradually escalated to two tablets (twice daily) by week 4. The most common TEAEs in the naltrexone sustained-release/bupropion sustained-release group were nausea (42.3%), constipation (17.7%), vomiting (18.3%), diarrhea (15.6%), and headache (13.8%). Nausea led to discontinuation in 9.6% of the naltrexone sustained-release/bupropion sustained-release group. Nausea was also higher in subjects taking metformin (46.2% compared with 26% not taking metformin) [59C].

Phentermine [SEDA-15, 2804; SEDA-32, 17; SEDA-33, 13; SEDA-34, 8; SEDA-36, 1]

Cases

• A 45-year-old woman taking phentermine (37.5 mg/daily) arrived at the emergency room complaining of a "worsen headache" over the last 24 hours. She typically took phentermine intermittently, two to three times a week. However, for the last 2 weeks she increased the medication to two to three times daily. She had a 20-pack-year history of smoking tobacco. Upon arrival her vital signs were within the normal range but CT scans reveal a subarachnoid hemorrhage (SAH) in the basal cistern. Phentermine was discontinued and the patient began a regiment of nimodipine (60 mg) and atorvastatin (80 mg) for 21 days. Patient remained stable during her 9-day hospitalization. At her 6-week follow-up she was stable and had resumed a normal routine. The authors suggest the cause of SAH was likely secondary to a suddenly escalation in phentermine [60A].

Phentermine/Topiramate Extended Release

In 2012, the US Food and Drug Agency (FDA) approved a combinational formulation of a fixed dose of phentermine (3.75 or 7.5 mg) and topiramate (23 or 46 mg) extended release (Qysmia®; VIVUS, Mountview, CA) for weight loss in obese (Body Mass Index; BMI > 30 kg/m^2) or overweight (BMI > 27 kg/m^2) individuals with a related comorbidity (e.g., type II diabetes mellitus, hypertension, or dyslipidemia) [61S]. Because of the potential for abuse the DEA has labeled phentermine/topiramate as a controlled substance (schedule IV). Topiramate has a teratogenic potential for oral clefts [62M] and the use of phentermine/topiramate extended release is restricted in women of childbearing years. Women with reproductive potential must have a negative pregnancy test before initiation of treatment as well as monthly while being prescribed phentermine/topiramate extended release [61S].

Studies

A randomized placebo-controlled study was performed in obese adults to evaluate phentermine (PHE)/topiramate extended release (TPM ER) (7.5 mg/46 mg or 15 mg/92 mg), PHE alone (7.5 or 15 mg), or TPM ER alone (46 or 92 mg). Subjects ($n = 756$) were obese adults (BMI > 30 and <45 kg/m^2) who were divided into 7 treatment groups for duration of 28 weeks. Overall, there were 7 subjects (0.9%) that had a serious AE, but unlikely a result of the treatment conditions. A discontinuation rate of 12.5% was due to one TEAE. More subjects in the PHEN/TPM ER 7.5/46 (15.1%) and PHEN/TPM ER 15/92 (21.3%) than placebo (7.5%) discontinued the study due to a TEAE. The most common TEAEs in the two PHE/TPM ER groups (7.5/46 and 15/92 mg) were paresthesia (16% and 23.1%), dry mouth (13.2% and 18.5%), headache (15.1% and 15.7%), constipation (6.6% and 15.7%), dysgeusia (8.5% and 14.8%) and upper respiratory tract infection (13.2% and 13%). Topiramate is the likely causative component for paresthesia, since it was reported in 11.3% and 22.4% of subjects taking topiramate alone (46 and 92 mg, respectively). Paresthesia rates were similar in placebo (3.7%) and phentermine [2.8% (7.5 mg) and 4.6% (15 mg), respectively]. Except for constipation (reported in 8.3% of the placebo group), the percentage of subjects reporting a TEAE was either the same or higher in the combinational dose groups compared with each individual monotherapy [63C]. A similar distribution of TEAE was reported in a 56-week randomized placebo-controlled Phase III trials in obese adults with type II diabetes mellitus population ($n = 518$). In this study, placebo was compared to PHE/TPM ER 15 mg/92 mg (daily) or PHE/TPM ER 7.5 mg/46 mg (daily). There were 58 hypoglycemic events in 17 subjects (placebo, $n = 5$; PHE/TPM ER 15 mg/92 mg, $n = 12$). In 56 of 58 hypoglycemic events, subjects were taking sulfonylurea concomitantly. Ten of the hypoglycemic events in 3 subjects were considered related to PHE/TPM ER [64C].

PARASYMPATHOMIMETICS [SEDA-32, 19; SEDA-33, 15; SEDA-34, 9]

Rivastigmine [SEDA-15, 3072; SEDA-32, 20; SEDA-33, 16; SEDA-34, 10; SEDA-36, 1]

Studies

In a placebo-controlled, double-blind, randomized study to examine the efficacy and safety of rivastigmine

(transdermal patch 9.5 mg/day) in Parkinson's disease (PD) subjects with moderate to severe apathy without dementia ($n = 30$). During the 6-month study, the percentage of subjects experiencing TEAEs in the placebo (36%) and rivastigmine (44%) groups was similar. The commonly reported TEAEs in the rivastigmine group were asthenia/drowsiness (18.75%), faintness (18.75%), and transient worsening of painful dyskinesia (6.25%) [65c]. In an open-label, randomized study the safety of rivastigmine capsules (12 mg/daily) compared with transdermal patch (9.5 mg/day) was evaluated for motor effects in PD subjects ($n = 295$ capsules; $n = 288$ patch). During the 76-week study, the percentage of subjects with worsening PD motor symptoms was similar between capsules and transdermal patch (36.1% vs. 31.9%, respectively). Tremor was the most commonly reported worsening PD symptom with capsules (24.5%), while a smaller percentage of subjects reported tremors with the patch (9.7%) leading to discontinuation in 2.4% of capsule subjects and 0.7% of patch subjects. The most commonly reported TEAEs with the capsule formulation were nausea (40.5%), Parkinsonian rest tremor (24.5%), fall (17%), vomiting (15.3%), dizziness (9.2%), diarrhea (9.2%), hypotension (8.2%), somnolence (8.2%), and confused state (7.8%). In contrast, the most common reported TEAE with the transdermal patch were fall (20.1%), application site erythema (13.9%), Parkinsonian rest tremor (9.7%), confused state (9.4%), hallucinations (8.7%), dizziness (8%), anxiety (8%), insomnia (8%), and depression (8%) [66C].

Cases

- A 78-year-old male who had gradual cognitive decline and mildly impaired daily life ability began oral rivastigmine (gradual dosage increase over 4 weeks). Oral rivastigmine (3 mg; twice daily) was transitioned to a transdermal patch (5 mg/cm^2). After 3 days the patient developed a psychotic episode with hallucinations and delusional thoughts. Symptoms subsided after patch was removed. Patient was returned to oral rivastigmine for 4 months without further psychotic episodes [67A].
- A 75-year-old female with gradual cognitive decline and memory loss for 1 year developed acute dystonia reaction (characterized by neck twisting, voluntary movement of limbs, and restlessness) 3 hours after increasing the dosage of her transdermal patch (5–10 mg/cm^2). Previously she tolerated the 5 mg/cm^2 transdermal patch for 1 month without issue. Acute dystonia resolved after removal of patch (10 mg/cm^2). One week later the patch (10 mg/cm^2) was reapplied and a similar acute reaction occurred [68A].

Donepezil [SEDA-15, 1179; SEDA-32, 19; SEDA-33, 15; SEDA-34, 10; SEDA-36, 1]

Studies

A 52-week open-label trial to investigate the safety and efficacy of donepezil (3 mg/day for 2 weeks; 5 mg/day for 50 weeks) was conducted in subjects with Lewy bodies dementia ($n = 108$). Approximately 94.4% of subjects experiencing TEAEs; there were 27 serious TEAE in 25 patients. Four events (myocardial infarction, subarachnoid hemorrhage, asphyxia, and acute pancreatitis) resulted in death in 3 subjects. Myocardial infarction and acute pancreatitis were result of donepezil. The most commonly reported TEAEs were elevated blood creatine phosphokinase (CPK; 11.1%), contusion (11.1%), nasopharyngitis (10.2%), increased blood pressure (10.2%), fall (10.2%), diarrhea (9.3%), constipation (7.4%), Parkinsonian tremors (7.4%), blood in urine (6.5%), and protein in urine (6.5%). Elevation in blood pressure and blood CPK appeared to be transient since they were reported in more subjects during the first 12 weeks than in the last 6 months of treatment [69C]. Electrocardiogram parameters were evaluated in patients ($n = 18$) with dementia or cognitive disorder before and after receiving donepezil (mean dose 7.5 ± 2.6 mg/day). Both the PR interval and RR interval were significantly increased ($P < 0.001$ and 0.014, respectively). Mean difference in PR interval was 9.5 ± 17.1 with 4 patients exhibited a PR interval of >200 ms (upper limit) after donepezil treatment. For the electrocardiogram data set, the mean donepezil duration was 16.5 ± 11.5 weeks [70c].

Cases

- A 44-year-old male with probable behavioral-variant fronto-temporal dementia (bvFTD) began a gradual dosing escalation of donepezil (up to 10 mg over 4 weeks). Impairments in sustained attention, processing speed, and executive function became worse as treatment progressed. Neuropsychiatric evaluation at 5 weeks following the initiation of donepezil confirmed impairments. Donepezil was discontinued over a 2-week period. Re-examination after 1 month demonstrated marked improved in attention and executive functions to pre-treatment baseline. Patient died at 47 years old and confirmed bvFTD by autopsy [71A].
- Two patients presented with donepezil-induced mania (a 28-year-old male and a 64-year-old male) after displaying erratic behaviors, reduced sleep, and excessive spending patterns. The 28-year-old male self-initiated donepezil (up to 15 mg/day) to increase cognitive performance while writing his graduate thesis. Upon arrival to the emergency room the patient was treated with risperidone (0.5 mg; twice daily). Symptoms resolved after 4 days of treatment and he was gradually taken off of risperidone after 3 months.

The 64-year-old male had been taking his wife's prescription of donepezil for 4 weeks while his wife took the patient's nonsteroidal anti-inflammatory medication due to a medication mix-up. The patient was treated with risperidone (0.25 mg; twice daily) for 2 months. Donepezil-induced mania resolved in 2 days [72A].

- A 79-year-old female with PD progressively developed a forward flexion of the head a few weeks after an increase in donepezil treatment (5–10 mg/day). Symptoms of antecollis markedly improved following the cessation of donepezil [73A]. A similar presentation and resolution of antecollis was noted in 81-year-old female with Alzheimer's disease after 10 months of donepezil (5 mg/day). Cervical dystonia completed resolved 6 weeks after cessation on donepezil [74A].
- An 80-year-old female was administered an accidental high dose of donepezil (30 mg/day) for 25 days. She developed myoclonus jerks in upper and lower extremities. After 36 hours of cessation of donepezil the frequency of her myoclonic jerks was reduced. Patient resumed 10 mg/day dose of donepezil without issue at 6-month follow-up [75A].
- A 72-year-old male with Alzheimer's disease had an increase in donepezil dosage (from 5 to 10 mg/day) 2 weeks prior to being admitted to the emergency room for episodes lightheadedness and fainting, in addition to two episodes of syncope in the past week. Patient had bradycardia (30 bpm with 10-second sinus pause) with atrial fibrillation. Donepezil was discontinued and cardiac function was restored. Enhanced peripheral parasympathetic actions resulting from recently escalated donepezil dose was suspected for abnormal cardiac function [76r]. Similarly, a 77-year-old female with Alzheimer's disease was receiving oral doses of telmisartan (40 mg/day), nifedipine (40 mg/day) and pravastatin (5 mg/day). After she was hospitalized for dementia-related issues, she was administered donepezil (3 mg/day, which gradually increased to 10 mg/day on day 24). On day 30 her electrocardiogram showed a PR prolongation. Because her dementia-related symptoms were not improved, memantine (5 mg/day) was added on day 33. Her PR prolongation worsened and her heart rate dropped (56 bpm). Memantine treatment was discontinued on day 36. Following discharge donepezil was reduced to 5 mg/day [77A].
- An interaction between fluoxetine (80 mg/day) and donepezil (dose not specified) was suspected in 79-year-old male with Alzheimer's disease. The patient was also being treated with lamivudine (dose not specified) for hepatitis B cirrhosis with Child-Pugh (severity A). Elevated transaminases were noted 6 weeks after starting donepezil; patient had been taking

fluoxetine continuously for 4 years. Fluoxetine and donepezil were discontinued and a normal liver function test was noted 6 weeks later. Patient was switched to sertraline and memantine without issue [78A].

Galantamine [SEDA-36, 1]

Studies

In a 36-month, open-label trial subjects with mild Alzheimer's disease ($n = 75$) received galantamine (up to 24 mg/day based on tolerability). Approximately 72% of the study population experienced at least one TEAE by 36 months. The most common TEAEs were nausea (17.3%), skin condition not otherwise specified (NOS; 13.3%), rhinitis (13.3%), musculoskeletal condition NOS (12%), dizziness (12%), depression (12%), urinary tract infection (12%), fall with injury (12%), vomiting (10.7%), cold/influenza (10.7%), and nervous system condition NOS (9.3%). It was also noted there was a decrease in systolic blood pressure (-5 mm Hg; $P = 0.003$) and decrease in diastolic blood pressure (-3 mm Hg; $P = 0.007$). The clinical relevance of the blood pressure decrease is unknown [79c]. In a double-blind, placebo-controlled study, the effect of galantamine on cognitive aversion to electroconvulsive therapy (ECT) was evaluated in subjects with psychiatric disorders ($n = 39$). One subject discontinued the study as a result of galantamine-induced intolerable nausea [80c].

Cases

- An 81-year-old female with a history of hypertension, dyslipidemia, and spondyloarthropathy was recently diagnosed with Alzheimer disease. She was started on galantamine (dose not specified) in the preceding month and developed acute generalized exanthematous pustulosis (AGEP). Galantamine was discontinued and within 2 weeks the edematous pustules and plaques completely resolved [81A].
- A 74-year-old male with Alzheimer disease was being treated with rivastigmine (9.5 mg transdermal patch) for 1 year. Pruritus and allergic rash developed and oral galantamine was initiated. After a 4 days treatment with oral galantamine, the patient developed a rash in the same area as where rivastigmine transdermal patch was previously located [82r].

References

[1] Martin PT, Corcoran M, Zhang P, et al. Randomized, double-blind, placebo-controlled, crossover study of the effects of lisdexamfetamine dimesylate and mixed amphetamine salts on cognition throughout the day in adults with attention-deficit/hyperactivity disorder. Clin Drug Investig. 2014;34(2):147–57 [c].

[2] Lee WJ, Lee TA, Pickard AS, et al. Drugs associated with adverse events in children and adolescents. Pharmacotherapy. 2014;34(9):918–26 [M].

[3] Morasco BJ, ME O' Neil, Duckart JP, et al. Comparison of health service use among veterans with methamphetamine versus alcohol use disorders. J Addict Med. 2014;8(1):47–52 [C].

[4] Akindipe T, Wilson D, Stein DJ. Psychiatric disorders in individuals with methamphetamine dependence: prevalence and risk factors. Metab Brain Dis. 2014;29(2):351–7 [c].

[5] Fasihpour B, Molavi S, Shariat SV. Clinical features of inpatients with methamphetamine-induced psychosis. J Ment Health. 2013;22(4):341–9 [c].

[6] Lin SS, Chen YC, Chang YL, et al. Crystal amphetamine smoking-induced acute eosinophilic pneumonia and diffuse alveolar damage: a case report and literature review. Chin J Physiol. 2014;57(5):295–8 [A].

[7] Fowler AH, Majithia V. Ultimate mimicry: methamphetamine-induced pseudovasculitis. Am J Med. 2014;128(4):364–6 [A].

[8] Muller CP, Homberg JR. The role of serotonin in drug use and addiction. Behav Brain Res. 2015;277:146–92 [H].

[9] Yubero-Lahoz S, Kuypers KP, Ramaekers JG, et al. Changes in serotonin transporter (5-HTT) gene expression in peripheral blood cells after MDMA intake. Psychopharmacology (Berl). 2015;232(11):1921–9 [c].

[10] Peters NF, Gosselin R, Verstraete KL. A rare case of diffuse alveolar hemorrhage following oral amphetamine intake. JBR-BTR. 2014;97(1):42–3 [A].

[11] Pauwels S, Lemmens F, Eerdekens K, et al. Ecstasy intoxication as an unusual cause of epileptic seizures in young children. Eur J Pediatr. 2013;172(11):1547–50 [A].

[12] Clause AL, Coche E, Hantson P, et al. Spontaneous pneumomediastinum and epidural pneumatosis after oral ecstasy consumption. Acta Clin Belg. 2014;69(2):146–8 [A].

[13] Payance A, Scotto B, Perarnau JM, et al. Severe chronic hepatitis secondary to prolonged use of ecstasy and cocaine. Clin Res Hepatol Gastroenterol. 2013;37(5):e109–13 [A].

[14] Adjei A, Teuscher NS, Kupper RJ, et al. Single-dose pharmacokinetics of methylphenidate extended-release multiple layer beads administered as intact capsule or sprinkles versus methylphenidate immediate-release tablets (Ritalin®) in healthy adult volunteers. J Child Adolesc Psychopharmacol. 2014;24(10):570–8 [c].

[15] Wigal SB, Greenhill LL, Nordbrock E, et al. A randomized placebo-controlled double-blind study evaluating the time course of response to methylphenidate hydrochloride extended-release capsules in children with attention-deficit/hyperactivity disorder. J Child Adolesc Psychopharmacol. 2014;24(10):562–9 [c].

[16] Huss M, Ginsberg Y, Arngrim T, et al. Open-label dose optimization of methylphenidate modified release long acting (MPH-LA): a post hoc analysis of real-life titration from a 40-week randomized trial. Clin Drug Investig. 2014;34(9):639–49 [C].

[17] Johnson KA, Barry E, Lambert D, et al. Methylphenidate side effect profile is influenced by genetic variation in the attention-deficit/hyperactivity disorder-associated CES1 gene. J Child Adolesc Psychopharmacol. 2013;23(10):655–64 [c].

[18] Song J, Kim SW, Hong HJ, et al. Association of SNAP-25, SLC6A2, and LPHN3 with OROS methylphenidate treatment response in attention-deficit/hyperactivity disorder. Clin Neuropharmacol. 2014;37(5):136–41 [c].

[19] Kim SW, Lee JH, Lee SH, et al. ABCB1 c.2677G>T variation is associated with adverse reactions of OROS-methylphenidate in children and adolescents with ADHD. J Clin Psychopharmacol. 2013;33(4):491–8 [c].

[20] Ramasamy R, Dadhich P, Dhingra A, et al. Case report: testicular failure possibly associated with chronic use of methylphenidate, F1000Res. 2014;3:207. http://f1000research.com/articles/3-207/v1#reflist [A].

[21] Mattison DR, Plant TM, Lin HM, et al. Pubertal delay in male nonhuman primates (Macaca mulatta) treated with methylphenidate. Proc Natl Acad Sci USA. 2011;108(39):16301–6 [E].

[22] Hole LD, Schjott J. Myocardial injury in a 41-year-old male treated with methylphenidate: a case report. BMC Res Notes. 2014;7:480 [A].

[23] Gahr M, Kolle MA. Methylphenidate intoxication: somnolence as an uncommon clinical symptom and proof of overdosing by increased serum levels of ritalinic acid. Pharmacopsychiatry. 2014;47(6):215–8 [A].

[24] Karapinar U, Saglam O, Dursun E, et al. Sudden hearing loss associated with methylphenidate therapy. Eur Arch Otorhinolaryngol. 2014;271(1):199–201 [A].

[25] Kim JY, Baik JS. Adult onset methylphenidate induced dyskinesia after stroke. Parkinsonism Relat Disord. 2014;20(7):789–91 [A].

[26] Waugh JL. Acute dyskinetic reaction in a healthy toddler following methylphenidate ingestion. Pediatr Neurol. 2013;49(1):58–60.

[27] Chen LW, Wu Y, Neelakantan N, et al. Maternal caffeine intake during pregnancy is associated with risk of low birth weight: a systematic review and dose–response meta-analysis. BMC Med. 2014;12:174 [M].

[28] Salinero JJ, Lara B, Abian-Vicen J, et al. The use of energy drinks in sport: perceived ergogenicity and side effects in male and female athletes. Br J Nutr. 2014;112(9):1494–502 [c].

[29] Campana C, Griffin PL, Simon EL. Caffeine overdose resulting in severe rhabdomyolysis and acute renal failure. Am J Emerg Med. 2014;32(1):111. e3-4 [A].

[30] Eichner ER. Fatal caffeine overdose and other risks from dietary supplements. Curr Sports Med Rep. 2014;13(6):353–4 [r].

[31] Schwartz S, Correll CU. Efficacy and safety of atomoxetine in children and adolescents with attention-deficit/hyperactivity disorder: results from a comprehensive meta-analysis and metaregression. J Am Acad Child Adolesc Psychiatry. 2014;53(2):174–87 [M].

[32] Dittmann RW, Cardo E, Nagy P, et al. Efficacy and safety of lisdexamfetamine dimesylate and atomoxetine in the treatment of attention-deficit/hyperactivity disorder: a head-to-head, randomized, double-blind, phase IIIb study. CNS Drugs. 2013;27(12):1081–92 [C].

[33] Garg J, Arun P, Chavan BS. Comparative short term efficacy and tolerability of methylphenidate and atomoxetine in attention deficit hyperactivity disorder. Indian Pediatr. 2014;51(7):550–4.

[34] Green EA, Raj V, Shibao CA, et al. Effects of norepinephrine reuptake inhibition on postural tachycardia syndrome. J Am Heart Assoc. 2013;2(5):e000395 [C].

[35] Bahali K, Yalcin O, Avci A. Atomoxetine-induced wake-time teeth clenching and sleep bruxism in a child patient. Eur Child Adolesc Psychiatry. 2014;23(12):1233–5 [A].

[36] Bhattacharya A, Praharaj SK, Sinha VK. Persistent camptocormia associated with atomoxetine in a child with attention-deficit/hyperactivity disorder. J Child Adolesc Psychopharmacol. 2014;24(10):596–7 [A].

[37] Baweja R, Petrovic-Dovat L. A case of severe akathisia with atomoxetine. J Child Adolesc Psychopharmacol. 2013;23(6):426–7 [A].

[38] Yamaguchi H, Nagumo K, Nakashima T, et al. Life-threatening QT prolongation in a boy with attention-deficit/hyperactivity disorder on atomoxetine. Eur J Pediatr. 2014;173(12):1631–4 [A].

[39] Madias JE. Atomoxetine resulting in Takotsubo syndrome: is the locally-released norepinephrine from the autonomic sympathetic cardiac nerves or the blood-borne catecholamines the cause? Eur J Pediatr. 2014;173(8):1119–20 [A].

[40] Gokcen C, Kutuk MO, Coskun S. Dose-dependent Raynaud's phenomenon developing from use of atomoxetine in a girl. J Child Adolesc Psychopharmacol. 2013;23(6):428–30 [A].

[41] Liu CC, Lan CC, Chen YS. Atomoxetine-induced mania with auditory hallucination in an 8-year-old boy with attention-deficit/hyperactivity disorder and tic disorder. J Child Adolesc Psychopharmacol. 2014;24(8):466–7 [A].

[42] Goetz M, Surman CB. Prolonged penile erections associated with the use of atomoxetine and aripiprazole in an 11-year-old boy. J Clin Psychopharmacol. 2014;34(2):275–6 [r].

[43] Chapman JL, Kempler J, Chang CL, et al. Modafinil improves daytime sleepiness in patients with mild to moderate obstructive sleep apnoea not using standard treatments: a randomised placebo-controlled crossover trial. Thorax. 2014;69(3):274–9 [c].

[44] Inoue Y, Takasaki Y, Yamashiro Y. Efficacy and safety of adjunctive modafinil treatment on residual excessive daytime sleepiness among nasal continuous positive airway pressure-treated japanese patients with obstructive sleep apnea syndrome: a double-blind placebo-controlled study. J Clin Sleep Med. 2013;9(8):751–7 [c].

[45] Kpaeyeh Jr. J, Mar PL, Raj V, et al. Hemodynamic profiles and tolerability of modafinil in the treatment of postural tachycardia syndrome: a randomized, placebo-controlled trial. J Clin Psychopharmacol. 2014;34(6):738–41 [c].

[46] Dauvilliers Y, Bassetti C, Lammers GJ, et al. Pitolisant versus placebo or modafinil in patients with narcolepsy: a double-blind, randomised trial. Lancet Neurol. 2013;12(11):1068–75 [C].

[47] Menn SJ, Yang R, Lankford A. Armodafinil for the treatment of excessive sleepiness associated with mild or moderate closed traumatic brain injury: a 12-week, randomized, double-blind study followed by a 12-month open-label extension. J Clin Sleep Med. 2014;10(11):1181–91 [c].

[48] Calabrese JR, Ketter TA, Youakim JM, et al. Adjunctive armodafinil for major depressive episodes associated with bipolar I disorder: a randomized, multicenter, double-blind, placebo-controlled, proof-of-concept study. J Clin Psychiatry. 2014;71(10):1363–70 [C].

[49] Saraf G, Viswanath B, Narayanaswamy JC, et al. Modafinil for the treatment of antipsychotic-induced excessive daytime sedation: does it exacerbate tics? J Neuropsychiatry Clin Neurosci. 2013;25(4):E35–6 [A].

[50] Rudhran V, Manjunatha N, John JP. High-dose, self-administered modafinil-related psychosis: is it the pedal in the prodrome of psychosis? J Clin Psychopharmacol. 2013;33(4):576–7 [A].

[51] Bavle A, Phatak A. Armodafinil induced mania in schizophrenia. Aust N Z J Psychiatry. 2014;48(4):381 [A].

[52] Arena Belviq (Locaserin) Package Insert. http://www.belviq.com/documents/Belviq_Prescribing_information.pdf, 2012 [S].

[53] Bello NT, Liang NC. The use of serotonergic drugs to treat obesity—is there any hope? Drug Des Devel Ther. 2011;5:95–109 [H].

[54] Brashier DB, Sharma AK, Dahiya A, et al. Lorcaserin: a novel antiobesity drug. J Pharmacol Pharmacother. 2014;5(2):175–8 [H].

[55] Aronne L, Shanahan W, Fain R, et al. Safety and efficacy of lorcaserin: a combined analysis of the BLOOM and BLOSSOM trials. Postgrad Med. 2014;126(6):7–18 [C].

[56] Orexigen Contrave- Package Insert. http://www.accessdata.fda.gov/drugsatfda_docs/label/2014/200063s000lbl.pdf, 2014 [S].

[57] Verpeut JL, Bello NT. Drug safety evaluation of naltrexone/bupropion for the treatment of obesity. Expert Opin Drug Saf. 2014;13(6):831–41 [H].

[58] Smith SR, Fujioka K, Gupta AK, et al. Combination therapy with naltrexone and bupropion for obesity reduces total and visceral adiposity. Diabetes Obes Metab. 2013;15(9):863–6 [C].

[59] Hollander P, Gupta AK, Plodkowski R, et al. Effects of naltrexone sustained-release/bupropion sustained-release combination therapy on body weight and glycemic parameters in overweight and obese patients with type 2 diabetes. Diabetes Care. 2013;36(12):4022–9 [C].

[60] Bain JA, Dority JS, Cook AM. Subarachnoid hemorrhage in a patient taking phentermine for weight loss. J Am Pharm Assoc (2003). 2014;54(5):548–51 [A].

[61] VIVUS Qsymia- Package Insert. http://vivus.com/docs/QsymiaPI.pdf, 2013 [S].

[62] Margulis AV, Mitchell AA, Gilboa SM, et al. Use of topiramate in pregnancy and risk of oral clefts. Am J Obstet Gynecol. 2012;207(5):405. e1-e7 [M].

[63] Aronne LJ, Wadden TA, Peterson C, et al. Evaluation of phentermine and topiramate versus phentermine/topiramate extended-release in obese adults. Obesity (Silver Spring). 2013;21(11):2163–71 [C].

[64] Garvey WT, Ryan DH, Bohannon NJ, et al. Weight-loss therapy in type 2 diabetes: effects of phentermine and topiramate extended release. Diabetes Care. 2014;37(12):3309–16 [C].

[65] Devos D, Moreau C, Maltete D, et al. Rivastigmine in apathetic but dementia and depression-free patients with Parkinson's disease: a double-blind, placebo-controlled, randomised clinical trial. J Neurol Neurosurg Psychiatry. 2014;85(6):668–74 [c].

[66] Emre M, Poewe W, De Deyn PP, et al. Long-term safety of rivastigmine in Parkinson disease dementia: an open-label, randomized study. Clin Neuropharmacol. 2014;37(1):9–16 [C].

[67] Ku SC, Hsu CC, Chang HA, et al. Psychotic episode in a patient with Alzheimer's dementia while shifting from the oral to patch form of rivastigmine. J Neuropsychiatry Clin Neurosci. 2014;26(3): E51–2 [A].

[68] Dhikav V, Anand KS. Acute dystonic reaction with rivastigmine. Int Psychogeriatr. 2013;25(8):1385–6 [A].

[69] Ikeda M, Mori E, Kosaka K, et al. Long-term safety and efficacy of donepezil in patients with dementia with Lewy bodies: results from a 52-week, open-label, multicenter extension study. Dement Geriatr Cogn Disord. 2013;36(3–4):229–41 [C].

[70] Igeta H, Suzuki Y, Tajiri M, et al. Cardiovascular pharmacodynamics of donepezil hydrochloride on the PR and QT intervals in patients with dementia. Hum Psychopharmacol. 2014;29(3):292–4 [c].

[71] Arciniegas DB, Anderson CA. Donepezil-induced confusional state in a patient with autopsy-proven behavioral-variant frontotemporal dementia. J Neuropsychiatry Clin Neurosci. 2013;25(3):E25–6 [A].

[72] Tourian Jr L, Margolese HC, Gauthier S. Donepezil-associated mania in two patients who were using donepezil without a prescription. J Clin Psychopharmacol. 2014;34(6):753–5 [A].

[73] Oh YS, Kim JS, Ryu DW, et al. Donepezil induced antecollis in a patient with Parkinson's disease dementia. Neurol Sci. 2013;34(9):1685–6 [A].

[74] Ikeda K, Yanagihashi M, Sawada M, et al. Donepezil-induced cervical dystonia in Alzheimer's disease: a case report and literature review of dystonia due to cholinesterase inhibitors. Intern Med. 2014;53(9):1007–10 [A].

[75] Bougea A, Gerakoulis S, Anagnostou E, et al. Donepezil-induced myoclonus in a patient with Alzheimer disease. Ann Pharmacother. 2014;48(12):1659–61 [A].

[76] Shahani L. Donepezil-associated sick sinus syndrome. J Neuropsychiatry Clin Neurosci. 2014;26(1):E5 [r].

[77] Igeta H, Suzuki Y, Motegi T, et al. Deterioration in donepezil-induced PR prolongation after a coadministration of memantine in a patient with Alzheimer's disease. Gen Hosp Psychiatry. 2013;35(6):680. e9-10 [A].

[78] Chew AP, Lim WS, Tan KT. Donepezil-induced hepatotoxicity in an elderly adult taking fluoxetine. J Am Geriatr Soc. 2014;62(10):2009–11 [A].

[79] Richarz U, Gaudig M, Rettig K, et al. Galantamine treatment in outpatients with mild Alzheimer's disease. Acta Neurol Scand. 2014;129(6):382–92 [c].

[80] Matthews JD, Siefert CJ, Blais MA, et al. A double-blind, placebo-controlled study of the impact of galantamine on anterograde memory impairment during electroconvulsive therapy. J ECT. 2013;29(3):170–8 [c].

[81] Perez-Garcia MP, Sanchez-Motillas JM, Mateu-Puchades A, et al. Acute generalized exanthematous pustulosis induced by galantamine. Actas Dermosifiliogr. 2013;104(10):930–1.

[82] Goluke NM, van Strien AM, Dautzenberg PJ, et al. Skin lesions after oral acetylcholinesterase inhibitor therapy: a case report. J Am Geriatr Soc. 2014;62(10):2012–3.

2

Antidepressants

Jonathan Smithson[*,†], *Philip B. Mitchell*[*,†,1]

*School of Psychiatry, University of New South Wales, Sydney, NSW, Australia
†Black Dog Institute, Sydney, NSW, Australia
1Corresponding author: phil.mitchell@unsw.edu.au

GENERAL

Hematological

While increased bleeding risk with serotonergic antidepressants has been recognised for many years, the incidence and severity of this have been uncertain—issues of particular pertinence in those patients having surgical procedures. The underlying mechanism involves inhibition of platelet serotonin uptake, resulting in defective platelet aggregation and impaired hemostasis [1R,2R].

Perioperative Bleeding

Several studies have found that SSRIs are associated with increased perioperative bleeding. A large retrospective cohort study of 530 416 adult patients was conducted across 375 hospitals, examining a wide range of perioperative bleeding outcomes in patients on SSRIs and controls. Patients receiving SSRIs had a higher likelihood of both in-hospital mortality (adjusted OR (aOR), 1.20 [95% CI, 1.07–1.36]), and bleeding (aOR 1.09 [95% CI, 1.04–1.15]) [3C]. In an 11-year study of 2285 cosmetic breast surgery patients, 33 (1.4%) experienced a bleeding event (i.e. hematoma requiring surgical draining). Of the 196 patients (8.6%) in the SSRI group, 9 (4.6%) experienced a bleeding event, compared to 24 (1.2%) of those in the "non-use" group; patients using SSRIs had a greater than fourfold risk of breast hematoma (OR, 4.14; 95% CI, [1.90–9.04]) [4c]. Gahr et al. examined spontaneous reports of ADRs from 2 pharmacovigilance databases using a case–control methodology, examining for associations between SSRI/SNRI usage and hemorrhages [5C]. They found that none of the SSRIs was associated with heightened risk of hemorrhage. A further systematic review and meta-analysis of the bleeding risk associated with SSRIs in surgical settings included 13 studies across differing surgical procedures. Both an increased risk of perioperative bleeding (ORs of 1.21–4.14) and need for blood transfusions (ORs of up to 3.71) were found [6R].

Perioperative Bleeding and Hip Surgery

Three studies have examined the specific association between the use of SSRIs and bleeding after hip surgery. Hip surgery is frequently associated with significant bleeding due to the highly vascular anatomy of the hip and the nature of injury and operative management. Schutte et al. studied the risk of blood transfusion in patients using SSRIs in a 15-year retrospective cohort study of patients admitted for planned or emergency hip surgery [7c]. They compared 114 SSRI users to 1773 non-users, finding an increased risk for blood transfusion in SSRI users (OR 1.7 [95% CI, 1.1–2.5]). Dall et al. reported on the association between SSRIs and perioperative bleeding in patients undergoing hip replacement in a 5½-year retrospective study of 1318 consecutive patients, of whom 83 (6%) were taking a serotonergic antidepressant. They found increased rates of observed blood loss in users of serotonergic antidepressants compared to non-serotonergic antidepressants and non-users, after adjusting for potential confounders [8c]. A third study examined the risk of blood transfusions and postoperative complications with serotonergic antidepressants among 11 384 adults aged 66 years or older who were undergoing hip fracture surgery [9C]. Patients currently taking serotonergic antidepressants had an increased risk of blood transfusion compared with recent former users of these medications (OR 1.28; 95% CI, [1.14–1.43]). Furthermore, they found also greater blood loss in patients taking non-serotonergic antidepressants (OR, 1.17; 95% CI, [1.03–1.33]).

© 2015 Elsevier B.V. All rights reserved.

Although SSRIs appear to be associated with a small but significant increased risk of bleeding in intraoperative and postoperative settings, the clinical consequences of this increased tendency of bleeding seem limited, with routine discontinuation of antidepressant before surgery generally unwarranted in most cases.

Combination with Anticoagulation Therapies

The increased risk of bleeding with SSRIs is greater when co-prescribed with medications such as nonsteroidal anti-inflammatory drugs (NSAIDs), aspirin and Cox-2 inhibitors. However, the association between warfarin and SSRIs with bleeding risk is less clear. The effect of this combination was examined in a study of 9186 patients taking warfarin [10C]. The authors identified 461 major hemorrhages during the 32 888 person-years of follow-up, with 45 events during SSRI use, 12 during TCA-only use, and 404 in patients on neither medication. They found that hemorrhage rates were higher with SSRI exposure when compared to periods on no antidepressants (2.32 vs 1.35 per 100 person-years, $p < 0.001$) and that TCA exposure was not associated with increased risk of hemorrhage. The increased risk of hemorrhage with SSRIs persisted after adjusting for supra-therapeutic INR (international normalized ratio) levels. After adjustment for underlying bleeding risk and time in INR range >3, SSRIs were still associated with an increased rate of hemorrhage compared with no antidepressants (relative risk 1.41, 95% CI, [1.04–1.92], $p = 0.03$), confirming previous findings that SSRIs were associated with higher major hemorrhagic risk in patients also taking warfarin [11M].

Gastrointestinal (GI) Bleeding

There have been consistent prior reports of an increased risk of bleeding—including upper GI bleeding (UGIB)—associated with SSRIs, with a greater risk noted when these are co-prescribed with NSAIDs, anticoagulants or antiplatelet agents. The clinical implications of these observations have been unclear due to a lack of prospective randomized controlled trials and uncertainty as to the magnitude of the risk. While the main mechanism underlying SSRI-induced UGIB is inhibition of platelet serotonin uptake, there has also been some speculation that this may also result from increased gastric acid secretion, with evidence for this arising from animal studies [12E,13E] and an increase in peptic ulceration risk [14C] with SSRIs ameliorated by proton pump inhibitors [15C].

The association between SSRIs and UGIB has been the subject of recent intense scrutiny in the literature, with several meta-analyses conducted. Results have been remarkably consistent as to both the magnitude of the association and the size of the additional risk from co-prescribed drugs such as NSAIDs and aspirin. This association between SSRIs and the occurrence of UGIB was examined in a meta-analytic review of 22 cohort and case–control studies conducted by Jiang et al. [16M]. A significant association between SSRIs and UGIB was found (OR 1.55; 95% CI, [1.35–1.78]; $p < 0.001$). Furthermore, concomitant use of NSAIDs or antiplatelet agents increased the magnitude of the association. The investigators concluded that the risk of UGIB attributable to SSRI was minimal in "low-risk" SSRI users with a 'number needed to harm' (NNH) of 760 due to the low baseline risk of developing UGIB. They noted, however, that the risk might be greater in those patients with other risk factors for UGIB, for example, finding a NNH of 160 if SSRIs and NSAIDs were used concurrently.

A second meta-analysis examining the relationship between SSRIs and UGIB was performed by Anglin et al. [17M]. The authors also found a significant association between SSRI use and UGIB (OR 1.66, 95% CI, [1.44–1.92]) in 15 case–control studies, with a similar association being found in 5 cohort studies (OR 1.68, 95% CI, [1.13–2.50]). Furthermore, they found that the risk of UGIB was further increased when SSRIs and NSAIDs were used concurrently (OR = 4.25, 95% CI [2.82–6.42]). The NNH for UGIB with SSRIs was 3177 in a "low-risk" population and 881 in a "high-risk" population. In another meta-analysis of studies published in the 13 years to 2012, Oka et al. evaluated differences in risk of UGIB when SSRIs, NSAIDs, or both, were used [18M]. They found ORs for the risk of UGIB in association with SSRIs, NSAIDs, or SSRIs and NSAIDs in combination, to be 1.73 (95% CI, [0.65–2.82]), 2.55 (95% CI, [1.51–3.59]), and 4.02 (95% CI, [2.89–5.15]), respectively; i.e., SSRIs alone did not increase risk, while NSAIDs alone did, with the latter risk increased substantially on co-prescription with SSRIs.

A pooled case–control study examined the risk of UGIB with the concomitant use of NSAIDs and low-dose aspirin with other drugs including SSRIs [19C]. SSRI monotherapy increased the risk of UGIB by a factor of 1.59 (95% CI, [1.20–2.12]). When NSAIDs or aspirin were used concomitantly with SSRIs the risk increased to 4.58 (95% CI, [2.73–7.69] $p < 0.001$) and 3.86 (95% CI, [2.75–5.42] $p < 0.001$), respectively. The increase in risk for Cox-2 inhibitors with SSRIs did not achieve significance. In a study of the short-term use of SSRIs and risk of UGIB, Wang et al. examined data for 5377 UGIB patients [20C]. The adjusted odds ratio for the risk of UGIB after SSRI exposure was 1.67 (95% CI, [1.23–2.26]) for the first 7-day window after commencement of the antidepressant, 1.84 (95% CI, [1.42–2.40]) for the 14-day window and 1.67 (95% CI, [1.34–2.08]) for the 28-day window. Interestingly, only SSRIs with a high or intermediate affinity for the serotonin transporter (fluoxetine and sertraline) were found to be associated with UGIB (AOR, 1.68 (95% CI, [1.10–2.57]) and AOR,

1.87 (95% CI, [1.16–3.02]), respectively). No increased risk was found in patients taking tricyclic antidepressants.

Brain Hemorrhage

Eighty-seven percent of strokes are ischemic, caused by either a thrombotic or embolic event, while 13% are hemorrhagic—10% due to intracerebral hemorrhage and 3% to subarachnoid hemorrhage. The relationship between SSRIs and stroke, either ischemic or hemorrhagic, remains complex and controversial.

Shin et al. performed a meta-analysis of 13 studies (three case–controls, six nested case–control, and four cohorts). Interestingly, they found the use of SSRIs to be associated with an increased risk of *all* types of stroke [adjusted odds ratio (aOR), 1.40; 95% CI 1.09–1.80], including ischemic (aOR 1.48; 95% CI 1.08–2.02) and hemorrhagic (aOR 1.32; 95% CI 1.02–1.71) [21M]. Further analysis of the two subtypes of hemorrhagic stroke, i.e., intracerebral and subarachnoid hemorrhage, showed an increased risk of intracerebral hemorrhage to be associated with SSRIs (aOR 1.30; 95% CI 1.02–1.67). As most strokes are ischemic, given that SSRIs *reduce* platelet aggregation, there is at least the theoretical possibility that treatment with such an agent might reduce the incidence of ischemic stroke. Aarts et al. undertook a population-based study of 4945 patients in whom brain MRI was available [22c]. The authors found that the use of antidepressants with strong serotonin reuptake inhibition were not associated with greater rates of microbleeds or ischemic vascular brain damage. In contrast, a recent meta-analysis of 16 observational studies involving 506 411 participants reported that SSRIs were associated with an increased risk of intracerebral hemorrhage (ICH); adjusted risk ratio, 1.42; (95% CI, [1.23–1.64]) [23M]. Considering the usual incidence of ICH of about 25 per 100 000 person-years [24M], this meta-analysis has been interpreted as suggesting that SSRIs may "realize one additional ICH per 10 000 persons (0.01%) treated for 1 year" [25R].

Mortensen and coworkers examined the association between pre- and post-stroke use of SSRIs with stroke severity, clinical outcome and mortality in two studies [26C,27c]. They sought to examine the effects of pre-stroke SSRIs among first-ever patients with hemorrhagic and ischemic stroke in a national registry-based follow-up study. Considering 1252 *hemorrhagic* strokes (626 pre-stroke SSRI users and 626 propensity score-matched nonusers), they found that *pre-stroke* SSRI use was associated with greater severity (aOR, 1.41; 95% CI; [1.08–1.84]) and a higher mortality risk within 30 days (aOR, 1.60; 95% CI; [1.17–2.18]). In the 8956 patients with *ischemic* stroke (4478 pre-stroke SSRI users and 4478 propensity score-matched nonusers), *pre-stroke* SSRI use was not associated with either greater severity or higher 30-day

mortality risk. The same authors performed a nationwide follow-up study of the effects of SSRIs administered *after ischemic* stroke [27c]. They found that SSRI users had a *lower* risk of the combined outcome of acute myocardial infarction (AMI) and recurrent ischemic stroke (adjusted HR, 0.77; 95% CI, [0.62–0.96]), although the risk of either individually did not reach significance. They reported that SSRI users had a higher risk of overall major bleeding (adjusted HR, 1.33; 95% CI, [1.14–1.55]).

Although anticoagulant therapies are used to reduce the risk of recurrence of ischemic events such as acute myocardial infarction (AMI) and ischemic stroke, their use involves the risk of a greater likelihood, or increased severity, of hemorrhage. SSRIs may further exacerbate this risk. Addressing this issue, Lopponen et al. examined for any differential fatality rate following primary intracerebral hemorrhage (PICH) in patients receiving warfarin alone, or with either aspirin, SSRIs or SNRIs [28C]. 1983 patients with PICH were initially identified; of those, 176 with warfarin-associated PICH were eligible for analysis. Nineteen patients had taken SSRI or SNRI antidepressants with warfarin, and 17 aspirin with warfarin. Considering those taking warfarin alone, with aspirin, or with a SSRI or SNRI, the 30-day case fatality rates were 50.7%, 58.8%, and 78.9%, respectively; the rate for warfarin plus an SSRI or SNRI compared with warfarin alone was significant ($p = 0.03$). Furthermore, warfarin combined with an SSRI or SNRI was a significant independent predictor of case fatality [adjusted HR 2.10, 95% CI, (1.13–3.92), $p = 0.02$].

Also noting the previously inconsistent results regarding the role of SSRIs in stroke, Lee et al. examined for any association between different types of antidepressants (SSRIs and TCAs) and the risk of cerebrovascular events in patients with either depression or anxiety. They performed a retrospective nationwide population-based cohort study of patients with depression or anxiety who commenced SSRIs and TCAs [29C]. Compared with TCAs, SSRIs significantly reduced risk of stroke, with an adjusted hazard ratio of 0.67 (95% CI; [0.47–0.96]).

In contrast to the findings of the Lee et al. study, Hung et al., using the same National Health Insurance claims database over the same time period, analyzed 28 145 subjects older than 65 years. Their survival analysis showed a greater probability of stroke in those with SSRI exposure (hazard ratio: 2.66, 95% [CI; 2.21–3.20]); this was independent of depression-related stroke risk [30C].

Postpartum Hemorrhage

A study by Palmsten et al. of 106 000 low income women found that women with exposure to SSRIs at delivery had a 1.47-fold increased risk of PPH (95% CI [1.33–1.62]). Those with only a recent SSRI or past non-SSRI antidepressant exposures showed lesser associations, albeit still significant, with PPH, with adjusted relative risks of 1.19 (95% [CI, 1.03–1.38]) and 1.26 (95% CI, [1.00–1.59]), respectively. This study suggested that there may be one additional case of PPH for every 80–100 women using antidepressants around the time of delivery [31C]. A hospital-based cohort study examining the association between SSRI use in pregnancy and PPH and post-partum anemia involved all women who gave birth at Karolinska University Hospital over a 5-year period [32C]. Five hundred women were identified as being exposed to an SSRI. The investigators found that the absolute risks of PPH and post-partum anemia for the 1.2% of women exposed to SSRIs were 18.0% and 12.8%, respectively. Women who reported use of SSRI during pregnancy and had a vaginal non-surgical delivery had an approximately twofold increased risk of both PPH (OR, 2.6; 95% CI, [2.0–3.5]) and postpartum anemia (OR, 2.1; 95% CI, [1.5–2.9]). Using a national birth registry and data from a Mother and Child Cohort (MoBa) study, Lupatelli et al. examined obstetric bleeding outcomes following exposure during pregnancy to four classes of antidepressants: SSRIs, SNRIs, TCAs, and other antidepressant drugs (OADs) [33C]. Of these patients, 527 (0.92%) used either an SSRI or a SNRI. Compared with non-exposed subjects, no overall increased risk of vaginal bleeding in pregnancy or PPH was found among women exposed to antidepressants. Although there are some inconsistent reports, there appears to be growing consensus for a slightly increased risk of PPH in women exposed to SSRIs at delivery, although the absolute risk is small and the clinical significance uncertain.

Reproductive System (Pregnancy, Development and Infancy)

Spontaneous Abortion/Miscarriage

Several studies have further examined for the association between SSRIs in early pregnancy and risk of miscarriage. These studies have variously reported either a small increased risk, no additional risk [34C], or a risk associated with discontinuation of SSRI treatment before pregnancy. A meta-analysis of three studies reporting on spontaneous abortion lacking a depressed control group found no significant association between antidepressant medication exposure and spontaneous abortion [35M]. A nationwide cohort study correlated SSRI use with risk of miscarriage. The authors found that of 22 884 mothers exposed to an SSRI during the first 35 days of their pregnancy, 12.6% (2883) had a miscarriage. This compared with 11.1% among mothers unexposed to SSRIs. The adjusted hazard ratio for miscarriage following exposure to an SSRI was 1.27 (95% CI, [1.22–1.33]). Importantly, women who discontinued SSRI treatment 3–12 months before pregnancy had a comparable increased hazard

ratio for miscarriage of 1.24 (95% CI, [1.18–1.30]) [36C]. A multi-nation population-based cohort study of women with singleton births examined the association between maternal SSRI use during pregnancy and stillbirth, neonatal death, and post-neonatal death. After accounting for potential confounding variables, SSRI use was not found to be associated with greater rates of any of these outcomes [37C].

Teratogenesis—General Findings

A cohort study of singleton pregnancies in women aged 15–45 years identified 3276 women who took either a TCA or SSRI during the first trimester of pregnancy. There was no increase in the risk of congenital anomalies in the offspring of mothers exposed to these medications [38C].

Teratogenesis—Cardiac Malformations

Huybrechts et al. performed a large population-based cohort study of women enrolled in a national health insurance scheme. The rate of cardiac defects was 90.1 per 10 000 in the 580 exposed to antidepressants *in utero* compared to 72.3 per 10 000 in the 6403 infants who were not exposed to antidepressants—a relative risk of 1.25 (95% CI, [1.13–1.38]). However, after adjustment for multiple factors including maternal depression, there was no significant increase in risk [39C]. Bérard et al. examined the relationship between exposure to sertraline during the first trimester of pregnancy and the risk of subsequent congenital malformations in a population-based cohort of depressed women from 1998 to 2010 [40C]. Sertraline was not found to be associated with an increased risk of overall major malformations when compared to non-use of antidepressants but was associated with an increased risk of atrial/ventricular defects (RR 1.34, 95% CI [1.02–1.76]) and craniosynostosis (RR 2.03, 95% CI [1.09–3.75]). Craniosynostosis was also associated with exposure to SSRIs other than sertraline during the first trimester of pregnancy (RR: 2.43, 95% CI, [1.44–4.11]) as were musculoskeletal defects (RR: 1.28, 95% CI, [1.03–1.58]). Ban et al. sought to estimate risks of major congenital anomaly (MCA) in children whose mothers were prescribed antidepressants during early pregnancy or who received a diagnosis of depression but did not receive antidepressants. They conducted a large population-based cohort study of 349 127 singleton live births [41C]. The overall risk of a MCA was not increased in children of mothers with unmedicated depression, SSRIs or TCAs when compared with women without depression. However, paroxetine was associated with increased heart anomalies compared with both women without depression (aOR 1.78, 95% CI, [1.09–2.88]) and those with unmedicated depression (aOR 1.67, 95% CI, [1.00–2.80]). Despite a growing and substantial literature regarding the use of SSRIs in pregnancy, there are major inconsistencies in the findings of studies examining for cardiac teratogenic effects. Recent studies have reported that an additional risk for cardiovascular malformations may also occur also in offspring of women with untreated depression.

Teratogenesis—Neurological Abnormalities

Munch et al. conducted a nationwide, register based, cohort study to investigate potential maternal and pregnancy-related risk factors for congenital hydrocephalus (CHC) [42C]. From their cohort of 1 928 666 live-born children, 1193 cases of isolated CHC were identified (0.062/1000 born children). The authors found that first trimester exposure to maternal antidepressants was associated with a significantly increased risk of isolated CHC (RR 2.52, 95% CI, [1.47–4.29]). In this study, the association between isolated CHC and maternal use of antidepressants was based on small case numbers. Of the 14 affected cases identified, 13 were on SSRIs. The authors specifically estimated the risk of isolated CHC following maternal SSRI use and found a relative risk of 2.7 (95% CI, [1.5–4.6]). The authors noted that it could not be determined whether the observed association was reflective of a direct causal relationship, or whether a range of comorbidities or subject behaviors (such as a lower ultrasound screening rate) associated with the use of antidepressants may have affected the risk.

Teratogenesis—Talipes Equinovarus ("Clubfoot")

The authors of a population-based case–control study performed logistic regression on 622 clubfoot cases compared with 2002 non-cases [43c]. They found that SSRI use, for a period of more than 30 days in the second and third month of pregnancy (the relevant gestational period), was higher in "case" mothers (5%) than control mothers (3%). This corresponded to an OR for any SSRI use and clubfoot of 1.8 (95% CI=1.1–2.8). For escitalopram the OR was 2.8 (95% CI, [1.1–7.2]), however, the authors noted that due to the small numbers the OR estimates for other individual SSRIs were unstable.

Preterm Birth and Low Birth Weight

Jensen et al. [44C] undertook a national register study on 673 853 pregnant women to investigate the effect of antidepressants on rates of 'small for gestational age' (SGA) pregnancies and further, to differentiate the effect of in utero antidepressant exposure from that of maternal depression. The authors found that antidepressant use during pregnancy was only weakly associated with SGA (hazard ratios (HR)=1.19; 95% CI, [1.11–1.28]), but a psychiatric diagnosis before or during pregnancy was not (HR=1.02; 95% CI, [0.92–1.13]). Sub-analysis showed that the association with SGA for antidepressant use during pregnancy was found only for SSRI and newer antidepressants. Noting a recent meta-analysis which showed that antidepressant use in pregnancy

was not associated with spontaneous abortion but was significantly associated with preterm birth (PTB) and low birth weight (LBW) [45M], Huang et al. conducted a further meta-analysis adding eight more recent studies [46M]. In this updated analysis, they found antidepressant use during pregnancy to be significantly associated with LBW (RR: 1.44, 95% CI: [1.21–1.70]) and PTB (RR: 1.69, 95% CI: [1.52–1.88]).

Apgar Scores

In an national registry study of psychiatric patients, Jensen et al. sought to estimate the effects of both maternal depression and exposure to antidepressants in utero on low (<7) Apgar scores 5 min after delivery [47C]. While confirming that infants exposed to antidepressants were at increased risk (OR=1.72, 95% CI, [1.34–2.20]), the authors found that maternal depression per se (i.e. in the absence of antidepressants) was not associated with a low Apgar score. The increased risk of a low Apgar was only found among infants exposed to SSRIs (OR=1.96, 95% CI, [1.52–2.54]). The authors concluded that the use of SSRIs during pregnancy increases the risk of a low Apgar score by more than 70%, independent of maternal depression, however, noted that the absolute prevalence of a low Apgar score was still low at 1.14%.

Persistent Pulmonary Hypertension of the Newborn

Grigoriadis and coworkers conducted a meta-analysis of seven studies to examine the risk for PPHN associated with antenatal exposure to antidepressants. They found that exposure to SSRIs in late pregnancy was associated with PPHN (OR 2.50, 95% CI, [1.32–4.73]; $p=0.005$), but that exposure to SSRIs in early pregnancy was not [48M]. The authors estimated the number needed to harm (NNH) for PPHN in late pregnancy to be between 286 and 351.

Respiratory Distress

A meta-analysis of six randomized controlled trials and 15 observational studies found that maternal SSRI treatment, compared with untreated maternal depression, was associated with a significantly increased risk of respiratory distress in infants with a pooled odds ratio of 1.91 (95% CI [1.63–2.24]) [49M].

Poor Neonatal Adaptation (PNA)

In the largest of risk factors for PNA in infants exposed to antidepressants, the authors performed a single center cohort study of 247 infants exposed to an antidepressant during the last trimester of fetal life. 157 (64%) were assessed as developing PNA [50C]. SSRIs were associated with an increased risk of PNA compared to SNRIs (OR 2.52 95% CI, [1.07–5.95] $p=0.04$).

Infant Neurodevelopment/Development

A small study of the effect of prenatal antidepressant exposure (mostly SSRIs) on infant neurodevelopment compared 35 antidepressant exposed and 25 non-exposed infants at 18 months of age on a range of neurodevelopmental domains. There was no difference in any of the neurodevelopmental assessments, which included cognitive, motor and language outcomes [51c]. A further study by Santucci et al. examined the impact of prenatal exposure to both SSRIs and maternal major depressive disorder (MDD) on infant development. They conducted a longitudinal study of 166 mother and infant dyads, of which 68 of the mothers had MDD [52c]. Using the Bayley Scales of Infant Development, the authors found that there was no effect of maternal depression, irrespective of whether they were treated with an SSRI, compared with non-exposed controls. A large national register was used to investigate the relationships between prenatal SSRIs and childhood weight at 7 years of age [53C]. While overall there was no effect of antidepressants on weight in the total sample, an increased risk of being above the 85 percentile for weight was observed among males (adjusted prevalence ratio, aPR 1.78; 95% CI, 1.01–3.12) but not females.

Autism

A number of research groups continue to examine the association between exposure to SSRIs *in utero* and Autism Spectrum Disorders (ASD). Although some agreement for an association between SSRIs in pregnancy and childhood ASD appears to be emerging, the findings in this area remain inconsistent [54c]. The authors of a recent critical analysis of this association found an increased risk, albeit with uncertain causality [55M]. Four case–control studies were included in their meta-analysis and the adjusted odds ratios from these studies were 1.81 (95% CI, [1.47–2.24]). The findings of this meta-analysis support an increased risk of ASD in children of mothers exposed to SSRIs during pregnancy; however, the nature of the association remains unclear. In a large population-based case–control study of the risk of ASD in children following *in utero* exposure to SSRIs, Gidaya and coworkers found 1.5% of cases and 0.7% of controls exposed to SSRIs. In addition, they found a greater effect with longer *in utero* exposure, with the effect present in all 'exposure windows' (i.e. early, middle and late pregnancy). Notably the strongest associations were for the highest prenatal exposure, and persisted after adjustment for possible confounding by indication [56C]. El Marroun et al. prospectively examined whether *in utero* SSSRI exposure was associated with childhood autistic symptoms in a population of 376 children exposed to maternal depressive symptoms (with no SSRI exposure), 69 children prenatally exposed to SSRIs, and 5531 unexposed

children. They found that prenatal exposure to maternal depressive symptoms without SSRIs was associated with both pervasive developmental difficulties (odds ratio (OR) = 1.44, 95% CI, [1.07–1.93]) and affective problems (OR = 1.44, 95% CI, [1.15–1.81]). Children with prenatal exposure to SSRIs were at higher risk for developing pervasive developmental problems (OR = 1.91, 95% CI, [1.13–3.47]) compared with unexposed children. Children with prenatal SSRI exposure had more autistic traits (B = 0.15, 95% CI, [0.08–0.22]) when compared with those exposed to depressive symptoms only [57C]. Hviid et al. performed a cohort study of all single live births over a 10-year period in Denmark involving 626 875 births. When they compared the use of SSRI during pregnancy with no use of SSRIs both before and during pregnancy the authors found no significant increase in risk. However, among women who received SSRIs before, but not during pregnancy, there was a significantly increased risk compared to those who had not used SSRIs at any stage [1.46, 95% CI, (1.17–1.81)]. Sorenson et al. also examined the association between prenatal exposure to antidepressant medication and. They found that children with prenatal exposure to antidepressants had an adjusted hazard ratio of 1.5 (95% CI, [1.2–1.9]) for ASD compared with unexposed children. However, they found that the risk of ASD was not significantly different when exposed children were compared with their unexposed siblings, leading them to conclude that, after controlling for relevant confounding factors, no significant association between prenatal exposure to antidepressant medication and ASDs in the offspring could be determined. While the relationship between ASD and *in utero* exposure to SSRIs during pregnancy remains uncertain, there is some evidence for an approximate doubling of risk, with the risk being greater with first trimester exposure and longer exposure *in utero*. Some studies, however, suggest that this apparent effect may reflect rather the impact of maternal depression.

Attention Deficit Hyperactivity Disorder

A study of 1377 children diagnosed with ASD and 2243 with attention deficit hyperactivity disorder (ADHD), matched 3:1 with healthy controls, examined for the risk to each disorder associated with SSRI exposure *in utero* [58C]. SSRI antidepressant exposure, both before and during pregnancy, was associated with risk for ASD; however, this was no longer significant after controlling for maternal major depression. In contrast, exposure to SSRIs *in utero*, but not before pregnancy, was associated with greater risk of ADHD (OR 1.81 (1.22–2.70)), with this association remaining significant after adjustment for maternal depression. In contrast, however, a national register study of 877 778 children, of whom 1.7% were exposed to antidepressants either 30 days before or during pregnancy, with a median follow up of 8 years, found no evidence for an increased risk of developing ADHD [59C].

Cardiovascular

Coronary Heart Disease (CHD)

A meta-analysis of seven case–control studies and eight cohort studies examined the relationship between SSRIs and the risk of CHD among subjects with no prior history of this condition; no association was found between SSRIs and CHD [60M].

Mortality Rates/Cardiac Arrest

A prospective study of 956 patients with coronary heart disease (CHD) found that TCAs were associated with increased mortality compared to both SSRIs and no antidepressants. The death rate after follow up of up to 7 years was 52.3% for the TCA users, compared with 38.2% with SSRIs and 37.3% for those on no antidepressants (hazard ratio 1.74 [95% confidence interval (CI), [1.12–2.69], $p = 0.01$]), though this association was no longer significant after adjustment for measures of autonomic function [61C]. A second paper reported on a nationwide out-of hospital cardiac arrest (OHCA) study which examined the association between specific antidepressants and OHCA. An association between cardiac arrest and antidepressants was observed, with a significant (albeit small) increased risk being observed only for citalopram (OR = 1.29, CI: 1.02–1.63) and nortriptyline (OR = 5.14, 95% CI: [2.17–12.2]) [62C].

Idiopathic Pulmonary Arterial Hypertension

A nested case control study using national primary care and hospital databases examined the relationship between antidepressants and idiopathic pulmonary arterial hypertension (IPAH). The authors found that the use of *any* antidepressant was associated with a significantly increased risk of IPAH (RR, 1.67; 95% CI, [1.17–2.37]) [63C].

Takotsubo Cardiomyopathy (TTC)

A small retrospective descriptive study [64c] examined the association between SSRIs and TTC. Seventy-eight inpatients with TTC, of whom 15 were taking a SSRI, were followed for up to 6 months. Patients on SSRIs had a lower survival rate compared with those not taking SSRIs ($p = 0.04$).

Sensory Systems

Eye—Cataract

A population-based case–control study investigated for any potential association between SSRIs and new cases of first-eye cataract surgery [65M]. SSRI use of 12 months or more was associated with an increased risk of cataract surgery (OR, 1.36; 95% CI, [1.23–1.51]; $p < 0.001$). The risk of cataract surgery was highest with citalopram (OR 1.53; 95% CI, [1.33–1.77]; $p < 0.001$).

Metabolism

Weight Gain

Uguz et al. examined weight gain in patients taking newer antidepressants in a cross-sectional study of 362 consecutive psychiatric patients taking antidepressants for 6–36 months. Over half of the patients studied (55.2%) gained weight with 40.6% gaining 7% or more of their initial weight. Citalopram, escitalopram, sertraline, paroxetine, venlafaxine, duloxetine and mirtazapine, but not fluoxetine, were all associated with significant weight gain [66c]. Blumenthal et al. [67C] identified 22 610 adult patients who had commenced an antidepressant and for whom weight data were available in a regional health care system, assessing the association between individual antidepressants and weight change over 12 months after treatment initiation. They found the greatest weight gain in patients taking mirtazapine and paroxetine, which was similar in magnitude to that observed with citalopram. Compared with citalopram, a significantly decreased rate of weight gain was observed in patients treated with bupropion, amitriptyline and nortriptyline. Noting limited empirical data on antidepressant use and weight change in younger patients, Cockerill et al. performed a historical cohort study assessing change in BMI associated with antidepressant use in overweight adolescents with a depressive disorder [68c]. They found that BMI significantly increased only in those adolescents treated with SSRIs.

Musculoskeletal

Fracture/Bone Loss

A large prospective randomly selected population-based community cohort of subjects aged 50 years and over was conducted, assessing the association between SSRIs and SNRIs and fracture [69C]. SSRI/SNRI use was associated with increased risk of 'fragility fracture' (hazard ratio (HR), 1.88; 95% CI [1.48–2.39]). Diem and coworkers examined annual BMD changes in new users of antidepressants (SSRIs and TCAs) and nonusers in a prospective cohort study [70C]. The authors found no evidence that SSRI or TCA users had an increased rate of bone loss at the total hip and femoral neck.

Psychiatric

Suicide Risk

A population-based cohort study from a national primary care database examined the association between initiation of SSRIs, TCAs and other antidepressants, and the risk of suicide or attempted suicide. Current use of any of the SSRIs, TCAs or other antidepressants was not associated with increased risk of suicide compared to past use of any antidepressants [71C]. Another retrospective cohort study of 36842 children compared the risk of suicide attempts among new users of non-fluoxetine SSRIs and venlafaxine to that of new users of fluoxetine [72C]. The adjusted rate of suicide attempts did not differ between current users of non-fluoxetine SSRI and SNRI antidepressants compared with current users of fluoxetine. Miller et al. investigated this issue in the largest US cohort study of children and adults to date [73C]. They found that, regardless of age, rates of deliberate self-harm were similar in patients initiating SSRIs and SNRIs. In a further study, Miller and coworkers examined the relationship between risk of suicidal behavior and antidepressant dose [74C]. They found that the rate of deliberate self-harm among subjects 24 years of age or younger who were treated with high-dose SSRIs was approximately twice that of matched patients on "modal-dose" therapy (hazard ratio [HR], 2.2 [95% CI, 1.6–3.0]). There was no such dosage effect for adults 25–64 years of age. Interestingly, a prospective naturalistic study in France similarly found that high commencing doses of SSRIs doubled the risk of worsening suicidal intent during the first 6 weeks of treatment [75C].

Gastrointestinal

Microscopic Colitis (MC)

Tong et al. conducted a meta-analysis of 25 published epidemiological studies of MC, finding an increased risk of MC associated with SSRIs (OR 2.41, 95% CI, [1.64–3.53]) [76R]. An elegant case–control study using national patient, pathology and prescription registries examined the relationship between MC and exposure to SSRIs [77C]. The authors found a significant association between SSRIs and both lymphocytic colitis (adjusted OR = 2.89; 95% CI, [2.61–3.20]) and collagenous colitis (adjusted OR = 1.59 95% CI, [1.45–1.74]).

SELECTIVE SEROTONIN RE-UPTAKE INHIBITORS (SSRIs) [SED-15, 3109; SEDA-31, 18; SEDA-32, 33; SEDA-33, 26; SEDA-34, 17; SEDA-35, 30; SEDA-36, 14]

Citalopram and Escitalopram

Cardiovascular

QTc INTERVAL AND TORSADE DE POINTES

A cross-sectional study of 38397 patients who had an ECG following prescription of an antidepressant confirmed the effect of citalopram on the QTc interval.

A significant dose–response relationship for QTc prolongation was identified for citalopram, escitalopram and amitriptyline [78C]. Beach et al. have reported the first meta-analysis of the relationship between SSRIs and corrected QT interval (QTc). They considered 16 prospective controlled studies, finding that SSRIs as a group were associated with a modest, statistically significant, dose-dependent increase in QTc interval compared to placebo (+6.10 ms; 95% CI, [3.47–8.73]; $p < 0.001$) [79M]. In this study, the analysis of individual SSRIs on the QTc interval showed that citalopram (10.58 ms; 95% CI, [3.93–17.23]), escitalopram (7.27 ms; 95% CI, [3.78–10.83]) and sertraline (3.00 ms; 95% CI, [2.95–3.05]) all led to statistically greater QTc prolongation than placebo; neither fluoxetine nor paroxetine were associated with QTc prolongation. Citalopram was associated with significantly greater QTc prolongation compared to fluoxetine, sertraline, paroxetine or fluvoxamine. A retrospective cohort study of depressed patients who received either citalopram ($n = 618450$) or sertraline ($n = 365898$) found that citalopram—at a dose above 40 mg—was not associated with a higher risk of ventricular arrhythmia, or cardiac or non-cardiac death. Rather, this higher dose was associated with a statistically significantly *reduced* risk of ventricular arrhythmia, all-cause mortality and non-cardiac mortality when compared to doses of 20 mg or less [80C]. A cross-sectional study of 6790 inpatients at admission found that 27.3% had an abnormal ECG, 107 (1.6%) had a long QT interval, and 62 (0.9%) fulfilled criteria for drug-induced long QT interval cases. Although citalopram and escitalopram were associated with QTc >500 ms (aOR 4.38, 95% CI, [1.45–13.3]), these antidepressants were not associated with the more serious outcomes of TdP or sudden cardiac death [81C]. With regard to the effect of escitalopram on the QTc interval, Thase et al. examined the cardiovascular effects of this SSRI in large double-blind, randomized, placebo-controlled studies of short-term (8–12 weeks) and long term treatment [82C]. Initial and final ECG assessments for 2407 escitalopram patients and 1952 placebo patients showed no clinically meaningful changes in ECG values.

Fluoxetine

Dermatological

Angioedema   A further report of angioedema in association with fluoxetine at therapeutic doses has been published [83A]:

An 11-year-old depressed male was commenced on fluoxetine 10 mg/day and 4 days later presented to the ED with edema of hands, face, tongue, periorbital areas and scrota along with respiratory distress. Following dermatological consultation and routine biochemical, hematological and complement investigations a diagnosis of angioedema with mild symptoms of anaphylaxis was made. Pollens, foodstuffs, insect bites, cold, and light were excluded as etiological agents. There was no history of stressors or infectious illness and the patient had not used any other drugs or food supplements except fluoxetine. There was no family history of angioedema no previous history of allergies or intestinal colic. Complement levels also supported exclusion of hereditary angioedema. Fluoxetine was ceased and the patient was commenced on prednisolone and pheniramine. The signs and symptoms completely remitted within 48 hours, and the patient was restarted on sertraline 12.5 mg/day without incident.

Chronic Angle-Closure Glaucoma
There has been a recent case report of chronic angle-closure glaucoma which presented after 4 months of treatment with paroxetine [84A].

A 33-year-old woman who had been taking paroxetine for 4 months presented to the ER with acute unilateral visual loss due to chronic angle-closure glaucoma. She described a sudden loss of visual acuity in the left eye. Examination revealed a narrow anterior chamber and an intraocular pressure of 42 mm Hg in the left eye and 29 mm Hg in the right eye. Examination of her fundi revealed a cup to disc ratio of 0.9–1 for the left eye and 0.1–0.2 for the right eye. Paroxetine was ceased and 48 hours later the IOP was 10 mm Hg in both eyes. Bilateral laser iridotomy was performed. At follow up intraocular pressure was 41 mm Hg in the left eye and 25 mg in the right, history revealed that the patient had resumed paroxetine therapy on her own. The patient was asked to cease paroxetine after which intraocular pressure in both eyes returned to 10 mm Hg after 48 hours.

Acute Generalized Exanthematous Pustulosis (AGEP)
Recently, a further report of AGEP in association with SSRI treatment has been published, the first involving paroxetine [85A].

A 16-year-old girl with anorexia nervosa, with no personal or family history of psoriasis, was reviewed on account of a generalized pruritic pustular eruption which was first noticed 12 days after commencing 20 mg daily of paroxetine at which time she was observed to have erythematous papules and pustules on her neck and face, which spread to both her extremities and trunk over the next three days. On examination she was afebrile and had bilateral symmetrical confluent patches of erythema on all four limbs and trunk which were studded with numerous scattered non-follicular pustules. There was no involvement of her scalp or mucous membranes. She was afebrile with no lesions of the scalp; Routine investigations revealed a neutrophilic leukocytosis, with C-reactive protein within normal limits. Histology of the lesions revealed spongiform pustulation, subcorneal pustules and a perivascular and diffuse dermal infiltrate of lymphocytes and eosinophils with a mild dermal edema was also noted. Culture of pustules failed to lead to identification of a responsible microorganism. On account of the clinical presentation, its temporal association with paroxetine administration, and histopathological features, a diagnosis of AGEP attributable to paroxetine was made. Following discontinuation of paroxetine and treatment with prednisone 50 mg daily the patient's cutaneous eruptions gradually improved and resolved within a fortnight.

Sertraline

Ophthalmic

Acute Angle-Closure Glaucoma
The first case of acute angle-closure glaucoma related to sertraline has been reported [86A]:

A 64-year-old Chinese female with no history of mental disorder presented with a 2 month history of depression and sertraline 50 mg daily commenced. Her medical history was negative except for osteoporosis treated with hormone replacement therapy. She denied previous eye problems or family history of glaucoma. After a first dose of 50 mg sertraline around midday, the patient reported ocular pain and blurring of vision in her right eye within 12 hours however the symptoms resolved the following day, and she continued sertraline for 2 more days when she experienced a recurrence ocular pain and blurred vision in her right eye of much greater intensity but now also associated with vomiting. On the fourth day the patient stopped the sertraline and saw her family practitioner as her symptoms had not abated. Urgent referral to an ophthalmologist revealed that visual acuity of her right and left eyes were 1/80 and 20/30, respectively. Slit lamp examination of her right eye, revealed corneal injection and edema. Her pupil was mid-dilated and sluggish. The anterior chamber was shallow with evidence of inflammation. Her lens showed minimal cataract. Intraocular pressure (IOP) of her right eye was markedly elevated at 56 mm Hg. The optic discs were pink with normal cup–disc ratios for both fundi. Automated refraction found bilateral mild hypermetropia (of +2 to +3D) with minimal astigmatism. She was diagnosed with acute angle closure glaucoma (AACG) of her right eye. Topical anti-glaucoma medications and steroids were commenced and Argon laser peripheral iridoplasty performed the same day. Her right eye IOP was lowered to 20 mm Hg 1 hour after iridoplasty. The next day, the visual acuity in the right eye returned to 20/30 with resolution of corneal edema and IOP was 8 mm Hg for each eye. Gonioscopy revealed quadrants of closed iridocorneal angles in both eyes and bilateral laser peripheral iridotomy was performed as a definitive treatment. Topical medications were tapered and ceased after 1 month with normal IOP maintained. Visual acuity was 20/30 for each eye, and the patient received ongoing ophthalmological follow-up.

Dermatological

Acneiform Eruption
SSRIs are recognized as potentially associated with a wide range of cutaneous side effects such as spontaneous bruising, pruritus, urticaria, angioedema, erythema multiforme, Stevens–Johnson syndrome, toxic epidermal necrolysis, erythema nodosum, alopecia, hypertrichosis, leukocytoclastic vasculitis, and acneiform eruption [87R]. A degree of cross-reactivity is observed within the class of SSRIs with respect to cutaneous adverse reactions. In SEDA 36 we reported a case of escitalopram-induced acneiform eruption which remitted but recurred after commencement of another SSRI [88A]. Although acneiform eruption is listed in the product information as an infrequent side effect of sertraline [89S], there have been no previous published reports of this reaction. A case in a 38-year-old woman has been reported [90A].

A 38-year-old woman, diagnosed with paranoid schizophrenia, who was maintained on risperidone 8 mg/day and treated with topiramate 50 mg/day for migraine, was commenced on sertraline 50 mg daily for depressive symptoms. Twelve days later she was distressed by the development of acneiform papulopustular eruptions lesions over her face which were not preceded by comedones. There was no medical or dermatological history of note and routine biochemical and hematological investigations were within normal limits. After the cessation of sertraline, acneiform lesions disappeared over 5 days without any other intervention.

SEROTONIN AND NORADRENALINE RE-UPTAKE INHIBITORS (SNRIs)

Venlafaxine and Desvenlafaxine [SED-15, 3614; SEDA-31, 22; SEDA-32, 35; SEDA-33, 32; SEDA-34, 20; SEDA-35, 32; SEDA-36, 19]

Venlafaxine

PERIPHERAL EDEMA

A case of venlafaxine-associated edema and weight gain has been reported [91A].

A 38-year-old woman, with no previous psychiatric history, presented with increasing depressive symptoms over 4 weeks, not involving changes in appetite or a history of weight gain and was commenced on venlafaxine 75 mg daily, increasing to 150 mg after 1 week. Two weeks after commencing venlafaxine she reported a weight gain of 15 kg and a marked swelling particularly of her legs and hands, but involving almost all regions of her body. She denied any increase in appetite. Examination and routine laboratory tests were within normal limits. Following the cessation of venlafaxine her weight gain and edema resolved within 1 week.

SEIZURES IN A NEONATE

A case of neonatal seizures following maternal venlafaxine during pregnancy and breastfeeding has been reported [92A].

A 31-year-old woman with a history of depression and anxiety who had been taking 150 and 75 mg venlafaxine on alternate days during pregnancy was delivered of her first baby at term by normal vaginal delivery after an uncomplicated pregnancy. The infant weighed 3789 grams and his Apgar scores were 8, 9 and 9 at 1, 5 and 10 minutes respectively. The mother breastfed her baby, and except for mild respiratory distress, there were no obvious signs of withdrawal or toxicity. The infant was observed by nursing staff to have short episodes of jerks of his arms on the third day of life and the following day episodes with myoclonic fits were also observed. Despite these observations, physical examination was normal, including muscular tone, movement patterns and normal primitive reflexes. The modified Finnegan score was four and SNRI withdrawal syndrome was considered most likely. Breast feeding was ceased. A continuous multichannel EEG monitoring showed normal background activity for a term infant however during one observed seizure, a short period of EEG amplitude suppression over the right hemisphere was seen. Other seizures occurred without obvious changes in EEG. Repeated standard EEG registrations were also found with sharp activity, suspicious for epilepsy in the same area, unrelated to seizures observed clinically. The infant responded well to a single dose of 20 mg/kg of phenobarbitone, followed by 5 mg/kg daily and antibiotics and antiviral treatment were continued for 5 days until bacterial and viral etiologies could be excluded. After abnormalities persisted on EEG fosphenytoin was given however this was associated with the baby becoming hypotonic, with diminished reflexes, leading to the withdrawal of fosphenytoin and phenobarbitone. Clinical seizures returned and phenobarbitone was reinstated. Exhaustive investigation including CSF and blood culture, metabolic screening, blood count, CRP, calcium and magnesium levels, ammonium and anion gap, blood glucose concentration and acid base status were with normal limits. No signs of toxic or hypoxic-ischemic injury were seen on repeated (three) Tesla cerebral MRI scans performed on days 4 and 10 at which time venlafaxine and O-desmethylvenlafaxine serum levels were nil.

Duloxetine

ACUTE ANGLE-CLOSURE GLAUCOMA

Several reports have linked Acute Angle-Closure Glaucoma (AACG) to SSRI treatment, especially with paroxetine [84A]. Venlafaxine has also been implicated in Acute Angle-Closure Glaucoma in four case reports [93A,94A,95A,96A], but there have been no prior reports associating duloxetine with AACG. The first case of duloxetine-induced AACG has recently been reported [97A].

An 81-year-old Caucasian woman with hyperopia and cataract developed ocular symptoms 2 days after starting duloxetine, and was diagnosed with AACG. Her elevated intraocular pressure (IOP) was lowered with medical treatment, and she discontinued duloxetine, subsequently underwent bilateral laser iridotomy in both eyes, after which time her IOP remained adequately controlled.

SPONTANEOUS ABORTION

A recent review by Andrade noted that the safety of duloxetine during pregnancy and breastfeeding remains to be established [98R]. Studying a national register of 1005319 pregnancies, Kjaersgaard et al. found that 114721 (11.4%) ended in a spontaneous abortion [99C]. 22061 of these pregnancies involved exposure to antidepressants, and 1843 involved a hospital-based diagnosis of depression but no treatment with antidepressants. The investigators found that, compared with no exposure, antidepressant exposure was associated with an aRR of 1.14 (95% CI, [1.10–1.18]) for spontaneous abortion. There was no increase in risk for those with untreated depression. While no individual SSRI was associated with spontaneous abortion, 3 antidepressants with both serotonergic and nor-adrenergic effects were associated with increased risk of this complication venlafaxine (RR 1.80; 95% CI [1.19–2.72]), duloxetine (RR 3.12; 95% CI [1.55–6.31]) and mirtazapine (RR 2.23; 95%, [1.34–3.70]). A separate safety and surveillance study noted an absolute risk of 18% in pregnancies exposed to duloxetine compared to a background risk of 12–15% [100c].

NEUROLOGICAL

Paresthesias The majority of cases of sensory disturbances related to antidepressants have been in association with SSRIs. Reports of paresthesia or distinct disturbance to sensation with SNRIs are relatively rare. The first case of paresthesia associated with duloxetine has been reported [101A].

A 50-year-old woman with depression was treated with duloxetine 30 mg. Although there was an improvement in her mood after 2 weeks, she reported an episodic "unpleasant tingling or burning sensation in the sole of her foot", which occurred for up to 2 hours at a time, several times a day. Physical examination revealed no abnormality and she denied taking other medications or preparations. At the second follow up after 2 weeks, the burning sensation was reported as being worse and continuing throughout the day. Duloxetine was ceased and tianeptine 12.5 mg twice daily started; subsequently the burning or tingling sensation disappeared within 7 days. The patient refused the offer of duloxetine re-challenge.

Galactorrhoea and Restless Legs Syndrome A case of galactorrhoea and restless legs in association with duloxetine was reported [102A].

A 46-year-old woman presented with depression which was treated with duloxetine 30 mg daily, increasing to 60 mg daily after 4 weeks. There was no medical history of note and her menstrual periods had ceased. She denied taking other medications or preparations. After 6 weeks of treatment at this dose she presented complaining of a milky discharge from her breasts, and sensations of fullness and pain in both breasts. In addition she described "distressing sensations deep inside the limbs occurring at bedtime" and "an irresistible urge to move her legs". She denied any previous experience of these symptoms. A general physical examination and neurological examination were normal as were laboratory investigations which included blood chemistry, thyroid function test TFT/TSH, FSH and LH levels. A cranial MRI revealed no abnormality and, in particular, her pituitary gland was not enlarged. Her serum prolactin level was measured as 37.9 ng/mL (normal <20 ng/ml). Duloxetine was ceased and bupropion commenced at 150 mg daily, gradually increasing to 300 mg daily over 4 weeks. Within 2 weeks, the galactorrhoea and RLS symptoms had improved considerably. Six weeks following the cessation of duloxetine, her serum prolactin was 20.2 ng/mL.

Milnacipran

TOLERABILITY

In an open-label, flexible-dosing, phase 3 study conducted in 110 study centers with 1227 subjects, 642 subjects discontinued milnacipran, 256 (20.9%) due to adverse events. The mean duration of treatment was 19 months. Treatment-emergent adverse events were reported in 88.3% of subjects, with nausea and headache the most common, occurring in 25.9% and 13.4% of patients, respectively [103A]. Of the patients who withdrew from the trial due to adverse effects, the most common were nausea (2.9%), hypertension (1.7%), hyperhidrosis (1.5%), hot flushes (1.3%), depression (1.3%), palpitations (1.3%) and headache (1.1%). Serious adverse events occurred in 109 (8.9%) patients, with the most serious being cholelithiasis, which occurred in 7 patients (0.6%).

Levomilnacipran

Levomilnacipran, the levo-enantiomer of milnacipran, is a selective serotonin-norepinephrine reuptake inhibitor (SNRI) with greater potency for inhibition of norepinephrine than serotonin reuptake. It was approved by the FDA in the United States in July 2013, following one 10-week phase II and four 8-week phase III clinical trials.

The most commonly reported adverse effects—occurring in at least 5% of subjects, and at least twice the rate found with placebo—were nausea, hyperhidrosis, constipation, increased heart rate, erectile dysfunction (in men), vomiting, tachycardia, and palpitations [104R]. Urinary hesitancy and erectile dysfunction were dose-related. Discontinuation rates were triple those reported on placebo (9% vs 3%). with the commonest reason for discontinuation being nausea which occurred in 1.5% of subjects [105S]. In the short term trials of 1583 patients with major depressive disorder who were treated with between 40 and 120 mg of levomilnacipran daily, both urinary hesitation and testicular pain were observed in 4% of patients on levomilnacipran compared with zero, or less than 1%, respectively, on the 1040 patients assigned to placebo. Hypertension, hypotension, reduced appetite and hot flushes, all occurred in about 3% of patients receiving levomilnacipran compared to 1% of patients receiving placebo [106R].

OTHER ANTIDEPRESSANTS

Agomelatine

Hepatotoxicity

Agomelatine is a relatively new antidepressant with known potential for dose-dependent hepatic effects. In SEDA 36, we noted six reports of hepatic failure associated with agomelatine and updated warnings guidance for agomelatine, including the monitoring of liver function tests at initiation of treatment and at weeks 3, 6, 12 and 24 as well as with increased doses of agomelatine [107S]. There have been further reports associating agomelatine and liver injury. Montastruc et al., using data from four national (Spanish, French, Italian and Portuguese) pharmacovigilance databases, used a case/non-case approach to assess the strength of the association between antidepressants and hepatotoxicity [108C]. Over the survey period, 3300 cases of hepatotoxicity were recorded for all antidepressants including agomelatine. 63 cases of hepatotoxicity associated with agomelatine were identified. Agomelatine was statistically associated with hepatotoxicity in Spain [reporting odds ratio (ROR), 4.9 (95% CI, 2.4–9.7)], France (ROR, 2.4 [95% CI, 1.5–3.7]) and Italy (ROR, 5.1 [95% CI, 1.7–14.0]).

Gynecomastia

A case of gynecomastia induced by agomelatine has been reported [109A].

A 19-year-old male presented to a general medical clinic with a 2-month history of progressive bilateral breast swelling and tenderness. He had been taking agomelatine 25 mg daily for depression for about 4 months and denied using alcohol, illicit drugs, anabolic steroid or any other preparation. There was no medical history of note, including no history of thyroid, liver or renal disease. Physical examination revealed bilateral tender gynecomastia, without galactorrhoea. Laboratory tests revealed a mildly increased serum prolactin of 443 mIU/L (normal range 86–324 mIU/L). Testosterone, luteinizing hormone, estradiol and human chorionic gonadotropin (HCG) levels were normal. Agomelatine was discontinued; 2 months later, significant improvement was reported with reduced breast swelling and no tenderness. At 4 months after the cessation of agomelatine, the gynecomastia had completely resolved and prolactin normalized (263 mIU/L).

Bupropion (Amfebutamone) [SED-15, 108; SEDA-31, 22; SEDA-32, 35; SEDA-33, 33; SEDA 34, 21; SEDA-35, 34; SEDA-36, 21]

Neurological

STUTTERING

A case of bupropion induced stuttering, believed to be the first in the literature, has been reported [110A].

A 59-year-old African-American woman with a history depression presented to the ER with acute speaking difficulty. One hour earlier when speaking to her daughter on the telephone she became unable to form words. Her speech defect included sound prolongations, silent blocking, word production with excess physical tension, and monosyllabic whole-word repetitions. Her stuttering was exacerbated when stressful topics were discussed at interview. There was no dysarthria or aphasia. A potential stroke was excluded by neurological consultation who determined that, except for some slight finger dysdiadochokinesia, neurologic examination and head CT were normal. The patient was alert and oriented, without signs of psychosis or encephalopathy. She described her mood was "good", with affect appearing appropriate. Cognition was unimpaired as per a Mini Mental Status Exam, 30/30. Results of laboratory investigations, including urine toxicology, were within normal limits. Initially, somatization was suspected and the patient transferred to inpatient psychiatry service. A review of the patient's medication history, however, revealed that she was started bupropion sustained release (SR) 150 mg bid 4 days prior to assessment and a medication effect was considered. Bupropion was ceased and 2 days later her speech had normalized.

Hyponatremia

Although hyponatremia has been repeatedly reported with tricyclic antidepressants, SSRIs, venlafaxine and mirtazapine [111R], bupropion has hitherto only been linked to hyponatremia in two previous case reports. A third case has been reported [112A].

A 75-year-old man presented with a 4-month history of depression. He had a 10-year history of hypertension, treated with amlodipine 5 mg/day and atenolol 50 mg/day, and a 3-year history of Parkinson's disease treated with carbidopa 37.5 mg/day and levodopa 150 mg/day. There was no past history of hyponatremia. Investigations in the form of hemogram, serum electrolytes, renal function tests, liver function tests, thyroid function test, fasting blood glucose level and lipid profile were within normal limits. Before starting bupropion, the serum sodium level was 148 mEq/L. Bupropion was commenced, initially at 75 mg/day, and gradually increased to 300 mg/day, with continuous monitoring of serum sodium and potassium levels. After 2 weeks of bupropion treatment, a sodium level of 126.4 mEq/L was noted but without clinical

manifestations on either mental status or physical examination of hyponatremia. Specifically there was no suggestion of confusion, fluid loss, nausea, vomiting, headache, muscle weakness, muscle spasms or seizures. Further, there was no worsening of fatigue, lethargy and restlessness. Physical examination revealed no evidence of pedal edema or dehydration. No change was made in any of his previously continued medications (levodopa, carbidopa, amlodipine and atenolol). Following advice to reduce his fluid intake, increase his salt intake, serum sodium levels were repeated after 4 days and showed a serum sodium level of 119.5 mEq/L. Bupropion was ceased; four days later the serum sodium level was 125.6 mEq/L returning, to 138 mEq/L after 3 days.

Renal Impairment

The first case of serum creatinine elevation in association with bupropion has been reported [113A].

A 34-year-old male was commenced on bupropion 150 mg daily day for 3 days, thence 150 mg twice daily after 3 days, following admission to a clinic for smoking cessation. On initial evaluation, serum creatinine was 1.09 mg/dl, serum urea level was 32.6 mg/dl and other routine laboratory results were within normal limits. After the second week of treatment serum creatinine was found to be elevated at 1.31 mg/dl and the patient was referred to a nephrology clinic. The patient was asymptomatic and other laboratory findings, including serum lipids, albumin, total protein, creatine phosphokinase, C-reactive protein, anti-nuclear antibody, anti-neutrophil cytoplasmic antibody, C3, C4, immunoglobulin (Ig) G, IgA, IgM and urine analysis, were all within normal limits. At review, no potential causes of an elevation in serum creatinine, such as gastroenteritis, the use of new drugs or herbal preparation, extreme exercise, polyuria or other urinary problems were found. On examination blood pressure was normal, and physical examination unremarkable. Urinary and renal ultrasonography in pre and post void phase was normal. At the end of the third week of bupropion treatment, serum creatinine level was 2.12 mg/dl. Repeated urinalysis with sediment revealed no suggestion of renal injury, and the spot urine protein/creatinine ratio was 0.1. In the absence of other causes, bupropion was ceased. Following cessation of bupropion, the patient's serum creatinine levels gradually decreased to normal over 9 days.

Hematologic

Bupropion has been twice previously linked to eosinophilia [114A,115A]. A third case of bupropion-related eosinophilia has been recently reported [116A].

A 48-year-old woman with depression was prescribed bupropion 150 mg/day by a psychiatrist. After 19 days of bupropion the patient consulted her general practitioner complaining of myalgia and a nonproductive cough. Investigation 5 days later showed a hemoglobin 11.7 g/dL (reference range 12.1–16). All sub fractions were normal except her eosinophils which were elevated at 4.7×10^9/L (0–0.5). Blood tests performed in the previous 9 months were within normal range including eosinophils: (0.2×10^9/L). A comprehensive physical examination, paying special attention to skin, soft tissues, lungs, liver and spleen, and a complete patient interview regarding diet, drug and toxic exposure was performed. Consultation with the regional Pharmacovigilance Unit suggested bupropion as being responsible for the eosinophilia. Following gradual discontinuation of bupropion there was a significant decrease in the eosinophil count (from 4.7 to 1.0×10^9/L). The myalgia and non-productive cough also resolved.

Drug Abuse

Although early research did not suggest that bupropion had psychostimulant properties [117R] and was considered a drug of low abuse potential [118R], there has been growing evidence of its abuse [119R], with one review describing bupropion as "the most commonly cited misused antidepressant" of the last decade [120R]. In SEDA 36 we reported cases of nasal insufflation [121A] and intravenous misuse [122A], noting its popularity in correctional settings [123A]. A recent review has detailed a second case of intravenous bupropion abuse and seven case reports of nasal insufflation [124R]. Moreover, there is increasing anecdotal evidence of a greater extent of abuse, particularly in correctional settings [125R,126R,127,128R].

Seizures

Lewis et al. [129R] conducted an 11-year retrospective review of cases of nasal insufflation and seizures reported to a state poison control authority. There were 2270 bupropion related cases, of which 67 (3%) involved insufflation. Of the 67, 20 (30%) experienced a seizure before arrival at the health care facility. Tachycardia was present in almost all patients who had seizures.

Mirtazapine [SED-15, 2536; SEDA-32, 36; SEDA-33, 33; SEDA-34, 22; SEDA-35, 34; SEDA-36, 21]

Peripheral Edema

A case of tender, pitting pedal edema in association with mirtazapine, in a patient also taking venlafaxine, has been reported [130A]. A case of non-pitting, non-tender peripheral edema in association with venlafaxine has been previously reported [131A].

A 48-year-old female, who had been receiving venlafaxine for the prior 2 years, was admitted as an inpatient with a relapse of her depressive illness with suicidal ideation. She had no medical or surgical history of note, nor other medical problems. Physical and neurological examination was unremarkable. Comprehensive metabolic and hematologic investigations and urine testing were normal. Mirtazapine 15 mg/day was added to the venlafaxine and increased after 1 week to 30 mg/day, after which she complained of swollen and tender feet. Physical examination was normal except for bilateral tender pitting pedal oedema to the level of her ankles. Reduction of mirtazapine to 15 mg daily only partially reduced the edema but did not resolve it. Complete cessation of mirtazapine was followed by the complete resolution of the pitting edema within 48 hours. Repeat investigations were normal.

Sleep-Related Movement Disorder

A recent review described seven cases of restless legs syndrome (RLS) associated with mirtazapine, and a small prospective study in which 15 of 57 patients (28%) prescribed mirtazapine experienced new or worsening of RLS, especially during the initiation phase of treatment [132R]. A possible case of mirtazapine-induced periodic limb movement disorder (PLMD) has been reported [133A].

A 28-year-old male presented for treatment of opioid dependence of 6 years duration. In an effort to promote sleep, mirtazapine 15 mg was added, and following this, for 4 consecutive nights the patient complained of involuntary repetitive movements of both legs during sleep. These were associated with severe pricking pain in the distal half of his leg and the sole of his foot. The movements would start about 30 min after commencement of sleep, last for 3–5 seconds on each occasion and recurred every 10 min, continuing for 2 to 3 hours after retiring. The leg movements, over which he claimed no control, relieved the pain he experienced, but disturbed his sleep. The patients on adjacent beds confirmed seeing these movements at night. The patient denied any history of similar movements in childhood or adolescence, or during previous episodes of opiate withdrawal. With the discontinuation of mirtazapine, the pain and leg movements ceased and his sleep was no longer disturbed. Over the next 12 days of admission, and at follow up at 9 months, he denied any return of symptoms.

Vortioxetine

Vortioxetine is a new antidepressant approved by the FDA for the treatment of adult major depression in September 2013 [134S], and regulatory bodies in Europe later the same year. Vortioxetine selectively inhibits reuptake of serotonin (5-HT), enhances serotonergic activity, agonizes the 5-HT1A receptor, partially agonizes the 5-HT1B receptor, and antagonizes the 5-HT3, 5-HT1D, and 5-HT7 receptors [135R,136R]. Apart from the company-sponsored clinical trials preceding registration, there is limited data yet available on the adverse effects of vortioxetine. As yet, there have been no case reports of adverse reactions. In the registration trials, nausea, vomiting and constipation were common (occurring in more than 5% of subjects) and drug-related (occurring at twice the rate found with placebo). Nausea was the most common adverse effect, and was dose-related, occurring in 32% of patients. In a meta-analysis of 7 published and 5 unpublished short-term (6–12 week) RCTs of vortioxetine, Pae et al. found that discontinuation owing to adverse events was significantly more common with vortioxetine than placebo (OR 1.530, 95% CI [1.144–2.047]) though less common than with the comparator antidepressants, duloxetine and agomelatine {OR 0.728, 95% CI, (0.554–0.957)} [137M].

In another systematic review and meta-analysis of all-available reports of clinical trials of vortioxetine for the treatment of major depressive disorder, Citrome concluded that the number needed to harm (NNH)—for discontinuation of vortioxetine due to an adverse event—was 36 (95% CI) [24–70]. The most common adverse effects (incidence 5%, and at least twice the rate of placebo) were nausea, constipation and vomiting, with NNH values vs placebo of 6 (95% CI, [6–7]), 64 (95% CI,

[37–240]), and 28 (95% CI, [23–28]), respectively [138M]. Llorca performed meta-regression analyses to indirectly compare vortioxetine to seven other antidepressants with different mechanisms of action, using only experimental drug and placebo arms from placebo-controlled registration studies to ensure comparability [139C]. With regard to tolerability (as assessed by withdrawal rates) only agomelatine [1.77 ($p = 0.03$)] showed significantly better tolerability. Vortioxetine was significantly less likely to result in withdrawal compared with desvenlafaxine, 0.58 ($p = 0.04$), venlafaxine, 0.47 ($p = 0.01$), and sertraline, 0.30 ($p = 0.01$).

References

[1] Halperin D, Reber G. Influence of antidepressants on hemostasis. Dialogues Clin Neurosci. 2007;9:47–59 [R].
[2] Li N, Wallen NH, Ladjevardi M, et al. Effects of serotonin on platelet activation in whole blood. Blood Coagul Fibrinolysis. 1997;8:517–23 [R].
[3] Auerbach AD, Vittinghoff E, Maselli J, et al. Perioperative use of selective serotonin reuptake inhibitors and risks for adverse outcomes of surgery. JAMA Intern Med. 2013;173(12):1075–81 [C].
[4] Basile FV, Basile AR, Basile VV. Use of selective serotonin reuptake inhibitors antidepressants and bleeding risk in breast cosmetic surgery. Aesthetic Plast Surg. 2013;37(3):561–6 [c].
[5] Gahr M, Zeiss R, Lang D, et al. Risk of bleeding related to selective and non-selective serotonergic antidepressants: a case/non-case approach using data from two pharmacovigilance databases. Pharmacopsychiatry. 2015;48(1):19–24 [C].
[6] Mahdanian AA, Rej S, Bacon SL, et al. Serotonergic antidepressants and perioperative bleeding risk: a systematic review. Expert Opin Drug Saf. 2014;13(6):695–704 [R].
[7] Schutte HJ, Jansen S, Schafroth MU, et al. SSRIs increase risk of blood transfusion in patients admitted for hip surgery. PLoS One. 2014;9(5):e95906 [c].
[8] Dall M, Primdahl A, Damborg F, et al. The association between use of serotonergic antidepressants and perioperative bleeding during total hip arthroplasty—a cohort study. Basic Clin Pharmacol Toxicol. 2014;115(3):277–81 [c].
[9] Seitz DP, Bell CM, et al. Risk of perioperative blood transfusions and postoperative complications associated with serotonergic antidepressants in older adults undergoing hip fracture surgery. J Clin Psychopharmacol. 2013;33(6):790–8 [C].
[10] Quinn GR, Singer DE, Chang Y, et al. Effect of selective serotonin reuptake inhibitors on bleeding risk in patients with atrial fibrillation taking warfarin. Am J Cardiol. 2014;114(4):583–6 [C].
[11] Hackam DG, Mrkobrada M. Selective serotonin reuptake inhibitors and brain hemorrhage: a meta-analysis. Neurology. 2012;79(18):1862–5 [M].
[12] Abdel Salam OM. Fluoxetine and sertraline stimulate gastric acid secretion via a vagal pathway in anaesthetised rats. Pharmacol Res. 2004;50:309–16 [E].
[13] Yamaguchi T, Hidaka N, Suemaru K, et al. The coadministration of paroxetine and low-dose aspirin synergistically enhances gastric ulcerogenic risk in rats. Biol Pharm Bull. 2008;31:1371–5 [E].
[14] Dall M, Schaffalitzky de Muckadell OB, Lassen AT, et al. There is an association between selective serotonin reuptake inhibitor use and uncomplicated peptic ulcers: a population-based case–control study. Aliment Pharmacol Ther. 2010;32(11–12):1383–91 [C].
[15] Targownik LE, Bolton JM, Metge CJ, et al. Selective serotonin reuptake inhibitors are associated with a modest increase in the risk of upper gastrointestinal bleeding. Am J Gastroenterol. 2009;104(6):1475–82 [C].
[16] Jiang HY, Chen HZ, Hu XJ, et al. Use of selective serotonin reuptake inhibitors and risk of upper gastrointestinal bleeding: a systematic review and meta-analysis. Clin Gastroenterol Hepatol. 2015;13(1):42–50 [M].
[17] Anglin R, Yuan Y, Moayyedi P, et al. Risk of upper gastrointestinal bleeding with selective serotonin reuptake inhibitors with or without concurrent nonsteroidal anti-inflammatory use: a systematic review and meta-analysis. Am J Gastroenterol. 2014;109(6):811–9 [M].
[18] Oka Y, Okamoto K, Kawashita N, et al. Meta-analysis of the risk of upper gastrointestinal hemorrhage with combination therapy of selective serotonin reuptake inhibitors and non-steroidal anti-inflammatory drugs. Biol Pharm Bull. 2014;37(6):947–53 [M].
[19] Masclee GMC, Valkhoff VE, Coloma PM, et al. Risk of upper gastrointestinal bleeding from different drug combinations. Gastroenterology. 2014;147(4):784–92 [C].
[20] Wang YP, Chen YT, Tsai CF, et al. Short-term use of serotonin reuptake inhibitors and risk of upper gastrointestinal bleeding. Am J Psychiatry. 2014;171(1):54–61 [C].
[21] Shin D, Oh YH, Eom CS, et al. Use of selective serotonin reuptake inhibitors and risk of stroke: a systematic review and meta-analysis. J Neurol. 2014;261(4):686–95 [M].
[22] Aarts N, Akoudad S, Noordam R, et al. Inhibition of serotonin reuptake by antidepressants and cerebral microbleeds in the general population. Stroke. 2014;45(7):1951–7 [c].
[23] Hackam DG, Mrkobrada M. Selective serotonin reuptake inhibitors and brain hemorrhage: a meta-analysis. Neurology. 2012;79(18):1862–5 [M].
[24] van Asch CJ, Luitse MJ, Rinkel GJ, et al. Incidence, case fatality, and functional outcome of intracerebral haemorrhage over time, according to age, sex, and ethnic origin: a systematic review and meta-analysis. Lancet Neurol. 2010;9(2):167–76 [M].
[25] Hankey GJ. Selective serotonin reuptake inhibitors and risk of cerebral bleeding. Stroke. 2014;45(7):1917–8 [R].
[26] Mortensen JK, Larsson H, Johnsen SP, et al. Post stroke use of selective serotonin reuptake inhibitors and clinical outcome among patients with ischemic stroke: a nationwide propensity score-matched follow-up study. Stroke. 2013;44(2):420–6 [C].
[27] Mortensen JK, Larsson H, Johnsen SP, et al. Impact of prestroke selective serotonin reuptake inhibitor treatment on stroke severity and mortality. Stroke. 2014;45(7):2121–3 [c].
[28] Lopponen P, Tetri S, Juvela S, et al. Association between warfarin combined with serotonin-modulating antidepressants and increased case fatality in primary intracerebral hemorrhage: a population-based study. J Neurosurg. 2014;120(6):1358–63 [C].
[29] Lee YC, Lin CH, Lin MS, et al. Effects of selective serotonin reuptake inhibitors versus tricyclic antidepressants on cerebrovascular events: a nationwide population-based cohort study. J Clin Psychopharmacol. 2013;33(6):782–9 [C].
[30] Hung CC, Lin CH, Lan TH, et al. The association of selective serotonin reuptake inhibitors use and stroke in geriatric population. Am J Geriatr Psychiatry. 2013;21(8):811–5 [C].
[31] Palmsten K, Hernandez-Diaz S, Huybrechts KF, et al. Use of antidepressants near delivery and risk of postpartum hemorrhage: cohort study of low income women in the United States. BMJ. 2013;347:f4877 [C].
[32] Lindqvist PG, Nasiell J, Gustafsson LL, et al. Selective serotonin reuptake inhibitor use during pregnancy increases the risk of postpartum hemorrhage and anemia: a hospital-based cohort study. J Thromb Haemost. 2014;12(12):1986–92 [C].

[33] Lupattelli A, Spigset O, Koren G, et al. Risk of vaginal bleeding and postpartum hemorrhage after use of antidepressants in pregnancy: a study from the Norwegian Mother and Child Cohort Study. J Clin Psychopharmacol. 2014;34(1):143–8 [C].

[34] Jimenez-Solem E, Andersen JT, Petersen M, et al. SSRI use during pregnancy and risk of stillbirth and neonatal mortality. Am J Psychiatry. 2013;170(3):299–304 [C].

[35] Ross LE, Grigoriadis S, Mamisashvili L, et al. Selected pregnancy and delivery outcomes after exposure to antidepressant medication: a systematic review and meta-analysis. JAMA Psychiatry. 2013;70(4):436–43 [M].

[36] Andersen JT, Andersen NL, Horwitz H, et al. Exposure to selective serotonin reuptake inhibitors in early pregnancy and the risk of miscarriage. Obstet Gynecol. 2014;124(4):655–61 [C].

[37] Stephansson O, Kieler H, Haglund B, et al. Selective serotonin reuptake inhibitors during pregnancy and risk of stillbirth and infant mortality. JAMA. 2013;309(1):48–54 [C].

[38] Vasilakis-Scaramozza C, Aschengrau A, Cabral H, et al. Antidepressant use during early pregnancy and the risk of congenital anomalies. Pharmacotherapy. 2013;33(7):693–700 [C].

[39] Huybrechts KF, Hernandez-Diaz S, Avorn J. Antidepressant use in pregnancy and the risk of cardiac defects. N Engl J Med. 2014;371(12):1168–9 [C].

[40] Bérard A, Zhao JP, Sheehy O. Sertraline use during pregnancy and the risk of major malformations. Am J Obstet Gynecol. 2015;212(6):795.e1–795.e12 [C].

[41] Ban L, Gibson JE, West J, et al. Maternal depression, antidepressant prescriptions, and congenital anomaly risk in offspring: a population-based cohort study. BJOG. 2014;121(12):1471–81 [C].

[42] Munch TN, Rasmussen ML, Wohlfahrt J, et al. Risk factors for congenital hydrocephalus: a nationwide, register-based, cohort study. J Neurol Neurosurg Psychiatry. 2014;85(11):1253–9 [C].

[43] Yazdy MM, Mitchell AA, Louik C, et al. Use of selective serotonin-reuptake inhibitors during pregnancy and the risk of clubfoot. Epidemiology. 2014;25(6):859–65 [c].

[44] Jensen HM, Gron R, Lidegaard O, et al. The effects of maternal depression and use of antidepressants during pregnancy on risk of a child small for gestational age. Psychopharmacology (Berl). 2013;228(2):199–205 [C].

[45] Ross LE, Grigoriadis S, Mamisashvili L, et al. Selected pregnancy and delivery outcomes after exposure to antidepressant medication: a systematic review and meta-analysis. JAMA Psychiatry. 2013;70(4):436–43 [M].

[46] Huang H, Coleman S, Bridge JA, et al. A meta-analysis of the relationship between antidepressant use in pregnancy and the risk of preterm birth and low birth weight. Gen Hosp Psychiatry. 2014;36(1):13–8 [M].

[47] Jensen HM, Gron R, Lidegaard O, et al. Maternal depression, antidepressant use in pregnancy and Apgar scores in infants. Br J Psychiatry. 2013;202(5):347–51 [C].

[48] Grigoriadis S, Vonderporten EH, Mamisashvili L, et al. Prenatal exposure to antidepressants and persistent pulmonary hypertension of the newborn: systematic review and meta-analysis. BMJ. 2014;348:f6932 [M].

[49] McDonagh MS, Matthews A, Phillipi C, et al. Depression drug treatment outcomes in pregnancy and the postpartum period: a systematic review and meta-analysis. Obstet Gynecol. 2014;124(3):526–34 [M].

[50] Kieviet N, Hoppenbrouwers C, Dolman KM, et al. Risk factors for poor neonatal adaptation after exposure to antidepressants in utero. Acta Paediatr. 2015;104(4):384–91 [C].

[51] Austin MP, Karatas JC, Mishra P, et al. Infant neurodevelopment following in utero exposure to antidepressant medication. Acta Paediatr. 2013;102(11):1054–9 [c].

[52] Santucci AK, Singer LT, Wisniewski SR, et al. Impact of prenatal exposure to serotonin reuptake inhibitors or maternal major depressive disorder on infant developmental outcomes. J Clin Psychiatry. 2014;75(10):1088–95 [c].

[53] Grzeskowiak LE, Gilbert AL, Sorensen TI, et al. Prenatal exposure to selective serotonin reuptake inhibitors and childhood overweight at 7 years of age. Ann Epidemiol. 2013;23(11):681–7 [C].

[54] Källén B, Nilsson E, Olausson PO. Antidepressant use during pregnancy: comparison of data obtained from a prescription register and from antenatal care records. Eur J Clin Pharmacol. 2011;67:839e45 [c].

[55] Man KK, Tong HH, Wong LY, et al. Exposure to selective serotonin reuptake inhibitors during pregnancy and risk of autism spectrum disorder in children: a systematic review and meta-analysis of observational studies. Neurosci Biobehav Rev. 2015;49:82–9 [M].

[56] Gidaya NB, Lee BK, Burstyn I, et al. In utero exposure to selective serotonin reuptake inhibitors and risk for autism spectrum disorder. J Autism Dev Disord. 2014;44(10):2558–67 [C].

[57] El Marroun H, White TJ, van der Knaap NJ, et al. Prenatal exposure to selective serotonin reuptake inhibitors and social responsiveness symptoms of autism: population-based study of young children. Br J Psychiatry. 2014;205(2):95–102 [C].

[58] Clements CC, Castro VM, Blumenthal SR, et al. Prenatal antidepressant exposure is associated with risk for attention-deficit hyperactivity disorder but not autism spectrum disorder in a large health system. Mol Psychiatry. 2015;20(6):727–34 [C].

[59] Laugesen K, Olsen MS, Telen Andersen AB, et al. In utero exposure to antidepressant drugs and risk of attention deficit hyperactivity disorder: a nationwide Danish cohort study. BMJ Open. 2013;3(9):e003507 [C].

[60] Oh SW, Kim J, Myung SK, et al. Antidepressant use and risk of coronary heart disease: meta-analysis of observational studies. Br J Clin Pharmacol. 2014;78(4):727–37 [M].

[61] Zimmermann-Viehoff F, Kuehl LK, Danker-Hopfe H, et al. Antidepressants, autonomic function and mortality in patients with coronary heart disease: data from the heart and soul study. Psychol Med. 2014;44(14):2975–84 [C].

[62] Weeke P, Jensen A, Folke F, et al. Antidepressant use and risk of out-of-hospital cardiac arrest: a nationwide case-time-control study. Clin Pharmacol Ther. 2012;92(1):72–9 [C].

[63] Fox BD, Azoulay L, Dell'Aniello S, et al. The use of antidepressants and the risk of idiopathic pulmonary arterial hypertension. Can J Cardiol. 2014;30(12):1633–9 [C].

[64] Dias A, Franco E, Figueredo VM, et al. Occurrence of Takotsubo cardiomyopathy and use of antidepressants. Int J Cardiol. 2014;174(2):433–6 [c].

[65] Erie JC, Brue SM, Chamberlain AM, et al. Selective serotonin reuptake inhibitor use and increased risk of cataract surgery: a population-based, case–control study. Am J Ophthalmol. 2014;158(1):192–7 [M].

[66] Uguz F, Sahingoz M, Gungor B, et al. Weight gain and associated factors in patients using newer antidepressant drugs. Gen Hosp Psychiatry. 2015;37(1):46–8 [c].

[67] Blumenthal SR, Castro VM, Clements CC, et al. An electronic health records study of long-term weight gain following antidepressant use. JAMA Psychiatry. 2014;71(8):889–96 [C].

[68] Cockerill RG, Biggs BK, Oesterle TS, et al. Antidepressant use and body mass index change in overweight adolescents: a historical cohort study. Innov Clin Neurosci. 2014;11(11–12):14–21 [c].

[69] Moura C, Bernatsky S, Abrahamowicz M, et al. Antidepressant use and 10-year incident fracture risk: the population-based Canadian Multicentre Osteoporosis Study (CaMoS). Osteoporos Int. 2014;25(5):1473–81 [C].

[70] Diem SJ, Ruppert K, Cauley JA, et al. Rates of bone loss among women initiating antidepressant medication use in midlife. J Clin Endocrinol Metab. 2013;98(11):4355–63 [C].

[71] Cheung K, Aarts N, Noordam R, et al. Antidepressant use and the risk of suicide: a population-based cohort study. J Affect Disord. 2014;174c:479–84 [C].

[72] Cooper WO, Callahan ST, Shintani A, et al. Antidepressants and suicide attempts in children. Pediatrics. 2014;133(2):204–10 [C].

[73] Miller M, Pate V, Swanson SA, et al. Antidepressant class, age, and the risk of deliberate self-harm: a propensity score matched cohort study of SSRI and SNRI users in the USA. CNS Drugs. 2014;28(1):79–88 [C].

[74] Miller M, Swanson SA, Azrael D, et al. Antidepressant dose, age, and the risk of deliberate self-harm. JAMA Intern Med. 2014;174(6):899–909 [C].

[75] Courtet P, Lopez-Castroman J, Jaussent I, et al. Antidepressant dosage and suicidal ideation. JAMA Intern Med. 2014;174(11):1863–5 [C].

[76] Tong J, Zheng Q, Zhang C, et al. Incidence, prevalence, and temporal trends of microscopic colitis: a systematic review and meta-analysis. Am J Gastroenterol. 2015;110(2):265–76 [R].

[77] Bonderup OK, Fenger-Gron M, Wigh T, et al. Drug exposure and risk of microscopic colitis: a nationwide Danish case–control study with 5751 cases. Inflamm Bowel Dis. 2014;20(10):1702–7 [C].

[78] Castro VM, Clements CC, Murphy SN, et al. QT interval and antidepressant use: a cross sectional study of electronic health records. BMJ. 2013;346:f288 [C].

[79] Beach SR, Kostis WJ, Celano CM, et al. Meta-analysis of selective serotonin reuptake inhibitor-associated QTc prolongation. J Clin Psychiatry. 2014;75(5):e441–9 [M].

[80] Zivin K, Pfeiffer PN, Bohnert AS, et al. Evaluation of the FDA warning against prescribing citalopram at doses exceeding 40 mg. Am J Psychiatry. 2013;170(6):642–50 [C].

[81] Girardin FR, Gex-Fabry M, Berney P, et al. Drug-induced long QT in adult psychiatric inpatients: the 5-year cross-sectional ECG Screening Outcome in Psychiatry study. Am J Psychiatry. 2013;170(12):1468–76 [C].

[82] Thase ME, Larsen KG, Reines E, et al. The cardiovascular safety profile of escitalopram. Eur Neuropsychopharmacol. 2013;23(11):1391–400 [C].

[83] Tuman TC, Demir N, Topal Z, et al. Angioedema probably related to fluoxetine in a preadolescent being followed up for major depressive disorder. J Child Adolesc Psychopharmacol. 2013;23(10):697–8 [A].

[84] Sierra-Rodriguez MA, Saenz-Frances F, Santos-Bueso E, et al. Chronic angle-closure glaucoma related to paroxetine treatment. Semin Ophthalmol. 2013;28(4):244–6 [A].

[85] Mameli C, Tadini G, Cattaneo D, et al. Acute generalized exanthematous pustulosis induced by paroxetine in an adolescent girl. Acta Derm Venereol. 2013;93(6):733–4 [A].

[86] Ho HY, Kam KW, Young AL, et al. Acute angle closure glaucoma after sertraline. Gen Hosp Psychiatry. 2013;35(5):575.e1–575.e2 [A].

[87] Krasowska D, Szymanek M, Schwartz RA, et al. Cutaneous effects of the most commonly used antidepressant medication, the selective serotonin reuptake inhibitors. J Am Acad Dermatol. 2007;56(5):848–53 [R].

[88] Khanna S, Chirinos RE, Venna S. Escitalopram oxalate (Lexapro)-induced acneiform eruption. J Am Acad Dermatol. 2012;67(6):e261–3 [A].

[89] Summary of product characteristics. Zoloft: prescribing information. Available at: http://labeling.pfizer.com/ ShowLabeling.aspx?id5517. Accessed April 22, 2015 [S].

[90] Sinha S, Udupa S, Bhandary RP, et al. Sertraline-induced acneiform eruption. J Neuropsychiatry Clin Neurosci. 2014;26(2):E56–7 [A].

[91] Uguz F. Rapid weight gain associated with edema after use of paroxetine and venlafaxine: 2 case reports. Clin Neuropharmacol. 2014;37(1):34–5 [A].

[92] Haukland LU, Kutzsche S, Hovden IA, et al. Neonatal seizures with reversible EEG changes after antenatal venlafaxine exposure. Acta Paediatr. 2013;102(11):e524–6 [A].

[93] Aragona M, Inghilleri M. Increased ocular pressure in two patients with narrow angle glaucoma treated with venlafaxine. Clin Neuropharmacol. 1998;21(2):130–1 [A].

[94] Ng B, Sanbrook GM, Malouf AJ, et al. Venlafaxine and bilateral acute angle closure glaucoma. Med J Aust. 2002;176(5):241 [A].

[95] de Guzman MH, Thiagalingam S, Ong PY, et al. Bilateral acute angle closure caused by supraciliary effusions associated with venlafaxine intake. Med J Aust. 2005;182(3):121–3 [A].

[96] Ezra DG, Storoni M, Whitefield LA. Simultaneous bilateral acute angle closure glaucoma following venlafaxine treatment. Eye (Lond). 2006;20(1):128–9 [A].

[97] Shifera AS, Leoncavallo A, Sherwood M. Probable association of an attack of bilateral acute angle-closure glaucoma with duloxetine. Ann Pharmacother. 2014;48(7):936–9 [A].

[98] Andrade C. The safety of duloxetine during pregnancy and lactation. J Clin Psychiatry. 2014;75(12):e1423–e1427 [R].

[99] Kjaersgaard MI, Parner ET, Vestergaard M, et al. Prenatal antidepressant exposure and risk of spontaneous abortion—a population-based study. PLoS One. 2013;8(8):e72095 [C].

[100] Hoog SL, Cheng Y, Elpers J, et al. Duloxetine and pregnancy outcomes: safety surveillance findings. Int J Med Sci. 2013;10(4):413–9 [c].

[101] Woo YS, Bahk WM. Burning paresthesia related to duloxetine therapy. J Clin Psychopharmacol. 2014;34(3):392–4 [A].

[102] Belli H, Akbudak M, Ural C. Duloxetine-related galactorrhea and restless legs syndrome: a case report. Psychiatr Danub. 2013;25(3):266–7 [A].

[103] Arnold LM, Palmer RH, Ma Y. A 3-year, open-label, flexible-dosing study of milnacipran for the treatment of fibromyalgia. Clin J Pain. 2013;29(12):1021–8 [A].

[104] Citrome L. Levomilnacipran for major depressive disorder: a systematic review of the efficacy and safety profile for this newly approved antidepressant—what is the number needed to treat, number needed to harm and likelihood to be helped or harmed? Int J Clin Pract. 2013;67(11):1089–104 [R].

[105] Forest Pharmaceuticals, Inc. FETZIMA (levomilnacipran extended-release capsules). United States Prescribing information. Revised July 2014. Available from: http://pi.actavis.com/data_stream.asp?product_group=1903&p=pi&language=E [Last accessed 20 April 2015] [S].

[106] Mago R, Mahajan R, Thase ME. Levomilnacipran: a newly approved drug for treatment of major depressive disorder. Expert Rev Clin Pharmacol. 2014;7(2):137–45 [R].

[107] Servier. Updated liver function monitoring recommendations. December 2013. Available at: http://www.servier.co.uk/sites/default/files/media/2014-12_valdoxan_-_liver_function_monitoring_scheme.pdf [accessed 20.04.15] [S].

[108] Montastruc F, Scotto S, Vaz IR, et al. Hepatotoxicity related to agomelatine and other new antidepressants: a case/noncase approach with information from the Portuguese, French, Spanish, and Italian pharmacovigilance systems. J Clin Psychopharmacol. 2014;34(3):327–30 [C].

[109] Tan HL. Agomelatine-induced gynaecomastia. Aust N Z J Psychiatry. 2013;47(12):1211–2 [A].

[110] Fetterolf F, Marceau M. A case of bupropion-induced stuttering. Gen Hosp Psychiatry. 2013;35(5):574.e7–574.e8 [A].

[111] De Picker L, Van Den Eede F, Dumont G, et al. Antidepressants and the risk of hyponatremia: a class-by-class review of literature. Psychosomatics. 2014;55(6):536–47 [R].

[112] Kate N, Grover S, Kumar S, et al. Bupropion-induced hyponatremia. Gen Hosp Psychiatry. 2013;35(6):681.e11–681.e12 [A].

[113] Kinalp C, Kurultak I, Ceri M, et al. Serum creatinine elevation caused by bupropion. Wien Klin Wochenschr. 2014;126(3–4):138–9 [A].

[114] Malesker MA, Soori GS, Malone PM, et al. Eosinophilia associated with bupropion. Ann Pharmacother. 1995;29:867–9 [A].

[115] Bagshaw SM, Cload B, Gilmour J, et al. Drug induced rash with eosinophilia and systemic symptoms syndrome with bupropion administration. Ann Allergy Asthma Immunol. 2003;90:572–5 [A].

[116] García M, Ruiz B, Aguirre C, et al. Eosinophilia associated with bupropion. Int J Clin Pharm. 2013;35(4):532–4 [A].

[117] Dwoskin LP, Rauhut AS, King-Pospisil KA, et al. Review of the pharmacology and clinical profile of bupropion, an antidepressant and tobacco use cessation agent. CNS Drug Rev. 2006;12:178–207 [R].

[118] Stahl SM, Pradko JF, Haight BR, et al. A review of the neuropharmacology of bupropion, a dual norepinephrine and dopamine reuptake inhibitor. Prim Care Companion J Clin Psychiatry. 2004;6:159–66 [R].

[119] Stall N, Godwin J, Juurlink D. Bupropion abuse and overdose. CMAJ. 2014;186(13):1015 [R].

[120] Evans EA, Sullivan MA. Abuse and misuse of antidepressants. Subst Abuse Rehabil. 2014;5:107–20 [R].

[121] Yoon G, Westermeyer J. Intranasal bupropion abuse: case report. Am J Addict. 2013;22(2):180 [A].

[122] Baribeau D, Araki KF. Intravenous bupropion: a previously undocumented method of abuse of a commonly prescribed antidepressant agent. J Addict Med. 2013;7(3):216–7 [A].

[123] Hilliard WT, Barloon L, Farley P, et al. Bupropion diversion and misuse in the correctional facility. J Correct Health Care. 2013;19(3):211–7 [A].

[124] Oppek K, Koller G, Zwergal A, et al. Intravenous administration and abuse of bupropion: a case report and a review of the literature. J Addict Med. 2014;8(4):290–3 [R].

[125] Del Paggio D. Psychotropic medication abuse in correctional facilities. Bay Area Psychopharmacol Newslett. 2005;8(2):1–6 [R].

[126] Hilliard WT, Barloon L, Farley P, et al. Bupropion diversion and misuse in the correctional facility. J Correct Health Care. 2013;19(3):211–7 [R].

[127] Phillips D. Wellbutrin(R): misuse and abuse by incarcerated individuals. J Addict Nurs. 2012;23(1):65–9 [R].

[128] McKee J, Penn JV, Koranek A. Psychoactive medication misadventuring in correctional health care. J Correct Health Care. 2014;20(3):249–60 [R].

[129] Lewis JC, Sutter ME, Albertson TE, et al. An 11-year review of bupropion insufflation exposures in adults reported to the California Poison Control System. Clin Toxicol (Phila). 2014;52(9):969–72 [R].

[130] Saddichha S. Mirtazapine associated tender pitting pedal oedema. Aust N Z J Psychiatry. 2014;48(5):487 [A].

[131] Lin CE, Chen CL. Repeated angioedema following administration of venlafaxine and mirtazapine. Gen Hosp Psychiatry. 2010;32(3):341.e1–341.e2 [A].

[132] Rottach KG, Schaner BM, Kirch MH, et al. Restless legs syndrome as side effect of second generation antidepressants. J Psychiatr Res. 2008;43(1):70–5 [R].

[133] Mattoo SK, Mahajan S, Sarkar S, et al. PLMD-like nocturnal movements with mirtazapine. Gen Hosp Psychiatry. 2013;35(5):576.e7–576.e8 [A].

[134] FDA NEWS RELEASE. http://www.fda.gov/NewsEvents/Newsroom/PressAnnouncements/ucm370416.htm dated 30 Sep 2013. Accessed 20/04/2015 [S].

[135] Lincoln J, Wehler C. Vortioxetine for major depressive disorder. Curr Psychiatry. 2014;13(2):67 [R].

[136] Schatzberg AF, Blier P, Culpepper L, et al. An overview of vortioxetine. J Clin Psychiatry. 2014;75(12):1411–8 [R].

[137] Pae CU, Wang SM, Han C, et al. Vortioxetine: a meta-analysis of 12 short-term, randomized, placebo-controlled clinical trials for the treatment of major depressive disorder. J Psychiatry Neurosci. 2014;39(6):140120 [M].

[138] Citrome L. Vortioxetine for major depressive disorder: a systematic review of the efficacy and safety profile for this newly approved antidepressant—what is the number needed to treat, number needed to harm and likelihood to be helped or harmed? Int J Clin Pract. 2014;68(1):60–82 [M].

[139] Llorca PM, Lancon C, Brignone M, et al. Relative efficacy and tolerability of vortioxetine versus selected antidepressants by indirect comparisons of similar clinical studies. Curr Med Res Opin. 2014;30(12):2589–606 [C].

3

Lithium

Thomas R. Smith*,[1], Mei T. Liu[†], Megan E. Maroney[†]

*Manchester University College of Pharmacy, Fort Wayne, IN, USA
[†]Ernest Mario School of Pharmacy at Rutgers, The State University of New Jersey, Piscataway, NJ, USA
[1]Corresponding author: trsmith03@manchester.edu

INTRODUCTION

Lithium is considered a first line treatment option for bipolar disorder in many treatment guidelines [1R,2R,3R,4R,5R]. It is effective in the prevention of both manic and depressive episodes [6r,7M]. A recently published naturalistic study conducted in Austria over the course of 4 years in 300 patients with bipolar disorder found that lithium monotherapy was the only treatment to demonstrate a relapse prevention effect ($p=0.002$). Treatment with anticonvulsants, atypical antipsychotics, antidepressants, or combination therapy did not appear to provide a significant benefit in preventing relapse in this study. Overall, relapse rates in this trial were high, with 68% of patients relapsing into a mood episode during the 4-year period; this appears to be consistent with other published naturalistic bipolar studies [8C]. Additionally, results from a recently completed large pragmatic trial of quetiapine versus lithium treatment are highly anticipated. Thus far only the description of the study design [9C] and a brief report on the effect of adjunctive use of benzodiazepines have been published [10C]. It is hoped that this trial will elucidate the comparative benefits and harms of this second generation antipsychotic compared to lithium. The authors anticipate that lithium will demonstrate a more favorable overall benefit relative to harm as compared to quetiapine [9C].

Lithium is also recommended as a first line augmentation option for patients with treatment-resistant major depressive disorder (MDD) [11R]. However, a recently published meta-analysis of add-on treatment for patients with MDD who have not responded to treatment with an antidepressant found that add-on lithium did not produce a statistically significant difference from add-on placebo in terms of depressive response [12M]. A systematic review of 12 randomized controlled trials

of treatment-resistant MDD was recently funded by the National Institute for Health Research Health Technology Assessment Programme in the UK. These investigators found that there was no statistically significant difference between augmentation of a selective serotonin reuptake inhibitor (SSRI) with an atypical antipsychotic or augmentation with lithium in terms of efficacy. Cost-effectiveness analyses, however, found that lithium was less expensive and more effective than augmentation with an antipsychotic, resulting in a cost savings of £ 905 per year and 0.03 more quality-adjusted life-years. The clinical significance of this finding is unclear, particularly given the heterogeneity of the studies included in the analysis [13R].

Lithium was recently used as the active comparator in a study of quetiapine extended release as an add-on to antidepressant treatment. This 6-week, single-blinded study randomized 658 patients with MDD who had failed treatment with an adequate trial of an antidepressant to either add-on quetiapine extended release (XR), add-on lithium, or quetiapine XR monotherapy. Quetiapine, monotherapy or adjunct, was found to be non-inferior to lithium treatment in terms of improvement of depressive scores, response and remission. The overall incidence of adverse effects was lower in the add-on lithium treatment group, than in the add-on quetiapine or quetiapine monotherapy groups (rates of 51.5%, 67.1% and 66.7%, respectively). The rates of serious adverse events and rates of discontinuation due to adverse events were also lowest in the lithium group (serious adverse events: lithium 0.4%, add-on quetiapine 2.2%, quetiapine monotherapy 1.8%; discontinuation: 7.9% lithium, 10.0% add-on quetiapine, 12.3% quetiapine monotherapy). Six patients (2.6%) treated with lithium experienced vomiting, three (1.3%) experienced diarrhea, and three (1.3%) experienced nausea that led them to discontinue their

© 2015 Elsevier B.V. All rights reserved.

lithium treatment. Other side effects in the lithium-treated group included somnolence, fatigue, dry mouth, sedation, headache, vertigo, dizziness, tremor, elevated fasting blood glucose and weight gain. Significant weight gain ($\geq 7\%$ increase from baseline) occurred less often in the lithium-treated group (3.2%) than in the quetiapine groups (8.7% with add-on quetiapine and 7.6% with quetiapine monotherapy). Adverse changes in fasting lipids occurred more often in the quetiapine groups than the lithium group; however, changes in fasting glucose occurred more often with lithium [14C].

Aside from its beneficial effects on mood, lithium may also have positive effects in patients with neurologic disorders. A recently published pilot study evaluated the effects of lithium when given immediately (within 48 hours) post-stroke. Patients experiencing their first ischemic stroke who were not eligible to receive antithrombotic therapy were randomized to receive routine stroke treatment plus either lithium carbonate 300 mg twice daily or placebo. Eighty patients total, 40 in each group, were evaluated for improvements in motor recovery for the following 30 days. Overall there were not statistically significant differences in motor function rating scales between the two groups; however, further analysis based on stroke location found that patients with cortical stroke (involving gray matter) showed a significantly better improvement when treated with lithium as compared to placebo. Lithium was well-tolerated in this trial with dry mouth reported in three patients (7.5%) and mild transient muscle twitches reported in one patient (2.5%). No serious adverse events were reported [15C].

Another trial conducted by Boll and colleagues examined the effect of lithium and valproic acid combination treatment on survival in patients with amyotrophic lateral sclerosis (ALS). Eighteen patients with ALS were treated with valproic acid 200 mg three times daily plus lithium titrated to a plasma lithium concentration between 0.3 and 0.75 mEq/L. These patients were matched by age, gender and deterioration rate to a group of historical controls and followed for 18 months. Rates of functional decline and survival were significantly better in the treatment group than the control group. Lithium was found to be safe in this trial with no nephrotoxicity or hypothyroidism observed. Adverse events attributed to lithium included nausea, a metallic taste and anorexia. These generally occurred during the second year of treatment and led to discontinuation in three patients (16.7%), mostly due to weight loss and nausea [16C].

Lithium has also been studied recently in Machado-Joseph disease. It failed to show a significant effect on the primary outcome, modification of disease progression, but some secondary outcomes such as ataxia scores and coordination scores were significantly better in the lithium as compared to the control group after 48 weeks. There were no statistically significant differences in the

severity or types of adverse events reported in the lithium versus the placebo group [17c].

The clinical benefits of lithium need to be weighed against its potential adverse effects. Major adverse effects of lithium include tremor, gastrointestinal effects such as nausea, vomiting and diarrhea, polyuria, polydipsia renal failure, hypothyroidism, hyperparathyroidism, hypercalcemia, acne, psoriasis, alopecia, cognitive decline, decreased libido and weight gain [6r,18R,19R]. The burdensome adverse effect profile of lithium may affect adherence rates. Murru and colleagues evaluated various clinical factors related to adherence in patients with bipolar I disorder and schizoaffective disorder. Use of lithium was significantly associated with poor treatment adherence ($p = 0.003$) in this naturalistic study. However, this was not significant after controlling for diagnostic subtypes. The authors speculate that there could be several reasons for this finding. Clinicians may preferentially use lithium in patients with poor adherence due to the ease of monitoring for adherence with serum lithium levels, or, perhaps patients are less likely to adhere to lithium due to its troublesome side effects [20C].

Monitoring of lithium levels is important to minimize the risk of toxicity and adverse effects. Treatment guidelines and package inserts for lithium recommend obtaining serum lithium levels every 2–6 months. A recently published study from Japan reported the percentage of outpatients on lithium that had a serum lithium level measured during a 1-month period in 2006. Only 2.2% of their sample had documentation of a lithium level being drawn during that time, indicating a seemingly very low rate of compliance with monitoring [21C].

Lithium has less overall evidence in the child and adolescent population. Peruzzolo and colleagues recently published a review on the treatment of bipolar disorder in children and adolescents. Adverse effects cited in trials conducted in this age population were similar to those seen in adults and include polyuria, polydipsia, enuresis, nausea vomiting, rash, weight gain increased appetite, sedation, tremor, restlessness, fatigue, cognitive dulling, flu-like symptoms, muscle stiffness, headache, abdominal cramps, and alopecia [22R].

ORGANS AND SYSTEMS

Nervous System

Tremor is a classic and common side effect caused by lithium, with an estimated rate of 27%. While usually benign, this adverse effect may lead to nonadherence or, in some cases, may be an initial sign of lithium toxicity. Commonly, it presents in the hands or upper limbs at rest, oscillating at 8–12 Hz, and worsens during activity. Compiled results from a literature search on this side effect reveal that it usually manifests upon initiation of lithium, is not progressive, and decreases over time. Other characteristics include its symmetric nature and correlation with dose. Its mechanism has never been closely examined but may be related to effects on brainstem serotonergic neurons [23M].

While tremor with lithium therapy is common, it is crucial to differentiate it from more severe extrapyramidal symptoms resulting from toxicity, drug-induced Parkinsonism or Parkinson's disease itself [24A,25A]. This clinical picture was recently described in two reports. A 67-year-old male with a history of bipolar disorder presented with a bilateral resting tremor in both hands. Symptom appearance correlated with starting lithium therapy and increased in severity over a period of 6 months. Additionally, rigidity and bradykinesia were noted and the patient was initially diagnosed with drug-induced Parkinsonism. However, after evaluation with a dopamine transporter (DAT) scan and findings of abnormal functioning of the presynaptic dopaminergic neurons, the patient was diagnosed with Parkinson's disease. The authors concluded that lithium may have unmasked the preclinical stage of Parkinson's disease [24A].

Despite having a therapeutic lithium level of 0.67 mEq/L, a 33-year-old male with bipolar disorder developed acute rigidity, tremors, and confusion on 1200 mg per day of lithium therapy. MRI of the brain displayed bilateral symmetric T2-weighted hyperintensities. The patient's symptoms resolved by 1 month after replacing lithium with valproate. These cases highlight the potential of lithium neurotoxicity beyond that of a benign tremor that may occur with therapeutic doses [25A].

Lastly, a case of a 19-year-old male with a drug profile consisting of valproate, lithium, olanzapine, risperidone, and clonazepam developed both serotonin syndrome and neuroleptic malignant syndrome simultaneously. This case highlights the rare possibility for these syndromes to manifest together and the possibility of lithium contributing to both [26r].

Psychiatric

Delirium

Both lithium and electroconvulsive therapy (ECT) have been reported to cause delirium independently; however, Sadananda and colleagues reported a patient who developed delirium while being concurrently treated with both therapies. This 30-year-old male with a history of traumatic brain injury was being treated for manic symptoms. He had previously been treated with various medications including divalproate sodium, oxcarbazepine and olanzapine, as well as adjunctive ECT without significant side effects. Three years after his original

diagnosis of organic mania, he was hospitalized due to aggression and symptom exacerbation. At this time, lithium was added to his treatment regimen. One week following the addition of lithium, adjunctive ECT was ordered, since he had responded well to this treatment in the past. After receiving 6 ECT treatments over the course of 2 weeks, the patient began to develop delirium, with a Mini Mental State Examination score of 18, indicating moderate cognitive impairment. The patient's serum lithium level was 0.9 mEq/L and his valproate level was 92 ng/ml at the time. Computed tomography scan showed no lesions or acute bleeding. ECT-induced delirium was diagnosed and his symptoms gradually resolved over the following 2 weeks. The authors caution the use of ECT with lithium, particularly in patients with pre-existing brain damage [27A].

Mild Cognitive Impairment

A case of mild cognitive impairment possibly related to lithium treatment was recently documented. In this case, a 62-year-old male with a history of multiple depressive episodes and suicide attempts related to bipolar disorder was treated over a number of years with antidepressants and two separate courses of ECT. At the age of 59, lithium was initiated after his last ECT treatment, along with quetiapine. After some time, the patient began to note tremors of the hands, short-term memory loss and lack of motivation. The patient was seen by a neurologist who diagnosed quetiapine-induced Parkinsonism. At age 60, he was diagnosed as suffering from mild cognitive impairment and was subsequently followed up at yearly intervals with memory assessments. At age 62, he began treatment with levodopa for probable Parkinson's disease, at which time his cognitive symptoms greatly improved. Several factors could have contributed to this patient's mild cognitive impairment including a history of encephalitis, depression, Parkinson's disease, ECT treatment and medications, including lithium [28A].

Endocrine

Thyroid

Lithium accumulates in the thyroid gland where its concentration is three to four times higher compared to plasma levels. Lithium has been shown to decrease production and release of thyroid hormones, decrease the clearance of free serum thyroxine (FT4), and reduce activity of type I 5' deiodinase. Along with other mechanisms on the thyroid gland and hypothalamic–pituitary–thyroid axis, lithium can cause various thyroid dysfunctions such as hypothyroidism, goiter, and increase antithyroid antibodies [29R].

Although rare, hyperthyroidism induced by lithium has also been reported. The mechanism of lithium-induced hyperthyroidism could be due to direct toxic effect in which lithium destroys the thyroid cells and causes release of thyroglobulin and thyroid hormones into the circulation [29R]. The incidence of lithium-associated silent thyroiditis is estimated to be 1.3 cases per 1000 person-years and the incidence of lithium-associated thyrotoxicosis is estimated to be 2.7 cases per 1000 person-years [30c].

A 51-year-old female patient with an 18-year history of bipolar disorder presented with symptoms of generalized myalgia, palpitations, hair loss, anxiety, excessive sweating, restlessness, insomnia, and hot flushes. She was maintained on lithium carbonate 1350 mg per day with a serum lithium level of 0.4–0.6 mEq/L. Laboratory tests revealed low thyroid-stimulating hormone (TSH) and a normal FT4 level. No thyroid mass was detected by ultrasound and thyroid nuclear scan showed faint radiotracer uptake. A diagnosis of hyperthyroidism due to silent thyroiditis was made by the endocrinologist. This patient received 3 months of carbimazole but subsequently developed hypothyroidism. Use of antithyroid medications is usually not indicated in silent thyroiditis as it is commonly transient in nature, presents with spontaneously resolving thyrotoxicosis and very low radioiodine uptake, and is usually followed by hypothyroidism. Continuation of lithium therapy is usually encouraged to avoid worsening of thyrotoxicosis upon lithium discontinuation [31R].

Another case of lithium-induced hyperthyroidism was reported in a 27-year-old male with schizoaffective disorder. He was admitted to the hospital with symptoms of auditory hallucinations and agitation for the previous 3 weeks. The patient denied any diaphoresis, intolerance of heat, eye protrusion, or tremor. He was tachycardic with a heart rate of 110 beats per minute but did not have a goiter upon examination. His medication regimen included lithium at a dose of 1350 mg per day, risperidone, hydroxyzine, trazodone, and asenapine. Laboratory tests revealed normal FT4 level, mildly elevated T3 level, and low TSH. The patient also had decreased thyroid uptake and increased thyroglobulin which implicated the diagnosis of acute thyroiditis with resultant hyperthyroidism. Lithium was discontinued and his psychiatric symptoms resolved. His thyroid panel returned to normal at his follow-up visit 2 months later [32A].

A case of lithium-induced transient euthyroid hyperthyroxinemia was reported in a 24-year-old female patient with schizoaffective disorder [33A]. This patient was started on lithium carbonate 900 mg per day for the treatment of mania and psychosis. FT4 elevation and a slight decrease in TSH levels were found 2.5 months after lithium initiation. However, the patient was clinically euthyroid and had no symptoms of thyrotoxicosis. Further workup revealed elevated serum total thyroglobulin levels over 180 ng/mL (normal range 1.2–35 ng/mL) and low I^{123} uptake at 4 hours and at 24 hours on thyroid scan. Thyroid antibody levels were normal and no thyroid nodule was detected. Lithium was continued and thyroid function was monitored. The FT4 remained elevated and the decreased TSH persisted for another 2 months. However, the patient's FT4 level returned to normal limits spontaneously during the fourth month of treatment. The incidence of transient euthyroid hyperthyroxinemia in acute psychiatric inpatients has been reported to be 9–18% but the mechanism as it relates to lithium is unclear [33A].

Two cases of lithium-induced thyrotoxicosis have been reported recently. A 19-year-old female patient with treatment-resistant bipolar type 1 affective disorder presented to the emergency department with a 2-week history of headaches, lethargy, a 2 kg weight loss and tremor [34A]. The patient was tachycardic with a heart rate of 120 beats per minute. She had a small, diffuse, non-tender goiter, and was positive for lid lag, and tremor. She was maintained on lithium 1250 mg per day with a therapeutic lithium level of 0.72 mEq/L. The patient had a history of subclinical hypothyroidism 2 years prior while taking lithium that resolved spontaneously within months. It was noted that she had not been taking thyroxine or ingested excessive amounts of iodine or kelp recently. The result of her thyroid levels showed hyperthyroidism with an elevated FT4 level and a decreased TSH. The patient was prescribed propranolol 10 mg three times a day with continued lithium therapy. Her thyroid function improved significantly within 2 days of discharge. Repeat thyroid function tests 2 months later showed hypothyroidism and the patient was prescribed thyroxine 50 mcg once daily [34A]. In the second case, a 61-year-old female patient with bipolar disorder developed thyrotoxicosis after being on lithium for 18 years [35A]. The patient was started on carbimazole while lithium was continued during the thyrotoxicosis. Her symptoms and thyroid function gradually improved over the next several months. After 5 months of carbimazole, her TSH level increased beyond normal range and the patient was diagnosed with acquired hypothyroidism possibly due to carbimazole and lithium. Thyroxine was started and her thyroid function returned to normal after 7 months. She did not have any further episodes of thyrotoxicosis during the 5-year follow-up period [35A].

Parathyroid

Lithium has been associated with hypercalcemia and hyperparathyroidism. The rate of hypercalcemia and hyperparathyroidism range from 25–42.3% and 2.7–23.2%, respectively [36c]. Possible mechanisms include increased threshold of the calcium sensing receptor within the parathyroid gland, increased parathyroid hormone (PTH), decreased intracellular calcium uptake, inhibition of glycogen synthase kinase 3b action, and reduction of PTH gene transcription. A case–control cross-sectional study of 112 patients was conducted to compare PTH and calcium levels in lithium-exposed bipolar patients and patients who have never been exposed to lithium. PTH levels were significantly higher in the lithium-exposed patients with an 8.6% rate of hyperparathyroidism while no patient in the control group developed hyperparathyroidism. Higher rates of hypercalcemia were seen in lithium-exposed patients compared to the control group when ionized calcium was measured (24.1% vs. 5.6%, respectively). This study also found a relationship between the duration of exposure to lithium and the increase in ionized calcium [36c].

Renal/Urinary Tract

Nephrotoxicity

Lithium's potential for nephrotoxicity is well established, with a spectrum of effects ranging from nephrogenic diabetes insipidus (NDI) to end-stage renal disease [27M,37c]. Lithium-induced nephropathy, usually occurring only after many years of therapy, may result from tubular dysfunction and manifest with a decreased glomerular filtration rate (GFR). Histopathological findings may include a chronic tubule-interstitial nephritis, tubular atrophy, and glomerular sclerosis [38M,39R]. While end-stage renal disease induced by lithium therapy is a well-established outcome, the incidence is rare and the rates of this occurrence have decreased in recent years. One Swedish study attributes this to the modern utilization of lithium differing from decades ago, mainly a lower target serum lithium level and an increase in renal monitoring [40c,41c]. Conflicting data, however, was found in Roxanas's examination of lithium. This study conducted in Australia analyzed the rates of renal replacement therapy for lithium nephrotoxicity. It found a marked increase in the number of cases of lithium nephrotoxicity leading to use of this intervention. From 1992 to 1996, 0.14 cases per million individuals per year were recorded. This increased to 0.78 between 2007 and 2011. The authors concluded that lithium nephrotoxicity is an increasing cause of end-stage renal disease. Clinicians should consider an alternative mood stabilizer if a decrease in two consecutive calculations of the GFR is seen [42C].

Nephrogenic Diabetes Insipidus

Nephrogenic diabetes insipidus, characterized by polyuria and polydipsia, is more common with lithium therapy and may occur in up to 20% or more lithium-treated patients [43C]. The actions of vasopressin are diminished and aquaporin insertion in the collecting duct is reduced [44R]. These effects lead to diluted urine [39R]. A 47-year-old female developed NDI while on lithium therapy after a laparoscopic total abdominal colectomy. Her serum lithium level was found to be 1.8 mEq/L and associated symptoms of lithium toxicity such as confusion were evident. She was managed successfully with hemodialysis which reduced the lithium level to 0.5 mEq/L after 24 hours [41c].

After chronic lithium therapy, renal effects may persist even after discontinuation, as evident in a case of a 64-year-old female who developed NDI after a lymph node biopsy. She had not taken lithium for 14 years, but was prescribed the drug for 30 years prior. Despite years of being off lithium therapy, the author concluded that her NDI was induced by lithium and could not identify other causative factors [41c].

Lithium-induced NDI and associated hypernatremia has been reported to produce the neurological effect of aphasia. An 84-year-old female prescribed 600 mg of lithium daily was found alert but with a reduction in spontaneous language and related symptoms. Classic symptoms including polydipsia and polyuria as well as typical laboratory values for diabetes insipidus, including hypernatremia, were documented. The mechanism for the neurological deficit of this case is thought to be related to the hyperosmolarity of the plasma subsequent to NDI and the passage of water into the interstitium of the brain [45A].

Biomarkers of Kidney Injury

The effects of lithium on the kidney continue to be examined. Researchers analyzed 120 patients with bipolar disorder for biomarkers indicative of kidney injury associated with lithium. Long-term (mean 16 years) lithium-treated patients were found to have higher levels of serum neutrophil gelatinase-associated lipocalin (NGAL) and urinary β_2 microglobulin (β2-MG), lower urinary specific gravity, and a decreased GFR compared to patients not on lithium therapy. These biomarkers may correlate with the severity of damage to the kidney in chronic kidney disease, the degree of tubular solute reabsorption impairment, and may offer a future method for assessing lithium-induced renal insufficiency [46c].

In the first large-scale, population-based study of renal function in lithium-treated subjects, a population of 330 patients prescribed lithium was found to have a higher serum creatinine compared to matched controls (87.1 μmol/L compared to 81.3 μmol/L, $p < 0.001$). Additionally, the authors identified that lithium's renal effects were appropriately monitored in about 70% of the cases, indicating a deviation from recommended monitoring in a large number of patients [43C].

Skin

Acne

The incidence of lithium-related skin conditions is estimated to be anywhere between 3% and 45%. Acne tends to occur within the first 6 months of lithium treatment and typically presents as a monomorphic, papulopustular eruption on the trunk and extremities without the presence of comedones. An atypical case was described by Scarfi and Arunachalam in a 40-year-old female patient being treated with lithium for the previous 4 months. This patient had severe eruptions of cysts, papules, nodules and comedones on her face, but no other location on her body. Skin biopsy in this case revealed a follicular obstruction and cystic dilatation of the pilosebaceous duct which was diagnosed as lithium-related acne. Her skin condition improved 6 months after stopping lithium and completely resolved by 9 months post-discontinuation [47A].

Another recently published case illustrates an earlier-onset lithium-related skin reaction. In this case, a 39-year-old female was treated with lithium for 7 days when it was noticed that she had non-itching, erythematous, maculopapular eruptions on her face, trunk and all four limbs. The rash covered 70% of her total body surface area. Complete blood counts were normal and a lithium level was noted to be within normal range at 0.92 mEq/L. The patient was treated with the antihistamines hydroxyzine and chorampheniramine, but her condition remained unchanged after 12 hours. At this time all of her medications were discontinued. The rash reduced in size to 30% of her body surface within 36 hours of stopping medications, and was completely resolved within 72 hours [48A].

Respiratory

Acute Respiratory Distress Syndrome

A 46-year-old female with bipolar disorder suffered acute respiratory distress syndrome (ARDS) related to lithium toxicity. She presented with a supratherapetuic lithium level (3.3 mEq/L), generalized weakness, and hemodynamic instability. Despite hemodialysis, the patient developed hypoxic respiratory failure and required intubation. After three total dialysis sessions over 5 days, the patient was extubated. This is the fifth documented case of lithium-associated ARDS and therefore this outcome should be included in the possible sequela of lithium toxicity when evaluating the patient [49A].

Metabolism

Weight Gain

Obesity and obesity-related metabolic problems are common in patients with mental illness. Many psychotropic medications, including lithium, can contribute to weight gain and metabolic risk. The extent and likelihood of weight gain is estimated to be high with lithium treatment, with weight gain of up to 12 kg (mean of 2–6 kg) in around one-third of patients. Combining treatment with antipsychotics typically results in greater weight gains than with monotherapy. Once alternative causes of weight gain, such as hypothyroidism, another potential side effect of lithium, have been ruled out, switching to an alternate mood stabilizing medication should be considered [50R].

The mechanism behind lithium-induced weight gain remains unknown. A recently published study sought to examine this mechanism by evaluating plasma levels of the adipokines leptin, resistin, and adiponectin in bipolar depressed patients being treated with lithium. Twenty-five patients were treated with flexibly-dosed lithium for 6 weeks. These patients were matched with 23 healthy controls. Blood samples were collected from the lithium group at baseline and week 6, while healthy controls had one sample collected at baseline. Baseline adiponectin, leptin, and resistin levels were similar between the two groups. Adiponectin levels decreased significantly in the lithium treatment group ($p < 0.05$). This is potentially important, since lower levels of adiponectin have been reported in patients with metabolic syndrome. However, patients who experienced weight gain while on lithium had similar post-treatment levels of adiponectin relative to patients who did not gain weight. There were no significant differences in levels of leptin or resistin from baseline to endpoint [51c].

Electrolyte Balance

Interactions between lithium and various electrolytes, including calcium, have been documented [52R,53A]. Changes in intracellular calcium signaling in patients with bipolar disorder have been theorized and confirmed. Dubovsky and colleagues found increased platelet calcium concentrations in patients with bipolar disorder. Because lithium attenuates increases in intracellular calcium ion concentrations, response to the drug may be tracked with concentration monitoring. However, this approach is unlikely to be practical in routine practice [54C].

SECOND-GENERATION EFFECTS

Lithium is a known teratogen and its place in therapy in treating pregnant patients with bipolar disorder is complex. Its effects during the prenatal period include Ebstein's abnormality, a significant yet probably overestimated effect of lithium on the fetus [18R,55R]. This anomaly is rare, accounting for <1.5% of all congenital heart diseases as reported in Osiro's review of the complication. The tricuspid valve and right ventricle are affected with apical displacement of the attachments of the septal and posterior valve leaflets. This produces tall, broad, right atrial P waves, prolonged PR intervals, and deep Q waves. Repair of the tricuspid value is one possible strategy for long-term management [56R].

The risk of major abnormalities following lithium exposure was evaluated in a prospective, comparative study of 183 lithium-exposed pregnancies compared with 72 disease-matched and 745 nonteratogenic-exposed cases. The authors found significantly more miscarriages (adjusted odds ratio 1.94, 95% CI 1.08–3.48) and elective terminations of pregnancy (9.3% versus 2.0%) in the lithium-exposed group compared to the control group. Only cardiovascular abnormalities occurred more frequently in the lithium-exposed group. The authors concluded that women should be given echocardiography and level-2 ultrasound if exposed to lithium during pregnancy, specifically during organogenesis [57C].

SUSCEPTIBILITY FACTORS

Gender

The prevalence of hypothyroidism is reported to be two to seven times higher in female than in male patients and the prevalence increases with age with up to 20% of postmenopausal women suffering subclinical hypothyroidism. Additionally, the prevalence of thyroid autoimmunity and hyperthyroidism are also higher in females [58R,59C]. In the retrospective, cross-sectional, naturalistic study by Ozerdem and colleagues, patients with bipolar disorder were more likely to develop thyroid dysfunction than patients with unipolar disorder or other psychiatric diagnoses. Hyperthyroidism was more likely to develop in patients on lithium and in the female population. The study also found a larger percentage of female patients with abnormal TSH levels (normal range 0.4–5 μIU/mL) compared to males when lithium levels are equal or greater than 0.8 mEq/L (40.8% vs. 11.1%, respectively) [59C].

Elderly

Lithium's renal toxicity is a concern in the elderly population since renal dysfunction occurs commonly secondary to aging. Long-term use of low dose lithium (target lithium level 0.25–0.5 mEq/L) did not affect the renal function in the elderly patients with mild cognitive impairment in the study conducted by Aprahamian and colleagues. However, lithium patients had more significant weight gain and higher incidences of arrhythmia and diabetes mellitus during the follow-up [60C].

There is little information regarding the rate of NDI in the elderly. In a retrospective study of 55 lithium-treated geriatric patients, 4% of patients discontinued lithium due to polyuria and an additional 4% were both hospitalized for and died due to hypernatremia [61C]. A cross-sectional study was conducted by Rej to determine the prevalence of NDI in 100 geriatric and adult lithium patients [60]. Although the rates of decreased urine osmolality were similar between geriatric and adult patients (12.5% vs. 17.9%, respectively, $p=0.74$), geriatric patients were less likely to report severe urinary and thirst symptoms (13.3% vs. 43.6%, respectively, $p=0.001$). Routine monitoring of urine osmolality may be useful in preventing NDI [61C].

Renal Transplant

There is limited safety data to describe the effects of lithium post-renal transplant. A 56-year-old female patient with bipolar disorder received a standard criteria deceased donor kidney transplant for end-stage renal disease. The patient was on dialysis for 6 years and maintained on lithium 300 mg per day prior to the transplant. Alemtuzumab, methylprednisolone rapid taper, tacrolimus, and mycophenolate mofetil were initiated post-transplant and lithium therapy was resumed at the previous dose. A progressive improvement in serum creatinine (SCr) was shown and the patient was discharged home on postoperative day (POD) 7 with a SCr of 5.44 mg/dL. She was readmitted on POD 10 with a lithium level of 1.33 mEq/L, tacrolimus level of 8.5 ng/mL, SCr 6.14 mg/dL, nausea, diarrhea, altered mental status, coarse tremor, and hyperreflexia. Lithium and tacrolimus were discontinued and risperidone and cyclosporine were initiated. Symptoms resolved and renal function improved 5 days later without additional intervention. This case illustrates the possibility of more pronounced adverse effects of lithium in transplant patients. Thus, lithium should be avoided and other mood stabilizers such as anticonvulsants or atypical antipsychotics are preferred in these individuals [62A].

INTERACTIONS

Antidepressants and Antipsychotics

Lithium is commonly used in combination with antidepressants and antipsychotics for the treatment of various psychiatric illnesses such as depression or bipolar disorders. Although studies suggest that the combination of lithium and antipsychotics may offer better efficacy compared to using a mood stabilizer alone, this strategy could also result in a decrease in tolerability [63R]. Combination of lithium with first generation antipsychotics can increase the risk of extrapyramidal side effects

(EPS). Combination of lithium with second generation antipsychotics can increase the risk of weight gain, sedation, somnolence, tremor and EPS [63R]. When used together with antidepressants, lithium may increase the risk for developing serotonin syndrome and when used with antipsychotics, the risk for neuroleptic malignant syndrome may also be higher [26r].

Muscle Blockers and Anesthesia

Electroconvulsive therapy (ECT) is a procedure that is used for the treatment of multiple psychiatric symptoms. Cardiovascular adverse effects should be monitored in patients undergoing ECT while taking lithium and antidepressants. A 48-year-old female with bipolar disorder had been prescribed lithium for 18 years [64A]. At the time of admission, the patient was also on duloxetine 120 mg per day and her baseline lithium level was 0.77 mEq/L. ECT was initiated with propofol and succinylcholine. After the first ECT session, ventricular tachycardia (heart rate >200 beats per minute) was observed. Her lithium and duloxetine doses were reduced (lithium level 0.4 mEq/L) and the patient received rocuronium and sugammadex for the third ECT session. Despite this, the patient again developed ventricular tachycardia (polymorphic ventricular tachycardia) after the treatment. Duloxetine was discontinued and the lithium dose was further reduced (lithium level 0.2 mEq/L). The patient received rocuronium during the fourth ECT session and no cardiac adverse effects were observed. The lithium level remained low at 0.2 mEq/L during the fifth session and succinylcholine was administered. This resulted in an increase in blood pressure (>200/150 mm Hg) and the ECT session was interrupted. The lithium dose was further reduced (lithium level 0.1 mEq/L) prior to the next ECT treatment which resulted in no further complications with succinylcholine or rocuronium. The authors suspected that the combination of lithium and duloxetine and the interaction with succinylcholine are possible causes of the cardiac arrhythmia. The nondepolarizing muscle relaxant rocuronium may be a better option for patients maintained on lithium undergoing ECT [64A].

A case of prolonged curarisation due to lithium interaction with succinylcholine was reported in a 65-year-old male patient with congenital butyrylcholinesterase deficiency. Although most patients with butyrylcholinesterase deficiency can experience prolonged curarisation for up to 2 hours after administration of succinylcholine, this patient had persistent coma and absence of triggering of the respirator such that extubation was only possible 7 hours after the administration of succinylcholine [65A].

Peripheral nerve block with local anesthesia is used for oral surgery and dental implantology. An *in vitro* rat model showed that if the concentration of extracellular lithium ion increases, the potency of local anesthetic conduction block increases concomitantly [66E]. Two cases of prolonged anesthesia in patients who were taking lithium were described by Patil and colleagues [67A]. Both patients had normal lithium levels at baseline (0.85 and 0.5 mEq/L and lithium was discontinued 2 days prior to the procedure. The effects of the local anesthetic, which typically last 1.5–6 hours, were increased to 16 and 18 hours for these two patients [67A].

Non-Steroidal Anti-Inflammatory Drugs

Since lithium is excreted almost exclusively through the kidney, medications that affect renal clearance can alter lithium concentration. Two cases of lithium toxicity due to drug interactions with non-steroidal anti-inflammatory drugs (NSAIDs) were described by De Winter and colleagues [68A]. Both cases involved elderly female patients who were previously stabilized on lithium. They presented to the emergency department with signs and symptoms of anorexia, confusion, dysarthria, ataxia, tremor, coma, hypercalcemia, and renal insufficiency shortly after starting treatment with NSAIDs. Both cases scored six points on the Drug Interaction Probability Scale which indicate a probable adverse drug event due to the combination of lithium and NSAIDs. NSAIDs increase lithium retention by inhibition of prostaglandin synthesis and reduction of blood flow affecting GFR. However, sulindac in particular has been shown to have minimal effects on lithium clearance [68A].

DIAGNOSIS OF ADVERSE DRUG REACTIONS

Renal Imaging

Due to lithium's potential to cause nephropathy, particularly with long-term use, recent research has focused on identifying effective ways to use imaging technology to detect changes in kidney morphology in patients on lithium therapy. Approximately 33–62.5% of patients on lithium are found to have renal microcysts. Magnetic resonance imaging (MRI) is thought to be superior to ultrasonography (US) and computed tomography (CT) in detecting and visualizing small renal microcysts. Farschcian and colleagues recently performed a study to evaluate the relationship of MRI-detected microcysts and renal function in patients being treated with lithium for at least the past 2 years. Thirty-five patients with a mean duration of lithium therapy of 7.7 years and with normal renal function underwent MRI. Each renal microcyst measuring at least 1 mm was recorded. Serum creatinine level and blood urea nitrogen level were also measured and GFR was calculated using the Cockcroft-Gault equation. Seventeen patients in the sample were found to have renal microcysts and the mean number of microcysts in each kidney was 6.2. The general adult population is found to have an average of 1.87 microcysts, thus this finding was significantly higher than expected for a typical adult. Although there was a positive correlation between the duration of lithium treatment and the number of renal microcysts ($p = 0.03$), there was no statistically significant correlation found between the MRI findings and renal function tests. The authors concluded that MRI should not be used as a first line method for assessing renal function in patients on long-term lithium treatment and should not take the place of regularly measuring serum creatinine and GFR [69A].

A recent review on various imaging studies used to detect lithium-induced nephropathy described US as the most popular imaging modality for detecting abnormal kidney function. US together with Doppler technology may be particularly helpful for detecting other possible underlying causes of kidney dysfunction to help rule out lithium as the cause. Renal size is thought to be a good indicator used to differentiate lithium-induced nephropathy from other types of parenchymal diseases as the kidney size is usually preserved in the case of lithium, but generally is reduced in size with other diseases. This review also mentions that MRI is the most sensitive in detecting the very small microcysts that tend to be seen in patients on long-term lithium therapy. These cysts are much smaller than the cysts that are detected in patients with polycystic kidney disease. Cysts can also be detected with the use of CT; however, MRI is more effective in viewing these smaller cysts. One finding that the authors of this review highlighted, in particular, is that increased echogenicity of the kidney parenchyma, as detected via US, seems to correlate well with serum creatinine levels and the degree of parenchymal injury. They propose that even in patients with normal serum creatinine, increased echogenicity may represent a subclinical level of renal injury. Although studies with more patients are needed to confirm the usefulness of these imaging technologies, US, CT, and MRI may be helpful alone, or in combination with each other, in the early detection and possibly prevention of lithium-induced nephropathy [70R].

MANAGEMENT OF ADVERSE DRUG REACTIONS

Dols and colleagues, citing the high rates of nonadherence possibly related to adverse effects, conducted a review of the management of side effects of lithium therapy in bipolar disorders. General measures to target and reduce side effects include patient education and dosage reduction. Interestingly, no differences were found between single or multiple daily dosing patterns with lithium and adverse effect burden [18R]. Treatments for tremor involve eliminating contributing factors such as caffeine, reducing the lithium dose, changing

formulations, or the use of beta blockers, primidone, gabapentin, or other drugs. In many cases, lithium-induced tremor resolves spontaneously without intervention [18R,23M]. Gastrointestinal side effects can be attenuated with long acting preparations or histamine-2 antagonists. Hypothyroidism, even subclinical forms, may benefit from thyroid-stimulating hormone or free T4. Acne is a common side effect and may be treated with topical salicylic acid or tretinoin preparations [18R].

The treatment of sexual dysfunction with lithium is not well documented and until recently no published study had examined a possible intervention in patients with bipolar disorder who were stable on lithium therapy. Saroukhani and colleagues proposed that aspirin may represent an effective therapy. Lithium may cause erectile dysfunction through impairment of the nitric oxide pathway. Inhibiting the cyclooxygenase (COX) enzyme may reverse these effects. Aspirin was selected over other COX inhibitors because of its decreased likelihood for interaction compared to NSAIDs. Patients received aspirin 80 mg three times daily for 6 weeks. Patients receiving aspirin showed significant differences in the total International Index for Erectile Function score ($p = 0.010$) as well as trends toward significance in intercourse satisfaction ($p = 0.081$) and orgasmic function ($p = 0.067$) [71c].

The management of lithium-induced NDI was described in a report of a 37-year-old male presenting with a long history of polyuria, polydipsia, and nocturia while on lithium for 10 years. He was diagnosed with NDI in addition to destructive thyroiditis and primary hyperparathyroidism. The patient was given 600 μg of desmopressin three times daily which resulted in symptom improvement [53A].

Hyperparathyroidism (HPT) associated with lithium use has been reported. Although it may resolve after cessation of lithium, some patients may require surgical resection of the parathyroid gland. In a previous study on surgical intervention for lithium-associated hyperparathyroidism (LiHPT), 42% of patients had recurrence of HPT [72C]. In a study by Norlen and colleagues, the long-term outcome after parathyroidectomy for the management of LiHPT was evaluated in a retrospective cohort study that included 48 patients who received open-four-gland parathyroid exploration or focused parathyroidectomy [73C]. The median time for follow-up was 5.9 years and a 10-year cumulative combined rate of persistent and recurrent HPT was 16%. Seven patients had temporary complications after primary surgery for LiHPT but no permanent complications were found in this study. The lower recurrence rate seen in this study could be attributed to the higher number of parathyroid glands identified and therefore better detection of diseased gland compared to a previous study by Jarhult and colleagues. Recently, Papier commented on the use of bilateral neck exploration as a preferred surgical technique for patients on lithium therapy who develop primary hyperparathyroidism and are not eligible for minimally invasive parathyroidectomy [74C].

PHARMACOGENOMICS

Due to lithium's long history in the treatment of bipolar disorder, consistent observations of distinct features that are common to responders versus non-responders have surfaced. These include an episodic clinical course that does not demonstrate rapid cycling, and a family history of bipolar disorder. Because lithium efficacy follows this familial pattern, a genetic link to positive outcomes with lithium therapy is naturally hypothesized [75E]. A recent study examined responders and non-responders to lithium maintenance therapy for bipolar disorder using genome-wide expression profiling of lymphoblasts. Insulin-like growth factor 1 (IGF-1) was found to be over-expressed in the responder group. This represents a potential marker for positive response to lithium in maintenance therapy of bipolar disorder [75E].

Additional studies to elucidate the pharmacogenomic relationship between lithium and treatment response include an attempt to identify changes in genes expressed in peripheral blood in patients with bipolar disorder who responded or failed to respond to lithium therapy. After 6 months of therapy, patients who responded to lithium showed changes in BCL2L1 expression which were not seen in non-responders or those who did not receive lithium. This finding adds to the growing evidence of gene–drug interactions that will hopefully lead to a more personalized and precise treatment of bipolar disorder [76E].

References

[1] American Psychiatric Association. Practice guideline for the treatment of patients with bipolar disorder (revision). Am J Psychiatry. 2002;159:1 [R].

[2] Crismon ML, Argo TR, Bendele SD, et al. Texas Medication Algorithm Project procedural manual: bipolar disorder algorithms, Austin, TX: Texas Department of State Health Services; 2007. Accessed February 1, 2015, www.pbhcare.org/pubdocs/upload/documents/TIMABDman2007.pdf [R].

[3] Grunze H, Vieta E, Goodwin GM, et al. The world federation of societies of biological psychiatry (WFSBP) guidelines for the biological treatment of bipolar disorders: update 2009 on the treatment of acute mania. World J Biol Psychiatry. 2009;10(2):85–116 [R].

[4] Grunze H, Vieta E, Goodwin GM. The world federation of societies of biological psychiatry (WFSBP) guidelines for the biological treatment of bipolar disorders: update 2012 on the long-term treatment of bipolar disorder. World J Biol Psychiatry. 2013;14:154–219 [R].

[5] Yatham LN, Kennedy SH, Schaffer A, et al. Canadian network for mood and anxiety treatments (CANMAT) and international society for bipolar disorders (ISBD) collaborative update of CANMAT guidelines for the management of patients with bipolar disorder: update 2009. Bipolar Disord. 2009;11:225–55 [R].

[6] Mitchell PB. Bipolar disorder. Aust Fam Physician. 2013;42(9):616–9 [r].

[7] Bschor T, Bauer M. Side effects and risk profile of lithium: critical assessment of a systematic review and meta-analysis. Nervenarzt. 2013;84(7):860–3 [M].

[8] Simhandl C, König B, Amann BL. A prospective 4-year naturalistic follow-up of treatment and outcome of 300 bipolar I and II patients. J Clin Psychiatry. 2014;75(3):254–62 [C].

[9] Nierenberg AA, Sylvia LG, Leon AC, et al. Clinical and health outcomes initiative in comparative effectiveness for bipolar disorder (bipolar CHOICE): a pragmatic trial of complex treatment for a complex disorder. Clin Trials. 2014;11(1):114–27 [C].

[10] Bobo WV, Reilly-Harrington NA, Ketter TA, et al. Effect of adjunctive benzodiazepines on clinical outcomes in lithium- or quetiapine-treated outpatients with bipolar I or II disorder: results from the bipolar CHOICE trial. J Affect Disord. 2014;161:30–5 [C].

[11] Bauer M, Pfenning A, Severus E, et al. World federation of societies of biological psychiatry (WFSBP) guidelines for biological treatment of unipolar depressive disorders, part 1: update 2013 on the acute and continuation treatment of unipolar depressive disorders. World J Biol Psychiatry. 2013;14:334–85 [R].

[12] Turner P, Kantaria R, Young AH. A systematic review and meta-analysis of the evidence base for add-on treatment for patients with major depressive disorder who have not responded to antidepressant treatment: a European perspective. J Psychopharmacol. 2014;28(2):85–98 [M].

[13] Edwards SJ, Hamilton V, Nherera L, et al. Lithium or an atypical antipsychotic drug in the management of treatment-resistant depression: a systematic review and economic evaluation. Health Technol Assess. 2013;17(54):1–190 [R].

[14] Bauer M, Dell'osso L, Kasper S, et al. Extended-release quetiapine fumarate (quetiapine XR) monotherapy and quetiapine XR or lithium as add-on to antidepressants in patients with treatment-resistant major depressive disorder. J Affect Disord. 2013;151(1):209–19 [C].

[15] Mohammadianinejad SE, Majdinasab N, Sajedi SA, et al. The effect of lithium in post-stroke motor recovery: a double-blind, placebo-controlled, randomized clinical trial. Clin Neuropharmacol. 2014;37(3):73–8 [C].

[16] Boll MC, Bayliss L, Vargas-Cañas S, et al. Clinical and biological changes under treatment with lithium carbonate and valproic acid in sporadic amyotrophic lateral sclerosis. J Neurol Sci. 2014;340(1–2):103–8 [C].

[17] Saute JA, de Castilhos RM, Monte TL, et al. A randomized, phase 2 clinical trial of lithium carbonate in Machado-Joseph disease. Mov Disord. 2014;29(4):568–73 [c].

[18] Dols A, Sienaert P, van Gerven H, et al. The prevalence and management of side effects of lithium and anticonvulsants as mood stabilizers in bipolar disorder from a clinical perspective: a review. Int Clin Psychopharmacol. 2013;28:287–96 [R].

[19] Watanabe K, Kikuchi T. Adverse events of psychotropic drugs. Seishin Shinkeigaku Zasshi. 2014;116(4):323–31 [R].

[20] Murru A, Pacchiarotti I, Amann BL, et al. Treatment adherence in bipolar I and schizoaffective disorder, bipolar type. J Affect Disord. 2013;151(3):1003–8 [C].

[21] Inagaki A, Takeshima T. Metabolic and lithium monitoring in Japanese psychiatric outpatient clinics. Seishin Shinkeigaku Zasshi. 2014;116(2):130–7 [C].

[22] Peruzzolo TL, Tramontina S, Rohde LA, et al. Pharmacotherapy of bipolar disorder in children and adolescents: an update. Rev Bras Psiquiatr. 2013;35(4):393–405 [R].

[23] Baek JH, Kinrys G, Nierenberg AA. Lithium tremor revisited: pathophysiology and treatment. Acta Psychiatr Scand. 2014;129(1):17–23 [M].

[24] Bhattacharjee S, Yela R, Chadwick G. Can lithium unmask the preclinical Parkinsonian features? Ir Med J. 2013;106(8):254 [A].

[25] Vishnu VY, Kesav P, Goval MK, et al. Teaching neuroimages: reversible paradoxical lithium neurotoxicity. Neurology. 2013;81(14):e110 [A].

[26] Dosi R, Ambaliya A, Joshi H, et al. Serotonin syndrome versus neuroleptic malignant syndrome: a challenging clinical quandary. BMJ Case Rep. 2014; http://dx.doi.org/10.1136/bcr-2014-204154. PMID: 24957740 [r].

[27] Sadananda SK, Narayanaswamy JC, Srinivasaraju R, et al. Delirium during the course of electroconvulsive therapy in a patient on lithium carbonate treatment. Gen Hosp Psychiatry. 2013;35(6):678.e1–2 [A].

[28] Seshadri M, Mazi-Kotwal N, Aguis M. Reversible mild cognitive impairment-a case report. Psychiatr Danub. 2013;25(Suppl 2):S358–61 [A].

[29] Kraszewska A, Abramowicz M, Chłopocka-Woźniak M, et al. The effect of lithium on thyroid function in patients with bipolar disorder. Psychiatr Pol. 2014;48(3):417–28 [R].

[30] Miller KK, Daniels GH. Association between lithium use and thyrotoxicosis caused by silent thyroiditis. Clin Endocrinol. 2001;55(4):501–8 [c].

[31] Tan LH, Dhillon R, Mohan T, et al. Lithium-associated silent thyroiditis: clinical implications. Aust N Z J Psychiatry. 2013;47(10):965–6 [R].

[32] Siyam FF, Deshmukh S, Garcia-Touza M. Lithium-associated hyperthyroidism. Hosp Pract. 2013;41(3):101–4 [A].

[33] Chekuri L, Lange JR, Thapa PB. Lithium-induced transient euthyroid hyperthyroxinemia: a case report. Prim Care Companion CNS Disord. 2014;16(2); http://dx.doi.org/10.4088/PCC.13l01604. PMID: 25133055. PMCID: PMC4116284 [A].

[34] Chalasani S, Benson KA. Lithium-induced thyrotoxicosis in a patient with treatment-resistant bipolar type I affective disorder. Med J Aust. 2014;201(9):541–2 [A].

[35] Kar N, Hullumane SR, Williams C. Thyrotoxicosis followed by hypothyroidism in a patient on lithium. Ment Illn. 2014;6(2):5415 [A].

[36] Albert U, De Cori D, Aguglia A, et al. Lithium-associated hyperparathyroidism and hypercalcaemia: a case–control cross-sectional study. J Affect Disord. 2013;151(2):786–90 [c].

[37] Hoekstra R, van Alphen AM, Bosch TM. Lithium: only acceptable with careful monitoring. Ned Tijdschr Geneeskd. 2014;158:A7207 [c].

[38] Gahr M, Freudenmann RW, Connemann BJ, et al. Nephrotoxicity and long-term treatment with lithium. Psychiatr Prax. 2014;41(1):15–22 [M].

[39] Carter L, Zolezzi M, Lewczyk A. An updated review of the optimal lithium dosage regimen for renal protection. Can J Psychiatry. 2013;58(10):595–600 [R].

[40] Aiff H, Attman PO, Aurell M, et al. The impact of modern treatment principles may have eliminated lithium-induced renal failure. J Psychopharmacol. 2014;28(2):151–4 [c].

[41] Irefin SA, Sonny A, Harinstein L, et al. Postoperative adverse effects after recent or remote lithium therapy. J Clin Anesth. 2014;26(3):231–4 [c].

[42] Roxanas M, Grace BS, George CR. Renal replacement therapy associated with lithium nephrotoxicity in Australia. Med J Aust. 2014;200(4):226–8 [C].

[43] Minay J, Paul R, McGarvey D, et al. Lithium usage and renal function testing in a large UK community population; a case–control study. Gen Hosp Psychiatry. 2013;35(6):631–5 [C].

[44] Kortenoeven ML, Fenton RA. Renal aquaporins and water balance disorders. Biochim Biophys Acta. 2014;1840(5):1533–49 [R].

[45] Golimstok Á, Pigretti S, Rojas JI, et al. Aphasic syndrome associated with severe hypernatremia secondary to lithium treatment. Rev Psiquiatr Salud Ment. 2013;6(4):187–8 [A].

[46] Rybakowski JK, Abramowicz M, Chłopocka-Wozniak M, et al. Novel markers of kidney injury in bipolar patients on long-term lithium treatment. Hum Psychopharmacol. 2013;28(6):615–8 [c].

[47] Scarfi F, Arunachalam M. Lithium acne. CMAJ. 2013;185(17):1525 [A].

[48] Wang EH, Yang AC. Reversible skin rash in a bipolar disorder patient on first use of lithium. Psychiatry Clin Neurosci. 2013;67(5):365 [A].

[49] Kansagra AJ, Yang E, Nambiar S, et al. A rare case of acute respiratory distress syndrome secondary to acute lithium intoxication. Am J Ther. 2014;21(2):e31–4 [A].

[50] Hasnain M, Vieweg WV. Weight considerations in psychotropic drug prescribing and switching. Postgrad Med. 2013;125(5):117–29 [R].

[51] Soeiro-de-Souza MG, Gold PW, Brunoni AR, et al. Lithium decreases plasma adiponectin levels in bipolar depression. Neurosci Lett. 2014;564:111–4 [c].

[52] Matikainen N. Hypercalcemia. Duodecim. 2014;130(14):1404–12 [R].

[53] Kamath Govindan J, Premawardhana AD, et al. Nephrogenic diabetes insipidus partially responsive to oral desmopressin in a subject with lithium-induced multiple endocrinopathy. Clin Med. 2013;13(4):407–10 [A].

[54] Dubovsky SL, Daurignac E, Leonard KE. Increased platelet intracellular calcium ion concentration is specific to bipolar disorder. J Affect Disord. 2014;164:38–42 [C].

[55] Vinçotte I, Huguelet P. Can we prescribe lithium during pregnancy? Summary of a controversy. Rev Med Brux. 2014;35(1):17–21 [R].

[56] S1 Osiro, Tiwari KJ, Mathenge N, et al. When lithium hurts: a look at Ebstein anomaly. Cardiol Rev. 2013;21(5):257–63 [R].

[57] Diav-Citrin O, Shechtman S, Tahover E, et al. Pregnancy outcome following in utero exposure to lithium: a prospective, comparative, observational study. Am J Psychiatry. 2014;171(7):785–94 [C].

[58] Bauer M, Glenn T, Pilhatsch M, et al. Gender differences in thyroid system function: relevance to bipolar disorder and its treatment. Bipolar Disord. 2014;16(1):58–71 [R].

[59] Ozerdem A, Tunca Z, Cimrin D, et al. Female vulnerability for thyroid function abnormality in bipolar disorder: role of lithium treatment. Bipolar Disord. 2014;16(1):72–82 [C].

[60] Aprahamian I, Santos FS, dos Santos B, et al. Long-term, low-dose lithium treatment does not impair renal function in the elderly: a 2-year randomized, placebo-controlled trial followed by single-blind extension. J Clin Psychiatry. 2014;75(7):e672–8 [C].

[61] Rej S, Looper K, Segal M. Do antidepressants lower the prevalence of lithium-associated hypernatremia in the elderly? A retrospective study. Can Geriatr J. 2013;16(2):38–42 [C].

[62] Moss MC, Kozlowski T, Dupuis R, et al. Lithium use for bipolar disorder post renal transplant: is mood stabilization without toxicity possible? Transplantation. 2014;97(3):e23–e24 [A].

[63] Buoli M, Serati M, Altamura AC. Is the combination of a mood stabilizer plus an antipsychotic more effective than mono-therapies in long-term treatment of bipolar disorder? A systematic review. J Affect Disord. 2014;152–154:12–8 [R].

[64] Heinz B, Lorenzo P, Markus R, et al. Postictal ventricular tachycardia after electroconvulsive therapy treatment associated with a lithium-duloxetine combination. J ECT. 2013;29(3):e33–5 [A].

[65] Huynh-Moynot S, Moynot JC, Thill C, et al. Prolonged curarisation following succinylcholine injection on butyrylcholinesterase deficiency and potentiated by a lithium treatment: a case report. Ann Biol Clin. 2013;71(4):485–8 [A].

[66] Gold MS, Thut PD. Lithium increases potency of lidocaine-induced block of voltage-gated Na$^+$ currents in rat sensory neurons in vitro. J Pharmacol Exp Ther. 2001;299(2):705–11 [E].

[67] Patil PM. Prolonged peripheral nerve blockade in patients using lithium carbonate. J Craniomaxillofac Surg. 2014;42(3):e33–5 [A].

[68] De Winter S, Meersseman W, Verelst S, et al. Drug-related admissions due to interaction with an old drug, lithium. Acta Clin Belg. 2013;68(5):356–8 [A].

[69] Farshchian N, Farnia V, Aghaiani MR, et al. MRI findings and renal function in patients on lithium therapy. Curr Drug Saf. 2013;8(4):257–60 [A].

[70] Karaosmanoglu AD, Butros SR, Arellano R. Imaging findings of renal toxicity in patients on chronic lithium therapy. Diagn Interv Radiol. 2013;19(4):299–303 [R].

[71] Saroukhani S, Emami-Parsa M, Modabbernia A, et al. Aspirin for treatment of lithium-associated sexual dysfunction in men: randomized double-blind placebo-controlled study. Bipolar Disord. 2013;15(6):650–6 [c].

[72] Jarhult J, Ander S, Asking B, et al. Long-term results of surgery for lithium-associated hyperparathyroidism. Br J Surg. 2010;97:1680–5 [C].

[73] Norlén O, Sidhu S, Sywak M, et al. Long-term outcome after parathyroidectomy for lithium-induced hyperparathyroidism. Br J Surg. 2014;101(10):1252–6 [C].

[74] Papier A, Kenig J, Barczyński M. Bilateral neck exploration with intraoperative iPTH assay in patients not eligible for minimally invasive parathyroidectomy. Przegl Lek. 2014;71(2):66–71 [C].

[75] Squassina A, Costa M, Congiu D, et al. Insulin-like growth factor 1 (IGF-1) expression is up-regulated in lymphoblastoid cell lines of lithium responsive bipolar disorder patients. Pharmacol Res. 2013;73:1–7 [E].

[76] Beech RD, Leffert JJ, Lin A, et al. Gene-expression differences in peripheral blood between lithium responders and non-responders in the lithium treatment-moderate dose Use study (LiTMUS). Pharmacogenomics J. 2014;14(2):182–91 [E].

4

Drugs of Abuse

*Ashakumary Lakshmikuttyamma**,[1], *Abigail Kay*[†]

*Department of Pharmaceutical Sciences, Jefferson College of Pharmacy, Thomas Jefferson University Hospital, Philadelphia, PA, USA

[†]Department of Psychiatry and Human Behavior-Division of Substance Abuse, Thomas Jefferson University Hospital, Philadelphia, PA, USA

[1]Corresponding author: ashakumary.lakshmikuttyamma@jefferson.edu

INTRODUCTION

Misuse of drugs and/or alcohol is a significant problem worldwide. In the United States alone 9.4% of the population (24.6 million people) had used drugs within the past month in 2013, with 8.2 million of them meeting criteria for a substance use disorder [1R]. The cost of this misuse is estimated at more than $600 billion each year ($193 billion—illicit drugs, $163 billion—tobacco, and $235 billion—alcohol) [2R]. With the significant morbidity, mortality, and cost to society, due to substance misuse, it is clear that all medical practitioners must be cognizant of the medical signs and symptoms of substance use, including atypical presentations so as to be able to treat this devastating illness.

CANNABINOID

Cannabis is a very old drug and its various medicinal values such as healing powers, anti-inflammatory activity and pain relieving property are well documented [3R,4R,5R]. Currently, many people utilize marijuana to deal with chronic neuropathic pain, glaucoma, multiple sclerosis, and other conditions associated with chronic pain [6R,7R, 8R]. Different countries, 23 states and the District of Columbia in the United States have permitted the use of marijuana for medicinal purposes. In addition to the legalization in some states, recreational cannabis use has become as common as tobacco or alcohol use in young adults. Recreational cannabis use has spread globally in both developed and developing countries [6R,7R]. However, there is considerable evidence demonstrating the adverse effect of cannabinoid usage and it has been clearly established that long-term usage can lead to addiction [8R].

Nervous Systems

Prenatal and adolescent exposure of cannabinoids interferes with cytoskeletal dynamics, which are critical for the formation of neuronal connection in the brain. Regular cannabis use results in impairment of the neuronal connectivity in the brain [9C], including the hippocampus, an area for learning and memory [10C]. Since brain development continues up to young adulthood, chronic cannabis exposure in teenagers and in young adults may have far-reaching consequences. Various neuroimaging analyses on the impact of chronic cannabis use on brain structure and function in adolescents and adults demonstrate morphological brain alterations in the medial temporal and frontal cortices, as well as the cerebellum [11R]. This data supports of the hypothesis that cannabis use may result in long-term brain alterations.

Psychiatric

Cannabis use has been associated with very severe psychotic symptoms [10C]. The relationship between substance abuse and the development of acute psychosis or different types of psychotic disorder is well established [12R]. The following recent case reports are consistent with the assumption that cannabis usage may induce psychosis.

A study conducted by Australian researchers explored the relationship between cannabinoid use and age of onset of psychotic disorders. They carried out the studies in a large number of patients with psychosis in which

© 2015 Elsevier B.V. All rights reserved.

data on cannabinoid usage in the 12 months prior to onset of illness was available. The Phase 1 participants were aged 18–64 and were in contact with public mental health services and non-government organizations supporting patients with mental illness. After the initial screening, 7955 were categorized as psychosis positive. From this group 1642 participants with an established ICD-10 diagnosis of SSD (schizophrenia, schizoaffective, delusional and other non-organic psychotic disorder) or APD (bipolar disorder, depressive disorder with Psychotic features) were selected. In Phase 2, 1825 were randomly selected by assessing the DIP (Diagnostic Interview for Psychosis), a standardized, semi-structured interview for psychosis. Three classes according to substance use were identified: non-users ($n = 803$), cannabis predominant users ($n = 582$), and polysubstance users ($n = 257$). For participants with schizophrenia spectrum disorders, cannabis predominant users had a higher hazard of earlier age at onset than for non-users (adjusted HR = 1.38, 95% CI = 1.2–1.6); poly substance users had an even higher hazard (adjusted HR = 1.95, 95% CI = 1.5–2.4). In contrast, for participants with affective psychosis, cannabis predominant users (adjusted HR = 1.10, 95% CI = 0.8–1.4) and poly substance users (adjusted HR = 0.87, 95% CI = 0.6–1.3) did not have a higher hazard of earlier age at onset compared with non-users. The authors concluded that their findings are in agreement with the conception that cannabinoid usage results in earlier onset schizophrenia spectrum disorders but not affective psychotic disorders [13C]. In another Australian study, authors were aimed to evaluate the influence of cannabis use on the transition to psychosis in those at ultra-high risk (UHR) of developing psychosis. They examined the extent to which this depends on age at initial cannabis use, pattern of use, and genetic vulnerability for psychosis. Of the 155 lifetime cannabis users, 76.5% reported unpleasant experiences with cannabis usage. Different psychotic-like experiences such as paranoia, hearing voices, having visions were the most common, found among 67.5% of the cannabis users. Development of psychosis was higher among those who initiated cannabinoids in their early teens (before the age of 15 years) and went on to use regularly [14C].

There are different kinds of synthetic cannabinoids which were originally developed as therapeutic agents. These are sprayed on different herbal products and available under many names including Spice, K2, Spice Gold, Spice Silver, Spice Diamond, Black Mamba, Bombay Blue, Dark Matter, Magic, Mojo, and Galaxy [15C]. The adverse side effects of these cannabinoids are not well established. These synthetic cannabinoids are functionally similar to, but structurally different from delta-9-tetrahydrocannabinol (THC), the active compound in marijuana. Recently, health professional have witnessed an increase in the use of synthetic cannabinoids among patients with psychiatric disorders. This report is based on four schizophrenic patients who presented with synthetic cannabinoid intoxication. All four patients had smoked an unknown substance and then experienced adverse psychiatric effects. This substance was later identified as synthetic cannabinoid AM-2201. Although they used same cannabinoid the psychiatric symptoms exhibited were different in various patients. The most common psychiatric experience occurred in all four patients were mood changes, anxiety, and prominent behavioral changes. The authors hypothesized that the acute effects of synthetic cannabinoids are different in different patients, with or without schizophrenia; however, the reasons for these differences are not yet clearly understood [16C]. Another case study was reported regarding the development of manic episode in a 18-year-old boy who consumed a synthetic cannabinoid. The patient never had any psychiatric disorders prior to synthetic cannabinoid usage. The patient was consuming cannabis powder for 2 years and he switched from cannabis powder to synthetic cannabinoids. When he was admitted in the hospital, his mania rating scale (YMRS) score was 30/60. According to the DSM-V, his diagnosis was compatible with substance-induced bipolar disorder. After psychiatric treatment, on the 30th day of hospitalization, his YMRS score was 6/60 and his psychiatric condition was very close to normal. *Authors claimed that this is the first case of manic episode with psychotic symptoms induced by synthetic cannabinoid published in the literature* [17C].

Studies were also conducted to analyze driving under the influence (DUI) of synthetic cannabinoid. In all cases of study, synthetic cannabinoid use can lead to complications similar to typical performance deficits caused by cannabis use which are not compatible with safe driving [18R]. UR-144 [(1-pentyl-1H-indol-3-yl)(2,2,3,3-tetramethylcyclopropyl)-methanone] is a synthetic cannabinoid which has been on the market since 2012. A study was undertaken to confirm if UR-144 is pharmacologically similar to THC and to test whether UR-144 can produce effects incompatible with safe driving. Blood from the driver after the collision was analyzed by liquid chromatography–tandem mass spectrometry (LC–MS/MS). UR-144 (14.6 ng/mL) and its major pyrolysis product [1-(1-pentyl-1H-indol-3-yl)-3-methyl-2-(propan-2-yl)but-3-en-1-one] were detected. Analysis suggested that UR-144 produces effects and impairment similar or even more dangerous to THC and ingestion of this drug is unsafe for driving [19C].

Cardiovascular Disease

Cannabis usage is associated with higher heart rates, cardiac output, blood pressure, and venous carboxyhemoglobin levels than seen with heavy cigarette smoking

[20R]. Several cases of cannabinoid triggered arrhythmias and myocardial infarctions have been described [18R]. Marijuana appears to be more dangerous in those with pre-existing cardiovascular complications [21R]. Also, evidence suggests an increase in the risk of cardiovascular complications in young people associated with marijuana usage. It is therefore key that health care professionals consider marijuana usage as one of the possible causes of cardiovascular disorders in younger patients.

A study was carried out in France in order to analyze the clinical characteristics of cases collected by the French Addictovigilance Network from 2006 to 2010 on cardiovascular complications related to cannabis use. This study determined that 85.7% of patients affected by cardiac problems with cannabinoid use were men with an average age of 34.3 years [22M]. The following case studies are discussed on young adults presented to the emergency rooms with cardiovascular abnormalities after marijuana, or other forms of cannabinoid use. In this recent paper authors reported the cases of two young men, who died unexpectedly, with cannabinoid use. Both men, who were in their twenties, did not have history of cardiovascular complications or other illness. The toxicological examination revealed acute influence of cannabis, as measured by the concentration in the blood and in the brain tissue. The THC levels in case 1 (femoral blood: THC 5.2 ng/mL, 11-OH-THC 1.8 ng/mL, THC-COOH 12.9 ng/mL; brain tissue: THC 13.4 ng/g, 11-OH-THC 7.0 ng/g, THC-COOH 4.3 ng/g), in case 2 (femoral blood: THC 1.9 ng/mL, 11-OH-THC 0.8 ng/mL, THC-COOH 10.1 ng/mL; brain tissue: THC 6.3 ng/g, 11-OH-THC 2.3 ng/g, THC-COOH 2.3 ng/g). The other common drugs were absent in their system with the exception of nicotine and caffeine. The autopsy reports suggested that the cause of death, in both cases, may have been due to cardiac failure under the influence of cannabis [23C].

In another article, the authors reported on a case of a 16 year old, who suffered from cardiac abnormalities after synthetic cannabinoid use. This patient presented to the emergency department with 24 hours of continuous substernal chest pressure, and non-radiating pain, that was associated with dyspnea, nausea, and vomiting. The patient had a past medical history of exercise-induced asthma and attention deficit hyperactivity disorder (ADHD). The patient reported non-radiating pain that was associated with dyspnea, nausea, and vomiting. He was a daily cigarette smoker and had a history of marijuana use. He denied recent use of marijuana, because he was on judicial probation and subjected to frequent urine drug testing. However, he admitted to smoking "K2" (a synthetic cannabinoid) 60–90 min prior to the onset of his symptoms. When admitted the electrocardiogram (EKG) showed ST segment elevations in leads II, III, AVF, and

V4-V6. The initial troponin and creatine kinase MB (CKMB) levels were 1.47 and 17.5 ng/mL, respectively. The patient was admitted to the hospital where his EKG content persistent to show ST elevations with a higher troponin and CKMB concentration 8.29 and 33.9 ng/mL, respectively. After 4 days of treatment the patient recovered and studies showed normal coronary arteries, no wall motion abnormalities, and normal systolic function [24C].

The following study reported three cases in which marijuana usage resulted in severe cardiac abnormalities. Each patient was found collapsed in their home, where cardiopulmonary resuscitation (CPR) was performed, and there was a restoration of spontaneous circulation (ROSC). The first patient (a 52-year-old man), who was a heavy tobacco smoker developed coronary vasospasm after 2 hours of marijuana smoking. The other two patients (a 23-year-old and a 28-year-old), chronic marijuana users were admitted to the hospital with an acute ST-elevation myocardial infarction (STEMI). The drug screen was positive only for cannabis, not for other drugs. These lead the authors conclude that cannabis use can result in severe cardiovascular abnormalities and sudden death [25C].

Recent studies have revealed that different substances that are added to cannabis increase its psychotropic effect, and also able to develop toxic effects in multiple organs including the heart. In this study, authors reported an exceptional case of recurrent myopericarditis after the consumption of contaminated marijuana. The authors stated that this is the first report, and such a case has not been reported in the literature. A 29-year-old man was presented to the emergency department with chest pain which is increased with coughing or deep inspiration. His WBC count, C-reactive protein and troponin I levels (2.99 ng/mL) were elevated and his EKG showed ST-segment elevation in the inferior leads with PR-segment depression. The patient revealed that he had been admitted to a hospital 2 months prior with the same symptoms and in both cases he had marijuana from Mexico, which was presumably contaminated. In the first episode the chest pain started 48 hours after consuming the cannabis and the second episode was 72 hours after consumption. The authors concluded that recurrent myopericarditis in this young patient was due to the consumption of the contaminated marijuana [26C].

All these cases emphasized that the cardiovascular complications due to cannabis usage can develop not only in those at increased cardiovascular risk, but also in young people without any medical history, or risk factors for cardiovascular problems. The mortality rate due to cardiovascular disease associated with cannabis use in young adult is 25.6% [27M]. Given the legalization of cannabis use for medical purpose clearly require studies to determine its further safety.

Urinary Tract

Another study described the epidemiology of a toxicologic syndrome of acute kidney injury associated with synthetic cannabinoids [28C]. This study included nine patients with acute kidney injury (creatinine >1.3 mg/dL) from Oregon and southwestern Washington, who reported smoking synthetic cannabinoids. Analysis of the patient specimens for synthetic cannabinoids, their metabolites, and known nephrotoxins by liquid chromatography and time-of-flight mass spectrometry revealed the presence of a novel synthetic cannabinoid, XLR-11 ([1-(5-fluoropentyl)-1H-indol-3-yl] (2,2,3,3-tetramethylcyclopropyl)methanone). This study reinforces the association between synthetic cannabinoid exposure and acute kidney injury [28C].

ALCOHOL

Alcoholism is a major health problem not only in developed countries but also in developing countries. Alcohol abuse is responsible for 1400 disease-related deaths, 17 000 motor vehicle fatalities and 500 000 injuries in the US each year. The severity of the effects depending upon the individual, and also relies on the length of abuse [29R,30R]. Chronic alcohol abuse affects every major organ in the body, and can result in diabetes, obesity, liver disease, heart disease, dementia and some forms of cancer.

Liver

Acute and heavy alcohol consumption is common in all levels of society and liver cirrhosis due to chronic alcohol consumption is a common cause of death among heavy alcohol users [31R,32R]. Various studies have described the direct hepatotoxic effects of chronic alcohol abuse which leads to fibrosis, liver failure, and death [33M,34R]. The following randomized clinical trial was designed to investigate the immediate effects of moderate alcohol consumption on gut wall integrity and hepatocytes. Fifteen healthy volunteers consumed water on 1 day and alcohol on the other. A blood sample was collected pre-consumption, five every hour post-consumption, and one after 24 hours. Alcohol consumption resulted in a significant increase in serum, intestinal, and liver fatty acid binding protein levels compared to water consumption. Levels increased directly post-consumption and returned to normal levels within 4 hours. Lipopolysaccharide binding protein, soluble CD14, and interleukin-6 were used to assess the acute inflammatory response to endotoxemia. The authors concluded that moderate, acute alcohol consumption results

in immediate damage to the enterocytes, but did not appear to cause endotoxemia [35C].

Tumorigenecity

Cancer is one of the major causes of death world-wide. The World Cancer Research Fund (WCRF)/American Institute of Cancer Research (AICR) identified that alcohol consumption is related to an increased risk of certain cancers, oral cavity, pharynx, larynx, esophagus, colorectal, female breast, and liver [36M,37M,38R,39M,40M]. Colorectal cancer, the third most common cancer world-wide, is the fourth most common cause of cancer death, and is fatal in approximately half of all cases [40M]. Previous studies suggested that the increased risk of colorectal cancer associated with alcohol intake is stronger in men as compared to women. A systemic review and meta-analysis on epidemiological studies was performed to quantify the risk for colorectal cancer mortality at different levels of alcohol consumption. The authors used all relevant studies published from January 1966 to June 2013 for their analysis. The pooled relative risk (RR) and the corresponding 95% confidence interval (CI) were estimated by categorical meta-analysis. Nine cohort studies exploring the association between colorectal cancer mortality and alcohol use were identified. Compared with non/occasional drinkers, the pooled RR was 1.03 (95% CI, 0.93–1.15) for any intake, 0.97 (95% CI, 0.86–1.10) for light intake ($\leq$12.5 g/day of ethanol), 1.04 (95% CI, 0.94–1.16) for moderate intake (12.6–49.9 g/day of ethanol), and 1.21 (1.01–1.46) for heavy intake ($\geq$50 g/day of ethanol). Additionally, this study also confirmed that the risk of colorectal cancer associated with alcohol consumption is higher in men [41C].

Another study undertaken last year in Korea also emphasized that alcohol intake was associated with a higher prevalence of colorectal adenoma in male drinkers compared to non-drinkers. Though there was a possible increase in the prevalence of colorectal cancer in women, the association of alcohol intake for women users is weaker than men [41C]. The following study identified a molecular epigenetic alteration in colon cancer patients who consumed alcohol. Using a molecular pathologic epidemiology database in two prospective cohort studies (the Nurses' Health Study and Health Professionals Follow-up Study) revealed the association between alcohol intake and incidence of colorectal cancer is based on the methylation level of insulin like growth factor 2 (IGF2). The authors identified that, compared with no alcohol consumption, the intake of 15 g alcohol per day was associated with an elevated risk of colorectal cancer and lower levels of IGF2 methylation. The study concluded that higher alcohol consumption was associated with the risk of colorectal cancer with IGF2 hypomethylation, but not the risk of cancer with high-level IGF2 methylation. The association between alcohol intake and colorectal cancer risk may differ based on IGF2 methylation status [42C].

Breast cancer is a heterogeneous disease. However, several subtypes based on hormone receptor status and histological types have different etiological and clinical features. Strong evidence is available which links alcohol consumption to estrogen receptor–positive (ER+)/progesterone receptor–positive (PR+) tumors, but not to estrogen receptor–negative (ER−)/progesterone receptor–negative (PR−) tumors [43M]. A recent study carried out by National Cancer Institute evaluated the association between alcohol consumption and breast cancer risk in 54 562 women aged 55–74 years recruited at 10 US screening centers between 1993 and 2001. This study identified that alcohol consumption was not associated with all breast cancer subtypes. However, higher risks were seen only for those with ER+/PR+ disease. Also, the risks were observed for ductal and mixed ductal/lobular cancers, in women consuming 7 or more drinks per week [44M]. Another study was carried out in France to obtain an overview of the associations between alcohol consumption and breast cancer risk at adulthood, by type of alcohol and subtype of breast cancer. The authors carried out a follow up of 66 481 women from the French E3N-EPIC cohort (between 1998 and 2003) who were asked to report their alcohol consumption, by type of alcohol, through a 208-item diet-history questionnaire. This study confirmed approximate 2812 cases of breast cancer, and found no association between high alcohol consumption and increased risk for breast cancer in premenopausal women. However, a linear association between total alcohol consumption and breast cancer risk was found in postmenopausal women [45C].

Second Generation Effects

Alcohol is a known teratogen, which causes life-long complications [46R,47C]. Prenatal exposures to alcohol, and other drugs of abuse, are associated with various postnatal adverse effects [48C]. Alcohol intake during pregnancy seems to occur more often in those with a family history of alcohol dependence [49C]. A systemic review of 128 articles regarding the association of substance abuse on the development of congenital anomalies, and the long-term implications in exposed offspring identified that the major alcohol abuse associated fetal abnormalities are facial dysmorphisms and alterations in the central nervous system development [46R]. It is therefore advisable that women abstain from alcohol intake when planning to conceive and throughout pregnancy in order to avoid the fetal abnormalities.

BENZODIAZEPINES

Drug misuse and abuse are major public health problems in the United States. The number of emergency department visits has increased more each year in relation to prescription drug abuse than to illicit drugs abuse [50C]. Since their approval in 1960, Benzodiazepines (BZD) are the most widely used drug worldwide to treat insomnia and anxiety. The long-term use of BZD, which represent the main risk factor for tolerance and dependence, affects 2–7.5% of the population in developed countries. Even now BZD are among the most widely prescribed drugs in developed countries. However, the chronic use of BZD has a number of serious side effects, i.e., cognitive impairment, falls, traffic accidents. The quality of life was evaluated in 62 high-dose BZD-dependent patients seeking a BZD detoxification. Significant weakening was observed in physical and social functioning by long-term BZD abuse and mostly affected to female patients [51C]. Many drug users combine different types of drugs which may work synergistically leading to drug interactions and cause unwanted severe side effects. The following study was carried out to compare the severity of buprenorphine and methadone toxicity with concomitant use of BZD. Clinical effects, treatments, disposition and final medical outcomes were evaluated in 692 methadone–BZD cases and in 72 buprenorphine–BZD cases. Clinical effects in methadone–BZD and BUP–BZD groups included lethargy (71.1%, 59.7%), respiratory depression (29.0%, 15.3%), coma (22.4%, 5.6%), respiratory arrest (4.5%, 0%), hypotension (11.8%, 2.8%) and cardiac arrest (1.9%, 0%), respectively. Hospitalization and ICU utilization rates were higher for nonmedical use of BZD with methadone compared to BZD with buprenorphine [52M]. Recently, there has been a great deal of clinical concern regarding alprazolam abuse, alone or with alcohol and other drugs. A study conducted by Australian investigators analyzed the association of alprazolam with sudden or unnatural deaths in 412 cases presented to the New South Wales Department of Forensic Medicine. Circumstances of death identified were accidental drug toxicity (57.0%), deliberate drug toxicity (10.4%), suicide by means other than drug overdose (12.6%), disease (10.0%), accident (5.1%), and homicide (2.4%). In 94.9% of cases, drugs other than alprazolam and its metabolites were present. Commonly detected drugs included opioids (64.6%), other BZD (44.4%), and alcohol (34.5%). This study highlights the deleterious effect of combined exposure of alprazolam and alcohol/opioids [53C]. Earlier, as well as the recent studies, highlighted that BZD abuse alone or in combination with other drugs, could result in very serious complications, including sudden death. The health professionals must take extensive caution when prescribing BZD to patients with a current or previous history of substance abuse.

SYMPATHOMIMETICS—COCAINE

According to the Substance Abuse and Mental Health Administration (SAMHSA)-USA, in 2013 a staggering 601 000 people, aged 12 and older, had tried cocaine, a sympathomimetic agent, for the first time in the past year [54] and worldwide, over 14 million people use cocaine [55C]. As cocaine is the second most common reason for emergency department visits amongst those who have drug-related complaints [55C] it is vital that clinicians have knowledge of both common and rare side effects of this drug. The sympathomimetic effects of the cocaine are a result of its inhibition of monoamine reuptake transporters via the presynaptic transporters. Normally, these transporters cause neurons to uptake dopamine in order to be broken down by monoamine oxidase. Blockage of reuptake by cocaine results in the buildup of dopamine, which can now bind to the receptors in the post-synaptic membrane, which results in the "high" experienced by users of this agent [56]. Multiple medical sequelae have been seen due to the use of cocaine (e.g. cerebral vascular accidents, dilated cardiomyopathy, dysrhythmias, endocarditis, hypertension, myocardial infarctions, and myocarditis) [55C].

℞ *More recently, new side effects have been seen in cocaine secondary to adulteration with levamisole. It has been suggested that levamisole is used as an adulterant as it both potentiates cocaine's stimulant properties in addition to having metabolites, which have their own stimulatory effects [57C]. It is known that levamisole acts as a monoamine oxidase inhibitor (MAOi), a mechanism of action used in a class of antidepressant agents to result in elevated levels of monoamines, including dopamine, but it also results in enhancing cocaine's stimulant effects [58R,59C,60R]. An additional reason for its use is that levamisole is its ability to increase endogenous opioid levels [58R]. Another proposed reason for its use is that it is not detected when it is exposed to chlorine bleach, which is used to detect adulterants in cocaine, and therefore artificially increases the perceived amount of cocaine being purchased [57C].*

Levamisole was initially used as an anthelminthic agent (anti-parasitic worms), but later was discovered to have significant immune modulatory effects. In 1999 it was withdrawn in the United States due to serious side effects (e.g. agranulocytosis, cutaneous vasculopathy, leukoencephalopathy, and neutropenia) [57C,58R,59C,60R]. Also Levamisole is present in European cocaine specimens and severe adverse health effects are reported [58R]. Cocaine adulterated with levamisole has a much higher rate of cutaneous vasculopathy than seen with levamisole by itself [60R]. Estimates, of the amount of illicit cocaine adulterated with Levamisole, have ranged from 69% to 88% [57C,59C,60R]. This adulteration has, understandably, resulted in the presentation of patients, who have used

cocaine, with leukoencephalopathy, vasculitis, and skin necrosis which have been described in recent literature, and will be summarized in this chapter. The skin manifestations are described as a "distinctive vasculopathic purpura", which tend to be stellate with a bright erythematous border and necrotic center. These ulcerations can be complicated by a secondary infection, but generally resolve in less than 1 month, if the drug exposure is discontinued [57C, 59C].

In addition to a urine drug screen positive for cocaine, laboratory findings which aid in the diagnosis of a levamisole-induced syndrome include elevated perinuclear anti-neutrophil antibodies (p-ANCA), seen in 86–100% of presenting patients, positive cytoplasmic anti-neutrophil cytoplasmic antibody (c-ANCA), which was noted to be found in approximately half of the cases of patients presenting with this syndrome, and finally leukopenia, which is seen 50–60% [57C]. In almost every presentation of this syndrome, myeloperoxidase antibodies (anti-MPO) were found [57C]. Anti-human neutrophil elastase (anti-HNE) is useful as it is not found in patients with anti-neutrophil antibody-induced vasculitis but is seen in the majority of patients with the midline lesions from cocaine [57C]. Any patient with a urine drug screen positive for, or a history of, cocaine should be screened for neurologic, immune, and skin disorders as these can all be the result of adulteration with levamisole [60R].

One paper described levamisole-induced vasculitis in two African American women, both of whom had findings of positive c-ANCA, anti-HNE, and anti-cardiolipin antibody (IgM). The first patient presented with a recurrent necrotizing vasculitis in her ears, whereas the second patient, who subsequently died, presented with a much more severe case that included her ears, nose, cheeks, and a significant portion of her skin. The authors noted that steroids have been used for treatment but felt that it was not clear if they provide any benefit and may, in fact, result in harm [57C].

Levamisole-induced vasculitis and skin necrosis was described in a 39-year-old man, with a history of methicillin-resistant Staphylococcus aureus (MRSA), "[He] presented with painful lesions on his right hand, left food, and bilateral ears. Onset was 3 days prior to presentation where he started to have constant burning sensations, most severely on the superior aspect of his ears. He had last smoked cracked cocaine 1 day prior to presentation and he was snorting it the day before." It was noted that his vitals were normal with the exception of an elevated heart rate of 110 beats per minute. On physical exam he was noted to have new blisters on the dorsum of his right hand, "scaly lesion" on his left foot, and "black necrotic bilateral auricular lesions with 1–2 mm blisters noted on both ears. The tongue had a hard non-erythematous nodule on the center, tender to the touch." The physical symptoms expanded over the lateral aspect of his nose as well as the buccal area. The patient was admitted with a presumptive diagnosis of septic vasculitis due to MRSA, and therefore vancomyocin was initiated. His white blood count was elevated at 15.4 K/µL, his ANA was positive, titer 1:40, as was his p-ANCA at 1.1U, and his c-ANCA was negative. He was treated with supportive wound care and levamisole was on the differential diagnosis as the cause of his vasculitis. These authors highlight the fact that levamisole has a short half-life (5.6 hours), which emphasizes the importance of having this adulterant on the differential diagnosis early on. They too commented upon the lack of clarity in using steroids, noting the importance of supportive care, with the exception of severe cases in which surgical treatments may be necessitated [59C].

A third case report described the following: "a 48-year-old woman with a history of cocaine dependence and idiopathic neutropenia, presented to the emergency department with the complaint of 4 days of fevers, cough, rhinorrhea, shortness of breath, and diffuse body aches." In addition she had a chest X-ray with stable hilar adenopathy. Her vital signs were within normal limits with the exception of her blood pressure, which was 83/44. Her laboratory results were significant for a urine drug screen positive for cocaine, a decreased white blood count of 2.3 K/μL, absolute neutrophil count of 1.0 K/μL. As an aside, she reported her last use of cocaine was 6 days prior to admission; however, this is inconsistent with her positive toxicology screen, which would be unlikely to be positive if this were the case.

She was admitted for observation, the authors noting her history of severe pneumonia, reported fevers, as well as her neutropenia. She was started on broad spectrum antibiotics after becoming febrile and subsequently transferred to the ICU as sepsis was suspected. It was at this time that it was noted that she had "large, non-blanching purpuric batches on both forearms" biopsy of which showed vaso-occlusive vasculitis. Further laboratory work-up demonstrated positive p-ANCA 1:1280, but negative for c-ANCA or anti-cardiolipin antibodies. Her dermatologic condition evolved into bullae after which they were described to have necrosed and sloughed. Her skin manifestations were thought to be due to a levamisole-induced cutaneous vasculopathy [60R].

In the next case report, unlike the others, the patient, a 40-year-old woman who used cocaine daily, presented with neurological symptoms, rather than skin manifestations, that were also thought to be due to use of levamisole adulterated cocaine [61C]. The patient presented "for acute onset of confusion, altered language and mild fever." She was febrile with a temperature of 38.5 °C and had a motor aphasia. Her lumbar puncture (LP) results included leucocytes, 200 cells/mm^3 (75% PMN and 25% MN), a glucose value of 85 mg/dL, proteins 35 mg/dL, and whose gram and fungal stains were negative. Her "T2 and FLAIR sequences of the brain MRI displayed areas of hyperintense signal in the white matter of the left parietal lobe." She was treated for a possible brain abscess, but a search for a cause came up negative, and she was her baseline 2 days later. A repeat LP, 10 days later, demonstrated leucocytes 10 cells/mm^3, glucose 72 mg/dL, and protein of 17 mg/dL. The MRI results, however, showed only a small improvement of her lesion. She was status post 14 days of antibiotics, at which time she was no longer showing any

neurological symptoms. She was re-admitted 10 days later after she developed "sudden visual changes and weakness of the left arm". Although her initial lesion was demonstrated to have resolved, her MRI showed a lesion in her right frontal lobe. She was given IV imipenem, linezolid, and dexamethasone. Her laboratory results were negative for anti-phospholipid and antinuclear antibodies, as were serum antibodies against Borrelia and Hystoplasma. A week later she presented again, this time with motor and speech aphasia, in addition to being unable to read or write. Her MRI now demonstrated a new lesion in her left frontal lobe, and resolution of the prior two lesions. Although they were unable to obtain consent for a brain biopsy, there was no evidence of an autoimmune demyelinating disease or lymphoma, and she returned to baseline within 2 weeks. During this admission she reported that she had used cocaine. As multiple other causes of immune leukoencephalopathy had been ruled out, including PRES, MS, ADEM, SLE, Sjogren's, and anti-phospholipid syndrome, it was thought that her leukoencephalopathy was due to levamisole adulteration of the cocaine that she had been using. It was hypothesized that the serial MRI findings were "similar to other spongiform encephalopathies, where fluid entrapment is found in small vacuoles within the myelin lamellae" [61R].

Unadulterated cocaine has long been known to be a risk factor for kidney disease/injury, including ischemic acute tubular necrosis and direct proximal tubular toxicity. A case report of cocaine-induced acute interstitial nephritis (AIN) described as an "idiosyncratic allergic response" as a rare cause of acute kidney injury (AKI) [62C]. "A 49-year-old African American man presented to the emergency department with a 4-day history of diffuse abdominal pain associated with fatigue, anorexia and malaise. He had smoked marijuana and snorted cocaine within the 2 weeks prior to his presentation." The patient's physical exam was significant for elevated vital signs (170/95, 92, 18), and an abdomen which was diffusely tender upon palpitation; however, there were no fundoscopic exam findings, edema, petechiae, or rashes. Laboratory values showed elevated blood urea nitrogen (BUN 69 mg/dL) as well as an elevated creatinine (Cr) of 10.8 mg/dL. The authors noted that his Cr values had been 0.8 mg/dL 6 months prior and 2.3 mg/dL 2 weeks prior. His urinalysis demonstrated moderate blood, 10–14 white blood cells/HPF, and proteinuria (with a protein/creatinine ratio <0.5). His total CK was 621 U/L, but his ANA, ANCA, HIV, and GMB antibodies were negative. His urine drug screen (UDS) was significant for both cocaine and marijuana (authors note: although a person who uses marijuana chronically can test positive for this substance for up to 1 month's time after cessation, cocaine is usually only present in the UDS for approximately 2 days after the most recent use, suggesting recent use in this case). The patient's serum creatinine reached a high of 11.2 mg/dL and a kidney biopsy was done which demonstrated "patchy areas of interstitial edema with interstitial lymphocytic and eosinophilic infiltrates with tubulitis and focal acute tubular injury with granular casts consistent with AIN. Mild interstitial fibrosis, mild thickening *of the tunica media and hyalinosis of arterioles was also present." The patient's kidney function improved without treatment. His serum creatinine returned to 2.1 mg/dL on day 8, and 1.0 mg/dL 2 months later [62C].*

The authors looked at the three other case reports of AIN secondary to cocaine use and observed that in all four cases patients had abdominal pain, hematuria, and slight proteinuria. They noted that the significantly increased creatinine levels implied kidney injury. Although the patient in this case did not have low urine output, the other three cases did which resulted in a need for renal replacement therapy. Although all four patients had restored kidney function after a few weeks, the authors underscore the importance of determining the cause of the AIN, as the treatment requires discontinuation of the instigating cause, cocaine in this case. The authors were unable to conclusively comment upon the usage of steroids in shortening the recovery time for this patient population [62C]. The authors note that this diagnosis may be more common than previously thought as autopsy biopsies of this patient population shows possible chronic interstitial nephritis, which could mean that they could have had a previous episode of AIN [62C].

Use of cocaine is a known cause of cardiac and cardiovascular disorders [55C]. A 38-year-old man with a past medical history of hypertension and an 18-year history of weekly cocaine use, presented with new onset of dyspnea. He had been hospitalized a month prior with community acquired pneumonia, which also had initially presented with dyspnea. Other symptoms included a productive cough that was associated with a whitish/blood-tinged sputum, frontal headache as well as mid-sternal chest discomfort. Upon presentation his vitals were elevated with a heart rate of 104–110 beats per minute, an oxygen saturation of 86–89% on 2 L via nasal cannula, and a blood pressure of 179/121 mmHg. His physical exam was significant for jugular vein distention, a 2/6 systolic murmur at the mitral valve, which radiated to the left axilla, and bilateral diffuse coarse crackles. His studies were significant for left atrial enlargement; left ventricular hypertrophy and nonspecific T wave abnormalities in the anterior wall leads. His chest X-ray demonstrated patchy opacities, which were thought to be either pulmonary edema or a hemorrhage. A chest CT showed bilateral peribronchovascular airspace consolidation, ground-glass opacity with interlobular septal thickening, and small bilateral pleural effusions. A later chest X-ray showed marked improvement. It was determined that the onset of his initial presentation was after he had used cocaine and cardiomyopathy secondary to ischemia was determined not to be the cause via cardiac catheterization. The patient followed up 5 months after discharge and showed significant cardiac improvement. At this point it was felt that his diagnosis of congestive heart failure was due to his cocaine use [55C].

The authors noted that cardiomyopathy secondary to cocaine use does not present with symptoms prior to full onset, but does have symptoms which are consistent with those that are generally seen with cardiomyopathy. What makes this case unusual is the later reversal of the cardiomyopathy, as the authors note this has rarely been presented in the literature.

Key points from this paper include that a patient who presents with evidence of left ventricular dysfunction, adrenergic excess, and/or heart failure, especially those without other risk factors, should have cocaine included in the differential diagnosis of their cardiomyopathy. Secondly they remind us that beta-blockers should not be used in this situation, as this will allow there to be no blockage of the alpha-adrenergic receptors, and coronary vasoconstriction will result, followed by a hypertensive crisis [55C].

Sympathomimetics—Pediatric Exposure

A case study examined causes of drug-induced seizures in children, who presented to the ED, sympathomimetics were the primary inducer of seizures in both infants and toddlers. Amongst this group, in a subset of six children, the seizures were due to synthetic cannabinoids (whose mechanism of action for causing seizures is unknown) with three of them additionally exposed to methamphetamine (via "bath salts"), or dextromethorphan. Additional possible side effects include agitation, confusion, and loss of consciousness [63M].

OPIOIDS—HEROIN

Although the United States only represents 4.6% of the world's population, it consumes 80% of all opioids, including 99% of all hydrocodone [64R]. The National Survey on Drug Use and Health reported that in 2012, 669 000 people reported having used heroin in the prior year and that 156 000 had tried it for the first time (vs 90 000 in 2006) [65]. The Unites States has a significant problem with prescription opioids with 2.1 million people using it as an illicit substance. This is a reflection of the large increase in the prescription of opioids which has almost tripled from 76 000 000 in 1991 to 207 000 000 in 2013. It is not unusual that a person abusing prescription opioids will switch over to heroin, due it generally being a cheaper, or a more easily accessible option [66].

Heroin, a μ-opioid receptor agonist, creates multiple sensations in the user. Initially, the user has a strong experience of a rewarding/pleasurable feeling (often referred to as "a rush"). This feeling is increased with increasing amounts of heroin used and also depends upon how quickly the heroin binds to the μ-receptors. Some people experience negative symptoms including nausea, vomiting, and profound itching. After use, patients will present with drowsiness, decreased heart rate, decreased respiratory drive, and dulled mental processes. Medically a key concern is the respiratory depression as it can be so severe as to result in death [67]. There are common medical conditions seen in patients who are intravenous users of heroin, including abscesses and endocarditis, but more recently a case of AA amyloidosis, a form of amyloidosis, was reported.

Urinary Tract

AA amyloidosis, or secondary amyloidosis, is characterized by abnormal protein deposits, which can result in damage to an organ, as well as its ability to function normally. Cooper et al. [68C] present a patient who was determined to have developed AA renal amyloidosis due to subcutaneous injection (i.e. "skin popping") of heroin. The patient was a 37-year-old woman with a medical history significant for heroin use, cocaine use, HCV, DVT, and a recent admission 2 weeks earlier for a left axilla abscess of her breast. She represented with continued pain from her abscess and a bilateral lower extremity edema since her last admission. She had dysuria, fever, flank pain, shortness of breath, and urinary frequency. On physical exam she had evidence of multiple lesions due to her injection drug use, bilateral edema, which extended to knee level, but no evidence of lymphadenopathy. Her lab results demonstrated multiple abnormalities including a hemoglobin of 8.5 g/dL, a hematocrit of 26.7%, a blood urea nitrogen of 33 mg/dL, a C reactive protein of 5.47 mg/L, an erythrocyte sedimentation rate of 137 mm/h, and greater than 300 mg/dL of protein in her urinalysis. Her abscess was cultured and determined to be methicillin-resistant *Staphylococcus aureus* and her blood cultures were negative. She was started on anti-microbial therapy and a renal biopsy was done, whose pathology was consistent with secondary amyloidosis. The authors conclude that AA amyloidosis should be considered in the differential diagnosis of any patient with heroin use disorder with proteinuria and renal impairment.

ELECTRONIC CIGARETTES (E-CIGARETTES)

As approximately 48 100 people in the United States alone die each year from tobacco-related illnesses (one out of every five deaths), including 41 000 non-smokers, having new, effective, options to recommend to aid patients in their endeavors to quit are key [69]. But more importantly, these new options must be demonstrated to be safe, as well as effective.

E-cigarettes, initially created and now primarily made in China, have come to market with advertisements of being a healthier option to cigarettes or as an aid in smoking cessation. E-cigarettes are battery-powered devices designed to produce a vaporized form of the extremely addictive nicotine (hence the term "vaping") produced from heating it with propylene glycol and added flavor which is then inhaled [70C,71]. Although they are considered safer than standard cigarettes, current research does not support the statements that are made in regard to their effects on health or effectiveness for smoking cessation [70C]. One challenge is that, with the exception of E-cigarettes which are sold specifically as a medical aid for smoking cessation, in the United States the FDA does not regulate these devices, although they have put forth a proposal that they would have authority over all forms of tobacco, including E-cigarettes [71,72R]. The FDA notes that "E-cigarettes have not been fully studied, so consumers currently don't know the potential risks of E-cigarettes when used as intended". It is not yet identified "how much nicotine or other potentially harmful chemicals are being inhaled during use, or whether there are any benefits associated with using these products". Additionally, it is not known whether E-cigarettes may lead young people to try other tobacco products, including conventional cigarettes, which are known to cause disease and lead to premature death [71]. The FDA has received reports of multiple adverse events, which resulted in hospitalizations, thought to be due to E-cigarettes and those include congestive heart failure, disorientation, hypotension, pneumonia, and seizures [71]. In the United Kingdom, however, electronic nicotine products will be categorized as medications and thus be regulated beginning in 2016 [72R,73R]. This action is being taken due to an investigation in response to concerns about the E-cigarettes, including their safety, the consistency of the ingredients and their delivery. It was determined that the nicotine level was not consistent with what was stated on the product, nor was it consistent between different batches of the product, in addition to containing contaminants. One result of the future regulation is that added flavors, which are intended to attract children as flavored versions are used at a higher level by them, will not be permitted [72R,73R]. There is research which suggests that fluids from E-cigarettes, possibly due to the added flavors, may be more cytotoxic to stem cells than adult cells. This is worrisome when we consider the potential dangers on a developing fetus [72R]. Use of E-cigarettes is increasing with a doubling of users in the U.K. from 700 000 to 1.3 million in a 1-year period [73R]. Other concerns include that, unlike with cigarettes, many states do not have an age minimum for their usage, and/or they are easily accessible for purchase online, thus making them available to children [74M].

A recent review on E-cigarettes suggested that the exposure to particles from E-cigarettes is comparable to that of cigarettes, with higher particle exposure resulting from higher levels of nicotine in the fluid [72R]. They also noted that the exposures to toxins are lower than seen in cigarettes, but it is unclear what the health risks are at this time [72R]. One study, which looked at the risk of heavy metals being incorporated into the aerosol, found that levels of exposure were significantly higher than would be seen with cigarettes, due to liquid contents being exposed to the metal in the heating elements [72R]. These studies are especially important as they dispel the myth that the aerosol from the E-cigarette is just water vapor, and thus harmless [72R]. Another important finding, contrary to earlier studies, demonstrated that those who have "more puff intervals" with the E-cigarette had similar absorption of nicotine as cigarette smokers [72R].

The propylene glycol and glycerin, which are components of the fluid in the E-cigarettes, have existing warnings about the dangers of inhalation due to possible effects on the central nervous system, the respiratory system and its irritating effects on the eye [74M]. Another serious risk is the formation of propylene oxide from propylene glycol, which is a known class 2B carcinogen [72R].

Four studies, two of which looked at the effect of having used an E-cigarette within 30 days of the initiation of the study, and two others, which looked at the effect of ever having used E-cigarettes, individually showed that smokers who used E-cigarette was associated with smokers being less likely to quit smoking. When the authors compared all four studies they found a pooled odds ratio of 0.61 (95% CI, 0.50–0.75) for those who used E-cigarettes as an aid to smoking cessation. A limitation, not taken into account, in these studies was identified, and it turned out to be the severity of the participants' nicotine dependence [72R].

There are specific concerns with the availability, and accessibility, of E-cigarettes to children as ingestion of the e-liquid can be toxic, and is potentially lethal [74M]. The numbers of cases of reports to poison control centers has increased each year. In one state nearly half of the reports were in children who were 5 years or younger and overall 80% of the exposures were not purposeful [74M]. Symptoms which were documented in a minimum of 5% of the cases included dizziness, headache, nausea, and vomiting [74M].

CONCLUSION

Although many of the side effects of substance use that we described in the substance abusing population are rare, it is important that medical providers are aware of these "zebras" as they may see them in their practice. Although most practitioners will not be called upon to be the primary provider for the patient's addiction disorder, having knowledge of these issues will allow for better patient care.

References

[1] Alcohol, Tobacco, and Other Drugs. http://www.samhsa.gov/atod.
[2] National Institute on Drug Abuse. Understanding drug abuse and addiction: 2015. Retrieved from, http://www.drugabuse.gov/publications/drugfacts/understanding-drug-abuse-addiction [R].
[3] Baron EP. Comprehensive review of medicinal marijuana, cannabinoids, and therapeutic implications in medicine and headache: what a long strange trip it's been···. Headache. 2015;55(6):885–916 [R].
[4] Hadland SE, Knight JR, Harris SK. Medical marijuana: review of the science and implications for developmental-behavioral pediatric practice. J Dev Behav Pediatr. 2015;36(2):115–23 [R].
[5] Ostadhadi S, Rahmatollahi M, Dehpour AR, et al. Therapeutic potential of cannabinoids in counteracting chemotherapy-induced adverse effects: an exploratory review. Phytother Res. 2015;29(3):332–8 [R].
[6] Hill KP. Medical marijuana: more questions than answers. J Psychiatr Pract. 2014;20(5):389–91 [R].
[7] Pacula RL, Hunt P, Boustead A. Words can be deceiving: a review of variation among legally effective medical marijuana laws in the United States. J Drug Policy Anal. 2014;7(1):1–19 [R].
[8] Volkow ND, Baler RD, Compton WM, et al. Adverse health effects of marijuana use. N Engl J Med. 2014;370(23):2219–27 [R].
[9] Filbey F, Yezhuvath U. Functional connectivity in inhibitory control networks and severity of cannabis use disorder. Am J Drug Alcohol Abuse. 2013;39(6):382–91 [C].
[10] Cousijn J, Goudriaan AE, Ridderinkhof KR, et al. Neural responses associated with cue-reactivity in frequent cannabis users. Addict Biol. 2013;18(3):570–80 [C].
[11] Batalla A, Bhattacharyya S, Yücel M, et al. Structural and functional imaging studies in chronic cannabis users: a systematic review of adolescent and adult findings. PLoS One. 2013;8(2):e55821 [R].
[12] van Winkel R, Kuepper R. Epidemiological, neurobiological, and genetic clues to the mechanisms linking cannabis use to risk for nonaffective psychosis. Annu Rev Clin Psychol. 2014;10:767–91 [R].
[13] Vinkers CH, Van Gastel WA, Schubart CD, et al. The effect of childhood maltreatment and cannabis use on adult psychotic symptoms is modified by the COMT Val[158]Met polymorphism. Schizophr Res. 2013;150(1):303–11 [C].
[14] Valmaggia LR, Day FL, Jones C, et al. Cannabis use and transition to psychosis in people at ultra-high risk. Psychol Med. 2014;44(12):2503–12 [C].
[15] Harris CR, Brown A. Synthetic cannabinoid intoxication: a case series and review. J Emerg Med. 2013;44(2):360–6 [C].
[16] Celofiga A, Koprivsek J, Klavz J. Use of synthetic cannabinoids in patients with psychotic disorders: case series. J Dual Diagn. 2014;10(3):168–73 [C].
[17] Ustundag MF, Ozhan Ibis E, Yucel A, et al. Synthetic cannabis-induced mania. Case Rep Psychiatry. 2015;2015:310930 [C].
[18] Musshoff F, Madea B, Kernbach-Wighton G, et al. Driving under the influence of synthetic cannabinoids ("Spice"): a case series. Int J Legal Med. 2014;128(1):59–64 [R].
[19] Adamowicz P, Lechowicz W. The influence of synthetic cannabinoid UR-144 on human psychomotor performance—a case report demonstrating road traffic risks. Traffic Inj Prev. 2015;20:1–6 [Epub ahead of print] PMID: 25794331 [C].
[20] Katsiki N, Papadopoulou SK, Fachantidou AI, et al. Smoking and vascular risk: are all forms of smoking harmful to all types of vascular disease? Public Health. 2013;127(5):435–41 [R].
[21] Kicman AT, King LA. The current situation with cannabinoids. Drug Test Anal. 2014;6(1–2):1–6 [R].
[22] Jouanjus E, Lapeyre-Mestre M, Micallef J, et al. Cannabis use: signal of increasing risk of serious cardiovascular disorders. J Am Heart Assoc. 2014;3(2):e000638 [M].
[23] Hartung B, Kauferstein S, Ritz-Timme S, et al. Sudden unexpected death under acute influence of cannabis. Forensic Sci Int. 2014;237:e11–3 [C].
[24] Casier I, Vanduynhoven P, Haine S, et al. Is recent cannabis use associated with acute coronary syndromes? An illustrative case series. Acta Cardiol. 2014;69(2):131–6 [C].

[25] Rodríguez-Castro CE, Alkhateeb H, Elfar A, et al. Recurrent myopericarditis as a complication of Mari juana use. Am J Case Rep. 2014;15:60–2 [C].

[26] Bick BL, Szostek JH, Mangan TF. Synthetic cannabinoid leading to cannabinoid hyperemesis syndrome. Mayo Clin Proc. 2014;89(8):1168–9 [C].

[27] Murakami Y, Iwami T, Kitamura T, et al. Outcomes of out-of-hospital cardiac arrest by public location in the public-access defibrillation era. J Am Heart Assoc. 2014;3(2):e000533 [M].

[28] Buser GL, Gerona RR, Horowitz BZ, et al. Acute kidney injury associated with smoking synthetic cannabinoid. Clin Toxicol (Phila). 2014;52(7):664–73 [C].

[29] Zorumski CF, Mennerick S, Izumi Y. Acute and chronic effects of ethanol on learning-related synaptic plasticity. Alcohol. 2014;48(1):1–17 [R].

[30] de la Monte SM, Kril JJ. Human alcohol-related neuropathology. Acta Neuropathol. 2014;127(1):71–90 [R].

[31] Addolorato G, Mirijello A, Leggio L, et al. Management of alcohol dependence in patients with liver disease. CNS Drugs. 2013;27(4):287–99 [R].

[32] Streba LA, Vere CC, Streba CT, et al. Focus on alcoholic liver disease: from nosography to treatment. World J Gastroenterol. 2014;20(25):8040–7 [R].

[33] Damgaard Sandahl T. Alcoholic hepatitis. Dan Med J. 2014;61(10):B4755 [M].

[34] Liu J. Ethanol and liver: recent insights into the mechanisms of ethanol-induced fatty liver. World J Gastroenterol. 2014;20(40):14672–85 [R].

[35] de Jong WJ, Cleveringa AM, Greijdanus B, et al. The effect of acute alcohol intoxication on gut wall integrity in healthy male volunteers; a randomized controlled trial. Alcohol. 2015;49(1):65–70 [C].

[36] Cai S, Li Y, Ding Y, et al. Alcohol drinking and the risk of colorectal cancer death: a meta-analysis. Eur J Cancer Prev. 2014;23(6):532–9 [M].

[37] Testino G, Leone S, Borro P. Alcohol and hepatocellular carcinoma: a review and a point of view. World J Gastroenterol. 2014;20(43):15943–54 [M].

[38] Castro GD, Castro JA. Alcohol drinking and mammary cancer: pathogenesis and potential dietary preventive alternatives. World J Clin Oncol. 2014;5(4):713–29 [R].

[39] Huang Q, Luo K, Yang H, et al. Impact of alcohol consumption on survival in patients with esophageal carcinoma: a large cohort with long-term follow-up. Cancer Sci. 2014;105(12):1638–46 [M].

[40] Park S, Shin HR, Lee B, et al. Attributable fraction of alcohol consumption on cancer using population-based nationwide cancer incidence and mortality data in the Republic of Korea. BMC Cancer. 2014;14:420 [M].

[41] Park YM, Cho CH, Kim SH, et al. Alcohol intake, smoking, and colorectal adenoma. J Cancer Prev. 2014;19(2):137–43 [C].

[42] Nishihara R, Wang M, Qian ZR, et al. Alcohol, one-carbon nutrient intake, and risk of colorectal cancer according to tumor methylation level of IGF2 differentially methylated region. Am J Clin Nutr. 2014;100(6):1479–88 [C].

[43] Bao PP, Shu XO, Gao YT, et al. Association of hormone-related characteristics and breast cancer risk by estrogen receptor/progesterone receptor status in the shanghai breast cancer study. Am J Epidemiol. 2011;174(6):661–71 [M].

[44] Falk RT, Maas P, Schairer C, et al. Alcohol and risk of breast cancer in postmenopausal women: an analysis of etiological heterogeneity by multiple tumor characteristics. Am J Epidemiol. 2014;180(7):705–17 [M].

[45] Fagherazzi G, Vilier A, Boutron-Ruault MC, et al. Alcohol consumption and breast cancer risk subtypes in the E3N-EPIC cohort. Eur J Cancer Prev. 2014;24(3):209–14 [C].

[46] Viteri OA, Soto EE, Bahado-Singh RO, et al. Fetal anomalies and long-term effects associated with substance abuse in pregnancy: a literature review. Am J Perinatol. 2014;32(5):405–16 [R].

[47] May PA, Baete A, Russo J, et al. Prevalence and characteristics of fetal alcohol spectrum disorders. Pediatrics. 2014;134(5):855–66 [C].

[48] Cannon MJ, Dominique Y, O'Leary LA, et al. Characteristics and behaviors of mothers who have a child with fetal alcohol syndrome. Neurotoxicol Teratol. 2012;34(1):90–5 [C].

[49] O'Brien JW, Hill SY. Effects of prenatal alcohol and cigarette exposure on offspring substance use in multiplex, alcohol-dependent families. Alcohol Clin Exp Res. 2014;38(12):2952–61 [C].

[50] Feinstein JA, Feudtner C, Kempe A. Adverse drug event-related emergency department visits associated with complex chronic conditions. Pediatrics. 2014;133(6):e1575–85 [C].

[51] Lugoboni F, Mirijello A, Faccini M, et al. Quality of life in a cohort of high-dose benzodiazepine dependent patients. Drug Alcohol Depend. 2014;142:105–9 [C].

[52] Lee SC, Klein-Schwartz W, Doyon S, et al. Comparison of toxicity associated with nonmedical use of benzodiazepines with buprenorphine or methadone. Drug Alcohol Depend. 2014;138:118–23 [M].

[53] Darke S, Torok M, Duflou J. Circumstances and toxicology of sudden or unnatural deaths involving alprazolam. Drug Alcohol Depend. 2014;138:61–6 [C].

[54] Substance Abuse and Mental Health Services Administration. Results from the 2013 National Survey on Drug Use and Health: Summary of National Findings. Rockville, MD: Substance Abuse and Mental Health Services Administration; 2014. NSDUH Series H-48, HHS Publication No. (SMA) 14–4863.

[55] Cooper CJ, Said S, Alkhateeb H, et al. Dilated cardiomyopathy secondary to chronic cocaine abuse: a case report. BMC Res Notes. 2013;6:536 [C].

[56] The neurobiology of drug addiction. National Institute on drug abuse, National Institutes of Health. https://www.cnsforum.com/educationalresources/imagebank/substance_abuse/mao_cocaine.

[57] Abdul-Karim R, Ryan C, Rangel C, et al. Levamisole-induced vasculitis. Proc (Bayl Univ Med Cent). 2013;26(2):163–5 [C].

[58] Eiden C, Diot C, Mathieu O, et al. Levamisole-adulterated cocaine: what about in European countries? Psychoactive Drugs. 2014;46(5):389–92 [R].

[59] Souied O, Baydoun H, Ghandour Z, et al. Levamisole-contaminated cocaine: an emergent cause of vasculitis and skin necrosis. Case Rep Med. 2014;2014:434717 [C].

[60] Auffenberg C, Rosenthal LJ, Dresner N. Levamisole: a common cocaine adulterant with life-threatening side effects. Psychosomatics. 2013;54(6):590–3 [R].

[61] González-Duarte A, Williams R. Cocaine-induced recurrent leukoencephalopathy. Neuroradiol J. 2013;26(5):511–3 [C].

[62] Alfaro R, Vasavada N, Paueksakon P, et al. Cocaine-induced acute interstitial nephritis: a case report and review of the literature. J Nephropathol. 2013;2(3):204–9 [C].

[63] Finkelstein Y, Hutson JR, Freedman SB, et al. Drug-induced seizures in children and adolescents presenting for emergency care: current and emerging trends. Clin Toxicol (Phila). 2013;51(8):761–6 [M].

[64] Fishbain D, Johnson S, Webster L, et al. Review of regulatory programs and new opioid technologies in chronic pain management: balancing the risk of medication abuse with medical need. J Manag Care Pharm. 2010;16(4):276–87 [R].

[65] http://www.drugabuse.gov/publications/research-reports/heroin/scope-heroin-use-in-united-states [accessed 3/11/15].

[66] http://www.drugabuse.gov/about-nida/legislative-activities/testimony-to-congress/2014/ prescription-opioid-heroin-abuse [accessed 3/11/15].

[67] http://www.drugabuse.gov/publications/research-reports/heroin/what-are-immediate-short-term-effects-heroin-use.

[68] Cooper C, Bilbao JE, Said S, et al. Serum amyloid A renal amyloidosis in a chronic subcutaneous ("skin popping") heroin user. J Nephropathol. 2013;2(3):196–200 [C].

[69] Treating tobacco use and dependence. An evidence based clinical practice guideline for tobacco cessation. CDC: http://www.cdc.gov/tobacco/data_statistics/fact_sheets/fast_facts/.

[70] Goniewicz ML, Knysak J, Gawron M, et al. Levels of selected carcinogens and toxicants in vapour from electronic cigarettes. Tob Control. 2014;23(2):133–9 [C].

[71] Electronic Cigarettes (e-Cigarettes) www.fda.gov/newsevents/publichealthfocus/ucm172906.htm [accessed 3/3/15].

[72] Grana R, Benowitz N, Glantz SA. E-cigarettes: a scientific review. Circulation. 2014;129(19):1972–86 [R].

[73] Torjesen I. E-cigarettes are to be regulated as medicines from 2016. BMJ. 2013;346:f3859 [R].

[74] Durmowicz EL. The impact of electronic cigarettes on the paediatric population. Tob Control. 2014;23(Suppl 2):ii41–6 [M].

5

Hypnosedatives and Anxiolytics

Stephen Curran*, Shabir Musa*, Amir Sajjadi[†,1]

*Fieldhead Hospital, South West Yorkshire Partnership NHS Foundation Trust, Wakefield, United Kingdom
[†]St Mary's House, St Mary's Road, Leeds and York Partnerships-NHS Foundation Trust, Leeds, West Yorkshire, United Kingdom
[1]Corresponding author: a.sajjadi@nhs.net

BENZODIAZEPINES

Alprazolam

Psychological

Circumstances and toxicology of sudden or unnatural deaths involving alprazolam was investigated in 412 cases of sudden or unnatural deaths presenting to the New South Wales Department of Forensic Medicine (DOFM) between 1997 and 2012 [1C]. There was a significant increase in the annual number of cases, from 3 in 1997 to 86 in 2012. Circumstances of death were: accidental drug toxicity (57.0%), deliberate drug toxicity (10.4%), suicide by means other than drug overdose (12.6%), disease (10.0%), accident (5.1%), and homicide (2.4%). The study concluded that cases involving alprazolam increased markedly, driven mostly by toxicity deaths amongst people with known drug and alcohol problems. Caution in prescribing alprazolam would appear appropriate, particularly to those with known drug dependence.

Psychiatric

A population-based study examined the rate of detection of alprazolam among cases of heroin-related death (HRD) in Victoria, Australia from January 1990 to December 2010 [2C]. There were 2392 HRDs in Victoria from 1990 to 2010. The association between the detection of alprazolam in HRDs and alprazolam supply was strong and significant. The proportion of cases of HRD in which alprazolam was detected increased at an incidence rate ratio of 2.4 (95% CI, 2.1–2.8; $P < 0.001$). Alprazolam was detected among increasing proportions of HRDs, from 5.3% in 2005 to a peak of 35.3% in 2009. Alprazolam use increased from 8% in 2005 to 69% in 2011 in Victoria. The use of benzodiazepines by opioid-dependent people is widespread and alprazolam is now the most commonly injected benzodiazepine.

Central Nervous System

A study evaluated effects of alprazolam on cortical activity and tremors in eight patients with essential tremor [3c]. Eight patients from a general neurology out-patient clinic with diagnosis of essential tremor were included in the study. They had no other neurological or psychiatric disorder apart from essential tremor. Their hand tremors and contralateral cortical activity were recorded before and after a single dose of alprozolam (between 0.5 and 0.75 mg). The authors observed that alprazolam significantly attenuated tremors, decreased cortical activity in the tremor frequency range and increased cortical beta activity in all patients. At the same time, the cortico-muscular coherence at the tremor frequency became non-significant. They also found a significant correlation ($r = 0.757$, $P < 0.001$) between the reduction in tremor severity and the increased ratio of cortical activity in the beta band to the activity observed in the tremor frequency range.

Benzodiazepines

Psychological

A review of benzodiazepine dependence and its treatment with low dose flumazenil was published [4M]. This study found that continuous intravenous or subcutaneous flumazenil, a benzodiazepine receptor antagonist/partial agonist of GABA-A infusion for 4 days significantly reduces acute benzodiazepine withdrawal. It was also suggested that delivery of low dose flumazenil

© 2015 Elsevier B.V. All rights reserved.

either via subcutaneous implant or transdermal delivery via creams or patches may be able to manage some of the adverse iatrogenic effects and development of tolerance which occur with long-term use revolutionizing the way this class of drugs is used and prescribed.

Clobazam

Drug–Drug Interaction

Effects of sulthiame (STM) on the pharmacokinetics of clobazam (CLB) were investigated in five patients [5c]. Patients' serum CLB and of N-desmethyl-clobazam (DMCLB) concentrations were monitored after the addition or discontinuation of STM. There was an increase in the mean concentration to dose (CD) ratio of DMCLB by 82.6–248.5% when patients were taking STM (100–275 mg/day), this was higher than when they were not using STM. The CD ratio of CLB remained stable after addition or discontinuation of STM. This study suggested that sulthiame has the potential to inhibit the metabolism of clobazam, possibly via an action on CYP2C19 enzyme activity.

Diazepam

Central Nervous System

A study evaluated long-term response to high-dose diazepam treatment in continuous spikes and waves during sleep in 29 patients, age 1–21 years [6A]. Patients had 48 high-dose nocturnal diazepam treatment cycles. An overnight reduction of at least 50% occurred in 15 cycles (13 patients), and persisted within 6 months in eight of 15 cycles (eight patients), but returned to baseline in three cycles (three patients). Twenty of 29 cycles that responded in the short term had persistent response on follow-up. It was reported that treatment with high-dose diazepam reduced epileptiform activity in continuous spikes and waves during sleep in the short term, and improvement persisted for several months in most cycles.

Flubromazepam

Pharmacokinetics

A study investigated metabolism and pharmacokinetics of the designer benzodiazepine flubromazepam [7A]. Flubromazepam started to be sold as a recreational drug in late 2012. One of the authors of this study consumed 4 mg of flubromazepam to gain preliminary data on the pharmacokinetic properties and the metabolism of this compound. For this purpose, serum as well as urine samples were collected for up to 31 days post-ingestion and analyzed. On the basis of this study, flubromazepam appears to have an extremely long elimination half-life of more than 100 hours. One monohydroxylated compound

and the debrominated compound could be identified as the predominant metabolites, the first allowing a detection of a consumption for up to 28 days post-ingestion when analyzing urine samples in our case. Additionally, various immunochemical assays were evaluated, showing that the cross-reactivity of the used assay seems not to be sufficient for safe detection of the applied dose in urine samples, bearing the risk that it could be misused in drug-withdrawal settings or in other circumstances requiring regular drug testing. Furthermore, it may be used in drug-facilitated crimes without being detected.

Lorazepam

Ophthalmologic

A case report of a 21-year-old man admitted to a psychiatric ward with a provisional diagnosis of depression and Obsessive Compulsive Disorder (OCD) who developed diplopia following Lorazepam 4 mg IV [8A]. Diplopia started 8 hours post administration of lorazepam and resolved 12 hours of onset. Ophthalmologic and Neurologic examinations were non-significant. The patient had no previous history of similar condition. World Health Organisation probability scale indicated "probable" association between diplopia and Lorazepam.

Midazolam

Drug–Drug Interaction

Effect of netupitant, on the pharmacokinetics of midazolam was studied in 20 healthy subjects [9C]. Netupitant is a new highly selective neurokinin-1 receptor antagonist being studied for the prevention of nausea and vomiting in patients undergoing chemotherapy. Netupitant inhibiting the CYP3A4 increased the Cmax and AUCinf of midazolam by 40% and 144%, respectively. The results of this study suggest that netupitant is a moderate inhibitor of CYP3A4 and therefore, co-administration with drugs that are substrates of CYP3A4 like midazolam may require dose adjustments.

Drug–Drug Interaction

Pharmacokinetic interaction between PA-824, a novel antitubercular nitroimidazo-oxazine, and midazolam, a CYP3A4 substrate, was evaluated in 14 healthy adult male and female subjects [10C]. The total study duration for each subject from check-in through study termination (including a 2-day washout) spanned 18 nights and 19 days, with follow-up evaluation over 3 months. Subjects received a single oral dose of midazolam (2 mg), followed by a 2-day washout. After the washout, all subjects received PA-824 (400 mg) once daily for 14 consecutive days. On day 14, all subjects received the final PA-824 dose coadministered with a 2-mg oral dose of midazolam. This study demonstrated that PA-824 at the 400-mg dose does not produce changes in midazolam exposure that would require dose adjustment. Any changes in midazolam exposure that occur for the 100- and 200-mg PA-824 doses are likely to be even less than that observed for the 400-mg dose, PA-824.

HYPNOSEDATIVES AND BENZODIAZEPINE-LIKE DRUGS

Buspirone

Drug Formulation

A pharmacokinetic study evaluated bioavailability of buspirone hydrochloride via cup and core buccal tablets compared to Buspar® tablets [11c, E]. The tablets were prepared according to 5×3 factorial design where polymer type was set at five levels (carbopol, hydroxypropyl methylcellulose, sodium alginate, sodium carboxymethyl cellulose and guar gum), and polymer to drug ratio at three levels (1:1, 2:1 and 3:1). Mucoadhesion force, *ex vivo* mucoadhesion time, percent BH released after 8 hours (Q8h) and time for release of 50% BH ($T_{(50\%)}$) were chosen as dependent variables. The *in vitro* release studies showed that the cup and core buccal tablet CA10 released 97.91% of the drug at the end of 8 hours. The *in vivo* evaluation, in four healthy human volunteers, of formula CA10 revealed a 5.6-fold increase in bioavailability compared to the oral commercial Buspar®.

Chloral Hydrate

Paediatrics

A case-report indicated a 14-month-old female developed drug rash with eosinophilia and systemic symptoms (DRESS) syndrome after administration of chloral hydrate [12A]. The patient underwent operation for correction tetralogy of Fallout. Chloral hydrate was administered 3 weeks prior to her visit for preoperative echocardiography. There was no history of adverse reactions or hypersensitivity. On postoperative day 7, she had a good condition and there were not abnormal laboratory findings. She was administered 500 mg of chloral hydrate for echocardiography. The rash appeared abruptly 10 hours later and spread from the face and trunk to the extremities within 4 days. On the fifth day after administration of chloral hydrate, the fever persisted and oliguria and generalized oedema progressed. She was found with hepatosplenomegaly and interstitial pneumonia was observed on the chest radiography. Laboratory findings showed hepatitis, hyperbilirubinemia, leukocytosis, atypical lymphocytosis, hyper-eosinophilia, and proteinuria. Oral prednisolone (1 mg/kg/day) was administered daily

for 14 days and was then tapered for 7 days. During a 2-month follow-up period, clinical symptoms, laboratory tests and chest radiography returned to normal. Chloral hydrate is a sedative and hypnotic drug frequently used in paediatric patients. DRESS, also known as drug-induced hypersensitivity syndrome (DIHS), is a rare, acute and severe life-threatening systemic disease. DRESS syndrome is characterized by fever, lymphadenopathy, rash, hyper-eosinophilia and involvement of systemic organs.

Paediatric

Three cases of paediatric chloral hydrate poisoning, all occurred following procedural sedation in outpatient clinic settings, presented to the emergency department. The ages ranged from 15 months to 4 years of age and all required resuscitation. Unfortunately, the 4 year old died [13A].

Case 1: A 4-year-old girl weighting 12.8 kg was prescribed chloral hydrate 900 mg (70 mg/kg) by her dentist, given orally at home prior to a dental extraction. She was fasting as instructed for the procedure. She was sedated upon arrival at the office and underwent a successful tooth extraction without any additional sedation. She remained somnolent but arousable 6 hours following the procedure; she then became unresponsive and not breathing. In the emergency department, she had a Glasgow coma score (GCS) of 3 and was asystolic. CPR and intubation were not successful and she was announced dead later.

Case 2: A 3-year-old boy weighing 10 kg was prescribed chloral hydrate 500 mg (50 mg/kg) prior to a dental procedure. However, he had mistakenly much higher dose of 6000 mg (400 mg/kg) of chloral hydrate. He vomited en route in the ambulance. On arrival to the emergency department, he was afebrile with a GCS 3 and emergently intubated. An esmolol infusion was initiated with complete resolution of ventricular irritability. He was extubated, 30 hours after the ingestion and discharged to home without apparent neurologic sequelae.

Case 3: A 15-month-old girl weighing 12.4 kg with panhypopituitarism, hydrocephalus, with ventriculo-peritoneal shunt, and septal optic dysplasia was given 1200 mg chloral hydrate (100 mg/kg) at an outpatient ophthalmology clinic for sedation prior to evaluation. Within 25 min of dosing, she vomited and had stridorous respirations with a decrease in heart rate to 101 bpm and respiratory rate of 18 bpm followed by obtundation, cyanosis, and apnoea with oxygen desaturation to 64%. Resuscitation was begun and was put on oxygen. As she improved effectively, endotracheal intubation was not performed. She was able to be weaned to room air over 45 min and monitored for 12 hours and discharged to home without sequelae.

Eszopiclone

Central Nervous System

The U.S. Food and Drug Administration (FDA) has issued a new warning that the insomnia drug eszopiclone, a sedative-hypnotic sleep medicine used to treat insomnia in adults, can cause next-day impairment of driving and other activities that require alertness [14S]. Patients were often unaware they were impaired. FDA recommends a decreased starting dose of Lunesta (eszopiclone) to 1 mg at bedtime. The starting dose can be increased to 2 or 3 mg if needed, but the higher doses are more likely to result in next-day impairment of driving and other activities that require full alertness.

Melatonin

Drug–Drug Interaction

The effect of melatonin on metabolic side effects of olanzapine was evaluated in a randomized double-blind placebo-controlled trial of 48 patients with first episode schizophrenia who were eligible for olanzapine treatment [15C]. Patients were randomly assigned to olanzapine plus either melatonin 3 mg/day or matched placebo and were followed for 8 weeks. Metabolic parameters including weight, waist circumference, triglyceride, cholesterol, insulin, and blood sugar were assessed at baseline, week 4, and week 8. The study found that melatonin was associated with significantly less weight gain, increase in waist circumference and triglyceride than the placebo. Changes in cholesterol, insulin, and blood sugar did not differ significantly between the two groups.

Sodium Oxybate

Psychological

A case report of a 39-year-old female diagnosed with narcolepsy and cataplexy who revealed central sleep apnoea in a Cheyne–Stokes pattern when under constant treatment with Sodium oxybate (γ-hydroxybutyric acid, GHB) [16A]. GHB is used therapeutically in the treatment of narcolepsy. The female patient had no pre-existing sleep-disordered breathing. Current safety recommendations have been formulated for the use of GHB in patients with pre-existing breathing disorders. Patient developed sudden sleep apnoea which disappeared following discontinuation of GHB.

Psychiatric

A case report described a 18-year-old girl who acutely developed psychotic agitation and suicidal ideation, culminating in a near fatal suicide attempt, while taking sodium oxybate for narcolepsy [17A]. Little is known about potential adverse effects of sodium oxybate in younger populations [18C]. A young female was admitted to a psychiatric hospital due to self-harm; she had a diagnosis of narcolepsy, but had no prior psychiatric diagnoses. She was then started on sodium oxybate 1.5 g titrated up to 4.5 g twice nightly. She was not taking any other medications. Three days after the last dose increase, she was observed to be "sluggish" and incoherent at times, and began making vague suicidal comments. She exhibited paranoid thoughts, and experienced auditory hallucinations and symptoms of derealisation. On the same day, in a state of acute agitation, she unexpectedly stabbed herself multiple times in the chest with a kitchen knife, resulting in significant cardiopulmonary injury and cardiac arrest. Her subsequent hospital course, lasted 4 months.

Zolpidem

Psychological

A case report was published by Sing et al. on somnambulism following zolipem exposure [19A]. A 46-year-old male, who had subdural hematoma extraction through burr hole surgery following a traffic accident developed somnambulism, sleep-walking after 2 weeks of initiation of zolpidem 10 mg [19A]. Somnambulism was observed to be associated with staring expression and some incoherent speech. The patient had no memory of this event in the morning. The patient had no personal or family history of sleep-walking and there were no new changes to his medication apart from zolpidem. Somnambulism stopped following discontinuation of zolpidem.

Driving

Residual effects of low-dose sublingual zolpidem on highway driving performance the morning after middle-of-the-night use was evaluated in a randomized, double-blind, placebo-controlled, crossover study in 40 healthy volunteers (20 females) [20C]. Single dose of zolpidem 3.5 mg administered in the middle of the night at 3 and 4 hours before driving, zopiclone 7.5 mg at bedtime 9 hours before driving, and placebo. Driving performance was assessed using a standardized highway driving test. The morning after zopiclone, 45% of the drivers were classified as impaired however zolpidem 3.5 mg in a buffered sublingual formulation had a minimal risk of impairing driving performance in the morning ≥4 hours after middle-of-the night use. When taken 3 hours before driving, the drug may have impairing effects. The use of healthy volunteers instead of patients with insomnia could be seen as a limitation of this study.

Head Injury

The relationship between the use of zolpidem and risk of head injury or fracture requiring hospitalization was evaluated in a large scale population cohort study [21C]. 8188 Adult patients who had received a first prescription for zolpidem between January 1, 2000, and December 31, 2009, were compared with 32 752 age- and sex-matched patients who had not used sedative-hypnotic agents. They were followed up for at least 1 year or until hospitalization for head injury or fracture (major injury) accrued. The result of the study indicated a significantly greater risk of head injury or fracture requiring hospitalization in patients who used zolpidem ($P < 0.001$), particularly in the younger (aged 18–54 years) patients. The adjusted hazard ratio for major injury in zolpidem users was 1.67 (95% CI, 1.19–2.34).

Zopiclone

Psychological

Effects of withdrawal from the long-term use of temazepam, zopiclone and zolpidem on cognition were evaluated in 92 older adults with primary insomnia [22]. Participants had 1 month medically supported withdrawal attempt followed by 5-month follow-up. The findings of this study suggested that long-term use of temazepam, zopiclone and zolpidem by older adult is associated with impairment of attention and psychomotor cognitive functioning, these effects lasted for the total duration of the study after withdrawal from hypnotics.

References

[1] Darke S, Torok M, Duflou J. Circumstances and toxicology of sudden or unnatural deaths involving alprazolam. Drug Alcohol Depend. 2014;138:61–6 [C].

[2] Rintoul AC, Dobbin MD, Nielsen S, et al. Recent increase in detection of alprazolam in Victorian heroin-related deaths. Med J Aust. 2013;198(4):206–9 [C].

[3] Ibáñez J, González de la Aleja J, Gallego JA, et al. Effects of alprazolam on cortical activity and tremors in patients with essential tremor. PLoS One. 2014;9(3):e93159 [c].

[4] Hood SD, Norman A, Hince DA, et al. Benzodiazepine dependence and its treatment with low dose flumazenil. Br J Clin Pharmacol. 2014;77(2):285–94 [M].

[5] Yamamoto Y, Takahashi Y, Imai K, et al. Interaction between sulthiame and clobazam: sulthiame inhibits the metabolism of clobazam, possibly via an action on CYP2C19. Epilepsy Behav. 2014;34:124–6 [c].

[6] Sánchez Fernández I, Peters JM, An S, et al. Long-term response to high-dose diazepam treatment in continuous spikes and waves during sleep. Pediatr Neurol. 2013;49(3). 163–170.e4 [C].

[7] Moosmann B, Huppertz LM, Hutter M, et al. Detection and identification of the designer benzodiazepine flubromazepam and preliminary data on its metabolism and pharmacokinetics. J Mass Spectrom. 2013;48(11):1150–9 [A].

[8] Lucca JM, Ramesh M, Parthasarathi G, et al. Lorazepam-induced diplopia. Indian J Pharmacol. 2014;46(2):228–9 [A].

[9] Lanzarotti C, Rossi G. Effect of netupitant, a highly selective NK1 receptor antagonist, on the pharmacokinetics of midazolam, erythromycin, and dexamethasone. Support Care Cancer. 2013;21(10):2783–91 [C].

[10] Winter H, Egizi E, Erondu N, et al. Evaluation of pharmacokinetic interaction between PA-824 and midazolam in healthy adult subjects. Antimicrob Agents Chemother. 2013;57(8):3699–703 [C].

[11] Kassem MA, Elmeshad AN, Fares AR. Enhanced bioavailability of buspirone hydrochloride via cup and core buccal tablets: formulation and in vitro/in vivo evaluation. Int J Pharm. 2014;463(1):68–80 [c, E].

[12] Yoo SD, Kim SG, Kim SH, et al. Drug rash with eosinophilia and systemic symptoms syndrome induced by chloral hydrate in early childhood. Allergy Asthma Immunol Res. 2014;6(3):270–2 [A].

[13] Nordt SP, Rangan C, Hardmaslani M, et al. Pediatric chloral hydrate poisonings and death following outpatient procedural sedation. J Med Toxicol. 2014;10(2):219–22 [A].

[14] FDA Drug Safety Communication. FDA warns of next-day impairment with sleep aid Lunesta (eszopiclone) and lowers recommended dose, http://www.fda.gov/Drugs/DrugSafety/ucm397260.htm [accessed 05/02/2015] [S].

[15] Modabbernia A, Heidari P, Soleimani R, et al. Melatonin for prevention of metabolic side-effects of olanzapine in patients with first-episode schizophrenia: randomized double-blind placebo-controlled study. J Psychiatr Res. 2014;53:133–40 [C].

[16] Frase L, Schupp J, Sorichter S, et al. Sodium oxybate-induced central sleep apneas. Sleep Med. 2013;14(9):922–4 [A].

[17] Chien J, Ostermann G, Turkel SB. Sodium oxybate-induced psychosis and suicide attempt in an 18-year-old girl. J Child Adolesc Psychopharmacol. 2013;23(4):300–1 [A].

[18] Alshaikh MK, Gacuan D, George S, et al. Long-term follow-up of patients with narcolepsy-cataplexy treated with sodium oxybate (Xyrem). Clin Neuropharmacol. 2011;34(1):1–4 [C].

[19] Singh H, Thangaraju P, Natt NK. Sleep-walking a rarest side effect of zolpidem. Indian J Psychol Med. 2015;37(1):105–6 [A].

[20] Vermeeren A, Vuurman EF, Leufkens TR, et al. Residual effects of low-dose sublingual zolpidem on highway driving performance the morning after middle-of-the-night use. Sleep. 2014;37(3):489–96 [C].

[21] Lai MM, Lin CC, Lin CC, et al. Long-term use of zolpidem increases the risk of major injury: a population-based cohort study. Mayo Clin Proc. 2014;89(5):589–94 [C].

[22] Puustinen J, Lähteenmäki R, Polo-Kantola P, et al. Effect of withdrawal from long-term use of temazepam, zopiclone or zolpidem as hypnotic agents on cognition in older adults. Eur J Clin Pharmacol. 2014;70(3):319–29 [C].

6

Antipsychotic Drugs

P. Chue[1], G. Baker

University of Alberta, Edmonton, AB, Canada
[1]Corresponding author: pchue@ualberta.ca; glen.baker@ualberta.ca

GENERAL [SEDA-15, 2438; SEDA-32, 83; SEDA-33, 89; SEDA-34, 51; SEDA-35, 85; SEDA-36, 59]

Comparative Studies

A 12-month, randomised study of aripiprazole, quetiapine and ziprasidone in first-episode patients (FEP) reported a *discontinuation rate* of 16.3% due to adverse events (AEs) [1C]; the most common AEs were *weight gain*, *fatigue* and *sedation*.

In a randomised, controlled study of aripiprazole vs. risperidone in acute bipolar mania ($n=50$) the most common AE was *headache* (risperidone, $n=2$; aripiprazole, $n=1$) [2C].

A randomised, controlled study of clozapine vs. ziprasidone in schizophrenia and cannabis use disorder ($n=30$) reported a high *discontinuation rate* due to AEs [3C]; these included *sedation* ($n=7$), *sialorrhea* ($n=1$) and *fever* ($n=1$) with clozapine, and *agitation* ($n=2$) and *lack of efficacy* ($n=7$) with ziprasidone.

A 2-month, double-blind, randomised clinical trial of aripiprazole and risperidone was conducted in children and adolescents (6–18 years) with tic disorder ($n=60$) [4C]; AEs included *increased appetite* (25.8%), *drowsiness* (25.8%), and *decreased appetite* (12.9%) for aripiprazole; and *increased appetite* (27.6%), *drowsiness* (17.2%), and *urinary incontinence* (13.8%) for risperidone.

Observational Studies

A cross-sectional study of olanzapine, clozapine, quetiapine and ziprasidone in patients with schizophrenia ($n=218$) found that olanzapine was associated with the least AEs overall [5C]. There were significant group differences between UKU Side Effect Rating Scale scores for *memory difficulties* (ziprasidone vs. quetiapine), *tension/restlessness* (ziprasidone vs. quetiapine), *tremor*

(ziprasidone vs. risperidone, olanzapine), *seizures* (clozapine/quetiapine vs. olanzapine/risperidone/ziprasidone), *sialorrhea* (quetiapine vs. ziprasidone), *orthostatic dizziness* (risperidone vs. olanzapine), *sweating* (quetiapine vs. ziprasidone), *rash* (risperidone vs. olanzapine), *weight gain* (quetiapine vs. ziprasidone), *galactorrhea* (risperidone vs. olanzapine, ziprasidone, quetiapine, clozapine), *increased libido* (quetiapine vs. olanzapine), *decreased libido* (quetiapine vs. olanzapine), *erectile dysfunction* (quetiapine vs. olanzapine) and *orgasmic dysfunction* (quetiapine vs. olanzapine).

A 20-year open-label study ($n=62$) reported fewer *metabolic alterations* in *lipids* and *glucose* with haloperidol and aripiprazole vs. clozapine, olanzapine and quetiapine [6C].

A study of patients receiving antipsychotics ($n=517$) reported an AE incidence rate of 42% (289 AEs in 217 patients) [7c]. *Central and peripheral nervous system* was the most commonly affected system ($n=59$) and *weight gain* ($n=30$) was the most commonly observed AE; olanzapine was most commonly implicated ($n=92$) followed by risperidone ($n=59$).

A 12-month, prospective, observational study of antipsychotics in delirium ($n=2453$) reported AEs that included *aspiration pneumonia* ($n=17$), followed by *cardiovascular events* ($n=3$) that included *hypotension* (quetiapine, $n=2$), *bradycardia* (blonanserin, $n=1$), and *venous thromboembolism* ($n=1$) [8c].

A 12-week study evaluated adolescents and young adults (16–19 years) with schizophrenia spectrum disorders ($n=79$) treated with aripiprazole, olanzapine, quetiapine, risperidone, or ziprasidone [9c]. Overall, 30.8% had at least mild extrapyramidal symptoms (*EPS*) during the course of the study (increased in early non-responders vs. early responders); 7.8% developed *akathisia* and 64.5% gained at least 7% of their *body weight*.

A 24-month study ($n=110$) of children and adolescents (9–17 years) found that at 6 (but not 12 or 24)

© 2015 Elsevier B.V. All rights reserved.

months, there were significant differences in *Body Mass Index (BMI)* increase (olanzapine > risperidone > quetiapine) and in *neurological AEs* (most frequent with risperidone group) [10c].

A retrospective analysis of second generation antipsychotic (SGA) poisoning (clozapine, olanzapine, quetiapine, risperidone) in young children (<6 years) found the most common AEs included *minor reduction in vigilance* (62%), *miosis* (12%) and *mild tachycardia* (10%) and 1 case of *EPS* with risperidone [11c].

Adjunctive aripiprazole was found to be significantly better tolerated than haloperidol for the first 3 months when added to clozapine in a 12-month, randomised, naturalistic trial based on Liverpool University Neuroleptic Side Effect Rating Scale scores [12c].

In a study of agitated patients no significant differences were found in AEs including *QTc prolongation*, between haloperidol ($n=314$) and droperidol ($n=218$) given by intramuscular (im) or intravenous routes (iv) [13c]. One droperidol patient with a history of congenital heart disease suffered a *cardiopulmonary arrest* (successfully resuscitated).

In a prospective study of parenteral sedation (droperidol, haloperidol, midazolam monotherapy and combination) for acute behavioural disturbance ($n=171$) AEs included *hypotension* ($n=14$), *oxygen desaturation* ($n=1$), and *hypotension* and *oxygen desaturation* ($n=1$); more AEs were seen with higher doses [14c].

A study of im olanzapine, haloperidol, and levomepromazine in acutely, agitated patients ($n=122$) found that mean changes from baseline on *movement disorder* scales were significantly better for olanzapine and levomepromazine vs. haloperidol, and significantly better for olanzapine vs. levomepromazine [15c].

Haloperidol, risperidone, olanzapine and aripiprazole were compared in elderly patients with delirium ($n=21$) [16c]; *EPS* were most frequent with haloperidol (followed by risperidone), and *sedation* most frequent with olanzapine.

A retrospective analysis of quetiapine-, olanzapine- and risperidone-related ambulance attendances found that quetiapine was consistently associated with *higher rates of ambulance attendances* [17c].

Systematic Reviews

A systematic review of mood stabilizer–antipsychotic combinations (19 studies) found all combinations were associated with increased AEs [18R]. These included *motor side effects* with haloperidol, *weight gain* with olanzapine, risperidone and quetiapine, *tremor* and *akathisia* with aripiprazole and *tremor* with ziprasidone. Additionally, *encephalopathy, Steven–Johnson syndrome, neutropenia,* and *neuroleptic malignant syndrome* (NMS) were described in case reports with all agents except ziprasidone.

Two reviews of SGAs in the treatment of psychosis in adolescents (13 randomised controlled trials [RCTs], $n=1112$) reported *weight gain* with clozapine, olanzapine and risperidone, *elevated prolactin* with risperidone, olanzapine, and molindone (vs. first generation antispsychotics [FGAs]) and *lower serum cholesterol* with aripiprazole (vs. placebo) [19r,20r].

A meta-analysis examined *weight gain* stratified according to duration of antipsychotic use (≤6 weeks, 6–16 weeks, 16–38 weeks >38 weeks) [21R]. With the exception of amisulpride, aripiprazole and ziprasidone, there was a mean *increase* in *body weight*, *BMI* and clinically relevant *weight gain* with increased duration of antipsychotic use. These effects were greatest in antipsychotic-naive patients with the proportion of clinically relevant *weight gain* ≥20% for all antipsychotics. The proportion of patients showing clinically relevant *weight loss* was approximately 10%, except aripiprazole which was >15%.

A meta-analysis examined the comparative efficacy and tolerability of 15 antipsychotic drugs in schizophrenia (9212 studies, $n=43\,049$) [22R]. *EPS* was greatest with haloperidol and least with clozapine; *sedation* was greatest with clozapine and least with amisulpride; *weight gain* was greatest with olanzapine and least with haloperidol; *prolactin increase* was greatest with paliperidone and least with aripiprazole; and *QTc prolongation* was greatest with sertindole and least with lurasidone.

A meta-analysis of SGA augmentation of antidepressants in major depressive disorder (MDD) (17 studies, $n=3870$) found that SGA augmentation was associated with a higher *discontinuation rate* due to AEs [23R].

A review of the literature reported that all SGAs can induce *prolactin elevations*, especially at the beginning of treatment [24r]. The highest rates of *prolactin elevation* were reported with amisulpride, risperidone and paliperidone; aripiprazole and quetiapine had the least effect. Another review reported that 18% of men and 47% of women treated with antipsychotics for severe mental illness had an elevated *prolactin level* [25r].

A review of antipsychotics and safety in breast-feeding infants reported no *developmental problems* with aripiprazole, haloperidol, perphenazine, or trifluoperazine [26r]. Olanzapine, quetiapine, and risperidone were reported as safe although *mental* and *motor delay* was reported with paroxetine ($n=1$) and quetiapine ($n=1$) and *developmental delay* with chlorpromazine ($n=1$) and haloperidol ($n=1$). *Sedation, decreased suckling, restlessness, irritability, seizures,* and *cardiovascular instability* were reported with clozapine.

A systematic review and meta-analysis of FGAs vs. SGAs (13 studies, $n=2509$) in FEP found that compared to FGAs, *EPS* were significantly less frequent but *weight gain* was significantly greater with clozapine, olanzapine and risperidone [27R].

A systematic review and meta-analysis of antipsychotics in alcohol dependence found increased *drowsiness*, *appetite* and *dry mouth* for the pooled antipsychotics (amisulpride, aripiprazole, flupenthixol, olanzapine, quetiapine, tiapride) vs. placebo [28R].

A systematic review compared the tolerability of the latest SGAs [29R]. *QT prolongation* was greater for iloperidone than for asenapine with no effect observed with lurasidone; *akathisia* was noted with cariprazine, lurasidone, and asenapine but not with iloperidone, and *sedation* noted with asenapine.

A review of short-acting im antipsychotics for the management of acute agitation found that olanzapine (14 studies), ziprasidone (13 studies) and aripiprazole (5 studies) had less *EPS* than haloperidol [30R]. The most common AE with aripiprazole was *headache*; ziprasidone was associated with a non-significant increase in *QTc*.

A review of SGAs in children and adolescents with pervasive developmental disorders commented on the risks of *metabolic disruption, hyperprolactinemia* and *movement disorder* [31r]. Another review and meta-analysis of SGAs in autistic disorders found that the majority of studies reported *weight gain* as an AE [32R].

A review (71 intervention trials, 42 observational studies, 14 literature reviews) of children and adolescents treated with antipsychotics reported a greater risk of *weight gain* and *increased BMI* for SGAs vs. FGAs; olanzapine caused the most *weight gain* and ziprasidone the least [33r]. A review of antipsychotics in the treatment of delirium reported more *EPS* with haloperidol vs. olanzapine, more *sedation* but less *abnormal involuntary movements* with quetiapine vs. placebo, and comparable but mild *EPS* with olanzapine vs. risperidone [34r].

A review of the use of SGAs (risperidone, olanzapine, quetiapine, aripiprazole, ziprasidone) in the treatment of generalized anxiety disorder (17 studies) reported that serious AEs including *EPS* were infrequent but *weight gain* was a concern with olanzapine [35r].

A review of genetics, epigenetics, and biomarkers for antipsychotic-induced *weight gain* reported that the most consistently replicated findings were in the melanocortin 4 receptor (MC4R), serotonin 2C receptor (HTR2C), leptin, neuropeptide Y (NPY) and cannabinoid receptor 1 (CNR1) genes [36r].

Cardiovascular

A claims database study compared aripiprazole, olanzapine ($n=9917$), quetiapine ($n=14935$), risperidone ($n=10192$) and ziprasidone ($n=5696$) in matched non-diabetic adults [37c]. Increased risk of *stroke* and any *cardiovascular event* was reported with olanzapine, quetiapine, and risperidone, while ziprasidone showed no difference from aripiprazole.

A case–crossover study in elderly patients (>64 years) found an increased risk of *ischemic stroke* with risperidone

and quetiapine, but not with olanzapine, during the 30 days prior to stroke [38C]. However, the increased *stroke* risk in demented patients was also observed with olanzapine within 30 days after exposure.

A study of the risk of *out-of-hospital cardiac arrest* ($n=2205$) found that treatment with any antipsychotic was associated with increased risk (odds ratio (OR)= 1.53, 95% confidence interval (CI): 1.23–1.89) [39c]. The use of FGAs was associated with *increased risk* (OR=1.66, CI: 1.27–2.17) but not SGAs (OR=1.29, CI: 0.90–1.85). Haloperidol (OR=2.43, CI: 1.20–4.93), levomepromazine (OR=2.05, CI: 1.18–3.56), and quetiapine (OR=3.64, CI: 1.59–8.30) were all associated with *increased risk*.

A study of ECG parameters, including mean QTc and QT dispersion in children ($n=60$) treated with risperidone or aripiprazole did not find significant changes with either drug [40c]. Risperidone was associated with a slight increase of both *mean QTc* and *QT dispersion* and aripiprazole was associated with a slight increase of *QT dispersion*.

A study of antipsychotic drugs (FGA, $n=9777$; SGA, $n=21164$) in patients ≥65 years found that FGAs were associated with slightly higher risks of *stroke* (risk ratio=1.24, 95% CI: 1.01, 1.53) and *death* (risk ratio=1.15, 95% CI: 1.08, 1.22) vs. SGAs [41c]. However, only 2.7% of the observed difference in overall *mortality risk* between FGAs and SGAs was attributable to *stroke*.

A nested, case–control analysis of 30-day *mortality* associated with antipsychotics in patients with ischemic stroke ($n=47225$) vs. controls ($n=37780$) found that antipsychotic use prior or after was associated with decreased *mortality rate* [42c].

A cohort study of patients initiated with oral/im olanzapine ($n=15774$), oral quetiapine ($n=18717$), and oral/im risperidone ($n=14134$) found that the crude rate of any *major cardiovascular event* was 5.3 per 1000 person-years for olanzapine, 3.4 for quetiapine, and 5.2 for risperidone [43c]. The risk of any *major cardiovascular event* was not significantly different for olanzapine or quetiapine vs. risperidone.

A case–control study ($n=1546$) examined patients with a first recorded *myocardial infarction* and antipsychotic [44c], found an association for FGAs (incidence rate ratio (IRR) 2.82, 95% CI: 2.0–3.9) and SGAs (IRR: 2.5, 95% CI: 1.18–5.32) for the first 30 days after first prescription.

Nervous System

A study compared iv chlorpromazine ($n=75$) to iv prochlorperazine ($n=274$) in the treatment of migraine in adolescents and young adults (12–21 years) [45c]. The most common AEs were *hypotension* with chlorpromazine and *akathisia* with prochlorperazine.

An analysis of drug safety data examined type and frequency of severe AEs for flupentixol vs. haloperidol, clozapine, olanzapine, quetiapine, risperidone and amisulpride ($n = 56861$) [46c]. For severe *EPS*, haloperidol (0.55%) and amisulpride (0.52%) were the most associated, flupentixol (0.27%) and risperidone (0.28%) were intermediate, and olanzapine/quetiapine (<0.1%) the least.

Endocrine

A 12-month, prospective study ($n = 163$) in FEP found *that bone mineral density* was significantly lower with antipsychotics vs. healthy controls and for FGAs (perphenazine, sulpiride, and chlorpromazine) vs. SGAs (clozapine, quetiapine, and aripiprazole) [47c]. *Prolactin levels* were significantly higher with FGAs vs. SGAs.

Metabolism

A randomised, open-label study compared aripiprazole, ziprasidone and quetiapine in medication-naïve, FEP ($n = 202$) [48c]. Mean *weight gain* was greatest with aripiprazole and this was significant vs. ziprasidone group. However, patients stayed on aripiprazole for significantly longer. Mean *prolactin levels* were significantly increased with quetiapine and ziprasidone, but not with aripiprazole. A significant increase in *total cholesterol* and *LDL-cholesterol* was seen with quetiapine and aripiprazole, and there was a significantly higher increase in *LDL-cholesterol* with quetiapine vs. ziprasidone.

A study of FEP ($n = 394$) found that antipsychotic treatment duration correlated significantly with higher *non-HDL-cholesterol, triglycerides,* and *triglycerides: HDL-total cholesterol ratio,* and lower *HDL-cholesterol* and *systolic blood pressure* [49c]. Olanzapine was significantly associated with higher *triglycerides* and *insulin levels,* and *insulin resistance,* while quetiapine was associated with significantly higher *triglycerides.*

A metabolomic profiling of patients with schizophrenia ($n = 60$) treated with high (clozapine, olanzapine), medium (quetiapine, risperidone), or low (ziprasidone, aripiprazole) risk for developing *metabolic syndrome* vs. healthy controls ($n = 20$) was conducted [50c]. *Insulin* and *TNF-α* were significantly higher and *adiponectin* was significantly decreased in patients at medium and high risk for *metabolic syndrome,* compared to controls. In the patient group *diacylglycerides, triacylglycerides* and *cholestenone* were increased and *α-Ketoglutarate* and *malate* were significantly decreased vs. controls.

A 6-month study of children and adolescents (4–17 years) on a SGA ($n = 279$) vs. Unmedicated controls ($n = 15$) found that olanzapine, quetiapine, and risperidone all increased *body weight* (olanzapine > risperidone > quetiapine) but had different *cardiometabolic side effect profiles* and different temporal side effect patterns [51c]. At 6 months, *fasting glucose, insulin, homeostasis model assessment of insulin resistance,* and *triglycerides* had increased

significantly with risperidone; *fasting glucose, total cholesterol,* and *LDL cholesterol* had increased significantly with olanzapine.

A study of children and adolescents FEP ($n = 36$) found a significant increase in *BMI, serum triglycerides* and *cholesterol* with SGAs (olanzapine, risperidone, quetiapine) treatment [52c]. Olanzapine and quetiapine were associated with a greater increase in *serum triglycerides.*

A multicentre, retrospective, administrative health data cohort study ($n = 725489$) [53c] found there was no significant difference between olanzapine and risperidone and the risk of *hyperglycemic* emergencies, but the risk was significantly lower with quetiapine vs. risperidone in the older patients.

A retrospective cohort study of children and youth (6–24 years) ($n = 28858$) vs. matched controls ($n = 14429$) found antipsychotics were associated with a threefold increased risk for *type 2 diabetes* (HR = 3.03 [95% CI = 1.73–5.32]), in the first year of follow-up [54c]. The risk increased with cumulative dose and remained elevated for up to 1 year following discontinuation (HR = 2.57 [95% CI = 1.34–4.91]). The risk was elevated in younger patients (6–17 years) (HR = 3.14 [95% CI = 1.50–6.56]), and for SGAs (HR = 2.89 [95% CI = 1.64–5.10]) including risperidone (HR = 2.20 [95% CI = 1.14–4.26]).

Post hoc analyses of data from 17 asenapine trials (13 schizophrenia; 4 bipolar mania) vs. placebo ($n = 1748$) and/or olanzapine ($n = 3430$) were conducted [55c]. Mean *weight gain* was significantly greater with asenapine vs. placebo but significantly less than with olanzapine. Mean changes for *triglycerides* and fasting *glucose* were significantly greater for asenapine vs. placebo but significantly lower than vs. olanzapine including also for *total* and *LDL-cholesterol.*

A cross-sectional study in adolescents (8–18 years) treated with quetiapine ($n = 16$) or risperidone ($n = 20$) found that quetiapine was associated with decreased *insulin secretion* compared with a neuroleptic-naïve group ($n = 18$) [56c].

A chart review ($n = 307$) investigated *metabolic* risk for clozapine vs. other antipsychotics [57c]. On all *metabolic* measures, there were no statistically significant differences for clozapine vs. other antipsychotics (mean *BMI,* 31 vs. 32; *type 2 diabetes,* 17% vs. 18%; *dyslipidemia,* 35% vs. 38%; *hypertension,* 32% vs. 39%; and *obesity,* 48% vs. 54%, all respectively).

Gastrointestinal

A retrospective chart review of cancer patients receiving oxycodone and treated with either prochlorperazine ($n = 50$) or perospirone ($n = 50$) found an increased incidence of *EPS* with prochlorperazine, particularly *akathisia* in the first week [58c].

Hematologic

A case of chronic and benign *neutropenia/agranulocytosis* associated with multiple non-clozapine antipsychotics (fluphenazine, olanzapine, flupenthixol, haloperidol, and paliperidone) is reported [59c].

Susceptibility Factors

A significant association was found between the incidence of *neurological AEs* and specific polymorphisms in genes (DRD2 and SCL6A4) in healthy volunteers given a single dose of risperidone (1 mg), olanzapine (5 mg) or quetiapine (25 mg) [60c].

A study of patients with schizophrenia switched to either aripiprazole or ziprasidone ($n=115$) reported significant associations with reduction in *BMI* at 6 months with polymorphisms of ADRA2A (rs1800544) and MTHFR (rs1801131) genes [61c].

A study of single-nucleotide polymorphisms in or near peroxisome proliferator-activated receptor gamma (PPARG) and adiponectin (ADIPOQ) genes ($n=216$) in patients receiving antipsychotics for up to 14 weeks found no association with *weight gain* [62c].

Data from a drug surveillance programme examined the frequency of antipsychotic AEs ($n=699$) with age [63c]. Logistic regression analyses showed a significantly negative relationship with age for *weight gain*, *EPS*, increased *liver enzymes* and *galactorrhoea*.

Toxicity

A retrospective case analysis ($n=106$) of SGA (clozapine, quetiapine, olanzapine, risperidone) intoxication in children (<6 years) reported *decreased alertness* as the most common symptom, followed by *miosis* and *tachycardia* [64c], with one case of *EPS* and no *deaths*.

Susceptibility Factors

A 3-month, controlled study examined patients with schizophrenia randomised to perazine, olanzapine or ziprasidone monotherapy and genotyped for polymorphisms of DRD2, DAT1, COMT, MAOA, SERT, 5HT2A, and GRIK3 [65c]. *Weight gain* was significantly greater with olanzapine and significantly less with ziprasidone. Perazine treatment was significantly associated with the greatest severity of *EPS*. No relationship of AEs to any of the polymorphisms was found.

A study ($n=25$) after 3–6 months of treatment with antipsychotic monotherapy (risperidone, paliperidone, clozapine, olanzapine) [66c] found that baseline weight and leptin levels were predictive of *weight gain* during follow-up, with an inverse association. Patients showed significant increases in *BMI* and *total cholesterol* and *apolipoprotein B* levels.

A case of a 16-year-old male with a history of dextromethorphan and pseudoephedrine abuse who developed *NMS* while on olanzapine (10 mg/day) and who received injections of levomepromazine (37.5 mg/day), and a single injection of haloperidol (2.5 mg) is reported [67A]. The patient was found to be homozygous for a non-functional CYP2D6*4 allele.

A study of olanzapine, clozapine, risperidone, paliperidone, quetiapine or amisulpride for 4 weeks ($n=341$) showed that carriers homozygous for the rs489693 A-allele had 2.2 times higher *weight gain* (+2.2 kg) than those with the CC-genotype (+1 kg) [68c].

A study of polymorphisms of protein kinase cAMP-dependent regulatory type II beta (PRKAR2B) gene in patients on olanzapine or clozapine ($n=99$) found that patients with the minor allele at rs9656135 vs. those without, had a mean *weight increase* of 4.1% compared with a *weight increase* of 3.4% (non-significant) [69c].

A study of polymorphisms of the methylenetetrahydrofolate reductase (MTHFR) gene found a significant association between C677T (rs1801133) and A1298C (rs1801131) polymorphisms with serum HDL-*cholesterol* levels [70c]. Although there was a trend for the 677-C allele to be associated with *weight gain* in the total, this was driven by the FEP in which those carrying the C-allele gained, on average, twice as much *weight*.

Drug–Drug Interactions

An increased risk of *AEs* in bipolar disorder was reported due to pharmacokinetic and pharmacodynamic drug–drug interactions between valproic acid in combination with quetiapine or olanzapine [71c].

Obsessive Compulsive Symptoms

The SGAs (amisulpride, aripiprazole, olanzapine, paliperidone, quetiapine and risperidone) have been implicated in cases of *pathological gambling*, *hypersexuality*, *compulsive eating* and *compulsive shopping* [72r]. A review of *obsessive compulsive symptoms* and SGAs found that the greatest risk was with clozapine, with 20–28% of patients experiencing *de novo* symptoms and 10–18% experiencing an exacerbation of pre-existing symptoms [73r]. Secondary *obsessive compulsive symptoms* were reported in 11–20% of olanzapine patients, but there were insufficient data for the other SGAs.

INDIVIDUAL DRUGS

Amisulpride [SEDA-32, 92; SEDA-33, 99; SEDA-34, 60; SEDA-35, 85; SEDA-36, 59]

Observational Studies

Full-dose amisulpride was compared to a combination of low-dose amisulpride and low-dose sulpiride in combination [74c]. There were no significant between-group differences and no patient had a *QTc interval* >500 ms; *prolactin levels* were increased particularly in females.

Controlled Studies

A randomised, double-blind, dose-finding study ($n = 215$) investigating amisulpride in postoperative nausea and vomiting (PONV) prophylaxis found no difference to placebo at all doses [75c]. There were no significant *CNS* or *cardiac* AEs.

Nervous System

Three cases of *akathisia*, acute *dystonia*, and drug-induced *Parkinsonism* with low doses of amisulpride are reported [76A].

Metabolic

A case series of violent patients on clozapine ($n = 5$) treated with adjunctive amisulpride reported no increase in metabolic parameters except for 1 patient who experienced an increase in *BMI* [77A].

Aripiprazole [SEDA-32, 93; SEDA-33, 99; SEDA-34, 60; SEDA-35, 96; SEDA-36, 59]

Controlled Studies

A randomised, placebo-controlled study of aripiprazole LAI in acute schizophrenia reported increased *weight, headache,* and *akathisia* vs. placebo [78C].

A 6-week, double-blind, randomised, parallel study ($n = 279$) compared aripiprazole to risperidone in Chinese patients with schizophrenia [79c]. The incidence of clinically significant *weight gain* and *hyperprolactinemia* was significantly less for aripiprazole compared with risperidone. The incidence of *EPS* was similar for both (25% aripiprazole; 24% risperidone).

Systematic Reviews

A Cochrane review compared aripiprazole with clozapine, quetiapine, risperidone, ziprasidone and olanzapine (174 studies, $n = 17\,244$) [80R]. Aripiprazole caused fewer *EPS* than risperidone, significantly more *weight gain* than ziprasidone but significantly less than olanzapine.

Reviews

A review of aripiprazole in children and adolescents with bipolar disorder reported lower rates of *sedation, weight gain, hyperprolactinemia, EPS* and *cardiac effects* than with other antipsychotic but more *sedation, gastrointestinal disturbance* and *EPS/akathisia* than placebo [81r].

A review of real-world data (21 studies) found that, compared with other SGAs aripiprazole, was either less likely to have an impact or had a comparable impact on *weight gain* and *dyslipidemia*; the degree of effect appeared to be dependent on study design [82r]. In addition, there was less risk of *diabetes mellitus* with aripiprazole compared with most other SGAs.

Observational Studies

A retrospective, disproportionality analysis extracted from the FDA Adverse Event Reporting System for Reports ($n = 2.7$ million) of *impulse control disorders (pathological gambling, hypersexuality, compulsive shopping)* reported an association for strong dopamine agonists and a signal for aripiprazole [83c].

In a study patients with schizophrenia were switched to aripiprazole LAI while continuing with oral supplementation with olanzapine ($n = 3$), quetiapine ($n = 28$), risperidone ($n = 24$) or ziprasidone ($n = 5$) for 0–15 days [84c]. Most AEs occurred in the first 8 days and included *injection-site pain* and *toothache* (each 6.7%), followed by *dystonia, fatigue, increased blood creatine phosphokinase, insomnia* and *restlessness* (each 5.0%).

A *post hoc* analysis evaluated adjunctive aripiprazole to either bupropion ($n = 47$) or SSRIs/SNRIs antidepressants ($n = 245$) in patients with MDD [85c]. The most common AEs were *fatigue* and *somnolence* with aripiprazole plus bupropion, and *fatigue* and *akathisia* with aripiprazole plus a SSRI/SNRI. Mean change in *body weight* at week 52 was greater for aripiprazole plus bupropion, but mean change from baseline in *fasting glucose* and *fasting total cholesterol abnormalities* were greater for aripiprazole plus a SSRI/SNRI.

Nervous System

A case of TD persisting over 2 years is reported in a 52-year-old neuroleptic-naive female with bipolar disorder who developed TD after 2 months of treatment (30 mg/day) [86A].

Psychiatric

In a cohort of pathological gamblers with schizophrenia or bipolar disorder comorbidities ($n = 166$) the use of aripiprazole was felt to be related to *pathological gambling* in 7 patients [87A].

Metabolism

A case of normalization of olanzapine-induced *elevations in triglyceride* and *cholesterol levels* and *liver transaminase enzymes* after switching to aripiprazole is reported [88A].

Endocrine

A case of *hypersexuality* in a male subject treated with aripiprazole is reported [89A]. A case of *prolonged penile erections* in an 11-year-old male with Apergers, ADHD and tic disorder and taking aripiprazole and atomoxetine is described [90A].

- Patient had previously been on atomoxetine and risperidone, but experienced *sedation* with the latter; aripiprazole was restarted without the atomoxetine with no recurrence.

Psychiatric

A case of *worsening of psychosis* with aripiprazole is reported in a 33-year-old female with history of alcohol abuse and psychosis [91A].

Gastro-Intestinal

A case of *hiccups* in a 29-year-old female switched from olanzapine to aripiprazole is reported [92A]. The *hiccups* resolved on discontinuation and resumed on rechallenge.

A case of *partial bowel obstruction* after aripiprazole addition to clozapine in a 25-year-old male is reported [93A].

- One week after the addition of aripiprazole to clozapine the patient presented with *partial bowel obstruction* which did not resolve until 2 weeks after the discontinuation of aripiprazole. The authors postulated that although aripiprazole is devoid of anticholinergic effects it does possess significant activity at 5-HT receptors including 5-HT3.

Drug–Drug Interactions

A case of *non-cardiogenic pulmonary edema* in a 35-year-old female on sertraline following the addition of aripiprazole was attributed to the inhibition of CYP2D6 by sertraline leading to increased exposure to aripiprazole [94A].

Asenapine [SEDA-37, 69]

Observational Studies

A 12-week, prospective study in older adults with bipolar disorder (≥60 years) with sub-optimal previous response ($n = 15$) reported that there was a high *discontinuation rate* due to AEs [95c]. The most common reported AEs were *gastrointestinal discomfort, restlessness, tremors, cognitive difficulties*, and *sluggishness*.

Metabolism

A retrospective analysis of *metabolic risk* found a significantly lower risk of *type 2 diabetes* with asenapine than compared with olanzapine (2.2% vs. 3.5%, respectively) and a significantly lower risk of developing *dyslipidemia* (2.8% vs. 6.8%, respectively) [96c].

A study of asenapine in patients with borderline personality disorder reported no serious AEs and there was significant *weight loss* [97c].

Skin

A case of a Pityriasis rosea-like drug reaction to asenapine is reported [98A].

Blonanserin

Systematic Reviews

A systematic review and meta-analysis (4 studies) found that blonanserin ($n = 1080$) produced less *weight gain* than risperidone but there were no differences in *metabolic parameters* or *QTc* between blonanserin and risperidone or haloperidol [99R].

Nervous System

Two cases of blonanserin improving *dystonia* induced by risperidone and olanzapine are reported [100A].

Chlorpromazine [SEDA-35, 85; SEDA-36, 59]

Observational Studies

In a study of iv chlorpromazine for status migrainosus ($n = 21$) [101A], one patient experienced *tachycardia, palpitation, flushing* and *hypertension*.

Systematic Reviews

A Cochrane review (55 studies) reported that chlorpromazine was associated with *sedation, acute movement disorder* (*Parkinsonism* but not akathisia), *hypotension, dizziness* and *weight gain* [102r].

Clozapine [SEDA-32, 94; SEDA-33, 102; SEDA-34, 6; SEDA-35, 99; SEDA-36, 59]

Observational Studies

A study of rapid ($n = 44$) vs. slow titration ($n = 23$) of clozapine in bipolar patients reported that 1 patient in each group discontinued due to *sedation* [103c]. In the rapid titration group there were discontinuations due to *hypotension* ($n = 1$) and *pneumonia* ($n = 1$).

A study of geriatric patients ($n = 48$) on clozapine for 1 month to 8 years found that 7 (12.5%) experienced *neutropenia* [104c]; 5 patients discontinued.

A 5-year cohort study modeled the effect of clozapine on *mortality* ($n = 14\,754$) in individuals with serious mental illness [105c]; there was a strong association between clozapine and lower *mortality* despite the presence of many confounding risk factors.

Clozapine ($n = 17$) was compared to non-clozapine antipsychotics ($n = 19$) in children (<13 years) with very early onset schizophrenia [106c]. AEs reported with clozapine included *transient moderate neutropenia* (12%), *mild neutropenia* (6%), *hyperlipidemia* (6%) and *tachycardia* (47%). There were no cases of *agranulocytosis* or *severe infection*. For the non-clozapine antipsychotics AEs included *hematological abnormalities* (11%) and *tachycardia* (5%).

A retrospective chart review study ($n = 320$) found that AEs accounted for 28% of clozapine discontinuations;

45% were due to *hematological AEs* and 35% were due to *CNS AEs* (*somnolence, seizures*) with 2 of 24 *deaths* due to *agranulocytosi*s and *constipation/aspiration* [107c].

Systematic Reviews

A systematic review of youth with early onset schizophrenia reported no *deaths* and a low *discontinuation rate* (3–6%) [108r]. The most common AEs were *sedation* and *hypersalivation* (>90%), followed by *enuresis, constipation, weight gain*, and *non-specific EEG changes* (10–60%), and *akathisia, tachycardia* and *changes in blood pressure* (10–30%). *Neutropenia* was usually transient (6–15%) but *agranulocytosis* was rare (<0.1%). *Seizures* were also uncommon (<3%). Emergent *diabetes* was infrequent (<6%) but *metabolic changes* were relatively common (8–22%).

A systematic review of *cardiomyopathy* associated with clozapine (28 articles) reported that symptoms developed a mean 14.4 months after initiation and included *heart failure, shortness of breath* (60%) and *palpitations* (36%), with echocardiography demonstrating *dilated cardiomyopathy* (39%) [109r].

Reviews

A review evaluated clozapine-induced *hypersalivation, constipation, tachycardia*, and *nocturnal enuresis* [110r].

Cardiovascular

A case of a 34-year-old male who developed *recurrent pulmonary thromboembolism* during 4 years of treatment with clozapine is reported [111A].

A case of *myocarditis* in a 42-year-old male approximately 3 weeks after starting clozapine is reported [112A]. Another case of successful and rapid rechallenge with clozapine after *myocarditis* in patient with treatment resistant schizophrenia is reported [113A].

A case of *cardiomyopathy* in 20-year-old male is reported [114A].

- The patient developed a *fever* after 9 days and *dyspnea, sinus tachycardia* and *hypotension* after 18 days. Cardiac ultrasound showed *left ventricular hypokinesia*, and *decreased ejection fraction* with improvement within 4 days of discontinuing clozapine and steroid treatment.

Nervous System

A study of patients with treatment resistant schizophrenia (*n* = 26) found that 38.5% developed *EEG abnormalities* and 23.1% went on to experience *seizures* [115c].

A case of a 26-year-old female who experienced *seizures* on clozapine despite dose reduction (300 mg from 450 mg) and who was subsequently successfully treated with ECT is reported [116A].

A study of polymorphisms of CYP1A2 (*1C and *1F) in patients with schizophrenia (*n* = 108) found the *1F/ *1F genotype to be significantly associated with *seizures*,

but there was no relationship with combinations of *1F and *1C alleles [117c].

Psychiatric

A case of clozapine-induced *obsessive–compulsive symptoms* in a patient with bipolar disorder is reported [118A].

Metabolism

A study of the long-term risk of *metabolic disturbance* found no statistically significant differences between clozapine (*n* = 96) and non-clozapine (*n* = 211) groups (mean *BMI* body mass, 31 vs. 32; *diabetes type 2*, 17% vs. 18%; *dyslipidemia*, 35% vs. 38%; *hypertension*, 32% vs. 39%; and *obesity*, 48% vs. 54%) [119c].

A case of *elevated triglycerides* is reported with clozapine [120A].

Hematologic

A retrospective, chart review study (*n* = 147) found an increased incidence of *blood dyscrasias* in Saudi Arabs including *agranulocytosis, neutropenia* and *leukopenia* (10.9%), *lymphocytopenia, thrombocytopenia*, and *eosinophilia*, especially in the first 18 weeks of treatment [121c].

A study reported that in Australia (1993–2011) there were 141 recorded cases of *agranulocytosis* and four *deaths* attributable to clozapine [122c].

A case of late-onset (>6 months) *agranulocytosis* in a patient with comorbid multiple sclerosis successfully treated with granulocyte stimulating factor (GSF) is reported [123A]. A case of successful treatment of *neutropenia* with GSF of a 53-year-old male with chronic lymphocytic lymphoma on chemotherapy is reported [124A]. A case of successful treatment with GSF of a *low white cell count* in a 46-year-old male with B-cell lymphoma on chemotherapy is reported [125A]. A case of unsuccessful treatment of *agranulocytosis* with GSF after clozapine rechallenge is reported [126A].

A study of genome-wide genotyping and whole-exome sequencing (*n* = 163) found two loci of the major histocompatibility complex (126Q in HLA-DQB1 and 158T HLA-B) were independently associated with clozapine-induced *agranulocytosis* [127c]. A case of *pancytopenia* reported in a 57-year-old malnourished male was detected on hospitalisation (no blood monitoring in previous year) and improved after discontinuation of clozapine and treatment with ECT [128A].

A case of pure *red cell aplasia* is reported [129A].

Salivary Glands

A study of clozapine-induced *sialorrhea* (*n* = 45) found a significant association with a 120 base-pairs tandem duplication polymorphism in the dopamine receptor subtype D4 (DRD4) gene [130c]. Another study (*n* = 237) found a polymorphism in the adrenoceptor alpha 2A gene (ADRA2A) to be associated with *sialorrhea* [131c].

A case of a 46-year-old male who developed severe *sialorrhea* at a dose of 400 mg/day of clozapine successfully treated with hyoscine hydrobromide and sublingual atropine solution is reported [132A]. A case of *recurrent parotid swelling* in a 35-year-old female with clozapine leading to discontinuation is reported [133A].

Gastrointestinal

Death due to *ischemic colitis* is reported in a 28-year-old male after 3 months treatment with clozapine [134A]. A case of 46-year-old male on clozapine who developed *perforation* of the *large intestine* and *partial embolism* of the *pulmonary artery* is reported [135A].

A case of clozapine-induced *severe constipation* leading to pneumonia with a subsequent *respiratory arrest* is reported [136A]. A case of clozapine-induced *constipation* responding to treatment with bethanechol is reported [137A]. A case is reported of a 53-year-old male with a history of *small bowel obstruction* secondary to clozapine who was successfully treated with lubiprostone and able to continue clozapine [138A].

A case of *severe sudden haematemesis* requiring transfusion is reported in a 46-year-old male after treatment with clozapine for 6 weeks [139A].

Hepatitis is reported in a 48-year-old woman due to clozapine *toxicity* at a dose of 325 mg/day (clozapine level 5019 nmol/L) after 28 days treatment but with full recovery after discontinuation [140A]. A case of *acute liver injury* with *elevated liver function tests* and *pleural effusion* is reported in a 47-year-old female 30 days after clozapine initiation, and resolving after discontinuation [141A]. Another case of a 21-year-old male who developed *fulminant liver toxicity* after 3 weeks treatment with clozapine is reported [142A].

Musculoskeletal

A case of *burning bone pain* is reported in a 43-year-old male which developed after several months of treatment with clozapine, stopped on cessation and returned on rechallenge [143A].

Sexual

A case of *priapism* in a 30-year-old male is reported [144A].

- The patient had been treated with clozapine for 12 years. He experienced *priapism* requiring surgical intervention on two occasions before responding to prophylactic goserline acetate injections.

Body Temperature

A case of a 22-year-old male treated with clozapine, who developed a *fever* (up to 40.1 °C) after 14 days treatment, is reported [145A].

Susceptibility Factors

A case series ($n = 3$) of clozapine *toxicity* as a result of an infectious or inflammatory process (possibly through cytokine-mediated inhibition of cytochrome P450 1A2) is reported [146A]. A case of 62-year-old male who experienced *life-threatening toxicity* on clozapine attribute to a respiratory infection impairing CYP1A2 function is described [147A].

Drug Overdose

A case of extended *coma* (70 hours) due to clozapine intoxication is reported [148A].

Cyamemazine

Gastrointestinal

A case of *gastric dilatation* in a 76-year-old male treated for several years with cyamemazine is reported [149A].

Droperidol [SEDA-36, 59]

Cardiovascular

A prospective study of patients with aggression ($n = 46$) treated with droperidol found *abnormal QT* measurements in 4 patients who received doses of 10–20 mg (with concomitant medications); no patient given >30 mg had *QT prolongation* and there were no *arrhythmias* [150c].

Nervous System

A case of *NMS* is reported in a 75-year-old male who received epidural droperidol post surgery [151A]. Two cases of *acute EPS* misdiagnosed as psychiatric disorders after droperidol administration for PONV are reported [152A].

- An *acute dystonic reaction* in a 23-year-old female with agitation, *difficulty speaking and moving her limbs* and *eyes* was diagnosed with a seizure.
- *Akathisia* in a 39-year-old female who complained of *inner tension, anxiety and motor restlessness* was diagnosed with an anxiety disorder.

Flupenthixol

Observational Studies

An analysis of a drug safety program ($n = 56861$) [153c] found that flupenthixol ranked the lowest for *SAEs* overall; for *severe EPS* it was comparable to risperidone, but less than haloperidol or amisulpride and more than olanzapine or quetiapine.

Systematic Reviews

A Cochrane review (1 study) reported that flupenthixol was associated with more *dizziness, dystonia, unsteady gait, decreased facial expression, rigidity,* and *tremor* but less *dry mouth* than chlorpromazine [154R].

Fluphenazine

Systematic Reviews

A Cochrane review (7 studies) reported that fluphenazine was associated with more *akathisia* and *rigidity* than placebo [155R].

Haloperidol [SEDA-35, 107; SEDA-36, 59]

Sytematic Reviews

A Cochrane review (25 studies) reported that haloperidol was associated with *Parkinsonism, akathisia,* and *acute dystonia* [156R]. Another Cochrane review (19 studies) reported lower doses of haloperidol (>3 to 7.5 mg/day) had a lower rate of *EPS* than higher doses [157R].

Nervous System

Two cases of *EPS* with haloperidol for agitated delirium are reported, with resolution after switch to high-dose chlorpromazine and high-dose olanzapine; but both agents were more *sedative* than haloperidol [158A].

Iloperidone [SEDA-33, 103; SEDA-35, 109; SEDA-36, 59]

Reviews

A review of iloperidone (121 articles) reported *lower EPS* and *akathisia* rates compared to haloperidol and risperidone [159]. *Clinically significant weight gain* was comparable to risperidone (12.9% vs. 11.9%) with most *weight gain* occurring after initiation. *QTc prolongation* was comparable to ziprasidone at 10 ms and increased in the presence of CYP2D6 and 3A4 inhibitors. *Orthostatic hypotension* (13%) with statistically significant *BP changes* occurred primarily in the first week of treatment and more than with ziprasidone (2%).

Sexual Function

A case of *refractory priapism* in a 42-year-old male 24 hours after the addition of iloperidone to lithium and paroxetine is reported [160A].

Levomepromazine (Methotrimeprazine) [SEDA-36, 59]

Observational Studies

A study in children and infants ($n=18$) for palliative symptom relief reported *sedation* as the only AE [161c].

Levosulpiride

Cardiovascular

A case of an 89-year-old female on citalopram who developed *polymorphic ventricular tachycardia* secondary to *QT prolongation* (650 ms) after the addition of levosulpiride is reported [162A].

Loxapine [SEDA-35,108; SEDA-36, 59]

Controlled Studies

A randomised, placebo-controlled, double-blind crossover study ($n=48$) found no effect of inhaled loxapine on *QT* [163c].

Lurasidone

Controlled Studies

A randomised, double-blind, placebo controlled study of add-on lurasidone to lithium or valproate in bipolar depression was conducted [164C]. The most frequent AEs were *nausea, somnolence, tremor, akathisia,* and *insomnia*. There were minimal changes in weight, lipids, and glucose; the *discontinuation* rate due to AEs was 6.0% for lurasidone and 7.9% for placebo.

Observational Studies

The most common AEs in a 6-month, open-label, flexible-dose, extension study ($n=148$) were *insomnia* (8.8%), *nausea* (18.8%), *akathisia* (8.1%), and *anxiety* (6.1%); 10.8% of patients discontinued due to an AE [165c].

Reviews

A *post-hoc* analysis of data from two, 6-week multicenter, randomised, double-blind, placebo-controlled, studies found the most frequently occurring AEs were *nausea, akathisia,* and *somnolence* [166c]. The Number Needed to Harm (NNH) for lurasidone vs. placebo ranged from 11 (*nausea* with lurasidone monotherapy) to 130 (*somnolence* with lurasidone monotherapy). Lurasidone was not associated with any clinically meaningful mean *weight* or *metabolic changes* compared to placebo; NNH vs. placebo for *weight gain* ≥7% was 29–5550 for monotherapy, and 42 for add-on lurasidone.

Olanzapine [SEDA-32, 99; SEDA-33, 104; SEDA-34, 66; SEDA-35, 108; SEDA-36, 59]

Controlled Studies

An 8-week, randomised, double-blind, placebo-controlled study ($n = 68$) found that mean *weight* and *total cholesterol, triglyceride,* and *LDL-cholesterol levels* increased significantly with olanzapine [167C]. Another 6-week, randomised, double-blind, placebo-controlled study followed by open-label olanzapine (≤48 weeks) in Japanese patients ($n = 165$) found the most common AE was *weight increase* (47.9%) [168C]. Significant increases were seen in *weight, fasting glucose, total cholesterol,* and *triglycerides.*

Observational Studies

A retrospective case study ($n = 91$) of high-dose olanzapine (45–160 mg/day) reported *EPS* (27%), *sedation* (25%), *weight gain* (14%), *hypotension* (2%), and *QTc prolongation* (1%) [169c]. Five patients died and 2 *deaths* possibly related to olanzapine.

A study of olanzapine pamoate in the management of violent male patients ($n = 8$) reported an increase in *BMI* ($n = 2$) and an *increase in glucose* ($n = 2$) [170c].

A study of olanzapine and chemotherapy ($n = 46$) reported mild AEs that included *dizziness, fatigue,* and *dyspepsia* [171c].

The addition of low-dose olanzapine to duloxetine and ($n = 103$) compared with duloxetine alone ($n = 165$) was found to reduce *nausea* and *vomiting* [172c].

A 10-week study of olanzapine in combination with atomoxetine in children and adolescents ($n = 11$) reported significant *weight gain* (mean = 3.9 kg) [173c].

Systematic Reviews

A systematic review and meta-analysis (47 studies, $n = 387$) in children (0.6–18 years) [174R] reported *weight gain* (78%), *sedation* (48%), *EPS* (9%), *electrocardiogram abnormalities* (14%), *elevation in liver function tests* (7%) and *blood glucose abnormalities* (4%); there were no *deaths* attributed to olanzapine.

Reviews

A drug safety evaluation of olanzapine and fluoxetine examined *weight gain* and *metabolic symptoms* [175R].

Nervous System

A 3-year study found that the short-term incidence of *EPS* was 5.6% during treatment with olanzapine LAI (45–405 mg every 2–4 weeks) and 5.0% with oral olanzapine (5–20 mg/day) [176c]. The incidences of *akathisia* (2.6% LAI, 1.2% oral) and *Parkinsonism* (1.8% LAI, 3.7% oral) were overall similar. The long-term incidence of *EPS* was 9.2% for olanzapine LAI.

A case report of a 22-year-old male who developed *tardive dystonia* after 12 months treatment is reported [177A]. Another case of *tardive dystonia* in a 21-year-old female after 6 months treatment is reported [178A].

- The patient had shown movement disorder with other antipsychotics including trifluoperazine.

A case of *NMS* after the addition of the valproate in a 60-year-old female on olanzapine for 2 years is reported [179A].

Psychiatric

A case of a 46-year-old male with schizoaffective disorder treated with olanzapine 20 mg/day who experienced an *exacerbation of psychosis* is reported [180A].

Metabolism

A study of a weight management program ($n = 100$) found no effect on *weight* but there was a significantly smaller increase in *waist circumference* and impact on *glucose dysregulation* after 48 weeks [181c].

A case of *rapid weight gain* with *metabolic disruption* including *hypertriglyceridemia* in a 33-year-old male is reported [182A].

- *Weight gain* (6 kg) and elevations of *triglycerides, total cholesterol, non-HDL-cholesterol, glucose,* and *liver function* tests were observed after 1 week.

A case of *hypoglycemia* in a patient with anorexia is reported [183A].

Fluid Balance

A case of *hyponatremia* in a patient with autism is reported [184A].

Gastrointestinal

A case of *acute necrotizing pancreatitis* with olanzapine is reported [185A].

Susceptibility Factors

A study found that patients with SULT4A1-1-positive status experienced significantly less *weight gain* [186c].

Toxicity

A case of a male in his twenties on olanzapine who died of *hyponatremia* associated with *water intoxication* and high serum levels of olanzapine (610 ng/mL) is reported [187].

Two cases of *postinjection delirium/sedation syndrome* are reported [188A], including a 46-year-old male 4 hours post injection [189A].

Paliperidone [SED-33, 108, SEDA-35, 85; SEDA-36, 59]

Controlled Studies

A 24-month, double-blind, randomised, controlled study [190c] found paliperidone LAI patients had greater *weight gain* and *prolactin elevation* but *lower akathisia* than haloperidol LAI.

Observational Studies

A 12-month, open-label study in FEP ($n=80$) [191c] found the most common AEs were *insomnia* (17.9%), *nausea* (8.3%), *akathisia* (4.8%), *anxiety* (4.8%) and *depression* (4.8%). *Body weight* at endpoint was significantly higher compared with baseline.

A 12-week, open-label switch study ($n=17$) from risperidone to paliperidone ER in elderly patients with schizophrenia found a reduction in *movement disorder* [192c].

A 1-year follow-up study ($n=210$) reported that 5% discontinued due to AEs that included *sexual dysfunction* ($n=7$), *EPS* ($n=2$) and *TD* ($n=1$) [193c].

Cardiovascular

Two cases of *pulmonary thromboembolism* attributed to paliperidone are reported [194A].

- A 28-year-old neuroleptic-naïve male on paliperidone for 8 weeks developed a *PE*; after treatment with anticoagulants he continued with paliperidone for a further 6 months with no recurrence.
- A 40-year-old male smoker switched from risperidone to paliperidone developed a *PE* after 4 days; after treatment with anticoagulants he continued with paliperidone for a further 3 years with no recurrence.

Nervous System

A case of *motor tics* in a 30-year-old male on paliperidone ER (15 mg/day) is reported [195A].

Metabolic

A case of better *appetite control* and lower risk of *weight gain* in a patient switched from risperidone is reported [196A].

Gastrointestinal

A study of paliperidone ER in patients with hepatic disease did not show any significant change in *liver function* [197A].

Perazine [SEDA-36, 59]

Systematic Reviews

A Cochrane review (7 studies, $n=479$) of perazine reported that compared with zotepine and amisulpride there was no greater risk of *akathisia, dyskinesia, parkinsonism* or *tremor* [198R].

Pericyazine

Systematic Reviews

A Cochrane review (5 studies) reported a higher incidence of *EPS* compared to other FGAs and SGAs [199R].

Perospirone [SEDA-36, 59]

Systematic Reviews

A systematic review and meta-analysis (5 studies) found that perospirone ($n=256$) had lower *EPS* scores compared to pooled antipsychotics (olanzapine, quetiapine, risperidone, aripiprazole, haloperidol, mosapramine) [200R].

Nervous System

Two cases of *serotonin toxicity*, in a 64-year-old woman, and an 81-year-old woman, both on perospirone and Paroxetine, are reported [201A].

Perphenazine [SEDA-32, 104; SEDA-35, 85; SEDA-36, 59]

Observational Studies

A retrospective case study of patients treated with perphenazine for PONV ($n=45766$) reported 5 cases of *akathisia* and 1 *dystonic reaction* [202c].

Systematic Reviews

A Cochrane review (4 studies, $n=365$) found that perphenazine was more likely to cause *akathisia* and less likely to cause severe *toxicity* than other low-potency FGAs [203R].

Prochlorperazine [SEDA-35, 85; SEDA-36, 59]

Susceptibility Factors

A study of cancer patients on oxycodone and prochlorperazine found that a genetic polymorphism (OPRM1 A118G) and female sex increased *prolactin levels* [204c]. Similarly, the presence of DRD2 TaqIA and female sex was associated with increased *nausea*.

Quetiapine [SEDA-32, 104; SEDA-33, 110; SEDA-34, 69; SEDA-35, 85; SEDA-36, 59]

Observational Studies

A study of quetiapine (150–300 mg) in patients ($n=111$) with borderline personality disorder found that the risk of *sedation, change in appetite,* and *dry mouth* were elevated for the 300 mg dose vs. placebo, while for the 150 mg dose only risk of *dry mouth* was elevated [205c].

The 300 mg dose was associated with a significant increase in *heart rate* while the 150 mg dose was associated with a *significant decrease in BP*. In contrast, a study of quetiapine XR (300–600 mg) in acute bipolar depression ($n = 21$) found that there was a significant increase in *hypotension* with the higher dose [206c].

A study of quetiapine as add-on therapy in bipolar patients with concurrent alcohol dependence ($n = 90$) found a significant increase in *weight* and *akathisia* scores at 6 but not 12 weeks [207c].

A study of quetiapine in cannabis dependence ($n = 15$) found that the most common AEs reported were *fatigue* and *somnolence* [208c].

A study of quetiapine XR ($n = 45$) vs. amitriptyline ($n = 45$) in the treatment of fibromyalgia found that the *discontinuation rate* due to AEs was greater with quetiapine XR [209c].

Systematic Reviews

A Cochrane review found that compared with olanzapine, quetiapine induced slightly fewer *movement disorders*, less *weight gain* and *glucose elevation*, but increased *QTc prolongation* [210R]; compared with risperidone, quetiapine induced slightly fewer *movement disorders* and less *prolactin* increase but greater *cholesterol* increase; compared with paliperidone, quetiapine induced less *EPS* and less *prolactin* increase and *weight gain*; and compared with ziprasidone, quetiapine induced slightly less *EPS* and less *prolactin* increase, but more *sedation* and *weight gain* and *cholesterol* increase.

Nervous System

A case of *TD* is reported in a female (age not recorded) after 2 years of treatment with quetiapine and duloxetine [211A].

A case of a 35-year-old male with schizoaffective disorder who developed paradoxical agitation after the addition of quetiapine is reported [212A]

* Within 48 hours of the addition of quetiapine (to long-term zuclopenthixol and lithium) the patient presented with severe *agitation* which recurred after a further trial.

Gastrointestinal

A case of a 58-year-old male who developed *pancreatitis* after 10 years treatment with quetiapine is reported [213A].

Risperidone [SEDA-32, 107; SEDA-33, 111; SEDA-34, 70; SEDA-35, 85; SEDA-36, 59]

Cardiovascular

In a study of patients ($n = 21$) switched from olanzapine to risperidone there was a significant decrease in *PR interval* [214c]. In female, but not male patients, the *QTc interval* was significantly decreased.

Nervous System

A case of *Pisa syndrome* in a 31-year-old male with multiple sclerosis on risperidone resolved with lurasidone and recurred with chlorpromazine [215].

Endocrine

A case of premature thelarche in an 8-year-old female is reported [216A].

Susceptibility Factors

A genotyping study of healthy volunteers ($n = 70$) treated with risperidone found that both female sex and specific polymorphisms were associated with increased incidence of certain AEs; AGTR1 and NAT2 with *headache* and CYP2C19 with *neurological* AEs [217c]. Risperidone increased *prolactin* levels (iAUC and iCmax), which were higher in women than in men. The most common AEs were *somnolence* (47.1%), *headache* (21.4%), and *dizziness* (17.1%). Another study of CYP2D6, ABCB1 C3435T and G2677T/A genotypes in patients with schizophrenia ($n = 66$) found that *QTc* was significantly longer with ABCB1 3435CT + 3435TT than with 3435CC genotypes [218c]. Multiple regression analysis showed that C/T or T/T genotypes at the ABCB1 C3435T locus as well as lower weight and older age contributed to *QTc prolongation*.

Sertindole [SEDA-32, 110; SEDA-33, 114; SEDA-34, 73; SEDA-35, 85; SEDA-36,59]

Reviews

A review of the literature reported that, although generally well tolerated, sertindole is associated with a dose-related *QT prolongation* [219r].

Sulpiride [SEDA-35,115; SEDA-36]

Observational Studies

A prescription database study ($n = 5750$) found that sulpiride was associated with *EPS* and *hyperprolactinemia* [220c].

Ziprasidone [SEDA-32, 111; SEDA-33, 114; SEDA-34, 74; SEDA-35, 85; SEDA-36, 59]

Controlled Studies

A 6-week, double-blind, randomised, placebo-controlled study of ziprasidone added to clozapine schizophrenia ($n = 40$) [221C] found the most common AEs included *gastrointestinal symptoms, headache*, and dizziness; *QTc prolongation* from baseline was significant within-group but not vs. placebo.

An 8-week, randomised, double-blind, placebo-controlled, parallel group study of ziprasidone in bipolar and an anxiety disorder ($n = 49$) found a high *discontinuation rate* due to AEs and an increase in *movement disorder* [222C].

A 4 week, randomised, double-blind, placebo-controlled study followed by a 26 week open-label extension phase in children and adolescents (10–17 years) with bipolar I disorder found the most common AEs for ziprasidone (randomised phase) were *sedation* (32.9%), *somnolence* (24.8%), *headache* (22.1%), *fatigue* (15.4%), and *nausea* (14.1%); one subject had a *QTcF* $\geq$460 ms [223C]. The most common AEs in the extension phase were *sedation* (26.5%), *somnolence* (23.5%), *headache* (22.2%), and *insomnia* (13.6%).

Ziprasidone was studied with schizophrenia in A 6 week, randomised, double-blind, placebo-controlled study followed by a 26 week open-label extension phase in children and adolescents (13–17 years) [224C]. The most common AEs during the randomised phase were *somnolence* and *EPS*. The most common AEs during the open-label phase were *somnolence*. No subjects had a *QTcF* $\geq$500 ms in any phase. There was one *suicide* attributed to poor symptom control.

An 8-week, placebo-controlled, fixed-dose escalation trial compared ziprasidone 160 mg/day with 320 mg/day in patients with schizophrenia or schizoaffective disorder for 3 weeks ($n = 75$) [225C]. While the rate of AEs was not different between the groups, there was a correlation between ziprasidone serum concentration and *more negative symptoms*, i.e., *decreased diastolic BP* and *QTc*.

Observational Studies

In a 24-week, open-label study patients ($n = 213$) treated with clozapine for $\geq$2 years were switched to ziprasidone or the combination [226c]. *Triglyceride* levels for ziprasidone were significantly lower than baseline and compared with the combination group by week 4. *BMI* and *triglyceride* levels for ziprasidone and combination group were significantly lower than the baseline by week 24. *HDL-cholesterol* was significantly lower for the combination than ziprasidone.

Cardiovascular

A case of 23-year-old Chinese male who experienced a *QTc prolongation* of 83 ms after receiving 20 mg ziprasidone im is reported [227A, r]. A systematic review of ziprasidone im (19 trials, $n = 1428$) found a mean *QTc change* from baseline of -3.7 to 12.8 ms, but no significant differences between ziprasidone and haloperidol im [227A, r].

A case of transient, asymptomatic, fluctuating *bradycardia* is reported in an 80-year-old female with a history of hypertension, diabetes and schizophrenia [228A].

Nervous System

The addition of ziprasidone to tramadol in a 67-year-old male with Parkinson's disease and bipolar disorder resulted in the development of a *serotonin syndrome* [229A].

A case of a 28-year-old male who developed severe *EPS* (*dystonia, akathisia, parkinsonism*) on ziprasidone 80 mg/day with sertraline 25 mg/day is described [230A].

Metabolism

A 8-week, prospective, open-label study of patients with bipolar I disorder switched from olanzapine to ziprasidone demonstrated a statistically significant reduction in *weight, BMI, fasting triglycerides and total cholesterol* [231C].

Allergic

Drug hypersensitivity syndrome (DHS) has been described with ziprasidone [232A].

- A 33-year-old female with bipolar disorder initiated on lithium and ziprasidone developed a *pruritic rash, pyrexia* and *elevated LDH, ESR* and *CRP* initially attributed to the lithium, but rechallenge with ziprasidone resulted in a recurrence.

Zotepine [SEDA-33, 114; SEDA-35,116; SEDA-36, 59]

Observational Studies

A 12-week, prospective, randomised, rater-blinded study investigated switching from clozapine to zotepine ($n = 59$) [233c]. There was an increase in AEs including *EPS* (and increased use of propanolol and anticholinergics) and *prolactin* as well as *psychotic symptoms*.

Acknowledgements

The authors thank Sam Joshva for his editorial assistance.

References

[1] Crespo-Facorro B, Ortiz-García de la Foz V, Mata I, et al. Aripiprazole, ziprasidone and quetiapine in the treatment of first-episode nonaffective psychosis: a 12-week randomized, flexible-dose, open-label trial. Schizophr Res. 2013;147(2–3):375–82 [C].

[2] Rezayat AA, Hebrani P, Behdani F, et al. Comparison of the effectiveness of aripiprazole and risperidone for the treatment of acute bipolar mania. J Res Med Sci. 2014;19(8):733–8 [C].

[3] Schnell T, Koethe D, Krasnianski A, et al. Ziprasidone versus clozapine in the treatment of dually diagnosed (DD) patients with schizophrenia and cannabis use disorders: a randomised study. Am J Addict. 2014;23(3):308–12 [C].

[4] Ghanizadeh A, Haghighi A. Aripiprazole versus risperidone for treating children and adolescents with tic disorder: a randomized double blind clinical trial. Child Psychiatry Hum Dev. 2014;45(5):596–603 [C].

[5] de Araújo AA, de Araújo Dantas D, do Nascimento GG, et al. Quality of life in patients with schizophrenia: the impact of socio-economic factors and adverse effects of atypical antipsychotics drugs. Psychiatr Q. 2014;85(3):357–67 [C].

[6] Francesco F, Cervone A. Metabolic alterations associated with first and second generation antipsychotics: a twenty-years open study. Psychiatr Danub. 2014;26(Suppl 1):184–7 [C].

[7] Lucca JM, Madhan R, Parthasarathi G, et al. Identification and management of adverse effects of antipsychotics in a tertiary care teaching hospital. J Res Pharm Pract. 2014;3(2):46–50 [c].

[8] Hatta K, Kishi Y, Wada K, et al. Antipsychotics for delirium in the general hospital setting in consecutive 2453 inpatients: a prospective observational study. Int J Geriatr Psychiatry. 2014;29(3):253–62 [c].

[9] Stentebjerg-Olesen M, Jeppesen P, Pagsberg AK, et al. Early nonresponse determined by the clinical global impressions scale predicts poorer outcomes in youth with schizophrenia spectrum disorders naturalistically treated with second-generation antipsychotics. J Child Adolesc Psychopharmacol. 2013;23(10):665–75 [c].

[10] Noguera A, Ballesta P, Baeza I, et al. Twenty-four months of antipsychotic treatment in children and adolescents with first psychotic episode: discontinuation and tolerability. J Clin Psychopharmacol. 2013;33(4):463–71 [c].

[11] Meli M, Rauber-Lüthy C, Hoffmann-Walbeck P, et al. Atypical antipsychotic poisoning in young children: a multicentre analysis of poisons centres data. Eur J Pediatr. 2014;173(6):743–50 [c].

[12] Cipriani A, Accordini S, Nosè M, et al. Aripiprazole versus haloperidol in combination with clozapine for treatment-resistant schizophrenia: a 12-month, randomized, naturalistic trial. J Clin Psychopharmacol. 2013;33(4):533–7 [c].

[13] Macht M, Mull AC, McVaney KE, et al. Comparison of droperidol and haloperidol for use by paramedics: assessment of safety and effectiveness. Prehosp Emerg Care J. 2014;18(3):375–80 [c].

[14] Calver L, Drinkwater V, Isbister GK. A prospective study of high dose sedation for rapid tranquilisation of acute behavioural disturbance in an acute mental health unit. BMC Psychiatry. 2013;13:225 [c].

[15] Suzuki H, Gen K, Takahashi Y. A naturalistic comparison study of the efficacy and safety of intramuscular olanzapine, intramuscular haloperidol, and intramuscular levomepromazine in acute agitated patients with schizophrenia. Hum Psychopharmacol. 2014;29(1):83–8 [c].

[16] Boettger S, Jenewein J, Breitbart W. Haloperidol, risperidone, olanzapine and aripiprazole in the management of delirium: a comparison of efficacy, safety, and side effects. Palliat Support Care. 2014;13(4):1079–85 [c].

[17] Heilbronn C, Lloyd B, McElwee P, et al. Trends in quetiapine use and non-fatal quetiapine-related ambulance attendances. Drug Alcohol Rev. 2013;32(4):405–11 [c].

[18] Buoli M, Serati M, Altamura AC. Is the combination of a mood stabilizer plus an antipsychotic more effective than mono-therapies in long-term treatment of bipolar disorder? A systematic review. J Affect Disord. 2014;152–154:12–8 [R].

[19] Kumar A, Datta SS, Wright SD, et al. Atypical antipsychotics for psychosis in adolescents. Cochrane Database Syst Rev. 2013;10: CD009582 [r].

[20] Datta SS, Kumar A, Wright SD, et al. Evidence base for using atypical antipsychotics for psychosis in adolescents. Schizophr Bull. 2014;40(2):252–4 [r].

[21] Bak M, Fransen A, Janssen J, et al. Almost all antipsychotics result in weight gain: a meta-analysis. PLoS One. 2014;9(4): e94112 [R].

[22] Leucht S, Cipriani A, Spineli L, et al. Comparative efficacy and tolerability of 15 antipsychotic drugs in schizophrenia: a multiple-treatments meta-analysis. Lancet. 2013;382(9896):951–62 [R].

[23] Wen XJ, Wang LM, Liu ZL, et al. Meta-analysis on the efficacy and tolerability of the augmentation of antidepressants with atypical antipsychotics in patients with major depressive disorder. Braz J Med Biol Res. 2014;47(7):605–16 [R].

[24] Peuskens J, Pani L, Detraux J, et al. The effects of novel and newly approved antipsychotics on serum prolactin levels: a comprehensive review. CNS Drugs. 2014;28(5):421–53 [r].

[25] Besnard I, Auclair V, Callery G, et al. Antipsychotic-drug-induced hyperprolactinemia: physiopathology, clinical features and guidance. Encéphale. 2014;40(1):86–94 [r].

[26] Parikh T, Goyal D, Scarff JR, et al. Antipsychotic drugs and safety concerns for breast-feeding infants. South Med J. 2014;107(11):686–8 [r].

[27] Zhang JP, Gallego JA, Robinson DG, et al. Efficacy and safety of individual second-generation vs. first-generation antipsychotics in first-episode psychosis: a systematic review and meta-analysis. Int J Neuropsychopharmacol. 2013;16(6):1205–18 [R].

[28] Kishi T, Sevy S, Chekuri R, et al. Antipsychotics for primary alcohol dependence: a systematic review and meta-analysis of placebo-controlled trials. J Clin Psychiatry. 2013;74(7): e642–e654 [R].

[29] Citrome L. A review of the pharmacology, efficacy and tolerability of recently approved and upcoming oral antipsychotics: an evidence-based medicine approach. CNS Drugs. 2013;27(11):879–911 [R].

[30] Bosanac P, Hollander Y, Castle D. The comparative efficacy of intramuscular antipsychotics for the management of acute agitation. Australas Psychiatry. 2013;21(6):554–62 [R].

[31] Politte LC, McDougle CJ. Atypical antipsychotics in the treatment of children and adolescents with pervasive developmental disorders. Psychopharmacology (Berl). 2014;231(6):1023–36 [r].

[32] Sochocky N, Milin R. Second generation antipsychotics in Asperger's Disorder and high functioning autism: a systematic review of the literature and effectiveness of meta-analysis. Curr Clin Pharmacol. 2013;8(4):370–9 [R].

[33] Martínez-Ortega JM, Funes-Godoy S, Díaz-Atienza F, et al. Weight gain and increase of body mass index among children and adolescents treated with antipsychotics: a critical review. Eur Child Adolesc Psychiatry. 2013;22(8):457–79 [r].

[34] Wang HR, Woo YS, Bahk WM. Atypical antipsychotics in the treatment of delirium. Psychiatry Clin Neurosci. 2013;67(5):323–31 [r].

[35] Hershenberg R, Gros DF, Brawman-Mintzer O. Role of atypical antipsychotics in the treatment of generalized anxiety disorder. CNS Drugs. 2014;28(6):519–33 [r].

[36] Shams TA, Müller DJ. Antipsychotic induced weight gain: genetics, epigenetics, and biomarkers reviewed. Curr Psychiatry Rep. 2014;16(10):473 [r].

[37] Citrome L, Collins JM, Nordstrom BL, et al. Incidence of cardiovascular outcomes and diabetes mellitus among users of second-generation antipsychotics. J Clin Psychiatry. 2013;74(12):1199–206 [c].

[38] Shin JY, Choi NK, Jung SY, et al. Risk of ischemic stroke with the use of risperidone, quetiapine and olanzapine in elderly patients: a-based, case-crossover study. J Psychopharmacol. 2013;27(7):638–44 [C].

[39] Weeke P, Jensen A, Folke F, et al. Antipsychotics and associated risk of out-of-hospital cardiac arrest. Clin Pharmacol Ther. 2014;96(4):490–7 [c].

[40] Germanò E, Italiano D, Lamberti M, et al. ECG parameters in children and adolescents treated with aripiprazole and risperidone. Prog Neuropsychopharmacol Biol Psychiatry. 2014;51:23–7 [c].

[41] Jackson JW, VanderWeele TJ, Viswanathan A, et al. The explanatory role of stroke as a mediator of the mortality risk difference between older adults who initiate first- versus second-generation antipsychotic drugs. Am J Epidemiol. 2014;180(8):847–52 [c].

[42] Wang JY, Wang CY, Tan CH, et al. Effect of different antipsychotic drugs on short-term mortality in stroke patients. Medicine (Baltimore). 2014;93(25):e170 [c].

[43] Pasternak B, Svanström H, Ranthe MF, et al. Atypical antipsychotics olanzapine, quetiapine, and risperidone and risk of acute major cardiovascular events in young and middle-aged adults: a nationwide register-based cohort study in Denmark. CNS Drugs. 2014;28(10):963–73 [c].

[44] Brauer R, Smeeth L, Anaya-Izquierdo K, et al. Antipsychotic drugs and risks of myocardial infarction: a self-controlled case series study. Eur Heart J. 2015;36(16):984–92 [c].

[45] Kanis JM, Timm NL. Chlorpromazine for the treatment of migraine in a pediatric emergency department. Headache. 2014;54(2):335–42 [c].

[46] Grohmann R, Engel RR, Möller HJ, et al. Flupentixol use and adverse reactions in comparison with other common first- and second-generation antipsychotics: data from the AMSP study. Eur Arch Psychiatry Clin Neurosci. 2014;264(2):131–41 [c].

[47] Wang M, Hou R, Jian J, et al. Effects of antipsychotics on bone mineral density and prolactin levels in patients with schizophrenia: a 12-month prospective study. Hum Psychopharmacol. 2014;29(2):183–9 [c].

[48] Pérez-Iglesias R, Ortiz-Garcia de la Foz V, Martínez García O, et al. Comparison of metabolic effects of aripiprazole, quetiapine and ziprasidone after 12 weeks of treatment in first treated episode of psychosis. Schizophr Res. 2014;159(1):90–4 [c].

[49] Correll CU, Robinson DG, Schooler NR, et al. Cardiometabolic risk in patients with first-episode schizophrenia spectrum disorders: baseline results from the RAISE-ETP study. JAMA Psychiatry. 2014;71(12):1350–63 [c].

[50] Paredes RM, Quinones M, Marballi K, et al. Metabolomic profiling of schizophrenia patients at risk for metabolic syndrome. Int J Neuropsychopharmacol. 2014;17(8):1139–48 [c].

[51] Arango C, Giráldez M, Merchán-Naranjo J, et al. Second-generation antipsychotic use in children and adolescents: a six-month prospective cohort study in drug-naïve patients. J Am Acad Child Adolesc Psychiatry. 2014;53(11):1179–90 [c].

[52] O'Donoghue B, Schäfer MR, Becker J, et al. Metabolic changes in first-episode early-onset schizophrenia with second-generation antipsychotics. Early Interv Psychiatry. 2014;8(3):276–80 [c].

[53] Lipscombe LL, Austin PC, Alessi-Severini S, et al. Canadian Network for Observational Drug Effect Studies (CNODES) Investigators. Atypical antipsychotics and hyperglycemic emergencies: multicentre, retrospective cohort study of administrative data. Schizophr Res. 2014;154(1–3):54–60 [c].

[54] Bobo WV, Cooper WO, Stein CM, et al. Antipsychotics and the risk of type 2 diabetes mellitus in children and youth. JAMA Psychiatry. 2013;70(10):1067–75 [c].

[55] Kemp DE, Zhao J, Cazorla P, et al. Weight change and metabolic effects of asenapine in patients with schizophrenia and bipolar disorder. J Clin Psychiatry. 2014;75(3):238–45 [c].

[56] Ngai YF, Sabatini P, Nguyen D, et al. Quetiapine treatment in youth is associated with decreased insulin secretion. J Clin Psychopharmacol. 2014;34(3):359–64 [c].

[57] Kelly AC, Sheitman BB, Hamer RM, et al. A naturalistic comparison of the long-term metabolic adverse effects of clozapine versus other antipsychotics for patients with psychotic illnesses. J Clin Psychopharmacol. 2014;34(4):441–5 [c].

[58] Yomiya K, Takei D, Kurosawa H, et al. A study on the antiemetic effect and extrapyramidal symptoms of prochlorperazine versus perospirone for the control of nausea and vomiting due to opioid introduction. Gan To Kagaku Ryoho. 2013;40(8):1037–41 [c].

[59] Vila-Rodriguez F, Tsang P, Barr AM. Chronic benign neutropenia/agranulocytosis associated with non-clozapine antipsychotics. Am J Psychiatry. 2013;170(10):1213–4 [c].

[60] López-Rodríguez R, Cabaleiro T, Ochoa D, et al. Pharmacodynamic genetic variants related to antipsychotic adverse reactions in healthy volunteers. Pharmacogenomics. 2013;14(10):1203–14 [c].

[61] Roffeei SN, Reynolds GP, Zainal NZ, et al. Association of ADRA2A and MTHFR gene polymorphisms with weight loss following antipsychotic switching to aripiprazole or ziprasidone. Hum Psychopharmacol. 2014;29(1):38–45 [c].

[62] Brandl EJ, Tiwari AK, Zai CC, et al. No evidence for a role of the peroxisome proliferator-activated receptor gamma (PPARG) and adiponectin (ADIPOQ) genes in antipsychotic-induced weight gain. Psychiatry Res. 2014;219(2):255–60 [c].

[63] Greil W, Häberle A, Schuhmann T, et al. Age and adverse drug reactions from psychopharmacological treatment: data from the AMSP drug surveillance programme in Switzerland. Swiss Med Wkly. 2013;143:w13772 [c].

[64] Meli M, Rauber-Lüthy C, Hoffmann-Walbeck P, et al. Atypical antipsychotic poisoning in young children: a multicentre analysis of poisons centres data. Eur J Pediatr. 2014;173(6):743–50 [c].

[65] Tybura P, Trześniowska-Drukała B, Bienkowski P, et al. Pharmacogenetics of adverse events in schizophrenia treatment: comparison study of ziprasidone, olanzapine and perazine. Psychiatry Res. 2014;219(2):261–7 [c].

[66] Cortés B, Bécker J, Mories Álvarez MT, et al. Contribution of baseline body mass index and leptin serum level to the prediction of early weight gain with atypical antipsychotics in schizophrenia. Psychiatry Clin Neurosci. 2014;68(2):127–32 [c].

[67] Butwicka A, Krystyna S, Retka W, et al. Neuroleptic malignant syndrome in an adolescent with CYP2D6 deficiency. Eur J Pediatr. 2014;173(12):1639–42 [A].

[68] Czerwensky F, Leucht S, Steimer W. MC4R rs489693: a clinical risk factor for second generation antipsychotic-related weight gain? Int J Neuropsychopharmacol. 2013;16(9):2103–9 [c].

[69] Gagliano SA, Tiwari AK, Freeman N, et al. Protein kinase cAMP-dependent regulatory type II beta (PRKAR2B) gene variants in antipsychotic-induced weight gain. Hum Psychopharmacol. 2014;29(4):330–5 [c].

[70] Kao AC, Rojnic Kuzman M, Tiwari AK, et al. Methylenetetrahydrofolate reductase gene variants and antipsychotic-induced weight gain and metabolic disturbances. J Psychiatr Res. 2014;54:36–42 [c].

[71] Vella T, Mifsud J. Interactions between valproic acid and quetiapine/olanzapine in the treatment of bipolar disorder and the role of therapeutic drug monitoring. J Pharm Pharmacol. 2014;66(6):747–59 [c].

[72] Atypical neuroleptics: compulsive disorders. Prescrire Int. 2014;23(146):43–4 [r].

[73] Fonseka TM, Richter MA, Müller DJ. Second generation antipsychotic-induced obsessive-compulsive symptoms in schizophrenia: a review of the experimental literature. Curr Psychiatry Rep. 2014;16(11):510 [r].

[74] Lin CH, Wang FC, Lin SC, et al. Antipsychotic combination using low-dose antipsychotics is as efficacious and safe as, but cheaper, than optimal-dose monotherapy in the treatment of schizophrenia: a randomized, double-blind study. Int Clin Psychopharmacol. 2013;28(5):267–74 [c].

[75] Kranke P, Eberhart L, Motsch J, et al. APD421 (amisulpride) prevents postoperative nausea and vomiting: a randomized, double-blind, placebo-controlled, multicentre trial. Br J Anaesth. 2013;111(6):938–45 [c].

[76] Mandal N, Singh OP, Sen S. Extrapyramidal side effects with low doses of amisulpride. Indian J Psychiatry. 2014;56(2):197–9 [A].

[77] Hotham JE, Simpson PJ, Brooman-White RS, et al. Augmentation of clozapine with amisulpride: an effective therapeutic strategy for violent treatment-resistant schizophrenia patients in a UK high-security hospital. CNS Spectr. 2014;19(5):403–10 [A].

[78] Kane JM, Peters-Strickland T, Baker RA, et al. Aripiprazole once-monthly in the acute treatment of schizophrenia: findings from a 12-week, randomized, double-blind, placebo-controlled study. J Clin Psychiatry. 2014;75(11):1254–60 [C].

[79] Li H, Luo J, Wang C, et al. Efficacy and of aripiprazole in Chinese Han schizophrenia subjects: a randomized, double-blind, active parallel-controlled, multicenter clinical trial. Schizophr Res. 2014;157(1–3):112–9 [c].

[80] Khanna P, Suo T, Komossa K, et al. Aripiprazole versus other atypical antipsychotics for schizophrenia. Cochrane Database Syst Rev. 2014;1:CD006569 [R].

[81] Kirino E. Profile of aripiprazole in the treatment of bipolar disorder in children and adolescents. Adolesc Health Med Ther. 2014;5:211–21 [r].

[82] Citrome L, Kalsekar I, Baker RA, et al. A review of real-world data on the effects of aripiprazole on weight and metabolic outcomes in adults. Curr Med Res Opin. 2014;30(8):1629–41 [r].

[83] Moore TJ, Glenmullen J, Mattison DR. Reports of pathological gambling, hypersexuality, and compulsive shopping associated with dopamine receptor agonist drugs. JAMA Intern Med. 2014;174(12):1930–3 [c].

[84] Potkin SG, Raoufinia A, Mallikaarjun S, et al. Safety and tolerability of once monthly aripiprazole treatment initiation in adults with schizophrenia stabilized on selected atypical oral antipsychotics other than aripiprazole. Curr Med Res Opin. 2013;29(10):1241–51 [c].

[85] Clayton AH, Baker RA, Sheehan JJ, et al. Comparison of adjunctive use of aripiprazole with bupropion or selective serotonin reuptake inhibitors/serotonin-norepinephrine reuptake inhibitors: analysis of patients beginning adjunctive treatment in a 52-week, open-label study. BMC Res Notes. 2014;7:459 [c].

[86] Goyal R, Devi SH. A case of aripiprazole induced tardive dyskinesia in a neuroleptic-naïve patient with two years of follow up. Clin Psychopharmacol Neurosci. 2014;12(1):69–71 [A].

[87] Gaboriau L, Victorri-Vigneau C, Gérardin M, et al. Aripiprazole: a new risk factor for pathological gambling? A report of 8 case reports. Addict Behav. 2014;39(3):562–5 [A].

[88] Pawelczyk T, Pawelczyk A, Rabe-Jablonska J. Olanzapine-induced triglyceride and aminotransferase elevations without weight gain or hyperglycemia normalized after switching to aripiprazole. J Psychiatr Pract. 2014;20(4):301–7 [A].

[89] Vrignaud L, Aouille J, Mallaret M, et al. Hypersexuality associated with aripiprazole: a new case and review of the literature. Therapie. 2014;69(6):525–7 [A].

[90] Goetz M, Surman CB. Prolonged penile erections associated with the use of atomoxetine and aripiprazole in an 11-year-old boy. J Clin Psychopharmacol. 2014;34(2):275–6 [A].

[91] Eatt J, Varghese ST. Worsening of psychosis with aripiprazole. J Neuropsychiatry Clin Neurosci. 2014;26(2):E20 [A].

[92] Hori H, Nakamura J. Hiccups associated with switching from olanzapine to aripiprazole in a patient with paranoid schizophrenia. Clin Neuropharmacol. 2014;37(3):88–9 [A].

[93] Legrand G, May R, Richard B, et al. A case report of partial bowel obstruction after aripiprazole addition to clozapine in a young male with schizophrenia. J Clin Psychopharmacol. 2013;33(4):571–2 [A].

[94] Cetin M, Celik M, Cakıcı M, et al. Aripiprazole induced non-cardiogenic pulmonary edema: a case report. Turk Psikiyatri Derg. 2014;25(4):287–9 [A].

[95] Sajatovic M, Dines P, Fuentes-Casiano E, et al. Asenapine in the treatment of older adults with bipolar disorder. Int J Geriatr Psychiatry. 2014;30(7):710–9 [c].

[96] Maina G, Ripellino C. The risk of metabolic disorders in patients treated with asenapine or olanzapine: a study conducted on real-world data in Italy and Spain. Expert Opin Drug Saf. 2014;13(9):1149–54 [c].

[97] Martín-Blanco A, Patrizi B, Villalta L, et al. Asenapine in the treatment of borderline personality disorder: an atypical antipsychotic alternative. Int Clin Psychopharmacol. 2014;29(2):120–3 [c].

[98] Makdisi J, Amin B, Friedman A. Pityriasis rosea-like drug reaction to asenapine. J Drugs Dermatol. 2013;12(9):1050–1 [A].

[99] Kishi T, Matsuda Y, Iwata N. Cardiometabolic risks of blonanserin and perospirone in the management of schizophrenia: a systematic review and meta-analysis of randomized controlled trials. PLoS One. 2014;9(2):e88049 [R].

[100] Takaki M, Mizuki Y, Miki T. Blonanserin improved dystonia induced by risperidone or olanzapine in two patients with schizophrenia. J Neuropsychiatry Clin Neurosci. 2014;26(2):E14 [A].

[101] Utku U, Gokce M, Benli EM, et al. Intra-venous chlorpromazine with fluid treatment in status migrainosus. Clin Neurol Neurosurg. 2014;119:4–5 [A].

[102] Adams CE, Awad GA, Rathbone J, et al. Chlorpromazine versus placebo for schizophrenia. Cochrane Database Syst Rev. 2014;1:CD000284 [r].

[103] Ifteni P, Correll CU, Nielsen J, et al. Rapid clozapine titration in treatment-refractory bipolar disorder. J Affect Disord. 2014;166:168–72 [r].

[104] Guenette MD, Powell V, Johnston K, et al. Risk of neutropenia in a clozapine-treated elderly population. Schizophr Res. 2013;148(1–3):183–5 [c].

[105] Hayes RD, Downs J, Chang CK, et al. The effect of clozapine on premature mortality: an assessment of clinical monitoring and other potential confounders. Schizophr Bull. 2015;41(3):644–55 [c].

[106] Midbari Y, Ebert T, Kosov I, et al. Hematological and cardiometabolic safety of clozapine in the treatment of very early onset schizophrenia: a retrospective chart review. J Child Adolesc Psychopharmacol. 2013;23(8):516–21 [c].

[107] Davis MC, Fuller MA, Strauss ME, et al. Discontinuation of clozapine: a 15-year naturalistic retrospective study of 320 patients. Acta Psychiatr Scand. 2014;130(1):30–9 [c].

[108] Schneider C, Corrigall R, Hayes D, et al. Systematic review of the efficacy and tolerability of clozapine in the treatment of youth with early onset schizophrenia. Eur Psychiatry. 2014;29(1):1–10 [r].

[109] Alawami M, Wasywich C, Cicovic A, et al. A systematic review of clozapine induced cardiomyopathy. Int J Cardiol. 2014;176(2):315–20 [r].

[110] Sagy R, Weizman A, Katz N. Pharmacological and behavioral management of some often-overlooked clozapine-induced side effects. Int Clin Psychopharmacol. 2014;29(6):313–7 [r].

[111] Munoli RN, Praharaj SK, Bhat SM. Clozapine-induced recurrent pulmonary thromboembolism. J Neuropsychiatry Clin Neurosci. 2013;25(3):E50–E51 [A].

[112] Kontoangelos K, Loizos S, Kanakakis J, et al. Myocarditis after administration of clozapine. Eur Rev Med Pharmacol Sci. 2014;18(16):2383–6 [A].

[113] Ittasakul P, Archer A, Kezman J, et al. Rapid re-challenge with clozapine following pronounced myocarditis in a treatment-resistance schizophrenia patient. Clin Schizophr Relat Psychoses. 2013;1–11 [A].

[114] Kikuchi Y, Ataka K, Yagisawa K, et al. Clozapine-induced cardiomyopathy: a first case in Japan. Schizophr Res. 2013;150(2–3):586–7 [A].

[115] Kikuchi YS, Sato W, Ataka K, et al. Clozapine-induced seizures, electroencephalography abnormalities, and clinical responses in Japanese patients with schizophrenia. Neuropsychiatr Dis Treat. 2014;10:1973–8 [c].

[116] Park S, Lee MK. Successful electroconvulsive therapy and improvement of negative symptoms in refractory schizophrenia with clozapine-induced seizures: a case report. Psychiatr Danub. 2014;26(4):360–2 [A].

[117] Kohlrausch FB, Severino-Gama C, Lobato MI, et al. The CYP1A2 -163C > A polymorphism is associated with clozapine-induced generalized tonic-clonic seizures in Brazilian schizophrenia patients. Psychiatry Res. 2013;209(2):242–5 [c].

[118] Lemke NT, Bustillo JR. Clozapine-induced obsessive-compulsive symptoms in bipolar disorder. Am J Psychiatry. 2013;170(8):930 [A].

[119] Kelly AC, Sheitman BB, Hamer RM, et al. A naturalistic comparison of the long-term metabolic adverse effects of clozapine versus other antipsychotics for patients with psychotic illnesses. J Clin Psychopharmacol. 2014;34(4):441–5 [c].

[120] Kontoangelos K, Economou M, Kiriaki P, et al. Administration of clozapine and excessive elevated serum triglycerides: a case report. J Clin Psychopharmacol. 2014;34(3):387–8 [A].

[121] Abanmy NO, Al-Jaloud A, Al-Jabr A, et al. Clozapine-induced blood dyscrasias in Saudi Arab patients. Int J Clin Pharm. 2014;36(4):815–20 [c].

[122] Drew L. Clozapine and agranulocytosis: re-assessing the risks. Australas Psychiatry. 2013;21(4):335–7 [c].

[123] Raveendranathan D, Sharma E, Venkatasubramanian G, et al. Late-onset clozapine-induced agranulocytosis in a patient with comorbid multiple sclerosis. Gen Hosp Psychiatry. 2013;35(5):574.e5–e6 [A].

[124] Usta NG, Poyraz CA, Aktan M, et al. Clozapine treatment of refractory schizophrenia during essential chemotherapy: a case study and mini review of a clinical dilemma. Ther Adv Psychopharmacol. 2014;4(6):276–81 [A].

[125] Kolli V, Denton K, Borra D, et al. Treating chemotherapy induced agranulocytosis with granulocyte colony-stimulating factors in a patient on clozapine. Psychooncology. 2013;22(7):1674–5 [A].

[126] Hazewinkel AW, Bogers JP, Giltay EJ. Add-on filgrastim during clozapine rechallenge unsuccessful in preventing agranulocytosis. Gen Hosp Psychiatry. 2013;35(5):576.e11–e12 [A].

[127] Goldstein JI, Jarskog LF, Hilliard C, et al. Clozapine-induced agranulocytosis is associated with rare HLA-DQB1 and HLA-B alleles. Nat Commun. 2014;5:4757 [c].

[128] Jovanović N, Loveretić V, Kuzman MR. The use of electroconvulsive therapy and general anaesthesia in catatonic schizophrenia complicated by clozapine—induced pancytopenia—case report. Psychiatr Danub. 2014;26(3):285–7 [A].

[129] Kikuchi YS, Ataka K, Yagisawa K, et al. Clozapine administration and the risk of drug-related pure red cell aplasia: a novel case report. J Clin Psychopharmacol. 2014;34(6):763–4 [A].

[130] Rajagopal V, Sundaresan L, Rajkumar AP, et al. Genetic association between the DRD4 promoter polymorphism and clozapine-induced sialorrhea. Psychiatr Genet. 2014;24(6):273–6 [c].

[131] Solismaa A, Kampman O, Seppälä N, et al. Polymorphism in alpha 2A adrenergic receptor gene is associated with sialorrhea in schizophrenia patients on clozapine treatment. Hum Psychopharmacol. 2014;29(4):336–41 [c].

[132] Mustafa FA, Khan A, Burke J, et al. Sublingual atropine for the treatment of severe and hyoscine-resistant clozapine-induced sialorrhea. Afr J Psychiatry (Johannesbg). 2013;16(4):242 [A].

[133] Vohra A. Clozapine- induced recurrent and transient parotid gland swelling. Afr J Psychiatry (Johannesbg). 2013;16(4):236 238 [A].

[134] Baptista T. A fatal case of ischemic colitis during clozapine administration. Rev Bras Psiquiatr. 2014;36(4):358 [A].

[135] Ikai S, Suzuki T, Uchida H, et al. Reintroduction of clozapine after perforation of the large intestine—a case report and review of the literature. Ann Pharmacother. 2013;47(7–8):e31.

[136] Galappathie N, Khan S. Clozapine-associated pneumonia and respiratory arrest secondary to severe constipation. Med Sci Law. 2014;54(2):105–9.

[137] Poetter CE, Stewart JT. Treatment of clozapine-induced constipation with bethanechol. J Clin Psychopharmacol. 2013;33(5):713–4 [A].

[138] Meyer JM, Cummings MA. Lubiprostone for treatment-resistant constipation associated with clozapine use. Acta Psychiatr Scand. 2014;130(1):71–2.

[139] Adebayo KO, Ibrahim N, Mosanya T, et al. Life-threatening haematemesis associated with clozapine: a case report and literature review. Ther Adv Psychopharmacol. 2013;3(5):275–7 [A].

[140] Brown CA, Telio S, Warnock CA, et al. Clozapine toxicity and hepatitis. J Clin Psychopharmacol. 2013;33(4):570–1 [A].

[141] Kane JP, O'Neill FA. Clozapine-induced liver injury and pleural effusion. Ment Illn. 2014;6(2):5403 [A].

[142] Tucker P. Liver toxicity with clozapine. Aust N Z J Psychiatry. 2013;47(10):975–6 [A].

[143] Linton B, Fu R, MacDonald PA, et al. Burning pain secondary to clozapine use: a case report. BMC Psychiatry. 2014;14:299 [A].

[144] Kashyap GL, Nayar J, Bashier A, et al. Treatment of clozapine-induced priapism by goserline acetate injection. Ther Adv Psychopharmacol. 2013;3(5):298–300 [A].

[145] Martin N, Williams R. Management of clozapine-induced fever: a case of continued therapy throughout fever. J Psychiatry Neurosci. 2013;38(4):E9–E10 [A].

[146] Leung JG, Nelson S, Takala CR, et al. Infection and inflammation leading to clozapine toxicity and intensive care: a case series. Ann Pharmacother. 2014;48(6):801–5 [A].

[147] Matthews CJ, Hall TL. A clozapine conundrum: clozapine toxicity in an acutemedical illness. Australas Psychiatry. 2014;22(6):543–5 [A].

[148] Reddy SM, Khairkar PH, Jajoo U. 70 hours of coma by clozapine intoxication. J Neuropsychiatry Clin Neurosci. 2013;25(4):E22–E23 [A].

[149] Parent V, Popitean L, Loctin A, et al. Gastric dilation due to a neuroleptic agent in an elderly patient: a case report. Case Rep Med. 2014;2014:961048 [A].

[150] Calver L, Isbister GK. High dose droperidol and QT prolongation: analysis of continuous 12-lead recordings. Br J Clin Pharmacol. 2014;77(5):880–6 [c].

[151] Kishimoto S, Nakamura K, Arai T, et al. Postoperative neuroleptic malignant syndrome-like symptoms improved with intravenous diazepam: case report. J Anesth. 2013;27(5):768–70 [A].

[152] Berna F, Timbolschi ID, Diemunsch P, et al. Acute dystonia and akathisia following droperidol administration misdiagnosed as psychiatric disorders. J Anesth. 2013;27(5):803–4 [A].

[153] Grohmann R, Engel RR, Möller HJ, et al. Flupentixol use and adverse reactions in comparison with other common first- and second-generation antipsychotics: data from the AMSP study. Eur Arch Psychiatry Clin Neurosci. 2014;264(2):131–41 [c].

[154] Tardy M, Dold M, Engel RR, et al. Flupenthixol versus low-potency first-generation antipsychotic drugs for schizophrenia. Cochrane Database Syst Rev. 2014;9:CD009227 [R].

[155] Matar HE, Almerie MQ, Sampson S. Fluphenazine (oral) versus placebo for schizophrenia. Cochrane Database Syst Rev. 2013;7:CD006352 [R].

[156] Adams CE, Bergman H, Irving CB, et al. Haloperidol versus placebo for schizophrenia. Cochrane Database Syst Rev. 2013;11:CD003082 [R].

[157] Donnelly L, Rathbone J, Adams CE. Haloperidol dose for the acute phase of schizophrenia. Cochrane Database Syst Rev. 2013;8:CD001951 [R].

[158] Bascom PB, Bordley JL, Lawton AJ. High-dose neuroleptics and neurolepticrotation for agitated delirium near the end of life. Am J Hosp Palliat Care. 2014;31(8):808–11 [A].

[159] Dargani NV, Malhotra AK. Safety profile of iloperidone in the treatment of schizophrenia. Expert Opin Drug Saf. 2014;13(2):241–6.

[160] Rodriguez-Cabezas LA, Kong BY, Agarwal G. Priapism associated with iloperidone: a case report. Gen Hosp Psychiatry. 2014;36(4). 451.e5–451.e6 [R].

[161] Hohl CM, Stenekes S, Harlos MS, et al. Methotrimeprazine for the management of end-of-life symptoms in infants and children. J Palliat Care. 2013;29(3):178–85 [c].

[162] Agosti S, Casalino L, Bertero G, et al. Citalopram and levosulpiride: a dangerous drug combination for QT prolongation. Am J Emerg Med. 2013;31(11):1624.e1–e2 [A].

[163] Spyker DA, Voloshko P, Heyman ER, et al. Loxapine delivered as athermally generated aerosol does not prolong QTc in a thorough QT/QTc study in healthy subjects. J Clin Pharmacol. 2014;54(6):665–74 [c].

[164] Loebel A, Cucchiaro J, Silva R, et al. Lurasidone as adjunctive therapy with lithium or valproate for the treatment of bipolar I depression: a randomized, double-blind, placebo-controlled study. Am J Psychiatry. 2014;171(2):169–77 [C].

[165] Citrome L, Weiden PJ, McEvoy JP, et al. Effectiveness of lurasidone in schizophrenia or schizoaffective patients switched from other antipsychotics: a 6-month, open-label, extension study. CNS Spectr. 2014;19(4):330–9 [c].

[166] Citrome L, Ketter TA, Cucchiaro J, et al. Clinical assessment of lurasidone benefit and risk in the treatment of bipolar I depression using number needed to treat, number needed to harm, and likelihood to be helped or harmed. J Affect Disord. 2014;155:20–7 [c].

[167] Wang M, Tong JH, Huang DS, et al. Efficacy of olanzapine monotherapy for treatment of bipolar I depression: a randomized, double-blind, placebo controlled study. Psychopharmacology (Berl). 2014;231(14):2811–8 [C].

[168] Katagiri H, Tohen M, McDonnell DP, et al. Safety and efficacy of olanzapine in the long-term treatment of Japanese patients with bipolar I disorder, depression: an integrated analysis. Psychiatry Clin Neurosci. 2014;68(7):498–505 [C].

[169] Petersen AB, Andersen SE, Christensen M, et al. Adverse effects associated with high-dose olanzapine therapy in patients admitted to inpatient psychiatric care. Clin Toxicol (Phila). 2014;52(1):39–43 [c].

[170] Baruch N, Das M, Sharda A, et al. An evaluation of the use of olanzapine pamoate depot injection in seriously violent men with schizophrenia in a UK high-security hospital. Ther Adv Psychopharmacol. 2014;4(5):186–92 [c].

[171] Chanthawong S, Subongkot S, Sookprasert A. Effectiveness of olanzapine for the treatment of breakthrough chemotherapy induced nausea and vomiting. J Med Assoc Thai. 2014;97(3):349–55 [c].

[172] Zhong Z, Zhang Y, Han H, et al. Effects of low-dose olanzapine on duloxetine-related nausea and vomiting for the treatment of major depressive disorder. J Clin Psychopharmacol. 2014;34(4):495–8 [c].

[173] Holzer B, Lopes V, Lehman R. Combination use of atomoxetine hydrochloride and olanzapine in the treatment of attention-deficit/hyperactivity disorder with comorbid disruptive behavior disorder in children and adolescents 10-18 years of age. J Child Adolesc Psychopharmacol. 2013;23(6):415–8 [c].

[174] Flank J, Sung L, Dvorak CC, et al. The safety of olanzapine in young children: a systematic review and meta-analysis. Drug Saf. 2014;37(10):791–804 [R].

[175] Cristancho MA, Thase ME. Drug safety evaluation of olanzapine/fluoxetine combination. Expert Opin Drug Saf. 2014;13(8):1133–41 [R].

[176] Hill AL, Sun B, McDonnell DP. Incidences of extrapyramidal symptoms in patients with schizophrenia after treatment with long-acting injection (depot) or oral formulations of olanzapine. Clin Schizophr Relat Psychoses. 2014;7(4):216–22 [c].

[177] Sun Z, Wang X. Case report of refractory tardive dystonia induced by olanzapine. Shanghai Arch Psychiatry. 2014;26(1):51–3 [A].

[178] Gnanavel S, Thanapal S, Khandelwal SK, et al. Olanzapine-induced tardivedystonia: a case report. J Neuropsychiatry Clin Neurosci. 2014;26(2):E24–E25 [A].

[179] Verma R, Junewar V, Rathaur BP. An atypical case of neuroleptic malignant syndrome precipitated by valproate. BMJ Case Rep. 2014; Published online 6 March 2014, http://dx.doi.org/10.1136/bcr-2013-202578 [A].

[180] Volpe U, Vignapiano A, Gallo O, et al. Add-on oral olanzapine worsens hallucinations in schizoaffective disorder. BMJ Case Rep. 2014; Published online 21 October 2014, http://dx.doi.org/10.1136/bcr-2014-205805 [A].

[181] Cordes J, Thünker J, Regenbrecht G, et al. Can an early weight management program (WMP) prevent olanzapine (OLZ)-induced disturbances in body weight, blood glucose and lipid metabolism? Twenty-four- and 48-week results from a 6-month randomized trial. World J Biol Psychiatry. 2014;15(3):229–41 [c].

[182] Kimmel RJ, Levy MR. Profound hypertriglyceridemia and weight gain in the first week following initiation of olanzapine: a case report with implications for lipid monitoring guidelines. Psychosomatics. 2013;54(4):392–4 [A].

[183] Haruta I, Asakawa A, Inui A. Olanzapine-induced hypoglycemia in anorexia nervosa. Endocrine. 2014;46(3):672–3 [A].

[184] Gupta A, Ghoshal UC, Mohindra S, et al. Acute necrotizing pancreatitis following olanzapine therapy. Trop Gastroenterol. 2014;35(2):132–4 [A].

[185] Chiang CL, Lin YH, Hsieh MH. Olanzapine-induced hyponatremia in a patient with autism. J Child Adolesc Psychopharmacol. 2013;23(10):699–700 [A].

[186] Ramsey TL, Liu Q, Brennan MD. Replication of SULT4A1-1 as a pharmacogenetic marker of olanzapine response and evidence of lower weight gain in the high response group. Pharmacogenomics. 2014;15(7):933–9 [c].

[187] Nagasawa S, Yajima D, Torimitsu S, et al. Fatal water intoxication during olanzapine treatment: a case report. Leg Med (Tokyo). 2014;16(2):89–91 [A].

[188] Vodovar D, Malissin I, Deye N, et al. Olanzapine postinjection delirium/sedation syndrome: an unrecognized diagnosis in the emergency department. J Emerg Med. 2014;47(1):e23–e24 [A].

[189] Buts K, Van Hecke J. Post-injection delirium/sedation syndrome following injection of olanzapine pamoate: a new syndrome in emergency psychiatry. Tijdschr Psychiatr. 2014;56(4):273–6 [A].

[190] McEvoy JP, Byerly M, Hamer RM, et al. Effectiveness of paliperidone palmitate vs haloperidol decanoate for maintenance

treatment of schizophrenia: a randomized clinical trial. JAMA. 2014;311(19):1978–87 [c].

[191] Üçok A, Saka MC, Bilici M. Effects of paliperidone extended release on functioning level and symptoms of patients with recent onset schizophrenia: an open-label, single-arm, flexible-dose, 12-months follow-up study. Nord J Psychiatry. 2014;31:1–7 [c].

[192] Suzuki H, Gen K, Inoue Y, et al. The influence of switching from risperidone to paliperidone on the extrapyramidal symptoms and cognitive function in elderly patients with schizophrenia: a preliminary open-label trial. Int J Psychiatry Clin Pract. 2014;18(1):58–62 [c].

[193] Attard A, Olofinjana O, Cornelius V, et al. Paliperidone palmitate long-acting injection—prospective year-long follow-up of use in clinical practice. Acta Psychiatr Scand. 2014;130(1):46–51 [c].

[194] Şengül MC, Kaya K, Yilmaz A, et al. Pulmonary thromboembolism due to paliperidone: report of 2 cases. Am J Emerg Med. 2014;32(7):814.e1–e2 [A].

[195] Hsieh MH, Chiu NY. Paliperidone-associated motor tics. Gen Hosp Psychiatry. 2014;36(3):360.e7–e8 [A].

[196] Hou YC, Lai CH. Lower risk for body weight gain and better control of appetite after switching risperidone to paliperidone in a schizoaffective patient. J Neuropsychiatry Clin Neurosci. 2014;26(2):E36–E37 [A].

[197] Amatniek J, Canuso CM, Deutsch SI, et al. Safety of paliperidone extended-release in patients with schizophrenia or schizoaffective disorder and hepatic disease. Clin Schizophr Relat Psychoses. 2014;8(1):8–20 [A].

[198] Leucht S, Helfer B, Hartung B. Perazine for schizophrenia. Cochrane Database Syst Rev. 2014;1:CD002832 [R].

[199] Matar HE, Almerie MQ, Makhoul S, et al. Pericyazine for schizophrenia. Cochrane Database Syst Rev. 2014;5:CD007479 [R].

[200] Kishi T, Iwata N. Efficacy and tolerability of perospirone in schizophrenia: a systematic review and meta-analysis of randomized controlled trials. CNS Drugs. 2013;27(9):731–41 [R].

[201] Nakayama H, Umeda S, Nibuya M, et al. Two cases of mild serotonin toxicity via 5-hydroxytryptamine 1A receptor stimulation. Neuropsychiatr Dis Treat. 2014;10:283–7 [A].

[202] Henao JP, Peperzak KA, Lichvar AB, et al. Extrapyramidal symptoms following administration of oral perphenazine 4 or 8 mg: an 11-year retrospective analysis. Eur J Anaesthesiol. 2014;31(4):231–5 [c].

[203] Tardy M, Huhn M, Engel RR, et al. Perphenazine versus low-potency first-generation antipsychotic drugs for schizophrenia. Cochrane Database Syst Rev. 2014;10:CD009369 [R].

[204] Tashiro M, Naito T, Ohnishi K, et al. Impact of genetic and non-genetic factors on clinical responses to prochlorperazine in oxycodone-treated cancer patients. Clin Chim Acta. 2014;429:175–80 [c].

[205] Black DW, Zanarini MC, Romine A, et al. Comparison of low and moderate dosages of extended-release quetiapine in borderline personality disorder: a randomized, double-blind, placebo-controlled trial. Am J Psychiatry. 2014;171(11):1174–82 [c].

[206] Porcelli S, Balzarro B, de Ronchi D, et al. Quetiapine extended release: preliminary evidence of a rapid onset of the antidepressant effect in bipolar depression. J Clin Psychopharmacol. 2014;34(3):303–6 [c].

[207] Sherwood Brown E, Davila D, Nakamura A, et al. A randomized, double-blind, placebo-controlled trial of quetiapine in patients with bipolar disorder, mixed or depressed phase, and alcohol dependence. Alcohol Clin Exp Res. 2014;38(7):2113–8 [c].

[208] Mariani JJ, Pavlicova M, Mamczur AK, et al. Open-label pilot study of quetiapine treatment for cannabis dependence. Am J Drug Alcohol Abuse. 2014;40(4):280–4 [c].

[209] Calandre EP, Rico-Villademoros F, Galán J, et al. Quetiapine extended-release (Seroquel-XR) versus amitriptyline monotherapy for treating patients with fibromyalgia: a 16-week, randomized, flexible-dose, open-label trial. Psychopharmacology (Berl). 2014;231(12):2525–31 [c].

[210] Asmal L, Flegar SJ, Wang J, et al. Quetiapine versus other atypical antipsychotics for schizophrenia. Cochrane Database Syst Rev. 2013;11:CD006625 [R].

[211] Hou YC, Lai CH. Late-onset quetiapine-related tardive dyskinesia side effects in a patient with psychotic depression. Clin Psychopharmacol Neurosci. 2014;12(2):163–5 [A].

[212] Fond G, MacGregor A, Ducasse D, et al. Paradoxical severe agitation induced by add-on high-doses quetiapine in schizo-affective disorder. Psychiatry Res. 2014;216(2):286–7 [A].

[213] Chang TG, Chiu NY, Hsu WY. Acute pancreatitis associated with quetiapine use in schizophrenia. J Clin Psychopharmacol. 2014;34(3):382–3 [A].

[214] Suzuki Y, Sugai T, Ono S, et al. Changes in PR and QTc intervals after switching from olanzapine to risperidone in patients with stable schizophrenia. Psychiatry Clin Neurosci. 2014;68(5):353–6 [c].

[215] Iuppa CA, Diefenderfer LA. Risperidone-induced Pisa syndrome in MS: resolution with lurasidone and recurrence with chlorpromazine. Ann Pharmacother. 2013;47(9):1223–8 [A].

[216] White PA, Singh R, Rais T, et al. Premature thelarche in an 8-year-old girl following prolonged use of risperidone. J Child Adolesc Psychopharmacol. 2014;24(4):228–30 [A].

[217] Cabaleiro T, Ochoa D, López-Rodríguez R, et al. Effect of polymorphisms on the pharmacokinetics, pharmacodynamics, and safety of risperidone in healthy volunteers. Hum Psychopharmacol. 2014;29(5):459–69 [c].

[218] Suzuki Y, Tsuneyama N, Fukui N, et al. Effect of risperidone metabolism and P-glycoprotein gene polymorphism on QT interval in patients with schizophrenia. Pharmacogenomics J. 2014;14(5):452–6 [c].

[219] Muscatello MR, Bruno A, Micali Bellinghieri P, et al. Sertindole in schizophrenia: efficacy and safety issues. Expert Opin Pharmacother. 2014;15(13):1943–53 [r].

[220] Lai EC, Hsieh CY, Kao Yang YH, et al. Detecting potential adverse reactions of sulpiride in schizophrenic patients by prescription sequence symmetry analysis. PLoS One. 2014;9(2): e89795 [c].

[221] Muscatello MR, Pandolfo G, Micò U, et al. Augmentation of clozapine with ziprasidone in refractory schizophrenia: a double-blind, placebo-controlled study. J Clin Psychopharmacol. 2014;34(1):129–33 [C].

[222] Suppes T, McElroy SL, Sheehan DV, et al. A randomized, double-blind, placebo-controlled study of ziprasidone monotherapy in bipolar disorder with co-occurring lifetime panic or generalized anxiety disorder. J Clin Psychiatry. 2014;75(1):77–84 [C].

[223] Findling RL, Cavuș I, Pappadopulos E, et al. Efficacy, long-term safety, and tolerability of ziprasidone in children and adolescents with bipolar disorder. J Child Adolesc Psychopharmacol. 2013;23(8):545–57 [C].

[224] Findling RL, Cavuș I, Pappadopulos E, et al. Ziprasidone in adolescents with schizophrenia: results from a placebo-controlled efficacy and long-term open-extension study. J Child Adolesc Psychopharmacol. 2013;23(8):531–44 [C].

[225] Goff DC, McEvoy JP, Citrome L, et al. High-dose oral ziprasidone versus conventional dosing in schizophrenia patients with residual symptoms: the ZEBRAS study. J Clin Psychopharmacol. 2013;33(4):485–90 [C].

[226] Li CH, Shi L, Zhan GL, et al. A twenty-four-week, open-label study on ziprasidone's efficacy and influence on glucolipid

metabolism in patients with schizophrenia and metabolic disorder. Eur Rev Med Pharmacol Sci. 2013;17(16):2136–40 [c].

[227] Li XB, Tang YL, Zheng W, et al. QT interval prolongation associated with intramuscular ziprasidone in Chinese patients: a case report and a comprehensive literature review with meta-analysis. Case Rep Psychiatry. 2014;2014:489493 [A, r].

[228] Menon V, Ramamourthy P, Ayyanar S. Transient, asymptomatic, fluctuating bradycardia with oral ziprasidone in an older woman. Aust N Z J Psychiatry. 2014;48(2):201–2 [A].

[229] El-Okdi NS, Lumbrezer D, Karanovic D, et al. Serotonin syndrome after the use of tramadol and ziprasidone in a patient with a deep brain stimulator for Parkinson disease. Am J Ther. 2014;21(4):e97–e99 [A].

[230] Praharaj SK, Jana AK, Sarkhel S, et al. Acute dystonia, akathisia, and parkinsonism induced by ziprasidone. Am J Ther. 2014;21(2): e38–e40 [A].

[231] Lee HB, Yoon BH, Kwon YJ, et al. The efficacy and safety of switching to ziprasidone from olanzapine in patients with bipolar I disorder: an 8-week, multicenter, open-label study. Clin Drug Investig. 2013;33(10):743–53 [C].

[232] Kim MS, Kim SW, Han TY, et al. Ziprasidone-induced hypersensitivity syndrome confirmed by reintroduction. Int J Dermatol. 2014;53(4):e267–e268 [A].

[233] Lin CC, Chiu HJ, Chen JY, et al. Switching from clozapine to zotepine in patients with schizophrenia: a 12-week prospective, randomized, rater blind, and parallel study. J Clin Psychopharmacol. 2013;33(2):211–4 [c].

7

Antiepileptics

Brian Spoelhof*,[1], Lynn Frendak*, Lucia Rivera Lara[†]

*Department of Pharmacy, Johns Hopkins Bayview Medical Center, Baltimore, MD, USA
[†]Departments of Neurology, Anesthesiology, and Critical Care Medicine, Johns Hopkins Medicine, Baltimore, MD, USA
[1]Corresponding author: brian.spoelhof@jhmi.edu

Brivaracetam

Introduction

Brivaracetam is a structurally similar analog of levetiracetam with a high affinity for synaptic vesicle protein 2A ligand. Brivaracetam has a 10-fold higher affinity for SV2A compared to levetiracetam with additional voltage-dependent sodium inhibition [1R]. Brivaracetam is excreted as inactive metabolites in the urine. Metabolism is thought to be mediated by non-CYP hydrolysis and CYP2C19.

Placebo-Controlled Trials

A randomized, placebo-controlled trial evaluated the use of brivaracetam as adjunctive therapy for partial seizures. Treatment-emergent adverse events were present in 71.1%, 79%, and 75.2% in patients receiving 5, 20, and 50 mg, respectively. The reported adverse effects were somnolence, dizziness, and fatigue for all dose strengths. Influenza, nausea, and unitary tract infection occurred in the 20 mg group. Furthermore, diarrhea, insomnia, vomiting, and nasopharyngitis were seen in the 50 mg group. Serious adverse events occurred in 2.3% of brivaracetam treated patient compared to 0% in the placebo group [2C]. Two similar trials demonstrated headache, somnolence, dizziness, fatigue, and psychiatric events [3C,4C].

Pharmacogenomics

An evaluation of CYP2C19 polymorphism on brivaracetam was evaluated in a Japanese population. Those considered a poor metabolizer had a 29% decrease in brivaracetam metabolism [5c].

Drug–Drug Interactions

Brivaracetam was not found to have a significant difference in oral contraceptive metabolism or in break through bleeding at a dose of 100 mg/day [6c].

Carbamazepine [SEDA-31, 107; SEDA-32, 126; SEDA-33, 132; SEDA-34, 94; SEDA-35, 135; SEDA-36, 88]

Meta-Analysis

A meta-analysis confirmed the association between HLA-B* 15:02 genotype and Stevens–Johnson syndrome/toxic epidermal necrolysis in patients of Han-Chinese, Thai, and Malaysian decent [7M].

Cardiovascular

A cross-sectional study in children on carbamazepine or phenytoin monotherapy found a potential increased risk of preclinical atherosclerosis [8c]. Children on carbamazepine therapy had significantly higher total, HDL, and LDL cholesterol as well as higher right carotid, left carotid and overall average carotid intima media thickness compared to controls. Children on phenytoin therapy had significantly higher HDL cholesterol, right carotid, and overall average carotid intima media thickness compared to controls.

A case of ventricular ectopic beats was reported in an 8-year-old child taking carbamazepine 15 mg/kg/day for epilepsy [9A]. At the time of presentation, the patient was noted to have an irregularly irregular pulse; ectopic heart beats after every 8–10 beats, a heart rate of 70–80 beats per minute, and carbamazepine levels in the therapeutic range. Carbamazepine was replaced with valproate and the patient's EKG normalized; the patient showed no abnormality at 3 months and 1-year follow-up. Cardiac effects are thought to be due to its action as a sodium channel blocker.

Nutrition

A prospective study did not find a relationship between carbamazepine and serum levels of homocysteine, vitamin B12 and folic acid in children [10c].

ISSN: 0378-6080
http://dx.doi.org/10.1016/bs.seda.2015.06.008

© 2015 Elsevier B.V. All rights reserved.

Skin

A retrospective study found that carbamazepine was associated with increased severe cutaneous drug reactions in elderly Korean patients regardless of the indication for therapy [11c].

A case of drug rash with drug reaction with eosinophilia and systemic symptoms (DRESS syndrome) was reported in a 64-year-old male who was started on carbamazepine for pain management [12A]. The patient presented with maculopapules exanthema, fever, hepatitis, leukocytosis, and eosinophilia after 5 weeks of therapy. The report did not establish whether a causal relationship was confirmed and how quickly the patient recovered after discontinuing carbamazepine. A separate case of drug rash with DRESS syndrome was reported in a 14-year-old male who was started on carbamazepine for seizures 2 weeks prior [13A]. Symptoms continued to worsen even after discontinuation of carbamazepine and supportive therapy. The patient then received methylprednisolone 1 gram daily and oral ursodeoxycholic acid 900 mg daily for 3 days which resulted in rapid reversal of symptoms including liver function. DRESS syndrome has been identified in pediatric patients as well as adults and high dose IV steroids may be considered for refractory cases. A case of DRESS with skeletal muscle involvement was reported in a 61-year-old male taking carbamazepine for 3 months [14A]. Symptoms resolved with corticosteroids after stopping the carbamazepine. Carbamazepine was determined to be the cause although a drug-challenge was not done.

A case of neurophilic eccrine hidradenitis (NEH) was reported in a 40-year-old female who was had been initiated on carbamazepine for epilepsy 1 month prior [15A]. The patient presented with fever, puffiness of face, vomiting, and skin rash for 5 days. Other dermatologic conditions were ruled out and a diagnosis of NEH was made. Symptoms improved with oral corticosteroids after stopping carbamazepine. Due to the temporal relationship between symptoms and carbamazepine initiation a probable relationship with carbamazepine was suggested.

A case of carbamazepine induced lichen sclerosus et atrophicus was reported in a 73-year-old male treated with carbamazepine for epilepsy [16A]. The patient presented with multiple reddish-brown maculas on his trunk and limbs 6 months after starting carbamazepine 400 mg BID. Symptoms improved with corticosteroids after changing carbamazepine to oxcarbazepine. Carbamazepine was monotherapy for epilepsy, however it was not reported if the patient was on any other concurrent medications.

Drug Overdose

A retrospective study found that patients with acute carbamazepine poisoning may have therapeutic or even subtherapeutic carbamazepine blood concentrations at the time of presentation due to delayed or erratic absorption [17C]. These concentrations increased to toxic levels overtime, leading to the recommendation to measure serial concentrations until a downward trend is evident.

A case of fatal carbamazepine overdose was reported in a 23-month-old child with febrile and epileptic seizures [18A]. The child, who had been on phenytoin, was started on carbamazepine 127 days prior with serum levels in the therapeutic range. Twenty-nine days prior to presentation phenytoin was discontinued. Due to the carbamazepine–phenytoin drug interaction, the removal of phenytoin resulted in supratherapeutic carbamazepine serum levels, measured at 22 mcg/mL postmortem. Acute carbamazepine intoxication was ruled the cause of death.

Sexual and Reproductive Function

A placebo-controlled, cross-sectional study found that adult males taking carbamazepine for epilepsy had a significant increase in luteinizing hormones, sex hormone-binding globulin, and total testosterone; significant decreases in total testosterone and dehydroepiandrosterone; were more likely to experience erectile dysfunction; had altered sperm vitality and motility; and had a decreased frequency of sexual intercourse compared to controls [19C]. These effects are hypothesized to be due to such mechanisms as disturbance in cytochrome P450 enzyme system action, effect on neurotransmitters, or endocrine changes.

Pharmacogenomics

A study evaluated the strength of association of genetic markers HLA-A and HLA-B and carbamazepine-induced hypersensitivity reactions in patients of Han Chinese decent [20c]. Carbamazepine induced Stevens–Johnson syndrome/toxic epidermal necrolysis had a strong association with HLA-B*15:02. In patients >5% body surface area (BSA) involvement all patients were positive for HLA-B*15:02 poly morphism. Furthermore, the genetic polymorphism was present 85.1% of cases with <5% BSA involvement. HLA-B*40:01 showed a negative association with carbamazepine induced Stevens–Johnson syndrome (SJS)/toxic epidermal necrolysis (TEN). Carbamazepine-induced maculopapular exanthema/drug rash with eosinophilia and systemic symptoms had an association with HLA-A*31:01 and HLA-B*51:01 but no association with HLA-B*15:02.

A second study evaluated predictability of genetic markers HLA-B*15:02 and HLA-A*31:01 to SJS and drug-induced hypersensitivity syndrome in North American children with diverse ethnic backgrounds [21c], a previously unstudied population. Genetic marker HLA-B*15:02 was found to be associated with carbamazepine-induced Stevens–Johnson syndrome and HLA-A*31:01

was associated with carbamazepine-induced hypersensitivity syndrome. The study identified the predictability of genetic markers HLA-B*15:02 and HLA-A*31:01 across a diverse patient population including various ancestries and patient ages.

A third study demonstrated that the association between the HLA-B* 15:02 genotype and carbamazepine-induced SJS/TEN is evident in children as well as adults [22c]. The HLA-B*15:02 genotype was positive in all 5 cases of SJS/TEN, 0/6 cases of hypersensitivity syndrome, and in 1/10 controls.

Another study found that 8 of 35 patients (22.9%) of Han Chinese descent who carried the HLA-B*15:02 genotype developed SJS versus 2 of 125 control patients (1.6%) without the genotype [23c]. This shows an association between the genotype and carbamazepine induced SJS, but not necessary to develop TEN.

Due to the well documented close association of the HLA-B* 15:02 genotype and risk of SJS/TEN clinical guidelines were published by the Clinical Pharmacogenetics Implementation Consortium recommending that any patient testing positive for the genotype be started on a different agent, unless the benefit clearly outweighs the risk [24R].

Two studies found screening for the HLA-B*15:02 genotype before starting carbamazepine therapy in the Thai population to be cost effective [25c, 26c]. It is unclear if these results would hold true in other patient populations.

Eslicarbazepine [SEDA-34, 97; SEDA-35, 136; SEDA-36, 89]

Placebo-Controlled Trials

A randomized, double-blind, placebo-controlled trial was conducted to evaluate the safety and efficacy in patients with refractory partial onset seizures. Treatment emergent adverse effects occurred in 67% of patients taking 800 mg and 77.6% of patients taking 1200 mg compared to 55.8% of patented taking placebo. Dizziness was the most common adverse effect occurring in 8.5%, 15.7%, and 56.2% in the placebo, 800, and 1200 mg groups, respectively. Somnolence, nausea, headache, vomiting, diplopia, vertigo, and fatigue were the most commonly reported adverse effects. Adverse events leading to discontinuation occurred in 12% (800 mg) and 25.7% (1200 mg) vs 8% of the placebo group. Dizziness, nausea, vomiting, ataxia, and dysarthria were the most common events leading to discontinuation. Finally, serum sodium was evaluated due to risk of inappropriate antidiuretic hormone secretion associated with similar agents. One patient taking 800 mg and five patients taking 1200 mg had serum sodium <125 mEq/L, while nine patients in the 800 mg group and 12 patients in the 1200 mg group had a >10 mEq drop [27C].

Another randomized, historical-controlled trial was performed to assess antiepileptic withdrawal to eslicarbazepine monotherapy. Patients received either 1200 or 1600 mg. Greater than 10% of patients receiving either dose reported dizziness, headache, fatigue, somnolence, nausea, and nasopharyngitis. Severe adverse events were experienced in 8.8% of patients. Results from the study matched previous prospective trials [28C].

Observational

An observational 2-year follow-up study was performed with patients taking eslicarbazepine. Dizziness and somnolence were seen in 11.2% and 7.3%, respectively. Univariate analysis determined that adverse events were gender, diagnosis, number of concomitant antiepileptic drugs (AED), or final eslicarbazepine dosage. However, patients on carbamazepine inducing regimens vs non-inducing regimens, likely attributed to concurrent carbamazepine [29c]. Another follow-up study of patients on eslicarbazepine found an adverse event rate of 40.7% of which 16.2% lead to discontinuation. Dizziness, nausea, and somnolence were most common [30C].

Skin

A 41-year-old white female receiving 4000 mg of levetiracetam, 600 mg lacosamide was initiated on 400 mg eslicarbazepine and titrated to 800 mg. Following 25 days of therapy, the patient developed painful and itching cutaneous eruptions with the appearance of erythema multiforme. The lesions were on the trunk, soles, and palms. The rash also involved the conjunctiva, oral, and vaginal mucosa. Other signs and symptoms included pain, dysphagia, dyspnea, and elevated liver enzymes. Eslicarbazepine was withdrawn and the patient was treated with topical and systemic steroids, and gentamicin. Symptoms resolved after 2 weeks [31A].

Ethosuximide [SEDA-36, 90]

Neurologic

One case report of a 6-year-old child with recurrent absence seizures showed increase presences of Rolandic spikes following ethosuximide initiation. The authors of the study could not conclude whether ethosuximide contributed to a conversion between the conditions or if this represented a continuum [32A].

Felbamate [SEDA 33, 136; SEDA-34, 198; SEDA-35, 137; SEDA-36, 90]

Observational

A retrospective study reviewed the use of felbamate in pediatric patients with refractory epilepsy. The mean age was 5.5 years with a range from 4 months to 17 years. Forty-four percent of patients developed adverse effects. The most common effects were decreased appetite, insomnia, fatigue, irritability and leukopenia. None of the patients developed aplastic anemia or liver failure, which felbamate has US FDA-issued black box warnings [33c].

Systematic Review

A Cochrane review identified the most common reported adverse effects as ataxia, dizziness, fatigue, nausea, and somnolence. No further details or analysis was provided by the authors [34M].

Gabapentin [SEDA-31, 110; SEDA-32, 131; SEDA-33, 136; SEDA-34, 99; SEDA-35, 137; SEDA-36, 90]

Nervous System

A randomized placebo-controlled trial evaluated gabapentin enacarbil for migraine prophylaxis [35C]. A total of 526 patients were randomized to receive gabapentin enacarbil 1200, 1800, 2400, 3000 mg, or placebo daily. Use of gabapentin enacarbil did not differ significantly from placebo in headache prophylaxis. The most common side effects reported were dizziness, fatigue, nausea, and somnolence. Dizziness was the only side effect that occurred more frequently in all treatment groups compared to placebo; however, no statistical analyses were reported for side effects. Uniquely, one serious adverse effect was noted to be possibly caused by gabapentin enacarbil. A patient experienced moderate pseudoseizure (focal left upper extremity jerking, turning of the head to the left side) twice after sexual intercourse. The treatment was stopped and the side effect resolved without further action.

A 76-year-old female in good health who had been taking gabapentin 900 mg/day for 2 years for polyneuropathy abruptly discontinued therapy without medical advice. The day after discontinuation she experienced delirium with mental confusion, incoherent speech, and bizarre behavior. Delirium was responsive to treatment with haloperidol [36A].

Endocrine

A randomized placebo-controlled trial evaluated the effect of gabapentin on hot flashes in postmenopausal women [37c]. Sixty patients were randomized to receive gabapentin 300 mg three times a day for 3 months or placebo. At the end of therapy, the gabapentin group showed a difference in intensity, frequency, and duration of hot flashes compared to the control. The gabapentin group reported more drowsiness but no other significant difference in side effects was noted between the groups.

Urinary Tract

In a prospective study gabapentin was evaluated as an add-on therapy for refractory overactive bladder (OAB) in children [38c]. Thirty-one patients with OAB received oral gabapentin 10-20 mg/kg/day divided into three doses for a period of at least 12 weeks. Continence improved in 16 (53.3%) patients. Twenty-four (80%) of patients experienced mild side effects (concentration problems, mood swings, hyperactivity) and 5 (16.7%) of patients reported moderate side effects (somnolence, anxiety). All patients experiencing mild or moderate side effects continued with therapy. One (3.3%) patient experienced serious side effects (drowsiness, dizziness, headache, and fatigue) and discontinued therapy.

Drug Monitoring

A second prospective study evaluated the efficacy of gabapentin and usefulness of blood level measurements in children with partial seizures [39C]. Thirty children age 2.4–18 years were administered gabapentin titrated to a maximum of 40 mg/kg/day. Blood levels were monitored and effective cases (20) were compared to ineffective cases (10). No side effects were noted in either group; therefore, frequency and severity of side effects could not be correlated to blood levels.

Lacosamide [SEDA-33, 139; SEDA-34, 101; SEDA-35, 138; SEDA-36, 90]

Systematic Review

A systematic review of lacosamide use including 3899 patients confirmed that dizziness (21.2%), diplopia/blurred vision (10.1%), drowsiness/sedation/somnolence (7.3%), headache (6.8%), nausea (6.3%), and ataxia/balance/coordination problems (5.7%) were the most common adverse effects [40R].

Observational

A prospective observational study was performed evaluating the safety and efficacy of lacosamide in infants and children. Drowsiness, nervousness, vomiting, and gait instability were the only reported adverse effects, and occurred in 8 of the 24 patients. Drowsiness in two patients, vomiting in one patient and gait instability resolved after either dose reduction or drug discontinuation [41c]. Another study confirmed that lacosamide was well tolerated in pediatric patients with a 17.5% rate of adverse effects, none of which led to withdrawal [42c].

A retrospective observational study of lacosamide use at a tertiary referral epilepsy reviewed lacosamide safety and efficacy. One-third of patients experienced adverse effects, most commonly dizziness/ataxia, sedation, and diplopia. This risk was more likely to experience adverse effects when on other sodium channel blockers [43c].

A similar large retrospective observational study found similar adverse effects. However, there was no difference in adverse events in those taking concomitant sodium channel blockers [44c].

A retrospective observational study reviewed the use of lacosamide in pediatric patient with refractory partial epilepsy. Somnolence and dizziness were reported in two and three patients respectively. Depression and aggressive behavior was reported in one child each, leading to discontinuation of lacosamide [45c].

In a single-center retrospective observational study evaluated the long term use of lacosamide, 61.4% of patients experienced adverse events with 20.7% of patients discontinuing therapy. The most commonly reported adverse effects were dizziness, double/blurred vision, and digestive complaints [46c]. Other studies have demonstrated similar adverse effects and also demonstrated that adult patients may be more sensitive to lacosamide adverse effects [47c].

A retrospective analysis of lacosamide use in neurosurgical patients with brain tumors showed fatigues, dizziness, confusion, weakness, and nausea as adverse effects in more than one patient [48c].

An observational study evaluated the safety and efficacy of rapid intravenous lacosamide. Infusion times of 15, 30, or 60 minutes were well tolerated, with three patients experiencing diplopia, dizziness, and headache [49c]. Results of another trial evaluating rapid (15 minutes) infusions of lacosamide demonstrated similar results. The risk of adverse events appeared to be dose dependent, with the highest number and severity of events in the 400 mg cohort [50c].

Cardiac

A 56-year-old male presented in cardiac arrest following an intentional ingestion of 7 grams of lacosamide. The patient continued to demonstrates a widened QRS. He did not recover and passed away [51A].

A 49-year-old female developed sinus node dysfunction and bradycardia on 500 mg daily of lacosamide. Symptoms resolved 4 days after discontinuation of lacosamide. Bradycardia and intermittent asystole developed following reintroduction of lacosamide at 100 mg/day [52A].

Neurologic

Two cases are described with status epilepticus during lacosamide monotherapy. A 33-year-old male was receiving 400 mg/day of lacosamide and developed status epilepticus 2 months after a gradual carbamazepine withdrawal. A 56-year-old male on 400 mg of lacosamide daily presented with status epilepticus 2 months after abrupt withdrawal of oxcarbazepine [53A]. The majority of studies evaluated lacosamide as add-on therapy and rate of seizure worsening was 5.3% in a large systematic

review [40A]. Caution should be used with lacosamide as a monotherapy agent.

Psychiatric

A 43-year-old male with a history of phenytoin and lamotrigine use for refractory epilepsy was started on lacosamide. Following 7 days of treatment at 100 mg daily of lacosamide the patient began to have paranoid behavior and psychotic symptoms. Lacosamide was discontinued and the patient was treated with olanzapine. Symptoms resolved 3 days later and olanzapine treatment was continued for 2 weeks [54A]. One study evaluated lacosamide in patients with a history of depression and found no effect on mood or anxiety in most patients [55A].

Pharmacokinetics

No reports of significant adverse events were reported following a single dose of 100 mg intravenous lacosamide in patients with varying levels of renal dysfunction. However, pharmacokinetic data demonstrates that significant accumulation can occur as renal dysfunction decreased [56A].

Drug–Drug Interactions

A 4-year-old girl presented with presumed valproic acid toxicity after her lacosamide dose was increased from 25 to 50 mg twice daily. Previously, the patient was on high dose valproic acid (60 mg/kg/day), and several months earlier had been switched from carbamazepine to oxcarbazepine and initiated on lacosamide (3.8 mg/kg/day). Serum valproic concentration prior to dose increase was 148 mcg/mL which later increased to 199 mcg/mL. Symptoms included decrease appetite, dizziness, trouble walking, and increased somnolence. Laboratory assessments demonstrated hyperammonemic encephalopathy, leukopenia, and thrombocytopenia. The symptoms were consistent with valproate toxicity. Lacosamide and valproate were held and symptoms resolved. Though the timing is suspicious of a lacosamide interaction, the probability is low [57A]. A valproic acid and lacosamide interaction has not been previously demonstrated.

Lamotrigine [SEDA-31, 113, SEDA-32, 134, SEDA-33, 141; SEDA-34, 101; SEDA-35, 138; SEDA-36, 91]

Comparative Studies

A retrospective control study found the cognitive side effect profile of lacosamide and lamotrigine are similar and both are superior to topiramate [58c]. The study compared patients in the outpatient setting. Both subjective and objective measures were evaluated. No difference in memory, quality of life or mood was noted.

A prospective, unblinded, randomized control trial compared the efficacy and tolerability of lamotrigine compared to valproate in adult patients with Juvenile Myoclonic Epilepsy [59C]. The study found lamotrigine similarly efficacious and more tolerable compared to valproate. The most common adverse effects identified with lamotrigine were sleep disturbance and rash (including two cases of Stevens–Johnson syndrome).

Nervous System

A 15-year-old male experienced facial tics that started when lamotrigine was titrated to 150 mg/day for bipolar disorder [60A]. The frequency of tics increased to thousands of times per day when the dose was further increased to 200 mg/day. Symptoms resolved when therapy was switched to sodium valproate. The facial tics were attributed to lamotrigine although the patient was also taking risperidone at the time.

Psychiatric

A literature review evaluated the safety and efficacy of lamotrigine in psychiatric disorders [61M]. The review found the best evidence for lamotrigine in the maintenance treatment of bipolar disorder. Reported adverse effects were similar to patients taking lamotrigine for other indications and included headache, nausea, and rash. Only one case of serious rash was reported.

Skin

A case of pityriasis rosea was reported in a 33-year-old female when she was converted from valproic acid to lamotrigine for epilepsy [62A]. The reaction began as a single lesion on her breast that spread to her trunk and extremities within days, followed by cervical and axillary adenopathy without fever 2 months later. Symptoms resolved after changing lamotrigine back to valproic acid. However, a patch test with lamotrigine in 10% and 30% preparations were negative 3 months after the initial reaction.

A case of toxic epidermal necrolysis (TEN) was reported in a 72-year-old female [63A]. The patient was hospitalized for mucocutaneous erythema and erosion with optical neuromyelitis with concurrent limb spasticity. Treatment with methylprednisolone and lamotrigine was initiated. Symptoms of TEN developed on day 11 of hospitalization after methylprednisolone was stopped. The patient improved with resuming methylprednisolone and intravenous immunoglobulin.

A second case of TEN was reported in a 12-year-old female [64A]. The patient presented with skin eruption, oral mucosa erosion, and eyelid edema 14 days after lamotrigine 25 mg/day was added to her long standing regimen of levetiracetam 1500 mg/day for epilepsy. Both drugs were discontinued and the patient was treated with methylprednisolone 120 mg/day, ventilator and circulatory support, broad spectrum antibiotics, and wound care. By day 17, lesions were resolved and the patient was discharged. Patients should be monitored for dermatologic reactions when starting lamotrigine therapy, especially when prescribed in conjunction with another anticonvulsant medication.

An observational study found that patients with a past medical history of depression were more likely to develop skin rash when beginning lamotrigine for epilepsy compared to those patients without a history of depression [65c]. A possible mechanism could be an immune-mediated pathogenesis, including increased levels of inflammatory cytokines, provoking both depression and rash. The study was unable to exclude other possible risk factors for developing skin reaction such as age, history of rash with AEDs, or lamotrigine dose.

Pharmacogenomics

A case of lamotrigine-induced drug hypersensitivity syndrome was reported in a 32-year-old female of Han-Chinese descent with genotype HLA-B*5801 [66A]. The patient was admitted with fever, generalized erythema, and jaundice 4 weeks after lamotrigine titrated to 100 mg/day was added to her standing valproic acid 400 mg/day therapy for epilepsy. Both lamotrigine and valproic acid were discontinued and the patient improved after treatment with methylprednisolone 60 mg/day and discharged within 1 week.

Death

A review article evaluated the risk of sudden unexpected death in lamotrigine randomized-controlled trials [67R]. The study found 2.2 deaths per 1000 patient years. This was not a statistically significant difference compared to other antiepileptic drugs or controls; however, the researchers did not rule out possible clinical significance.

Levetiracetam [SEDA-31, 116; SEDA-32, 137; SEDA-33, 146; SEDA-34, 104; SEDA-35, 140; SEDA-36, 91]

Observational

A cohort study evaluated the efficacy of levetiracetam in children <16 years [68c]. The study found the primary reason for levetiracetam discontinuation in the patient population was insufficient efficacy followed by poor tolerance. The most common adverse events reported were behavioral or psychological symptoms followed by fatigue or somnolence. One patient was hospitalized secondary to adverse effects but no details were provided by the investigators.

A multicenter, retrospective, open-label study evaluated the efficacy of levetiracetam in electrical status epilepticus during sleep in children [69C]. The study found levetiracetam improved seizures both clinically and on electroencephalography. No patients discontinued therapy due to adverse effects; however, the most commonly reported adverse effects were somnolence, anorexia, and nausea. All symptoms appeared early after initiation.

An open-label study evaluated the efficacy of levetiracetam on seizure frequency and neuropsychological impairments in 11 children with refractory epilepsy with secondary bilateral synchrony [70c]. Eight of the 11 patients were considered responders. Only one patient reported any adverse effects, drowsiness that was not severe enough to warrant discontinuation.

Nervous System

A randomized, double-blind, placebo-controlled trial evaluated the efficacy and tolerability of levetiracetam for central post-stroke pain [71C]. The study did not find a difference in pain control in the levetiracetam group compared to placebo. In addition, patients in the levetiracetam group reported tiredness, pain increase, dizziness, pruritus, and headache more frequently than the control group. Withdrawals were more frequent in the levetiracetam group due to reported effects of fatigue and pain increase.

Psychiatric

A retrospective study evaluated the long-term efficacy and safety of levetiracetam use for epilepsy [72c]. Despite finding a 33.6% seizure-free rate, the study found 486 adverse effects occurring in 55.6% of patients. The most commonly reported adverse effects were irritability, dizziness, headache, and somnolence. Irritability, somnolence, and psychosis were associated with the highest rates of discontinuation. Patients with a history of mood disorders were more likely to develop irritability while patients with a history of psychosis or cognitive impairment were more likely to develop psychosis.

Skin

A case of levetiracetam-induced bullous pemphigoid was reported in a 70-year-old female [73A]. Two months after beginning levetiracetam 1000 mg/day to prevent seizures following stroke, the patient presented with diffuse vesicles on her trunk and proximal extremities. Symptoms improved spontaneously upon discontinuation of levetiracetam and on 2-month follow-up, the patient was lesion-free. The only past medical history besides recent stroke was Alzheimer's and the patient had been taking acetylsalicylate 300 mg daily for 5 years prior to starting levetiracetam.

A case of levetiracetam associated acute generalized exanthematous pustulosis was reported in a 91-year-old female [74A]. The patient with past medical history of hypertension and diabetes was started on levetiracetam for seizures associated with a previous stroke 8 weeks prior and benzyl hydrochlorothiazide for hypertension 6 weeks prior to presenting with skin lesions on the trunk and limbs. Both drugs were stopped and symptoms resolved with corticosteroids. After discharge, benzyl hydrochlorothiazide was restarted without recurrence of skin lesions; therefore, levetiracetam was thought to be the offending agent.

A case of levetiracetam induced erythema multiforme was reported in a 27-year-old female who was started on levetiracetam 1000 mg/day 15 days earlier for epilepsy [75A]. The patient presented with red and itchy eruptions on the dorsal areas of both hands. After the levetiracetam was changed to carbamazepine, her symptoms improved with IV prednisolone.

Renal

A case of levetiracetam to treat seizures following late-onset anticonvulsant hypersensitivity syndrome was reported in a 47-year-old male [76A]. The patient experienced nausea, vomiting, oliguria, and abdominal pain associated with severe renal failure and liver failure after taking phenytoin, lamotrigine, and clobazam for focal cryptogenic epilepsy for 7 years. Symptoms improved after the patient was treated with corticosteroids and hemodialysis and his long-standing anticonvulsant regimen was replaced with levetiracetam with renal dosing.

Liver

A case of acute pancreatitis and elevated liver transaminases was reported in a 25-year-old female after rapid titration of levetiracetam [77A]. The patient with past medical history of post-traumatic stress disorder, borderline hypertension, and prior history of gall stones was started on levetiracetam titrated to 3000 mg/day over 1 week after failing phenytoin for new onset convulsive seizures. On initiation of therapy she experienced abdominal discomfort, nausea, and decreased appetite, which progressed to fever, malaise, increased abdominal pain, vomiting, and diarrhea with increased liver transaminases and pancreatic and lipase enzymes 2 days after reaching the target dose. Symptoms improved with supportive care after levetiracetam was replaced with pregabalin.

A case of levetiracetam-induced encephalopathy in an 84-year-old female was reported [78A]. The patient had a history of epilepsy, arterial hypertension, and arthroplasty of both hips and knees; home medication regimen was lorazepam, furosemide, and valproate. Levetiracetam 1000 mg/day was added following two tonic-clonic seizures. Eleven months later levetiracetam was increased to 1250 mg/day and valproate was changed to lamotrigine 100 mg/day for continued seizures. The patient experienced confusion and electroencephalogram (EEG) changes. Encephalopathy induced by antiepileptic drugs was suspected. Levetiracetam was thought to be the culprit because symptoms improved after discontinued.

Hair

A series of five case reports demonstrated hair loss in adult patients started on levetiracetam for epilepsy [79A]. The 4 females and 1 male between the ages of 21 and 39 all developed hair loss within 2 months of starting levetiracetam treatment. Three were receiving levetiracetam monotherapy and two combination therapy (topiramate; valproate and oxcarbazepine). Symptoms improved with either discontinuation or dose reduction in four cases. The fifth patient continued treatment despite the adverse effect.

Drug Overdose

A case of overdose with levetiracetam in a 49-year-old male in a suicide attempt was reported [80A]. The patient presented to the emergency room 6.5 hours after ingesting 22–500 mg tablets of levetiracetam (358 mg/kg). All vital signs, physical exam, and laboratory results were normal at that time. He was transferred to the MICU for monitoring. All finding continued to be within normal limits except for a BUN of 7 mg/dL 24 hours after presentation. No lasting effects of levetiracetam were noted.

A retrospective chart-review evaluated the safety and tolerability of intravenous levetiracetam to treat seizures in intensive care unit patients [81c]. The study did not identify any adverse effects associated with levetiracetam use. The researchers hypothesized that this was because symptoms such as dizziness and somnolence would not be objectively assessed in a critically ill population.

Teratogenicity

A review of the UK and Ireland Epilepsy in Pregnancy Registers was conducted to evaluate the use of levetiracetam during the first-trimester [82c]. A total of 671 pregnancies were exposed to levetiracetam (304 monotherapy and 367 polytherapy). In the monotherapy group, two major congenital malformations were reported and 19 in the polytherapy group. In the polytherapy group, major congenital malformations were less common when levetiracetam was given in combination with lamotrigine than with valproate or carbamazepine. The study confirms a low risk for developing major congenital malformations when levetiracetam is used as monotherapy during pregnancy.

Drug–Drug Interaction

A case of drug–drug interaction between methotrexate and levetiracetam was reported in a 15-year-old male being treated for acute lymphoblastic leukemia [83A]. After seven intrathecal injections of methotrexate $5 \text{ g/m}^2/\text{day}$, the patient developed seizures and started on levetiracetam 15 mg/kg/day. After three more methotrexate infusions, the patient developed vomiting, renal failure, and hypertension. A rescue procedure was performed with alkaline hydration and administration of IV folinic acid; levetiracetam was changed to clonazepam. When renal function did not improve, the patient received carboxypeptidase G2 which resulted in a rapid decrease of methotrexate levels and improvement in renal function.

Oxcarbazepine [SEDA-31, 118; SEDA-32, 141; SEDA-33, 151; SEDA-34, 106; SEDA-35, 141; SEDA-36, 93]

Cardiovascular

A prospective open-label study evaluated oxcarbazepine's effect on the lipid profile and thyroid hormone concentrations in children with epilepsy [84C]. The study found significant increases of total cholesterol, LDL-C, lipoprotein a, and gamma-glutamyltransferase at 8 months of therapy and significant increases of LDL-C and gamma-glutamyltransferase at 18 months of therapy. In addition, free thyroxine was significantly decreased, while TSH was significantly increased at 8 and 18 months of therapy. No change was noted in HDL-C, triglycerides, or free triiodothyronine.

Nervous System

A case of oxcarbazepine-induced see-saw nystagmus was reported in a 43-year-old female [85A]. The patient presented with dizziness, drowsiness, and generalized urticarial 18 days after starting oxcarbazepine for epilepsy. Jerky see-saw nystagmus on the right eye was noted on exam. Symptoms improved after oxcarbazepine was converted to carbamazepine. Oxcarbazepine was thought to be the culprit due to the known adverse effect of nystagmus (although, not necessarily see-saw nystagmus) and the adverse effect time course.

Musculoskeletal

A prospective study looked at the effect of oxcarbazepine on bone mineral density and biochemical markers of bone metabolism [86c]. The study found that only serum calcium and bone specific alkaline phosphatase (ALP) was reduced significantly after oxcarbazepine use. Bone mineral density at the lumbar spine was significantly increased after oxcarbazepine use if confounders were corrected, but when evaluating gender specifically, it was only increased in female patients.

Electrolyte Balance

A retrospective study evaluated the safety and efficacy of oxcarbazepine for refractory status epilepticus [87c]. Thirteen patients were treated with oxcarbazepine after failed first and second line therapy. Addition of the drug resulted in status epilepticus cessation in eight patients; however, hyponatremia was seen in three patients.

A retrospective review wanted to identify the frequency and risk factors for oxcarbazepine-induced severe and symptomatic hyponatremia [88c]. Age, antiepileptic polytherapy, and concomitant diuretics were independent risk factors for oxcarbazepine-induced severe hyponatremia; age and concomitant diuretics were independent risk factors for oxcarbazepine-induced symptomatic hyponatremia.

Pharmacogenomics

A study investigated the association between oxcarbazepine-induced maculopapular eruptions and the presence of HLA-B alleles in Han Chinese patients. Results demonstrated that the HLA-B*3802 allele occurred significantly more and that there was no difference in the occurrence of HLA-B*1502 in patients taking oxcarbazepine who experienced a maculopapular eruption [89c].

Perampanel [SEDA-35, 142; SEDA-36, 93]

Systematic Review

A meta-analysis of nine studies comparing the use of perampanel to placebo for partial epilepsy or Parkinson's disease was performed to evaluate the adverse event profile of perampanel. The absolute rate of serious adverse effects was 5.7 vs 6.1 ($p = 0.65$) in the perampanel and placebo groups, respectively. Patients experienced a statistically significant increase in dizziness, somnolence, and weight gain. Patients also experienced ataxia, falls, fatigue, and irritability though not statistically significant due to a narrow confidence interval. The risk of ataxia and dizziness were specifically found to be dose dependent [90M]. A meta-analysis showed that both 8 and 12 mg of perampanel were associated with a significant increase in dizziness and 8 mg was associated with a significant increase in somnolence compared to placebo. The 4 mg dose did not demonstrate an increased risk of adverse effects [91M].

Psychiatric

Three observed cases of suicidality were observed in a three young adults: a 21-year-old female, a 22-year-old female, and a 22-year-old male. Patients doses were 8, 4 and 10 mg/day, respectively, and began to develop unreported symptoms between 3 and 8 weeks. Two cases were attributed to impulsive behavior and increased

sensitivity rather than depression; one of which had a history of a suicide attempt with levetiracetam [92c].

Liver

Two cases are reported of potential perampanel liver enzyme induction. The first patient, a 22-year-old male, was taking phenytoin and oxcarbazepine. The patient was initiated on perampanel 2 mg for ongoing epilepsy management. About 2 weeks later the patient presented with status epilepticus. The patient's phenytoin level decreased from 42.8 to 13.2 μmol/L. The patient continued to have decreases in total serum phenytoin levels following perampanel dose titration to 12 mg and required further dose titration of phenytoin. The second patient, a 29-year-old male, presented in status epilepticus 17 days after initiating perampanel. Serum phenobarbital levels were decreased from 150.9 to 65.8 μmol/L and serum rufinamide from 59 to 18 μmol/L. Perampanel induction is possible due to the time course of the patients. Prior phase II trials, however, have not demonstrated significant hepatic interactions. The observations indicate likely induction of CYP2C19 for phenobarbital/phenytoin and carboxylesterase for rufinamide [93c].

Drug Overdose

A case of perampanel toxicity was reported in a 34-year-old Caucasian woman. The patient reported ingesting the remaining trial medication which was estimated to be 204 mg, approximately 25.5 times her daily dose. She was evaluated 75 minutes after initial contact and was found to be in soporific state with a Glasgow Coma Scale of 8. She remained impaired for approximately for 2 days. Follow-up revealed mood instability and impaired impulse control following initiation of perampanel that resolved following psychiatric treatment [94A].

Phenobarbital, Primidone, and Other Barbiturates [SEDA-32, 145; SEDA-33, 154; SEDA-34, 107; SEDA-35, 142; SEDA-36, 93]

Cardiovascular

A case of thiopentone induced bradycardia was reported in a 30-year-old male with new onset tonic-clonic seizures [95A]. A thiopentone 100 mg bolus followed by 100 mg/hour infusion was started which resolved the seizures but resulted in sinus bradycardia within minutes. Thiopentone was stopped and the arrhythmia quickly normalized as well as the return of seizures. Thiopentone was retried at 50 mg/hour which again resulted in sinus bradycardia.

Skin

Two cases of erythema multiforme associated with phenytoin and cranial radiation therapy (EMPACT) were reported with phenobarbital use instead of phenytoin. Both patients were females in their early forties. In one case the rash began in the scalp and the other the trunk, but both spread throughout the body. Both patients had symptomatic improvement with discontinuation of phenobarbital and treatment with intravenous steroids [96c].

A case of phenobarbital-induced pellagra was reported in a 29-year-old female who was taking phenobarbital, levetiracetam, and carbamazepine for epilepsy. Skin eruptions started 1 year after adding phenobarbital to her antiepileptic regimen. Therapy was stopped and the patient was started on prednisolone. The patient was hospitalized and diagnosed with pellagra when dermatologic and neurologic symptoms worsened. Niacin treatment was started but the patient died of multiorgan failure [97A].

Immunologic

A case of hypersensitivity syndrome and Leukemoid reaction due to phenobarbital was reported in a 27-year-old female. The patient presented with erythema and fever in addition to a leukocyte count that peaked at $127.2 \times 109/L$ 3 weeks after beginning phenobarbital for epilepsy. The patient gradually improved with high dose intravenous methylprednisolone after the phenobarbital was discontinued [98A].

Pharmacogenomics

Thai children with the CYP2C19*2 allele were four times more likely to develop phenobarbital associated severe cutaneous adverse drug reactions than those without the allele; however, there was no association with the HLA-B*1520 allele [99c].

Therapeutic Drug Monitoring

A 7.5-year-old female, with nocturnal generalized tonic-clonic seizures and previous episodes of elevated phenobarbital levels, was admitted for lowered consciousness and a phenobarbital level that peaked at 534 μmol/L (65–170 μmol/L). The patient's serum primidone level was elevated to 81.5 μmol/L despite the patient never being previously exposed to primidone. The authors theorized that phenobarbital may have converted back to its prodrug primidone in the setting of severely elevated serum concentrations [100A].

Phenytoin and Fosphenytoin [SEDA-31, 120; SEDA-32, 145; SEDA-33, 155; SEDA-34, 108; SEDA-35, 143; SEDA-36, 94]

Neurologic

A 3-year-old male developed stuttering following initiation of phenytoin 5 mg/kg/day for generalized tonic-clonic seizure post minor head trauma. The patient had

no other symptoms and follow-up imaging revealed no acute abnormalities. Serum concentration was 0.85 mcg/mL (authors did not specify whether this was a free or total serum concentration). Phenytoin was discontinued and valproate was initiated. Ten days post intervention the patient no longer exhibited any symptoms. Dopaminergic activity of phenytoin was suspected; however, there is limited supportive evidence [101A].

A 51-year-old male developed pendular nystagmus 45 minutes after receiving a 1-gram fosphenytoin infusion (13.3 mg/kg). The nystagmus was present with both straight ahead and eccentric gaze and was characterized by both horizontal and vertical movements. There were minimal other neurologic changes. Serum phenytoin was measured at 19.3 mcg/mL. Symptoms resolved in 12 hours. Nystagmus has been reported with supratherapeutic and therapeutic levels of phenytoin; however, this case is unique for pendular eye movements [102A].

A 16-year-old male presented with fever and weakness. Further examination revealed gaze-evoked nystagmus and ataxia, and the MRI demonstrated cerebellar atrophy which was not consistent with prior MRIs. Total serum phenytoin concentration was elevated at 30 mcg/mL. Phenytoin was replaced with valproic acid. The authors did not provide any details on follow-up [103A].

Endocrine

A 40-year-old male presented to the emergency department with generalized tonic-clonic seizures. The patient had a 2-year history of chronic kidney disease and subarachnoid hemorrhage. The patient had been receiving phenytoin for seizure prophylaxis post subarachnoid hemorrhage but no epileptic history. Laboratory assessment demonstrated severe hypocalcemia (total calcium: 1.27 μmol/L; free ionized calcium: 0.77 μmol/L), vitamin D deficiency (13.4 nmol/L), elevated PTH (446 ng/L), and normal serum phosphate (1.34 μmol/L). The lab abnormalities were associated with vitamin D deficiency. Phenytoin was discontinued and calcium and vitamin D were initiated. The patient had resolution of symptoms. The interaction was likely due to phenytoin CYP24A induction, which leads to active vitamin D catabolism [104A].

Mouth and Teeth

A 30-year-old male presented with grade II gingival swelling. The patient had received phenytoin therapy for 11 years and was currently receiving 800 mg daily. Gingival hyperplasia is a commonly reported adverse effect of phenytoin [105A].

A 59-year-old female with a history of phenytoin 300 mg daily for 7 years presented with bilateral swelling in the sub-mandibular region. The swelling had been present for the last 4 years with no other symptoms.

Phenytoin was replaced with oxcarbazepine and biopsy of the submandibular lymph nodes was performed. The biopsy demonstrated multiple granulomas. The patients lymphadenopathy resolved with no other treatment [106A].

Skin

A 33-year-old male developed fever, diffuse rash, jaundice, back pain, dark urine, and oligoanuria after receiving phenytoin for the last 23 days. Hepatosplenomegaly was accompanied with elevated transaminases which peaked on day 6 of admission (AST: 1268; ALT: 1703 IU/I; total bilirubin of 11.74 mg/dL). The patient also had an elevated white blood cell count of 22.4 kcell/mL with 54% neutrophils, 16% eosinophils, and 23% lymphocytes. The presumed diagnosis of drug reaction with eosinophilia and systemic symptoms (DRESS) was diagnosed. The patient was treated with supportive measures, corticosteroids, and withholding phenytoin. Seven days after admission the patient improved significantly and was discharged [107A].

Drug Overdose

A 49-year-old male was admitted in a comatose state after intentional ingestion of 50 phenytoin pills of an unreported strength and developed acute respiratory failure. The patient has a total serum concentration of greater than 40 µg/mL. The following day the patient developed fever and bilateral pulmonary infiltrates and was intubated secondary to respiratory failure. The patient was extubated 5 days post ingestion, despite having a total serum phenytoin concentration >50 mcg/mL. Phenytoin has been associated with multiple pulmonary toxicities, but not acute respiratory failure. Due to the course of the symptoms, it would not be unreasonable to consider an aspiration pneumonitis [108A].

An 88-year-old female with a history of non-compliance on phenytoin was initiated on phenytoin 300 mg daily after head trauma. After 5 days of treatment with phenytoin the patient began to experience vertigo, gait imbalance, dysarthria, and constant involuntary movements. After 26 days of therapy the patient continued to show abnormal neurologic symptoms including orolingual dyskinetic movements and paroxysmal backward neck movements. Furthermore, nystagmus and with severe truncal and appendicular ataxia was observed. Total serum phenytoin levels were 34 mcg/mL. Phenytoin was discontinued and the symptoms completely resolved by day 4 [109A].

A 4-year-old female presented with generalized tonic-clonic seizures with history of vomiting, hypotonia, dysarthria, and dysphagia during the previous 4 days following unintentional ingestion of phenytoin. Further exam demonstrated a GCS of 9, irritability, neck stiffness, and horizontal nystagmus. Serum phenytoin concentrations were elevated at 80 mcg/mL. The patient was given supportive management and all symptoms except dysarthria resolved [110A].

Drug Administration Route

A 71-year-old male presented with purple hand syndrome of the upper right extremity for 2 days. The patient had received intravenous phenytoin 2 days prior. Assessment was negative for deep venous thrombosis or arterial clot; however, intravenous phenytoin was suspected. The patient underwent amputation of two digits and had no further complications. Intravenous phenytoin has been associated with purple glove syndrome and is thought to be attributed partially to phenytoin's poor solubility and potential for precipitation [111A].

A 16-year-old male was given intravenous phenytoin 1000 mg in normal saline in the lower left extremity following two episodes of generalized tonic-clonic seizures. Within 1 hour of infusion, the patient developed severe pain, bruising, and swelling. Distal pulses were diminished. A fasciotomy was performed due to increased compartmental pressure. Symptoms improved and skin closure was performed at 72 hours. The patient had no other complications [112A].

Pharmacogenomics

An observational cohort study reviewed the risk of cerebellar atrophy in patients with CYP2C9 polymorphisms. Nineteen individuals with CYP2C9*2 or *3 polymorphisms were matched to patients with wild-type CYP2C9*1. The mutant CYP2C9 group had a lower white matter normalized for cerebral volumes compared to the wild type group, 1.8% versus 2.3%, respectively ($p = 0.002$). There was no statistical difference in total brain volume (60.3% versus 60.5%, $p = 0.981$) between the groups. The mechanism by which white matter decreases in these patients is unknown; however, patients with altered CYP2C9 isozyme have a decreased metabolic clearance of phenytoin. Though increased serum concentration may be an explanation, the median daily exposure was similar between the two groups (315 mg vs 305 mg, $p = 0.55$). Patients had been stable and followed on phenytoin for greater than a year, though serum levels were not reported by the study [113c].

An observational cohort studied the risk of CYP2C9 polymorphisms on metabolic abnormalities. Patients with CYP2C9 polymorphisms had higher total phenytoin serum concentrations (19 mg/L vs 15.9 mg/L, $p = <0.01$). The patients with wild type CYP2C9 had lower, but clinical insignificant, fasting blood glucose (93.9 vs 97.8, $p = 0.04$) and had higher triglycerides and total, LDL, and HDL cholesterol. Prior studies have demonstrated that phenytoin leads to insulin resistance.

However, those with genetic polymorphisms were likely to have a more favorable lipid profile [114c].

Another observational study evaluated the effect of CYP2C9 polymorphisms on bone health. Those with mutant CYP2C9 had a higher total serum phenytoin concentration (18.9 vs 16.6 mg/L, $p=0.01$). Patients with CYP2C9 polymorphism had a higher femoral neck Z-score (-0.36 vs 0.77, $p=0.4$) and T-score (0.30 vs 0.86, $p=0.02$); no differences were seen in lumbar Z and T-scores. Though data has suggested phenytoin leads to lower vitamin D levels, patients with decreased clearance, had higher vitamin D and more favorable bone mineral density. Furthermore, all groups had a bone mineral density within normal range (-1 to $+1$) [115c].

A case–control study evaluated apolipoprotein E4 allele on several effects comparing newly diagnosed epileptic patients to those with a history of well-controlled epileptic patients. A mini-mental status exam was performed to assess cognitive status. Both newly started and long-term phenytoin users with apolipoprotein E4 allele had a poorer cognitive status with no differences in lipid panels. Furthermore, patients with long term phenytoin use were found to have lower lipid panel indices with the exception of LDL regardless of apolipoprotein E4 allele status [116c].

Drug–Drug Interactions

An 87-year-old male presented with progressive falling and gate instability over the prior 6 months. The patient was diagnosed with invasive tuberculosis cystitis and started on rifampin, isoniazid, ethambutol, and pyrazinamide. Ten days following admission the patient became icteric and developed bilateral nystagmus, intention tremor, and central ataxia. The patient's albumin decreased to 2.4 g/dL, bilirubin increased from 17 to 92 μmol/L, and his total serum phenytoin concentration was 20 mcg/mL. The daily phenytoin was decreased from 200 to 100 mg due to concern of phenytoin toxicity. The patient subsequently had resolution of symptoms. Though free phenytoin concentrations were not measured, the decrease in albumin could lead to increased free and, therefore, toxic phenytoin. The authors did not mention that several potential interactions exist between phenytoin and the patients tuberculosis regimen [117A].

Pregabalin [SEDA-32, 146; SEDA-33, 157; SEDA-34, 110; SEDA-35, 145; SEDA-36, 95]

Nervous System

A 70-year-old female diagnosed with herpes zoster was using pregabalin 150 mg twice daily for pain management [118A]. She experienced vertigo and unsteadiness. Examination revealed truncal ataxia, perverted head-shaking nystagmus and downbeat nystagmus. All symptoms resolved 5 days after discontinuation of pregabalin.

Psychiatric

A data base review evaluated the risk of pregabalin abuse and dependence [119c]. It found that pregabalin abuse or dependence is rare (3.5% rate). Some possible predisposing factors are male gender, history of abuse or dependence on psychotropic substances, and middle age (median age 36 years old.)

A 46-year-old male who was prescribed pregabalin in addition to continuation of milnacipran for treatment of conversion disorder [120A]. Five days after beginning pregabalin, the patient began experiencing manic symptoms including hyperthymia, increased activity, inflated self-esteem, and aggressiveness. Upon increasing the pregabalin the patient experienced grandiose delusion; a manic state was diagnosed and both pregabalin and milnacipran were discontinued. The manic symptoms improved within days of stopping therapy.

Sexual Function

Three case reports were described in which patients experienced anorgasmia during pregabalin use [121c]. All patients were male, age 24–35, and using pregabalin as add-on therapy for partial seizures. In all three cases pregabalin was gradually withdrawn and a different antiepileptic drug added resulting in resolution of side effect.

Retigabine/Ezogabine [SEDA-34, 112; SEDA-35, 146; SEDA-36, 96]

Skin

One patient developed a full body maculopapular rash 6 days following discontinuation. Another developed coma with a GCS of 3 while receiving retigabine 1200 mg with coadministration of citalopram, lamotrigine, and recently started lormetazepam [122c].

Two cases of retigabine induced blue-grey skin dyspigmentation were reported in two females in their early 30s, primarily in the face. Both patients had been on multiple antiepileptics for >2 years; however, the only commonality was retigabine doses at 300 and 350 mg three times daily. Examination ruled out metabolic and other causes of discoloration. Histologic examination demonstrated increased melanin accumulation, similar to other drug induced dyspigmentation. Retigabine was discontinued and patients had full resolution of symptoms within 4 months. Subsequent post-marketing surveillance found 6.3% of patients have skin discoloration [123A]. The US FDA has released updated prescribing information to include risk of retinal abnormalities, potential vision loss, and skin discoloration [124S].

Drug Dosage Regimens

The effect on dose titration was evaluated in a randomized trial conducted on patients with a history of seizure disorder. The most commonly reported adverse effects were somnolence, dizziness, and speech disorder. The three arms consisted of a fast, medium, and slow titration in which patients reached a maximum dose of 1200 mg in 13, 25, and 43 days, respectively. At least one adverse effect was reported in 93% of all patients with no statistically significant difference between the arms. Patients were, however, 5.9 times more likely to discontinue in the fast titration arm due to adverse effects ($p = 0.01$) [122c].

Drug–Drug Interactions

A double-blind, crossover study was performed to assess the effects of 1 g/kg ethanol and retigabine coadministration. Pharmacokinetic analysis demonstrated ethanol increased retigabine's C_{max} by 23% and AUC by 36%. There was no appreciable difference in any adverse effects except blurred vision [125c].

Pharmacokinetics

A pharmacokinetic analysis of two double-blind placebo-controlled trials demonstrated an exposure related increase in developing dizziness, somnolence, abnormal coordination, tremor, blurred vision, and dysarthria [126c].

Rufinamide [SEDA-33, 160; SEDA-34, 113; SEDA-35, 146; SEDA-36, 96]

Placebo-Controlled Trials

A randomized, placebo-controlled trial of rufinamide in patients with Lennox-Gastaut syndrome was performed. Decreased appetite, somnolence, and vomiting were the most commonly reported adverse effects in those taking rufinamide and mostly reported in patients 17 or older [127C].

Systematic Review

A meta-analysis of double-blind, placebo-controlled trials was performed to assess the safety of rufinamide. A total of 1262 patient were included in the analysis. Significant adverse events experienced were somnolence, dizziness, fatigue, and headache. The number needed to treat to experience each adverse event was 14, 6, 16, and 16, respectively. Furthermore, 1 out of 14 patients treated with rufinamide discounted due to an adverse event rate [128M].

Observational Studies

A retrospective observational study evaluated the use of rufinamide in 300 pediatric patients. Medication discontinuation was observed in 15.7% of patients. All discontinuation due to adverse events occurred within the first 3 months of initiation; discontinuation was independent of the number of concurrent antiepileptic, valproic use, or method of titration. This study may indicate that adverse events are most commonly seen early in rufinamide therapy [129c].

A retrospective observational study evaluated the use of rufinamide in children less than 4 years of age. A total of 15% of patients discontinued due to adverse events. The most commonly reported side effects were vomiting, drowsiness, nervousness, and anorexia/weight loss. Dose reduction improved tolerability. Other adverse event reports may have been limited due to patient age [130c].

A small single center study of 23 patients was performed evaluating rufinamide use in Korean patients with Lennox-Gastaut syndrome. Adverse events were minimal and included somnolence, aggressive behavior and aggravation of seizures in a total of six patients [131c].

Hematologic

A 10-year-old male developed agranulocytosis with a total white blood cell count of 5.3 kcell/mL. The patient had been started 200 mg of rufinamide during the prior 17 days, and recently increased to 400 mg/day. The patient also was febrile (40 °C) with a full body rash consistent with erythema multiforme. Work up revealed no other acute abnormalities other than elevated C-reactive protein and lactate dehydrogenase. Rufinamide was withdrawn and symptoms improved rapidly by the third day, and absolute neutrophil count returned to baseline on day 9. The patient had also been receiving lamotrigine, valproic acid, and clonazepam; however, he had been receiving the medications for more than a year, and therefore the time course favors a rufinamide reaction [132A].

Skin

A 10-year-old male developed DRESS. The patient had been initiated on 600 mg/day of rufinamide 1 month prior. The patient exhibited red, indurated papules and erythematous papules. Biopsy demonstrated eosinophils and was consistent with a drug hypersensitivity reaction. The patient also demonstrated lymphadenopathy and lymphopenia. The patient was treated with systemic corticosteroids which resolved the symptoms. Of note the patient had a history of Stevens–Johnson Syndrome associated with lamotrigine and unspecified rash on phenobarbital [133A].

Topiramate [SEDA-31, 124; SEDA-32, 148; SEDA-33, 161; SEDA-34, 114; SEDA-35, 147; SEDA-36, 96]

Psychiatric

A case of topiramate-induced hallucinations and renal tubular acidosis was reported in a 13-year-old female [134A]. The patient had been started on topiramate 150 mg/day and olanzapine 5 mg/day 3 months prior for mental disorder due to epilepsy. The patient improved with sodium bicarbonate and potassium supplementation after medication discontinuation. Olanzapine cannot be ruled out as a contributing factor in this case.

Sensory Systems

A case of topiramate-induced maculopathy was reported in a 22-year-old female [135A]. The patient presented with severe visual acuity deterioration in both eyes 6 days after starting topiramate 100 mg/day for migraine headaches. The patient recovered with steroid therapy after topiramate was discontinued.

Urinary Tract

A prospective study found an increased risk of renal stones in children taking topiramate with 4.8% of study patients developing stones [136C]. Patients also had frequent lithogenic abnormalities on spot urine testing which included hypercalciuria (51%), hypocitraturia (93%), and high urine pH (68%).

Skin

A case of granuloma annulare was reported in a 50-year-old female who was started on topiramate for migraine prophylaxis [137A]. Painless, purplish dermal nodules on the left ankle and leg appeared after 1 month of therapy with topiramate 50 mg/day and resolved after therapy was discontinued. Two years later, the patient had new granuloma annulare after resuming topiramate which again resolved spontaneously after discontinuation.

Pediatrics

A randomized, open-label study evaluating the pharmacokinetics and safety of adjunctive topiramate for refractory partial-onset seizures in infants found that 64% of infants experienced at least one treatment-emergent adverse event [138C]. Most common adverse effects were upper respiratory tract infection (15%), fever (15%), vomiting (13%), somnolence (11%), and anorexia (11%). Adverse effects were more common in patients taking high dose topiramate (25 mg/kg). Adverse effects that resulted in permanent discontinuation included viral infection, maculopapular rash, aggravated convulsions, and somnolence. All infants were taking at least one concurrent antiepileptic drug, therefore adverse effects could be related to the study drug alone or a drug–drug interaction.

A post hoc analysis evaluated the effect of topiramate monotherapy on height in children with newly diagnosed epilepsy [139c]. The study found a significant correlation between height velocity (centimeters per year) z score and change from baseline in height z score. Although continued growth was observed, the rate was slower compared to matched controls.

Drug–Drug Interactions

A case of coma with increased plasma gamma-hydroxybutyrate concentrations was reported in a 52-year-old woman taking gamma-hydroxybutyrate and topiramate for chronic cluster headaches [140A]. Topiramate 25 mg/day was added to the existing regimen of gamma-hydroxybutyrate 9 g/day which the patient had been maintained on for 6 years. After one dose of topiramate, the patient experienced confusion, myoclonic jerks, myiosis, and coma with gamma-hydroxybutyrate plasma concentration at 259 mg/L. Over the next 5 hours, the patient awoke from the coma, rapidly recovered, and plasma concentrations returned to normal. Patients should be monitored closely since both drugs are frequently used to treat headaches and the drug–drug interaction developed rapidly in this case.

A retrospective chart review of patients taking valproic acid with or without topiramate found that the combination of topiramate and valproic acid resulted in a 10-fold increase in the prevalence of valproic acid induced encephalopathy [141c].

Pharmacokinetics

An open-label study compared the pharmacokinetics and safety profiles of intravenous vs oral topiramate [142c]. Bioavailability for the oral formulation was 109%. There was not a statistically significant difference in mean volume of distribution, clearance, and half-life. Side effect profile was similar as well with mild cognitive adverse effects and ataxia occurring in both groups.

Body Temperature

A case of fatal heat stroke was reported in a 40-year-old male taking topiramate and divalproex sodium for seizures following history of gunshot wound to the head [143A]. Serum topiramate and valproate concentrations were within therapeutic range at the time of presentation.

A case of topiramate-induced heat stroke was reported in a 36-year-old male with history of alcohol abuse and head-trauma related epilepsy [144A]. The patient, who was maintained on topiramate 200 mg/day, presented in a comatose state with temperature 41 °C several hours after working in a hot environment. Aggressive treatment was provided in the ICU setting, however, 6 months after the event he was still experiencing some symptoms. Serial MRI images showed regression of signal alterations and restricted diffusion and atrophy.

Valproic Acid [SEDA-31, 126; SEDA-32, 153; SEDA-33, 167; SEDA-34, 116; SEDA-35, 149; SEDA-36, 97]

Liver

A 31-year-old male developed a case of valproate-induced hyperammonemic encephalopathy. Valproic acid was initiated at 500 mg daily after the patient experienced a tonic-clonic seizure and was subsequently diagnosed with a right temporal-insular lesion presumed to be a glioma. Over the course of the next 7 days, his dose was increased to 150 mg. The patient underwent neurosurgery on day 2. Day 6, the patients became lethargic with a GCS of 9. Follow-up diagnostics demonstrated normal imaging and lab values, except an elevated ammonia level of 204 μmol/L and a normal valproic acid of 95 μg/mL (reference 50–100 μg/mL). The valproic acid was discontinued and levetiracetam was initiated. Levocarnitine was given at 100 mg/kg bolus followed by 50 mg/kg every 8 hours for 24 hours. The patient improved rapidly within 24 hours. At 24 hours, the valproic acid level was 77 μg/mL and the ammonia level was 28 μg/mL. The patient did not have repeated symptoms or seizures at 3-month follow-up [145A].

A 57-year-old male developed lethargy that progressed to coma after receiving several doses of valproic acid 1000 mg every 12 hours which was later increased to 1500 mg every 12 hours. The serum valproate level was normal at 54 mg/L and serum ammonia level was elevated at 97 μmol/L. Valproic acid was discontinued and levocarnitine was started at 2.5 mg/kg/day. Despite supportive measures, the patients ammonia continued to increase to 459 μmol/L and hemodialysis was initiated. The patient became asymptotic and the serum ammonia level decreased to 47 μmol/L. The patient was later diagnosed with portosystemic shunt [146A].

A 28-year-old male was admitted after developing a subdural hematoma post-fall. The patient was on valproic acid outpatient but had ceased taking the medication 1 week earlier. Post-operative day 2 the patient was found to be subclinical status epilepticus. The patient was initiated on a valproic acid (0.05 mg/kg/h) and midazolam infusion. The following day the EEG revealed absence of any activity with intact brainstem reflexes. Serum valproic acid concentration was 117 μg/mL and subsequent serum ammonia was 1180 μmol/L. Valproic acid was discontinues and carbamazepine was initiated. Within 48 hours, serum ammonia had decreased to

104 μmol/L and the EEG normalized. The patient demonstrated no neurologic sequel [147A].

A pharmacovigilance study was performed to review all cases of valproate-induced hepatotoxicity. A total of 132 cases were reported; 34 of which were fatal. Analysis of the data demonstrated approximately 35% of cases were in patients with valproic acid monotherapy. Concurrent medication did not appear to affect mortality. Further analysis found that higher rates of non-fatal liver failure in children under age 11. Conclusions should be limited as collected data is dependent on historical reporting to a national database [148c].

Immunologic

A 53-year-old female was taking sodium valproate for a history of post-traumatic seizures for 5 years. The patient had been experiencing symmetrical polyarthritis of the hands, wrists, knees, and feet with concurrent pitting edema; lack of appetite; muscle weakness; and fatigue. Lab values were within normal limits except for normocytic anemia (Hgb 9.5 g/dL) lymphocytopenia (1 kcells/dL), elevated erythrocyte sedimentation rate (ESR) (700 mm/h) and C-reactive protein (CRP) (57 mg/dL). Immunologic testing was positive for antinuclear and antinucleosome antibodies. A clinical diagnosis of Systemic Lupus Erythematous was made. The patient experienced resolution of symptoms when sodium valproate was discontinued and chloroquine 200 mg/day was initiated [149A].

Neurologic

A 40-year-old Caucasian female was given a single IV dose of valproic acid 1000 mg for acute agitation and psychosis. The patient was subsequently intubated for acute altered mental status. Serum ammonia level was found to be 212 μmol/L which increased to 359 μmol/L 14 hours post dose. The patient had normal liver function tests and a serum valproate level of 50 mcg/mL. Serum ammonia levels dropped to 16 μmol/L after 24 hours. The patient returned to baseline at follow-up and was found to have a serum carnitine level of 24 μmol/L [150A].

Hematologic

A 41-year-old male developed cerebral hemorrhage 12 days post-neurosurgical intervention. The patient was initiated on 20 mg/kg/day post-op day 0. An analysis of coagulation laboratory values demonstrated normal function with the exception of hypofibrinogenemia (0.8–1.6 g/L). The patient continued to require daily fibrinogen supplementation for 5 days. On follow-up the patient was found to have a fibrinogen level of 0.53 g/L. Valproic acid induced hypofibrinogenemia was suspected and valproic acid was discontinued; the patients had no further symptoms [151A].

Pancrease

A 15-year-old male presented with history of consistent pain radiant from the back for 6 days. Valproic acid had been initiated at 23 mg/kg 2 months prior. Laboratory analysis was significant for elevated serum and urine amylase, both 10 times the normal upper limit. The patient also had a slightly elevated serum valproic acid level (114.4 μg/mL). An abdominal ultrasound was performed and was consistent with pancreatitis. Potential etiologies were ruled out and valproate induced pancreatitis was suspected. Two days following discontinuation of valproic acid, the serum amylase level decreased to near normal. The patient continued to be asymptomatic at 3-year follow-up [152A].

Multi-organ Failure

A 6-year-old male complained of abdominal pain and vomiting after being initiated on valproic acid 20 mg/kg/day 3 months earlier. The patient demonstrated several lab abnormalities consistent with pancreatitis, acute kidney injury, acute liver dysfunction, thrombocytopenia, and decreased blood pressure. Valproic acid was stopped and supportive measures were initiated. The patient improved clinically by day 10 [153A]. Though acute pancreatitis is a rare reported adverse effect of valproic acid therapy, multi-organ failure may have been precipitated by comorbidities such as sepsis and dehydration.

Teratogenicity

A study found an association with valproate exposure and the risk of developing Autism Spectrum Disorder and Childhood Autism. The 14-year absolute risk is 1.53% (95% CI, 1.47–1.58%) for autism spectrum disorder and 0.48% (95% CI, 0.46–0.51%) for childhood autism. Maternal valproate exposure was associated with a 2.9-fold increase (95% CI, 1.7–4.9) in Autism Spectrum Disorder and a 5.2-fold increase (2.7–10.0) in Childhood Autism adjusted for multiple factors. This association was not found with other antiepileptics [154C].

A retrospective study reviewing fetal malformations and valproic exposure demonstrated a dose-dependent correlation and risk of abnormalities at birth. Spina bifida and hypospadias were associated with maternal exposure of 2000 and 2417 mg daily doses, respectively. Other malformations were associated with significant lower doses of 740–1527 mg. Furthermore, mean maternal daily exposure decreased over time with a corresponding decrease in spina bifida and hypospadias, but not in other malformations. Of note, direct correlation cannot be inferred from the above findings. However, the authors did note that the correlation may be stronger with spina bifida than hypospadias because 85% of spina bifida cases were associated with valproic acid [155c].

Drug Overdose

A case of pediatric valproate toxicity was reported for a 2-year-old female admitted for accidental ingestion of 4-grams of sodium valproate (330 mg/kg). The patient was intubated for a GCS of 8 and had a QTc of 500 ms. Serum valproate levels were 611 mg/L 8 hours post ingestion and the patient was initiated on CVVH. Repeat valproate levels were found to be 97 mg/L 19 hours of dialysis. Both her mental status and QTc had normalized [156A, 157A].

A 7-year-old female with severe developmental delay and cerebral palsy has been receiving valproate for seizure disorder. The patient's valproic acid dose had changed from 250 to 200 mg/mL. However, the same total volume was given leading to a 4-fold increase in dose. The patient presented with 2 months of progressive deterioration and significant lethargy. Upon examination the patient was hypoxic with oxygen saturations of 80%, jugular congestion and slight edema of the peripheral exterminates. Laboratory assessment revealed a chronic respiratory acidosis (pH: 7.32; PCO_2: 76 mmHg; HCO_3: 39 μmol/L), thrombocytopenia (42 kcell/mL), and hypoalbuminemia (3.3 g/dL). The patient's serum valproic acid level was 700 mg/dL. Valproic acid was held and the patient returned to baseline within 5 days [158A].

Vigabatrin [SEDA-31, 136; SEDA-32, 160; SEDA-33, 176; SEDA-34, 121; SEDA-35, 154; SEDA-36, 99]

Neurologic

A retrospective observational study was performed to assess magnetic resonance imaging changes and movements disorders in pediatric patients with infantile spasms. Ten of the 124 patients developed a movement disorder. A likely association was established in two patients. Furthermore, two patients had changes in the globus pallidus, similar to other reports of vigabatrin-induced MRI changes. A link between MRI changes and movement disorders could not be established from this article [159c].

Sensory System

A long-term follow-up study of vigabatrin use was performed to evaluate visual field loss. Nine of the 14 patients on long term vigabatrin had some degree of visual field loss. At the 10-year follow-up, 13 of the 14 patients had visual field loss. Furthermore, each patients trended towards an increase visual field loss with cumulative vigabatrin doses. Visual loss is a well-known adverse effect of vigabatrin. Since this study only evaluated individuals on vigabatrin, the degree of loss compared to those not exposed to vigabatrin cannot be established [160c].

A separate observational study evaluating long-term vigabatrin use found a sharp increased risk of visual field loss for those with a cumulative exposure of 5-grams and 6 years. Furthermore, the risk did not appear to increase immediately, but only following 6 months to 1 year of therapy [161c]. An observational cohort of children receiving vigabatrin demonstrated a 5.3% risk of retinal disease at 6 months, 13.3% at 12 months, and 38% of children at 30 months. This further supports that long term or cumulative exposure of vigabatrin increases risk of eye disease [162c].

Zonisamide [SEDA-31, 137; SEDA-32, 161; SEDA-33, 179; SEDA-34, 123; SEDA-35, 154; SEDA-36, 100]

Meta-Analysis

A meta-analysis was conducted to review the adverse effects profile of zonisamide [163M]. The analysis did not find any major safety concerns but identified the adverse effects occurring most frequently were weight loss and headache.

Observational

An observational study was conducted to evaluate the long term efficacy and tolerability of zonisamide [164c]. Twenty-five percent of patients reported at least one adverse effect; the most common effects were somnolence, fatigue, weight decrease, and asthenia. Adverse effects most often appeared early after starting zonisamide and were not dose-dependent. Three severe adverse effects occurred: acute psychotic disorder requiring hospitalization for delirium, agranulocytosis, and weight loss >12 kg.

Psychiatric

A retrospective chart review evaluated psychiatric adverse effects in patients with a history of mental disorders taking zonisamide for epilepsy [165c]. Twenty-three patients with psychiatric histories including attention-deficit hyperactivity disorder, pervasive development disorder, non-epileptic attack disorder, generalized anxiety disorder, major depressive disorder, obsessive-compulsive disorder, or Tourette's disorder were reviewed. Of those cases the only reported adverse effect of zonisamide was depression in one patient who discontinued therapy due to the adverse effect.

An open-label prospective study evaluated the efficacy and safety of zonisamide for bulimia nervosa [166c]. Zonisamide was associated with decreased frequency of binge-purge episodes while weight remained unchanged. The most common reported adverse effects were fatigue, dry mouth, word finding difficulties, and rash.

Urinary Tract

A case of bilateral urolithiasis with zonisamide in a 10-year-old female was reported [167A]. The patient, who was taking zonisamide for 9 years to treat epilepsy, developed microscopic hematuria while being treated for ventriculoperitoneal shunt infection. Zonisamide was discontinued, a left ureteral stent was placed, ureteral calculi stones were discharged, and symptoms improved. The acute urolithiasis was attributed to zonisamide use in the setting of dehydration.

Lactation

Two cases of nursing mothers taking zonisamide were reviewed [168c]. In the first case, the mother was taking 300 mg/day and milk concentration was found to be 18 μg/mL (44%). By partial breastfeeding (2 of 10 feedings per day), the infant serum level was reduced to below detectable levels. In the second case the mother was taking zonisamide 100 mg/day and the milk concentration was found to be 5.1 μg/mL (36%). The mother chose not to breastfeed in this case. No adverse effects were noted in either infant.

References

[1] Mula M. Emerging drugs for focal epilepsy. Expert Opin Emerg Drugs. 2013;18:87–95. http://dx.doi.org/10.1517/14728214.2013. 750294 [R].

[2] Biton V, Berkovic SF, Abou-Khalil B, et al. Brivaracetam as adjunctive treatment for uncontrolled partial epilepsy in adults: a phase III randomized, double-blind, placebo-controlled trial. Epilepsia. 2014;55:57–66. http://dx.doi.org/10.1111/epi.12433 [C].

[3] Kwan P, Trinka E, Van Paesschen W, et al. Adjunctive brivaracetam for uncontrolled focal and generalized epilepsies: results of a phase III, double-blind, randomized, placebo-controlled, flexible-dose trial. Epilepsia. 2014;55:38–46. http://dx. doi.org/10.1111/epi.12391 [C].

[4] Ryvlin P, Werhahn KJ, Blaszczyk B, et al. Adjunctive brivaracetam in adults with uncontrolled focal epilepsy: results from a double-blind, randomized, placebo-controlled trial. Epilepsia. 2014;55:47–56. http://dx.doi.org/10.1111/epi.12432 [C].

[5] Stockis A, Watanabe S, Rouits E, et al. Brivaracetam single and multiple rising oral dose study in healthy Japanese participants: influence of CYP2C19 genotype. Drug Metab Pharmacokinet. 2014;29:394–9 [c].

[6] Stockis A, Watanabe S, Fauchoux N. Interaction between brivaracetam (100 mg/day) and a combination oral contraceptive: a randomized, double-blind, placebo-controlled study. Epilepsia. 2014;55:e27–31. http://dx.doi.org/10.1111/ epi.12535 [c].

[7] Tangamornsuksan W, Chaiyakunapruk N, Somkrua R, et al. Relationship between the HLA-B*1502 allele and carbamazepine-induced Stevens-Johnson syndrome and toxic epidermal necrolysis: a systematic review and meta-analysis. JAMA Dermatol. 2013;149:1025–32 [M].

[8] Sankhyan N, Gulati S, Hari S, et al. Noninvasive screening for preclinical atherosclerosis in children on phenytoin or carbamazepine monotherapy: a cross sectional study. Epilepsy Res. 2013;107:121–6. http://dx.doi.org/10.1016/j.eplepsyres. 2013.08.011 [c].

[9] Mishra D, Juneja M. Ventricular ectopic beats in a child receiving carbamazepine. Indian Pediatr. 2013;50:612–3 [A].

[10] Kumar V, Aggarwal A, Sharma S, et al. Effect of carbamazepine therapy on homocysteine, vitamin B12 and folic acid levels in children with epilepsy. Indian Pediatr. 2013;50:469–72 [c].

[11] Kim JY, Lee J, Ko YJ, et al. Multi-indication carbamazepine and the risk of severe cutaneous adverse drug reactions in Korean elderly patients: a Korean health insurance data-based study. PLoS One. 2013;8:e83849. http://dx.doi.org/10.1371/journal.pone.0083849 [c].

[12] Werber A, Schiltenwolf M, Barie A. DRESS syndrome. Rare and potentially lethal allergic reaction to carbamazepine - a case report. Schmerz. 2013;27:395–400. http://dx.doi.org/10.1007/s00482-013-1328-8 [A].

[13] Teng P, Tan B. Carbamazepine-induced DRESS syndrome in a child: rapid response to pulsed corticosteroids. Dermatol Online J. 2013;19:18170 [A].

[14] Matsuda H, Saito K, Takayanagi Y, et al. Pustular-type drug-induced hypersensitivity syndrome/drug reaction with eosinophilia and systemic symptoms due to carbamazepine with systemic muscle involvement. J Dermatol. 2013;40:118–22. http://dx.doi.org/10.1111/1346-8138.12028 [A].

[15] Bhanu P, Santosh KV, Gondi S, et al. Neutrophilic eccrine hidradenitis: a new culprit-carbamazepine. Indian J Pharmacol. 2013;45:91–2. http://dx.doi.org/10.4103/0253-7613.106445 [A].

[16] Pranteda G, Muscianese M, Grimaldi M, et al. Lichen sclerosus et atrophicus induced by carbamazepine: a case report. Int J Immunopathol Pharmacol. 2013;26:791–4 [A].

[17] Patel VH, Schindlbeck MA, Bryant SM. Delayed elevation in carbamazepine concentrations after overdose: a retrospective poison center study. Am J Ther. 2013;20:602–6. http://dx.doi.org/10.1097/MJT.0b013e3182258e51 [C].

[18] Venci JV, Rowcliffe MM, Wollenberg L, et al. Pharmacokinetic simulation of fatal carbamazepine intoxication in 23-month old child following phenytoin discontinuation. Forensic Sci Med Pathol. 2013;9:73–6. http://dx.doi.org/10.1007/s12024-012-9373-7 [A].

[19] Reis RM, de Angelo AG, Sakamoto AC, et al. Altered sexual and reproductive functions in epileptic men taking carbamazepine. J Sex Med. 2013;10:493–9. http://dx.doi.org/10.1111/j.1743-6109.2012.02951.x [C].

[20] Hsiao YH, Hui RC, Wu T, et al. Genotype-phenotype association between HLA and carbamazepine-induced hypersensitivity reactions: strength and clinical correlations. J Dermatol Sci. 2014;73:101–9. http://dx.doi.org/10.1016/j.jdermsci.2013.10.003 [c].

[21] Amstutz U, Ross CJ, Castro-Pastrana LI, et al. HLA-A 31:01 and HLA-B 15:02 as genetic markers for carbamazepine hypersensitivity in children. Clin Pharmacol Ther. 2013;94:142–9. http://dx.doi.org/10.1038/clpt.2013.55 [c].

[22] Chong KW, Chan DW, Cheung YB, et al. Association of carbamazepine-induced severe cutaneous drug reactions and HLA-B*1502 allele status, and dose and treatment duration in paediatric neurology patients in Singapore. Arch Dis Child. 2014;99:581–4. http://dx.doi.org/10.1136/archdischild-2013-304767 [c].

[23] He XJ, Jian LY, He XL, et al. Association between the HLA-B*15:02 allele and carbamazepine-induced Stevens-Johnson syndrome/toxic epidermal necrolysis in Han individuals of northeastern China. Pharmacol Rep. 2013;65:1256–62 [c].

[24] Leckband SG, Kelsoe JR, Dunnenberger HM, et al. Clinical Pharmacogenetics Implementation Consortium guidelines for HLA-B genotype and carbamazepine dosing. Clin Pharmacol Ther. 2013;94:324–8. http://dx.doi.org/10.1038/clpt.2013.103 [R].

[25] Rattanavipapong W, Koopitakkajorn T, Praditsitthikorn N, et al. Economic evaluation of HLA-B*15:02 screening for carbamazepine-induced severe adverse drug reactions in Thailand. Epilepsia. 2013;54:1628–38. http://dx.doi.org/10.1111/epi.12325 [c].

[26] Tiamkao S, Jitpimolmard J, Sawanyawisuth K, et al. Cost minimization of HLA-B*1502 screening before prescribing carbamazepine in Thailand. Int J Clin Pharm. 2013;35:608–12. http://dx.doi.org/10.1007/s11096-013-9777-9 [c].

[27] Sperling MR, Abou-Khalil B, Harvey J, et al. Eslicarbazepine acetate as adjunctive therapy in patients with uncontrolled partial-onset seizures: results of a phase III, double-blind, randomized, placebo-controlled trial. Epilepsia. 2015;56(2):244–53. http://dx.doi.org/10.1111/epi.12894. Epub 2014 Dec 22 [C].

[28] Sperling MR, Harvey J, Grinnell T, et al. Efficacy and safety of conversion to monotherapy with eslicarbazepine acetate in adults with uncontrolled partial-onset seizures: a randomized historicalcontrol phase III study based in North America. Epilepsia. 2015;56(4):546–55. http://dx.doi.org/10.1111/epi.12934. Epub 2015 Feb 16 [C].

[29] Correia FD, Freitas J, Magalhães R, et al. Two-year follow-up with eslicarbazepine acetate: a consecutive, retrospective, observational study. Epilepsy Res. 2014;108:1399–405. http://dx.doi.org/10.1016/j.eplepsyres.2014.06.017 [c].

[30] Villanueva V, Serratosa JM, Guillamón E, et al. Long-term safety and efficacy of eslicarbazepine acetate in patients with focal seizures: results of the 1-year ESLIBASE retrospective study. Epilepsy Res. 2014;108:1243–52. http://dx.doi.org/10.1016/j.eplepsyres.2014.04.014 [C].

[31] Massot A, Gimenez-Arnau A. Cutaneous adverse drug reaction type erythema multiforme major induced by eslicarbazepine. J Pharmacol Pharmacother. 2014;5:271–4. http://dx.doi.org/10.4103/0976-500X.142456 [A].

[32] Anyanwu C, Ghavami F, Schuelein M, et al. Ethosuximide-induced conversion of typical childhood absence to Rolandic spikes. J Child Neurol. 2013;28:111–4. http://dx.doi.org/10.1177/0883073812439250 [A].

[33] Heyman E, Levin N, Lahat E, et al. Efficacy and safety of felbamate in children with refractory epilepsy. Eur J Paediatr Neurol. 2014;18:658–62. http://dx.doi.org/10.1016/j.ejpn.2014.05.005 [c].

[34] Shi LL, Dong J, Ni H, et al. Felbamate as an add-on therapy for refractory epilepsy. Cochrane Database Syst Rev. 2011;19(1): CD008295. http://dx.doi.org/10.1002/14651858.CD008295.pub2 [M].

[35] Silberstein S, Goode-Sellers S, Twomey C, et al. Randomized, double-blind, placebo-controlled, phase II trial of gabapentin enacarbil for migraine prophylaxis. Cephalalgia. 2013;33:101–11. http://dx.doi.org/10.1177/0333102412466968 [C].

[36] Di Fabio R, D'Agostino C, Baldi G, et al. Delirium after gabapentin withdrawal. Case report. Can J Neurol Sci. 2013;40:126–7 [A].

[37] Saadati N, Mohammadjafari R, Natanj S, et al. The effect of gabapentin on intensity and duration of hot flashes in postmenopausal women: a randomized controlled trial. Glob J Health Sci. 2013;5:126–30. http://dx.doi.org/10.5539/gjhs.v5n6p126 [c].

[38] Ansari MS, Bharti A, Kumar R, et al. Gabapentin: a novel drug as add-on therapy in cases of refractory overactive bladder in children. J Pediatr Urol. 2013;9:17–22. http://dx.doi.org/10.1016/j.jpurol.2011.10.022 [c].

[39] Nonoda Y, Iwasaki T, Ishii M. The efficacy of gabapentin in children of partial seizures and the blood levels. Brain Dev. 2014;36:194–202. http://dx.doi.org/10.1016/j.braindev.2013.04.006 [C].

[40] Paquette V, Culley C, Greanya ED, et al. Lacosamide as adjunctive therapy in refractory epilepsy in adults: a systematic review. Seizure. 2015;25C:1–17. http://dx.doi.org/10.1016/j.seizure.2014.11.007 [R].

[41] Grosso S, Parisi P, Spalice A, et al. Efficacy and safety of lacosamide in infants and young children with refractory focal epilepsy. Eur J Paediatr Neurol. 2014;18:55–9. http://dx.doi.org/10.1016/j.ejpn.2013.08.006 [c].

[42] Gulati P, Cannell P, Ghia T, et al. Lacosamide as adjunctive therapy in treatment-resistant epilepsy in childhood. J Paediatr Child Health. 2015; http://dx.doi.org/10.1111/jpc.12850 [c].

[43] Kamel JT, DeGruyter MA, D'Souza WJ, et al. Clinical experience with using lacosamide for the treatment of epilepsy in a tertiary centre. Acta Neurol Scand. 2013;127:149–53. http://dx.doi.org/10.1111/j.1600-0404.2012.01704.x [c].

[44] Villanueva V, Garcés M, López-Gomáriz E, et al. Early add-on lacosamide in a real-life setting: results of the REALLY study. Clin Drug Investig. 2015;35:121–31. http://dx.doi.org/10.1007/s40261-014-0255-5 [c].

[45] Kim JS, Kim H, Lim BC, et al. Lacosamide as an adjunctive therapy in pediatric patients with refractory focal epilepsy. Brain Dev. 2014;36:510–5. http://dx.doi.org/10.1016/j.braindev.2013.07.003 [c].

[46] Novy J, Bartolini E, Bell GS, et al. Long-term retention of lacosamide in a large cohort of people with medically refractory epilepsy: a single centre evaluation. Epilepsy Res. 2013;106:250–6. http://dx.doi.org/10.1016/j.eplepsyres.2013.05.002.

[47] Verrotti A, Loiacono G, Pizzolorusso A, et al. Lacosamide in pediatric and adult patients: comparison of efficacy and safety. Seizure. 2013;22:210–6. http://dx.doi.org/10.1016/j.seizure.2012.12.009 [c].

[48] Saria MG, Corle C, Hu J, et al. Retrospective analysis of the tolerability and activity of lacosamide in patients with brain tumors: clinical article. J Neurosurg. 2013;118:1183–7. http://dx.doi.org/10.3171/2013.1.JNS12397 [c].

[49] Li W, Stefan H, Matzen J, et al. Rapid loading of intravenous lacosamide: efficacy and practicability during presurgical video-EEG monitoring. Epilepsia. 2013;54:75–80. http://dx.doi.org/10.1111/j.1528-1167.2012.03651.x [c].

[50] Fountain NB, Krauss G, Isojarvi J, et al. Safety and tolerability of adjunctive lacosamide intravenous loading dose in lacosamide-naive patients with partial-onset seizures. Epilepsia. 2013;54:58–65. http://dx.doi.org/10.1111/j.1528-1167.2012.03543.x [c].

[51] Malissin I, Baud FJ, Deveaux M, et al. Fatal lacosamide poisoning in relation to cardiac conduction impairment and cardiovascular failure. Clin Toxicol. 2013;51:381–2. http://dx.doi.org/10.3109/15563650.2013.778993 [A].

[52] Chinnasami S, Rathore C, Duncan JS. Sinus node dysfunction: an adverse effect of lacosamide. Epilepsia. 2013;54:e90–3. http://dx.doi.org/10.1111/epi.12108 [A].

[53] Papacostas SS. Status epilepticus developing during lacosamide monotherapy. BMJ Case Rep. 2015;2015 http://dx.doi.org/10.1136/bcr-2014-206354. pii: bcr2014206354 [A].

[54] Chatzistefanidis D, Karvouni E, Kyritsis AP, et al. First case of lacosamide-induced psychosis. Clin Neuropharmacol. 2013;36:27–8. http://dx.doi.org/10.1097/WNF.0b013e3182748ecb [A].

[55] Moseley BD, Cole D, Iwuora O, et al. The effects of lacosamide on depression and anxiety in patients with epilepsy. Epilepsy Res. 2015;110:115–8. http://dx.doi.org/10.1016/j.eplepsyres.2014.12.007 [A].

[56] Cawello W, Fuhr U, Hering U, et al. Impact of impaired renal function on the pharmacokinetics of the antiepileptic drug lacosamide. Clin Pharmacokinet. 2013;52:897–906. http://dx.doi.org/10.1007/s40262-013-0080-7 [A].

[57] Jones GL, Popli GS, Silvia MT. Lacosamide-induced valproic acid toxicity. Pediatr Neurol. 2013;48:308–10. http://dx.doi.org/10.1016/j.pediatrneurol.2012.12.039 [A].

[58] Helmstaedter C, Witt JA. The longer-term cognitive effects of adjunctive antiepileptic treatment with lacosamide in comparison with lamotrigine and topiramate in a naturalistic outpatient setting. Epilepsy Behav. 2013;26:182–7. http://dx.doi.org/10.1016/j.yebeh.2012.11.052 [c].

[59] Machado RA, Garcia VF, Astencio AG, et al. Efficacy and tolerability of lamotrigine in juvenile myoclonic epilepsy in adults: a prospective, unblinded randomized controlled trial. Seizure. 2013;22:846–55. http://dx.doi.org/10.1016/j.seizure.2013.07.006 [C].

[60] Lu D, Lin X, Liu X, et al. Lamotrigine-induced facial tic in a pediatric bipolar disorder patient. J Child Adolesc Psychopharmacol. 2013;23:583–4. http://dx.doi.org/10.1089/cap.2013.0057 [A].

[61] Reid JG, Gitlin MJ, Altshuler LL. Lamotrigine in psychiatric disorders. J Clin Psychiatry. 2013;74:675–84. http://dx.doi.org/10.4088/JCP.12r08046 [M].

[62] Papadavid E, Panayiotides I, Makris M, et al. Pityriasis rosea-like eruption associated with lamotrigine. J Am Acad Dermatol. 2013;68:e180–1. http://dx.doi.org/10.1016/j.jaad.2012.10.031 [A].

[63] Haoxiang X, Xu Y, Baoxi W. Lamotrigine-associated with toxic epidermal necrolysis: a case report and Chinese literature review. Int J Dermatol. 2014;53:e231–2. http://dx.doi.org/10.1111/j.1365-4632.2012.05800.x [A].

[64] Calka O, Karadag AS, Bilgili SG, et al. A lamotrigine induced toxic epidermal necrolysis in a child. Cutan Ocul Toxicol. 2013;32:86–8. http://dx.doi.org/10.3109/15569527.2012.662253 [A].

[65] Park SP. Depression in patients with newly diagnosed epilepsy predicts lamotrigine-induced rash: a short-term observational study. Epilepsy Behav. 2013;28:88–90. http://dx.doi.org/10.1016/j.yebeh.2013.03.028 [c].

[66] Chow JC, Huang CW, Fang CW, et al. Lamotrigine-induced hypersensitivity syndrome in a Han Chinese patient with the HLA-B 5801 genotype. Neurol Sci. 2013;34:117–9. http://dx.doi.org/10.1007/s10072-012-0947-7 [A].

[67] Tomson T, Hirsch LJ, Friedman D, et al. Sudden unexpected death in epilepsy in lamotrigine randomized-controlled trials. Epilepsia. 2013;54:135–40. http://dx.doi.org/10.1111/j.1528-1167.2012.03689.x [R].

[68] Dureau-Pournin C, Pedespan JM, Droz-Perroteau C, et al. Continuation rates of levetiracetam in children from the EULEVp cohort study. Eur J Paediatr Neurol. 2014;18:19–24. http://dx.doi.org/10.1016/j.ejpn.2013.07.003 [c].

[69] Chen XQ, Zhang WN, Yang ZX, et al. Efficacy of levetiracetam in electrical status epilepticus during sleep of children: a multicenter experience. Pediatr Neurol. 2014;50:243–9. http://dx.doi.org/10.1016/j.pediatrneurol.2013.10.015 [C].

[70] Kanemura H, Sano F, Sugita K, et al. Effects of levetiracetam on seizure frequency and neuropsychological impairments in children with refractory epilepsy with secondary bilateral synchrony. Seizure. 2013;22:43–7. http://dx.doi.org/10.1016/j.seizure.2012.10.003 [c].

[71] Jungehulsing GJ, Israel H, Safar N, et al. Levetiracetam in patients with central neuropathic post-stroke pain—a randomized, double-blind, placebo-controlled trial. Eur J Neurol. 2013;20:331–7. http://dx.doi.org/10.1111/j.1468-1331.2012.03857.x [C].

[72] Kang BS, Moon HJ, Kim YS, et al. The long-term efficacy and safety of levetiracetam in a tertiary epilepsy centre. Epileptic

Disord. 2013;15:302–10. http://dx.doi.org/10.1684/epd.2013.0599 [c].

[73] Karadag AS, Bilgili SG, Calka O, et al. A case of levetiracetam induced bullous pemphigoid. Cutan Ocul Toxicol. 2013;32:176–8. http://dx.doi.org/10.3109/15569527.2012.725444 [A].

[74] Lee YY, Ko JH, Chung WH. Acute generalized exanthematous pustulosis induced by levetiracetam. Int J Dermatol. 2014;53:e5–6. http://dx.doi.org/10.1111/j.1365-4632.2012.05549.x [A].

[75] Yesilova Y, Turan E, Sonmez A, et al. A case of erythema multiforme developing after levetiracetam therapy. Dermatol Online J. 2013;19:12 [A].

[76] Rodriguez-Osorio X, Pardo J, Lopez-Gonzalez FJ, et al. Levetiracetam following liver and kidney failure in late-onset anticonvulsant hypersensitivity syndrome. J Clin Neurosci. 2014;21:859–60. http://dx.doi.org/10.1016/j.jocn.2013.06.022 [A].

[77] Azar NJ, Aune P. Acute pancreatitis and elevated liver transaminases after rapid titration of oral levetiracetam. J Clin Neurosci. 2014;21:1053–4. http://dx.doi.org/10.1016/j.jocn.2013.08.016 [A].

[78] Hommet C, Beaufils E, Roubeau V, et al. Encephalopathy induced by levetiracetam in an elderly woman. Aging Clin Exp Res. 2013;25:111–3. http://dx.doi.org/10.1007/s40520-013-0009-x [A].

[79] Zou X, Hong Z, Zhou D. Hair loss with levetiracetam in five patients with epilepsy. Seizure. 2014;23:158–60. http://dx.doi.org/10.1016/j.seizure.2013.11.007 [A].

[80] Larkin TM, Cohen-Oram AN, Catalano G, et al. Overdose with levetiracetam: a case report and review of the literature. J Clin Pharm Ther. 2013;38:68–70. http://dx.doi.org/10.1111/j.1365-2710.2012.01361.x [A].

[81] Burakgazi E, Bashir S, Doss V, et al. The safety and tolerability of different intravenous administrations of levetiracetam, bolus versus infusion, in intensive care unit patients. Clin EEG Neurosci. 2014;45:89–91. http://dx.doi.org/10.1177/1550059413496777 [c].

[82] Mawhinney E, Craig J, Morrow J, et al. Levetiracetam in pregnancy: results from the UK and Ireland epilepsy and pregnancy registers. Neurology. 2013;80:400–5. http://dx.doi.org/10.1212/WNL.0b013e31827f0874 [c].

[83] Parentelli AS, Phulpin-Weibel A, Mansuy L, et al. Drug-drug interaction between methotrexate and levetiracetam in a child treated for acute lymphoblastic leukemia. Pediatr Blood Cancer. 2013;60:340–1. http://dx.doi.org/10.1002/pbc.24371 [A].

[84] Garoufi A, Koemtzidou E, Katsarou E, et al. Lipid profile and thyroid hormone concentrations in children with epilepsy treated with oxcarbazepine monotherapy: a prospective long-term study. Eur J Neurol. 2014;21:118–23. http://dx.doi.org/10.1111/ene.12262 [C].

[85] Adamec I, Nankovic S, Zadro I, et al. Oxcarbazepine-induced jerky see-saw nystagmus. Neurol Sci. 2013;34:1839–40. http://dx.doi.org/10.1007/s10072-013-1315-y [A].

[86] Koo DL, Hwang KJ, Han SW, et al. Effect of oxcarbazepine on bone mineral density and biochemical markers of bone metabolism in patients with epilepsy. Epilepsy Res. 2014;108:442–7. http://dx.doi.org/10.1016/j.eplepsyres.2013.09.009 [c].

[87] Kellinghaus C, Berning S, Stogbauer F. Use of oxcarbazepine for treatment of refractory status epilepticus. Seizure. 2014;23:151–4. http://dx.doi.org/10.1016/j.seizure.2013.11.002 [c].

[88] Kim YS, Kim DW, Jung KH, et al. Frequency of and risk factors for oxcarbazepine-induced severe and symptomatic hyponatremia. Seizure. 2014;23:208–12. http://dx.doi.org/10.1016/j.seizure.2013.11.015 [c].

[89] Lv YD, Min FL, Liao WP, et al. The association between oxcarbazepine-induced maculopapular eruption and HLA-B alleles in a northern Han Chinese population.

BMC Neurol. 2013;13:75. http://dx.doi.org/10.1186/1471-2377-13-75 [c].

[90] Zaccara G, Giovannelli F, Cincotta M, et al. The adverse event profile of perampanel: meta-analysis of randomized controlled trials. Eur J Neurol. 2013;20:1204–11. http://dx.doi.org/10.1111/ene.12170 [M].

[91] Hsu WW, Sing CW, He Y, et al. Systematic review and meta-analysis of the efficacy and safety of perampanel in the treatment of partial-onset epilepsy. CNS Drugs. 2013;27:817–27. http://dx.doi.org/10.1007/s40263-013-0091-9 [M].

[92] Huber B. Increased risk of suicidality on perampanel (Fycompa(R))? Epilepsy Behav. 2014;31:71–2. http://dx.doi.org/10.1016/j.yebeh.2013.11.017 [c].

[93] Novy J, Rothuizen LE, Buclin T, et al. Perampanel: a significant liver enzyme inducer in some patients? Eur Neurol. 2014;72:213–6. http://dx.doi.org/10.1159/000362446 [c].

[94] Hoppner AC, Fauser S, Kerling F. Clinical course of intoxication with the new anticonvulsant drug perampanel. Epileptic Disord. 2013;15:362–4. http://dx.doi.org/10.1684/epd.2013.0598 [A].

[95] Sharma S, Nair PP, Murgai A, et al. Transient bradycardia induced by thiopentone sodium: a unique challenge in the management of refractory status epilepticus. BMJ Case Rep. 2013. http://dx.doi.org/10.1136/bcr-2013-200484. pii: bcr2013200484 [A].

[96] Fabbrocini G, Panariello L, Pensabene M, et al. EMPACT syndrome associated with phenobarbital. Dermatitis. 2013;24:37–9. http://dx.doi.org/10.1097/DER.0b013e31827ede32 [c].

[97] Pancar Yuksel E, Sen S, Aydin F, et al. Phenobarbital-induced pellagra resulted in death. Cutan Ocul Toxicol. 2014;33:76–8. http://dx.doi.org/10.3109/15569527.2013.800546 [A].

[98] Zeng Q, Wu Y, Zhan Y, et al. Leukemoid reaction secondary to hypersensitivity syndrome to phenobarbital: a case report. Int J Clin Exp Pathol. 2013;6:100–4 [A].

[99] Manuyakorn W, Siripool K, Kamchaisatian W, et al. Phenobarbital-induced severe cutaneous adverse drug reactions are associated with CYP2C19*2 in Thai children. Pediatr Allergy Immunol. 2013;24:299–303. http://dx.doi.org/10.1111/pai.12058 [c].

[100] Tanoshima R, t Jong GW, Merlocco A, et al. A child exposed to primidone not prescribed for her. Ther Drug Monit. 2013;35:145–9. http://dx.doi.org/10.1097/FTD.0b013e3182843206 [A].

[101] Ekici MA, Ekici A, Ozdemir O. Phenytoin-induced stuttering: an extremely rare association. Pediatr Neurol. 2013;49:e5. http://dx.doi.org/10.1016/j.pediatrneurol.2013.03.011 [A].

[102] Shaikh AG. Fosphenytoin induced transient pendular nystagmus. J Neurol Sci. 2013;330:121–2. http://dx.doi.org/10.1016/j.jns.2013.04.013 [A].

[103] Kumar N, Chakraborty A, Suresh SH, et al. Phenytoin-induced cerebellar atrophy in an epileptic boy. Indian J Pharmacol. 2013;45:636–7. http://dx.doi.org/10.4103/0253-7613.121388 [A].

[104] Nseir G, Golshayan D, Barbey F. Phenytoin-associated severe hypocalcemia with seizures in a patient with a TSC2-PKD1 contiguous gene syndrome. Ren Fail. 2013;35:866–8. http://dx.doi.org/10.3109/0886022X.2013.801300 [A].

[105] Mohan RP, Rastogi K, Bhushan R, et al. Phenytoin-induced gingival enlargement: a dental awakening for patients with epilepsy. BMJ Case Rep. 2013. http://dx.doi.org/10.1136/bcr-2013-008679. pii: bcr2013008679 [A].

[106] Ovallath S, Remya RK, Kumar C, et al. Granulomatous lymphadenopathy secondary to phenytoin therapy. Seizure. 2013;22:240–1. http://dx.doi.org/10.1016/j.seizure.2012.12.005 [A].

[107] Velasco MJ, McDermott J. Drug rash with eosinophilia and systemic symptoms (DRESS) syndrome and hepatitis induced by

phenytoin. Int J Dermatol. 2014;53:490–3. http://dx.doi.org/10.1111/j.1365-4632.2012.05547.x [A].

[108] Kang CK, Kim MK, Kim MJ, et al. Acute respiratory failure caused by phenytoin overdose. Korean J Intern Med. 2013;28:736–8. http://dx.doi.org/10.3904/kjim.2013.28.6.736 [A].

[109] Gunduz T, Kocasoy-Orhan E, Hanagasi HA. Orolingual dyskinesia and involuntary neck movements caused by phenytoin intoxication. J Neuropsychiatry Clin Neurosci. 2013;25:E51. http://dx.doi.org/10.1176/appi.neuropsych.12120396 [A].

[110] Shukla A, Sankar J, Verma A, et al. Acute phenytoin intoxication in a 4-year-old mimicking viral meningoencephalitis. BMJ Case Rep. 2013. http://dx.doi.org/10.1136/bcr-2013-009492. pii: bcr2013009492 [A].

[111] Scumpia AJ, Yahsou J, Cajina J, et al. Purple glove syndrome after intravenous phenytoin administration presenting in the emergency department. J Emerg Med. 2013;44:e281–3. http://dx.doi.org/10.1016/j.jemermed.2012.07.057 [A].

[112] Chhabra P, Gupta N, Kaushik A. Compartment syndrome as a spectrum of purple glove syndrome following intravenous phenytoin administration in a young male: a case report and review of literature. Neurol India. 2013;61:419–20. http://dx.doi.org/10.4103/0028-3886.117611 [A].

[113] Twardowschy CA, Werneck LC, Scola RH, et al. The role of CYP2C9 polymorphisms in phenytoin-related cerebellar atrophy. Seizure. 2013;22:194–7. http://dx.doi.org/10.1016/j.seizure.2012.12.004 [c].

[114] Phabphal K, Geater A, Limapichart K, et al. Role of CYP2C9 polymorphism in phenytoin-related metabolic abnormalities and subclinical atherosclerosis in young adult epileptic patients. Seizure. 2013;22:103–8. http://dx.doi.org/10.1016/j.seizure.2012.10.013 [c].

[115] Phabphal K, Geater A, Limapichat K, et al. The association between CYP 2C9 polymorphism and bone health. Seizure. 2013;22:766–71. http://dx.doi.org/10.1016/j.seizure.2013.06.003 [c].

[116] Palanisamy A, Rajendran NN, Narmadha MP, et al. Association of apolipoprotein E epsilon4 allele with cognitive impairment in patients with epilepsy and interaction with phenytoin monotherapy. Epilepsy Behav. 2013;26:165–9. http://dx.doi.org/10.1016/j.yebeh.2012.11.005 [c].

[117] Robertson K, von Stempel CB, Arnold I. When less is more: a case of phenytoin toxicity. BMJ Case Rep. 2013. http://dx.doi.org/10.1136/bcr-2012-008023. pii: bcr2012008023 [A].

[118] Choi JY, Park YM, Woo YS, et al. Perverted head-shaking and positional downbeat nystagmus in pregabalin intoxication. J Neurol Sci. 2014;337:243–4. http://dx.doi.org/10.1016/j.jns.2013.12.007 [A].

[119] Gahr M, Freudenmann RW, Hiemke C, et al. Pregabalin abuse and dependence in Germany: results from a database query. Eur J Clin Pharmacol. 2013;69:1335–42. http://dx.doi.org/10.1007/s00228-012-1464-6 [c].

[120] Yukawa T, Suzuki Y, Fukui N, et al. Manic symptoms associated with pregabalin in a patient with conversion disorder. Psychiatry Clin Neurosci. 2013;67:129–30. http://dx.doi.org/10.1111/pcn.12012 [A].

[121] Calabro RS, De Luca R, Pollicino P, et al. Anorgasmia during pregabalin add-on therapy for partial seizures. Epileptic Disord. 2013;15:358–61. http://dx.doi.org/10.1684/epd.2013.0592 [c].

[122] Biton V, Gil-Nagel A, Brodie MJ, et al. Safety and tolerability of different titration rates of retigabine (ezogabine) in patients with partial-onset seizures. Epilepsy Res. 2013;107:138–45. http://dx.doi.org/10.1016/j.eplepsyres.2013.08.021 [c].

[123] Shkolnik TG, Feuerman H, Didkovsky E, et al. Blue-gray mucocutaneous discoloration a new adverse effect of ezogabine. JAMA Dermatol. 2014;150:984–9. http://dx.doi.org/10.1001/jamadermatol.2013.8895 [A].

[124] United States. Food an Drug Administration. FDA drug safety communication: FDA approves label changes for anti-seizure drug potiga (ezogabine) describing risk of retinal abnormalities, potential vision loss, and skin discoloration. FDA; 31 Oct. 2013. Web.

[125] Crean CS, Tompson DJ. The effects of ethanol on the pharmacokinetics, pharmacodynamics, safety, and tolerability of ezogabine (retigabine). Clin Ther. 2013;35:87–93. http://dx.doi.org/10.1016/j.clinthera.2012.12.003 [c].

[126] Tompson DJ, Crean CS, Reeve R, et al. Efficacy and tolerability exposure-response relationship of retigabine (ezogabine) immediate-release tablets in patients with partial-onset seizures. Clin Ther. 2013;35:1174–85. http://dx.doi.org/10.1016/j.clinthera.2013.06.012 [c].

[127] Ohtsuka Y, Yoshinaga H, Shirasaka Y, et al. Rufinamide as an adjunctive therapy for Lennox-Gastaut syndrome: a randomized double-blind placebo-controlled trial in Japan. Epilepsy Res. 2014;108:1627–36. http://dx.doi.org/10.1016/j.eplepsyres.2014.08.019 [C].

[128] Alsaad AMS, Koren G. Exposure to rufinamide and risks of CNS adverse events in drug-resistant epilepsy: a meta-analysis of randomized, placebo-controlled trials. Br J Clin Pharmacol. 2014;78:1264–71. http://dx.doi.org/10.1111/bcp.12479 [M].

[129] Thome-Souza S, Kadish NE, Ramgopal S, et al. Safety and retention rate of rufinamide in 300 patients: a single pediatric epilepsy center experience. Epilepsia. 2014;55:1235–44. http://dx.doi.org/10.1111/epi.12689.

[130] Grosso S, Coppola G, Dontin SD, et al. Efficacy and safety of rufinamide in children under four years of age with drug-resistant epilepsies. Eur J Paediatr Neurol. 2014;18:641–5. http://dx.doi.org/10.1016/j.ejpn.2014.05.001.

[131] Lee EH, Yum MS, Ko TS. Effectiveness and tolerability of rufinamide in children and young adults with Lennox-Gastaut syndrome: a single center study in Korea. Clin Neurol Neurosurg. 2013;115:926–9. http://dx.doi.org/10.1016/j.clineuro.2012.09.021.

[132] Ide M, Kato T, Nakata M, et al. A granulocytosis associated with rufinamide: a case report. Brain Dev. 2015. http://dx.doi.org/10.1016/j.braindev.2014.12.010. pii: S0387-7604(15)00002-9. [Epub ahead of print].

[133] Shahbaz S, Sivamani RK, Konia T, et al. A case of Drug Rash with Eosinophilia and Systemic Symptoms (DRESS) related to rufinamide. Dermatol Online J. 2013;19:4 [A].

[134] Cheng M, Wen S, Tang X, et al. Hallucinations and comorbid renal tubular acidosis caused by topiramate in a patient with psychiatric history. Gen Hosp Psychiatry. 2013;35:213.e1–3. http://dx.doi.org/10.1016/j.genhosppsych.2012.04.008 [A].

[135] Gualtieri W, Janula J. Topiramate maculopathy. Int Ophthalmol. 2013;33:103–6. http://dx.doi.org/10.1007/s10792-012-9640-3 [A].

[136] Corbin Bush N, Twombley K, Ahn J, et al. Prevalence and spot urine risk factors for renal stones in children taking topiramate. J Pediatr Urol. 2013;9:884–9. http://dx.doi.org/10.1016/j.jpurol.2012.12.005 [C].

[137] Cassone G, Tumiati B. Granuloma annulare as a possible new adverse effect of topiramate. Int J Dermatol. 2014;53:259–61. http://dx.doi.org/10.1111/ijd.12189 [A].

[138] Manitpisitkul P, Shalayda K, Todd M, et al. Pharmacokinetics and safety of adjunctive topiramate in infants (1-24 months) with refractory partial-onset seizures: a randomized, multicenter, open-label phase 1 study. Epilepsia. 2013;54:156–64. http://dx.doi.org/10.1111/epi.12019 [C].

[139] Ford LM, Todd MJ, Polverejan E. Effect of topiramate monotherapy on height in newly diagnosed children with

epilepsy. Pediatr Neurol. 2013;48:383–9. http://dx.doi.org/10.1016/j.pediatrneurol.2012.12.028 [c].

[140] Weiss T, Muller D, Marti I, et al. Gamma-hydroxybutyrate (GHB) and topiramate-clinically relevant drug interaction suggested by a case of coma and increased plasma GHB concentration. Eur J Clin Pharmacol. 2013;69:1193–4. http://dx.doi.org/10.1007/s00228-012-1450-z [A].

[141] Noh Y, Kim DW, Chu K, et al. Topiramate increases the risk of valproic acid-induced encephalopathy. Epilepsia. 2013;54:e1–4. http://dx.doi.org/10.1111/j.1528-1167.2012.03532.x [c].

[142] Clark AM, Kriel RL, Leppik IE, et al. Intravenous topiramate: comparison of pharmacokinetics and safety with the oral formulation in healthy volunteers. Epilepsia. 2013;54:1099–105. http://dx.doi.org/10.1111/epi.12134 [c].

[143] Borron SW, Woolard R, Watts S. Fatal heat stroke associated with topiramate therapy. Am J Emerg Med. 2013;31:1720.e5–6. http://dx.doi.org/10.1016/j.ajem.2013.07.013 [A].

[144] Muccio CF, De Blasio E, Venditto M, et al. Heat-stroke in an epileptic patient treated by topiramate: follow-up by magnetic resonance imaging including diffusion-weighted imaging with apparent diffusion coefficient measure. Clin Neurol Neurosurg. 2013;115:1558–60. http://dx.doi.org/10.1016/j.clineuro.2013.01.005 [A].

[145] Rigamonti A, Lauria G, Grimod G, et al. Valproate induced hyperammonemic encephalopathy successfully treated with levocarnitine. J Clin Neurosci. 2014;21:690–1. http://dx.doi.org/10.1016/j.jocn.2013.04.033 [A].

[146] Nzwalo H, Carrapatoso L, Ferreira F, et al. Valproic acid-induced hyperammonaemic coma and unrecognised portosystemic shunt. Epileptic Disord. 2013;15:207–10. http://dx.doi.org/10.1684/epd.2013.0575 [A].

[147] Belze O, Remerand F, Pujol A, et al. Hyperammonaemic encephalopathy and a flat electroencephalogram caused by valproic acid. Acta Anaesthesiol Scand. 2013;57:1084. http://dx.doi.org/10.1111/aas.12136 [A].

[148] Schmid MM, Freudenmann RW, Keller F, et al. Non-fatal and fatal liver failure associated with valproic acid. Pharmacopsychiatry. 2013;46:63–8. http://dx.doi.org/10.1055/s-0032-1323671 [c].

[149] Boussaadani Soubai R, Lahlou M, Tahiri L, et al. Valproate-induced systemic lupus erythematous: a case report. Rev Neurol. 2013;169:278–9. http://dx.doi.org/10.1016/j.neurol.2012.09.012 [A].

[150] Sofi A, Herial NA, Ali II. Valproate-induced hyperacute hyperammonemic coma in a patient with hypocarnitinemia. Am J Ther. 2013;20:e703–5. http://dx.doi.org/10.1097/MJT.0b013e3181d56671 [A].

[151] Chen HF, Xu LP, Luo ZY, et al. Valproic acid-associated low fibrinogen and delayed intracranial hemorrhage: case report and mini literature review. Drug Des Devel Ther. 2013;7:767–70. http://dx.doi.org/10.2147/DDDT.S47718 [A].

[152] Veri K, Uibo O, Talvik I, et al. Valproic acid-induced pancreatitis in a 15-year-old boy with juvenile myoclonic epilepsy. Medicina. 2013;49:487–9 [A].

[153] Yaman A, Kendirli T, Odek C, et al. Valproic acid-induced acute pancreatitis and multiorgan failure in a child. Pediatr Emerg Care. 2013;29:659–61. http://dx.doi.org/10.1097/PEC.0b013e31828ec2d5 [A].

[154] Christensen J, Gronborg TK, Sorensen MJ, et al. Prenatal valproate exposure and risk of autism spectrum disorders and childhood autism. JAMA. 2013;309:1696–703. http://dx.doi.org/10.1001/jama.2013.2270 [C].

[155] Vajda FJ. Effect of anti-epileptic drug therapy on the unborn child. J Clin Neurosci. 2014;21:716–21. http://dx.doi.org/10.1016/j.jocn.2013.09.022 [c].

[156] Ray S, Skellett S. Valproate toxicity in a child: two novel observations. Clin Toxicol. 2013;51:60. http://dx.doi.org/10.3109/15563650.2012.746694 [A].

[157] Ray S, Skellett S. Valproate toxicity in a child. Clin Toxicol. 2013;51:194. http://dx.doi.org/10.3109/15563650.2013.776070 [A].

[158] Weiner D, Nir V, Klein-Kremer A, et al. Chronic valproic acid intoxication. Pediatr Emerg Care. 2013;29:756–7. http://dx.doi.org/10.1097/PEC.0b013e318294f558 [A].

[159] Fong CY, Osborne JP, Edwards SW, et al. An investigation into the relationship between vigabatrin, movement disorders, and brain magnetic resonance imaging abnormalities in children with infantile spasms. Dev Med Child Neurol. 2013;55:862–7. http://dx.doi.org/10.1111/dmcn.12188 [c].

[160] Clayton LM, Stern WM, Newman WD, et al. Evolution of visual field loss over ten years in individuals taking vigabatrin. Epilepsy Res. 2013;105:262–71. http://dx.doi.org/10.1016/j.eplepsyres.2013.02.014 [c].

[161] Wild JM, Fone DL, Aljarudi S, et al. Modelling the risk of visual field loss arising from long-term exposure to the antiepileptic drug vigabatrin: a cross-sectional approach. CNS Drugs. 2013;27:841–9. http://dx.doi.org/10.1007/s40263-013-0100-z [c].

[162] Westall CA, Wright T, Cortese F, et al. Vigabatrin retinal toxicity in children with infantile spasms: an observational cohort study. Neurology. 2014;83:2262–8. http://dx.doi.org/10.1212/WNL.0000000000001069 [c].

[163] Verrotti A, Loiacono G, Di Sabatino F, et al. The adverse event profile of zonisamide: a meta-analysis. Acta Neurol Scand. 2013;128:297–304. http://dx.doi.org/10.1111/ane.12147 [M].

[164] Dupont S, Biraben A, Lavernhe G, et al. Management and monitoring of patients treated with zonisamide: the OZONE study. Epileptic Disord. 2013;15:278–88. http://dx.doi.org/10.1684/epd.2013.0591 [c].

[165] Cavanna AE, Seri S. Psychiatric adverse effects of zonisamide in patients with epilepsy and mental disorder comorbidities. Epilepsy Behav. 2013;29:281–4. http://dx.doi.org/10.1016/j.yebeh.2013.08.024 [c].

[166] Guerdjikova AI, Blom TJ, Martens BE, et al. Zonisamide in the treatment of bulimia nervosa: an open-label, pilot, prospective study. Int J Eat Disord. 2013;46:747–50. http://dx.doi.org/10.1002/eat.22159 [c].

[167] Sato S, Nishinaka K, Takahashi S, et al. Bilateral urolithiasis with zonisamide developed for a short period of time in a 10-year-old girl with intractable epilepsy. Nihon Hinyokika Gakkai Zasshi. 2013;104:674–7 [A].

[168] Ando H, Matsubara S, Oi A, et al. Two nursing mothers treated with zonisamide: should breast-feeding be avoided? J Obstet Gynaecol Res. 2014;40:275–8. http://dx.doi.org/10.1111/jog.12143 [c].

8

Opioid Analgesics and Narcotic Antagonists

Alicia G. Lydecker, Matthew K. Griswold, Peter R. Chai[1]

Division of Medical Toxicology, Department of Emergency Medicine, University of Massachusetts Medical School, Worcester, MA, USA

[1]Corresponding author: peter.chai@umassmemorial.org

Low-Dose Ketamine as an Analgesia Adjunct

Pain is a common ailment amongst those seeking medical care. The proportion of emergency department visits with a chief complaint of pain has been reported as high as 78% [1C,2c]. Medical practitioners have a variety of methods to help control pain, although these may be complicated by allergies, side effects, ineffectiveness, and so forth.

Ketamine is a phencyclidine derivative used as an anesthetic and induction agent first reported in 1965 [3E,4R]. Its main mechanism of action is through noncompetitive NMDA receptor antagonism producing dissociative, anesthetic and analgesic effects [5E]. Subdissociative dosing of ketamine has been used since 1971; however, there has been increased interest over the past few years regarding its use as an analgesic [6c]. Analgesic properties of ketamine are found at lower dosing that induction dosing. Current recommendations suggest a range of 0.1–0.3 mg/kg of ketamine—termed "low dose ketamine"—is adequate to achieve analgesia [7c,8C,9R]. Recent studies have demonstrated efficacy of low dose ketamine during labor, war injuries, burns, and significant limb entrapment during motor vehicle accident extrication [10c,11A,12C,13M]. Low dose ketamine has also been described to mitigate severe pain in the postoperative period [14M]. A recent review of postoperative low dose ketamine use for pain relief showed that intravenous administration of ketamine was able to reduce opioid consumption by 40% [15M,3E,5E,9R,10c,11A, 12C,13M,14M].

An emergency department-based study in 2007 showed low-dose ketamine was able to reduce the amount of morphine needed for analgesia by as much as 26% in patients with severe acute traumatic pain (0.149 versus 0.202 mg/kg) [16c]. A recent study comparing the efficacy of morphine to low dose (0.15–0.3 mg/kg) ketamine showed patients had equivalent and longer pain relief when administered ketamine [8C]. There is a growing body of support that suggests that low dose ketamine may be a useful adjunct for acute pain in the emergency department [7c,17M].

Low dose ketamine is well tolerated with minimal side effects. A large retrospective case series examining use of low dose ketamine for pain control in 530 emergency department patients reported an adverse event rate of 6%, with no serious adverse effects defined apnea, laryngospasm, hypertensive emergency, or cardiac arrest [7c]. Another double-blind, randomized, placebo-controlled trial using low dose ketamine combined with morphine for pain control in 60 emergency department patients found dysphoria and dizziness as major side effects [8C].

Low dose ketamine appears to be an effective, safe option for management of acute pain. In a 2013 study, 96% of physicians felt low dose ketamine was underused in the emergency department [17M]. Despite a majority of data demonstrating its effectiveness in achieving analgesia, a recent meta-analysis of low dose ketamine for analgesia examined four randomized controlled trials comprising a total of 428 patients and found a significant reduction in mean pain scores in only two of the studies [18R]. With increased focus on safe prescribing and appropriate use of opioids for pain control, low dose ketamine appears to be an interesting adjunct for achieving analgesia.

Side Effects of Drugs Annual, Volume 37
ISSN: 0378-6080
http://dx.doi.org/10.1016/bs.seda.2015.07.012

© 2015 Elsevier B.V. All rights reserved.

OPIOID RECEPTOR AGONISTS

General Opioid Receptor Agonists

No new information for the current year.
No additional information to add.

ALFENTANIL [SED-15, 72; SEDA-34, 152; SEDA-35, 173; SEDA-36, 108]

Neurological

A review article described the rapid onset and offset of alfentanil (0.96 and 5–20 minutes, respectively) and its short half time (50–55 minutes) which makes it advantageous for general anesthesia [19A]. A small double-blind study assessed the effects of opioid induced hyperanalgesia by comparing cold pain tolerance between two small groups of males who were given either alfentanil or a diphenhydramine placebo. This small study showed a reduction in cold pain tolerance from baseline in the alfentanil group; however, this was not a significant difference [20c].

CODEINE [SED-15, 880; SEDA-34, 152; SEDA-35, 174; SEDA-36, 108]

Pharmacogenetics

A Chinese study sampled bloods from Mongolian volunteers to determine the pharmacokinetics of codeine in populations with variation in CYP2D6 expression. The study assessed the metabolism of codeine and its metabolites, morphine, morphine 3-glucuronide (M3G), morphine 6-glucuronide (M6G) after one oral dose of 30 mg Codeine. The authors showed a significant difference in the area under the curve of CYP2D6 *1/*1 compared to CYP2D6*1/*10 and *10/*10 in the metabolism of morphine, M3G and M6G, revealing that CYP2D6 plays an important role in the pharmacokinetics of the O-demethylated metabolites of codeine after oral administration [21C].

Respiratory

A meta-analysis of randomized control trials from 1994 to 2012 addressing post-surgical pain management using opioids versus non-opioids in pediatric patients. The analysis showed that in 15 of the 16 reports there was no difference in respiratory depression, where as in 1 study there was a relative risk of 1.63 for respiratory depression [22M].

Long-Term Effects
DRUG ABUSE

A retrospective analysis of data from 2004–2011 taken from two drug abuse reporting databanks showed that the drug misuse rate for codeine increased 39% from 2004 to 2011 [23C].

DEXTROMETROPHAN [SED-15, 1088; SEDA-34, 153; SEDA-35, 174; SEDA-36, 108]

Psychiatric

A case report described a 40-year-old male who presented to an emergency department with acute psychosis and irritable mood after ingesting 30 tablets of Coricidin HBP (30 mg dextromethorphan and 4 mg chlorpheniramine per tablet). He was admitted to the intensive care unit, treated with IV benzodiazepines, and had complete resolution of his symptoms within 2 days [24c].

DIAMORPHINE [SED-15, 1096; SEDA-34, 153; SEDA-35, 175; SEDA-36, 108]

Ear, Nose, Throat

A pharmacovigilance study examining 0.1 mg/kg intranasal diamorphine administration in 226 pediatric patients demonstrated nasal irritation, most commonly itching and/or sneezing, in 46 patients (20.4%). All but one case were classified as mild, and most cases (76%) resolved within 1 hour of use. There were no severe or serious adverse effects [25c].

Nervous System

A case report described a 42-year-old male who developed a severe sensory–motor axonal neuropathy in his bilateral lower extremities following an intravenous heroin overdose, thought to be due to an opioid-induced Guillain–Barré Syndrome. He also presented with renal failure secondary to rhabdomyolysis and went on to develop a gluteal compartment syndrome [26A]. Another case study reported a 33-year-old male who presented with amnesia and indirect evidence of seizure 48 hours after his first heroin inhalation. MRI demonstrated cortical laminar necrosis of the left hippocampus in the absence of vascular abnormality. It is unknown if the stroke was due to direct toxicity or as a complication of seizure [27A].

Death

The CDC reported an increase in the death rate from heroin overdose from 1779 to 3635 patients (1.0–2.1 per 100000) between 2010 and 2012. These data were collected from 28 states (56% of the US population) [28C].

Long-Term Effects

DRUG WITHDRAWAL

A case report described a 40-year-old male who developed transient Takotsubo cardiomyopathy 1 day after entering a heroin detoxification unit. He had a 30-year history of inhaled heroin use and had been using approximately 15–20 bags of heroin per day [29A].

Susceptibility Factors

GENETIC FACTORS

A genetic analysis of 828 former heroin users and 232 healthy controls confirmed a negative association of *CSNK1E* SNP rs1534891 with heroin addiction [30c]. A meta-analysis consisting of 20 studies and 9419 participants demonstrated a significant association of the *BDNF* rs6265 polymorphism with heroin dependence in Chinese subjects, suggesting this allele may be a risk factor for heroin addiction in this population [31M].

No additional information to add.

DIHYDROCODEINE [SED-15, 1125; SEDA-34, 154; SEDA-35, 175; SEDA-36, 108]

No new information for the current year.

FENTANYL [SED-15, 1346; SEDA-34, 154; SEDA-35, 176; SEDA-36, 109]

Psychiatric

A case report describes a 73-year-old female who was receiving outpatient palliative treatment for metastatic cancer of unknown origin with 100 μg transdermal fentanyl patch for pain and 10 mg of metoclopramide hydrochloride for nausea who was admitted to an emergency department for auditory and visual hallucinations. The patient had experienced a recent 10 kg weight loss with concurrent hypoalbuminemia. It was determined that the patient suffered a fentanyl overdose and her condition improved following a dose adjustment [32A].

Nervous System

A case report describes a 50-year-old woman with idiopathic pulmonary fibrosis who developed pruritis 30 minutes after receiving intrathecal fentanyl and bupivacaine for regional anesthesia who having a fallopian tube abscess removed. The pruritis resolved immediately following the administration of pentazocine. [33A].

Abuse

A MMWR report found that between November 2013 and March 2014 there was a doubling of drug overdose deaths in Rhode Island compared the same period in previous years. Many of the deaths were among injection drug users and involved the adulteration of the injection drug supply with fentanyl or fentanyl analogs [34C].

The state of Rhode Island reported 10 overdose deaths between March 7 and April 11, 2013 which were confirmed to be the fentanyl analog, acetyl fentanyl. These were the first cases documented of acetyl-fentanyl use as an illicit drug, as well as overdose deaths [35C]. Fentanyl has been associated with 190 confirmed deaths from October 2013 to October 2014 in Southern Ohio [36C].

Musculoskeletal

A case report described the death of a 33-year-old male who was found to have pyomyositis after injecting a combination of morphine and fentanyl "painkillers." It was thought that the pyomyositis might have been caused by skin lesions in the patient's legs, which contributed to an overdose with fentanyl and morphine [37A].

Cardiovascular

A case report of a female patient suffering from recurrent ovarian cancer developed severe symptomatic bradycardia 36 hours after being switched from hydromorphone to transdermal fentanyl without any evidence of opioid toxicity or poor pain control. The patient's symptoms improved following the removal of the fentanyl patch without the administration of atropine [38A].

HYDROCODONE [SED-15, 1702; SEDA-34, 156; SEDA-35, 177; SEDA-36, 109]

Cardiovascular

A 56-year-old female experienced multiple episodes of spontaneously resolving ventricular standstill preceded by nausea after first time oral administration of hydrocodone/acetaminophen. Her cardiac workup was negative and symptoms resolved following cessation of the drug. It was suspected that this arrhythmia was secondary to extreme vasovagal response to hydrocodone [39A].

DEATH

A 48-week drug safety trial ($n = 638$) of hydrocodone bitartrate extended release demonstrated no unexpected adverse effects. One subject died 13 months after study completion by intentional overdose on multiple medications including hydrocodone. Diversion of extended release hydrocodone bitartrate may have occurred [40c].

Susceptibility Factors

GENETIC FACTORS

An observational study of 156 post-Cesarean section patients given hydrocodone/acetaminophen demonstrated a significant relationship with CYP2D6 genotype and plasma concentrations of hydromorphone, a metabolite of hydrocodone. It also showed a significant correlation between pain relief and plasma hydromorphone concentration, but not with hydrocodone concentration. This suggests that the CYP2D6 genotype may impact degree of pain relief experienced following hydrocodone administration [41c].

METHADONE [SED-15, 2270; SEDA-34, 157; SEDA-35, 177; SEDA-36, 110]

Nervous System

A double-blinded randomized control study using 30 subjects who were chronic substance abusers dependent on cocaine and opioids showed that subjects treated with both methadone (96 mg) and topiramate (300 mg) developed cognitive impairment compared to a population that only received methadone [42c].

Skin

A case report describes a male patient receiving methadone for chronic back pain and scrotal pain who developed bilateral peripheral edema. The edema resolved following the cessation of methadone [43A].

Gastrointestinal

A cross-sectional study of drug users with chronic hepatitis C infection observed that patients who were undergoing methadone treatment had a higher likelihood of having a dilated common bile duct—a sign of pancreatobiliary malignancy—on screening abdominal ultrasound. There was no correlation between methadone use and pancreatobiliary cancer [44c].

Cardiac

A large genetics study in Taiwan showed that functional polymorphisms in CYP2C12 increases the metabolism of methadone and the subsequent plasma R-methadone/methadone levels increases the risk of cardiac side effects [45C]. A study of chronic pain patients taking low-dose methadone showed that 5% of patients had a corrected QT interval greater than 500 ms and were therefore at a greater risk for torsades de pointes [46C].

MORPHINE [SED-15, 2386; SEDA-34, 159; SEDA-35, 181; SEDA-36, 111]

Susceptibility Factors

A study of children undergoing tonsillectomies that received intraoperative intravenous morphine found that caucasian girls have increased incidence of postoperative nausea and vomiting, respiratory depression and

prolonged PACU stays when compared to caucasian boys [47C].

Metabolism

A study of pharmacokinetics in 220 children undergoing outpatient adenotonsillectomies found that patients with ABCC3-211C > T polymorphism C/C genotype had approximately 40% higher levels of morphine-6-glucuronide and morphine-3-glucuronide compared to the C/T and T/T genotypes. Patients with OCT1 homozygous genotypes have reduced morphine clearance [48C].

OXYCODONE [SED-15, 2651; SEDA-34, 161; SEDA-35, 182; SEDA-36, 111]

ENT

A case-report described a 41-year-old female with a history of chronic oxycodone nasal insufflation who presented with severe nasal pain and difficulty with nasal breathing and was found to have nasal septal necrosis with abscess formation [49A].

Neuro

A case-report described a 14-year-old female who ingested 75 mg of oxycodone and was found pulseless and apneic by EMS. CPR was initiated and the patient was given naloxone and intubated. The patient was extubated in the intensive care unit, made a completed recovery, and was discharged home. Seven days following the initial ingestion, the patient developed new onset ballism, akathesia, and encephalopathy. Results from magnetic resonance imaging and spectrometry support the notion of oxycodone causing an acute insult with subsequent development of a delayed opioid toxic leukoencephalopathy. Symptoms resolved over the course of 3 months [50A].

Susceptibility Factors

A retrospective study ($n = 280$) examining nausea and vomiting following first time oxycodone use in patients with cancer found significant associations between the development of nausea and male gender (OR = 0.429), use of steroid (OR = 0.417), and history of lung cancer (OR = 2.049). When examining the occurrence of vomiting, the study found significant associations with male gender (OR = 0.4) and use of dopamine D2 receptor antagonists (OR = 2.778) [51c].

Interactions

DRUG–DRUG INTERACTIONS

A self-controlled case series ($n = 513$) demonstrated that coadministration of vitamin K antagonists with oxycodone had a significant association with an elevated INR [52c]. A case report described an 80-year-old hospitalized female who developed myoclonus after completing 7 days of oral ciprofloxacin with a concomitant increase in oxycodone dose from 5 to 10 mg 2 days prior. The ciprofloxacin course ended the day the movement disorder started and the oxycodone was fully discontinued 6 days later. Myoclonus resolved within 2 days of oxycodone discontinuation, leading the authors to suggest that one or both of the above mentioned drugs were likely the causative factor(s) [53A].

Long-Term Effects
DRUG ABUSE

A retrospective cohort study examining two different databases ($n = 13\,814$ and $25\,553$) found the risk of developing opioid abuse was higher with oxycodone than tapentadol [54C].

PAPAVERINE [SED-15, 2678; SEDA-34, 162; SEDA-35, 183; SEDA-36, 112]

Cardiac

A case report described a 64-year-old female who acutely developed QTc prolongation, torsade de points, and ventricular fibrillation following intracoronary administration of 12 mg papaverine during a cardiac study. She had a history of drug-induced QTc prolongation 10 months prior, suggesting this may be a risk factor for papaverine-induced arrhythmia [55A]. A prospective observational study of twenty-five patients who received 20 mg intracoronary papaverine demonstrated transient ST elevation without adverse sequelae in 56% of participants. All of those affected had a history of either diabetes, hypertension, and/or left ventricular hypertrophy [56c].

PETHIDINE (MEPERIDINE) [SED-15, 2791; SEDA-34, 163; SEDA-35, 183; SEDA-36, 112]

No new information for the current year.

REMIFENTANYL [SED-15, 3030; SEDA-34, 163; SEDA-35, 184; SEDA-36, 112]

Gastrointestinal

A double-blinded randomized cross-over trial showed use of remifentanyl is associated with increased risk for gastroesophageal reflux by causing esophagogastric junction impairment due to diaphragm contractions with inspiration. Further research is needed to determine if the swallowing mechanism is affected by remifentantyl [57c]. A second double-blinded cross-over trial study showed that the use of remifentanyl in the monitored anesthesia care setting can cause an increased incidence of aspiration in otherwise healthy individuals [58c].

Neurological

A meta-analysis of literature regarding remifentanyl opioid induced hyperalgesia (OIH) in the surgical setting found conflicting results. Sixteen articles supported the finding of remifentanyl OIH, while 6 articles disproved this finding. There were 22 articles which only discussed the prevention of OIH, however, neither confirmed nor denies the finding of OIH. Further research into OIH is necessary to determine whether remifentanyl causes OIH [59M].

TRAMADOL [SED-15, 3469; SEDA-34, 165; SEDA-35, 184; SEDA-36, 112]

Psychiatric

A study of 79 patients with at least 5 years of high dose (675 mg/day) tramadol dependence found that patients who were dependent showed increased levels of hostility, aggression, and anger. Three months following treatment for dependence patients were found to have significant increases in anxiety, depressive and obsessive-compulsive symptoms [60c].

PARTIAL OPIOID RECEPTOR AGONISTS

Buprenorphine [SED-15, 571; SEDA-34, 166; SEDA-35, 185; SEDA-36, 113]

Drug Administration
OVERDOSE

A review of a nationally representative adverse drug event database showed that buprenorphine was involved in 7.7% of the 1513 surveillance cases of unintentional prescription medication ingestions by children less than 6 years of age. Unsupervised ingestions of buprenorphine accounted for much higher rates of hospitalization of pediatric patients compared to other opioid medications [61C].

A root cause analysis of unintentional buprenorphine exposures to children ages 28 days to 6 years old found that children were more likely to be exposed to buprenorphine tablets in comparison to buprenorphine–naloxone films. There was a higher risk of exposure if the medications were stored not in their original packaging or if it was stored in plain sight [62C].

Allergic Reaction

There is a case report of two women who experienced fatal anaphylactic reactions after injecting buprenorphine. One patient suffered an anaphylactic reaction immediately after injecting a solution containing a crushed buprenorphine tablet. The other patient dissolved a Suboxone (buprenorphine/naloxone) 8 mg/2 mg strip and was found unresponsive and in cardiac arrest 5 minutes later in her room. Autopsies of both patients found elevated serum tryptase levels, eosinophilic infiltration, interstitial hemorrhage and other evidence of anaphylactic reaction [63A].

OPIOID RECEPTOR ANTAGONISTS

Methylnaltrexone [SED-15, 2307; SEDA-34, 168; SEDA-35, 186; SEDA-36, 114]

Nervous System

A randomized, double-blinded, placebo-controlled trial (*n* = 29) showed that administration of methylnaltrexone alone (0.45 mg/kg) resulted in a slight degree of miosis. The authors concluded this is evidence of methylnaltrexone crossing the blood–brain barrier [64c].

Gastrointestinal

A 66-year-old female on an oral morphine pain regimen developed intractable vomiting without preceding nausea following administration of 8 mg subcutaneous methylnaltrexone. The vomiting ceased when the patient's pain medication was switched to hydromorphone [65A].

NALOXONE [SED-15, 2421; SEDA-35, 186; SEDA-36, 114]

Drug–Drug Interaction

Neurologic

A study of 70 young, non-obese patients being treated with buprenorphine and naloxone showed that over half the study population (63%) developed mild sleep disorder breathing based on the apnea/hypoxia index. This shows that naloxone/buprenorphine may alter breathing during a patient's sleep cycle [66c].

NALTREXONE [SED-15, 2423; SEDA-34, 168; SEDA-35, 186; SEDA-36, 114]

Psychiatric

A randomized, double-blind study (*n* = 6) showed that participants who ingested 50 mg naltrexone 1 hour prior to sleep had increased stage 2 sleep, decreased REM sleep, and increased REM latency compared with placebo [67c]. A case report describes 63-year-old male with alcoholism who experienced a "high-like" euphoria after taking placebo capsules. This euphoria was attenuated shortly after ingestion of naltrexone, suggesting naltrexone may block the placebo effect [68A].

References

[1] Cordell WH, Keene KK, Giles BK, et al. The high prevalence of pain in emergency medical care. Am J Emerg Med. 2002;20(3):165–9 [C].

[2] Tanabe P, Buschmann M. A prospective study of ED pain management practices and the patient's perspective. J Emerg Nurs. 1999;25(3):171–7 [c].

[3] Domino EF, Chodoff P, Corssen G. Pharmacologic effects of CI-581, a new dissociative anesthetic, in man. Clin Pharmacol Ther. 1965;6:279–91 [E].

[4] Craven R. Ketamine. Anaesthesia. 2007;62(Suppl 1):48–53 [R].

[5] Lodge D, Anis NA, Burton NR. Effects of optical isomers of ketamine on excitation of cat and rat spinal neurones by amino acids and acetylcholine. Neurosci Lett. 1982;29(3):281–6 [E].

[6] Sadove MS, Shulman M, Hatano S, et al. Analgesic effects of ketamine administered in subdissociative doses. Anesth Analg. 1971;50(3):452–7 [c].

[7] Ahern TL, Herring AA, Anderson ES, et al. The first 500: initial experience with widespread use of low-dose ketamine for acute pain management in the ED. Am J Emerg Med. 2015;33(2):197–201 [c].

[8] Beaudoin FL, Lin C, Guan W, et al. Low-dose ketamine improves pain relief in patients receiving intravenous opioids for acute pain in the emergency department: results of a randomized, double-blind, clinical trial. Acad Emerg Med. 2014;21(11):1193–202 [C].

[9] Persson J. Ketamine in pain management. CNS Neurosci Ther. 2013;19(6):396–402 [R].

[10] Bion JF. Infusion analgesia for acute war injuries. A comparison of pentazocine and ketamine. Anaesthesia. 1984;39(6):560–4 [c].

[11] Cottingham R, Thomson K. Use of ketamine in prolonged entrapment. J Accid Emerg Med. 1994;11(3):189–91 [A].

[12] Joel S, Joselyn A, Cherian VT, et al. Low-dose ketamine infusion for labor analgesia: a double-blind, randomized, placebo controlled clinical trial. Saudi J Anaesth. 2014;8(1):6–10 [C].

[13] McGuinness SK, Wasiak J, Cleland H, et al. A systematic review of ketamine as an analgesic agent in adult burn injuries. Pain Med. 2011;12(10):1551–8 [M].

[14] Yang L, Zhang J, Zhang Z, et al. Preemptive analgesia effects of ketamine in patients undergoing surgery. A meta-analysis. Acta Cir Bras. 2014;29(12):819–25 [M].

[15] Jouguelet-Lacoste J, La Colla L, Schilling D, et al. The use of intravenous infusion or single dose of low-dose ketamine for postoperative analgesia: a review of the current literature. Pain Med. 2015;16(2):383–403 [M].

[16] Lester L, Braude DA, Niles C, et al. Low-dose ketamine for analgesia in the ED: a retrospective case series. Am J Emerg Med. 2010;28(7):820–7 [c].

[17] Richards JR, Rockford RE. Low-dose ketamine analgesia: patient and physician experience in the ED. Am J Emerg Med. 2013;31(2):390–4 [M].

[18] Sin B, Ternas T, Motov SM. The use of subdissociative-dose ketamine for acute pain in the emergency department. Acad Emerg Med. 2015;22(3):251–7 [R].

[19] Mandel JE. Considerations for the use of short-acting opioids in general anesthesia. J Clin Anesth. 2014;26(1 Suppl):S1–7 [A].

[20] Tompkins DA, Smith MT, Bigelow GE, et al. The effect of repeated intramuscular alfentanil injections on experimental pain and abuse liability indices in healthy males. Clin J Pain. 2014;30(1):36–45 [c].

[21] Wu X, Yuan L, Zuo J, et al. The impact of CYP2D6 polymorphisms on the pharmacokinetics of codeine and its metabolites in Mongolian Chinese subjects. Eur J Clin Pharmacol. 2014;70(1):57–63 [C].

[22] Whittaker MR. Opioid use and the risk of respiratory depression and death in the pediatric population. J Pediatr Pharmacol Ther. 2013;18(4):269–76 [M].

[23] Atluri S, Sudarshan G, Manchikanti L. Assessment of the trends in medical use and misuse of opioid analgesics from 2004 to 2011. Pain Physician. 2014;17(2):E119–28 [C].

[24] Aytha SK, Dannaram S, Moorthy S, et al. A case of acute psychosis secondary to coricidin overdose. Prim Care Companion CNS Disord. 2013;15(6) [c]. http://www.ncbi.nlm.nih.gov/pubmed/?term=A+case+of+acute+psychosis+secondary+to+coricidin+overdose.

[25] Kendall J, Maconochie I, Wong IC, et al. A novel multipatient intranasal diamorphine spray for use in acute pain in children: pharmacovigilance data from an observational study. Emerg Med J. 2015;32(4):269–73 [c].

[26] Adrish M, Duncalf R, Diaz-Fuentes G, et al. Opioid overdose with gluteal compartment syndrome and acute peripheral neuropathy. Am J Case Rep. 2014;15:22–6 [A].

[27] Benoilid A, Collongues N, de Seze J, et al. Heroin inhalation-induced unilateral complete hippocampal stroke. Neurocase. 2013;19(4):313–5 [A].

[28] Rudd RA, Paulozzi LJ, Bauer MJ, et al. Increases in heroin overdose deaths—28 states, 2010 to 2012. MMWR Morb Mortal Wkly Rep. 2014;63(39):849–54 [C].

[29] Revelo AE, Pallavi R, Espana-Schmidt C, et al. 'Stoned' people can get stunned myocardium: a case of heroin withdrawal precipitating Tako-Tsubo cardiomyopathy. Int J Cardiol. 2013;168(3):e96–8 [A].

[30] Levran O, Peles E, Randesi M, et al. Dopaminergic pathway polymorphisms and heroin addiction: further support for association of CSNK1E variants. Pharmacogenomics. 2014;15(16):2001–9 [c].

[31] Haerian BS. BDNF rs6265 polymorphism and drug addiction: a systematic review and meta-analysis. Pharmacogenomics. 2013;14(16):2055–65 [M].

[32] Colak S, Erdogan MO, Afacan MA, et al. Neuropsychiatric side effects due to a transdermal fentanyl patch: hallucinations. Am J Emerg Med. 2015;33(3):477.e1–2. http://dx.doi.org/10.1016/j.ajem.2014.08.051 [A].

[33] Hirabayashi M, Imamachi N, Sakakihara M, et al. Treatment of intrathecal fentanyl-induced itch with pentazocine: a case report. Masui. 2014;63(6):696–9 [A].

[34] Mercado-Crespo MC, Sumner SA, Spelke MB, et al. Notes from the field: increase in fentanyl-related overdose deaths—Rhode Island, November 2013–March 2014. MMWR Morb Mortal Wkly Rep. 2014;63(24):531 [C].

[35] Centers for Disease Control and Prevention. Acetyl fentanyl overdose fatalities—Rhode Island, March–May 2013. MMWR Morb Mortal Wkly Rep. 2013;62(34):703–4 [C].

[36] Marinetti LJ, Ehlers BJ. A series of forensic toxicology and drug seizure cases involving illicit fentanyl alone and in combination with heroin, cocaine or heroin and cocaine. J Anal Toxicol. 2014;38(8):592–8 [C].

[37] Kubat B. Drugs, muscle pallor, and pyomyositis. Forensic Sci Med Pathol. 2013;9(4):564–7 [A].

[38] Hawley P. Case report of severe bradycardia due to transdermal fentanyl. Palliat Med. 2013;27(8):793–5 [A].

[39] Sudhakaran S, Surani SS, Surani SR. Prolonged ventricular asystole: a rare adverse effect of hydrocodone use. Am J Case Rep. 2014;15:450–3 [A].

[40] Nalamachu S, Rauck RL, Hale ME, et al. A long-term, open-label safety study of single-entity hydrocodone bitartrate extended release for the treatment of moderate to severe chronic pain. J Pain Res. 2014;7:669–78 [c].

[41] Stauble ME, Moore AW, Langman LJ, et al. Hydrocodone in postoperative personalized pain management: pro-drug or drug? Clin Chim Acta. 2014;429:26–9 [c].

[42] Rass O, Umbricht A, Bigelow GE, et al. Topiramate impairs cognitive function in methadone-maintained individuals with concurrent cocaine dependence. Psychol Addict Behav. 2015;29:237–46 [c].

[43] Dawson C, Paterson F, McFatter F, et al. Methadone and oedema in the palliative care setting: a case report and review of the literature. Scott Med J. 2014;59(2):e11–3 [A].

[44] Leopold SJ, Grady BP, Lindenburg CE, et al. Common bile duct dilatation in drug users with chronic hepatitis C is associated with current methadone use. J Addict Med. 2014;8(1):53–8 [c].

[45] Wang SC, Ho IK, Tsou HH, et al. Functional genetic polymorphisms in CYP2C19 gene in relation to cardiac side effects and treatment dose in a methadone maintenance cohort. OMICS. 2013;17(10):519–26 [C].

[46] van den Beuken-van Everdingen MH, Geurts JW, Patijn J. Prolonged QT interval by methadone: relevance for daily practice? A prospective study in patients with cancer and noncancer pain. J Opioid Manag. 2013;9(4):263–7 [C].

[47] Sadhasivam S, Chidambaran V, Olbrecht VA, et al. Opioid-related adverse effects in children undergoing surgery: unequal burden on younger girls with higher doses of opioids. Pain Med. 2015;16:985–97 [C]. http://www.ncbi.nlm.nih.gov/pubmed/?term=pioid-related+Q10+Q11+adverse+effects+in+children+undergoing+surgery%3A+unequal+burden+on+younger+girls+with+higher+doses+of+opioids.

[48] Venkatasubramanian R, Fukuda T, Niu J, et al. ABCC3 and OCT1 genotypes influence pharmacokinetics of morphine in children. Pharmacogenomics. 2014;15(10):1297–309 [C].

[49] Pulia MS, Reiff C. Oxycodone insufflation resulting in nasal septal abscess. J Emerg Med. 2014;46(6):e181–2 [A].

[50] Beatty CW, Ko PR, Nixon J, et al. Delayed-onset movement disorder and encephalopathy after oxycodone ingestion. Semin Pediatr Neurol. 2014;21(2):160–5 [A].

[51] Kanbayashi Y, Hosokawa T. Predictive factors for nausea or vomiting in patients with cancer who receive oral oxycodone for the first time: is prophylactic medication for prevention of opioid-induced nausea or vomiting necessary? J Palliat Med. 2014;17(6):683–7 [c].

[52] Pottegard A, dePont Christensen R, Wang SV, et al. Pharmacoepidemiological assessment of drug interactions with vitamin K antagonists. Pharmacoepidemiol Drug Saf. 2014;23(11):1160–7 [c].

[53] Kango Gopal G, Hewton C, Pazhvoor SK. Myoclonus associated with concomitant ciprofloxacin and oxycodone in an older patient. Br J Clin Pharmacol. 2014;77(5):906–7 [A].

[54] Cepeda MS, Fife D, Ma Q, et al. Comparison of the risks of opioid abuse or dependence between tapentadol and oxycodone: results from a cohort study. J Pain. 2013;14(10):1227–41 [C].

[55] Goto M, Sato M, Kitazawa H, et al. Papaverine-induced QT interval prolongation and ventricular fibrillation in a patient with a history of drug-induced QT prolongation. Intern Med. 2014;53(15):1629–31 [A].

[56] Jain RK, Chitnis NS, Hygriv Rao B. ST elevation after intracoronary administration of Papaverine for fractional flow reserve estimation. Indian Heart J. 2014;66(3):289–93 [c].

[57] Savilampi J, Ahlstrand R, Magnuson A, et al. Effects of remifentanil on the esophagogastric junction and swallowing. Acta Anaesthesiol Scand. 2013;57(8):1002–9 [c].

[58] Savilampi J, Ahlstrand R, Magnuson A, et al. Aspiration induced by remifentanil: a double-blind, randomized, crossover study in healthy volunteers. Anesthesiology. 2014;121(1):52–8 [c].

[59] Rivosecchi RM, Rice MJ, Smithburger PL, et al. An evidence based systematic review of remifentanil associated opioid-induced hyperalgesia. Expert Opin Drug Saf. 2014;13(5):587–603 [M].

[60] El-Hadidy MA, Helaly AM. Medical and psychiatric effects of long-term dependence on high dose of tramadol. Subst Use Misuse. 2015;50(5):582–9. http://dx.doi.org/10.3109/10826084.2014. 991406 [c].

[61] Lovegrove MC, Mathew J, Hampp C, et al. Emergency hospitalizations for unsupervised prescription medication ingestions by young children. Pediatrics. 2014;134(4):e1009–16 [C].

[62] Lavonas EJ, Banner W, Bradt P, et al. Root causes, clinical effects, and outcomes of unintentional exposures to buprenorphine by young children. J Pediatr. 2013;163(5):1377–83 e1–3 [C].

[63] Boggs CL, Ripple MG, Ali Z, et al. Anaphylaxis after the injection of buprenorphine. J Forensic Sci. 2013;58(5):1381–3 [A].

[64] Zacny JP, Wroblewski K, Coalson DW. Methylnaltrexone: its pharmacological effects alone and effects on morphine in healthy volunteers. Psychopharmacology (Berl). 2015;232(1):63–73 [c].

[65] Stettler A, Zulian GB. Unexpected side effect of methylnaltrexone. J Palliat Med. 2013;16(10):1168 [A].

[66] Farney RJ, McDonald AM, Boyle KM, et al. Sleep disordered breathing in patients receiving therapy with buprenorphine/naloxone. Eur Respir J. 2013;42(2):394–403 [c].

[67] Sramek J, Andry JM, Ding H, et al. The effect of naltrexone on sleep parameters in healthy male volunteers. J Clin Psychopharmacol. 2014;34(1):167–8 [c].

[68] Samokhvalov AV, Gamaleddin I, Sproule B, et al. Naltrexone may block euphoria-like placebo effect. BMJ Case Rep. 2013; http://dx.doi.org/10.1136/bcr-2013-010098 pii: bcr2013010098 [A]. http://www.ncbi.nlm.nih.gov/pubmed/?term=Naltrexone+may+Q12 +block+euphoria-like+placebo+effect.

9

Anti-Inflammatory and Antipyretic Analgesics and Drugs Used in Gout

H. Raber*,1, A. Ali†, A. Dethloff*, K. Evoy*, J. Helmen*, L. Lim‡,
D. Nguyen§, E. Sheridan*

*Saint Joseph Regional Medical Center, Mishawaka, IN, USA
†Campbell University College of Pharmacy and Health Sciences, Buies Creek, NC, USA
‡Purdue University, West Lafayette, IN, USA
§Baylor College of Medicine, Houston, TX, USA
1Corresponding author: hanna.raber@gmail.com

AMIDOPYRINE AND RELATED COMPOUNDS [SEDA-34, 184; SEDA-35, 197]

Metamizole (Dipyrone, Normalidopyrine, Noraminosulfone) [SED-15, 226; SEDA-34, 184; SEDA-35, 197]

Hematologic

Metamizole was withdrawn from the market in several countries due to its potential for agranulocytosis [1R]. The mechanism behind this effect is unclear but thought to be immune mediated.

Renal

A case of acute renal failure alongside severe thrombocytopenia with metamizole was reported [2A].

- A 70-year-old male was admitted and found to have a creatinine of 9.42 mg/dL and platelets of 14 000/μL after metamizole use. He reported taking metamizole within 15 days prior to admission with the last dose administered 4 days prior. Ten days after metamizole discontinuation, the creatinine decreased to 1.4 mg/dL and platelet levels normalized.

Drug–Drug Interaction

In an observational study, metamizole was associated with a reduction in the antiplatelet effects of aspirin in older adults with coronary artery disease (CAD) [3r].

Platelet function was measured by arachidonic (AA) induced light transmission aggregometry and thromboxane (TX) formation by immunoassay. Patients in whom aspirin was withdrawn due to cardiac surgery (group A, $n = 10$) demonstrated AA induced TX formation. TX formation was completely inhibited in patients taking aspirin (group B; $n = 20$). In subjects taking aspirin and dipyrone (group C; $n = 36$), 50% of patients had platelets in which TX formation was fully restored. Randomized controlled trials with clinical endpoints are needed to fully establish the impact of this interaction and generalizability.

ANILINE DERIVATIVES [SED-15, 2679; SEDA-34, 184; SEDA-35, 197]

Paracetamol (Acetaminophen) [SED-15, 2679; SEDA-34, 185; SEDA 35, 197]

Cardiovascular

A single-center prospective observational cross-over study of six ventilated adults investigated the mechanism of intravenous paracetamol-induced hypotension [4c]. After 1 g of paracetamol administration, mean arterial pressure dropped by 7% ($p < 0.001$) with a nadir at the 19th minute. The authors concluded that paracetamol associated hypotension may be due to reduction of both cardiac index and systemic vascular resistance. Small

© 2015 Elsevier B.V. All rights reserved.

sample size, selection bias, and other intrinsic weaknesses limit clinical applicability.

Respiratory

Current evidence continues to be inadequate to justify the association between paracetamol use during pregnancy and in children with the development of asthma or atopic disease [5R].

Metabolism

A systematic review examining the clinical significance of 5-oxoproline in high anion gap metabolic acidosis following paracetamol exposure was conducted [6M]. No clear dose relationship between paracetamol and mortality with 5-oxoproline concentrations was observed and concurrent use of flucloxacilline confounded several of the cases. The cases varied considerably by paracetamol dose, duration, circumstances of exposure, and degree of liver enzyme elevations [6M,7A]. In rare cases, lactic acidosis was found to be associated with 5-oxoprolinemia.

Gastrointestinal

A multicenter prospective study of 402 infants investigated the risk factors associated with pediatric functional constipation (FC) [8C]. The use of acetaminophen as a potential risk factor for FC at 12 months was found to be significant with 79.1% constipated infants ($p = 0.005$) with a trend towards significance at 6 months ($p = 0.06$). No significant association was found between acetaminophen formulations. The mechanism of these effects is unknown but may be serotoninergic in nature.

Liver

The mortality rate of paracetamol-induced acute liver failure is as high as 50% [9H]. One time acetaminophen administration exceeding 15 g may cause severe liver injury that is fatal in 25% of cases [10R]. Acetaminophen associated acute liver damage may occur at therapeutic does and may be more likely in the following circumstances: chronic alcohol use, medications (i.e. CYP2E1 inducers and hepatic glucuronidation competitors), Gilbert syndrome, malnutrition, fasting state, chronic liver disease, and age. Recent literature suggests that protein binding, mitochondrial damage, and possibly apoptotic and necrotic cell deaths in the liver are central to acetaminophen toxicity [11R,12E].

Skin

Several cases of paracetamol induced hypersensitivity skin eruptions have been documented.

- A 33-year-old man presented with symmetrical drug related intertriginous and flexural exanthema (SDRIFE), previously coined "baboon syndrome" after

a single dose of paracetamol 500 mg [13A]. The rash resolved after 10 days.
- A 10-year-old child with a history of atopic dermatitis presented with hypersensitivity vasculitis after paracetamol use for 4 days. A notable increase in rash growth and severity was observed with dose administrations. The rash persisted for 2 months after paracetamol discontinuation [14r].

Teratogenicity

Exposure to paracetamol alone or in combination with nonsteroidal anti-inflammatory drugs (NSAIDs) during the 1st and 2nd trimesters of gestation is associated with an increased risk of cryptorchidism [15c]. A probable mechanism is analgesic-induced inhibition of insulin-like factor 3 levels during gestation.

ARYLALKANOIC ACID DERIVATIVES
[SED-15, 2555; SEDA-34, 185; SEDA-35, 200; SEDA-36, 119–120]

Diclofenac [SEDA-34, 185; SEDA-35, 200; SEDA-36, 119]

Cardiovascular

The UK Medicines and Healthcare Products Regulatory Agency released a warning stating that diclofenac is now contraindicated in patients with ischemic heart disease, peripheral arterial disease, cerebrovascular disease, and congestive heart failure (NYHA class II–IV) [16S]. This warning was in response to the publication of a meta-analysis describing the risk of acute myocardial infarction with use of individual nonsteroidal anti-inflammatory medications which included 25 observational studies published between 1990 and 2011 [17M]. In this analysis, diclofenac use was associated with an increased risk of myocardial infarction (OR 1.38, 95% CI 1.26–1.52). Since this meta-analysis included observational studies only, further research is needed to validate this study.

A 51-year-old man experienced coronary spasm in the absence of anaphylaxis after injection of 75 mg of diclofenac [18A]. The patient was being treated in the emergency department for lower back pain and had no history of drug allergies. Approximately 15 minutes after receiving the injection, the patient became restless and dyspneic and complained of epigastric pain. The patient's blood pressure dropped to 60/40 mmHg for about 5 minutes but he maintained a regular pulse. The ECG showed ST-segment elevation in antero-lateral leads which resolved spontaneously within 30 minutes. The patient had no signs of skin rash, angioedema or pruritus.

Skin

A 40-year-old male was prescribed diclofenac 50 mg three times daily for psoriatic arthritis [19A]. He developed thin and scarred skin on both hands and was diagnosed with diclofenac-induced pseudoporphyria. This patient did have significant sun exposure along with the ingestion of diclofenac, both risk factors for pseudoporphyria. Upon discontinuation of diclofenac, the skin fragility subsided and upon re-initiation it returned.

A 65-year-old male presented with a severe rash on his lower back after applying topical diclofenac to treat backache the previous day [20A]. The rash developed into a severe macular rash with blistering covering his upper and lower back and abdomen. This patient had previously used topical diclofenac without any rash development. This reaction was attributed to the combination of topical diclofenac application and sun exposure.

Pregnancy

A prospective cohort study of 90 417 pregnant women in Norway, including 6511 who used diclofenac, ibuprofen, naproxen, or piroxicam ($n = 5325, 491, 354$, and 150, respectively) during pregnancy and 83,906 women who did not use any of these medications, sought to determine the risk of adverse effects with exposure to the individual NSAID during specific trimesters of pregnancy [21c]. Utilizing multiple surveys and the Medical Birth Registry of Norway, the authors assessed the risk of stillbirth, any congenital malformations, major congenital malformations, patent *ductus arteriosus*, low birth weight, premature birth, Apgar score less than seven, neonatal respiratory depression, intracranial hemorrhage, intraventricular hemorrhage, vaginal bleeding during pregnancy, postpartum hemorrhage >500 milliliter, structural heart defects, and asthma within 18 months of birth. While there was no effect on infant survival, congenital malformation, or structural heart defects with any study medication, the following associations were found to be significant: second trimester ibuprofen use and low birth weight (adjusted OR 1.7, 95% CI 1.3–2.3); second and third trimester ibuprofen use and asthma at 18 months (adjusted OR 1.5, 95% CI 1.2–1.9 and adjusted OR 1.5, 95% CI 1.1–2.1, respectively); second trimester diclofenac use and low birth weight (adjusted OR 3.1, 95% CI 1.1–9.0); third trimester diclofenac use and maternal vaginal bleeding (adjusted OR 1.8, 95% CI 1.1–3.0). Additionally, while patient ductus arteriosus was not statistically significantly correlated with any of the four study medications, three cases were seen with third trimester diclofenac use (1.3% vs. 0.3%, 95% CI not provided). No other outcome measured showed statistically significant differences with the use of these medications during pregnancy versus unexposed women. When analyzing the results of this trial, it is important to consider potential limitations in external validity as this study was conducted solely in Norway. In addition, as this was survey-based research, the potential impact of recall bias must also be noted. Additionally, while a large number of patients were included in the study, there were relatively few patients exposed to naproxen or piroxicam, and thus it would be difficult to detect significant differences in rare adverse events with their use.

Two cases of diclofenac-induced intrauterine ductal closure were reported.

- A 28-year-old woman was unaware she was pregnant and had been taking diclofenac sodium 75 mg for back pain as needed for about 2 weeks while 7 months pregnant [22A]. A fetal echocardiogram 6 hours postnatally showed a dilated right atrium and ventricle with marked right ventricular hypertrophy and impaired function.
- Another case of intrauterine ductal closure was identified in a 31-year-old woman who also took diclofenac during pregnancy [23A]. This patient had only taken a single dose of diclofenac for a headache at 37 weeks gestation. Fetal echocardiogram showed mild right ventricular hypertrophy and moderate tricuspid valve regurgitation.

Ibuprofen [SEDA-34, 185; SEDA-35, 200; SEDA-36, 119]

Renal

A small study (52 patients, 26 receiving ibuprofen and 26 not receiving ibuprofen) was designed to determine the impact of chronic (at least 1 year) ibuprofen use in cystic fibrosis patients between the ages of 3 and 25 on markers of kidney injury. Patients with cystic fibrosis often are administered multiple renal toxic medications, but chronic use of 20–30 mg/kg of ibuprofen twice daily may be desirable as it has been shown to delay progression of pulmonary disease [24c]. This study displayed no difference in three markers of kidney injury (kidney injury molecule-1, N-acetyl-beta-glucosaminidase, or urinary protein levels) in patients receiving ibuprofen versus those not receiving ibuprofen. The authors concluded that chronic ibuprofen use may be safely administered in carefully selected cystic fibrosis patient populations without causing significant kidney injury. However, due to the very small number of patients in this trial, the assessment of kidney injury based on surrogate markers from a single blood draw, and the inclusion of patients from a single practice site, more evidence needs to be collected to validate this conclusion.

Oral

Three reports of a burning sensation in the mouth while consuming ibuprofen (two cases during ingestion of ibuprofen oral suspension and one following improper chewing of an oral gel cap which also resulted in edema and a burning in the throat) were described based on reports submitted via post-marketing surveillance from a Polish manufacturer of ibuprofen [25c]. Neither drug dose nor patient demographics were reported. These reactions resolved spontaneously and are likely of no clinical consequence.

Gastrointestinal

A case of ibuprofen-induced small bowel stricture was reported adding to the limited number of reports of this rare adverse effect of NSAIDs and was likely incurred due to abuse of codeine co-formulated with ibuprofen in a codeine-dependent patient [26A].

- A 35-year-old Australian man presented with 3 months of abdominal pain, acutely worsening, in the setting of codeine and ibuprofen abuse. Imaging revealed a small bowel obstruction due to fibrous stricture with extensive reactive and inflammatory changes consistent with prolonged NSAID abuse. Based on patient account, he had been using codeine/ibuprofen for 10 years and reported ingestion of up to 90 tablets (equivalent to between 450–1153 mg of codeine and 18000 mg of ibuprofen) per day.

A pooled analysis of two previously conducted clinical trials comparing single-tablet ibuprofen/famotidine versus ibuprofen alone provided further confirmation that the addition of acid-suppressing medications like famotidine reduces the incidence of upper gastrointestinal ulcers, displaying a 44% reduction in the ibuprofen/famotidine group versus those receiving ibuprofen alone amongst the 776 patients included in the study [27C].

Dependence

Based on the author's search, this case describes the first report of ibuprofen dependence [28A].

- A 17-year-old female was taking ibuprofen 400 mg eight times daily, originally for knee pain, over a relatively short time-frame (less than 1 year). Upon abrupt discontinuation, she developed withdrawal signs of tremor, sweating, and anxiety with symptoms resolved by resuming ibuprofen. After slowly weaning, the patient remained sober for 3 weeks before resuming ibuprofen dosing at 400 mg four to five times per day based on self-described fear of withdrawal, as well as anxiolysis and stimulation received from ibuprofen that made it impossible for her to wait 6 hours for her next dose. Under the treatment of a physician specializing in addiction, she

made several attempts to wean the drug without success and would continue to report similar withdrawal symptoms with reduced consumption. She was eventually diagnosed with ibuprofen dependence, meeting the most recent Diagnostic and Statistical Manual of Mental Disorders (DSM-V) criteria. The authors note that this is different from previous reports of NSAID abuse in that she was not using the medication to treat unresolved pain. The authors acknowledged conflicting evidence on COX-inhibitors' ability to produce dependence, but postulate that its actions on the cannabinoid system and dopamine level modulation could potentially produce this effect.

Pregnancy

This is discussed under 'Diclofenac'.

Ketorolac [SEDA-34, 186; SEDA-35, 200]

Cardiovascular

See Special Section.

Otolaryngological

See Special Section.

Pulmonary

A case of diffuse alveolar hemorrhage (DAH) attributed to ketorolac tromethamine was reported [29A]. According to the authors, there have been multiple reports of NSAID-induced DAH, but only one previous report of ketorolac tromethamine as the causative agent.

- A 39-year-old male experienced non-fatal DAH following appendectomy determined to be due to intramuscular ketorolac tromethamine administration (30 mg perioperatively and 30 mg postoperatively), as the event occurred the day of surgery with no other potential causes identified and resolved with conservative management.

Loxoprofen

Endocrine

A case of insulin autoimmune syndrome (IAS) attributed to loxoprofen sodium patch was reported [30A]. According to the authors, two cases of loxoprofen-induced IAS have been previously reported.

- A non-diabetic 62-year-old woman displayed repeated hypoglycemic events and a markedly elevated plasma insulin level and impaired glucose tolerance in response to a 75-g oral glucose tolerance test. She also displayed a high anti-insulin autoantibody plasma level. The hypoglycemic episodes ceased after discontinuation of her loxoprofen sodium patch but recurred following readministration of the medication, subsequently terminating after a second discontinuation of this medication.

Special Review - Controversial use of Ketorolac

℞ Ketorolac tromethamine is a NSAID that is indicated for the management of moderately severe acute pain requiring analgesia at the opioid level. Oral ketorolac is recommended for use after therapy with intravenous or intramuscular therapy. The total duration of therapy with oral and intravenous or intramuscular therapy should not extend beyond 5 days.

Though effective, there are a number of instances in which the use of ketorolac is not currently recommended, including in pediatrics and certain situations peri-operatively [31S]. For example, based on prescribing recommendations ketorolac is not recommended for use in the pediatric population since safety and efficacy studies have not been established in patients 17 years and younger. Additionally, in clinical trials, an increase in the risk of cardiovascular thrombotic events, myocardial infarction, and stroke have been observed with the use of some COX-2 selective and nonselective NSAIDs. Though not specifically displayed in clinical trials involving each specific NSAID, these risks theoretically may be possible with all NSAIDS and COX-2 selective agents and, therefore, cardiovascular thrombotic events may be possible with ketorolac therapy. Prophylactic use of ketorolac prior to major surgery is contraindicated, as well, as is ketorolac for peri-operative pain in coronary artery bypass graft (CABG) surgery. Postmarketing evidence demonstrates peri-operative use of intravenous or intramuscular ketorolac has been associated with postoperative hematomas and bleeding. Since ketorolac inhibits platelet function, the risk of bleeding is increased and ketorolac is also contraindicated in those with cerebrovascular bleeding, hemorrhagic diathesis, incomplete hemostasis, and those at a high risk of bleeding. Despite these warnings, ketorolac is still commonly used peri- or post-operatively in a number of hospitals (including in pediatric populations) as it provides effective pain relief while limiting the use of opioids. Within the past year, a number of well-conducted reviews have been conducted and published assessing the safety of ketorolac in this peri- and/or post-operative setting.

Otolaryngological

A well-conducted systematic review and meta-analysis including seven studies conducted in children under age 18 and 3 studies in adults identified a fivefold greater risk of post-tonsillectomy hemorrhage in adults administered perioperative ketorolac versus those not receiving ketorolac (RR 5.64, 95% CI 2.08–15.27), but no statistical difference in children under the age of 18 (RR 1.39, 95% CI 0.84–2.30). Including all studies together, the relative risk of ketorolac administration was statistically significant (RR 2.04, 95% CI 1.32–3.15) [32M].

Cardiovascular

In 2005, a black box warning was issued by the United States Food and Drug Administration (FDA) recommending against the use of NSAIDs immediately following coronary artery bypass graft surgery due to cardiovascular safety concerns. A retrospective observational study was conducted within a single hospital to compare the outcomes of patients who had received intravenous ketorolac within 72 hours of cardiac surgery (CABG, valve surgery, atrial fibrillation procedures, or pericardial window surgery) versus patients not receiving ketorolac [3r]. Among the 1309 patients (n = 408 receiving ketorolac; n = 821 not receiving ketorolac), no statistically significant difference was noted in perioperative myocardial infarction (1% in ketorolac group versus 0.6% in control group, p = 0.51), stroke or transient ischemic attack (1% versus 1.7%, p = 0.47), while the ketorolac group had a significantly lower mortality rate (0.4% versus 5.8%, p < 0.0001). However, at baseline the patients in the ketorolac group were younger, had better preoperative renal function, and underwent less complex operations compared with the non-ketorolac patients, though a risk-adjusted model also showed no difference in cardiac outcomes. Additionally, this study may not have been large enough to assess a small difference in cardiac events between the groups. The authors concluded that this study demonstrates the safety of ketorolac when "selectively administered after cardiac surgery", however this is likely insufficient evidence to make such claims and further data should be collected before advising the use of this product despite the black box warning [33c].

Prolonged Bleeding Time

A meta-analysis involving 27 double-blind, randomized, controlled studies demonstrated no increased risk of postoperative bleeding associated with ketorolac versus other analgesic medications when used for postoperative pain [34M]. Ketorolac was given intraoperatively in 18 of the 27 studies and postoperatively in nine of the 27 studies. The duration of therapy with ketorolac ranged from 24 hours to 4 days postoperatively. Five of the 27 studies reported prolonged bleeding time. Three of these studies found an increase in bleeding with no significant difference, while two found no clinically significant bleeding associated. The increased bleeding time varied among the studies. One found bleeding time increased an average of 1 minute 46 seconds after treatment with 60 mg of ketorolac intramuscularly. In another study, a ketorolac dose of 30 mg intramuscularly four times per day for 5 days resulted in an increased bleeding time from 4.9 to 7.8 minutes. A third study found ketorolac increased bleeding time by 106 seconds, which was postulated to be due to a decrease in platelet aggregation. Although studies reported a *change in the bleeding time, ketorolac did not lead to an increase in clinically significant bleeding.*

Postoperative Bleeding

Of the 1304 ketorolac patients within the 27 study meta-analysis discussed above, 33 patients (2.5%) experienced postoperative bleeding whereas 21 out of 1010 patients (2.1%) in the control group experienced postoperative bleeding (OR 1.1, 95% CI 0.61–2.06, p=0.72) [34M]. When comparing those patients who received a dose greater than 30 mg (OR 0.76, p=0.71) versus those who received a dose of 30 mg or less (OR 1.24, p=0.55), there was no difference in bleeding events between either of these groups and placebo. Nine of the 27 studies reported higher incidences of postoperative bleeding with ketorolac than the control treatments; however, the difference was not statistically significant ranging from 2% to 3.5%. One post marketing surveillance cohort study within the meta-analysis found an increase in bleeding with higher doses of ketorolac in older patients with treatment for more than 5 days. When comparing ketorolac and opiates, the odds ratio of bleeding at the operative site increased (OR 1.02) with ketorolac use. Subjects 75 years and older demonstrated an odds ratio that was significant for operative site bleeding at 1.12. Neither p-values nor 95% CI were provided in the meta-analysis. However, this cohort study does include biases such as selection, information, and misclassification bias. Additionally, this study was conducted in medical and surgical patients, which could potentially decrease the difference observed between the cohorts studied. This cohort study determined eight cases of increased operative site bleeding would be required for every 1000 patients treated with ketorolac in order to have one clinically significant increase in bleeding.

Increased Use of Additional Hemostatic Measures

In eight of 25 studies, the ketorolac groups were found to require additional hemostatic measures than the control groups (one of 25 studies) [34M]. Even though extra hemostatic measures were required, there was no significant increase in bleeding episodes observed.

Thus, while caution should still be promoted when using ketorolac peri- or post-operatively, recent large-scale meta-analyses support the notion that the risk may be less than previously purported in certain clinical situations [34M].

COX-2 SELECTIVE INHIBITORS [SEDA-34, 186; SEDA-35, 201; SEDA 36, 120]

Celecoxib [SEDA-34, 186; SEDA-35, 201; SEDA-36, 124]

Cardiovascular

A large prospective study assessing the cardiovascular risk between celecoxib and nonselective NSAIDs in patients with rheumatoid and osteoarthritis was conducted [35C]. The incidence of the composite endpoint (cardiovascular events of myocardial infarction (MI), angina pectoris, heart failure, cerebral infarction, and cerebral hemorrhage) was 1.2% (n=66) in the celecoxib group and was 1.3% (n=65) in the NSAID group (p=0.58). A higher incidence of MI was observed in the celecoxib group than the NSAID group (adjusted HR 1.41, 95% 0.39–5.04) and although statistical significance was not reached, clinical significance should be considered. A meta-analysis examining the safety profile of celecoxib found that over 41 000 patients reported that celecoxib was not associated with significant increases in non-fatal MI, non-fatal stroke, and cardiovascular death when compared with placebo and NSAIDs [36M]. The mechanism of cardiovascular effect of celecoxib may be related to inhibition of aldosterone glucuronidation [37E].

Gastrointestinal

There is more literature demonstrating improved gastrointestinal tolerability of celecoxib when compared with nonselective NSAIDs [35C]. Conversion from nonselective NSAIDs to celecoxib may be useful in protecting patients with rheumatoid arthritis from small bowel injury [38c]. Accessibility and affordability may improve given recent FDA approval for generic formulations [39r].

Etoricoxib [SEDA-34, 187; SEDA-35, 201; SEDA-36, 126]

Immunologic

In a retrospective study of 74 Asian patients with history of intolerance to at least one NSAID, etorixcoxib was found to be well tolerated. Four patients had mild reactions consisting of facial edema, urticaria, and transient giddiness [40c]. Cumulative dosages associated with reactions ranged from 30 to 120 mg.

Rofecoxib [SEDA-34, 187; SEDA-35, 201; SEDA-36, 126]

Cardiovascular

In 2004, rofecoxib was removed the market due to increased risk of myocardial infarctions and strokes based on results from the VIGOR study [41C]. In the APPROVe study, the increased cardiovascular risks were determined to be unanticipated. However this has been since contradicted in multiple Alzheimer studies discussed in further detail in SEDA-36 [42c].

Valdecoxib

In 2005, valdecoxib was removed from the market due to potential increased risk for serious cardiovascular adverse events, increased risk of serious skin reactions (e.g., toxic epidermal necrolysis, Stevens–Johnson syndrome, erythema multiforme) compared to other NSAIDs [43S].

Hematological

A case report of death potentially related to valdecoxib was reported [44r].

- A 28-year-old female with no past medical history of kidney disease, hypertension, diabetes, vasculitis, systemic lupus erythematis, or rheumatic fever developed hypertension after ibuprofen use (on day 10) and was subsequently prescribed valdecoxib (days 76 to 139). She ultimately died due to cerebral hemorrhage.

INDOLEACETIC ACIDS [SEDA-34, 187]

Indomethacin [SEDA-34, 187]

Nervous System

A 34-year-old female was diagnosed with hemicrania continua and treated with indomethacin 50 mg three times a day [45A]. Upon increase of indomethacin dose to 75 mg three times daily, the patient experienced a severe pulsating bilateral headache with migrainous features. This was the first occurrence of this nature experienced by the patient. After the dose was decreased back to 50 mg three times daily the migraine resolved. Several trials of the higher indomethacin dose again resulted in migrainous bilateral headache.

Teratogenicity

The exposure of human fetal testes to indomethacin between 7 and 12 weeks of gestation stimulated testosterone production (+16% at 48 hours and +32% at 72 hours) [14r]. Stimulation was higher at earlier gestation (+50% for 8–9.86 weeks gestation vs. +29% at 10–12 weeks gestation).

Drug Formulations

In a phase 3 trial, the safety and efficacy of indomethacin submicron particle capsules in patients following bunionectomy was evaluated [46c]. The most frequently reported adverse effects included nausea, postprocedural edema, dizziness, and headache.

OXICAMS [SEDA-34, 187; SEDA-35, 201; SEDA-36, 126]

Piroxicam [SEDA-36, 127]

Pregnancy

This is discussed under 'Diclofenac'.

Skin

The first case of acute generalized exanthematous pustulosis (AGEP) induced by oral oxicams was reported [47A]. A 61-year-old woman with no history of psoriasis or other skin disorder was given oral piroxicam 20 mg/day for treatment of renal colic. She presented with generalized itchy eruption consisting of multiple papules that coalesced to larger plaques with widespread erythema, and histology of a skin biopsy was consistent with AGEP. Resolution began within 1 week of drug withdrawal.

PROPIONIC ACID DERIVATIVES [SEDA-36, 127]

Naproxen [SEDA-35, 200; SEDA-36, 127]

Pregnancy

This is discussed under 'Diclofenac'.

Comparative Study

In the Infliximab as First-Line Therapy in Patients with Early Active Axial Spondyloarthritis Trial (INFAST) Part 1 study, 158 patients were randomized to evaluate whether combination therapy with intravenous infliximab 5 mg/kg and oral naproxen 1000 mg was superior to treatment with naproxen alone [48c]. Generally, the pattern of adverse events (AEs) in the infliximab group was similar to that reported in the literature for other tumor-necrosis factor antagonists. The INFAST Part 2 was a follow-up study that randomized 83 patients from Part 1 who achieved partial remission in a placebo-controlled study to explore whether biologic-free remission can be achieved and to determine whether continued treatment with naproxen was superior to discontinuing all treatments in order to maintain disease control for 6 months [49c]. The most frequently reported treatment-emergent adverse events (TEAEs) in the naproxen group were rhinitis and intervertebral disc protrusion (each $n=1$), and one TEAE led to early withdrawal (fatigue).

Systematic Reviews

This meta-analysis examining naproxen use for acute migraine headaches in adults found mostly mild/moderate AEs, and the incidence of any specific event was less than 5% and too low for useful analysis [50M].

Hematologic

A 42-year-old woman with a history of alcohol-dependence was hospitalized and diagnosed with acute, severe methemoglobinemia after taking naproxen [51A]. Although the specific mechanism is unknown, it is hypothesized that the combined action of naproxen and alcohol as oxidative stressors in a reduced glucose-6-phosphate dehydrogenase (G6PD) activity state induced by alcohol consumption led to methemoglobinemia.

Immunologic

A 74-year-old man stabilized on losartan 50 mg reported developing angioedema on two occasions following naproxen use [52A]. It is suggested that naproxen administration impaired renal function, precipitating a dose-dependent reaction in a patient who had multiple existing risk factors for angioedema.

Drug–Drug Interactions

Three phase 1 studies conducted to evaluate the safety of co-administrating naproxen 500 mg/day and edoxaban 60 mg, an oral factor Xa inhibitor, showed no clinically important pharmacokinetic interactions [53c]. Concurrent administration was well tolerated, and limited doses of naproxen were recommended with edoxaban in the phase 3 study ENGAGE AF-TIMI 48 for stroke prevention in atrial fibrillation population.

SALICYLATES [SED-15, 15; SEDA-34, 188; SEDA-35, 202; SEDA-36, 127]

Acetylsalicylic Acid (Aspirin) [SED-15, 15; SEDA-34, 188; SEDA-35, 202; SEDA-36, 127]

Sensory Systems

Two meta-analysis studies evaluated the association between aspirin use and neovascular age-related macular degeneration (AMD). Sobrin et al. pointed out the high possibilities for confounding variables, sampling bias and recall bias in the studies looking at the relationship between aspirin use and the development of AMD [54M]. Results of these studies have been inconsistent and currently do not warrant a change in practice. There is poor evidence to suggest stopping aspirin therapy for risk of developing AMD in patients taking aspirin for primary or secondary prevention of cardiovascular disease. The Canadian Journal of Ophthalmology meta-analysis from early 2014 reviewed many of the same studies [55M]. They combined the studies and the pooled OR was 1.43 (95% CI 1.09–1.95) with a risk ratio of 1.35 (95% CI 1.02–1.78). Publication bias was noted to be a limitation as well as the high heterogeneity between studies ($I_2 = 73\%$). This meta-analysis suggests a small statistically significant association between using aspirin and the onset of early AMD, but clinical relevance has yet to be determined.

Genetic Factors

A meta-analysis of 21 articles discussing the association of four polymorphisms mapped on four candidate genes (cyclooxygenase-1 (COX-1), cyclooxygenase-2 (COX-2), integrin alpha 2B (ITGA2B), and integrin alpha 2 (ITGA2)) noted to have an association with aspirin insensitivity were reviewed. Weng et al. found that COX-2 and ITGA2 genetic defects may increase the risk for aspirin insensitivity, especially noted in the Chinese populations which were found to be as high as 58.58% for the ITGA2 gene compared to 40.77% in Caucasian patients [56M]. This analysis supports the need for further investigation into the specific mechanism of COX-2 and ITGA2 genes as they pertain to aspirin insensitivity.

Drug–Drug Interaction

This is discussed under Metamizole.

Sensory Systems

Bilateral vestibulopathy (BV) causes gait unsteadiness and difficulty stabilizing gaze during movements. Aminoglycoside treatment is a frequent cause of BV (10–20%). A 71-year-old female developed BV 2 weeks after being treated with amoxicillin-clavulanate 875/125 mg twice daily for 10 days along with her regular dose of aspirin 100 mg daily for which she had been taking for the past 4 years [57A]. This patient had longlasting bilateral vestibular deficit for at least 6 months. It is known that high dose aspirin (5–6 g per day) can cause BV and topical application of ticarcillin into the middle ear causes ototoxicity, but neither of these matched with this particular patient. The authors proposed a mechanism by which penicillin and aspirin had an additive effect on prostaglandin function. Prostaglandins in the inner ear are otoprotective. Penicillin may have aggravated the ototoxic capability of aspirin by also inhibiting the COX enzyme. Penicillin may also increase the free serum concentrations of aspirin due to protein binding competition. This case report may induce a need for a larger prospective investigational study to occur on this subject.

Salsalate

Cardiovascular

In a randomized, placebo-controlled, double-blind crossover trial, healthy patients, those with metabolic syndrome and those with atherosclerosis were given high dose (4.5 g) salsalate therapy to determine its effect on endothelial function [58c]. Vascular function was evaluated after each treatment period. The purpose was to compare brachial artery flow-mediated dilation (FMD) response in those taking placebo against those who took salsalate therapy. The mean age of the subjects was 56 years old while the oldest subjects tended to be the ones with atherosclerosis ($p = 0.005$). Other patient parameters were not statistically significant. The patients with plasma salsalate concentrations within therapeutic ranges had impaired endothelium-dependent flow mediated vasodilation compared to placebo therapy ($n = 31$, $p < 0.02$) but this did not occur in subjects with subtherapeutic levels ($p > 0.2$). This endothelium-dependent impairment of vasodilation occurred in patients with therapeutic levels regardless of their health status suggesting that salsalate-induced impairment in endothelial function is independent of the current health of the endothelium. Caution should be taken when utilizing high-dose salsalate treatment to prevent or treat cardiovascular disease. More trials should be conducted to determine mechanism of action seen here since previous studies have had opposite effects [59c].

Metabolism

Stage two of TINSAL-T2D was a randomized, placebo-controlled, parallel trial conducted to assess the efficacy and safety of salsalate in patients with type 2 diabetes when taken for 1 year [60C]. The trial included 283 participants who were assigned randomly to placebo ($n = 137$) or salsalate 3.5 g per day ($n = 146$) therapy. Primary outcome was the change in hemoglobin A1c, followed by safety and efficacy. It was reported that weight and low-density lipoprotein (LDL) cholesterol levels increased with salsalate use. There was an increase in urinary albumin-creatinine ratio (ACR) by 2.3 mcg/mg (CI 2.0–2.7 mcg/mg, $p < 0.001$), but this reversed when salsalate was discontinued. Mild hypoglycemic events occurred more often with patients receiving salsalate than placebo ($p = 0.036$) along with a sixfold increased RR when salsalate was taken concomitantly with a sulfonylurea ($p < 0.001$). There were no major signs of cardiovascular risk, but the increase in weight (1.3 kg placebo-corrected increase $p < 0.001$), LDL cholesterol ($p < 0.001$), and urinary albumin levels may be of concern. Although this trial was conducted longer than previous trials and showed improvement of glycaemia along with decreased inflammatory mediators, the authors determined that long-term cardiorenal safety and outcomes should be evaluated further before salsalate is recommended in majority of patients with T2DM.

MISCELLANEOUS DRUGS

Nefopam [SED-15, 2433; SEDA-34, 188; SEDA-35, 207; SEDA-36, 128]

Drug Dosage Regimens

A study consisting of 48 elderly patients with ages ranging 65–99 years old was conducted to determine the pharmacology of nefopam in this patient population with or without renal impairment [61c]. Based on a two-compartment open model, researchers were able to determine the pharmacokinetics of nefopam in the elderly who have age-related reductions in renal and hepatic function. This study found that this patient population tended to have three times higher values of nefopam compared to previously reported values in younger subjects. Renal impairment was not associated with the development of tachycardia and postop nausea and vomiting, rather these adverse effects were related to the infusion duration. Nefopam 20 mg was better tolerated with infusion duration between 45 and 60 minutes versus the standard 20 mg over 30 minutes. This study was small, lacked external validity and could not determine the impact that renal impairment had on subsequent doses or accumulation of nefopam.

Nimesulide [SED-15, 2524; SEDA-33, 249; SEDA-36, 128]

Sensory Systems

A 59-year-old woman presented with a foreign body sensation and irritation of her left eye [62A]. Further evaluation revealed that vision and other ocular tests were within normal limits. The ocular symptoms began about 12 hours after ingestion of 100 mg nimesulide sachet used for low back pain. Six hours after the ocular symptoms, she developed a skin rash with circular erythematous maculae on the trunk, arms and legs. The patient had no other pertinent medical history or prior adverse drug reactions. Nimesulide was discontinued. Further tests revealed this reaction to be consistent with Fixed Drug Eruption (FDE). The patient's symptoms were clear within 3 weeks. The patient returned after 4 weeks to conduct a patch test with nimesulide placed on the back for 48 hours. Positive reactions were noted on days 2 and 4 and were negative by the day 6 reading. Eyelid involvement from nimesulide is rare and this report is the first case known to present with both ocular and skin involvement.

DRUGS USED IN THE TREATMENT OF GOUT

Allopurinol [SED-15, 80; SEDA-34, 189; SEDA-35, 207; SEDA-36, 129]

Skin

The first case of esophageal stricture secondary to allopurinol-induced toxic epidermal necrolysis (TEN) was reported in a 70-year-old man presenting with severe dysphagia secondary to TEN involving his mouth and esophagus [63A]. Another 73-year-old woman reported with allopurinol-induced TEN accompanied by human herpes virus 6 reactivation [64A].

Many risk factors for allopurinol hypersensitivity (AHS) have been documented [65M]. Additional cases of drug reactions with eosinophilia and systemic syndrome (DRESS) linked to allopurinol have been reported:

- A 45-year-old man presented with marked generalized erythema with multiple papules and plaques over the entire body, cervical lymphadenopathy, and liver and kidney dysfunction after taking allopurinol for 2 months [66r];
- An 80-year-old man who took allopurinol 300 mg/day had developed AHS with diffuse maculopapular rash; he had several risk factors including recent initiation of allopurinol, presence of HLA-B*58:01 allele in the Han Chinese ancestry, concurrent use of thiazide diuretic, and chronic kidney disease [67A];
- A 45-year-old man developed generalized erythematous maculopapular rash and fever 3 weeks after starting allopurinol 200 mg/day for asymptomatic hyperuricemia; improved after 2 weeks of removing allopurinol and giving steroid and supportive treatment [68A];
- A 41-year-old man experienced AHS exfoliative skin lesions with hemorrhage, fever, eosinophilia, and acute liver and renal failure, requiring a liver transplant, 4 weeks after starting treatment with allopurinol 300 mg/day for asymptomatic hyperuricemia; factors included heredity, kidney function, concomitant drugs, and the starting dose; authors suggested that starting with the lowest dose possible is most prudent [69A];
- An 81-year-old woman developed severe AHS after the first administration of allopurinol 150 mg/day for asymptomatic hyperuricemia and died a few days after hospital admission [70r].

Genetic

Studies have already established an association between HLA-B*58:01 allele and severe cutaneous adverse reactions (SCAR) that may underline ethnic differences in incidence [71R]. A study genotyped 25 Portuguese patients, all except one taking 300 mg/day allopurinol, who had developed a SCAR: 19 DRESS and 6 Stevens–Johnson syndrome (SJS)/TEN [72c]. HLA-B*58:01 was present in 12 of the 19 (OR 37.71, 95% CI 4.13–343.87) DRESS and 4 of the 6 (OR 44.0, 95% CI 3.18–608.19) SJS/TEN patients when compared with the allopurinol-tolerant patients. This suggested that Portuguese patients developing SCAR from allopurinol have a high incidence of HLA-B*58:01. A case-controlled study confirmed previous association of significant association between HLA-B*58:01 with allopurinol induced SCAR in the Japanese population [73r].

Hematologic Malignancy

A retrospective cohort study reviewed 463 patients who had taken allopurinol for the prevention of hyperuricemia prior to chemotherapy to prevent tumor lysis syndrome and had undergone serologic HLA typing for the incidence and risk factors of allopurinol-induced hypersensitivity [74c]. The incidence of maculopapular eruptions (MPE) was 2.9% ($n = 13$) and none experienced severe cutaneous adverse reactions (SCARs). There was no statistically significant association between reactions with HLA-B*58:01. However, there were two other serologic HLA typing significantly associated with MPE as compared with the allopurinol tolerant group: HLA-DR9 (38.5% (5/13) vs. 13.6% (53/443), $p = 0.019$) and HLA-DR14 (38.5% (5/13) vs. 15.6% (41/440), $p = 0.038$). Chronic myeloid leukemia was also found to be significantly higher in the allopurinol hypersensitivity group (23.1% (3/13) vs. 5.9% (26/440), $p = 0.044$).

Renal Disease

A review found studies assessing allopurinol use in patients with chronic kidney disease have reported inconsistent safety and efficacy findings [75R]. Weighing the risk of AHS, need for reducing starting dose and gradual titration are some factors to consider in using allopurinol to safely lower urate levels.

Colchicine [SEDA-34, 189; SEDA-35, 208]

Neuromuscular Function

Eighty-eight pediatric patients with familial Mediterranean fever currently taking colchicine for 11–45 months were assessed for neuromyopathy [76c]. Ten patients (11%) had side effects overall: Eight (9%) patients had diarrhea, one (1%) patient had leukopenia, and one (1%) patient developed alopecia. No elevated risk of neuromyopathy was found.

A 81-year-old white male with hypertension, valvular heart disease, pulmonary hypertension, chronic atrial fibrillation, GI bleed, myelodysplastic syndrome, chronic renal insufficiency, diabetes, and gout for which he had been taking colchicine 0.6 mg daily and propranolol presented with weakness starting in the lower legs, worsening over the next 4 weeks [77A]. He had mild pain in his arms and legs accompanied by arm weakness, hip and leg weakness, and sensory loss. He had elevated LFTs and CK. Colchicine was discontinued and the weakness subsided.

Drug–Drug Interaction

A 58-year-old female with a history of renal transplant, gout, and chronic kidney disease on colchicine 0.6 mg daily, therapeutic cyclosporine, bumetidine, clonazepam, mirtazapine, oxycodone, prednisone, conjugated estrogen, flurazepam, levothyroxine, and gabapentin, presented to the ER with weakness, hypotension, and altered mental status [78A]. She had taken 3.6 mg of colchicine, 3 mg of colchicine, and 1.2 mg of colchicine the 3 days, respectively, before the ER visit in divided doses. Labs revealed pancytopenia with a peripheral smear showing dysplastic neutrophils with vacuolization. In addition to the large dosage of colchicine, a cyclosporine/colchicine interaction was implicated by either inhibition of CYP3A4 or P-glycoprotein by cyclosporine.

Febuxostat [SEDA-34, 250; SEDA-35, 209; SEDA-36, 129]

Incidence

A systematic review of 34 trials assessed the difference in safety and efficacy of allopurinol and febuxostat [79M]. Five of these trials looked at differences in adverse events between the two medications. Febuxostat demonstrated a small reduction in adverse events compared to allopurinol (0.94); however, the information was not detailed enough to determine which adverse reactions were lessened. There was no difference between the cardiac and liver effects of both drugs.

A post hoc analysis of a randomized trial including 312 adult patients with diabetes and 1957 adult patients without diabetes demonstrated small reductions in serious adverse events in patients on febuxostat 40, 80 mg, and allopurinol 200 or 300 mg in patients with and without diabetes one patient (1%), eight patients (7%), and seven patients (7%), vs. 13 patients (3%), 20 patients (3%), and 23 patients (8%), respectively [80c].

Nephrology

A 73-year-old male with a past history of stroke, stage 3. CKD, gout, dyslipidemia, angina, and hypertension was seen in the ER for progressive weakness in his legs [81A]. Apart from a recent change to febuxostat 80 mg daily from allopurinol 200 mg daily, his medication regimen of colchicine 0.6 mg daily, rosuvastatin 10 mg daily, losartan 50 mg daily, and diltiazem SR 180 mg daily had remained the same for several years. Upon evaluation, his AST was 278 (0–37), ALT 285 (0–41), CK 7650 (0–170), LDH 711 (135–225), and nerve conduction was found to be abnormal. Other disease processes and drug interactions where ruled out.

Neurology

In a prospective open labeled 12 ± 2-month trial, the safety and efficacy of febuxostat was assessed in 22 adult renal transplant patients [82c]. Patients who were previously on allopurinol, benzbromarone, or treatment naive were started on febuxostat 20 mg, febuxostat 10 or 20 mg, or febuxostat 20 mg daily, respectively, to decrease urate

to <6. One patient (4.5%) experienced paresthesia and discontinued use of febuxostat (1 per patient year).

Leflunomide [SEDA-36, 131]

Pharmacogenomics

Leflunomide pharmacogenomics was discussed in a recent review article [83R]. CYP1A2 IF allele with CC genotype results in a 10-fold increase in toxicity compared to CA or AA allele. However, CYP2C19*2 increases clearance compared to noncarriers suggesting that an increased leflunomide dose may be necessary in this patient population.

Gastrointestinal

In a retrospective cohort of 65 adult patients evaluating the effectiveness of leflunomide added to corticosteroids for the treatment of henoch schoenlein nephritis, three patients developed anemia (1.5 per patient year), and four patients had increased AST (two per patient year) [84c]. The incidence of new diabetes mellitus, hypertension, or infection was similar in both groups. Leflunomide was taken as a 50 mg loading dose for 3 days followed by 20 mg daily.

The efficacy and safety of leflunomide was assessed in 16 patients (three on 10 mg, 13 on 20 mg progressing to six on 10 mg, and 10 on 20 mg by 6 weeks) with steroid dependent or resistant nephrotic syndrome [85c]. Fifty percent of patients experienced mild side effects: four patients (25%) had increases in AST, three (18.8%) developed hypertension requiring treatment in two of the cases, two (12.5%) developed alopecia, and one patient (6.3%) developed diarrhea.

Risk Factors for Infection

A retrospective study of 401 rheumatoid arthritis patients was conducted in South Korea to determine risk factors associated with severe infections [86c]. Thirty-three patients (8.2%, 24.7 per 100 patient years), 12 of whom were on leflunomide 20 mg and 21 who were on leflunomide 10 mg, developed infection requiring hospitalization: 15 (3.7%) cases of pneumonia (10.9 per 100 patient years), five (1.3%) cases of oral candidiasis and stomatitis (3.6 per 100 patient years), five (1.3%) cases of pyelonephritis (3.6 per 100 patient years), four (1%) cases of TB (2.9 per 100 patient years): one mortality. Of the 33 patients, 24 (72.7%) received oral corticosteroids. Once confounders were controlled, age greater than 65 (OR 1.89, 95% CI 1.16–3.11), corticosteroid dose >7.5 mg prednisone equivalent (OR 1.52, 95% CI 1.04–2.45), treatment with corticosteroids and methotrexate (OR 1.42, 95% CI 1.12–2.16), and diagnosis of diabetes mellitus (OR 1.39, 95% CI 1.09–1.96) were identified as independent predictors of infection.

Skin

A 78-year-old female with rheumatoid arthritis was started on leflunomide. She was also taking corticosteroids, alendronate, and etoricoxib, no dosages noted. One month after initiation and for a period of 2 years she developed 14 squamous cell carcinomas and keratoacanthomas [87A]. When leflunomide was stopped, no new lesions were noted. Though leflunomide is implicated in various skin reactions, this is the first incidence of keratoacanthomas reported.

References

[1] Jasiecka A, Maslanka T, Jaroszewki JJ. Pharmacological characteristics of metamizole. Pol J Vet Sci. 2014;17(1):207–14 [R].

[2] Redondo-Pachon MD, Enriquez R, Sirvent AE, et al. Acute renal failure and severe thrombocytopenia associated with metamizole. Saudi J Kidney Dis Transpl. 2014;25(1):121–5 [A].

[3] Polzin A, Zeus T, Schror K, et al. Dipyrone (metamizole) can nullify the antiplatelet effect of aspirin in patients with coronary artery disease. J Am Coll Cardiol. 2013;62(18):1725–6 [r].

[4] Krajcova A, Vojtech M, Duska F. Mechanism of paracetamol-induced hypotension in critically ill patients: a prospective observational cross-over study. Aust Crit Care. 2013;26:136–41 [c].

[5] Moral L, Torres-Borrego J, Murua JK, et al. Association between paracetamol exposure and asthma: update and practice guidelines. An Pediatr (Barc). 2013;79(3):188.e1–188.e5. [R] Spanish.

[6] Liss DB, Paden MS, Schwarz ES, et al. What is the clinical significant of 5-oxoproline (pyroglutamic acid) in high anion gap metabolic acidosis following parcetamol (acetaminophen) exposure? Clin Toxicol. 2013;51:817–27 [M].

[7] Luyasu A, Wamelink MMC, Galantic L, et al. Pyroglutamic acid-induced metabolic acidosis: a case report. Acta Clin Belg. 2014;69(3):221–3 [A].

[8] Turco R, Miele E, Russo M, et al. Early-life factors associated with pediatric functional constipation. J Pediatr Gastroenterol Nutr. 2014;58(3):307–11 [C].

[9] Larsen FS, Wendon J. Understanding paracetamol-induced liver failure. Intensive Care Med. 2014;40:888–90 [H].

[10] Buchornatvakul C, Reddy KR. Acetaminophen-related hepatotoxicity. Clin Liver Dis. 2013;15:587–607 [R].

[11] McGill MR, Jaeschke H. Metabolism and disposition of acetaminophen: recent advances in relations to hepatotoxicity and diagnosis. Pharm Res. 2013;30:2174–87 [R].

[12] Bulku E, Stohs SJ, Cicero L, et al. Curcumin exposure modulates multiple pro-apoptotic and anti-apoptotic signaling pathways to antagonize acetaminophen-induced toxicity, Curr Neurovasc Res. 2012;9(1):58–71. http://www.ncbi.nlm.nih.gov/pubmed/22272768 [E].

[13] Lugovic-Mihic L, Duvancic T, Vucic M, et al. SDRIFE (baboon syndrome) due to paracetamol: case report. Acta Dermatovenerol Croat. 2013;21(2):113–7 [A].

[14] Guerrero C, Perino F, Favoriti N, et al. Paracemtaol-induced hypersensitivity vasculitis in a 10-year-old child. Eur Rev Med Pharmacol Sci. 2013;17:3405–6 [r].

[15] Mazaud-Guittot S, Nicolaz CH, Desdoits-Lethimonier C, et al. Paracetamol, aspirin, and indomethacin induced endocrine disturbances in the human fetal testis capable of interfering with testicular descent. J Clin Endocrinol Metab. 2013;98(11): E1757–E1767 [c].

[16] Medicines and Healthcare Products Regulatory Agency. Drug safety update. 2013. https://www.gov.uk/drug-safety-update/diclofenac-new-contraindications-and-warnings [S].

[17] Varas-Lorenzo C, Riera-Guardia N, Calingaert B, et al. Myocardial infarction and individual nonsteroidal anti-inflammatory drugs meta-analysis of observational studies. Pharmacoepidemiol Drug Saf. 2013;22:559–70 [M].

[18] Mahamid M, Francis A, Khalaila W, et al. Diclofenac-induced coronary spasm in the absence of anaphylaxis or allergic manifestation. Isr Med Assoc J. 2013;15:590–1 [A].

[19] Turnbull N, Callan M, Staughton RCD. Diclofenac-induced pseudoporphyria; an under-recognized condition? Clin Exp Dermatol. 2014;39:348–50 [A].

[20] Akat PB. Severe photosensitivity reaction induced by topical diclofenac. Indian J Pharmacol. 2013;45(4):408–9 [A].

[21] Nezvalova-Henriksen K, Spigset O, Nordeng H. Effects of ibuprofen, diclofenac, naproxen, and piroxicam on the course of pregnancy and pregnancy outcome: a prospective cohort study. BJOG. 2013;120:948–59 [c].

[22] Shastri AT, Abdulkarim D, Clarke P. Maternal diclofenac medication in pregnancy causing in utero closure of the fetal ductus arteriosus and hydrops. Pediatr Cardiol. 2013;34:1925–7 [A].

[23] Karadeniz C, Ozdemir R, Kurtulmus S, et al. Diclofenac-induced intrauterine ductal closure. Fetal Diagn Ther. 2013;34:133–4 [A].

[24] Lahiri T, Guillet A, Diehl S, et al. High-dose ibuprofen is not associated with increased biomarkers of kidney injury in patients with cystic fibrosis. Pediatr Pulmonol. 2014;49:148–53 [c].

[25] Kuchar E, Han S, Karlowicz-Bocalska K, et al. Safety of oral ibuprofen – analysis of data from the spontaneous reporting system in Poland. Acta Pol Pharm. 2014;71(4):687–90 [c].

[26] Lake H. Ibuprofen belly: a case of small bowel stricture due to non-steroidal anti-inflammatory drug abuse in the setting of codeine dependence. Aust N Z J Psychiatry. 2014;47(12):1210–1 [A].

[27] Bello AE, Kent JD, Grahn AY, et al. Risk of upper gastrointestinal ulcers in patients with osteoarthritis receiving single-tablet ibuprofen/famotidine versus ibuprofen alone: pooled efficacy and safety analyses of two randomized, double-blind, comparison trials. Postgrad Med. 2014;126(4):82–91 [C].

[28] Etcheverrigaray F, Grall-Bronnec M, Blanchet MC, et al. Ibuprofen dependence: a case report. Pharmacopsychiatry. 2014;47:115–7 [A].

[29] Marak CP, Alappan N, Shim C, et al. Diffuse alveolar hemorrhage due to ketorolac tromethamine. Pharmacology. 2013;92:11–3 [A].

[30] Okazaki-Sakai S, Yoshimoto S, Yagi K, et al. Insulin autoimmune syndrome caused by an adhesive skin patch containing loxoprofen-sodium. Intern Med. 2013;52:2447–51 [A].

[31] Ketorolac Tromethamine [package insert]. Lake Forest, IL: Hospira, Inc.; 2011 http://www.accessdata.fda.gov/drugsatfda_docs/label/2013/019645s019lbl.pdf [S].

[32] Chan DK, Parikh SR. Perioperative ketorolac increases post-tonsillectomy hemorrhage in adults but not children. Laryngoscope. 2014;124:1789–93 [M].

[33] Oliveri L, Jerzewski K, Kulik A. Black box warning: is ketorolac safe for use after cardiac surgery? J Cardiothorac Vasc Anesth. 2014;28(2):274–9 [c].

[34] Gobble RM, Hoang HLT, Kachniarz B, et al. Ketorolac does not increase perioperative bleeding: a meta-analysis of randomized controlled trials. Plast Reconstr Surg. 2014;133:741–55 [M].

[35] Hirayama A, Tanahashi N, Daida H, et al. Assessing the cardiovascular risk between celecoxib and nonselective nonsterioidal anti-inflammatory drugs in patients with rheumatoid arthritis and osteoarthritis. Circ J. 2014;78:194–200 [C].

[36] Essex MH, Zhang RY, Berger MF, et al. Safety of celecoxib compared with placebo and non-selective NSAIDS: cumulative meta-analysis of 89 randomized controlled trials. Expert Opin Drug Saf. 2013;12(4):465–77 [M].

[37] Crilly MA, Mangoni AA, Knights KM, et al. Aldosterone glucoronidation inhibition as a potential mechanism for arterial dysfunction associated with chronic celecoxib and diclofenac use in

patients with rheumatoid arthritis. Clin Exp Rheumatol. 2013;31:691–8 [E].

[38] Inoue T, Lijima H, Arimitsu J, et al. Ameiloration of small bowel injury by switching from nonselective nonsteroidal anti-inflammatory drugs to celecoxib in rheumatoid arthritis patients: a pilot study. Digestion. 2014;89:124–32 [c].

[39] Kuehn BM. FDA approves first celecoxib generics. JAMA. 2014;311(24):2470 [r].

[40] Llanora GW, Ling Loo EX, Gerez IA, et al. Etoricoxib: a safe alternative for NSAID intolerance in Asian patients. Asian Pac J Allergy Immunol. 2013;31:330–3 [c].

[41] Bombardier C, Laine L, Reciin A, et al. Comparison of upper gastrointestinal toxicity of rofecoxib and naproxen in patients with rheumatoid arthritis. VIGOR Study Group. N Engl J Med. 2000;343(21):1520–8 [C].

[42] Madigan D, Sigleman DW, Mayer JW, et al. Under-reporting of cardiovascular events in th rofecoxib Alzhiemer disease studies. Am Heart J. 2012;164(2):186–93 [c].

[43] U.S. Food and Drug Administration. Postmarket Drug Safety Information: Information for Healthcare Professionals: Valdecoxib (Marketed as Bextra). U.S. Food and Drug Administration; 2015. Retrieved from http://www.fda.gov/Drugs/DrugSafety/PostmarketDrugSafetyInformatio nforPatientsandProviders/ucm124649.htm [S].

[44] Lohiya GS, Lohiya P, Krishna V, et al. Death related to ibuprofen, valdecoxib, and medical errors: case report and medicolegal issues. J Occup Environ Med. 2013;55(6):601–2. Comment in: Author's reply: NSAIDS and small kidneys in a workers' compensation death claim. J Occup Enviorn Med 2013; 55(12):1383–3 [r].

[45] Jurgens TP, Schulte LH, May A. Indomethacin-induced de novo headache in hemicranias continua-fighting fire with fire? Cephalalgia. 2013;33(14):1203–5 [A].

[46] Altman R, Daniels S, Young CL. Indomethacin submicron particle capsules provide effective pain relief in patients with acute pain: a phase 3 study. Phys Sportsmed. 2013;41(4):7–15 [c].

[47] Cherif Y, Jallouli M, Mseddi M, et al. Acute generalized exanthematous pustulosis induced by piroxicam: a case report. Indian J Pharmacol. 2014;46:232–3 [A].

[48] Sieper J, Lenaerts J, Wollenhaupt J, et al. Efficacy and safety of infliximab plus naproxen versus naproxen alone in patients with early axial spondyloarthritis: results from the double-blind, placebo-controlled INFAST study, part 1. Ann Rheum Dis. 2014;73:101–7 [c].

[49] Sieper J, Lenaerts J, Wollenhaupt J, et al. Maintenance of biologic-free remission with naproxen or no treatment in patients with early, active axial spondyloarthritis: results from a 6-month, randomized, open-label follow-up study, INFAST part 2. Ann Rheum Dis. 2014;73:108–13 [c].

[50] Law S, Derry S, Moore RA. Naproxen with or without an antiemetic for acute migraine headaches in adults. Cochrane Database Syst Rev. 2013;10. Art. No.: CD009455 [M].

[51] Lee WS, Lee JY, Sung WY, et al. Naproxen-induced methemoglobinemia in an alcohol-dependent patient. Am J Emerg Med. 2014;32(11):1439e9–1439e10 [A].

[52] Venci JV, Shamaskin JA. Recurrent angioedema after naproxen use in a patient stabilized with losartan. Ann Allergy Asthma Immunol. 2014;113(6):666–7 [A].

[53] Mendell J, Lee F, Chen S. The effects of the antiplatelet agents, aspirin and naproxen, on pharmacokinetics and pharmacodynamics of the anticoagulant edoxaban, a direct factor Xa inhibitor. J Cardiovasc Pharmacol. 2013;62(2):212–21 [c].

[54] Sobrin L, Seddon J. Regular aspirin use and risk of age-related macular degeneration. Am J Ophthalmol. 2013;156(2):213–7 [M].

[55] Kahawita SK, Casson RJ. Aspirin use and early age-related macular degeneration: a meta-analysis. Can J Ophthalmol. 2014;49(1):35–9 [M].

[56] Weng Z, Li X, Li Y, et al. The association of four common polymorphisms from four candidate genes (COX-1, COX-2, ITGA2B, ITGA2) with aspirin insensitivity: a meta-analysis. PLoS One. 2013;8(11):1–7 [M].

[57] Hertel S, Schwaninger M, Helmchen C. Combined toxicity of penicillin and aspirin therapy may elicit bilateral vestibulopathy. Clin Neurol Neurosurg. 2013;115(7):1114–6 [A].

[58] Nohria A, Kinlay S, Buck JS, et al. The effect of salsalate therapy on endothelial function in a broad range of subjects. J Am Heart Assoc. 2014;3:1–10 [c].

[59] Pierce GL, Lesniewski LA, Lawson BR, et al. Nuclear factor-{kappa} b activation contributes to vascular endothelial dysfunction via oxidative stress in overweight/obese middle-aged and older humans. Circulation. 2009;119:1284–92 [c].

[60] Goldfine AB, Fonseca V, Jablonski KA, et al. Salicylate (salsalate) in patients with type 2 diabetes: a randomized trial. Ann Intern Med. 2013;159(1):1–12 [C].

[61] Djerada Z, Fournet-Fayard A, Gozalo C, et al. Population pharmacokinetics of nefopam in elderly, with or without renal impairment, and its link to treatment response. Br J Clin Pharmacol. 2013;77(6):1027–38 [c].

[62] Rubegni P, Tognetti L, Tosi GM, et al. Ocular involvement in generalized fixed drug eruption from nimesulide. Clin Experiment Ophthalmol. 2013;41(9):896–8 [A].

[63] Njei B, Schoenfeld A, Vaziri H. Esophageal stricture secondary to drug-induced toxic epidermal necrolysis presenting in an adult: an unusual complication of a rare disease. Conn Med. 2013;77(9):541–4 [A].

[64] Watanabe Y, Matsukura S, Isoda Y. A case of toxic epidermal necrolysis induced by allopurinol with human herpesvirus-6 reactivation. Acta Derm Venereol. 2013;93(6):731–2 [A].

[65] Ramasamy SN, Korb-Wells CS, Kannangara DR, et al. Allopurinol hypersensitivity: a systematic review of all published cases, 1950–2012. Drug Saf. 2013;36(10):953–80 [M].

[66] Kim MS, Lee JH, Park K. Allopurinol-induced DRESS syndrome with a histologic pattern consistent with interstitial granulomatous drug reaction. Am J Dermatopathol. 2014;36(2):193–6 [r].

[67] Tyrell T, Gick J. Recent onset of rash, dehydration, and nonbloody diarrhea in an elderly man. J Fam Pract. 2013;62(9):E1–E5 [A].

[68] Sharma G, Govil DC. Allopurinol induced erythroderma. Indian J Pharmacol. 2013;45(60):627–8 [A].

[69] Miederer SE, Miederer KO. Allopurinol hypersensitivity syndrome: liver transplantation after treatment of asymptomatic hyperuricaemia. Deut Med Wochenschr. 2014;139(49):2537–40 [A].

[70] Carnovale C, Venegoni M, Clementi E. Allopurinol overuse in asymptomatic hyperuricemia: a teachable moment. JAMA Intern Med. 2014;174(7):1031–2 [r].

[71] Lam MP, Yeung CK, Cheung BM. Pharmacogenetics of allopurinol-making an old drug safe. J Clin Pharmacol. 2013;53(7):675–9 [R].

[72] Goncalo M, Coutinho I, Teixera V, et al. HLA-B*58:01 is a risk factor for allopurinol-induced DRESS and Stevens-Johnson syndrome/toxic epidermal necrolysis in a Portuguese population. Br J Dermatol. 2013;169(3):660–5 [c].

[73] Niihara H, Kaneko S, Ito T, et al. HLA-B*58:01 strongly associates with allopurinol-induced adverse drug reactions in a Japanese sample population. J Dermatol Sci. 2013;71(2):150–2 [r].

[74] Jung JW, Kim JY, Yoon SS, et al. HLA-DR9 and DR14 are associated with the allopurinol-induced hypersensitivity in hematologic malignancy. Tohoku J Exp Med. 2014;233(2):95–102 [c].

[75] Thurston MM, Phillips BB, Bourg CA. Safety and efficacy of allopurinol in chronic kidney disease. Ann Pharmacother. 2013;47(11):1507–16 [R].

[76] Isikay S, Yilmaz K, Yigiter R, et al. Colchicine treatment in children with familial Mediterranean fever: is it a risk factor for neuromyopathy? Pediatr Neurol. 2013;49:417–9 [c].

[77] Ghosh P, Emslie-Smith A, Dimberg E. Colchicine induced myoneuropathy mimicking polyradiculoneuropathy. J Clin Neurosci. 2014;21:331–2 [A].

[78] Stromberg P, Willis B, Rose S. Case report. J Fam Pract. 2014;63(8):455–6 [A].

[79] Faruque LI, Ehteshami-Afshar A, Wiebe N, et al. A systematic review and meta-analysis on the safety and efficacy of febuxostat versus allopurinol in chronic gout. Semin Arthritis Rheum. 2013;43:367–75 [M].

[80] Becker MA, MacDonald PA, Hunt BJ, et al. Diabetes and gout: efficacy and safety of febuxostat and allopurinol. Diabetes Obes Metab. 2013;15:1049–55 [c].

[81] Kang Y, Kim MJ, Jang HN, et al. Rhabdomyolysis associated with initiation of febuxostat therapy for hyperuricaemia in a patient with chronic kidney disease. J Clin Pharm Ther. 2014;39:328–30 [A].

[82] Tojimbara T, Nakajima I, Yashima J, et al. Efficacy and safety of febuxostat, a novel nonpurine selective inhibitor of xanthine oxidase for the treatment of hyperuricemia in kidney transplant recipients. Transplant Proc. 2014;46:511–3 [c].

[83] Keen H, Conaghan P, Tett S. Safety evaluation of leflunomide in rheumatoid arthritis. Expert Opin Drug Saf. 2013;12(4):581–8 [R].

[84] Zhang Y, Gao Y, Zhang Z, et al. Leflunomide in addition to steroids improves proteinuria and renal function in adult henoch-schoenlein nephritis with nephrotic proteinuria. Nephrology (Carlton). 2014;19:94–100 [c].

[85] Zhou J, Zhang Y, Liu G, et al. Efficacy and safety of leflunomide in treatment of steroid-dependent and steroid resistant adult onset minimal change disease. Clin Nephrol. 2013;80(2):121–9 [c].

[86] Yoo H, Yu H, Jun JB, et al. Risk factors of severe infections in patients with rheumatoid arthritis treated with leflunomide. Mod Rheumatol. 2013;23:709–15 [c].

[87] Frances L, Guijarro J, Marin I, et al. Multiple eruptive keratoacanthomas associated with leflunomide. Dermatol Online J. 2013;19(7):16 [A].

10

General Anaesthetics and Therapeutic Gases

Rebecca Gale, Alison Hall[1]

Anaesthesia and Critical Care, Royal Liverpool Hospital, Liverpool, United Kingdom
[1]Corresponding author: alison.hall@rlbuht.nhs.uk

INTRODUCTION

This review discusses the side effects documented in the recent literature associated with both traditional and newly emerging anaesthetic agents. It includes further information on commonly described side effects and adverse events associated with these drugs as well as detailing any newly discovered complications for the time period reviewed.

Etomidate

Trauma

A review article examined the most recent publications pertaining to the use of etomidate for critically ill septic and trauma patients. A prospective, randomised multicentre study compared patients induced with ketamine (2 mg/kg) with etomidate (0.3 mg/kg). The study found no significant difference in 3 or 28 day mortality although significantly more etomidate patients had adrenal insufficiency (OR 6.7, 95% CI 3.5–12.7). A further meta-analysis studied 21 articles and found patients who received etomidate had an increased risk of adrenal insufficiency (OR 1.64, $n = 2854$, $p < 0.0001$) and significantly higher mortality (RR 1.19, $n = 3516$, $p < 0.001$). The etomidate group also had significantly more ventilator days and greater length of intensive care and hospital stay [1R].

Sepsis

A recent retrospective cohort study of patients with sepsis or septic shock ($n = 2000$) found that hospital mortality for patients induced with etomidate ($n = 1102$) was similar to those induced with other agents (37.2% vs. 37.8%, $p = 0.77$). Mortality in intensive care, length of intensive care and hospital stay were all comparable between the two groups. More patients in the etomidate group received corticosteroids than the other induction agent group (52.9% vs. 44.5%, $p < 0.001$) but vasopressor requirement and number of ventilator days were similar. These results are opposed by a meta-analysis of etomidate versus non etomidate use for induction in critical care patients with and without a diagnosis of sepsis. 19 sets of data were included and the etomidate group had an increased risk ratio of 1.64 for adrenocortical suppression ($n = 2854$, $p < 0.0001$). The etomidate group had an increased risk ratio of death of 1.19 ($n = 3516$, $p < 0.0001$). This increase in risk ratio continued in the septic patients ($n = 1767$) but for non-septic patients the risk was not sustained [2R].

An electronic record review propensity matched 2144 patients who received etomidate for induction of general anaesthesia with 5233 patients who received propofol for non cardiac surgery. Patients who received etomidate had a 2.5 (98% CI 1.9–3.4) times the odds of dying than patients who received propofol. Patients receiving etomidate had a significantly increased odds of cardiovascular morbidity (OR 1.5, 98% CI 1.2–2.0) and longer hospital stay (Hazard ratio 0.82, 95% CI 0.78–0.87). Infectious morbidity and vasopressor use was similar between groups [3C].

Cardiovascular

Etomidate is known for its cardiovascular stability. A study randomised patients undergoing general anaesthesia for gynaecological surgery into 4 groups. Groups 1–3 received etomidate emulsion at 0.3 mg/kg for induction and then 10, 15 or 20 micrograms respectively, and group 4 received propofol at 6–10 mg/kg/hour. Groups 1–3 received remifentanil with an induction dose of 0.1–0.3 micrograms/kg/minute followed by infusion at 0.1, 0.2 or 0.3 micrograms/kg/minute for groups 1, 2 and 3, respectively, group 4 received propofol only. The groups receiving etomidate had greater cardiovascular stability in comparison to the propofol group. In the

© 2015 Elsevier B.V. All rights reserved.

etomidate groups, there were 7 cases of post-operative agitation, 20 of lethargy and 19 patients vomited compared to no adverse reactions observed in the propofol group. These effects appeared to be dose dependent with increasing incidence of side effects as the concentration of etomidate increased [4c].

A retrospective study of 100 patients by a helicopter emergency medical service compared patients intubated with etomidate ($n=50$) or ketamine ($n=50$) looking at clinical end points of successful intubation and complications, heart rate and blood pressure. All patients in both groups were successfully intubated but there was an increase in peri-intubation hypoxaemia in the ketamine group (16% vs. 10%) which did not reach statistical significance ($p=0.55$). Haemodynamic stability was equal between the two groups [5c].

Ketamine

Nervous System

Ketamine has been previously linked with schizophrenia like symptoms and a small study ($n=16$) looked at the cerebral microstructure in chronic ketamine users compared to 16 controls. There was a decrease in the right hemisphere white matter axial diffusivity profile in ketamine users and a significant increased association between the caudate nucleus and lateral prefrontal cortex connectivity profile. This suggests that ketamine can cause extensive disruption of the white matter and white matter pathways between sub and prefrontal cortical areas. This may account for the variety of dissociative experiences that individuals have to ketamine [6c].

A paediatric prospective randomised placebo controlled study compared a combination of intranasal midazolam (0.5 mg/kg) and ketamine (2 mg/kg) ($n=19$) with placebo (saline spray) ($n=17$) undergoing gastric aspirates. The mean Modified Objective Pain Score was 3.5 (range 1–8) in the sedation group versus 7.2 (range 4–9) in the placebo group ($p<0.0001$). Post-sedation agitation occurred in 10.5% of the sedation group compared with none observed in the placebo group [7c].

A small prospective observational study of 47 patients presenting to the emergency department with moderate or severe pain assessed the response to 0.5–0.75 mg/kg intranasal ketamine. Using visual analogue scores, 88% had a reduction in pain score by 13 mm or more within 30 minutes of ketamine administration. Median time to achieve a reduction of 13 mm in VAS score was 9.5 minutes (IQR 5–13 minutes, range 5–25 minutes). There were no reported serious adverse effects but minor effects were common and transient with 21 patients experiencing dizziness, 14 patients a feeling of unreality, 4 patients reported nausea and 3 patients a change in mood. 1 patient had an alteration in hearing. No minor effects required any treatment [8c].

Psychological

A small observational study of 25 paediatric patients looked at quality of sedation in a paediatric outpatient dental practice. Patients received oral ketamine (5 mg/kg) in combination with oral diazepam (0.2 mg/kg). They found sedation effectiveness to be 84% and all patients who required extra sedation needed this for procedures lasting in excess of 35 minutes. 12% of patients developed hyperthermia on the first post-operative night and 4% reported hallucinations. Unfortunately, there was no control group for comparison in this study [9c].

Psychiatric-1

Recreational ketamine use is known to stimulate psychological symptoms. In a survey of 1614 ketamine users symptoms such as anxiety, dysphoria and tremors were commonly reported in female users (16.2% of cohort were female). 76% of total ketamine users reported cognitive impairment and 51.6% reported urinary symptoms, again the severity of which was significantly higher in females [10R].

100 patients who used ketamine as part of mixed drug use were compared to 100 controls to establish any differences in mood or memory. The 100 ketamine users were subdivided into current users of ketamine and other drugs ($n=32$) and ex users ($n=64$). Patients who were currently still using ketamine had significantly higher depression ($p<0.001$) and anxiety scores ($p<0.02$) as assessed on the Beck Depression Inventory and the Hospital Anxiety Depression Scale compared to ex users and controls. The significantly higher depression score persisted when ex users were compared to controls ($p=0.006$). The ketamine group, both current and ex users had significantly poorer logical memory delayed recall scores and Rey Osterrieth Complex Figure delayed recall than controls indicating poorer verbal and visual memory even if not currently using ketamine. The presence of poly drug use could lend bias to this study [11C].

A small double blind, randomised study of 8 cocaine addicted patients to receive 3 separate infusions of lorazepam (2 mg) and ketamine (0.41 and 0.71 mg/kg), each separated by at least 48 hours. 15 minutes after each infusion the patients were assessed against the Clinician Administered Dissociative Symptoms Scale (CADSS) and Hoods Mysticism Scale (HMS). The ketamine significantly increased mystical effects and patients had significantly higher HMS scores which were dose dependent. At 24 hours post-infusion, these effects appeared to increase the desire to stop taking cocaine although there was no reduction in cue induced craving. There were no adverse effects from these infusions stated [12c].

Psychiatric-2

An editorial on two small randomised controlled trials using ketamine for treatment resistant depression found a 64% response rate in 47 patients given ketamine. Approximately, half of these responsive patients then relapsed the following week but without an increase in suicidal ideation. Anxiety on the day of ketamine treatment and the day following was the main side effect reported and eight patients reported dissociative feelings. Blood pressure during treatment with ketamine increased within acceptable clinical limits (122/72–141/81 mmHg, 40 minutes after infusion) and two patients had to have the infusion stopped for haemodynamic concerns, one patient had non responsive hypertension, the other had clinically significant hypotension and bradycardia. The applicability of the study was questioned as the inclusion criteria were tight and all patients were drug free for 7 days prior to ketamine. As such, there is no evidence on the safety or interactions of ketamine with other psychiatric medication [13r].

In a small double blind, placebo controlled, cross over study 27 patients hospitalised with depression received ketamine at a dose of 0.54 mg/kg over 30 minutes. Using the Brief Psychiatric Rating Scale to measure psychotomimetic symptoms, the study found that a higher level of psychotomimetic symptoms during the infusion of ketamine was associated with an improvement in mood in the subsequent week with a maximum effect on day 7. The action is thought to be mediated by the trough NMDA receptors. No side effects were reported [14c].

Further case reports however have documented variable response to intravenous ketamine for the relief of depressive symptoms. A case series of 4 patients (mean age 72 years) documented their response to intravenous ketamine for treatment of severe depression [15A].

Patient 1: A male terminated his ketamine treatment after 2 infusions as he had no relief of his depression but experienced confusion, depersonalisation and feeling cold.
Patient 2: A female had 5 ketamine infusions and had no benefit in reduction in depression but had side effects of a floating sensation, double vision, paraesthesia and tinnitus.
Patient 3: A male had 6 ketamine infusions and experienced fear, paraesthesia and changes in perception but no relief from his depressive symptoms.
Patient 4: A male had 6 infusions with some reduction in his depressive symptoms initially but his depression then increased back to baseline at the end of the ketamine therapy. His only reported side effect was tiredness.

A further case series of three patients detail a sustained anti-depressant response to ketamine. In these patients, 100 mg of ketamine was given intramuscularly with effects lasting approximately 1 hour [16A].

Patient 1: 43-year-old female experienced a total resolution of depressive symptoms which has persisted post-treatment. The only side effect reported was short lived motor incoordination post-injection which resolved within an hour.
Patient 2: 40-year-old female had an immediate response to ketamine which lasted 3 months (at time of publication). No side effects were described.
Patient 3: Female who received ketamine and while it did not resolve her depression post-treatment she was able to identify life stresses and ability to manage these to reduce their effect on her mood. No side effects were reported.

Liver

Case report 1

A 28-year-old female presented with raised liver function tests, specifically enzyme levels with a normal bilirubin. She had used ketamine recreationally for the 5 preceding years. An Endoscopic Retrograde Cholangiopancreatography was performed as a gallstone was visible in the gallbladder on ultrasound and it found strictures in the common bile duct and both intrahepatic ducts. A liver biopsy showed mild to moderate portal fibrosis in keeping with chronic cholestasis. The liver function tests improved after ketamine intake stopped but the strictures remained. This complication of ketamine use has been detailed previously, the only available treatment modalities are stenting and to cease ketamine intake [17A].

Case report 2

A 21-year-old obese patient with a past medical history of bilateral hydronephrosis and acute renal failure presented with acute pyelonephritis and was found to have deranged liver function tests. He revealed he had inhaled ketamine daily for the preceding 9 months. Ultrasound demonstrated an echogenic liver with normal blood flow and liver biopsy revealed concentric periductal fibrosis consistent with secondary sclerosing cholangitis. After drug rehabilitation, his liver function tests dramatically improved and follow up imaging showed normal intrahepatic and common bile duct [17A].

Urinary Tract

Case report 1

A 30-year-old male with dysuria, severe urinary frequency, nocturia and testicular pain was referred to a urology department. He had a history of recreational ketamine use for the past 10 years (1–2 g daily for 3 years then 2 g two to three times per week). He was treated with a 6-week course of intravesical chondroitin sulphate (Gepan 0.2% 40 mL once a week for 6 weeks). He had marked symptom improvement with a reduction in urinary frequency, nocturia and resolution of testicular pain and dysuria. The treatment was continued once a month for a year given symptom resolution [18A].

Case report 2

A 45-year-old male was admitted to the emergency department with a reduced level of consciousness and renal failure. He had been using intranasal ketamine for the preceding 3 years. He had a 12-month history of urinary frequency and discomfort which had improved with stopping ketamine and use of propiverine and tamsulosin. Blood tests revealed acute renal and liver impairment and an abdominal CT scan demonstrated bilateral hydronephrosis. He received haemodialysis and JJ stenting of his ureters plus a course of levofloxacin and oral silymarin (an antioxidant originating from milk thistle) for liver impairment and was discharged home with stable renal and liver function after 1 week [19A].

An online survey on a drug information website recruited 18 802 participants to answer questions regarding drug use and their health. 18.7% admitted ketamine use in the past with 5.8% using it within the preceding 6 months. Multivariate analysis was performed and found a significant association in reported lower urinary tract symptoms and recent ketamine use. For each extra day of ketamine use, the odds of urinary frequency increased by 1.6%, urinary urgency by 1.4%, dysuria by 1.7% and haematuria by 1.9%. For every 17 ketamine users, there was one extra case of urinary frequency [20A].

At a molecular level, a study looked at human epithelial cells of the proximal tubule and found ketamine at 24–48 hours produces a gross change in cellular morphology and alters the architecture of the cytoskeleton. The effect of ketamine is concentration dependent (0.1–1 mg/mL) and is due to a reduction in the adherens junction proteins, epithelial and neural cadherin and beta catenin. This is evidence that ketamine could have significant clinical implications on kidney function, particularly in the proximal kidney by reducing cell to cell adhesion and cell coupling [21E].

Death

Case 1.

A 25-year-old male with a past medical history of myelomeningocoele

A 25-year-old male with a past medical history of myelomeningocoele was admitted to hospital with abdominal pain and developed respiratory distress. He was cardiovascularly unstable with a heart rate of 160 bpm, a respiratory rate of 30 breaths/minutes

and temperature of 104 F. He received 2 mg/kg ketamine as induction for anaesthesia and had a cardiac arrest with initial rhythm of PEA. After resuscitation for 15 minutes, he had return of circulation and was found to have intestinal perforation. Despite treatment for this, he had suffered hypoxic brain damage and died in hospital.

Case 2.

An 11-year-old female with a 3-day history of vomiting, cough, temperature and myalgia

She had received radiotherapy for a craniopharyngioma in the past. She had a metabolic acidosis, raised white cell count and was haemodynamically unstable with a heart rate of 165 bpm and blood pressure of 76/32. Decision was made for intubation given her deteriorating clinical condition and ketamine 2.4 mg/kg and rocuronium 0.8 mg/kg was administered, 1 minute later she progressed to bradycardia and asystole. Following resuscitation she had a return of circulation rapidly but required significant inotropic support and had a pulseless ventricular tachycardia in paediatric intensive care from which she could not be resuscitated. The authors postulated the arrests could have been due to the negative inotropy of ketamine given to patients with depleted stores of endogenous catecholamines [22A].

Thiopentone

Nervous System

A cochrane review looked at all randomised controlled trials comparing the use of thiopentone and propofol for the treatment of refractory status epilepticus. One small single blind multicentre trial was reviewed and 14 patients received propofol and 7 received thiopentone. There was a significant increase in duration of mechanical ventilation in the thiopentone group but overall there was no difference in seizure control or functional outcome at 3 months. Incidence of infection and hypotension were not significantly different between groups. However, there was a wide confidence interval suggestive that there could be a difference between the drugs of up to two times in efficacy. The quality of the evidence was felt to be low. Further larger randomised controlled trials need to be conducted on this topic [23R].

Gastrointestinal

52 critically ill adults receiving thiopentone for intracranial hypertension were included in a study to evaluate the interaction of thiopentone with esomeprazole. The total mean dose of thiopentone given was 282.8 ± 172.7 mg/kg. The use of concurrent esomeprazole increased the volume of distribution of thiopentone

from a mean of 153.2–256.1 L and prolonged its half life. The authors conclude this could have a clinical impact on achieving a steady state thiopentone level in these patients [24c].

Methoxetamine

Psychological

A qualitative study looked at 33 anonymously written internet reports and analysed using the Empirical Phenomenological Psychological Method. From this, the authors found methoxetamine caused a heavily altered state of consciousness and appeared to have a high abuse potential. The main negative effects reported were anxiety and fear [25c].

Propofol

Uses

SEDATION

Propofol is a commonly used sedative outside anaesthetic practice. A 12-year retrospective observational study of 36 516 procedural sedations with propofol administered by paediatricians demonstrated a low rate of adverse events. There were six emergency calls (0.02%) for prolonged laryngospasm, bleeding and intestinal perforation. 0.05% of patients developed hypotension necessitating fluid resuscitation. 0.4% required face mask ventilation, 0.2% had laryngospasm and 0.04% had bronchospasm. Gastroscopy was associated with an increased incidence of minor complications. Thus, propofol given in this context is safe with a low incidence of adverse events; however, the majority were airway related and therefore administrators of propofol must be proficient in airway managements if they are to work in an isolated setting outside the theatre environment [26R].

156 patients were included in a prospective study of propofol sedation administered by a physician for therapeutic endoscopic retrograde cholangiopancreatography. This study looked at safety as its primary outcome. Mean propofol dose was 201 ± 132 mg (approx. 0.05 ± 0.04 mg/kg/minute). 2 patients developed respiratory compromise, 1 major requiring endotracheal intubation and 1 minor managed with bag mask ventilation. The authors concluded non anaesthetic sedation was safe in ASA 1 and 2 patients but advised the presence of an anaesthetist for patients with an ASA score of 3 or above [27c].

1008 cases receiving propofol sedation for manipulation of fractures or electrical cardioversion in an emergency department were reviewed against the World SIVA International Sedation Task Force adverse event tool. This tool is an internet based resource for reporting adverse events that occur under sedation. Overall, there were 73 events, 11 were defined as sentinel events with 5 cases of significant hypoxia and 6 cases of hypotension requiring boluses of vasopressor. There were 34 moderate risk cases identified, 28 needed bag mask ventilation and 6 required crystalloid infusion for hypotension. 25 minor cases were highlighted such as hypoxia requiring airway positioning or self-correcting hypotension. All patients who had an adverse event recovered fully which the authors felt demonstrated that adherence to sedation guidelines can result in safe practice [28C].

An observational study of 197 paediatric patients having transoesphageal echocardiography and percutaneous atrial septal defect closure had deep sedation rather than formal general anaesthesia. Median patient age was 6.1 years (range 0.5–18.8 years) and patients received a median ketamine dose of 2.7 mg/kg (range 0.3–7) and continuous propofol infusion rate of 5 mg/kg/hour (range 1.1–10.7). Device placement was successful in 92% of patients. 2 patients required intubation as a consequence of airway obstruction post-sedation initiation. 8% had minor respiratory complications needing frequent oral suctioning or temporary bag mask ventilation. Whilst there was no general anaesthesia or control group to compare to, complication rates were low and the procedure used was deemed safe [29c].

A retrospective case study analysis reviewed 37 480 colonoscopies performed with propofol sedation to 80 524 colonoscopies performed without sedation. Overall colonic perforation risk was 4.1 per 10 000. There was a 2.5 times increased risk for patients undergoing colonoscopy with propofol sedation compared to no sedation (6.9 vs. 2.7 per 10 000 procedures, $p = 0.0015$). This was further increased in patients undergoing therapeutic colonoscopies with propofol sedation where there was a 3.4 times increased risk of perforation (8.7 versus 2.6 per 10 000, $p = 0.0016$). There was no increase in risk due to patient sex but an independent increase with patient age and risk of perforation and biopsy or polypectomy increased the perforation risk. The authors postulated that propofol sedation improved tolerance of the procedure and removed feedback from patients, thus risking damage that would have been highlighted by awake patients [30R].

A retrospective study identified 309 patients with decompensated cirrhosis. They were divided into groups that received sedation with fentanyl (40 micrograms) and propofol (2 mg/kg) for oesphagogastroduodenoscopy ($n = 83$) or endoscopic ligation of varices ($n = 137$) and an unsedated group having endoscopic ligation of varices ($n = 83$). The control arm was 100 patients without cirrhosis undergoing sedation for endoscopy for gastritis. There were 19 patients who experienced complications in the control group (4 aspiration, 11 hypoxia, 2 hypotension and 2 bradycardia). This was not statistically different from the decompensated cirrhosis groups. (No minimal hepatic encephalopathy was observed in the two groups with cirrhosis that received sedation.) Propofol improved the tolerance of the variceal ligation procedure with 94.9% of procedures classed as easy in the propofol group versus only 47.2% in the unsedated group, $p < 0.05$ [31c].

Cardiovascular

237 patients who received propofol in two neurocritical care units were included in a multicentre retrospective study. Propofol initiation caused a maximum reduction in mean arterial pressure of 28.8% from baseline. 26.2% of patients developed severe hypotension to a mean arterial pressure of 56 mmHg resulting in a significantly increased duration of ventilation (5.0 vs. 3.6 days, $p = 0.01$) and mortality in hospital (38.7% vs. 24%, $p = 0.03$). Repeated propofol infusion rate changes, use of renal replacement therapy and baseline mean arterial pressure of 60–70 mmHg were identified as predictors of severe hypotension by multivariable logistic regression analysis [32c].

A small prospective parallel group study compared 14 young patients (age <65 years) with 14 older patients (age >65 years) to look at the effect of aging and propofol in combination on the autonomic nervous system. Heart rate variability analysis was used to evaluate the activity of the autonomic nervous system. Propofol had significant effects in the older age group in reducing cardiovascular activity in the autonomic nervous system. In younger patients, this effect was compensated for by increasing sympathetic activity but this did not occur in the older patient group [33c].

Forty patients undergoing thoracotomy for oesphagectomy were included in a randomised controlled trial looking at cardiovascular parameters with PiCCO2 and a Swan Ganz catheter when receiving propofol anaesthesia ($n = 20$) versus sevoflurane ($n = 20$). Propofol was inferior for preservation of right ventricular (RV) function with a significant reduction in cardiac index, RV ejection fraction, RV systolic work index and RV end diastolic volume index ($p < 0.05$) throughout surgery. In contrast to this, during one lung ventilation propofol significantly improved oxygen and reduced shunt fraction compared to sevoflurane ($p < 0.05$). Pulmonary vascular resistance index was significantly smaller in the sevoflurane group ($p < 0.05$). The authors suggested utilising the positives of both techniques to achieve the minimal effect on both right ventricular function and oxygenation [34c].

A prospective trial of 60 patients having off-pump coronary artery bypass grafting compared a group receiving only volatile (sevoflurane), a second group receiving only propofol for induction and maintenance and a third group that underwent IV propofol induction and then sevoflurane maintenance. The group that received only sevoflurane had significantly lower N terminal pro-brain natriuretic peptide (501 ± 280 pg/mL, $p < 0.05$) and troponin I (0.5 ± 0.4 ng/mL, $p < 0.05$) in comparison to the other two groups. The group that received propofol had higher myocardial markers of injury and required more support with inotropic drugs suggesting propofol has greater negative haemodynamic effects than volatile anaesthesia in this patient group [35c].

A randomised controlled trial included 91 patients with acute circulatory failure, 45 patients were sedated with propofol and 46 with dexmedetomidine. Preload was assessed prior to sedative infusion initiation using straight leg raising test and prior to a 250 mL crystalloid fluid bolus over 5 minutes. Central venous pressure and cardiac index were measured pre- and post-test. An increase of >10% in cardiac index was considered a positive for preload dependency. After the sedatives were started, there was significant reduction in cardiac index in both groups ($-9.5 \pm 6.6\%$ for propofol versus $-16.4\% \pm 8.5\%$ in the dexmedetomidine group) $p < 0.001$. There was a significant increase in cardiac index induced by the second straight leg raise test post-crystalloid bolus in the propofol group compared to initial values but not in the dexmedetomidine group suggesting that propofol infusion can cause an increase in preload dependency and response to fluid in patients with circulatory failure that does not occur in patients receiving dexmedetomidine [36c].

A single centre retrospective review looked at 582 patients who underwent cardiac surgery and received post-operative propofol versus dexmedetomidine sedation. The dexmedetomidine group were extubated earlier (68.7% vs. 58.1%, $p = 0.008$) with an average of 8.8 hours versus 12.8 hours ($p = 0.026$). Hospital length of stay was significantly reduced in the dexmedetomidine group (181.9 versus 221.3 hours, $p = 0.001$) but there were no significant difference between the groups for intensive care length of stay or in hospital mortality. This suggests that propofol sedation in this patient group could prolong time to recovery and discharge and in contrast dexmedetomidine sedation could improve patient throughput [37C].

A systematic review looked at all randomised controlled trials comparing dexmedetomidine with propofol for sedation in intensive care. 10 studies with 1202 patients were assessed. Propofol as a sedative agent was inferior, with dexmedetomidine sedation leading to a significant reduction in ICU length of stay by <1 day, the mean difference was -0.81 day 95% CI -1.48 to -0.15. In comparison to propofol, dexmedetomidine sedation significantly reduced delirium incidence (RR 0.40, 95% CI 0.22–0.77). There was no difference between dexmedetomidine and propofol with regards to ICU mortality or duration of ventilation. Adverse events between the groups were similar but dexmedetomidine was associated with an increased incidence of hypertension (RR 1.56, 95% CI 1.11–2.20) [38M].

Propofol has been investigated for its effects on microvascular flow. 16 patients initially sedated with propofol for septic shock were changed to midazolam infusion after 24 hours of intubation. Following the midazolam commencement, the microvascular flow index was greater than with propofol 2.8 (2.4–2.9) versus 2.3 (1.9–2.6) with $p < 0.05$. Flow heterogenicity index was greater with propofol than midazolam 0.49 versus 0.19, $p < 0.05$. The difference in the microcirculation was not reflected by systemic circulatory changes as there were no significant differences between the two groups haemodynamically [39c].

In a non-randomised study, 19 children receiving propofol sedation were compared to 18 children with no sedation who were undergoing cerebral MRI for infratentorial brain tumours. Blood flow was measured by dynamic susceptibility contrast perfusion. The cerebral blood flow in the anterior and middle cerebral artery was significantly less in the propofol group ($p < 0.05$). The age related reductions in cerebral blood flow in anterior cerebral and middle cerebral arteries described in the literature were reversed in children receiving propofol sedation ($r = 0.53$, $p = 0.02$ in the anterior cerebral artery and $r = 0.47$, $p = 0.04$ in the middle cerebral artery). The group receiving IV sedation with propofol was significantly younger in age than the group with no sedation and this could have had an impact on the results [40c].

Respiratory

A prospective study used a sleep apnoea monitor to detect oxygen desaturation events (defined as blood oxygen saturation drop below 94%) during sedation with propofol-remifentanil for dental extraction in 174 patients. There was an increase in desaturation events with increasing body mass index (81.8% vs. 20% in underweight patients). Odds of one desaturation event were 1.2 times higher for each BMI unit increase (OR 1.2, 95% CI 1.1–1.3). Males were 2.6 times as likely to desaturate than females for a given BMI (OR 2.6, 95% CI 1.2–5.25) [41c].

Case report

An 86-year-old on dabigatran for atrial fibrillation underwent percutaneous pinning of an impacted right femoral neck fracture at 28 hours post-injury. The dabigatran was a contraindication to neuroaxial anaesthesia and general anaesthesia was felt to be undesirable due to the patients' co-morbidities. The patient received 2 mg midazolam and 50 micrograms of fentanyl as a premed and then general anaesthesia was undertaken with this relates more to phenobarbitol side effects than propofol (145 mg), ketamine (25 mg) and lidocaine (50 mg) combined in a 20-mL syringe. Following the first 2-mL bolus of the mixture, the patient required a nasopharyngeal airway to maintain patency as the patient became obtunded to the point of snoring and supplementary ventilatory support was needed with a bag and mask for 5 minutes. Given the polypharmacy used in this technique, it is difficult to attribute the respiratory complication to one agent in particular [42A].

A study investigated cytokine release in the lung epithelial lining following one lung ventilation for oesophagectomy. This small prospective study randomly assigned 20 patients to receive either propofol or sevoflurane maintenance following an intravenous induction. Lung epithelial lining fluid was obtained by bronchoscopy before and after one lung ventilation with paired blood samples. The pro-inflammatory cytokine, IL-6 was significantly increased in both lungs following one-lung ventilation in the sevoflurane group but there were no changes in the propofol group. The pro-inflammatory chemokine, IL-8, was also increased in the sevoflurane group but only in the dependent, ventilated lung and there were no changes in the concentrations of IL-10 (anti-inflammatory) in either lung or group. Post-operatively, there were no differences in the clinical parameters of respiratory failure (P/F ratio) or in the duration of acute lung injury. This suggests that propofol may suppress the pro-inflammatory response to one lung ventilation and oesophagectomy; however, this study is too small to claim an effect of this on clinical outcome [43c]

Neurological

A review article discussed how the anticholinergic properties of propofol have been implicated in causing post-operative delirium. A number of case reports and a study of children ($n = 87$) undergoing surgery with propofol or halothane found a threefold increased incidence of emergence agitation with propofol. The mechanism postulated for this is via blockade of muscular acetylcholine receptors, specifically M1, M2 and M3 receptors [44r].

Pain

A retrospective observational study of 100 critically ill ventilated patients compared single agent sedation with fentanyl ($n = 50$) versus propofol ($n = 50$). An increased number of patients receiving propofol required rescue opioid therapy (56% versus 34%, $p = 0.04$) and significantly higher quantities of fentanyl equivalents (150 micrograms versus 100 micrograms, $p = 0.03$). There was no difference between groups in duration of mechanical ventilation, intensive care unit length of stay or delirium rate. Delirium in the propofol group was 27% versus 23% in the fentanyl group ($p = 0.80$) [45c].

Attempts to improve pain experienced on injection of propofol have again been investigated. A prospective, randomised, double blind, placebo controlled trial in 75 adult patients undergoing elective surgery looked at the use of lidocaine (2 mL 2%), dezocine (2 mg) or placebo (2 mL of saline) to reduce the pain of propofol injection. 6 patients in the placebo group reported severe pain on injection (using a 4 point verbal rating scale) compared to none in the two treatment arms. Overall 84% of the placebo group experienced pain in comparison to 40% in the lidocaine and 28% in the dezocine groups ($p = 0.05$). Local anaesthetic is superior to placebo in the reduction of the pain of propofol administration. There were no reported side effects of the local anaesthetic [46c].

50 patients undergoing anaesthesia with propofol at 2.5 mg/kg for gynaecological procedures had ketamine injected 15 seconds prior to propofol. The ketamine was increased from 0.175 to 0.275 mg/kg and ED_{50}, ED_{95} and 95% CI were calculated by probit analysis. A dose of ketamine of 0.3 mg/kg was effective in removing the pain associated with propofol injection [47c].

Psychiatric

A retrospective study of 3932 anaesthetics for electroconvulsive therapy used multivariate repeated measurement regression analyses to compare seizure quality and seizure parameters. Propofol accounted for a very small number of the anaesthetics included ($n = 42$, 1.07%) but produced seizures of lowest quality with reduced duration on EEG monitoring (43.7 seconds for propofol vs. 48.1 seconds for etomidate, $p = 0.009$). Propofol produced the lowest peak heart rate compared to etomidate ($p < 0.001$), thiopentone ($p = 0.001$) and ketamine ($p = 0.001$) [48C].

Emergence delirium (ED) in children is common and can result in longer length of stay. A prospective randomised controlled trial investigated ED in children undergoing a MRI scan. 120 Children were randomised to receive either propofol/remifentanil or sevoflurane. Post-operative emergence delirium was assessed by a blinded observer using the validated PAED (Paediatric Anaesthesia Emergence Delirium) score. The primary outcome was PAED score at 30 minutes. PAED scores were significantly higher in the sevoflurane group at time points up to 45 minutes post-operatively. Interestingly, there was a higher incidence of preoperative agitation in the sevoflurane group which may have contributed to this result. There were 5 episodes of bradypnoea and 1 desaturation observed in the propofol/remifentanil group but no adverse events reported in the sevoflurane group. 15 patients in the propofol group moved during the scan compared to no patients in the sevoflurane group [49c].

Liver

URINARY TRACT

Case 1

A 29-year-old male who was intubated for respiratory distress after near drowning developed pink sediment in his urine after sedation with 1.8g of propofol. It was negative for blood on screening. In addition he had received fentanyl, midazolam, pantoprazole, ceftriaxone, metronidazole, diazepam, thiamine and transcutaneous nicotine [50A].

Case 2

A 61-year-old male was sedated with 800 mg of propofol after reversal of Hartmanns procedure and appendicectomy. Other drugs he had received were fentanyl, heparin, thyroxine, paracetamol and cephazolin. The urine was discoloured pink and again the urine screen was negative for blood. The mechanism behind the discoloration is unknown but could be due to uric acid crystals [50A].

Endocrine

Case report

A 31-year-old male with multiple organ failure following trauma required renal replacement therapy. He was anticoagulated with citrate but had recurrent episodes of clotting in the dialysis filter and the blood appeared greasy on inspection. On measurement the patient had high triglycerides at 1772 mg/dL in his serum and 1667 mg/dL in the dialysis circuit. The patient was receiving propofol for sedation and this was felt to be the cause of the hypertriglyceridaemia. On discontinuation of propofol, the patients' triglyceride level fell to 534 mg/dL [51A].

Skin

Case report

A 75-year-old male patient with a past medical history of allergic rhinitis had received multiple propofol sedations for day case procedures and suffered penile blistering and oedema which worsened in severity each time propofol was used. The reaction usually began 6–7 hours post-propofol administration. A punch biopsy performed post-propofol challenge was used to confirm the drug reaction [52A].

Immunological

A 44 patient study compared 22 patients anaesthetised with thiopentone and sevoflurane to 22 patients induced and maintained on propofol infusion for one lung ventilation during thoracic surgery. The propofol group had significantly lower heart rate 1 minute prior to ventilating both lungs (65.05 ± 11.32 versus 73.95 ± 13.00, $p < 0.01$) and after 30 minutes of two lung ventilation than the sevoflurane group (62.91 ± 12.21 versus 72.05 ± 15.57, $p < 0.01$). The Ischaemia Modified Albumin (IMA) level indicating ischaemia-reperfusion injury was significantly higher in the group receiving propofol anaesthesia (0.83 ± 0.09 versus 0.76 ± 0.09, $p < 0.05$) [53c].

A randomised controlled trial compared 16 patients who received isoflurane anaesthesia to 18 patients who received propofol anaesthesia for minor surgery. Proinflammatory cytokine IL-6 was significantly increased in the isoflurane group at 120 minutes post-induction and on the first post-operative day ($p < 0.01$). In the propofol group, both IL-6 and IL-8 were significantly increased on the first post-operative day compared to preoperative levels. Both agents cause a significant increase in proinflammatory cytokines but suggest the inflammatory response may begin sooner with volatile anaesthesia. The clinical relevance of this is unknown as there were no medical or surgical complications recorded in either group post-operatively [54c].

Sixty patients undergoing anaesthesia for tongue cancer were randomised into three groups (propofol for induction and maintenance, propofol for induction and sevoflurane for maintenance and sevoflurane induction and maintenance). Blood samples were taken and analysed for T lymphocyte subsets at 30 minutes prior to induction, at 1, 3 and 5 hours post-induction, at the end of surgery, and at 24, 48 and 72 hours post-surgery. All T lymphocyte subsets except CD3 and CD8 were significantly reduced at 1, 3, 5 hours, end of surgery and 24 hours post-operatively compared to preoperative values ($p < 0.05$) in all 3 groups. Propofol had a reduced effect on immune responses at a cellular level compared to the sevoflurane group with significantly higher CD3, CD4, natural killer cells and CD3/CD4 ratios at 48 hours post operatively ($p < 0.05$) [55c].

Death

In Korea, recreational propofol abuse has been implicated in a number of deaths. A retrospective study examined 14 673 autopsy patients between 2005 and 2010 and detected blood levels of propofol in 131 cases (0.88%). It was the solitary agent in 49 fatal cases and in combination with other drugs in 82 cases. Propofol concentration detected varied from 0.05–8.83 mg/L in the heart and 0.08–8.65 mg/L in femoral blood. More patients who received a diagnosis of accidental death after self-administration were young (20–40 years), female and medical personnel [56C].

Fospropofol

Sixty patients received sedation with fospropofol (6.5 mg/kg with 1.6 mg/kg supplemental doses) or midazolam (0.05 mg/kg with 0.02 mg/kg supplemental doses) for oral outpatient surgery. Both groups received fentanyl at 1 microgram/kg prior to sedation. Patients in the fospropofol group demonstrated a non-significant decrease in recovery time from sedation (11.6 vs. 18.4 minutes, $p = 0.07$) with no difference in cognitive recovery. 90.4% of fospropofol patients had recall of local anaesthetic administration compared to 44.4% of midazolam patients ($p = 0.004$) and 40.6% of fospropofol patients experienced perineal discomfort versus 0% in the midazolam group ($p < 0.001$). Thus suggesting that fospropofol may be an inferior agent for sedation in oral outpatient surgery [57c].

A small prospective phase 1 open label, single centre randomised controlled trial randomised 16 patients to receive total intravenous anaesthesia with fospropofol ($n = 8$) or propofol ($n = 8$) plus alfentanil for cardiac surgery. Total dose of fospropofol used was 11.3 ± 2.5 mg/kg/hour and propofol was 4.4/-1.0 mg/kg/hour. There was no difference between the groups for bispectral index values so fospropofol was comparable in this patient group for anaesthesia. 4 patients in the fospropofol group reported a short lived perineal burning sensation on initiation of anaesthesia while 3 patients in the propofol group had pain related to the injection site [58c].

Dexmedetomidine

Sedation

A randomised controlled trial of 66 oral and maxillofacial patients compared the use of dexmedetomidine 1 mg/kg in recovery followed by infusion of 0.2–0.7 micrograms/kg/hour, with propofol 0.1 mg/kg in recovery and infusion of 1–2 mg/kg/hour. The propofol group had a higher number of oxygen desaturations at 30 minutes post-initiation and significantly lower blood pressure at 10 minutes post-initiation. The dexmedetomidine group had a significantly higher Ramsay sedation score at 3 hours ($p < 0.05$) suggestive of an improved sedation profile in comparison to propofol [59c].

Cardiovascular

In a small paediatric study, 40 patients undergoing ambulatory surgery were randomised to receive dexmedetomidine 1 microgram/kg at induction and then 0.1 microgram/kg intraoperatively or saline. Sevoflurane was used for maintenance of anaesthesia. The end tidal sevoflurane concentration was significantly reduced by 60% ($\pm 10\%$) in the dexmedetomidine group. Furthermore, emergence agitation was significantly less in the dexmedetomidine group (5% vs. 55% in the saline group, $p = 0.001$). The dexmedetomidine group had a significantly lower mean arterial pressure and heart rate and atropine was required for 6 patients ($p = 0.02$). There was no difference between the groups regarding pain, nausea or vomiting, urinary retention or time to recovery discharge [60c].

A small observational paediatric study investigated 22 patients (aged 5–17 years) undergoing an electrophysiological study and supraventricular tachycardia ablation. Patients received a loading dose of dexmedetomidine (1 microgram/kg) followed by an infusion of 0.7 micrograms/kg. This was followed by a bolus dose of ketamine (1 mg/kg) and a continuous infusion 1 mg/kg/hour. The hypothesis to be tested was ketamine's sympathomimetic qualities could counteract the bradycardia and hypertension that dexmedetomidine can cause. Haemodynamic variables such as mean arterial pressure, heart rate blood pressure and ECG variables (Sinus node recovery, QT interval, AV refractory period) were measured. Results show a significant mean arterial pressure rise, reduction in heart rate and prolonged sinus node recovery time and QTc interval after dexmedetomidine administration, all of which reversed back to baseline once the ketamine loading dose was given. This suggests the observed negative haemodynamic effects of dexmedetomidine can be compensated for by the concurrent administration of ketamine [61c].

Desflurane

Nervous System

Forty patients undergoing arthroscopic shoulder surgery in the sitting position were randomised to receive either a propofol based general anaesthetic or a desflurane (following intravenous induction) based anaesthetic to examine regional cerebral oxygenation. Maintenance of anaesthesia was measured using a bispectral index of 40–50. Using a cerebral oximeter, cerebral oxygenation was lower compared to baseline in both groups but was significantly higher in the desflurane group than the propofol group at 3, 5, 7 and 9 minutes following positioning. There were some small but statistically significant reductions in blood pressure which may have contributed to the reductions in cerebral oxygenation. In addition, the desflurane group received thiopentone as the induction agent and this may have contributed to the observed differences [62c].

The bispectral index of equipotent doses of volatile anaesthesia was carried out in 83 patients undergoing a partial or total thyroidectomy. Patients underwent an intravenous induction followed by randomisation to receive isoflurane, sevoflurane or desflurane at 1 MAC. All patients also received a remifentanil infusion titrated to maintain cardiovascular parameters within 20% of baseline. Desflurane anaesthesia resulted in lower BIS values (increased depth of anaesthesia) than the sevoflurane group. In addition, the time spent at a deeper plane of anaesthesia (BIS < 40) was longer in the desflurane group.

There were no differences between desflurane and isoflurane or isoflurane and sevoflurane. Although this study is limited by a lack of control group, these findings may be relevant to clinical practice as there is evidence to suggest that longer periods of deeper hypnosis may be related to increased post-operative morbidity, mortality and delirium [63c].

Ear, Nose and Throat

This small prospective study investigated the hypothesis that inhalational anaesthesia can increase middle ear pressure. They randomised 56 patients to receive either desflurane or sevoflurane in 50% oxygen/Air (MAC 1.25) following IV induction and measured middle ear pressure (MEP) by tympanometry at baseline and at 5, 15 and 30 minutes post-induction. At all time points in both groups, MEP was significantly higher than baseline. Values at 15 and 30 minutes post-induction for the patients in the desflurane group were significantly higher than those in the group receiving sevoflurane. Whilst a small study, the results are significant and may impact on the choice of anaesthesia for middle ear surgery [64c].

Immunologic

Inhalational anaesthesia is thought to impact on the immune system and the release of inflammatory cytokines. A small ($n = 24$) prospective trial randomly assigned patients undergoing elective prostatectomy to receive either general anaesthesia with desflurane (in oxygen and air) or a spinal anaesthetic with 0.5% bupivacaine. Bloods were taken pre-operatively and 24 hours post-operatively to investigate lymphocyte counts and cytokine release. Total numbers of lymphocytes did not alter in either group. In the spinal group, the numbers of interferon-λ and IL-10 producing T-cells reduced in equal numbers, thus not altering the ratio. In the GA group, however, interferon-λ producing cells increased whereas IL-10 producing cells were reduced post-operatively [65c].

Other

A retrospective database analysis investigated patients undergoing eye surgery comparing operating time between desflurane and propofol. They looked at 595 patients who had total intravenous anaesthesia (TIVA) versus 810 patients receiving desflurane maintenance anaesthesia in terms of surgical, anaesthetic extubation, operating room and recovery times. The desflurane group had longer extubation times by 1.85 minutes and a longer stay in the recovery area by 3.62 minutes but there were no other differences between the two groups in terms of times. There was an increased post-operative nausea and vomiting rate in the desflurane group [66r].

Isoflurane

Nervous System

It is known that isoflurane can affect the permeability of the blood brain barrier (BBB) through an effect on occludins, which maintains the integrity of BBB tight junctions. Following incubation with isoflurane at multiple concentrations, mRNA and protein expression of occludins was decreased in human brain vascular endothelial cells. In addition, this study demonstrated that isoflurane upregulated the expression of Vascular Endothelial Growth Factor and Transforming Growth Factor-β3. VEGF reduces the expression of occludins and TGF-β3 can enhance the endocytosis of occludins, both mechanisms that may contribute to the increased permeability of the BBB [67E].

Methoxyflurane

Psychological

A multicentre trial randomised 251 adults referred for colonoscopy to receive patient controlled inhaled methoxyflurane or conventional sedation practices to evaluate the efficacy, outcome and safety profile of methoxyflurane. Primary outcomes were pain, anxiety, time to discharge and patient willingness to undergo the same procedure. There were no differences in pain and anxiety scores between the two drugs but 8% of patients receiving methoxyflurane required IV sedation to complete the procedure. Wake up times in the methoxyflurane group were significantly shorter than the IV sedation group with patients being discharged on average 15 minutes earlier. Whilst the adverse event rate was the same between the two groups, most of them occurred in the group of patients who required IV sedation in addition to methoxyflurane to complete the procedure. General satisfaction of inhaled methoxyflurane was high with 93% of those with a successful procedure willing to use the same technique again [68C].

A small single centre observational study investigated the use of a handheld, patient controlled methoxyflurane inhaler for pain and anxiety relief in 15 patients undergoing during burns dressing changes. In this study, the analgesic effect of methoxyflurane was not observed with the primary outcome of post-dressing pain scores being significantly higher post-procedure but the anxiety scores were significantly lower. There were no serious adverse events but 2 patients describing self-limiting altered mood and taste [69c].

Nitrous Oxide

Nervous System

Case 1

A 21-year-old male, recreational user of nitrous oxide, presented with a 2-week history of ascending numbness involving all four limbs. Examination demonstrated diminished vibration and proprioception in fingers, toes and ankles with a high stepped gait and a positive Romberg sign. Vitamin B12 levels were at the lower end of the normal range (212 pg/mL) but homocysteine levels were very high (87 μmol/L). MRI spine showed abnormal T2-weighted hyperintensity along the posterior columns affecting C2–C7. There was some transient initial improvement observed but this was not complete during his acute in-patient stay [70A].

Case 2

A 35-year-old male with escalating nitrous oxide abuse attending the Emergency Department with recent onset generalised weakness, decreased sensation in a glove and stocking distribution and abnormally brisk reflexes. Vitamin B12 levels were normal but no other investigative bloods were performed. MRI identified increased T2 weighted signal within the dorsal columns from C2–C7. The patient was prescribed high dose vitamin B12 supplements but recovery was slow and not yet complete at time of publication [71A].

Case 3

A 16-year-old female recreational user of nitrous oxide presented with ascending numbness over all 4 limb, starting in the peripheries accompanied by an unsteady gait. Proprioception, vibration and pinprick sensation was reduced below the neck. She was ataxic with a positive Romberg test. Routine blood tests were normal including vitamin B12, homocysteine and folate. Somatosensory evoked potentials were also normal. MRI showed hyperintensity in the central and dorsal spinal columns from C1–C6 with additional abnormalities at T7/8. Following high dose vitamin B12 treatment, neurology had improved [72A].

Gastrointestinal

A meta-analysis of studies that randomised patients prospectively to nitrous oxide general anaesthetic or nitrous-free general anaesthetic was performed looking specifically at the rates of post-operative nausea and vomiting. 27 studies were included looking at the effect of duration of anaesthetic on 10 317 patients (N_2O $n=5179$/N_2O free $n=5138$). A significant relationship was demonstrated between duration of GA and the risk of PONV with the risk increasing by 20% per hour after 45 minutes exposure (RR 1.21, $p=0.014$) with the NNT to prevent PONV increasing from 128 (duration <1 hour) to 9 (duration >2 hour). Due to the nature of the study, there was no standardised anaesthetic method which will likely affect the results as propofol has inherent anti-emetic properties compared to emetogenic volatile based GA. There was no comment on the dose of nitrous oxide used. In addition, the duration and type of the surgery per se may have confounded the results as this may have significantly impacted on the risk of PONV irrespective of the modality of anaesthetic given [73M].

Immunological

A prospective randomised control trial investigated 52 patients undergoing elective mastectomy for the effect of sevoflurane or propofol with or without N_2O on the production of inflammatory cytokines in the airway epithelium. Subjects were evenly distributed between the four groups and underwent bronchoscopic microsampling pre- and post-procedure to obtain airway epithelial lining fluid for cytokine analysis. In the sevoflurane/N_2O group, levels of inflammatory cytokines (IL-1β, IL-8 and MCP-1) were elevated compared with baseline but these cytokines were unchanged from baseline in the sevoflurane/air group. There was no effect on IL-6, TNF-α or IL-10. Levels of anti-inflammatory cytokine, IL-12p70, were reduced in the sevoflurane/air group and not in the N_2O group. In the propofol group, only IL-6 and IL-8 were measured and there was no change in IL-8 and IL-6 was below the level of detection. Whilst difficult to draw specific conclusions, the inhalation of N_2O and sevoflurane clearly affect the inflammatory milieu of the airway peri-operatively and this will require further investigation [74c].

Psychological

Propofol is known to cause pain on injection. A prospective single centre study randomised 205 patients undergoing an elective general anaesthetic with propofol into 4 groups (C: control group, L: 0.5 mg/kg lignocaine pre-injection both preoxygenated for 1 minute with 100% oxygen, N: 67% N_2O/33% O_2 pre-oxygenation with no lignocaine and LN: 67% N_2O/33% O_2 pre-oxygenation with 0.5 mg/kg lignocaine) to assess effects. Pain scores were recorded by a blinded investigator at baseline, after pre-oxygenation, after propofol injection and before muscle relaxation using a 0–3 point scale. The incidence of pain was significantly lower in the L (22%), N (34%) and LN (6%) group compared to the control group (76%, $p < 0.001$). The incidence and severity of pain was lower in group LN (6% incidence, pain score 0.18) compared to groups L (22% incidence, pain score 1.12) and N (34% incidence, pain score 2.02) alone ($p < 0.01$). There were no cardiovascular complications or other adverse effects including an increased risk of nausea and vomiting; however, 2 patients were excluded due to side effects of nitrous oxide (oversedation and laughing) [75C].

Sevoflurane

Sensory Systems

A prospective observational study investigated 66 patients undergoing a robotic prostatectomy in the steep head down position looking at changes in intraocular pressure. Patients were randomised to receive a general anaesthetic either using sevoflurane or propofol TIVA. An ophthalmologist blinded to the anaesthetic technique measured intro-ocular pressure at pre-defined time points from baseline to 24 hours post-operatively. The primary outcome was a change in IOP from baseline to 30 minutes after pneumoperitoneum and trendelenburg position (T_3). IOP reduced on induction and the increased both on pneumoperitoneum and trendelenburg positioning, returning to baseline after 24 hours. Sevoflurane increased IOP significantly by 6 mmHg ($p < 0.001$) compared to the propofol group where there was no difference. This was also reflected at T_3 with a significantly higher IOP (23.5 vs. 19.9 mmHg). The patients in the sevoflurane group also had a higher incidence of individual IOP measurements above 24 mmHg (the treatment indication for glaucoma) (74% vs. 52%, $p = 0.002$). There were no ocular complications. Thus sevoflurane is not as effective at controlling IOP in the steep head down position as propofol [76c].

Other

A Proseal Laryngeal mask (pLMA) is larger than a standard LMA thus its removal can stimulate coughing, biting and other upper airway complications. A small observational study attempted to ascertain the optimal depth of anaesthesia for safe removal of the pLMA by randomising 39 fit gynaecology day case surgery patients to receive either desflurane (4–6%) or sevoflurane (1–1.5%). End tidal concentrations were increased/ decreased using the Dixon Massey up and down method in the next patient depending on previous patient's response (movement or no movement). Post-removal, patients were observed for 1 minute for movement, any signs of airway obstruction and recovery time. The EC_{50} and EC_{95} for successful removal of pLMA with sevoflurane was 1.5% and 2.26%, and 2.79% and 3.26% for desflurane, respectively. Successful removal of pLMA (patients with no coughing, clenching of teeth, breath holding, laryngospasm or purposeful movement within 1 minute of pLMA removal) was achieved in 58% and 52% of patient in the sevoflurane and desflurane groups, respectively, with recovery in under 3 minutes for all patients (no differences between the two groups). Adverse events were rare with 3 patients in each coughing, 4 patients biting (5 in desflurane group) and 1 incidence of laryngospasm in each group (no significant differences). There were no desaturations, episodes of hypoxia or recall of the event [77c].

Psychological

The effect of anaesthetic technique on post-operative and chronic pain has been examined. This prospective, double blind study randomised 80 adult patients undergoing an abdominal hysterectomy to receive propofol or sevoflurane as maintenance following IV induction titrated to a BIS of 40–60. They looked at pain scores immediately in recovery and also at 1 and 3 months post-operatively. In the sevoflurane group, pain scores were significantly higher both in the first 4 hours post-operatively (equalising with propofol group by 5 hours). 50% patients in the sevoflurane group compared to 20% in the propofol group were experiencing persistent post-operative pain at 1 and 3 months. The sevoflurane group had a significantly longer surgical time (94 vs. 83 minutes) which may have impacted on the pain scores. There were no cardiovascular complications in either group. Post-operative anxiety and depression scores were significantly higher in the sevoflurane group at 3 months compared to those patients receiving propofol. Unfortunately, there were no pre-operative anxiety and depression scores to compare to therefore this may be present pre-operatively or related to the persistence of surgical pain [78c].

A prospective, randomised, double blind study has investigated the effect of desflurane on a high risk group for emergence delirium, children (aged 2–6 years) undergoing cataract surgery. Following a gas induction, 88 children were randomised to receive either sevoflurane or desflurane at a MAC of 1–1.2 with a subtenon block. Following deep extubation, a blinded investigator used the validated PAED (Paediatric anaesthesia emergence delirium) score to assess the children every 10 minutes for 60 minutes. Emergence was much slower with sevoflurane (3.23 vs. 2.14 23 minutes, $p=0.001$) but there was no difference in the incidence of emergence delirium between the two groups (20.4% in the desflurane group vs. 18.1% in the sevoflurane group, $p=1.0$). In addition, there were no differences in the adverse events of PONV, secretions or cough reported between the two groups and there were no post-operative pain issues [79c].

Nervous System

Sevoflurane is known to produce asymptomatic epileptiform EEG changes but its pharmacological parameters make it an attractive agent for gas induction in children. The clinical relevance of these EEG changes is unknown. A prospective trial randomised 100 children (mean age 4.6 years) undergoing elective surgery to investigate EEG changes with varying concentrations of sevoflurane. The children were randomised to receive either 8% sevoflurane for 3 minutes or 6% sevoflurane for 5 minutes before reducing the dose to 4%, obtaining IV access and proceeding with TIVA maintenance anaesthesia. EEG electrodes were placed pre-operatively and the surgical time was divided into sections (A: start of sevoflurane to start of propofol, B: start of propofol to deep hypnosis on EEG and C: deep hypnosis to the end of the procedure). The time to loss of consciousness was the same in both groups however, the time to deep hypnosis was quicker in the patients receiving 8% propofol (64 vs. 77.9 seconds, $p=0.002$). During section A, a significantly higher proportion of patients had epileptiform activity in those receiving 8% sevoflurane compared to the 6% group (76% vs. 52%, $p=0.0106$). These changes reduced in frequency in section B and there were no differences between the two groups. In section C, only 3 patients per group had epileptiform activity lasting more than 60 seconds. This study thus concludes that 6% sevoflurane has a similar onset of action with reduced epileptiform activity than the higher induction dose of sevoflurane although it is unclear why different durations of sevoflurane were used for induction when the time to loss of consciousness was <45 seconds [80c].

A further case report identified a 21-year-old healthy male, who underwent a sevoflurane anaesthesia as part of a volunteer study. On induction with an ET_{sevo} of 1.24%, the patient developed convulsions without epileptiform EEG changes. On increasing the sevoflurane concentration to 4.15%, he underwent a tonic-clonic seizure with EEG changes consistent with seizure activity. Seizure stopped on cessation of sevoflurane and propofol was given as rescue medication. The patient recovered completely and there were no other adverse effects [81A].

Once again, the ideal anaesthesia for ECT has been investigated. A prospective randomised double blind study looking at patients with resistant depression undergoing ECT has been carried out. They randomised 12 patients having 120 ECT sessions to receive either propofol 0.5 mg/kg or 8% sevoflurane. All groups received 1 microgram/kg remifentanil. The patients receiving sevoflurane had a longer induction and recovery time ($p<0.05$) and a shorter duration of motor and EEG changes suggestive of convulsions. Although not elaborated on, side effects of nausea and vomiting were reported as the same in each group. This study identifies that the combination of propofol and remifentanil was, therefore, a more favourable drug regime for ECT than sevoflurane. This may be due to the addition of remifentanil allowing a lower dose of propofol to be utilised. Unfortunately sevoflurane concentrations were not available and therefore the depth of sevoflurane anaesthesia was unknown [82c].

Immunologic

A study randomised 80 women undergoing elective caesarean section to receive either sevoflurane or desflurane maintenance anaesthesia following IV induction. Blood samples were taken blood pre- and post-operatively and umbilical artery blood at time of delivery to examine to assess markers of oxidative stress. Despite comparable haemodynamic stability, the desflurane group, when compared to sevoflurane, had a higher lipid hydroperoxide, total oxidative status and oxidative stress index, indicating a greater degree of oxidative stress. This was also reflected in the umbilical artery blood taken at delivery. There were no changes in the concentration of free sulphydryl groups in the desflurane group. The lipid hydroperoxide and the sulphydryl groups actually decreased in the sevoflurane groups when compared to baseline [83c].

Respiratory

A well designed prospective randomised study has looked at the utility of TIVA for flexible fibreoptic bronchoscopy in children, a common procedure done to investigate paediatric respiratory disease. The study was undertaken in two phases; phase one to identify the ED_{99} of both propofol and sevoflurane and phase 2 to compare the ED_{99} of both drugs to assess efficacy and safety. In phase one, the study randomised 75 children in each group to receive either TIVA or sevoflurane and a number of doses and the results examined by probit analysis. Success of the technique was described as (1) no bucking, coughing, nausea, vomiting, bronchospasm or agitation and (2) no hypoxaemia or hypercapnia. The ED_{99} were 8.9 micrograms/mL and 6.8% for propofol and sevoflurane, respectively. Phase two then commenced using these doses for flexible fibreoptic bronchoscopy in a total of 50 further children. Induction time was quicker (34.8 vs. 81.6 seconds, $p < 0.001$) in the TIVA group but recovery time was significantly longer (44.9 vs. 15.4 seconds, $p < 0.001$). Most of the children in the TIVA group compared to only 40% of the sevoflurane group had apnoeic episodes, requiring airway support. Stress hormone levels and plasma glucose were also measured. Glucose, cortisol, adrenaline and noradrenaline levels were reduced from baseline in both groups but in the TIVA group were significantly lower than the volatile group. 92% of the children receiving volatile anaesthesia had coughing on emergence compared to 24% in the propofol group ($p < 0.001$). In addition, agitation on induction (96% vs. 12%) and on emergence (52% vs. 4%, $p < 0.001$) was both higher in the sevoflurane group. There were no differences in any other measured adverse event (laryngospasm, nausea, vomiting, bronchospasm) thus concluding that TIVA is superior to sevoflurane for paediatric FFB [84C].

Cardiovascular

The left atrium (LA) plays a key role in cardiac function both as a reservoir and conduit for passive LV filling and as an active booster pump, completing LV filling during late diastole. A retrospective study investigated the effects of volatile anaesthesia and positive pressure ventilation on the function of the left atrium. Pooled results of all volatile agents were included in this post hoc analysis. However, the authors examined a large range of echo parameters thus improving the validity of the study. They found that spontaneous ventilation with volatile anaesthesia reduced the LA pump function significantly (as measured by multiple TTE parameters). The addition of positive pressure ventilation reduced this further. The volume of the LA remained preserved throughout. Limited by its retrospective nature, there should be further prospective studies in patients with pre-existing cardiac dysfunction as this would be more clinically relevant [85c].

Case report

A 63-year-old female with a history of paroxysmal atrial fibrillation (AF) on anti-arrhythmic dofetilide, underwent an AF ablation due to increased symptoms. Pre-operative investigation including echocardiography, routine blood tests, nuclear perfusion test and a left heart catheterisation were all normal. ECG on the morning of the operation demonstrated a mildly prolonged QTc (477 ms) and she underwent a general anaesthetic with sevoflurane. Following catheterisation of the left atrium, she went spontaneously into ventricular fibrillation requiring a 200J DC shock. She continued to have frequent premature ventricular complexes and QTc interval was greatly prolonged (850 ms) but transthoracic echocardiogram was normal as were arterial blood gases, plasma electrolytes and coronary angiogram. An interaction between the patient's AF medications (dofetilide, a known QTc prolonger) and the sevoflurane was assumed and the volatile anaesthetic was stopped and converted to intravenous anaesthesia. Within 10 minutes, all arrhythmias disappeared and QTc interval started to normalise. This adverse event was attributed to an interaction between two QTc interval prolonging drugs [86A].

Neuromuscular Function

A number of studies have investigated the role of volatiles in the onset of malignant hyperthermia and rhabdomyolysis

Case report

A 6-year-old boy with Duchenne muscular dystrophy (DMD) required a general anaesthetic for debridement of a dog bite. He was mobile and had had three uneventful general anaesthetics in the past. Previous cardiology review was unremarkable. He underwent an inhalational induction as he would not allow IV access. Very soon after, he developed a broad complex bradycardia which was resistant to atropine. Sevoflurane was stopped and 100% oxygen delivered whilst CPR was commenced. Initial ABG showed a pH pf 7.01, PCO$_2$ 84 mmHg, HCO$_3$ 20 mmol/L and a K > 9 mmol/L. He received the appropriate resuscitation with calcium, dextrose, insulin and was intubated. Adrenaline infusion was commenced. Working diagnosis was acute rhabdomyolysis with hyperkalaemia. Despite 2 brief returns of spontaneous circulation, arrhythmias continued and after 1 hour, resuscitation was stopped, final blood tests showed a CK 45 300 IU/L and K$^+$ was 14.3 mmol/L. Post-mortem confirmed DMD and rhabdomyolysis. In DMD, the transition from histologically normal muscle to severe atrophy and fibrosis occurs over the first decade and hence provides a potential reason for the difference between this and the previous anaesthetics. Post-mortem histology demonstrated roughly equal proportions of healthy and diseased muscle, therefore hypothesising that in his younger years this preponderance was in favour of healthy muscle, therefore not causing a problem with general anaesthesia. This combined with a child not co-operating with IV access, thus requiring a gas induction, led to anaesthesia induced rhabdomyolysis with severity and speed of onset rarely observed [87A].

Reports of the symptoms of malignant hyperpyrexia being more delayed than previously thought have been published.

Case report

A 22-year-old male with an open femoral fracture requiring surgical fixation was reported. Pre-operative assessment identified no previous medical or surgical history or family history of reactions to general anaesthesia. Induction was uneventful, general anaesthesia was maintained with sevoflurane (2%) and total operative time was approximately 2 hours. Following an uneventful procedure, the patient became hypertensive, tachycardic and hyperthermic (T3 8.1 °C) with intense masseter spasm and increased abdominal rigidity. Venous blood gas showed mild hypercarbia (66 mmHg) and hyperkalaemia (5.5 mmol/L) which was treated with β-agonists and dextrose/insulin. A suspected diagnosis of malignant hyperthermia was made and 2.5 mg/kg dantrolene was administered which resulted in resolution of the hypercarbia and muscular rigidity. Twenty minutes later, observations were normal and temperature was reducing and he was stable enough to be transported to a higher level facility. He was extubated 9 hours later. The following day, he returned to theatre for definitive treatment of the injury, a non-triggering anaesthetic was given and the procedure was uneventful. There were no available facilities for further investigation of the suspected MH [88A].

DELAYED ONSET OF MALIGNANT HYPERTHERMIA

This has been examined further in two analyses of the North American registry of malignant hyperthermia looking at adults and children separately have been carried out.

The first identified 477 patients who fulfilled the criteria for possible or fulminant MH and divided them into four groups based on the presence or absence of volatile anaesthesia (halothane, sevoflurane, desflurane or isoflurane) and suxamethonium. They describe a delay in onset times with different volatile agents in the absence of suxamethonium with halothane being the quickest (median 15 minutes) increasing to isoflurane (median 135 minutes, p < 0.05) with sevoflurane and desflurane at intermediary times (45 and 113 minutes, respectively). The presence of suxamethonium reduced these times to 10, 30, 50 and 65 minutes for halothane, sevoflurane, desflurane and isoflurane, respectively. Of these cases, the first MH signs were hypercarbia (30.7%), masseter spasm (24.8%) and sinus tachycardia (21.1%) although these differed widely amongst the four groups. Following initial analysis, the patients were divided by age, those younger than 20 years had a shorter onset of MH symptoms and suxamethonium reduced this further (p < 0.005) [89R].

A second registry analysis looked at the 17% of cases on the North American registry who were under 18 years of age. The 264 cases deemed very likely or almost certain on a validated clinical score, were divided into age groups, 0–24 months (young), 25 months–12 years (middle) and 13–18 years (old). The variations in the groups (type of surgery and general anaesthetic were largely determined by age-based clinical practice and only 18% had a positive family history of MH). Clinical symptoms were largely dependent on age. The older group were more likely to develop a sinus tachycardia, hypercarbia, and hyperthermia, whereas the middle and younger age groups were more likely to develop masseter spasm and skin mottling, respectively. There were no differences in the incidence of muscle rigidity, tachypnoea, cyanosis, arrhythmias and hyperthermia between the groups. Master spasm was much more common if given suxamethonium (75/125 vs. 11/128, p < 0.001). The study concluded that older children have more severe symptoms related to MH which may be secondary to the increased muscle mass acquired during development. This may also account for the higher peak lactate and lower pH in younger individuals which may indicate a lower reserve to buffer the anaerobic metabolism [90R].

Liver

A retrospective study undertook an examination of case notes and results of patients undergoing volatile anaesthesia to ascertain the effect on hepatic function.

1556 patients were categorised in to groups dependent on their post-operative ALT (<120, 120–200, >200 U/L). A validated score (CIOMS/RUCAM) was then used to determine the hepatotoxicity of the anaesthetic agent with a score of ≥4 considered significant. The baseline groups were the same but there was a significant amount of missing data resulting in more than 50% of patients being excluded from analysis. The estimated incidence of anaesthetic induced liver injury was 3% (47/1556). No patient developed jaundice or fulminant liver injury [91c].

References

[1] Luedi MM, Koppenberg J, Stuber F. Etomidate for critically ill patients: still a matter for pro-con debates? Eur J Anaesthesiol. 2014;31:55–6 [R].

[2] van den Heuvel I, Wurmb TE, Bottiger BW, et al. Pros and cons of etomidate—more discussion than evidence? Curr Opin Anaesthesiol. 2013;26:404–8 [R].

[3] Komatsu R, You J, Mascha EJ, et al. Anesthetic induction with etomidate, rather than propofol, is associated with increased 30-day mortality and cardiovascular morbidity after noncardiac surgery. Anesth Analg. 2013;117:1329–37 [C].

[4] Weng D, Huang M, Jiang R, et al. Clinical study of etomidate emulsion combined with remifentanil in general anesthesia. Drug Des Devel Ther. 2013;7:771–6 [c].

[5] Price B, Arthur AO, Brunko M, et al. Hemodynamic consequences of ketamine vs. etomidate for endotracheal intubation in the air medical setting. Am J Emerg Med. 2013;31:1124–32 [c].

[6] Edward Roberts R, Curran HV, Friston KJ, et al. Abnormalities in white matter microstructure associated with chronic ketamine use. Neuropsychopharmacology. 2014;39:329–38 [c].

[7] Buonsenso D, Barone G, Valentini P, et al. A Utility of intranasal Ketamine and Midazolam to perform gastric aspirates in children: a double-blind, placebo controlled, randomized study. BMC Pediatr. 2014;14:67 [c].

[8] Andolfatto G, Willman E, Joo D, et al. Intranasal ketamine for analgesia in the emergency department: a prospective observational series. Acad Emerg Med. 2013;20:1050–4 [c].

[9] Folayan MO, Faponle AF, Oziegbe EO, et al. A prospective study on the effectiveness of ketamine and diazepam used for conscious sedation in paediatric dental patients' management. Eur J Paediatr Dent. 2014;15:132–6 [c].

[10] Chen WY, Huang MC. Lin SK Gender differences in subjective discontinuation symptoms associated with ketamine use. Subst Abuse Treat Prev Policy. 2014;9:39 [R].

[11] Liang HJ, Lau CG, Tang A, et al. Cognitive impairments in poly-drug ketamine users. Addict Behav. 2013;38:2661–6 [C].

[12] Dakwar E, Anerella C, Hart CL, et al. Therapeutic infusions of ketamine: do the psychoactive effects matter? Drug Alcohol Depend. 2014;136:153–7 [c].

[13] Rush AJ. Ketamine for treatment-resistant depression: ready or not for clinical use? Am J Psychiatry. 2013;170:1079–81 [r].

[14] Sos P, Klirova M, Novak T, et al. Relationship of ketamine's antidepressant and psychotomimetic effects in unipolar depression. Neuro Endocrinol Lett. 2013;34:287–93 [c].

[15] Szymkowicz SM, Finnegan N, Dale RM. Failed response to repeat intravenous ketamine infusions in geriatric patients with major depressive disorder. J Clin Psychopharmacol. 2014;34:285–6 [A].

[16] Atigari OV, Healy D. Sustained antidepressant response to ketamine. BMJ Case Rep. 2013;2013 [A].

[17] Lui KL, Lee WK, Li MK. Ketamine-induced cholangiopathy. Hong Kong Med J. 2014;20. 78 e1–e2 [A].

[18] Smart C, Kabir M, Pati J. Treatment of ketamine-associated cystitis with chondroitin sulphate. Br J Nurs. 2013;22:S4. S6, S8–9 [A].

[19] Jenyon T, Sole G. Bladder calcification secondary to ketamine. Urol J. 2013;10:912–4 [A].

[20] Pal R, Balt S, Erowid E, et al. Ketamine is associated with lower urinary tract signs and symptoms. Drug Alcohol Depend. 2013;132:189–94 [A].

[21] Hills CE, Jin T, Siamantouras E, et al. 'Special k' and a loss of cell-to-cell adhesion in proximal tubule-derived epithelial cells: modulation of the adherens junction complex by ketamine. PLoS One. 2013;8:e71819 [E].

[22] Dewhirst E, Frazier WJ, Leder M, et al. Cardiac arrest following ketamine administration for rapid sequence intubation. J Intensive Care Med. 2013;28:375–9 [A].

[23] Prabhakar H, Bindra A, Singh GP, et al. Propofol versus thiopental sodium for the treatment of refractory status epilepticus (Review). Evid Based Child Health. 2013;8:1488–508 [R].

[24] Marsot A, Goirand F, Milesi N, et al. Interaction of thiopental with esomeprazole in critically ill patients. Eur J Clin Pharmacol. 2013;69:1667–72 [c].

[25] Kjellgren A, Jonsson K. Methoxetamine (MXE)—a phenomenological study of experiences induced by a "legal high" from the internet. J Psychoactive Drugs. 2013;45:276–86 [c].

[26] Chiaretti A, Benini F, Pierri F, et al. Safety and efficacy of propofol administered by paediatricians during procedural sedation in children. Acta Paediatr. 2014;103:182–7 [R].

[27] Khan HA, Umar M, Tul-Bushra H, et al. Safety of non-anaesthesiologist-administered propofol sedation in ERCP. Arab J Gastroenterol. 2014;15:32–5 [c].

[28] Newstead B, Bradburn S, Appelboam A, et al. Propofol for adult procedural sedation in a UK emergency department: safety profile in 1008 cases. Br J Anaesth. 2013;111:651–5 [C].

[29] Hanslik A, Moysich A, Laser KT, et al. Percutaneous closure of atrial septal defects in spontaneously breathing children under deep sedation: a feasible and safe concept. Pediatr Cardiol. 2014;35:215–22 [c].

[30] Adeyemo A, Bannazadeh M, Riggs T, et al. Does sedation type affect colonoscopy perforation rates? Dis Colon Rectum. 2014;57:110–4 [R].

[31] Mao W, Wei XQ, Tao J, et al. The safety of combined sedation with propofol plus fentanyl for endoscopy screening and endoscopic variceal ligation in cirrhotic patients. J Dig Dis. 2014;15:124–30 [c].

[32] Jones GM, Doepker BA, Erdman MJ, et al. Predictors of severe hypotension in neurocritical care patients sedated with propofol. Neurocrit Care. 2014;20:270–6 [c].

[33] El Beheiry H, Mak P. Effects of aging and propofol on the cardiovascular component of the autonomic nervous system. J Clin Anesth. 2013;25:637–43 [c].

[34] Xu WY, Wang N, Xu HT, et al. Effects of sevoflurane and propofol on right ventricular function and pulmonary circulation in patients undergo esophagectomy. Int J Clin Exp Pathol. 2014;7:272–9 [c].

[35] Guerrero Orriach JL, Galan Ortega M, Ramirez Aliaga M, et al. Prolonged sevoflurane administration in the off-pump coronary artery bypass graft surgery: beneficial effects. J Crit Care. 2013;28:879. e13–8 [c].

[36] Yu T, Huang Y, Guo F, et al. The effects of propofol and dexmedetomidine infusion on fluid responsiveness in critically ill patients. J Surg Res. 2013;185:763–73 [c].

[37] Curtis JA, Hollinger MK, Jain HB. Propofol-based versus dexmedetomidine-based sedation in cardiac surgery patients. J Cardiothorac Vasc Anesth. 2013;27:1289–94 [C].

[38] Xia ZQ, Chen SQ, Yao X, et al. Clinical benefits of dexmedetomidine versus propofol in adult intensive care unit

patients: a meta-analysis of randomized clinical trials. J Surg Res. 2013;185:833–43 [M].

[39] Penna GL, Fialho FM, Kurtz P, et al. Changing sedative infusion from propofol to midazolam improves sublingual microcirculatory perfusion in patients with septic shock. J Crit Care. 2013;28:825–31 [c].

[40] Harreld JH, Helton KJ, Kaddoum RN, et al. The effects of propofol on cerebral perfusion MRI in children. Neuroradiology. 2013;55:1049–56 [c].

[41] Nagels AJ, Bridgman JB, Bell SE, et al. Propofol-remifentanil TCI sedation for oral surgery. N Z Dent J. 2014;110:85–9 [c].

[42] Hickel C. Early percutaneous pinning of hip fracture using propofol-ketamine-lidocaine admixture in a geriatric patient receiving dabigatran: a case report. AANA J. 2014;82:46–52 [A].

[43] Wakabayashi S, Yamaguchi K, Kumakura S, et al. Effects of anesthesia with sevoflurane and propofol on the cytokine/chemokine production at the airway epithelium during esophagectomy. Int J Mol Med. 2014;34:137–44 [c].

[44] Brown KE, Mirrakhimov AE, Yeddula K, et al. Propofol and the risk of delirium: exploring the anticholinergic properties of propofol. Med Hypotheses. 2013;81:536–9 [r].

[45] Tedders KM, McNorton KN, Edwin SB. Efficacy and safety of analgosedation with fentanyl compared with traditional sedation with propofol. Pharmacotherapy. 2014;34:643–7 [c].

[46] Lu Y, Ye Z, Wong GT, et al. Prevention of injection pain due to propofol by dezocine: a comparison with lidocaine. Indian J Pharmacol. 2013;45:619–21 [c].

[47] Wang M, Wang Q, Yu YY, et al. An effective dose of ketamine for eliminating pain during injection of propofol: a dose response study. Ann Fr Anesth Reanim. 2013;32:e103–6 [c].

[48] Hoyer C, Kranaster L, Janke C, et al. Impact of the anesthetic agents ketamine, etomidate, thiopental, and propofol on seizure parameters and seizure quality in electroconvulsive therapy: a retrospective study. Eur Arch Psychiatry Clin Neurosci. 2014;264:255–61 [C].

[49] Pedersen NA, Jensen AG, Kilmose L, et al. Propofol-remifentanil or sevoflurane for children undergoing magnetic resonance imaging? A randomised study. Acta Anaesthesiol Scand. 2013;57:988–95 [c].

[50] Sinnollareddy M, Marotti SB. Propofol-associated urine discolouration in critically ill patients—case reports. Anaesth Intensive Care. 2014;42:268–9 [A].

[51] Bassi E, Ferreira CB, Macedo E, et al. Recurrent clotting of dialysis filter associated with hypertriglyceridemia induced by propofol. Am J Kidney Dis. 2014;63:860–1 [A].

[52] Allchurch LG, Crilly H. Fixed drug eruption to propofol. Anaesth Intensive Care. 2014;42:777–81 [A].

[53] Erturk E, Topaloglu S, Dohman D, et al. The comparison of the effects of sevoflurane inhalation anesthesia and intravenous propofol anesthesia on oxidative stress in one lung ventilation. Biomed Res Int. 2014;2014:360936 [c].

[54] Mazoti MA, Braz MG, de Assis GM, et al. Comparison of inflammatory cytokine profiles in plasma of patients undergoing otorhinological surgery with propofol or isoflurane anesthesia. Inflamm Res. 2013;62:879–85 [c].

[55] Zhang T, Fan Y, Liu K, et al. Effects of different general anaesthetic techniques on immune responses in patients undergoing surgery for tongue cancer. Anaesth Intensive Care. 2014;42:220–7 [c].

[56] Han E, Jung S, Baeck S, et al. Deaths from recreational use of propofol in Korea. Forensic Sci Int. 2013;233:333–7 [C].

[57] Yen P, Prior S, Riley C, et al. S A comparison of fospropofol to midazolam for moderate sedation during outpatient dental procedures. Anesth Prog. 2013;60:162–77 [c].

[58] Fechner J, Ihmsen H, Schuttler J, et al. A randomized open-label phase I pilot study of the safety and efficacy of total intravenous anesthesia with fospropofol for coronary artery bypass graft surgery. J Cardiothorac Vasc Anesth. 2013;27:908–15 [c].

[59] Chen J, Zhou JQ, Chen ZF, et al. Efficacy and safety of dexmedetomidine versus propofol for the sedation of tube-retention after oral maxillofacial surgery. J Oral Maxillofac Surg. 2014;72. 285. e1–7 [c].

[60] Kim NY, Kim SY, Yoon HJ, et al. Effect of dexmedetomidine on sevoflurane requirements and emergence agitation in children undergoing ambulatory surgery. Yonsei Med J. 2014;55:209–15 [c].

[61] Char D, Drover DR, Motonaga KS, et al. The effects of ketamine on dexmedetomidine-induced electrophysiologic changes in children. Paediatr Anaesth. 2013;23:898–905 [c].

[62] Kim JY, Lee JS, Lee KC, et al. The effect of desflurane versus propofol on regional cerebral oxygenation in the sitting position for shoulder arthroscopy. J Clin Monit Comput. 2014;28:371–6 [c].

[63] Kim JK, Kim DK, Lee MJ. Relationship of bispectral index to minimum alveolar concentration during isoflurane, sevoflurane or desflurane anaesthesia. J Int Med Res. 2014;42:130–7 [c].

[64] Duger C, Dogan M, Isbir AC, et al. Comparison of the effects of desflurane and sevoflurane on middle ear pressure: a randomized controlled clinical trial. ORL J Otorhinolaryngol Relat Spec. 2013;75:314–9 [c].

[65] Koksoy S, Sahin Z, Karsli B. Comparison of the effects of desflurane and bupivacaine on Th1 and Th2 responses. Clin Lab. 2013;59:1215–20 [c].

[66] Wu ZF, Jian GS, Lee MS, et al. An analysis of anesthesia-controlled operating room time after propofol-based total intravenous anesthesia compared with desflurane anesthesia in ophthalmic surgery: a retrospective study. Anesth Analg. 2014;119:1393–406 [r].

[67] Zhao J, Hao J, Fei X, et al. Isoflurane inhibits occludin expression via up-regulation of hypoxia-inducible factor 1alpha. Brain Res. 2014;1562:1–10 [E].

[68] Nguyen NQ, Toscano L, Lawrence M, et al. Patient-controlled analgesia with inhaled methoxyflurane versus conventional endoscopist-provided sedation for colonoscopy: a randomized multicenter trial. Gastrointest Endosc. 2013;78:892–901 [C].

[69] Wasiak J, Mahar PD, Paul E, et al. Inhaled methoxyflurane for pain and anxiety relief during burn wound care procedures: an Australian case series. Int Wound J. 2014;11:74–8 [c].

[70] Arshi B, Shaw S. Subacute ascending numbness. Clin Toxicol (Phila). 2014;52:905–6 [A].

[71] Rheinboldt M, Harper D, Parrish D, et al. Nitrous oxide induced myeloneuropathy: a case report. Emerg Radiol. 2014;21:85–8 [A].

[72] Hu MH, Huang GS, Wu CT, et al. Nitrous oxide myelopathy in a pediatric patient. Pediatr Emerg Care. 2014;30:266–7 [A].

[73] Peyton PJ, Wu CY. Nitrous oxide-related postoperative nausea and vomiting depends on duration of exposure. Anesthesiology. 2014;120:1137–45 [M].

[74] Kumakura S, Yamaguchi K, Sugasawa Y, et al. Effects of nitrous oxide on the production of cytokines and chemokines by the airway epithelium during anesthesia with sevoflurane and propofol. Mol Med Rep. 2013;8:1643–8 [c].

[75] Kim E, Kim CH, Kim HK, et al. Effect of nitrous oxide inhalation on pain after propofol and rocuronium injection. J Anesth. 2013;27:868–73 [C].

[76] Yoo YC, Shin S, Choi EK, et al. Increase in intraocular pressure is less with propofol than with sevoflurane during laparoscopic surgery in the steep Trendelenburg position. Can J Anaesth. 2014;61:322–9 [c].

[77] Ghai B, Jain K, Bansal D, et al. End-tidal concentrations of sevoflurane and desflurane for ProSeal laryngeal mask airway removal in anaesthetised adults: a randomised double-blind study. Eur J Anaesthesiol. 2014;31:274–9 [c].

[78] Ogurlu M, Sari S, Kucuk M, et al. Comparison of the effect of propofol and sevoflurane anaesthesia on acute and chronic postoperative pain after hysterectomy. Anaesth Intensive Care. 2014;42:365–70 [c].

[79] Sethi S, Ghai B, Ram J, et al. Postoperative emergence delirium in pediatric patients undergoing cataract surgery—a comparison of desflurane and sevoflurane. Paediatr Anaesth. 2013;23:1131–7 [c].

[80] Kreuzer I, Osthaus WA, Schultz A, et al. Influence of the sevoflurane concentration on the occurrence of epileptiform EEG patterns. PLoS One. 2014;9:e89191 [c].

[81] Pilge S, Jordan D, Kochs EF, et al. Sevoflurane-induced epileptiform electroencephalographic activity and generalized tonic-clonic seizures in a volunteer study. Anesthesiology. 2013;119:447 [A].

[82] Ulusoy H, Cekic B, Besir A, et al. Sevoflurane/remifentanil versus propofol/remifentanil for electroconvulsive therapy: comparison of seizure duration and haemodynamic responses. J Int Med Res. 2014;42:111–9 [c].

[83] Yalcin S, Aydogan H, Yuce HH, et al. Effects of sevoflurane and desflurane on oxidative stress during general anesthesia for elective caesarean section. Wien Klin Wochenschr. 2013;125:467–73 [c].

[84] Chen L, Yu L, Fan Y, et al. A comparison between total intravenous anaesthesia using propofol plus remifentanil and volatile induction/maintenance of anaesthesia using sevoflurane in children undergoing flexible fibreoptic bronchoscopy. Anaesth Intensive Care. 2013;41:742–9 [C].

[85] Freiermuth D, Skarvan K, Filipovic M, et al. Volatile anaesthetics and positive pressure ventilation reduce left atrial performance: a transthoracic echocardiographic study in young healthy adults. Br J Anaesth. 2014;112:1032–41 [c].

[86] Saini A, Shah H, Saba S. QT prolongation and T-wave alternans during catheter ablation of atrial fibrillation: a case report. Ann Noninvasive Electrocardiol. 2014;19:190–2 [A].

[87] Simpson RS, Van K. Fatal rhabdomyolysis following volatile induction in a six-year-old boy with Duchenne Muscular Dystrophy. Anaesth Intensive Care. 2013;41:805–7 [A].

[88] Banek R, Weatherwax J, Spence D, et al. Delayed onset of suspected malignant hyperthermia during sevoflurane anesthesia in an Afghan trauma patient: a case report. AANA J. 2013;81:441–5 [A].

[89] Visoiu M, Young MC, Wieland K, et al. Anesthetic drugs and onset of malignant hyperthermia. Anesth Analg. 2014;118:388–96 [R].

[90] Nelson P, Litman RS. Malignant hyperthermia in children: an analysis of the North American malignant hyperthermia registry. Anesth Analg. 2014;118:369–74 [R].

[91] Lin J, Moore D, Hockey B, et al. Drug-induced hepatotoxicity: incidence of abnormal liver function tests consistent with volatile anaesthetic hepatitis in trauma patients. Liver Int. 2014;34:576–82 [c].

11

Local Anesthetics

Sujana Dontukurthy, Allison Kalstein, Joel Yarmush[1]

Department of Anesthesiology, New York Methodist Hospital, Brooklyn, NY, USA
[1]Corresponding author: joelyarmush@gmail.com

GENERAL INFORMATION

Adverse events of local anesthetics are often seen after an excessive dose of drug is given systemically. This is usually caused by either a non-excessive dose being inadvertently given intravenously or intra-arterially or an excessive dose being used and absorbed systemically. The age of a systemic overdose, especially when it is seen in regional anesthesia, ought to be coming to an end. The use of relatively inexpensive and easy to use ultrasound machines and widespread training in their use has led to a more precise technique thereby allowing lower volumes and concentrations of local anesthetics to be used. In other words, local anesthetic systemic toxicity (LAST) can now be minimized when ultrasound is used for traditional regional blocks. However, the increased use of the ultrasound has also led to new types of regional anesthesia such as the transverse abdominis plane (TAP) block where a large volume of local anesthetic is used and LAST may be seen in those blocks. While LAST should be minimized in many situations, treatment has also advanced with the use of lipid emulsions to reverse the cardiovascular and neurologic effects of the overdose. Our survey of the literature in the following pages shows that as well.

COMBINED ANESTHETICS

Cardiovascular

Benign Supraventricular Arrhythmias: Bupivacaine vs. Ropivacaine

A comparative study was done in 44 patients related to cardiovascular safety between ropivacaine and bupivacaine in brachial plexus blocks. Patients were randomized to receive 30 ml of either 0.5% bupivacaine with epinephrine 1:200000 or 0.5% ropivacaine with epinephrine 1:200000. Results showed similar efficacy between bupivacaine and ropivacaine for brachial plexus blockade with similar incidences of benign supraventricular arrhythmias [1c].

Cell Toxicity

A study in rat chondrocytes using different doses of bupivacaine and levobupivacaine found that local anesthetics have dose dependent cytotoxicity. The authors describe apoptosis seen on isolated, cleaned rat chondrocytes when exposed to very low concentrations of bupivacaine and levobupivacaine. The concentration of local anesthetic was much lower than seen in clinical applications. They showed that apoptosis was lessened at the least concentrations for the shortest time [2E].

A study was performed by exposing local anesthetics to human chondrocytes to further elucidate toxicity of intra-articular injections. The authors found that bupivacaine was greater than mepivacaine, which was greater than ropivacaine in inducing cytotoxicity. The toxicity increased with concentration and duration of drug. The local anesthetics were found to be more toxic in degenerative vs. intact cartilage [3E].

Nervous System

Delayed Manifestation of Local Anesthetic Local Toxicity After Combined Psoas Compartment and Sciatic Nerve Block

An elderly woman with multiple comorbidities (American Society of Anesthesiology (ASA) physical status IV) presented for emergency hip fracture repair. A combined psoas compartment and sciatic nerve block was utilized for anesthesia to avoid hemodynamic fluctuations seen in major neuraxial (i.e., spinal and/or epidural) or general anesthesia. The blocks were performed using bupivacaine and mepivacaine. Fifteen minutes after the conclusion of the block placement the patient became

© 2015 Elsevier B.V. All rights reserved.

unresponsive and was noted to have a fixed gaze. Given the patient's extensive history of vascular disease, cerebrovascular accident was entertained as the likely diagnosis. Approximately 5 minutes later, the patient had grand mal seizures which were treated with midazolam 2 mg and the airway was secured. The patient's course was further complicated by bradycardia after ~20 minutes, which initially responded to atropine but then progressed to pulseless electrical activity. ACLS was initiated, and the diagnosis was reevaluated. LAST was then diagnosed and a lipid emulsion was initiated. Resuscitation was unsuccessful and the patient was declared dead ~1.5 hours after the onset of her grand mal seizure [4A].

The authors present an enlightening discussion about recognizing and treating LAST. A fairly comprehensive review of LAST was also included. In a letter to the editor [5r], Petrar and Montemurro point out that the total dose of local anesthetic (in this case 450 mg of mepivacaine and 25 mg of bupivacaine) was excessive, especially for this frail, underweight (45 kg), elderly patient. In another letter to the editor [6r], Barrington and Weinberg, point out that fixation on technique without (implied) flexibility may have been the ultimate cause of LAST. In reply [7r], the authors of the case report acknowledge the salient points made in the letters and emphasize that clinical decision making of all types is the preeminent factor in LAST. The excessive local anesthetic needed for the regional anesthetic blocks chosen for this particular patient should have been noted *a priori* which would have given better direction in the clinical making decision and may have prevented LAST or at least have prompted earlier lipid treatment.

Toxicity After Spinal Anesthesia

A study with different intrathecal dosages of bupivacaine, levobupivacaine or ropivacaine in dogs showed that at clinical doses, there was no significant damage to the CSF, nerve roots or spinal cord. Damage might be more of a factor as concentration and volume of drug are increased [8E]. A study with an intrathecally administered combination of local anesthetics in rats showed that the combination of lidocaine and bupivacaine did not increase toxicity while the combination of lidocaine and ropivacaine did increase toxicity [9E].

A review article confirms that the incidence of reported neurologic damage after spinal anesthesia is very low [10R].

BENZOCAINE

Dermatologic

Acute Generalized Exanthematous Pustulosis After Benzocaine Spray

A case is presented of the first example of acute generalized exanthematous pustulosis (AGEP) in a patient given benzocaine spray for a dental extraction 24 hours before the eruption. The patient had exposure to benzocaine previously and in subsequent testing was found to have positive patch test consistent with an allergic contact dermatitis [11A]. This is a rare but significant new side effect of this topical ester local anesthetic. However, no mention is made of the extent of spraying (i.e., total amount of drug) or if there were any breaks in the skin or of any other possible local anesthetic absorption.

Hematologic

Methemoglobinemia After Benzocaine Administration

An 8-year-old boy was admitted to the hospital for an appendectomy. To facilitate placement of a nasogastric tube, benzocaine spray was used multiple times during multiple attempts. The patient subsequently became cyanotic, with an initial methemoglobin level of 32.9%. Methylene blue was administered and the patient promptly responded with resolution of cyanosis. The patient's serum was analyzed using liquid chromatography and mass spectrometry and a reference standard for N-hydroxy-*para*-amino benzoic acid (N-OH-PABA) was synthesized for comparison. The authors concluded that N-OH-PABA, an active metabolite of benzocaine was responsible for the oxidative stress after the topical application [12A]. The usual benzocaine instructions of a limit of two, 1 second bursts to avoid toxicity often make its use impractical. Substituting an alternative local anesthetic preparation such as a small amount of viscous lidocaine may be a preferred method of anesthetizing the pharynx.

Methemoglobinemia After Ingesting a Benzocaine Lollipop

Methemoglobinemia was diagnosed in a 71-year-old woman who received a hurricane lollipop (20% benzocaine gel impregnated on a stick) for transesophageal echocardiography done to rule out a cardioembolic etiology of stroke. The patient's arterial blood saturation fell to near venous levels (i.e., ~70%) 20 minutes after the uneventful procedure. An arterial blood gas revealed an oxygen saturation of 76% despite a PaO_2 of 252 mm Hg. Methemoglobin level was noted to be 44.2%. The patient responded to methylene blue treatment [13A].

Methemoglobinemia After Using Benzocaine Spray for Pain on Urination

A 29-year-old, 96.1 kg, woman had a complicated delivery with substantial blood loss eventually leading to a hysterectomy. Six days postoperatively she was found to have cyanosis and difficulty breathing. An arterial blood gas revealed a methemoglobin level of 16.7%. She was treated with methylene blue and her symptoms resolved. On questioning it was revealed that the patient used a full can of benzocaine spray (~56 g) per day to reduce the pain of urination [14A].

BUPIVACAINE

Anatomic

Bupivacaine Crystal Formation After Prolonged Epidural Infusion

A 45-year-old, 52 kg, man with recurrent gastric carcinoma had an epidural catheter placed at the T7–T8 interspace for long term use. The initial infusion was bupivacaine 0.25% and morphine 0.005% at 6 ml/h. After 3 months the concentration of solution was doubled and the volume flow rate halved. The patient died 6 months after the initiation of the epidural infusion without suffering any neurologic symptoms. An autopsy revealed extensive large white crystalline deposits in the epidural space extending from the T4 to T8 levels. The authors noted that the HCL salt of bupivacaine (weak base with pKa 8.05) was buffered to a pKa of between 5.5 and 6.0 for stability. They then postulated that the administered solution readjusted to near body pH of 7.4 ± 0.05, which caused the bupivacaine to precipitate [15A].

Cardiovascular

Efficacy of Resuscitation with Intralipid

Lipid emulsion was administered to rats with bupivacaine induced transient cardiovascular toxicity. The speed of recovery was seen in the following order: 30% lipid emulsion > 20% lipid emulsion > normal saline > no treatment. The authors applied pharmacokinetic and pharmacodynamic modeling to ascertain that the lipid emulsion had a primary cardiotonic effect on the heart as well as causing a secondary physical absorption of the local anesthetic (i.e., lipid sink theory) [16H]. This study complemented a previous modeling study that outlined the lipid sink theory and determined that the lipid sink theory was not the sole effect of lipid emulsion on local anesthetics [17H].

Lipid Resuscitation in a Pediatric Patient

A 3-year-old, 11 kg, child presented for excision of a calf mass. After induction of general anesthesia, a caudal block was placed using 10 ml of 0.25% bupivacaine administered in aliquots of ~3 ml at a time. The ECG showed a few ventricular ectopic beats, which rapidly progressed to pulseless ventricular tachycardia. Cardiopulmonary resuscitation (CPR) was initiated and epinephrine 0.3 mg was given intravenously. Pulses returned after 2 minutes with sustained tachycardia. The authors

postulated that the tachycardia was probably SVT with wide ventricular response, rather than sustained VT. Fifteen milliliter of a 20% lipid solution was given and the patient stabilized despite a V/Q mismatch [18A].

Ventricular Tachycardia After a Penile Block

An infant was given an overdose of bupivacaine in a penile block resulting in ventricular tachycardia. The authors then proceed to describe a root-cause analysis of the overdose [19H]. We agree with the author's presentation and feel that this paper's emphasis is how these cases should be presented. The actual overdose is presented briefly and the pathophysiology of the overdose is all but ignored, as it is well known. Discovering without specific blame why the overdose occurred and how to avoid the problem in the future enables the reader to ruminate over the topic and incorporate similar safety maneuvers into his or her practice.

Nervous System

Severe Flaccid Paralysis After Spinal Anesthesia

A 45-year-old, 74 kg, 164 cm, woman underwent spinal anesthesia for a 20-minute urologic procedure in the lithotomy position to correct her urinary stress incontinence. Hyperbaric bupivacaine was injected intrathecally without difficulty and the surgical intervention ended uneventfully. Six hours after the operation she was noted to be somnolent and have weakness of the lower limbs. She was unable to walk or stand erect independently. Imaging (CT and MRI) of the lumbar spine showed no pathological abnormalities. Somatosensory evoked potentials of the lower limbs were suggestive of a problem with the long somatosensory spinal tracts. The patient was treated with steroids and after 4 months of intensive rehabilitation her condition improved but not entirely [20A]. The authors suggest that either the bupivacaine acted as a neurotoxin or somehow a neurotoxic drug was inadvertently substituted for the bupivacaine. Other possibilities such as unobserved hypotension may have been a compounding factor in the deficit. This, as of yet, unexplained nervous system injury from an apparently uncomplicated intrathecal anesthetic should be further researched if possible. This may be one of the extremely rare cases where the nerves were damaged from a seemingly benign procedure without a suitable explanation.

Toxicity in a Parturient After a Transverse Abdominis Plane Block

A 25-year-old, 51 kg, 37-week gravida, woman presented in labor to the Labor & Delivery suite. She was thought to have symptoms consistent with acute fatty liver of pregnancy (AFLP). Because of fetal bradycardia the patient had a Caesarean section under general anesthesia, which was uneventful. A postoperative bilateral

TAP block was performed for pain management using 20 ml of 0.375% bupivacaine on each side. At ~15 hours after the initial TAP block, a subsequent one was performed using the same amount of bupivacaine bilaterally. The patient developed a seizure 30 minutes after the second TAP block and local anesthetic systemic toxicity (LAST) was diagnosed. The patient was treated with intralipid 1.5 ml/kg. The authors correctly state that pregnant as compared to non-pregnant patients have a greater free fraction of bupivacaine because of differences in protein binding. In AFLP, liver dysfunction may cause an even greater fraction of free bupivacaine. This greater free fraction of bupivacaine may have led to LAST. A lesser concentration (i.e., 0.25% bupivacaine) would be safer, especially in this small patient with compromised hepatic function [21A].

In contrast to problematic TAP blocks, an analysis of a large pediatric database [22M] revealed that TAP blocks in the pediatric population occasionally (~6.9%) used potentially toxic doses but the incidence of serious neurologic or cardiovascular adverse events was essentially zero.

EMLA

Nervous System

Seizures and Oxygen-Resistant Cyanosis After Application of EMLA Cream

An 8-year-old girl developed generalized tonic–clonic seizures and cyanosis attributed to methemoglobinemia after application of a 'large amount' of topical EMLA (i.e., eutectic mixture of lidocaine and prilocaine) cream was applied. The authors reviewed the literature over a nearly 30-year period with only 13 cases of methemoglobinemia with EMLA cream application. The authors state that methemoglobinemia more commonly presents with benzocaine use. They review methemoglobinemia in general and conclude with a warning about overdose of EMLA cream [23A]. All local anesthetics can cause methemoglobinemia in large doses. Usually these large doses are greater than the maximum allowable doses as described in the drug packaging. Prilocaine, in particular, had been associated with methemoglobinemia at doses that were often closer to the suggested clinical doses and its use had fallen out of favor until 'rediscovered' as EMLA, a eutectic mixture with lidocaine.

LEVOBUPIVACAINE

Cardiovascular

Technique of Block Makes a Difference

This study compared two different techniques for interscalene block to see if technique made a difference

in the often overlooked adverse event of hypertension presumably caused by blockade of the carotid sinus baroreceptor. The study compared ultrasound guided block with 20 ml of 0.5% levobupivacaine and neurostimulator guided block with 40 ml of 0.5% levobupivacaine. The authors, not surprisingly, found that the neurostimulator group had a much higher incidence of hypertension. Hypertension is often overlooked as an adverse event and may be problematic in patients who have cardiovascular issues. Certainly using an ultrasound machine and limiting the volume of local anesthetic should be favored [24c].

Efficacy of Resuscitation with Intralipid

A study to test the efficacy of 20% lipid solution combined with epinephrine to treat cardiac toxicity was performed. Fourteen rabbits were randomized to receive either 0.9% saline or a 20% lipid solution along with a 100 mcg/kg epinephrine bolus after levobupivacaine induced cardiac arrest. There was no statistical difference in eventual recovery. However, at 20 minutes, 3 subjects in the 20% lipid solution recovered while only one subject from the saline group recovered [25E].

Nervous System

Seizures After Transversus Abdominis Plane Blocks

Two cases of systemic toxicity leading to seizures were reported after postoperative bilateral ultrasound guided TAP blocks administered after Caesarian section. The first patient was a 36-year-old, 56 kg, woman who received 40 ml of 0.375% levobupivacaine. Ten minutes after the block she had tonic–clonic seizures. The second patient was a 33-year-old, 61 kg, woman who received 40 ml of 0.75% ropivacaine. Twenty-five minutes after the block, she too had tonic–clonic seizures. Both were successfully treated with intralipid. The authors speculate that the spinal anesthetics caused vasodilation and facilitated systemic absorption [26A]. The authors stated that lower concentration of drugs should be considered if large volume of drug is needed. Of note, is that, in both cases, the diagnosis of LAST was quickly embraced, and was successfully treated.

LIDOCAINE

Cardiovascular

Cardiac Arrest After Ingestion of Viscous Lidocaine

A 2-year-old, 12.5 kg, boy presented with convulsive status epilepticus and subsequent cardiac arrest after apparently ingesting a large amount of viscous lidocaine (estimated to be ~500 mg). Cardiopulmonary resuscitation was successful after ~8 minutes and the child seemed fine for 2 days. At that time he presented with progressive disorientation, dizziness, and visual neglect, which resolved after 2 more days. The diagnosis of posterior reversible encephalopathy syndrome was made [27A]. The viscous lidocaine was not contained in a child-proof package. The authors recommend that viscous lidocaine should be considered a potentially dangerous drug especially in the pediatric population. This is echoed in a non-attributed article [28r], where it is reported that the FDA is warning that 2% oral viscous lidocaine should not be used for teething pain as it can cause toxic effects.

Compounded Ointment and Toxicity in a Pediatric Patient

A mother of an 18-month-old child applied a topical pain cream belonging to the child's father on the child's diaper rash. The child developed respiratory distress after 20 minutes and became unresponsive. In the ER, the child was noted to be bradycardic and hypotensive. The cream was analyzed and found to have lidocaine amongst other drugs [29A]. Although easy to use, special warning should be placed on adult medicines and should never be administered to children.

Lidocaine Toxicity During Cardiac Intervention

A 56-year-old, 56 kg, woman with non-ischemic cardiomyopathy, hypertension and diabetes was scheduled for ICD placement under local anesthesia with monitored moderate sedation without the presence of an anesthesia team. A total of 30 ml of 2% lidocaine was injected subcutaneously in the left infraclavicular area. However, due to anatomical difficulty the procedure was abandoned on the left side and the right side was then prepared. A total of 30 ml of 2% lidocaine was injected subcutaneously in the right infraclavicular area. At the conclusion of the procedure, the patient developed generalized tonic–clonic seizures, followed by cardiac arrest. The patient regained her pulse 15 minutes after resuscitation and eventually recovered fully. A lidocaine level drawn during the resuscitation was 8.7 mcg/ml [30A]. The authors felt that the patient's heart disease was a major factor in her toxicity. They also felt that the dose may have been too large but is usually not the sole cause of LAST. The cardiomyopathy is probably a red herring and 1% rather than 2% lidocaine would have been sufficient for sensory anesthesia and would have been safer if limited to one side (i.e., 30 ml). Logistically, postponing the second attempt may have been problematic, but would certainly have been prudent.

Cell Toxicity

A study was performed by exposing human oral mucosa fibroblasts to differing concentrations of lidocaine. The authors found that cell damage was increased with lidocaine exposure with more damage being done at higher concentrations. Duration of exposure was found to be less of a factor in cell damage [31E].

A study was performed by exposing human corneal endothelial cells to differing concentrations of lidocaine. The authors found that cell damage was increased with lidocaine exposure with more damage being done at higher concentrations and greater duration of exposure [32E]. The relevance to clinical practice and whether the cell damage seen in both studies leads to disease needs further study.

Dermatologic

Lidocaine Contact Allergy is Becoming More Prevalent

Local anesthetics are often used to numb an area. Lidocaine is a very common local anesthetic in use. It is the archetypical amide anesthetic and has been thought to have a very modest allergic profile. Recent studies, however, suggest that there are a growing number of patients reporting lidocaine allergies. One suggestion for the increased incidence of the allergy is that over-the-counter products are now including lidocaine in their ingredients, which may be unmasking the true incidence of the allergy.

A retrospective chart review of over 1800 patients who underwent patch testing over a period of 4 years was completed in 2013. The study showed that there is an overall allergy to local anesthetics of 2.4%. The highest prevalence of local anesthetic allergy was to benzocaine, 45%, then lidocaine, 32%, and dibucaine 23%. The authors then suggest that products such as Polysporin complete ointment, which contain lidocaine, be avoided postoperatively. Risk of anaphylaxis is not of great concern in this allergic contact dermatitis because it is a Type IV hypersensitivity reaction [33R]. This retrospective study should be followed by a prospective study. Also, no mention was made of the concentrations or total amounts used which might be important factors in local anesthetics exhibiting contact dermatitis.

Infectious

Spinal Epidural Abscess After Continuous Epidural Block

An elderly woman received a continuous lidocaine epidural block placed for management of herpes zoster related pain. Four days later she developed cellulitis near the epidural insertion site. Ten days after discovering the cellulitis an epidural abscess was confirmed on MRI and the epidural catheter was removed. She was managed conservatively with antibiotics with complete resolution of her symptoms [34A]. Once cellulitis was observed, consideration should have been given to removing the epidural catheter as this foreign body probably allowed the infection to spread to the neuraxis with subsequent epidural abscess.

Nervous System

Superficial Skin Necrosis and Neurological Complications Following Lidocaine Administration for Dental Procedure

A healthy 22-year-old woman was given a left inferior alveolar block using 2.2 ml of 2% lidocaine with epinephrine 1:80 000 for a dental procedure. The procedure was uneventful, but 3 hours after its conclusion, the patient noticed blisters and erythema of her chin. Approximately 10 hours later, the patient developed neurological complications. After 24 hours, the symptoms subsided. Immunological testing with lidocaine and prilocaine were negative [35A]. The authors concluded that the mechanism behind this might be intra-arterial injection involving the maxillary artery and viral activation within the inferior alveolar nerve.

Neurologic Toxicity of Lidocaine During Awake Intubation in a Patient with a Tongue Base Abscess

A 55-year-old man presented with a deep neck abscess and airway edema. Due to the anticipated difficult intubation, an awake, fiberoptic intubation was planned. The patient received midazolam 4 mg IM premedication and lidocaine 1% applied to the nasal fossae, hypopharynx, and larynx for the procedure. The estimated total dose of lidocaine was 20 ml (i.e., 200 mg). Twenty minutes later the patient had psychomotor agitation and generalized tonic–clonic seizures. Immediately after securing the airway, a contrast enhanced computed tomography (CT) scan was done to rule out intracranial ischemic or hemorrhagic lesions as the cause of the seizures. The CT scan was negative. Serum lidocaine measured 20 minutes after the onset of seizures was 5.1 mcg/ml. The authors concluded that marked inflammatory changes in the oral mucosa and hypercarbia might have contributed to increased systemic absorption of the local anesthetic leading to systemic toxicity though the dosage was in the safe limit [36A].

Prolonged Local Anesthetic Duration of Action in Patients on Chronic Lithium Therapy

Two cases of a prolonged duration of action of peripheral nerve blockade was seen in patients receiving inferior alveolar, lingual and long buccal nerve block using ~2 ml of 2% lidocaine with adrenaline for dental procedures. The sensory loss persisted for 16–18 hours with eventual full recovery. The authors postulate that the lithium caused slowing of lidocaine clearance [37A].

OXYBUPROCAINE

Dermatologic

Toxic Epitheliopathy in a Patient with Sjogren's Syndrome

A 69-year-old woman with Sjogren's syndrome scheduled for cataract surgery had six drops of preservative free oxybuprocaine applied to the eye. Examination after 10 minutes identified a subepithelial peripheral ring infiltrate with conjunctival congestion. The patient was treated with topical dexamethasone (0.05%) without preservative, topical balanced salt solution eye drops and an eye patch, with eventual healing over the course of a week. The authors emphasize that patients with Sjogren's syndrome are susceptible to ocular complications from even low concentration of local anesthetic solutions. They postulated various possible mechanisms for epitheliopathy due to local anesthetics [38A].

ROPIVACAINE

Cardiovascular

Toxic Dose of Ropivacaine After a Paravertebral Block in a Patient with Severe Hypoalbuminemia

A 72-year-old, ASA physical status III, woman had a paravertebral catheter inserted by the surgeon at the end of a right superior lobectomy. The patient initially received a 30 ml bolus of 0.2% ropivacaine followed by a continuous infusion of 10 ml/h of 0.2% ropivacaine. Eleven hours later, the patient was noted to be hypotensive and unconscious. The patient died despite seemingly adequate resuscitation. Total plasma concentration of ropivacaine measured from the sample collected at the time of resuscitation was 3.21 mcg/ml. The authors concluded that the LAST may be due to severe hypoalbuminemia increasing the fraction of free local anesthetic leading to toxicity and recommended a lower dose of local anesthetics in patients with severe hypoalbuminemia and probable low serum cholinesterase activity [39A]. Hypoalbuminemia should indeed cause one to adjust the amount of local anesthetic used. If the initial bolus of 0.2% ropivacaine gave adequate analgesia, then the continuous infusion only needed to be 0.1% ropivacaine, which might have obviated or mitigated the problem.

Miscommunication Leads to a Local Anesthetic Overdose

A 25-year-old, 57 kg, woman had laparoscopic surgery performed under general anesthesia. At the end of the case, the surgeon, unbeknownst to the anesthesiologist, gave 20 ml of 0.75% ropivacaine intraperitoneally. After extubation the patient woke up with severe pain. The anesthesiologist, unbeknownst to the surgeon, performed a TAP block with 40 ml of 0.75% ropivacaine for pain management. The patient had a seizure and developed a ventricular arrhythmia 10 minutes after injection. A 20% lipid infusion was given (1.5 ml/kg) and the patient converted to sinus rhythm [40A].

Better communication was warranted and cannot be overemphasized. An editorial commenting on the miscommunication was presented [41r]. However, the dose of ropivacaine used during the TAP block alone (i.e., 30 mg) may have been large enough to cause toxicity and a lesser concentration (e.g., 0.25%) of drug should have been used by both the surgeon and anesthesiologist to minimize systemic toxicity. Also, since the patient awoke in a lot of pain, perhaps the surgeon's injection was partially intravascular.

LAST After Local Infiltration Analgesia Following a Polyethylene Tibial Insert Exchange

A 67-year-old woman who presented for a polyethylene tibial insert of a previous total knee arthroplasty received spinal anesthesia with 11 mg bupivacaine in 8% glucose and local anesthetic infiltration using a total of 400 mg of ropivacaine. Seventy minutes after the infiltration, she developed atrial fibrillation with a rapid ventricular response. She then developed tonic–clonic seizures. The patient responded successfully to midazolam and 20% lipid emulsion [42A].

Nervous System

Delayed Arousal After an Inadvertent Intravascular Epidural Catheter Placement

An epidural catheter was inserted at the T8–T9 interspace using a midline approach before the induction of general anesthesia in a 78-year-old man for gastrectomy. Blood was aspirated from the catheter. The epidural catheter was removed and a second catheter was placed at the T8–T9 level using a paramedian approach. Aspiration was negative for blood or CSF. During the procedure the patient received 15 ml of epidurally administered 0.375% ropivacaine over approximately 1 hour followed by an epidural infusion of 0.2% ropivacaine at a rate of 4 ml/h. The infusion was continued postoperatively for pain management. Two hours after the end of the procedure, the patient continued to be unarousable. Careful aspiration of the epidural catheter revealed fresh blood. The authors felt that this confirmed that the delayed arousal was from systemically administered ropivacaine [43A]. The epidural catheter should have been tested before inducing general anesthesia with a standard test dose such as 3 ml of 1.5% lidocaine with epinephrine 1:200 000. This would have revealed that the catheter was not working properly and might have been

misplaced (i.e., the catheter could have been inserted into or migrated into a vessel). Also, the unaccountable tachycardia, mild hypertension and greater than expected anesthetic requirements, observed persistently during the operation should have warned that the ropivacaine was being administered systemically rather than epidurally.

References

[1] Hamaji A, de Rezende MR, Mattar Jr R, et al. Comparative study related to cardiovascular safety between bupivacaine (S75-R25) and ropivacaine in brachial plexus block. Braz J Anesthesiol. 2013;63(4):322–6 [c].

[2] Gungor I, Yilmaz A, Ozturk AM, et al. Bupivacaine and levobupivacaine induce apoptosis in rat chondrocyte cell cultures at ultra-low doses. Eur J Orthop Surg Traumatol. 2014;24(3):291–5 [E].

[3] Breu A, Rosenmeier K, Kujat R, et al. The cytotoxicity of bupivacaine, ropivacaine and mepivacaine on human chondrocytes and cartilage. Anesth Analg. 2013;117(2):514–22 [E].

[4] Vadi MG, Patel N, Stiegler MP. Case scenario: local anesthetic systemic toxicity after combined psoas compartment–sciatic nerve block. Analysis of decision factors and diagnostic delay. Anesthesiology. 2014;120(4):987–96 [A].

[5] Petrar S, Montemurro T. Total local anesthetic administered is integral to the syndrome of local anesthetic systemic toxicity. Anesthesiology. 2014;121(5):1130–1 [r].

[6] Barrington MJ, Weinberg GL. Did preoperative fixation on choice of anesthetic confound assessment of alternative techniques? Anesthesiology. 2014;121(5):1131 [r].

[7] Vadi MG, Patel N, Stiegler MP. In reply. Anesthesiology. 2014;121(5):1131–2 [r].

[8] Guo J, Lv N, Su Y, et al. Effects of intrathecal anesthesia with different concentrations and doses on spinal cord, nerve roots and cerebrospinal fluid in dogs. Int J Clin Exp Med. 2014;7(12):5376–84 [E].

[9] Zhao G, Ding X, Guo Y, et al. Intrathecal lidocaine neurotoxicity: combination with bupivacaine and ropivacaine and effect of nerve growth factor. Life Sci. 2014;112(1–2):10–21 [E].

[10] Buowari OY. Permanent neurological damage after spinal anaesthesia. Niger J Med. 2014;23(4):330–4 [R].

[11] O'toole A, Lacroix J, Pratt M, et al. Acute generalized exanthematous pustulosis associated with 2 common medications: hydroxyzine and benzocaine. J Am Acad Dermatol. 2014;71(4): E147–9 [A].

[12] Spiller HA, Russell JL, Casavant MJ, et al. Identification of N-Hydroxy-para-aminobenzoic acid in a cyanotic child after benzocaine exposure. Clin Toxicol. 2014;52(9):976–9 [A].

[13] Aryal MR, Gupta S, Giri S, et al. Benzocaine-induced methaemoglobinaemia: a life-threatening complication after a transoesophageal echocardiogram (TEE). BMJ Case Rep. 2013. pii: bcr2013009398. http://dx.doi.org/10.1136/bcr-2013-009398. PubMed PMID: 24042203.

[14] Fittro K, Nichols W. Acute dyspnea in a postpartum patient. J Am Acad Physician Assist. 2014;27(1):29–31 [A].

[15] Balga I, Gerber H, Schorno XH, et al. Bupivacaine crystal deposits after long-term epidural infusion. Anaesthesist. 2013;62(7):543–8 [A].

[16] Fettiplace MR, Akpa BS, Ripper R, et al. Resuscitation with lipid emulsion: dose-dependent recovery from cardiac pharmacotoxicity requires a cardiotonic effect. Anesthesiology. 2014;120(4):915–25 [H].

[17] Kuo I, Akpa BS. Validity of the lipid sink as a mechanism for the reversal of local anesthetic systemic toxicity: a physiologically

based pharmacokinetic model study. Anesthesiology. 2013;118(6):1350–61 [H].

[18] Shenoy U, Paul J, Antony D. Lipid resuscitation in pediatric patients—need for caution? Paediatr Anaesth. 2014;24(3):332–4 [A].

[19] Buck D, Kreeger R, Spaeth J. Case discussion and root cause analysis: bupivacaine overdose in an infant leading to ventricular tachycardia. Anesth Analg. 2014;119(1):137–40 [H].

[20] Vyshka G, Vacchiano G. Severe flaccid paraparesis following spinal anaesthesia: a sine materia occurrence. BMJ Case Rep. 2014. pii: bcr2013202071. http://dx.doi.org/10.1136/bcr-2013-202071. PubMed PMID: 24832705.

[21] Naidu RK, Richebe P. Probable LAST in Postpartum patient with acute fatty liver of pregnancy after a transversus abdominus plane block. A A Case Rep. 2013;1(5):72–4 [A].

[22] Long JB, Birmingham PK, De Oliveira Jr GS, et al. Transversus abdominis plane block in children: a multicenter safety analysis of 1994 cases from the PRAN (Pediatric Regional Anesthesia Network) database. Anesth Analg. 2014;119(2):395–9 [M].

[23] Shamriz O, Cohen-Glickman I, Reif S, et al. Methemoglobinemia induced by lidocaine-prilocaine cream. Isr Med Assoc J. 2014;16(4):250–4 [A].

[24] Gianesello L, Magherini M, Pavoni V, et al. The influence of interscalene block technique on adverse hemodynamic events. J Anesth. 2014;28(3):407–12 [c].

[25] Karcioğlu M, Tuzcu K, Sefil F, et al. Efficacy of resuscitation with intralipid in a levobupivacaine-induced cardiac arrest model. Turk J Med Sci. 2014;44(2):330–6 [E].

[26] Weiss E, Jolly C, Dumoulin JL, et al. Convulsions in 2 patients after bilateral ultrasound-guided transversus abdominis plane blocks for cesarean analgesia. Reg Anesth Pain Med. 2014;39(3):248–51 [A].

[27] Kargl S, Hornath F, Rossegg U, et al. Status epilepticus, cardiac resuscitation, and posterior reversible encephalopathy syndrome after ingestion of viscous lidocaine: a plea for more childproof packaging of pharmaceuticals. Pediatr Emerg Care. 2014;30(3):185–7 [A].

[28] FDA. Don't use viscous lidocaine to treat teething pain. J Mich Dent Assoc. 2014;96(9):8 [r].

[29] Sullivan RW, Ryzewski M, Holland MG, et al. Compounded ointment results in severe toxicity in a pediatric patient. Pediatr Emerg Care. 2013;29(11):1220–2 [A].

[30] Tanawuttiwat T, Thisayakorn P, Viles-Gonzalez JF. LAST (local anesthetic systemic toxicity) but not least: systemic lidocaine toxicity during cardiac intervention. J Invasive Cardiol. 2014;26(1): E13–5 [A].

[31] Oliveira AC, Rodriguez IA, Garzon I, et al. An early and late cytotoxicity evaluation of lidocaine on human oral mucosa fibroblasts. Exp Biol Med. 2014;239(1):71–82 [E].

[32] Yu HZ, Li YH, Wang RX, et al. Cytotoxicity of lidocaine to human corneal endothelial cells in vitro. Basic Clin Pharmacol Toxicol. 2014;114(4):352–9 [E].

[33] Kossintseva ID, de Gannes G. Lidocaine contact allergy is becoming more prevalent. Dermatol Surg. 2014;40(12): 1367–72 [R].

[34] Miyamoto T, Nakatani T, Narai Y, et al. Case of spinal epidural abscess after continuous epidural block to manage the pain of herpes zoster. Masui. 2014;63(3):353–7 [A].

[35] Pattni N. Superficial skin necrosis and neurological complications following administration of local anaesthetic: a case report. Aust Dent J. 2013;58(4):522–5 [A].

[36] Giordano D, Panini A, Pernice C, et al. Neurologic toxicity of lidocaine during awake intubation in a patient with tongue base abscess. Am J Otolaryngol. 2014;35(1):62–5 [A].

[37] Patil PM. Prolonged peripheral nerve blockade in patients using lithium carbonate. J Craniomaxillofac Surg. 2014;42(3): E33–5 [A].

[38] Ansari H, Weinberg L, Spencer N. Toxic epitheliopathy from a single application of preservative free oxybuprocaine (0.4%) in a patient with Sjogren's syndrome. BMJ Case Rep. 2013. pii: bcr2013010487. http://dx.doi.org/10.1136/bcr-2013-010487. PubMed PMID: 24038291.

[39] Calenda E, Baste JM, Hajjej R, et al. Toxic plasma concentration of ropivacaine after a paravertebral block in a patient suffering from severe hypoalbuminemia. J Clin Anesth. 2014;26(2): 149–51 [A].

[40] Scherrer V, Compere V, Loisel C, et al. Cardiac arrest from local anesthetic toxicity after a field block and transversus abdominis plane block: a consequence of miscommunication between the anesthesiologist and the surgeon. A A Case Rep. 2013;1(5):75–6 [A].

[41] Wong CA. Editorial comment: cardiac arrest from local anesthetic toxicity after a field block and transversus abdominis plane block: a consequence of miscommunication between the anesthesiologist and the surgeon. A A Case Rep. 2013;1(5):77–8 [r].

[42] Fenten MG, Rohrbach A, Wymenga AB, et al. Systemic local anesthetic toxicity after local infiltration analgesia following a polyethylene tibial insert exchange: a case report. Reg Anesth Pain Med. 2014;39(3):264–5 [A].

[43] Akimoto K, Yamauchi C, Fujimoto K, et al. A case of delayed arousal after anesthesia due to aberrant epidural catheter placement in a blood vessel. Masui. 2014;63(7):814–6 [A].

12

Neuromuscular Blocking Agents and Skeletal Muscle Relaxants

Mona U. Shah[1]

Department of Pharmacy, Inova Fairfax Hospital, Falls Church, VA, USA
[1]Corresponding author: mona.shah@inova.org

DEPOLARIZING NEUROMUSCULAR BLOCKING AGENTS

Succinylcholine (Suxamethonium) (SEDA-28, 155; SEDA-31, 247; SEDA-32, 273; SEDA-33, 299; SEDA-34, 221; SEDA-35, 173, SEDA-36)

Organs and Systems

CARDIOVASCULAR

Succinylcholine can significantly prolong both QT and QTc intervals, especially when given in conjunction with thiopental. The underlying mechanism involves sympathoadrenal activation and an increase in norepinephrine concentrations. Pretreatment with opioids (alfentanil 25–75 µg/kg) or β_1-blockers (metoprolol, possibly esmolol) may help attenuate this response [1M].

Musculoskeletal

The Adverse Metabolic/Musculoskeletal Reaction to Anesthesia reports in the North American malignant Hyperthermia Registry contains the time to first sign of suspected malignant hyperthermia (MH) secondary to administration of anesthetics [2c]. Visoiu et al. examined these case reports and found that in the 394 patients exposed to only one of the four inhaled anesthetics, MH onset time was shorter with halothane compared to other anesthetics and shorter after succinylcholine in all anesthetics. In 14 cases (2.9%), succinylcholine was given without inhaled anesthetic. Eleven of these subjects (78.6%) experienced possible MH, and 3 (21.4%) experienced fulminant MH. The most frequent initial signs of MH in these patients were masseter spasm and tachycardia (both signs in 7 patients; 50%), hypercarbia ($n=5$; 35.7%), elevated temperature ($n=4$; 28.6%), and rapid increase in temperature ($n=4$; 28.6%). Ten of the 14 subjects had one unique first MH sign: masseter spasm ($n=6$; 60%), hypercarbia ($n=2$; 20%), cyanosis ($n=1$), and hyperkalemia ($n=1$).

Immunologic

HYPERSENSITIVITY REACTIONS

Reddy et al. reported a two-hospital, retrospective, observational cohort study confirming anaphylaxis is more common with rocuronium and succinylcholine than with atracurium [3C,4r]. The study included 92 858 new patient exposures to neuromuscular blocking agents (NMBAs) during the 7-year period from January 1, 2006 to December 31, 2012. Eighty-nine of these patients were referred to the Anesthetic Allergy Clinic for follow-up investigation of an intraoperative event thought to be anaphylaxis. After excluding non-IgE mediated allergic reactions and other causes, 21 cases of allergic anaphylaxis were attributed to muscle relaxants: succinylcholine ($n=12$), rocuronium ($n=6$), and atracurium ($n=3$). Results demonstrated that, in Auckland region, the use of succinylcholine and rocuronium was associated with a substantially higher rate of intraoperative anaphylaxis compared to atracurium. The incidence of anaphylaxis to rocuronium and succinylcholine was 1:2500 and 1:2000, respectively, whereas the rate of anaphylaxis to atracurium was substantially lower (1:22000). Due to geographical differences in sensitivity to NMBAs, the results of this study should be extrapolated to other regions with caution. The authors concluded that rocuronium is an useful alternative to succinylcholine in rapid sequence intubations where succinylcholine is contraindicated, but its routine use as a muscle relaxant in preference to atracurium or cisatracurium in regions

© 2015 Elsevier B.V. All rights reserved.

where pre-sensitization may be prevalent should be carefully considered.

ANAPHYLAXIS

NMBAs have a high cross-reactivity (63.4%) and the main antigenic determinants are thought to be the quaternary ammonium groups that are capable of bridging IgE antibodies [5M].

> There are a number of tests that can be used for the diagnosis of anaphylactic reactions: (1) plasma tryptase levels, when elevated, indicate mast cell activation and this test can be done at the time of the anaphylactic event; (2) skin prick tests help to identify the drug in question to prevent future events; (3) IgE tests are specific, but not readily available for all NMBAs; and (4) basophil activation tests use changes in cell phenotype CD63 to diagnose reactivity to various drugs, including NMBAs. A basophil activation test is considered positive if more than two dilutions of a drug produce greater than 10% basophil activation.

The authors used the French National Pharmacovigilance Database to retrieve reports of NMBA anaphylaxis that occurred between January 2000 and December 2011 [6C]. NMBAs included were atracurium, cisatracurium, mivacurium, pancuronium, rocuronium, succinylcholine, and vecuronium. Of the total 2022 cases of NMBA hypersensitivity reactions, 84 (4.1%) were fatal. Detailed information on outcome was provided for 31 cases, which showed a mean delay of 4 minutes to first symptom onset. Also, among the 1247 cases of severe NMBA anaphylaxis (grades 3 and 4), independent risk factors associated with a fatal outcome in a multivariate analysis were male gender (female gender: $OR = 0.4$; $P = 0.0004$), an emergency setting ($OR = 2.6$; 95% CI 1.5–4.6; $P = 0.0007$), a history of hypertension ($OR = 2.5$; $P = 0.0010$) or of other cardiovascular disease ($OR = 4.4$; $P < 0.0001$), obesity ($OR = 2.4$; $P = 0.0376$), and ongoing beta-blocker treatment ($OR = 4.2$; $P = 0.0011$). All 31 patients with a fatal outcome received epinephrine in a titrated manner according to international guidelines. However, there were several limitations in this study such as underreporting of mild/moderate cases; anaphylactic reaction ascribed to NMBAs when multiple agents were administered simultaneously, and absence of allergy testing to confirm the diagnosis.

Susceptibility Factors

GENETIC FACTORS

Succinylcholine's duration of action may be prolonged by genetic variants of butyrylcholinesterase enzyme (BChE). Kalow (K) variant is the most common mutation in the butyrylcholinesterase gene (BCHE), which is present in 25% Caucasians [7c]. Bretlau and colleagues enrolled 59 adult surgical patients (BCHE wild-type, $n = 38$; heterozygous for K-variant, $n = 21$) to determine the duration of action of succinylcholine (1 mg/kg) after

administration in rapid sequence intubation. The authors found that patients who were heterozygous for the K-variant had lower BChE activity compared with the wild-type group ($P = 0.0045$) and the duration of action of succinylcholine was inversely proportional with the BChE activity. The mean duration of action was prolonged by 4 minutes in the BChE heterozygous group compared to the wild-type [7c].

NON-DEPOLARIZING NEUROMUSCULAR BLOCKERS

Organs and Systems

CARDIOVASCULAR

Most non-depolarizing neuromuscular blockers have not been associated with QT or QTc prolongation. Clinical studies in patients without cardiovascular diseases indicate that pancuronium, vecuronium, and atracurium do not significantly affect QT and QTc intervals. Cisatracurium lacks any autonomic activity that could affect repolarization, and rocuronium has been safely used in patients with congenital or acquired long-QT syndrome (LQTS). When rocuronium or vecuronium was administered with sugammadex in healthy awake, non-intubated patients, QTc was not prolonged [1M].

NEUROMUSCULAR BLOCKERS: REVERSAL AGENTS

CALABADION 1

Calabadion 1 is an experimental agent that reverses the effects of steroidal (rocuronium) and benzylisoquinoline (cisatracurium) neuromuscular blockers, but its in vivo disposition and efficacy are unknown [8E]. Calabadion 1 doses of 30, 60, and 90 mg/kg (for rocuronium reversal) or 90, 120, and 150 mg/kg (for cisatracurium reversal) were administered to 60 anesthetized rats at maximum twitch depression. The result was resumption of spontaneous breathing and accelerated recovery of train-of-four ratio to 0.9 with 90 and 150 mg/kg of calabadion 1 in rats that were anesthetized with rocuronium and cisatracurium, respectively. Calabadion 1 did not affect heart rate, mean arterial blood pressure, pH, or arterial blood gas tension. More than 90% of the intravenously administered calabadion 1 appeared in the urine within 1 hour. Despite its ability to reverse all levels of steroidal neuromuscular blockade, sugammadex (Bridion) does not reverse residual neuromuscular blockade induced by benzylisoquinolines. Calabadion 1 may prove to be a promising new drug when rapid reversal of profound neuromuscular blockade is warranted.

Sugammadex

General Information

Sugammadex is a reversal agent for the aminosteroid-structured non-depolarizing neuromuscular blockers (NMBs), rocuronium and vecuronium. In a clinical study, the authors investigated the efficacy of sugammadex in 14 patients who experienced insufficient decurarization (train-of-four, TOF < 0.9) with neostigmine after general anesthesia [9C]. At the end of the operation, if patients were unable to open eyes, swallow, raise their head, and had TOF values <0.9 after 50 mcg/kg neostigmine administration, 2 mg/kg suggamadex was given intravenously. Following sugammadex administration, the time to reach TOF ≥0.9 was 2.1 ± 0.9 minutes, and the extubation time was 3.2 ± 1.4 minutes. There were no statistically significant differences in the hemodynamic parameters before and after sugammadex administration. Also, no side effects or complications were noted in patients from the time of sugammadex administration to the second postoperative hour and no patient exhibited acute respiratory failure or residual block [9C].

Immunologic

HYPERSENSITIVITY REACTIONS

The USA's Food and Drug Administration has not yet approved sugammadex due to concerns surrounding the potentially life-threatening, hypersensitivity reactions related to the drug. A database search of sugammadex (AND 'anaphylaxis' OR 'hypersensitivity') yielded a total of 157 results, of which 11 studies met inclusion criteria for the qualitative analysis: two case series of three patients each; six case reports; an abstract; and two clinical trials [10M]. The most frequently reported signs and symptoms were rash (80%), hypotension (53%) and tachycardia (47%). The World Anaphylaxis Organization (WAO) criteria were met in 73% cases. All patients eventually recovered from these adverse effects. The mean time to onset of reactions in 14 of the 15 patients was 1.9 minutes (1 minute and 52 s), with the earliest during administration and the latest 4 minutes after receiving a dose of sugammadex. Eleven patients underwent skin prick testing and/or intradermal testing, of which 10 had a positive confirmatory result. Some patients developed a hypersensitivity reaction to sugammadex with first exposure; one possible explanation is that these individuals could be sensitized by cyclodextrins found in their diet (average cyclodextrins consumption per person was 4 g/day).

Sugammadex-related literature, from 2013 to 2014, was recently reviewed by Ledowski [11R]. Based on current literature, sugammadex reverses neuromuscular blockade three to eight times faster than neostigmine. When administered in suspected cases of anaphylaxis to rocuronium, sugammadex improves hemodynamic parameters. There are case reports to suggest that sugammadex may be helpful in rescuing the lost airway by causing a rapid return of neuromuscular function, but in some cases, surgical airway may be required. However, in certain high-risk patients (e.g., myasthenia gravis), sugammadex might not always result in adequate extubation despite the administration of high dose (up to 12 mg/kg).

While sugammadex 1 mg/kg is effective in reversing a shallow rocuronium-induced block, the time to recovery could be slow (up to 8 minutes). In an obese patient, ideal or adjusted body weight may be safely used to reverse NMBs; however, quantitative neuromuscular monitoring may be necessary if lower than recommended doses of sugammadex are used.

The most important potential adverse effect is anaphylaxis. Sugammadex appears to be safe for neuromuscular blockade reversal in the presence of significant comorbidities (e.g., severe renal failure) and does not affect the QTc interval.

Interactions

DRUG–DRUG INTERACTIONS

The drugs identified with potential interactions with sugammadex include toremifene, flucloxacillin, fusidic acid and oral contraceptives [12r].

SKELETAL MUSCLE RELAXANTS

General Information

Skeletal muscle hypertonia can be caused by many conditions including multiple sclerosis, cerebral palsy, Parkinson's disease, and secondary to stroke. Hence, treatment options include agents with central and peripheral sites of action.

Baclofen, a gamma-amino butyric acid (GABA) receptor agonist, is a centrally acting agent used to treat spasticity. GABA receptors are classified into types A, B, and C. Type A is a target for most anesthetic agents. The GABA–GABA receptor system is inhibitory and the $GABA_B$ receptor (unlike A and C, which are ligand gated ion channels) is a G-protein coupled receptor family member. Activation of $GABA_B$ receptor with baclofen inhibits activation of spinal polysynaptic and monosynaptic motor neurons. Other centrally acting antispastic agents include tizanidine, which is an $alpha_2$-adrenoceptor agonist that produces presynaptic inhibition of motor neurons.

The peripherally acting agent, dantrolene, is a ryanodine receptor antagonist that inhibits the release of intracellular Ca^{2+} from the sarcoplasmic reticulum. It is used for the treatment of malignant hyperthermia, where there is unregulated sarcoplasmic reticulum Ca^{2+}

release in response to a number of triggering agents such as anesthetic gases and/or succinylcholine. There is some evidence (anecdotal and other) to suggest that cannabis-based medicines may have a role in controlling spasticity associated with multiple sclerosis.

Botulinum toxin, obtained from *Clostridium botulinum*, is a poison that causes botulism. Botulinum toxin is comprised of seven neurotoxins (types A–G). These toxins are endopeptidases that cause muscle contraction by attacking vesicle fusion proteins involved in the exocytosis of acetylcholine-containing vesicles. The botulinum toxin products available in the market are Botox, Xeomin and Dysport (toxin type A) and Myobloc (toxin type B). When these toxins are used at very low doses, they cause facial muscle paralysis, which helps to eliminate 'wrinkles'. In addition, these products are variably used for the treatment of cervical dystonia, strabismus, blepharospasm and severe axillary hyperhidrosis [13M].

Baclofen (SEDA-35, 173; SEDA-36)

General Information

Mechanism: Baclofen relieves spasticity and rigidity by activating presynaptic $GABA_B$ receptors, which causes slow synaptic inhibition by increasing the neuronal membrane's potassium ion conductance and by decreasing calcium influx into the presynaptic terminal. This leads to neuronal hyperpolarization and reduces the number and amplitude of excitatory postsynaptic potentials along the dendrites of motor neurons. When spasticity continues despite oral treatments and other alternatives, intrathecal baclofen (ITB) may be considered in selected patients.

ITB has a profound effect on spasticity for several reasons. Intrathecal administration produces at least four times higher cerebrospinal fluid (CSF) levels with only 1% of the systemic dose. In addition, infusion into the lumbar area concentrates baclofen at specific sites in the spinal cord where the $GABA_B$ receptors are located. By the time baclofen reaches the brain, it is in much lower concentrations; hence, the central side effects that occur in patients taking oral baclofen are much less likely [14M].

Organs and Systems

CARDIOVASCULAR

- A 41-year-old man receiving ITB pump for refractory spasticity developed hyperthermia, seizures, cognitive depression, acute hypoxemic respiratory failure and cardiovascular instability in less than 24 hours after first pump substitution. Patient was admitted to the ICU with multisystem organ failure that included hemodynamic instability despite fluids, vasopressor support, hyperlactatemia, EKG abnormalities, elevated cardiac enzymes, rhabdomyolysis, and acute renal failure with metabolic acidosis. Patient experienced cardiac arrest (pulseless electrical activity), but had return of spontaneous circulation after 4 minutes of resuscitation and 1 mg of epinephrine. Upon further investigation, the team found a leaky ITB catheter system, which was surgically fixed and ITB infusion was reinstituted. Patient recovered completely and was discharged to home 56 days later [15A].

CENTRAL NERVOUS SYSTEM AND URINARY TRACT

Baclofen accumulation and encephalopathy may occur when normal doses are administered to patients with impaired renal function. Baclofen-induced encephalopathy has been reported in patients with varying degrees of renal insufficiency. The authors report two cases of baclofen-induced encephalopathy secondary to chronic kidney disease: A 71-year-old-man on baclofen 10 mg every 8 hours was treated with hemodialysis and another patient, a 35-year-old woman on baclofen 10 mg twice daily was treated with peritoneal dialysis. There are case reports of baclofen-induced encephalopathy in patients with renal insufficiency where patient recovered consciousness after hemodialysis treatment [16A].

SENSORY SYSTEM: EAR

Baclofen is used off-label for the treatment of alcohol dependence and may be prescribed at much higher doses (up to 400 mg/day), but the safety and efficacy of high-dose baclofen (HDB) is unknown. The authors report two cases of tinnitus with HDB for alcohol dependence [17A].

- A 60-year-old man reported tinnitus when he reached a 180 mg daily dose of baclofen after 3 months of treatment. Tinnitus persisted until the dose was reduced to 90 mg daily.
- A 45-year-old woman presented with tinnitus at 210 mg daily of baclofen after 4 months of treatment. Tinnitus persisted until the dose was reduced to 60 mg daily.

Baclofen has been implicated in both the treatment and etiology of tinnitus. The reasons remain to be determined.

PSYCHOLOGICAL

Geoffroy and colleagues report a case of a 49-year-old white male who presented with no prior psychiatric history except for alcohol dependence [18A]. The patient reported a 20-year history of problematic alcohol use with an average daily consumption of 150–200 g of alcohol. Baclofen was initiated to reduce alcohol consumption, but it was introduced slowly to avoid dose-dependent drowsiness. After 5 months of baclofen use, the patient still consumed the same level of alcohol but since he tolerated the treatment well, the baclofen dose was progressively increased. Within a week of increasing the dose to 180 mg daily, the patient experienced behavioral disinhibition with inflated self-esteem, decreased need for sleep by approximately 3 hours per night, increased loquacity, flight of ideas, and distractibility. He was also caught stealing books from a library. He met the criteria of a manic episode and scored 24 of 60 on the Young Mania Rating Scale. Since the patient did not have a history of mood disorder, baclofen was identified as the causative agent. Baclofen treatment was tapered over 5 days to avoid withdrawal. The patient was also admitted to the hospital where baclofen was discontinued. The Young Mania Rating Scale score decreased to 10 of 60 after 1 week and then to zero after week 3. The mechanism through which baclofen may induce manic symptoms remain unclear.

Drug Administration

DRUG INTERACTION(S)

Baclofen doses of 30–60 mg have been evaluated in randomized controlled trials for the treatment of alcohol dependence. While there are no known reports of baclofen increasing triglyceride (TG) levels, risperidone increases TG levels but the increase is small, below 2 g/L. The authors describe a case of 39-year-old man with type 1 bipolar disorder and an alcohol dependence lasting for >10 years [19A]. The patient was started on baclofen 20 mg/day. At the time, the patient did not have diabetes, renal failure or signs of endocrine diseases. His BMI was 25.7. His serum triglyceride level was 0.94 g/L with total cholesterol level of 2.12 g/L. Patient's other medications included lithium 1200 mg/day. The baclofen dose was gradually increased to 180 mg/day (after 5 weeks). Seven weeks after the beginning of the treatment, lithium was switched to risperidone (1 mg/day during 1 week, then 2 mg/day) because the patient presented signs of lithium overdose. Patient's weight remained stable during this period and lipid levels were normal. One week after the introduction of risperidone, the dose of baclofen was gradually increased to 240 mg/day. One month later, the serum triglyceride level obtained was 6.56 g/L with total cholesterol of 1.78 g/L. Since the patient did not observe a strict diet and had elevated alcohol consumption, no pharmacological treatment was prescribed. The patient stopped drinking alcohol a few days later but started consuming sodas in large quantities. Due to persistence of manic symptoms, risperidone was increased to 4 mg/day 2 months later. Patient remained abstinent and his weight was stable. The dose of baclofen was still 240 mg/day. Risperidone dose was increased to 6 mg/day 45 days later. A week after risperidone dose increase, the serum triglyceride level was 41 g/L and total cholesterol was 7.81 g/L with induction

of hyponatremia (126 mmol/L). Risperidone and baclofen were discontinued and carbamazepine was initiated. Patient's triglyceride levels dropped rapidly to 10.1 g/L within 2 days and to 2 g/L after 15 days. Three months later, the patient had no mood symptoms and he was still abstinent. Triglycerides levels returned to a normal value. The above case suggests a strong correlation between increase in triglyceride levels in the presence of risperidone and high-dose baclofen [19A].

Botulinum Toxin (SEDA-35, 174; SEDA-36)

General Information

Although botulinum toxin is generally considered safe, its widespread use and the constantly expanded indications raise safety concerns. There are seven serologically distinct botulinum toxins. Botulinum toxin A is the most potent serotype, with one million-fold higher toxicity than cobra toxin and far higher than cyanide [20M].

Organs and Systems

NEUROMUSCULAR FUNCTION

The authors analyzed follow-up visit data on 89 patients who were treated with botulinum toxin for up to 26 years for dystonia [21R]. The mean ages at the time of the first and last injections were 49 and 68 years, respectively. The most common diagnoses were cervical dystonia ($n=51$), blepharospasm ($n=34$), and oromandibular dystonia ($n=26$). The total number of OnabotulinumtoxinA units received during the first injection was 140.3 versus 224.5 during the last injection ($P<0.0001$). From a total number of 4133 visits, adverse events were reported in 19% ($n=793$) of the visits. The most common side effects reported were dysphagia, ptosis, and neck weakness (Table 1).

Approximately 10% ($n=409$) of the visits were for complaint of cervical dystonia, 9.5% ($n=394$) for blepharospasm, and 7% ($n=291$) for oromandibular dystonia. A total of 47 botulinum toxin type A antibody tests were performed in 35 patients: 6 were positive and 41 were negative. Lack of response or recurrent decreased response was the most common reason for immunoresistance testing [21R].

Immunologic

HYPERSENSITIVITY REACTIONS

Botulinum toxin is contraindicated in patients with a known hypersensitivity to the components of the formulation or with disorders of the neuromuscular junction, in co-administration with aminoglycosides, streptomycin, or anticoagulant therapy, in presence of a bleeding disorder, and during pregnancy [20M].

TABLE 1 Different Type of Side Effects from Botulinum Toxin Injections from the Total Number of Reported Side Effects During the Entire Follow-Up Period (18.5 Years)

Side effects	Total number (793)	Percent (%)
Dysphagia	164	20.7
Ptosis	144	18.2
Neck weakness	71	9
Ocular side effects[a]	56	7
Injection site muscle weakness[b]	51	6.4
Injection site pain	44	5.5
Injection site hematoma	42	5.3
Flu-like symptoms	40	5
Hoarseness	36	4.5
Generalized weakness	31	3.9
Dry mouth	17	2.1
Dysarthria	14	1.8

[a]Includes: blurred vision, diplopia and dry eyes.
[b]Neck weakness not included.

Carisoprodol

Susceptibility Factors

AGE AND SEX

In a retrospective analysis of 14 965 patients, the authors measured carisoprodol and meprobamate urine concentrations via liquid chromatography–tandem mass spectrometry to determine the metabolic ratio (MR) of meprobamate to carisoprodol concentrations [22R]. The MR geometric mean of the young group was 47.4% higher than the middle-aged group and nearly two times higher than the elderly group. Females had a 20.7% higher MR compared with males.

References

[1] Staikou C, Stamelos M, Stavroulakis E. Impact of anaesthetic drugs and adjuvants on ECG markers of torsadogenicity. Br J Anaesth. 2014;112(2):217–30 [M].

[2] Visoiu M, Young MC, Wieland K, et al. Anesthetic drugs and onset of malignant hyperthermia. Anesth Analg. 2014;118(2):388–96 [c].

[3] Reddy JI, Cooke PJ, van Schalkwyk JM, et al. Anaphylaxis is more common with rocuronium and succinylcholine than with atracurium. Anesthesiology. 2015;122(1):39–45 [C].

[4] Mertes PM, Volcheck GW. Anaphylaxis to neuromuscular-blocking drugs: all neuromuscular blocking drugs are not the same. Anesthesiology. 2015;122(1):5–7 [r].

[5] Sadleir PH, Clarke RC, Bunning DL, et al. Anaphylaxis to neuromuscular blocking drugs: incidence and cross-reactivity in Western Australia from 2002 to 2011. Br J Anaesth. 2013;110(6):981–7 [M].

[6] Reitter M, Petitpain N, Latarche C, et al. Fatal anaphylaxis with neuromuscular blocking agents: a risk factor and management analysis. Allergy. 2014;69:954–9 [C].

[7] Bretlau C, Sørensen KM, Vedersoe AZ, et al. Response to succinylcholine in patients carrying the K-variant of the butyrylcholinesterase gene. Anesth Analg. 2013;116:596–601 [c].

[8] Hoffman U, Grosse-Sundrup M, Eikermann-Haerter K, et al. Calabadion: a new agent to reverse the effects of benzylisoquinoline and steroidal neuromuscular-blocking agents. Anesthesiology. 2013;119(2):317–25 [E].

[9] Dogan E, Akdemir MS, Guzel A, et al. A miracle that accelerates operating room functionality: sugammadex. BioMed Res Int. 2014;2014:1–4. http://dx.doi.org/10.1155/2014/945310 [C].

[10] Tsur A, Kalansky A. Hypersensitivity associated with sugammadex administration: a systematic review. Anaesthesia. 2014;69(11):1251–7 [M].

[11] Ledowski T. Sugammadex: what do we know and what do we still need to know? A review of the recent (2013 to 2014) literature. Anaesth Intensive Care. 2015;43(1):14–22 [R].

[12] Ortiz-Gómez JR, Palacio-Abizanda FJ, Fornet-Ruiz I. Failure of sugammadex to reverse rocuronium-induced neuromuscular blockade: a case report. Eur J Anaesth. 2014;31:708–21 [r].

[13] Lambert DG. Drugs used to treat joint and muscle disease. Anaesth Intensive Care Med. 2015;16(3):140–4 [M].

[14] Khurana SR, Garg DS. Spasticity and the use of intrathecal baclofen in patients with spinal cord injury. Phys Med Rehabil Clin N Am. 2014;25(3):655–69 [M].

[15] Calixto L, Quintaneiro C, Seabra H, et al. Cardiac arrest due to withdrawal baclofen syndrome: a clinical case report. Resuscitation. 2013;84:S92 [A].

[16] Lee J, Shin HS, Jung YS, et al. Two cases of baclofen-induced encephalopathy in hemodialysis and peritoneal dialysis patients. Ren Fail. 2013;35(6):860–2 [A].

[17] Auffret M, Rolland B, Deheul S, et al. Severe tinnitus induced by off-label baclofen. Ann Pharmacother. 2014;48(5):656–9 [A].

[18] Geoffroy PA, Auffret M, Deheul S, et al. Baclofen-induced manic symptoms: case report and systematic review. Psychosomatics. 2014;55(4):326–32 [A].

[19] Clarisse H, Imbert B, Belzeaux R, et al. Baclofen and risperidone association increases dramatically triglyceride level. Alcohol Alcohol. 2013;48(4):515–6 [A].

[20] Yiannakopoulou E. Serious and long-term adverse events associated with the therapeutic and cosmetic use of botulinum toxin. Pharmacology. 2015;95(1–2):65–9 [M].

[21] Ramirez-Castaneda J, Jankovic J. Long-term efficacy, safety, and side effect profile of botulinum toxin in dystonia: a 20-year follow-up. Toxicon. 2014;90:344–8 [R].

[22] Tse SA, Atayee RS, Ma JD, et al. Factors affecting carisoprodol metabolism in pain patients using urinary excretion data. J Anal Toxicol. 2014;38(3):122–8 [R].

13

Drugs that Affect Autonomic Functions or the Extrapyramidal System

Toshio Nakaki[1]

Department of Pharmacology, Teikyo University School of Medicine, Tokyo, Japan
[1]Corresponding author: nakaki@med.teikyo-u.ac.jp

DRUGS THAT STIMULATE BOTH ALPHA- AND BETA-ADRENOCEPTORS
[SEDA-33, 313; SEDA-34, 233; SEDA-35, 255; SEDA-36, 179]

Adrenaline (Adrenaline) and Noradrenaline (Noradrenaline) [SEDA-32, 281; SEDA-33, 259; SEDA-34, 233; SEDA-35, 255; SEDA-36, 179]

Reproductive System

It is widely accepted that local anesthetics with adrenaline should not be used in areas served by terminal vessels. There is no evidence in studies for this in penile surgery. A study was performed whether or not penile block using a local anesthetic with adrenaline is safe. Ninety-five patients received a penile ring block with subcutaneous infusion anesthesia, which consisted of ropivacaine and cocaine (0.11% and 0.21%) plus adrenaline. Short-term negative postoperative occurrences (<72 hours) were swelling (42%), problems with suture material (22%), pain (19%), hematoma and paresthesia (each 13%), erectile dysfunction (12%), small-area skin necrosis after wound healing without requiring further surgery (13%), micturition disorders (7%), and wound infection (6%). Supplementing a local anesthetic with adrenaline in penis operations has many advantages, including high patient satisfaction, relatively painless infiltration, low complication rates, improved view of the operating field, and an extended effect of anesthetics with a prolonged reduction in pain. There is no risk of necrosis related to using a subcutaneous penile ring block. Thus, the view that adrenaline should not be used in penis procedures may be obsolete [1R].

Randomized Clinical Trial

The effects of intravenous (i.v.) adrenaline on rhythm transitions during cardiac arrest with initial or secondary ventricular fibrillation/tachycardia were studied [2c]. Patients who received adrenaline had more rhythm transitions from return of spontaneous circulation and non-shockable rhythms to ventricular fibrillation/tachycardia.

Ephedrine [SEDA-32, 282; SEDA-33, 317; SEDA-34, 235; SEDA-35, 256; SEDA-37, 000]

Systematic Review

A large scale meta-analysis was performed to assess the effects and adverse effects of ephedrine in people with autoimmune myasthenia gravis, transient neonatal myasthenia gravis, and the congenital myasthenic syndromes. Reported adverse effects included tachycardia, sleep disturbances, nervousness, and withdrawal symptoms [3M].

Randomized Controlled Trial

Bolus and the combination of bolus and infusion of ephedrine for the treatment of maternal hypothermia under spinal anaesthesia prevent maternal and neonatal hypothermia during caesarean section under spinal anaesthesia compared to bolus administrations alone [4c].

DRUGS THAT PREDOMINANTLY STIMULATE ALPHA 1-ADRENOCEPTORS
[SEDA-33, 318; SEDA-34, 236; SEDA-35, 257; SEDA-36, 186]

Systematic Review

A systematic review was conducted to determine the harm and benefit associated with prophylactic

© 2015 Elsevier B.V. All rights reserved.

phenylephrine for caesarean section under spinal anaesthesia. The relative risk (95% CI) of hypotension with phenylephrine infusion as defined by authors before delivery was 0.36 (0.18–0.73) vs placebo, $p=0.004$; 0.58 (0.39–0.88) vs an ephedrine infusion, $p=0.009$; and 0.73 (0.55–0.96) when added to an ephedrine infusion, $p=0.02$. After delivery, the relative risks of hypotension and nausea and vomiting with phenylephrine compared with placebo were 0.37 (0.19–0.71), $p=0.003$ and 0.39 (0.17–0.91), $p=0.03$, respectively. There was no evidence that hypertension, bradycardia or neonatal endpoints were affected. Phenylephrine reduced the risk for hypotension and nausea and vomiting after spinal doses of bupivacaine generally exceeding 8 mg, but there was no evidence that it reduced other maternal or neonatal morbidities [5M].

DRUGS THAT STIMULATE β₁-ADRENOCEPTORS [SEDA-33, 265; SEDA-34, 285; SEDA-35, 257; SEDA-36, 187]

Dobutamine [SEDA-33, 319; SEDA-34, 285; SEDA-35, 257; SEDA-36, 187]

Adverse Effects During Dobutamine Stress Echocardiography

In patients with obstructive coronary artery disease, ST-segment elevation is frequently seen during dobutamine stress echocardiography in leads overlying previous transmural left ventricular myocardial infarction. The mechanism

and potential management of ST-segment elevation during dobutamine stress echocardiography are reviewed.

CARDIOVASCULAR

The authors retrospectively identified 28 adults (age 51–83 years) with ST-segment elevation and inducible myocardial ischemia in the same territory during dobutamine stress echocardiography. ST-segment elevation occurred in inferior, inferolateral, anterior, lateral, or anterolateral leads and was associated with ischemic symptoms in 17 patients (61%). Inducible left ventricular wall motion abnormality developed in left ventricular segments corresponding to ECG ST-segment elevation in all patients. Coronary arteriography showed severe luminal narrowing in the major epicardial coronary artery supplying the region with dobutamine stress ST-segment elevation and ischemia. Dobutamine-induced ST-segment elevation in left ventricular segments with normal baseline wall motion is a highly reliable marker of viable collateral-dependent myocardium [6R] (Figure 1).

HEMATOLOGIC

Intracranial haemorrhage resulting from dobutamine stress echocardiography is a rare complication in an otherwise relatively safe procedure. There had been one previously reported case of intracranial haemorrhage associated with dobutamine stress echocardiography in a patient who was fully anticoagulated. The authors reported a second case of intracranial haemorrhage associated with dobutamine stress echocardiography leading to a poor outcome. Unlike the previous report, this patient was not fully anticoagulated and bleeding resulted from uncontrolled hypertension. Clinicians should be attentive to

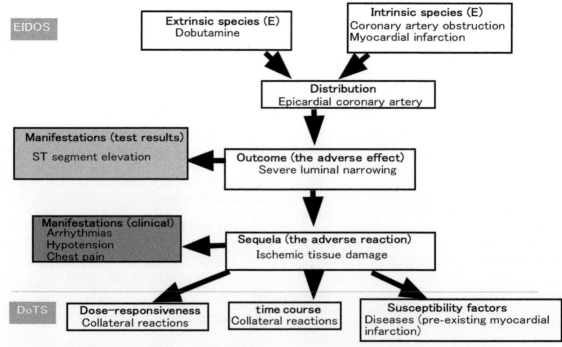

FIGURE 1   The EIDOS and DoTS descriptions of ST-segment elevation during dobutamine stress echocardiography.

the risk of intracranial haemorrhage associated with dobutamine stress echocardiography in the setting of uncontrolled hypertension [7A].

A 75-year-old man, who had a history of uncontrolled essential hypertension and coronary artery disease, underwent dobutamine stress echocardiography which showed ischemia in the right coronary artery territory. One month later, he again presented with atypical chest discomfort and he scheduled for a repeat dobutamine stress echocardiography. He was started on dobutamine infusion at a dose of 10 µg/kg/minute which increasing by 10 µg/kg/minute at the intervals of 3 minutes until either a maximum dose of 40 µg/kg/minute or heart rate of ≥85% of his maximum predicted heart rate (145 bpm) was achieved. During the procedure, his blood pressure increased to 199/115 mmHg and developed intraparenchymal haemorrhage and uncal herniation while receiving dobutamine and subsequently, followed by his death.

MANAGEMENT OF ADVERSE DRUG REACTIONS

Early injection of atropine during dobutamine stress echocardiography has been demonstrated in retrospective analyses to be effective to reduce the duration and dose of dobutamine infusion, while preserving a similar diagnostic accuracy with a lower incidence of adverse effects. In older patients undergoing dobutamine stress echocardiography, using atropine as a start drug is associated with shorter test duration, lower mean dobutamine infusion rate and consequently fewer adverse effects [8c].

Forty-five heart transplant patients (median age 62 years, 82% male) received 0.2–1 mg atropine during dobutamine stress echocardiography. Of these, 1 patient (2.2%) developed temporary complete heart block. No adverse events were identified in the control group of 154 patients who received dobutamine without atropine. Adverse events were defined as significant arrhythmias (sinus arrest, Mobitz type II heart block, complete heart block, ventricular tachycardia, or ventricular fibrillation), hypotension requiring hospitalization, syncope or presyncope, myocardial infarction, and death. These findings suggest that complete heart block can occur infrequently with the administration of atropine in heart transplant patients undergoing dobutamine stress echocardiography [9R].

Ivabradine is a heart rate-lowering agent acting by inhibiting the If-channel. A study evaluated whether ivabradine treatment blunts a dobutamine-induced increase in heart rate. In the control group, mean heart rate gradually and significantly increased at each step of dobutamine infusion, whereas no significant increase in heart rate was observed in the ivabradine group. Mean heart rate was also found to significantly increase during dobutamine infusion in the beta-blocker group. The median increase in heart rate from baseline was significantly higher in the control group compared to those in the ivabradine group. Therefore, Ivabradine treatment prevents dobutamine-induced

increase in heart rate and could be useful in reducing heart rate-related adverse effects of dobutamine [10c].

A case was reported, in which dobutamine induced cardiogenic shock due to systolic anterior motion after mitral valve repair [11A].

An adult male with severe eccentric mitral regurgitation caused by posterior leaflet prolapse underwent mitral valve repair by creation of new chordae at the posterior mitral leaflet. Mild basal septal hypertrophy was noted. Four hours later, his systolic blood pressure suddenly decreased from 80 to 40 mmHg. His left ventricular geometry was thought to have been affected by repair and intravenous dobutamine at 5 µg/kg/minute was initiated. The patient's systolic blood pressure rose to 100 mmHg temporarily, but decreased thereafter with progressive haemodynamic instability and a decrease in systolic blood pressure to 30–40 mmHg. The dobutamine was then increased up to 10 µg/kg/minute and noradrenaline of 0.01 µg/kg/minute was added. At that time, a loud systolic murmur was heard at the cardiac apex and an emergent transthoracic echocardiogram showed severe systolic anterior motion of mitral valve and dynamic obstruction of the left ventricular outflow tract with a mean pressure gradient of 64 mmHg. The physicians stopped intravenous dobutamine and noradrenaline immediately and infused large amounts of fluid to increase his left ventricular preload. His systolic murmur disappeared rapidly and the systolic anterior motion of mitral valve and the left ventricular outflow tract obstruction resolved [11A].

DRUGS THAT STIMULATE β₂-ADRENOCEPTORS

Indacaterol [SEDA-33, 361-2; SEDA-34, 318; SEDA-36, 188]

Randomized Controlled Trial

A randomized controlled pilot trial on acute exacerbations of chronic obstructive pulmonary disease, which enrolled 29 consecutive patients, was performed. All patients received a standard protocol consisting of ipratropium bromide aerosol 500 µg three times a day, intravenous methylprednisolone 20 mg twice daily and, if indicated, oral levofloxacin 500 mg once daily and they were randomly allocated to one of the two 5-day treatment groups (indacaterol maleate 300 µg once daily or salbutamol nebulizer 1250 µg three times a day). The administration of indacaterol 300 µg to patients admitted to emergency department for acute exacerbations of chronic obstructive pulmonary disease resulted in a greater improvement of pulmonary function compared with traditional therapy, without cardiovascular side effects. The results suggest that indacaterol could be a useful option in the treatment of acute exacerbations of chronic obstructive pulmonary disease [12c].

Data from clinical studies of 12–52 weeks duration in patients with chronic obstructive pulmonary disease receiving double-blind indacaterol at doses of 75 µg (449 patients), 150 µg (2611 patients), 300 µg (1157 patients), and 600 µg (547 patients) once daily compared with formoterol 12 µg twice daily (556 patients), salmeterol 50 µg twice daily (895 patients), tiotropium 18 µg once daily (1214 patients), or placebo (2012 patients) were screened. The incidence of adverse events was similar in the indacaterol and placebo groups and, in most cases, reflected the typical signs and symptoms of chronic obstructive pulmonary disease itself. Also, the risk of a "serious adverse event" (fatal or life-threatening, resulting in persistent or significant disability/incapacity, constituting a congenital anomaly/birth defect, requiring inpatient hospitalization or prolongation of existing hospitalization, or medically significant), including acute respiratory events, was similar in all indacaterol groups compared with placebo. Systemic β2-adrenoceptor-mediated effects on QTc interval, plasma potassium, and blood glucose were rare and showed no clinically significant changes with indacaterol treatment [13R].

Randomized Controlled Trial

The safety of indacaterol and tiotropium was investigated in 3444 patients with severe chronic obstructive pulmonary disease by multicentre, randomised, blinded, double-dummy, parallel group study. Tiotropium afforded greater protection from exacerbations, although the absolute number of events was small and the difference between treatments is of uncertain clinical importance [14c].

A Comparative study of salmeterol vs formoterol

A Comparative study of salmeterol vs formoterol assessed the efficacy and safety of combined long-acting β2-agonist and inhaled corticosteroid preparations, as measured by clinical endpoints and pulmonary function testing, compared with inhaled corticosteroids alone, in the treatment of adults with chronic obstructive pulmonary disease. The authors searched the Cochrane Airways Group Specialised Register of trials with a total of 7814 participants. Three preparations were used: fluticasone propionate/salmeterol, budesonide/formoterol, and mometasone furoate/formoterol. Adverse events were not significantly different between treatments [15M].

Systematic Review

The authors assessed the effects of β2-agonists given to women with preterm labour, and the authors searched the Cochrane Pregnancy and Childbirth Group's Trials Register. Results are based on the 20 trials involved 1367 women, compared β2-agonists with placebo. β2-Agonists were significantly associated with the following outcomes: withdrawal from treatment due to adverse effects, maternal chest pain, dyspnoea, palpitation, tremor, headaches, hypokalemia, hyperglycaemia, nausea or vomiting, nasal stuffiness, and fetal tachycardia [16M].

Salbutamol [SEDA-21, 182; SEDA-22, 190; SEDA-35, 318; SEDA-36, 189]

Systematic Review

The authors searched randomized control trials in continuous duodenal/jejunal levodopa/carbidopa pump infusion (1966 to January Week 2, 2014) and EMBASE (1998 to January 2014) and draw a conclusion; given the adverse side effects including tachycardia, oxygen desaturation and tremors and the expense associated with these treatments, bronchodilators such as albuterol or salbutamol are not effective in the routine management of bronchitis [17M].

Randomized Controlled Trial

β-Agonist overuse is associated with adverse outcomes in asthma, but the relationships between different metrics of salbutamol use and future risk are uncertain. Higher mean daily salbutamol use (per two actuations/day) [Odds ratio (OR) (95% CI) 1.24 (1.06–1.46)], higher days of salbutamol use (per 2 days in 2 weeks) [OR 1.15 (1.00–1.31)] and higher maximal 24-h use (per two actuations/day) [OR 1.09 (1.02–1.16)] were associated with future severe exacerbations. Higher mean daily salbutamol use was associated with future poor asthma control [OR 1.13 (1.02–1.26)]. Higher mean daily salbutamol use [OR 2.73 (1.84–4.07)], number of days of use [OR 1.46 (1.24–1.71)], and maximal daily use [OR 1.57 (1.31–1.89)] were associated with an increased risk of future extreme salbutamol overuse. Therefore, electronically recorded frequency of current salbutamol use is a strong predictor of risk of future adverse outcomes in asthma, with average daily use performing the best. These findings provide new information for clinicians considering metrics of salbutamol as predictors of future adverse outcomes in asthma [18c].

Randomized Controlled Trial
BACKGROUND

A previous randomised controlled Phase II trial suggested that an i.v. infusion of salbutamol may be beneficial, as it reduced extravascular lung water and plateau airway pressure. The Beta-Agonist Lung injury TrIal-2 (BALTI-2) was initiated to evaluate the effects of this intervention on mortality in patients with acute respiratory distress syndrome. Salbutamol increased 28-day mortality: 55 (34%) of 161 patients died in the salbutamol group compared with 38 (23%) of 163 in the placebo group (risk ratio 1.47, 95% confidence interval 1.03–2.08). Therefore, treatment with i.v. salbutamol early in the course of ARDS was poorly tolerated, is unlikely to be beneficial and could worsen outcomes. Further trials of beta-agonists in patients with acute respiratory distress syndrome are unlikely to be conducted. Some questions remain, such as whether or not there may be benefit at a different dose or in specific populations, but any studies investigating these would require a very strong rationale [19c].

DRUGS THAT STIMULATE DOPAMINE RECEPTORS [SEDA-33, 266; SEDA-34, 283; SEDA-35, 262; SEDA-36, 190]

Systematic Review

The risks for dyskinesia induced by dopamine receptor agonist monotherapy and the contribution of clinically significant factors in the development of this disorder were systematically assessed. Dopamine receptor agonist monotherapy resulted in an 87% lower risk for dyskinesia compared with treatment with levodopa (OR = 0.13, 95% confidence interval 0.09–0.19). The risk for dyskinesia was independent of the dose of dopamine receptor agonists, disease duration and treatment duration. A dose-related pattern was revealed between adjunct levodopa in the dopamine receptor agonist group and dyskinesia. Nevertheless, the odds for dyskinesia in the dopamine receptor agonist group were constantly lower than in the levodopa group. As the dose and treatment duration with dopamine receptor agonists are factors independent of the risk of dyskinesia, monotherapy with dopamine receptor agonists in early Parkinson's disease is suggested at doses that ensure efficacy and delay the need for levodopa [20M].

Pharmacogenetics

Maternal distress during pregnancy is linked to aggressive behavior in offspring. The 7-repeat (7r) allele of a variable number tandem repeat polymorphism in exon III of the human dopamine receptor D4 has consistently been associated with externalizing behavior problems, especially in the presence of adverse environmental factors. Under conditions of elevated prenatal maternal stress, children carrying one or two D4 receptor 7r alleles were at increased risk of a diagnosis of conduct disorder and/or oppositional defiant disorder. Moreover, homozygous carriers of the D4 receptor 7r allele displayed more externalizing behavior following exposure to higher levels of prenatal maternal stress, while homozygous carriers of the D4 receptor 4r allele turned out to be insensitive to the effects of prenatal stress. This study is

the first to report a gene–environment interaction related to D4 receptor [21R].

Cabergoline [SEDA-17, 169; SEDA-35, 262; SEDA-36, 190]

Systemic Review

Eight RCTs were considered to be eligible; data from seven studies could be extracted and included in the meta-analysis. Cabergoline reduces the risk of moderate–severe ovarian hyperstimulation syndrome (RR 0.38, 95% CI 0.29–0.51, 7 studies, 858 women) and probably has no clinically relevant negative impact on clinical pregnancy (RR 1.02, 95% CI 0.78–1.34, 4 studies, 561 women) or on the number of retrieved oocytes (MD 1.15, 95% CI −0.76 to 3.07, 5 studies, 628 women). However, our estimates were imprecise for distinguishing between substantial harm, no effect, and substantial benefit considering live birth (RR 1.03, 95% CI 0.71–1.48, 1 study, 200 women), and miscarriage (RR 0.69, 95% CI 0.27–1.76, 3 studies, 194 pregnant women). No studies reported congenital abnormalities. Cabergoline is unlikely to have a clinically relevant negative impact on clinical pregnancy or on the number of retrieved oocytes. However, it is still uncertain of its impact on live birth, miscarriage, and congenital abnormalities [22M].

Hematological

Dopamine agonists have been associated with adverse effects such as nausea, vomiting and psychosis. The first case with cabergoline-induced immune hemolytic anemia was reported.

A 16-year-old female patient had cabergoline treatment history for prolactinoma. She was started on cabergoline 0.5 mg twice per week and presented with weakness, fatigue, nausea, and paleness. Laboratory findings revealed severe anemia with a hemoglobin level of 4.7 g/dl. Her complete blood count results had been normal prior to cabergoline initiation. She received transfusions of erythrocyte suspension. However, her hemolytic anemia persisted. Carbergoline was then discontinued, as there was no other cause for the hemolytic anemia. There were no causes identified to explain hemolytic anemia except cabergoline. Therefore, cabergoline therapy was stopped and subsequently hemolytic anemia resolved and did not occur again [23A].

Rotigotine [SEDA-35, 264]

Systematic Review

A systematic review and meta-analysis of randomized controlled trials were performed to evaluate the efficacy, tolerability, and safety of rotigotine transdermal patch versus placebo in patients with Parkinson's disease. Six randomized controlled trials (1789 patients) were included in this meta-analysis. Rotigotine was associated with a significantly higher rate of withdrawals due to adverse events (relative risk [RR] 1.82, 95% CI 1.29-2.59), and higher rates of application site reactions (RR 2.92, 95% CI 2.29–3.72), vomiting (RR 5.18, 95% CI 2.25–11.93), and dyskinesia (RR 2.52, 95% CI 1.47–4.32) compared with placebo. No differences were found in the relative risks of headache, constipation, back pain, diarrhea, or serious adverse events [24M].

Randomized Controlled Trial

The efficacy and safety of transdermal rotigotine (2 and 3 mg/24 h) in 284 Japanese patients with restless legs syndrome were investigated. Overall, 80.0%, 86.2%, and 51.6% of patients in the rotigotine 2 mg/24 h, 3 mg/24 h, and placebo groups, respectively, experienced adverse events including application site reactions in 42.1%, 50.0%, and 7.4% of patients, respectively. None of the AEs were severe [25c].

Nervous System

'Dropped head sign' relates to a severe disproportionate antecollis in parkinsonism. It has also been described as a side effect of dopamine agonist medication with cabergoline and pramipexole. The first case of a rotigotine-induced dropped head sign was reported in a patient with suspected idiopathic Parkinson's disease, which was later defined as multiple system atrophy. The 'dropped head sign' is considered a rare symptom of unknown etiology.

A 64-year-old woman presented with a rapidly progressive two-and-a-half-year history of a hypokinetic Parkinson's syndrome with asymmetric development of symptoms and an initially good response to levodopa medication. Due to side effects of other dopamimetic medications, the patient was switched to rotigotine medication 5 weeks before clinical admission. Progressive antecollis without muscle weakness and prominent paraspinal muscle contraction developed within 2 weeks of treatment and resolved within a week after discontinuation of rotigotine and initiation of levodopa/cabergoline medication. The easily recognizable the 'dropped head sign' should prompt a thorough reevaluation of diagnosis and medication in patients with Parkinson's disease [26A].

Open-Label Study

Dopamine agonists are not often used in atypical Parkinson's disease because of inefficacy and in a minority of cases, side effects such as dyskinesias, impairment of extrapyramidal symptoms or the appearance of psychosis, and REM sleep behavioral disorders. An observational open-label study was carried out to evaluate the efficacy and tolerability of transdermal rotigotine in patients affected by atypical Parkinson's disease. Main adverse effects were hypotension, nausea, vomiting, drowsiness, and tachycardia. The electroencephalographic recording power spectra analysis showed a decrease of theta and an increase of low alpha power. In conclusion, transdermal transdermal rotigotine seems to be effective and well tolerated in patients with atypical Parkinson's disease [27c].

Apomorphine

Nervous System

In later stages of Parkinson's disease, treatment of 'off' periods with subcutaneous apomorphine is helpful but requires injection; inhaled apomorphine would be potentially more convenient. Reversal of 'off' episodes was significantly more likely for episodes treated with apomorphine than those treated with placebo: apomorphine 64.6% SD 32.3 of episodes versus placebo 11.1% SD 15.3 ($p < 0.0001$). During at-home treatment, 36% of apomorphine and 20% of placebo patients experienced adverse events. Therefore, daily 'off' time was not significantly reduced by the use of inhaled apomorphine [28c].

Psychiatric

Ninety-two patients who underwent deep brain stimulation surgery for Parkinson's disease were retrospectively analyzed for the safety of apomorphine. Main reason for omission of treatment was intolerable nausea (16/92, 17.3%). Apomorphine treatment was well tolerated and the most common side effect was nodular panniculitis. No severe complications were observed. No patient required ICU/IMC stay related to dopaminergic deprivation [29C].

Continuous subcutaneous apomorphine infusion therapy has proved to be effective in advanced Parkinson's disease. Contraindications to the use of continuous subcutaneous apomorphine infusion therapy are severe dementia or neuropsychiatric symptoms and severe biphasic dyskinesias; however, unlike deep brain stimulation, advanced age is not a contraindication [30R].

Gastrointestinal

Seventy-two out of 92 patients (78.3%) received apomorphine treatment in patients with Parkinson's disease; the main reason for omission of treatment was intolerable nausea (16/92, 17.3%). Apomorphine treatment was well tolerated and the most common side effect was nodular panniculitis. No severe complications were observed.

No patient required intensive care unit stay related to dopaminergic deprivation [29C].

Apomorphine vs Levodopa

Subcutaneous apomorphine infusion and intrajejunal levodopa infusion are two treatment options for patients with advanced Parkinson's disease and refractory motor complications, with varying cost of treatment. Adverse effects included peritonitis with intrajejunal levodopa infusion and skin nodules on subcutaneous apomorphine infusion [31R].

Dopamine Receptor Agonists [SEDA-34, 242; SEDA-35, 261; SEDA-36, 191]

Placebo-Controlled Study

In multicenter, randomized, double-blind, placebo-controlled, 667 patients admitted to intensive care units after cardiac surgery with early acute kidney injury were assigned to receive fenoldopam (338 patients) or placebo (329 patients). Treatment was continuous infusion of fenoldopam or placebo for up to 4 days with a starting dose of $0.1\,g/kg/minute$ (range, 0.025–$0.3\,\mu g/kg/minute$). The primary end point was the rate of renal replacement therapy. Mortality at 30 days was 78 of 338 (23%) in the fenoldopam group and 74 of 329 (22%) in the placebo group ($p = 0.86$). Hypotension occurred in 85 (26%) patients in the fenoldopam group and in 49 (15%) patients in the placebo group ($p = 0.001$). Among patients with acute kidney injury after cardiac surgery, fenoldopam infusion, compared with placebo, did not reduce the need for renal replacement therapy or risk of 30-day mortality but was associated with an increased rate of hypotension [32C].

Review

Apomorphine is likely effective at reducing daytime motor fluctuations and has a variable effect on dyskinesia, but existing evidence is too poor to permit firm conclusions. Off-time reduction with continuous duodenal/jejunal levodopa/carbidopa pump infusion is limited to the daytime; some nighttime effects have been reported. Although sometimes practiced, there are concerns about the safety of 24-h dopaminergic infusion therapy and uncertainty regarding nighttime dose adjustments required. Preliminary data suggest that continuous duodenal/jejunal levodopa/carbidopa pump infusion has a strong beneficial effect on dyskinesia [33R].

Psychiatric

Extended-release formulations of pramipexole and ropinirole and transdermal continuous delivery rotigotine patches are currently available. Despite a generally good safety profile, serious adverse events, such as impulse control disorder and sleep attacks, need to be routinely monitored. When treatment with dopamine receptor agonists is stopped abruptly, dopamine withdrawal syndrome may present. Suspending any dopamine receptor agonist, especially pramipexole, has been linked to onset of severe apathy [34R].

Piribedil [SEDA-35, 263]

Randomized Controlled Study

A study was carried out to investigate the effects of piribedil on vigilance and cognitive performance in patients with Parkinson disease experiencing excessive daytime sleepiness on pramipexole or ropinirole. In this 11-week randomized, active-controlled, rater-blinded phase III study, eligible 44 patients were randomly assigned to either receive piribedil or to continue on pramipexole or ropinirole. This study shows that switching from pramipexole or ropinirole to piribedil upholds the same therapeutic motor effect and reduces daytime sleepiness to a clinically relevant degree in patients with excessive daytime sleepiness [35c].

Psychiatric

A study based on the French national pharmacovigilance database identified and analysed seven reports of sleep attacks attributed to piribedil in patients without Parkinson's disease. The case reports are detailed and indicate that piribedil has a direct role in the onset of sleep attacks. To spare patients unnecessary exposure to the adverse effects of piribedil, it is better to avoid using piribedil and to choose drugs with demonstrated efficacy instead [36A].

Levodopa [SEDA-32, 285; SEDA-33, 320; SEDA-34, 286-8; SEDA-35, 259; SEDA-36, 192]

Systematic Reviews

Patients were randomized to receive levodopa therapy with levodopa/carbidopa/entacapone ($n = 373$) or levodopa/carbidopa ($n = 372$). Blinded assessments for dyskinesia and wearing-off were performed at 3-month intervals for the 134- to 208-week duration of the study. The patients were divided into four dose groups based on nominal levodopa dose at the time of onset of dyskinesia: group 1, $<400\,mg/day$ ($n = 157$); group 2, $400\,mg/day$ ($n = 310$); group 3, 401–$600\,mg/day$ ($n = 201$); and group 4, $>600\,mg/day$ ($n = 77$). The risk of developing dyskinesia and wearing-off increased in a levodopa dose-dependent manner ($p < 0.001$ for both). Factors that were predictive of dyskinesia, in rank order, were: young age at onset, higher levodopa dose, low body weight, North American geographic region, levodopa/carbidopa/entacapone treatment group, female gender, and more severe Unified Parkinson's Disease Rating Scale Part II. Multivariate analyses identified similar predictors for wearing-off but included baseline Unified Parkinson's Disease Rating Scale Part III and excluded weight and treatment allocation. The risk of developing dyskinesia or wearing-off was closely linked to levodopa dose. These results suggest that physicians should use the lowest dose of levodopa that provides satisfactory clinical control to minimize the risk of both dyskinesia and wearing-off [37c].

Medline and FDA searches were performed to gather information about the safety of the medications approved for the treatment of the motor symptoms of Parkinson's disease. The side effect and safety profiles of carbidopa/levodopa, dopamine agonists, selective monoamine oxidase inhibitors, catechol-O-methyltransferase inhibitors, anticholinergics and amantadine were reviewed. Though serious side effects may occur, as a group, the medications used for the treatment of Parkinson's disease motor symptoms tend to produce side effects that are mild to moderate in nature [38R].

Review

Dopamine receptor agonist monotherapy resulted in an 87% lower risk for dyskinesia compared with treatment with levodopa (OR = 0.13, 95% confidence interval 0.09–0.19, $p < 0.001$). The risk for dyskinesia was independent of the dose of dopamine receptor agonist, disease duration and treatment duration. A dose-related pattern was revealed between adjunct levodopa in the dopamine receptor agonist group and dyskinesia. Nevertheless, the odds for dyskinesia in the dopamine receptor agonist group were constantly lower than in the levodopa group [20M].

Dopamine agonist monotherapy can be used to delay the onset of levodopa therapy, and thus delays the development of levodopa-induced dyskinesia for a few years. The symptoms of levodopa-induced dyskinesia gradually appear. Most of the time, the symptoms of levodopa-induced dyskinesia correlate with the drug's optimal therapeutic window, and correspond to the maximal plasma and brain level of levodopa. These 'peak-dose levodopa-induced dyskinesia' are mainly choreiform and become more dystonic as the disease progresses. Levodopa-induced dyskinesia can also be observed during the rise and fall of levodopa plasma levels, with these 'diphasic dyskinesia' usually being more dystonic. Other forms of pure dystonia, in one foot for example, have also been reported in the absence of abnormal movement, in both 'on phase' and 'off phase' (high or low plasma level of levodopa, respectively). Patients do not always notice early levodopa-induced dyskinesia as they tend to affect facial muscles, usually manifesting as jaw movements and tongue protrusion,

but they are very heterogeneous and vary from patient to patient. However, they rapidly spread to the head and neck, usually in a wave-nodding movement, before affecting the limbs in a more dystonic and disabling manner. Levodopa-induced dyskinesia is also associated with weakening of the tendon reflexes and, more sporadically, toe flexion or panting respiration has also been described. Levodopa-induced dyskinesia also has a tendency to affect the side of the body that was first affected by the disease, which typically remains the worst side in terms of function. The main cited risk factors for levodopa-induced dyskinesia are the extent of dopaminergic denervation and the dose and duration of levodopa treatment, although early onset of the disease also significantly increases the risk of developing premature dyskinesia [39R].

Placebo-Controlled Studies

Several lines of evidence link the dopaminergic system to reward and punishment processing, but this evidence stems from studies in non-social contexts. A study investigated dopaminergic drug effects on individuals' reward seeking and punishment avoidance in social interaction. Two-hundred one healthy male participants were randomly assigned to receive 300 mg of levodopa or a placebo before playing an economic bargaining game. This game involved two conditions, one in which unfair behavior could be punished and one in which unfair behavior could not be punished. In the absence of punishment threats, levodopa administration led to more selfish behavior, likely mediated through an increase in reward seeking. In contrast, levodopa administration had no significant effect on behavior when faced with punishment threats. The results of this study broaden the role of the dopaminergic system in reward seeking to human social interactions. We could show that even a single dose of a dopaminergic drug may bring selfish behavior to the fore, which in turn may shed new light on potential causal relationships between the dopaminergic system and norm abiding behaviors in certain clinical subpopulations [40c].

Review

A complex relationship has been reported between impulse control disorders and obsessive–compulsive disorder. The concordance rates of obsessive–compulsive disorder in patients with trichotillomania have been found to be significantly higher (13–27%) when compared to that of the general community (1–3%). On the other hand, in regard to the co-occurrence of obsessive–compulsive disorder and pathological gambling, although inconsistent, studies revealed that in subjects with pathological gambling, rates of concurrent obsessive–compulsive disorder ranged from 1% to 20%, compared with the rate of 2% found in the general population. A functional MRI study revealed that pathological gamblers had lower activation in the thalamus, basal ganglia, and cortical regions compared to control subjects, and concluded that this pattern was different from those of obsessive–compulsive disorder patients who had increased activity in cortico-basal-ganglionic thalamic circuits. In association with this, patients with Parkinson's disease who developed pathological gambling had an abnormal resting state dysfunction of the mesocortico-limbic network possibly related to drug-induced overstimulation of relatively preserved reward-related neuronal systems.

A case control study investigated dopamine agonist-related brain activity changes that may differentiate Parkinson's disease patients with dopamine agonist-induced pathological gambling from those without a history of pathological gambling. PET studies showed dopamine agonists could be triggering pathological gambling and drug addiction in vulnerable patients with Parkinson's disease. On the other hand, Parkinson's disease patients with pathological gambling showed decreased raclopride binding potential in PET during the task, suggesting that patients on dopamine agonist treatment who had pathological gambling released more dopamine in the ventral striatal region when they gambled, just as in substance abusers. In a single case presentation, pathological gambling associated with modafinil, which releases dopamine in N. accumbens was reported in a patient at the age of 39 years with a 12-year history of narcolepsy and cataplexy, without any significant medical or psychiatric history. Modafinil increased desire to gamble, dis-inhibition, and risky decision making in people who have low impulsivity, whereas decreased these effects in people with high impulsivity. It has been demonstrated that modafinil inhibits dopamine transporter, enhances wakefulness and increases the dopamine levels in cortical areas and caudate nucleus. Since almost all the studies are on Parkinson's disease, it is possible that some clinical symptoms of impulse control disorders may be attributed to a primary problem or a personality feature rather than a drug-induced condition [41R].

Promising results coming from randomized clinical trials on selective serotonin reuptake inhibitors have been reported in patients with impulse control disorders without Parkinson's disease. Mood stabilizers such as valproic acid and lithium have been demonstrated to be effective in patients with pathological gambling not having Parkinson's disease. On the other hand, a double-blind, placebo-controlled trial of olanzapine for the treatment of video poker pathological gamblers but did not find any beneficial effect of olanzapine on pathological gambling. Valproate was shown to be effective in the management of impulse control disorders not associated with Parkinson's disease. Valproate's beneficial effects on impulse control disorders were linked to its action on both GABAergic and serotonergic neurotransmitter systems. Nalmefene at a dose of 40 mg/day in pathological gamblers and naltrexone for pathological gambling in Parkinson's disease were found to be beneficial. On the other hand, N-acetylcysteine, a glutamate modulator and precursor of glutathione, was shown to be effective in the treatment of trichotillomania and other compulsive behaviors [41R].

Management of Adverse Reactions

The extension of levodopa action without inducing levodopa-induced dyskinesia was realized by the novel monoamine oxidase B- and glutamate-release inhibitor safinamide; however, this had no obvious effect on existing levodopa-induced dyskinesia. To date, strategies of continuous dopaminergic stimulation seem the most promising to prevent or ameliorate levodopa-induced dyskinesia [42R].

Apomorphine is likely effective at reducing daytime motor fluctuations and has a variable effect on dyskinesia, but existing evidence is too poor to permit firm conclusions. Off-time reduction with continuous duodenal/jejunal levodopa/carbidopa pump infusion is limited to the daytime; some nighttime effects have been reported. Although sometimes practiced, there are concerns about the safety of 24-h dopaminergic infusion therapy and uncertainty regarding nighttime dose adjustments required. Preliminary data suggest that continuous duodenal/jejunal levodopa/carbidopa pump infusion has a strong beneficial effect on dyskinesia, but lack of formal evidence precludes firm conclusions [33R].

The available data for levodopa-induced dyskinesia do not allow firm conclusions on neuropsychiatric safety, but open label data suggest that it may be best tolerated of the options of intermittent injections of apomorphine, subcutaneous infusions of apomorphine or continuous duodenal/jejunal levodopa/carbidopa pump infusion in patients with a history of psychosis. Apomorphine and continuous duodenal/jejunal levodopa/carbidopa pump infusion may have positive effects on levodopa-sensitive gait and balance problems or on dyskinesia-related problems, but only weak supporting evidence exists [43R].

Drug Administration Route

All Parkinson's disease patients treated with levodopa/carbidopa intestinal gel over a 7-year period were analysed to determine the duration of treatment, retention rate, and reasons for discontinuation. The most common adverse events were dislocation and kinking of the intestinal tube [44c].

Drug–Device Interaction

Improvement of gait disorders following pedunculopontine nucleus area stimulation in patients with Parkinson's disease has previously been reported. However, it could have a deleterious effect on maximum phonation time and oral diadochokinesis, and mixed effects on speech intelligibility. Whereas levodopa intake and subthalamic nucleus stimulation alone had no and positive effects on speech dimensions, respectively, a negative interaction between the two treatments was observed both before and after pedunculopontine nucleus area surgery [45R].

Mechanism

Levodopa-induced dyskinesia is currently thought to relate to pre- and post-synaptic changes that result in dopaminergic imbalance. A recent report suggests that the development of levodopa-induced dyskinesia relates to the degree of dopaminergic denervation present at baseline in the putamen. This observation, if confirmed, strongly implicates presynaptic mechanisms in the development of levodopa-induced dyskinesia [46R].

Serotonergic mechanisms in levodopa-induced dyskinesia were investigated using PET to evaluate dopamine release. Parkinson's disease patients with levodopa-induced dyskinesia showed relative preservation of serotonergic terminals throughout their disease. Identical levodopa doses induced markedly higher striatal synaptic dopamine concentrations in Parkinson's disease patients with levodopa-induced dyskinesia compared with Parkinson's disease patients with stable responses to levodopa. Oral administration of the serotonin receptor type 1A agonist buspirone prior to levodopa reduced levodopa-evoked striatal synaptic dopamine increases and attenuated levodopa-induced dyskinesia. Parkinson's disease patients with levodopa-induced dyskinesia that exhibited greater decreases in synaptic dopamine after buspirone pretreatment had higher levels of serotonergic terminal functional integrity. Buspirone-associated modulation of dopamine levels was greater in Parkinson's disease patients with mild levodopa-induced dyskinesia compared with those with more severe levodopa-induced dyskinesia. These findings indicate that striatal serotonergic terminals contribute to levodopa-induced dyskinesia pathophysiology via aberrant processing of exogenous levodopa and release of dopamine. The results also support the development of selective serotonin receptor type 1A agonists for use as antidyskinetic agents in Parkinson's disease [47r].

Psychiatric

Mixed dopaminergic medication, comprising dopamine agonists and levodopa, may affect habit-learning in patients with Parkinson's disease. It was observed intact habit-learning in Parkinson's disease-patients off-medication. In contrast, the administration of 200 mg of levodopa impaired habit-learning. The authors conclude that potential deficits in habit-learning in Parkinson's disease may be attributed to the intake of levodopa [48c].

Drug Formulations

With conventional formulations of levodopa, irregular absorption and rapid catabolism are the basis for many of the problems associated with its chronic use. Extensive study of levodopa pharmacology has provided evidence that this drug behaves as more than just a transient metabolic intermediate in the pathway of catecholamine synthesis. Optimal dosing regimens can vary greatly among Parkinson's disease patients, as can the interplay of "short-duration" response and "long-duration" response. Several marketed levodopa products purport to offer more continuous dopaminergic stimulation than the immediate release formulation. However, pharmacokinetic analysis of several levodopa pharmaceuticals of worldwide major companies has shown that none of them provides reliable consistency of therapeutic concentrations of levodopa. These options include a new sustained-release oral carbidopa–levodopa formulation, two levodopa pro-drugs, two gastric-retentive slow-release levodopa formulations, an inhaled levodopa delivery system, and a subcutaneous infusion system using solubilized carbidopa–levodopa and levodopa. These products will join intestinally infused carbidopa–levodopa gel, a formulation currently marketed in Europe and elsewhere, and currently awaiting US regulatory approval. Although this levodopa formulation offers fine control of plasma levodopa concentration, drug administration by means of a tube through the stomach wall is not a practical treatment option for most patients experiencing motor fluctuations [49R].

DRUGS THAT AFFECT THE CHOLINERGIC SYSTEM [SEDA-31, 272; SEDA-32, 290; SEDA-33, 324; SEDA-34, 290-1, 318; SEDA-35, 266; SEDA-36, 199]

Anticholinergic Drugs [SEDA-31, 273; SEDA-32, 290; SEDA-33, 324; SEDA-34, 290-1,318; SEDA-35, 266; SEDA-36, 199]

Randomized Trial

A study was carried out to determine the effect of mydriatic drops on cognitive function, including memory, concentration, and orientation. The Montreal Cognitive Assessment test scores were shown to correlate with education, age, and race in patients with confirmed or suspected glaucoma. There was no significant difference in the Montreal Cognitive Assessment test scores of participants with confirmed or suspected glaucoma and participants without glaucoma. There was also no significant difference in the Montreal Cognitive Assessment scores of dilated participants and non-dilated participants as a whole. The results of this study suggest that physicians should spend more time with dilated glaucoma patients while explaining medical conditions and treatment instructions in order to ensure that patients have adequate time to comprehend instructions for glaucoma management [50C].

Genetic Factors

Anticholinergic activity was compared between metabolic phenotypes of the polymorphic enzymes cytochrome CYP2D6 and CYP2C19 in the elderly patients exposed to anticholinergic agents. Based on pharmacogenetic analyses of mutations encoding absent CYP2D6 or CYP2C19 metabolism, nursing home patients were divided into subgroups of poor metabolizers ($n=8$) and extensive metabolizers ($n=72$). The study population was represented by 78% women, 68% had mild to moderate dementia, and mean age was 86 years. More than 80% used more than one anticholinergic agent. The subpopulation of poor metabolizers had significantly higher median serum anticholinergic activity than the extensive metabolizers (10.3 versus 4.2 pmol atropine equivalents per milliliter, $p=0.012$). No significant differences in mouth dryness and cognitive function were observed between the subgroups ($p>0.3$). These findings suggest that elderly CYP2D6/CYP2C19 poor metabolizers with a high anticholinergic drug burden are at increased risk of elevated serum anticholinergic activity [51c].

Placebo-Controlled Study

In a two-center randomized, double-blind, placebo-controlled, parallel-group superiority trial, participants were allocated to receive 2 mg intramuscular benztropine or normal saline. Thirty participants were enrolled, 15 randomized to placebo and 15 to benztropine. Adverse events including blurred vision, dry mouth, drowsiness, dizzy, epigastric pain were more common in those receiving benztropine [52c].

The authors conducted a prospective, randomized study to compare the effects of oxybutynin at 10 mg daily and placebo in women with persistent plantar hyperhidrosis. Sixteen patients were included in each group (placebo and oxybutynin). The most common side effect was dry mouth (100% in the oxybutynin group vs 43.8% in the placebo group; $p=0.001$) [53C].

References

[1] Schnabl SM, Herrmann N, Wilder D, et al. Clinical results for use of local anesthesia with epinephrine in penile nerve block. J Dtsch Dermatol Ges. 2014;12(4):332–9 [R].

[2] Neset A, Nordseth T, Kramer-Johansen J, et al. Effects of adrenaline on rhythm transitions in out-of-hospital cardiac arrest. Acta Anaesthesiol Scand. 2013;57(10):1260–7 [c].

[3] Vrinten C, van der Zwaag AM, Weinreich SS, et al. Ephedrine for myasthenia gravis, neonatal myasthenia and the congenital myasthenic syndromes. Cochrane Database Syst Rev. 2014;12: Cd010028 [M].

[4] Gulhas N, Tekdemir D, Durmus M, et al. The effects of ephedrine on maternal hypothermia in caesarean sections: a double blind randomized clinical trial. Eur Rev Med Pharmacol Sci. 2013;17(15):2051–8 [c].

[5] Heesen M, Kolhr S, Rossaint R, et al. Prophylactic phenylephrine for caesarean section under spinal anaesthesia: systematic review and meta-analysis. Anaesthesia. 2014;69(2):143–65 [M].

[6] Shirani J, Pranesh S, Menhaji K, et al. Dobutamine-induced myocardial ischemia and st-segment elevation in collateral-dependent myocardium. Am J Cardiol. 2013;112(9):1293–7 [R].

[7] Bennin CL, Ramoutar V, Velarde G. Intraparenchymal haemorrhage and uncal herniation resulting from dobutamine stress echocardiography. BMJ Case Rep. 2014;2014: [A].

[8] Shehata M. Atropine first is safer than conventional atropine administration in older people undergoing dobutamine stress echocardiography. Ther Adv Cardiovasc Dis. 2014;8(5): 176–84 [c].

[9] Wang Ji J, Ye S, Haythe J, et al. The risk of adverse events associated with atropine administration during dobutamine stress echocardiography in cardiac transplant patients: a 28-year single-center experience. J Card Fail. 2013;19(11):762–7 [R].

[10] Cavusoglu Y, Mert U, Nadir A, et al. Ivabradine treatment prevents dobutamine-induced increase in heart rate in patients with acute decompensated heart failure. J Cardiovasc Med (Hagerstown). 2014; [c].

[11] Jeon YB, Park KY, Moon JK, et al. Dobutamine induced cardiogenic shock due to systolic anterior motion after mitral valve repair. Anaesth Intensive Care. 2013;41(4):551–2 [A].

[12] Segreti A, Fiori E, Calzetta L, et al. The effect of indacaterol during an acute exacerbation of COPD. Pulm Pharmacol Ther. 2013;26(6):630–4 [c].

[13] Ridolo E, Montagni M, Olivieri E, et al. Role of indacaterol and the newer very long-acting beta2-agonists in patients with stable COPD: a review. Int J Chron Obstruct Pulmon Dis. 2013;8:425–32 [R].

[14] Decramer ML, Chapman KR, Dahl R, et al. Once-daily indacaterol versus tiotropium for patients with severe chronic obstructive pulmonary disease (invigorate): a randomised, blinded, parallel-group study. Lancet Respir Med. 2013;1(7):524–33 [c].

[15] Nannini LJ, Poole P, Milan SJ, et al. Combined corticosteroid and long-acting beta(2)-agonist in one inhaler versus inhaled corticosteroids alone for chronic obstructive pulmonary disease. Cochrane Database Syst Rev. 2013;8:Cd006826 [M].

[16] Neilson JP, West HM, Dowswell T. Betamimetics for inhibiting preterm labour. Cochrane Database Syst Rev. 2014;2: Cd004352 [M].

[17] Gadomski AM, Scribani MB. Bronchodilators for bronchiolitis. Cochrane Database Syst Rev. 2014;6:Cd001266 [M].

[18] Patel M, Pilcher J, Reddel HK, et al. Metrics of salbutamol use as predictors of future adverse outcomes in asthma. Clin Exp Allergy. 2013;43(10):1144–51 [c].

[19] Gates S, Perkins GD, Lamb SE, et al. Beta-agonist lung injury trial-2 (balti-2): a multicentre, randomised, double-blind, placebo-controlled trial and economic evaluation of intravenous infusion of salbutamol versus placebo in patients with acute respiratory distress syndrome. Health Technol Assess. 2013;17(38): v–vi 1–87, [c].

[20] Chondrogiorgi M, Tatsioni A, Reichmann H, et al. Dopamine agonist monotherapy in parkinson's disease and potential risk factors for dyskinesia: a meta-analysis of levodopa-controlled trials. Eur J Neurol. 2014;21(3):433–40 [M].

[21] Zohsel K, Buchmann AF, Blomeyer D, et al. Mothers' prenatal stress and their children's antisocial outcomes—a moderating role for the dopamine d4 receptor (drd4) gene. J Child Psychol Psychiatry. 2014;55(1):69–76 [R].

[22] Leitao VM, Moroni RM, Seko LM, et al. Cabergoline for the prevention of ovarian hyperstimulation syndrome: systematic review and meta-analysis of randomized controlled trials. Fertil Steril. 2014;101(3):664–75 [M].

[23] Gurbuz F, Yagci-Kupeli B, Kor Y, et al. The first report of cabergoline-induced immune hemolytic anemia in an adolescent with prolactinoma. J Pediatr Endocrinol Metab. 2014;27(1–2):159–63 [A].

[24] Zhou CQ, Li SS, Chen ZM, et al. Rotigotine transdermal patch in parkinson's disease: a systematic review and meta-analysis. PLoS ONE. 2013;8(7):e69738 [M].

[25] Inoue Y, Shimizu T, Hirata K, et al. Efficacy and safety of rotigotine in Japanese patients with restless legs syndrome: a phase 3, multicenter, randomized, placebo-controlled, double-blind, parallel-group study. Sleep Med. 2013;14(11):1085–91 [c].

[26] Dohm CP, Groschel S, Liman J, et al. Dropped head sign induced by transdermal application of the dopamine agonist rotigotine in parkinsonian syndrome: a case report. J Med Case Rep. 2013;7:174 [A].

[27] Moretti DV, Binetti G, Zanetti O, et al. Behavioral and neurophysiological effects of transdermal rotigotine in atypical parkinsonism. Front Neurol. 2014;5:85 [c].

[28] Grosset KA, Malek N, Morgan F, et al. Inhaled apomorphine in patients with 'on-off' fluctuations: a randomized, double-blind, placebo-controlled, clinic and home based, parallel-group study. J Parkinsons Dis. 2013;3(1):31–7 [c].

[29] Slotty PJ, Wille C, Kinfe TM, et al. Continuous perioperative apomorphine in deep brain stimulation surgery for parkinson's disease. Br J Neurosurg. 2014;28(3):378–82 [C].

[30] Wenzel K, Homann CN, Fabbrini G, et al. The role of subcutaneous infusion of apomorphine in parkinson's disease. Expert Rev Neurother. 2014;14(7):833–43 [R].

[31] Martinez-Martin P, Reddy P, Katzenschlager R, et al. Euroinf: a multicenter comparative observational study of apomorphine and levodopa infusion in parkinson's disease. Mov Disord. 2014;30(4):510–6 [R].

[32] Bove T, Zangrillo A, Guarracino F, et al. Effect of fenoldopam on use of renal replacement therapy among patients with acute kidney injury after cardiac surgery: a randomized clinical trial. JAMA. 2014;312(21):2244–53 [C].

[33] Henriksen T. Clinical insights into use of apomorphine in parkinson's disease: tools for clinicians. Neurodegener Dis Manag. 2014;4(3):271–82 [R].

[34] Alonso Canovas A, Luquin Piudo R, Garcia Ruiz-Espiga P, et al. Dopaminergic agonists in parkinson's disease. Neurologia. 2014;29(4):230–41 [R].

[35] Eggert K, Ohlwein C, Kassubek J, et al. Influence of the nonergot dopamine agonist piribedil on vigilance in patients with Parkinson disease and excessive daytime sleepiness (pivicog-pd): an 11-week randomized comparison trial against pramipexole and ropinirole. Clin Neuropharmacol. 2014;37(4):116–22 [C].

[36] Piribedil: sleep attacks, also in patients without parkinson's disease. Prescrire Int. 2013;22(143):265 [A].

[37] Warren Olanow C, Kieburtz K, Rascol O, et al. Factors predictive of the development of levodopa-induced dyskinesia and wearing-off in parkinson's disease. Mov Disord. 2013;28(8):1064–71 [c].

[38] Faulkner MA. Safety overview of fda-approved medications for the treatment of the motor symptoms of parkinson's disease. Expert Opin Drug Saf. 2014;13(8):1055–69 [R].

[39] Breger LS, Lane EL. L-dopa and graft-induced dyskinesia: different treatment, same story? Exp Biol Med (Maywood). 2013;238(7):725–32 [R].

[40] Pedroni A, Eisenegger C, Hartmann MN, et al. Dopaminergic stimulation increases selfish behavior in the absence of punishment threat. Psychopharmacology (Berl). 2014;231(1):135–41 [c].

[41] Atmaca M. Drug-induced impulse control disorders: a review. Curr Clin Pharmacol. 2014;9(1):70–4 [R].

[42] Schaeffer E, Pilotto A, Berg D. Pharmacological strategies for the management of levodopa-induced dyskinesia in patients with parkinson's disease. CNS Drugs. 2014;28(12):1155–84 [R].

[43] Volkmann J, Albanese A, Antonini A, et al. Selecting deep brain stimulation or infusion therapies in advanced parkinson's disease: an evidence-based review. J Neurol. 2013;260(11):2701–14 [R].

[44] Zibetti M, Merola A, Artusi CA, et al. Levodopa/carbidopa intestinal gel infusion in advanced parkinson's disease: a 7-year experience. Eur J Neurol. 2014;21(2):312–8 [c].

[45] Pinto S, Ferraye M, Espesser R, et al. Stimulation of the pedunculopontine nucleus area in parkinson's disease: effects on speech and intelligibility. Brain. 2014;137(Pt. 10):2759–72 [R].

[46] Ko JH, Lerner RP, Eidelberg D. Effects of levodopa on regional cerebral metabolism and blood flow. Mov Disord. 2015;30(1):54–63 [R].

[47] Politis M, Wu K, Loane C, et al. Serotonergic mechanisms responsible for levodopa-induced dyskinesias in parkinson's disease patients. J Clin Invest. 2014;124(3):1340–9 [r].

[48] Fuhrer H, Kupsch A, Halbig TD, et al. Levodopa inhibits habit-learning in parkinson's disease. J Neural Transm. 2014;121(2):147–51 [c].

[49] LeWitt PA. Levodopa therapy for parkinson's disease: pharmacokinetics and pharmacodynamics. Mov Disord. 2015;30(1):64–72 [R].

[50] Dersu II, Spencer HT, Grigorian PA, et al. The effect of mydriatic solutions on cognitive function. Semin Ophthalmol. 2015;30(1):36–9 [C].

[51] Kersten H, Wyller TB, Molden E. Association between inherited cyp2d6/2c19 phenotypes and anticholinergic measures in elderly patients using anticholinergic drugs. Ther Drug Monit. 2014;36(1):125–30 [c].

[52] Asha SE, Kerr A, Jones K, et al. Benztropine for the relief of acute non-traumatic neck pain (wry neck): a randomised trial. Emerg Med J. 2014; [c].

[53] Costa Ada Jr. S, Leao LE, Succi JE, et al. Randomized trial—oxybutynin for treatment of persistent plantar hyperhidrosis in women after sympathectomy. Clinics (Sao Paulo). 2014;69(2):101–5 [C].

14

Dermatological Drugs, Topical Agents, and Cosmetics

Adrienne T. Black[*,†,1]

*3E Company, Carlsbad, CA, USA
†Institute of Public Health, New York Medical College, Valhalla, NY, USA
[1]Corresponding author: adrienne159@gmail.com

INTRODUCTION

This chapter provides a concise overview of drug-induced skin reactions or side effects reported in the literature from July 2013 to December 2014. The effects include those resulting from medications used to treat dermal disorders such as acne and psoriasis as well as drug-associated cutaneous reactions by antivirals, neurological treatments and chemotherapy. The information presented includes case reports, clinical trial results, pooled clinical trial analyses and literature reviews.

ACNE

Combination: Retinaldehyde, Glycolic Acid and Efectiose

A common combination therapy of 0.1% retinaldehyde, 6% glycolic acid and 0.1% efectiose is used to treat mild-to-moderate acne vulgaris. A retrospective study in 30 patients (aged 10–30 years old) with mild-to-moderate acne vulgaris was undertaken to determine the efficacy and tolerability of use of this medication in a cream formulation during sun exposure. The combination cream was applied once a day in the evening for 8 weeks, while in the morning SPF 50 sunscreen was applied. The Global Evaluation Scale grading system proposed by the FDA was used to evaluate efficacy at baseline, 30 and 60 days. Tolerability was also assessed at 30 and 60 days with few side effects such as erythema, dryness, desquamation, pruritus, burning reported [1c].

Combination: Dapsone Gel and Oral Isotretinoin

The combination of 5% dapsone gel plus oral isotretinoin for treatment of acne vulgaris was evaluated in a double-blind, randomized, placebo-controlled, study conducted with 58 patients (age range: 18–25 years) with moderate-to-severe facial acne. All subjects received oral isotretinoin 20 mg daily and topical gel twice a day for 8 weeks; the gel consisted of either 5% dapsone gel or vehicle gel. The Global Acne Assessment Score (GAAS) and side effects were noted at the start of the study, weeks 4, 8 and 12. The side effects on the dapsone-treated group occurred in 11 of the 58 subjects and were considered minor but tolerable; the effects consisted of mild burning sensation (7 patients), mild erythema (4 patients) and dryness of the skin (3 patients). A more serious adverse effect occurred in one patient who developed conjunctivitis when the dapsone gel was applied too close to the eye [2C].

ANTIFUNGALS

Antifungal Treatments: Literature Review

Tinea infections are fungal infections of the skin caused by dermatophytes that may affect up to 20% of the global population. These infections may be further classified as tinea corporis (ringworm) and tinea cruris (jock itch) and are generally diagnosed by appearance and confirmed with microscopy or culture. A literature review of 129 randomized controlled trials with 18 086 patients diagnosed with either tinea corporis or tinea cruris infections. The duration of treatments ranged from 1 week to

© 2015 Elsevier B.V. All rights reserved.

2 months, but the most common duration was 2–4 weeks. Follow-up also varied: from 1 week to 6 months. The adverse effects were minimal, occurred infrequently and were typically reports of irritation and burning. However, no conclusions could be made using the reported adverse effects as there was no clear differentiation between treatment versus placebo and between the different types of treatments. The authors concluded that terbinafine and naftifine treatments for tinea infections were the most effective with minimal side effects [3R].

HAIR LOSS TREATMENT

Minoxidil

Minoxidil is an approved drug for treatment for hair loss in men and women in the United States and Canada. However, while a 5% minoxidil foam once daily has been approved for men in both countries since 2006, a similar 5% minoxidil once daily product has only been approved for female pattern hair loss (FPHL) in the US and Canada since 2014. The approval of 5% once daily minoxidil foam for FPHL is the result of two recently completed randomized, double-blind, parallel, international multicenter Phase III trials. In the first trial, 404 patients used 5% minoxidil foam or vehicle once daily for 24 weeks and adverse events were evaluated every 6 weeks. In the second trial, patients used either 5% minoxidil foam once daily ($n=161$) or a 2% minoxidil solution twice daily ($n=161$) for 1 year with regular reporting of adverse effects. The number of adverse events was similar between the two trials and between the 5% foam and the 2% solution. The most common side effects reported were weight gain, headache, pruritus, and nasal and upper respiratory tract infections. Serious side effects were reported by six patients in the 5% minoxidil group in the first trial and included cardiac disorder, gastritis, dehydration, osteoarthritis, ovarian neoplasm, uterine leiomyoma, renal failure, and hypertensive crisis. In the second trial, 2 serious adverse effects were reported with the 5% foam (wrist fracture and anxiety) and 8 effects with the 2% solution (angina pectoris, abdominal pain, bile duct stone, anal abscess, influenza, metastatic neoplasm, menometrorrhagia, and asthma). However, these serious adverse effects were not considered clinically relevant to minoxidil use [4c].

PIGMENTATION DISORDERS

Tranexamic Acid

The current protocol for treatment of melasma is application of a hydroquinone and dexamethasone solution. It has been recently reported that tranexamic acid has whitening effects, particularly for ultraviolet-induced hyperpigmentation such as melasma. A prospective, randomized, double-blind, split-face trial of 12 weeks was recently completed with 50 adult females with moderate-to-severe epidermal melasma comparing a topical 3% solution of tranexamic acid with topical solution of 3% hydroquinone and 0.01% dexamethasone. Each subject served as their own control with one treatment applied to one side of the face and the other treatment applied to the other side; each treatment was applied twice daily. The Melasma Area and Severity Index (MASI) and side effects were evaluated at the start of the trial and every 4 weeks afterwards until the end of the trial. The reported side effects of tranexamic acid ($n=9$ patients) were erythema, skin irritation, xerosis, and scaling; similar side effects were reported for the hydroquinone and dexamethasone combination treatment including erythema, skin irritation, dryness of the skin, scaling, hypertrichosis, and inflammation ($n=20$ patients). No serious side effects were reported with tranexamic acid in comparison the combination treatment [5C].

Ozenoxacin

Ozenoxacin, available in a 1% cream formulation, is a new nonfluorinated quinolone for treatment of impetigo and has recently been evaluated in several clinical trials. In a randomized, double-blind, multicenter study, the protocol was treatment with 1% ozenoxacin cream or placebo cream or 1% received retapamulin twice daily for 5 days. The retapamulin ointment served as a control. No side effects were reported and all treatments were well tolerated [6C].

In a second trial, a Phase I open-label study, a 1% ozenoxacin cream was evaluated for 6 days in a total of 46 patients: children ($\geq$2 months of age) and adults with impetigo. Ozenoxacin was applied once on Day 1, twice daily for 4 days and once on Day 6. No patients withdrew from the study and ozenoxacin was reportedly well tolerated [7C].

Imiquimod

A recent report described a case of an imiquimod-induced vitiligo. A 28-year-old male presented with 3-year history of condylomata acuminata (genital warts); previous treatments included liquid nitrogen and electronic desiccation but his condition had relapsed and new warts had now appeared. After treatment with electronic desiccation to remove the condylomata acuminata, the patient was prescribed 5% imiquimod cream to prevent relapse; imiquimod is the FDA-only approved medication for condylomata acuminata. After 12 weeks of use, vitiligo-like depigmentation patches in the areas of imiquimod application were visible. A skin biopsy indicated an absence of melanocytes and melanin granules in the basal layer of the epidermis; the dermis appearance was normal. Imiquimod treatment was discontinued but, during the following 10 days, macules already present in the treated area became enlarged and the depigmented patches spread. A 0.1% tacrolimnus ointment was prescribed to treat the symptoms although repigmentation did not occur [8A].

PSORIASIS

Methotrexate

Methotrexate in low doses has been safely and effectively used for treatment of psoriasis for many years. This report describes two fatal cases of patients prescribed low dose methotrexate (MTX) for treatment of psoriasis where the individuals did not follow the prescribed administration protocol. First, a 50-year-old male was on intermittent treatment with methotrexate (7.5 mg once weekly) for psoriasis for 2 years. After a treatment-free period of 6 months, the patient self-medicated with methotrexate (7.5 mg once daily) and an analgesic for joint pain for 1 week. After 2 days, he developed ulceration of existing lesions and had an elevated fever and pulse rate. Upon hospitalization, a depressed white blood cell count with bone marrow suppression was found. Although he was treated with intravenous antibiotics and blood cell and platelet transfusion, he expired due to acute respiratory failure 10 days later. Second, a 37-year-old male with a history of psoriasis presented with painful ulcerated skin lesions and fever and chills. One week earlier, the patient had taken an unknown amount of methotrexate without having a medical examination. Upon hospitalization, bone marrow suppression was diagnosed along with a high creatinine level and an atrophied, nonfunctioning right kidney. Dialysis was begun with antibiotic and sodium bicarbonate therapy and platelet transfusion; however, the patient expired after 2 days. These reports demonstrate that strict adherence to the prescribing regimen is critical to ensure the safe use of methotrexate [9A].

Cyclosporin

Cyclosporin for the treatment of moderate-to-severe psoriasis vulgaris was evaluated in a prospective, open-label, multicenter study with 73 patients (aged 16–70) with chronic, moderate-to-severe plaque psoriasis that was unresponsive to corticosteroids and Vitamin D_3 analogs and having a Psoriasis Area and Severity Index (PASI) score of less than 20. The patients received 2.5 mg/kg per day twice daily of cyclosporin microemulsion in a gelatin capsule for 2–12 weeks; the duration was dependent upon a 75% reduction in the PASI score. Cyclosporin treatment was then stopped but restarted at the same dosage if relapse occurred; the relapse was defined as a less than 50% improvement from the baseline PASI score. The PASI score was evaluated at baseline, 12, 48 and 96 weeks after initial treatment with follow-up 2 weeks after the study conclusion and then monthly for 2 years. In 20 of 73 patients, the second course of cyclosporin was required and the interval between treatments was 94 days. Six patients required cyclosporin for the full 96 weeks. A total of 16 adverse events were reported in 14 patients during week 12, 2 events at week 48 ($n=2$) and 3 events at week 96 ($n=2$). The adverse events included facial nerve paralysis, general fatigue, polyuria, tinea corporis, decreased serum immunoglobulin M, proteinuria, hyperlipidemia, hypertension, elevated levels of creatinine and blood urea nitrogen, and elevated total bilirubin. Ten patients discontinued treatment and withdrew from the study due to facial nerve paralysis, elevated creatinine, hyperlipidemia, proteinuria or general fatigue. All adverse effects were resolved with discontinuation of cyclosporine [10C].

Tofacitinib

Tofacitinib is a Janus kinase (JNK) inhibitor currently under development for as an oral medication for treating inflammatory diseases. A multicenter, double-blind, vehicle-controlled Phase 2a trial was undertaken to determine the efficacy and safety of two topical tofacitinib ointment formulations for the treatment of chronic plaque psoriasis. The study included 71 adult patients with mild-to-moderate plaque psoriasis who were divided into four groups; a 1–2% tofacitinib ointment 1, vehicle 1, a 2% tofacitinib ointment 2 and vehicle 2. Each treatment or vehicle was applied twice daily for 4 weeks to a single 300 cm^2 area with an estimated dose of 3 mg/cm^2; the area remained constant throughout the study and contained a target plaque that could also contain nontarget plaques and normal skin. The ointment formulations were proprietary but contained standard excipients used in topical formulations with one exception, a penetration enhancer. Evaluations were based on the change from baseline in the Target Plaque Severity Score. Adverse events occurred in 25 patients and all adverse events were considered mild or moderate and similar across the groups and. No serious adverse events were reported and no patients discontinued the treatment. It was noted that the systemic absorption and exposure was greater for tofacitinib ointment 1 than for ointment 2 [11C].

Calcipotriol Plus Betamethasone Dipropionate Gel

The combination calcipotriol plus betamethasone dipropionate gel is generally the first medication prescribed for psoriasis vulgaris. A pooled analysis of the safety data from nine clinical trials was conducted to determine the safety and tolerability of the combination treatment. The patient inclusion criteria of the analyzed studies were adults with a diagnosis of mild psoriasis vulgaris on $\geq 10\%$ of the scalp or body. The treatments were once daily for 8 weeks in the following groups: combination gel (scalp: $n = 1953$; body: $n = 824$), betamethasone dipropionate gel alone (scalp: $n = 1214$; body: $n = 562$), calcipotriol gel alone (scalp: $n = 979$; body: $n = 175$), gel vehicle (scalp: $n = 824$; body: $n = 226$), calcipotriol scalp solution (scalp only: $n = 104$) and tacalcitol ointment (body only: $n = 184$). Most of the adverse side effects were of mild-to-moderate severity and included nasopharyngitis, pruritus and upper respiratory tract infections. Nasopharyngitis (4–5%) was reported in patients who used large amount of the combination gel (40 g per week) across the pooled data sets. The scalp psoriasis patients using the combination gel experienced the lowest number of side effects (approximately 35%) as compared to the other treatments. The incidence of side effects with the body psoriasis patients was similar: 32% with the combination gel, 24% with the betamethasone dipropionate gel and 29% with the calcipotriol gel. The combination treatment also resulted in the lowest incidence of adverse drug reactions in scalp psoriasis patients (8% versus 9–27% for other treatments) and second lowest to betamethasone dipropionate gel (6% versus 4%) for body psoriasis. Few serious adverse effects occurred (0–1%): for the combination treatment; these effects included psoriasis ($n = 5$) and alopecia, erythrodermic psoriasis, pruritus, skin atrophy and urticaria ($n = 2$ each). Two serious adverse effects were considered possibly related to comparator treatment: moderate sinus tachycardia (calcipotriol gel) and nephrolithiasis (betamethasone dipropionate gel). All adverse effects considered potentially related to the combination gel were resolved when treatment was discontinued [12M].

CUTANEOUS SIDE EFFECTS FROM ANTIVIRAL MEDICATIONS

Entecavir

Entecavir, an antiviral nucleoside drug, is used in the treatment of chronic hepatitis B. A number of entecavir-induced adverse effects were reported in patients with advanced cirrhosis in the clinical trials and the postmarket period including clinical chemistry changes, neuropathy, muscular weakness and pancreatitis. However, cutaneous reactions have rarely occurred and only two cases of cutaneous adverse drug effects as unspecified hypersensitivity allergic (type I) drug reaction ADR have been reported in the literature. A case of entecavir-induced delayed type IVb hypersensitivity skin reaction was recently reported in a 45-year-old woman with a 10-year history of chronic hepatitis B and assorted antiviral therapies. She presented with a generalized maculopapular rash following 7 days of entecavir treatment (1 mg, once daily) for lamivudine-resistant chronic hepatitis B. Symptoms included pruritic, erythematous macules with intermingled with papules, significantly increased lymphocytic and eosinophilic involvement in the dermis based on skin biopsy, and increased levels interleukin-4 (IL-4); these effects were consistent with a type IVb delayed hypersensitivity classification. The skin reaction was resolved upon discontinuation of entecavir treatment [13A].

Telaprevir and Boceprevir

Telaprevir and boceprevir are protease inhibitors that have been recently approved for the treatment of chronic hepatitis C infection. Both medications are widely used although skin rashes are known to occur frequently with telaprevir and, to a lesser extent, with boceprevir. A high incidence of telaprevir-related skin rash was also noted in clinical trials although this effect has not been reported fully in the literature. This report describes patients who have developed skin rashes when treated with telaprevir ($n = 6$) and boceprevir ($n = 3$). Telaprevir treatment also caused abnormal chemistry values and possible systemic symptoms in four patients. Five of the telaprevir patients discontinued treatment due to the adverse effects. Moreover, two of the patients that discontinued telaprevir treatment had symptoms that could be classified as Drug Reaction with Eosinophilia and Systemic Symptoms (DRESS). In contrast, the boceprevir patients had a milder rash and none discontinued treatment. It is of note that telaprevir may cause more severe symptoms and require more frequent discontinuation of the therapy [14A].

Antiretroviral Therapy: Ritonavir-Boosted Darunavir

An observational study was conducted in HIV-positive patients prescribed ritonavir-boosted darunavir (DRV/r), a protease inhibitor frequently used in treating HIV-1 infections. A well-known side effect of DRV treatment is development of a skin rash. A study consisted of 292 patients taking antiretroviral therapy containing DRV/r once daily was conducted. DRV-induced skin rashes developed in 31 patients 7–14 days after initiation of treatment. The rash was considered mild in most cases: one patient had a grade 3 rash, 24 patients had grade 2 and 6 rashes, and 6 patients had a grade 1 rash. Two patients discontinued the treatment due to skin rash development. The other patients continued DRV/r treatment; the rashes disappeared without further complication and symptoms were relieved through use of oral steroids or antihistamines. Of note, the drug-induced rash occurred more frequently in individuals with less advanced HIV-1 infection than in those with more advanced infection. Further analysis showed that the DRV-induced rash was not associated with sulfonamide allergy and that there was no significant difference in the incidence of the skin rash between patients with and without history of sulfonamide allergy [15c].

CUTANEOUS SIDE EFFECTS FROM CANCER MEDICATIONS

Mechlorethamine

Topical nitrogen mustard has been used for decades as a treatment for mycosis fungoides, a form of cutaneous T-cell lymphoma. Once diagnosed, mycosis fungoides is classified as early (IA-IIA) or late (IIB-IVB) stage disease. Topical mechlorethamine is known to several common adverse skin reactions including irritant contact dermatitis, allergic contact dermatitis and hyperpigmentation but these reactions are generally mild and reversible when treatment is stopped. It has been noted that treatment with nitrogen mustard may increase the risk of non-melanoma skin cancers if used in conjunction with other skin damaging therapies. Recently, a new topical nitrogen mustard drug, VALCHOR (0.016% mechlorethamine w/w, equivalent of 0.02% mechlorethamine hydrochloride), was approved for use in patients with IA or IB mycosis fungoides and previous skin-directed therapy (FDA approved in August 2013). The safety of VALCHOR was evaluated in a multi-center, randomized, observer-blinded, active controlled trial in 260 patients with IA, IB or IB mycosis fungoides with no mechlorethamine use in the previous 2 years and no history of carmustine therapy. The patients applied either a 0.02% mechlorethamine chloride gel (study drug) a 0.02% mechlorethamine chloride ointment (control drug) once daily to a specific area for 1 year. The adverse effects occurred at a similar prevalence between two treatments, were generally mild to moderate and were mostly skin-related and included skin irritation, pruritus, erythema, contact dermatitis, hyperpigmentation and folliculitis. No serious adverse effects were reported. There were no discontinuations and the symptoms were managed by decreasing the frequency of application [16C,17C].

Vemurafenib

Vemurafenib is a BRAF kinase inhibitor used to treat advanced metastatic melanoma in patients with a BRAF (V600) mutation. An open-label, multicenter study of patients ($n = 3222$) in 44 countries with untreated or previously treated melanoma and a BRAF (V600) mutation was conducted to evaluate the safety and efficacy of vemuranfenib. Vemurafenib, 960 mg, was administered orally twice a day. The most adverse effects were rash ($n = 1592$), arthralgia ($n = 1259$), fatigue ($n = 1093$), photosensitivity reaction ($n = 994$), alopecia ($n = 826$), and nausea ($n = 628$). More serious adverse events (grade 3 or 4) were also reported in a total of 1480 patients: cutaneous squamous cell carcinoma ($n = 389$), rash ($n = 155$), liver function abnormalities ($n = 165$), arthralgia ($n = 106$), and fatigue ($n = 93$). These grade 3 and 4 adverse events occurred more frequently in patients aged 75 years and older than in those younger than 75 years [18C].

Vismodegib

Upregulation of the Hedgehog (Hh) signaling pathway is important in the progression of basal cell carcinoma. In 2012, the FDA approved vismodegib for the treatment of local or metastatic advanced basal cell carcinoma (BCC) that cannot be treated with surgery or radiation. Vismodegib antagonizes the Smoothened (SMO) protein, thereby preventing propagation of the Hh pathway and subsequent downstream transcriptional activation of proliferation and survival genes. A Phase 2 clinical trial was conducted in 104 patients treated with vismodegib, 150 mg orally once daily, to determine the efficacy and safety of the medication. The most common adverse effects were mild to moderate and included muscle spasms, dysgeusia, decreased weight, fatigue, alopecia, and diarrhea. It was noted that a large number of patients discontinued treatment with vismodegib for non-disease related reasons [19C].

Hydroactive Colloid Gel

Dermatitis frequently occurs during radiation therapy for breast cancer. The dermatitis may progress to a more severe form such as moist desquamation that requires an interruption in the radiation treatment. A retrospective study was undertaken to compare the efficacy of two topical treatments, a dexpanthenol cream and a hydroactive colloid gel, in preventing the development of moist desquamation during radiation therapy. The study included patients with breast cancer who were undergoing radiotherapy following breast-sparing surgery. The first group ($n = 267$) used 5% dexpanthenol cream throughout the entire course of their radiotherapy. The second group ($n = 216$) applied 5% dexpanthenol cream for 11–14 days after starting radiotherapy and then used the hydroactive colloid gel for the remaining course of radiation. The incidence of moist desquamation was significantly lower with the hydroactive colloid gel than with dexpanthenol cream. In cases when moist desquamation occurred, the onset was significantly later in the radiotherapy course with the hydroactive colloid gel than with the dexpanthenol cream [20c].

Imiquimod

A multicenter, parallel-group, pragmatic, non-inferiority, randomized controlled trial was conducted in 501 patients with primary nodular or superficial basal-cell carcinoma to determine the efficacy 5% imiquimod cream versus surgical excision in patients with low-risk basal-cell carcinoma. Patients ($n = 254$) received either 5% imiquimod cream once daily for 6 weeks (superficial) or 12 weeks (nodular), or surgical excision ($n = 247$) with a 4 mm margin. No differences were observed between the groups in patient-assessed cosmetic outcomes. The most common adverse events were mild in nature: itching (211 patients in the imiquimod group and 129 in the surgery group) and weeping (160 patients in the imiquimod group and 81 in the surgery group). Serious adverse events occurred in 99 patients in the imiquimod group and 97 in the surgery group, although of these effects were considered related to the treatments. Although not treatment-related, 12 patients in the imiquimod group and 4 in the surgical group withdrew due to the adverse events. The authors concluded that, although excisional surgery was the optimal treatment option for low-risk basal-cell carcinoma, use of imiquimod cream might be useful for treatment of small low-risk superficial or nodular basal-cell carcinoma [21C].

CUTANEOUS SIDE EFFECTS FROM NEUROLOGICAL MEDICATIONS

Levetiracetam

Levetiracetam is an antiepileptic medication that has less cutaneous reactions as compared to other antiepileptics. A case was reported of a 64-year-old man presented with an altered mental status and aphasia. Upon hospitalization, levetiracetam (500 mg) was given intravenously twice a day, for seizure prophylaxis. After 13 doses, a diffuse, erythematous, warm, blanching, morbilliform rash developed. Levetiracetam was discontinued, methylprednisolone was started and the rash disappeared after 4 days. Only four other cases of skin reactions following levetiracetam administration have been reported in the literature: two were classified as Stevens–Johnson Syndrome, one as toxic epidermal necrolysis and one as

erythema multiforme. A Naranjo score of 7 indicated that levetiracetam therapy was the most likely cause of the skin reaction [22A].

Lacosamide

Many anti-seizure medications are known to have cutaneous side effects including eruptions and hypersensitivity. Lacosamide is a new-generation anti-seizure medication with few reports of cutaneous side effects. A recent case of diffuse skin eruption was reported in a patient with a history of epilepsy shortly after starting lacosamide therapy. Lacosamide was discontinued; the rash was treated and resolved using antihistamines and steroids [23A].

Antidepressants

Many antidepressant medications are known to have adverse cutaneous side effects, ranging from mild reactions to serious adverse events that may be life-threatening. A literature review was undertaken to evaluate the appearance and development of drug-induced skin reactions associated with the use of antidepressants. The most common adverse drug reactions were considered mild and included drug-induced rashes, phototoxic reactions, eczemas and urticarias; the majority of these reactions occurred upon beginning treatment. Serious adverse effects include erythema multiforme, Stevens–Johnson syndrome, Lyell's syndrome or toxic epidermal necrolysis, acute generalized exanthematous pustulosis and drug-induced hypersensitivity syndrome. The literature reports associations between the following medication and skin conditions: erythema multiforme (mianserin, trazodone, bupropion and the SSRI sertraline group); Stevens–Johnson syndrome and toxic epidermal necrolysis (fluoxetine, sertraline, paroxetine, bupropion and mirtazapine); acute generalized exanthematous pustulosis (amoxapine-tetracyclic antidepressant and sertraline, a selective serotonin reuptake inhibitor); drug-induced hypersensitivity syndrome (tricyclic antidepressants, selective serotonin reuptake inhibitors, sulfonamides, ant-inflammatory drugs, antiviral drugs, ACE-inhibitors and β-blockers) [24R].

INDIVIDUAL MEDICATIONS

Acyclovir and Hydrocortisone

Herpes labialis is a common viral infection of the lips and oral mucosa. A 5% acyclovir and 1% hydrocortisone cream (Xerese™) for treatment of herpes labialis has recently been approved in Canada (October 2013) and has been approved in the US since 2009. A Phase 3, open-label clinical trial with 131 patients using a 5% acyclovir and 1% hydrocortisone cream for treatment of recurrent herpes labialis reported only five adverse events. These effects were considered mild to moderate and included secondary herpes labialis recurrences ($n=2$), infectious rhinitis ($n=1$), application site inflammation ($n=1$) and bronchial asthma ($n=1$). Additional clinical trials have reported adverse effects in less than 1% patients; the most common reactions were drying or flaking of the skin, burning or tingling at the application sight, erythema, and pigmentation changes [25C].

Arsenic Sulfide

Arsenic sulfide or realgar has a long history of use in traditional medicine in China and is considered to be safe for use with very few side effects. A case was recently reported of fatality resulting from short-term use of a topical realgar-containing herbal medicine. A 24-year-old man with atopic dermatitis used an oral herbal medicine and realgar-containing herbal ointments over the whole body for 7 days. At this time, the patient had symptoms of diminished appetite, dizziness, abdomen discomfort, itching rash, and skin scaling and later developed generalized edema, nausea, vomiting, decreased urine amount, diarrhea, edematous exanthems, malodorous perspiration, fever, and shortness of breath. The patient was hospitalized on day 19 when the dyspnea worsened. Toxic epidermal necrolysis with soft tissue infection and sepsis was diagnosed; death occurred later due to septic shock and multiple organ failure. A postmortem blood arsenic level was 1225 µg/L and analysis of unlabeled realgar-containing ointments showed very high arsenic levels (4229–45 427 ppm). This report indicates that arsenic-containing herbal remedies may be systemically absorbed if repeatedly applied to compromised skin [26A].

Alternative Medicine: Panax Notoginseng Saponins

Panax notoginseng saponins (PNS) are a patented product and traditional medicine in China for treatment of cardiovascular disorders. Four case reports are presented describing the skin-related effects of PNS treatment. First, a 50-year-old female presented with erythema, nonfollicular pustules and itching and pain over her whole body. She received injections of 400 mg PNS and 40 mg sulfotanshinone sodium (for dizziness) a day before the rash appeared. Second, an 89-year-old male presented with a week-long generalized erythema, tiny pustules, pruritus and fever. A week prior to the appearance of the rash, he received an injection of PNS (4 g). Third, a 62-year-old female presented with generalized erythema and papules with itching, having received injections of PNS (800 mg) and oxiracetam (6 g) for dizziness a day earlier. Fourth, a 67-year-old female presented with generalized erythema, pruritus and fever. One week earlier, she received an injection of 500 mg PNS. In all cases, the symptoms were resolved with intravenous methylprednisolone. All PNS injections were produced under Good Manufacturing Practices (GMP) by different manufacturers [27A].

Ciprofloxacin

A 24-year-old female was prescribed ciproflaxcin after presenting with symptoms indicating a urinary tract infection. After 2 days of use, fever, diffuse rash, swelling of her face, arms and flanks appeared along with watery diarrhea and muscular pain. Five days later, her white blood cell and eosinophil counts were significantly increased and a peripheral blood smear showed immature eosinophilic myelocytes and metamyelocytes. A skin lesion was biopsied and showed superficial perivascular lymphocytic infiltration with dermal edema. A CT scan of the abdomen and pelvis indicated small bilateral pleural effusions with possible edema in the deep subcutaneous soft abdominal tissues. Further work-ups were negative for parasitic infestations, HIV and viral hepatitis infections, allergic diseases, hematologic and non-hematologic malignancies, vasculitides and autoimmune processes. Upon hospitalization, ciprofloxacin was discontinued; the patient shows rapid improvement and was completely asymptomatic at a 3-week follow-up. This report indicates that ciprofloxacin may cause Drug Reaction with Eosinophilia and Systemic Symptoms (DRESS), a rare potentially fatal drug reaction [28A].

Corticosteroids

The prolonged use of topical corticosteroids for chronic inflammatory skin disease has been reported to cause suppression of the pituitary–hypothalamic–adrenal axis. In two case reports, two men with chronic inflammatory skin disease presented with fatigue and cushingoid appearance after a long period of frequent self-medication of potent topical corticosteroids. Impairment of the skin barrier due to inflammation resulted in greatly increased absorption of the medications, resulting in systemic exposure with adrenal insufficiency [29A].

Dipeptidyl Peptidase IV Inhibitors

A 70-year-old male with a history of type 2 diabetes, chronic iron deficiency anemia, and hypertension presented with diffuse bullae. The patient had been taking sitagliptin, 50 mg daily, for at least 1 year prior to the appearance of the rash and it was discontinued by his physician 4 days before presentation. The eruptions were diagnosed as bullous pemphigoid following skin biopsy and blood work. The symptoms were significantly improved and eventually resolved with intravenous methylprednisolone for 3 days followed by oral prednisone for 3 months. Sitagliptin is a member of the gliptin family that function as dipeptidyl peptidase IV (DPP-IV) inhibitors. The enzyme DPP-IV is ubiquitously expressed in almost every organ system, including the skin. Other cases found in the Adverse Event Reports System database of the FDA have also demonstrated the potential link between dipeptidyl peptidase IV (DPP-IV) inhibitors (gliptins) and the development of bullous pemphigoid [30A].

Doxycycline

A case report described a patient using doxycycline for 2 years for the treatment of acne vulgaris. The symptoms included skin eruptions over the extremities, myalgias, fatigue, swelling of the face, hands, and feet, headache, and mood changes. Doxycycline was discontinued but similar symptoms returned rapidly upon rechallenge 1 year later [31A].

Dupilumab

Dupilumab is a fully human monoclonal antibody inhibitor of interleukin-4 (IL-4) and interleukin-13 (IL-13) approved for use in patients with asthma and elevated eosinophil levels. As both IL-4 and IL-13 are critical in the initiation of type 2 helper T-cell (Th2)-mediated inflammation, it was proposed that dupilumab may be beneficial in the treatment of atopic dermatitis. Accordingly, dupilumab was evaluated in four clinical trials designed to assess the safety of subcutaneous administration of dupilumab for treatment of atopic dermatitis as described below.

- Phase 1 study: dupilumab (75, 150 or 300 mg, $n=8$ each) or placebo ($n=6$), once per week for 4 weeks;
- Phase 1 study: dupilumab (150 mg, $n=14$, or 300 mg, $n=13$) or placebo ($n=10$), once per week for 4 weeks;
- Monotherapy trial: dupilumab (300 mg, $n=21$) or placebo ($n=10$), four doses per week for 12 weeks;
- Combination therapy: dupilumab (300 mg, $n=21$) or placebo ($n=10$), four doses per week for 12 weeks, all patients also received a standardized regimen of topical glucocorticoids.

Patients in all trials had moderate-to-severe atopic dermatitis and the drug or placebo was administered subcutaneously.

Similar adverse events were reported in all trials; they were generally mild to moderate in nature and were not dose-dependent. Skin infections occurred more frequently with the placebo while nasopharyngitis and headache were the most frequently reported with dupilumab treatment. The frequency of occurrence was similar between dupilumab and placebo. Thirteen serious adverse events were reported across the studies; however, almost all the events occurred in the placebo groups with only a facial fracture reported with dupilumab treatment [32C].

Hydralazine

A case report described a 75-year-old female presented with weakness, elevated blood pressure, anemia and nausea, and was diagnosed with hypertensive crisis. Hydralazine (50 mg, three times daily) was given followed by the appearance of an erythematous maculopapular rash that subsequently became a bullous rash with generalized edema of the extremities. After 16 days, the rash was diagnosed as drug-induced toxic epidermal necrolysis and hydralazine was discontinued All skin lesions were improved within 4 days and completely resolved in 20 days. Hydralazine (25 mg, three times daily) as prescribed 2 months later for resistant hypertension and identical skin lesions reappeared but were resolved after discontinuation of the medication [33A].

Infliximab

Although granulomas of the lungs, spleen, liver and skin may occur in 8–22% of common variable immunodeficiency (CVID) patients, there are currently limited treatment options. Five CVID patients with clinical symptoms secondary to granulomas were treated with infliximab, 5 mg/kg initially and at weeks 2 and 6 and every 4 weeks afterwards. All five patients showed significant improvement in their symptoms with four patients remaining on infliximab for 5–18 months (mean=9.4 months) without any reactions. One patient completed 6 months of treatment but discontinued therapy due to joint stiffness and rash; the patient stated her symptoms were due to the infliximab treatment [34A].

Isoniazid

Although anti-tuberculosis drugs are known to have a high incidence of adverse skin effects, isoniazid is considered to have the least potential for such reactions. A recent report described a case of isoniazid-induced cutaneous leucocytoclastic (hypersensitivity) vasculitis. A 64-year-old male diagnosed with Pott's spine with multiple vertebral body involvement (D8-12 vertebrae) was treated with the standard Anti Tuberculosis Treatment (ATT) consisting of isoniazid (300 mg), rifampicin (600 mg), pyrazinamide (1500 mg) and ethambutol (800 mg) once daily. On the fourth day of treatment, an erythematosus rash developed that was not associated with itching or pain, non-blanchable macules and papules, petechiae and a hyperpigmented, scaly rash. The diagnosis was cutaneous leukocytoclastic vasculitis based on skin biopsy. The anti-tuberculosis drugs were discontinued and an oral antihistamine and topical corticosteroids were administered with resolution of the rash. A rechallenge with each of the anti-tuberculosis drugs was conducted 9 days later; no skin reactions were found with rifampicin, pyrazinamide or ethambutol. Isoniazid exposure, however, resulted in new purpuric lesions that were resolved with antihistamine and corticosteroid use [35A].

Leflunomide

A case of leflunomide-associated eruptive keratoacanthomas was recently reported. A 78-year-old woman with rheumatoid arthritis and no history of skin tumors or immunosuppressive medication was prescribed leflunomide. After 1 month of initiating treatment and for the following 2 years, multiple crateriform nodules and papules developed that were diagnosed as keratoacanthomas and squamous cell carcinomas. The patient discontinued leflunomide treatment, suspecting that the drug may have caused development of the tumors. The patient was followed for additional 17 months and no new skin lesions appeared. This report is similar to those in the literature describing cases of multiple keratoacanthomas associated with immunosuppressive therapy, including sorafenib and imiquimod [36A].

Levamisole

Levamisole has been used for many years as an immune modulator and antihelmintic with generally mild and reversible side effects. A recent case report, however, describes a serious adverse effect attributed to levamisole administration. A 34-year-old female was prescribed levamisole, 100 mg daily for 5 days, recalcitrant warts. The patient later developed bilateral lower limb weakness with multiple painful and non-blanchable purpura; myopathy and leukocytoclastic vasculitis were diagnosed upon further testing. These symptoms resolved when levamisole was discontinued and a systemic steroid was administered [37A].

In a separate study, three cases in which use of cocaine contaminated with levamisole resulted in skin lesions and neutropenia. In 2009, it was found that approximately 69% of the cocaine seized at the US border was contaminated with levamisole. The cases include 45-, 40- and 43-year-old females who each presented on several successive occasions with necrotic skin lesions and ulcerations and neutropenia; in each case, toxicology screening was positive for cocaine and levamisole. The symptoms were resolved with methylprednisolone,

prednisone and methotrexate treatment. Upon follow-up, the first two patients have not used cocaine since their last bout of symptoms was resolved and have been asymptomic since that time [38A].

Lidocaine and Prilocaine (EMLA)

EMLA, a combination lidocaine and prilocaine mixture, is a widely used topical anesthetic cream. The majority of adverse side effects are generally mild local skin reactions such as edema, pallor and erythema. However, serious adverse reactions can occur and include methemoglobinemia, central nervous system toxicity, and cardiotoxicity. A literature review of 12 clinical trials was conducted to determine the risk of systemic toxicity from EMLA use in adults and children. Nine pediatric and three adult cases of systemic toxicity associated with EMLA have been reported. The authors suggest that development of the observed toxicity may affected by an excessive application amount of EMLA, large application area, prolonged application time, vascular malformations, eczema, abraded skin, patient age less than 3 months, and simultaneous use of a methemoglobin-inducing agent [39M].

Voriconazole

Voriconazole is an antifungal medication commonly used prophylactically and as treatment for fungal infection in lung and bone transplant patients. Although effective, significant dermal side effects have been reported with prolonged use of voriconazole. These effects include photosensitivity causing facial erythema and cheilitis, pseudoporphyria, discoid lupus erythematosus, and accelerated photoaging. Voriconazole has also been associated with development of skin cancer with several cases in lung transplant patients being associated with use of the medication. These findings were confirmed in a multicenter case study that reported 51 cases of cutaneous squamous cell carcinoma in 8 immunocompromised patients as well as four epidemiological studies that associated long-term use of voriconazole with the development of squamous cell carcinoma. Although not as well studied as the relationship with squamous cell carcinoma, cases of voriconazole-associated melanoma have also been reported. Prolonged use of voriconazole is considered independent risk factor for the development of skin cancer in lung transplant patients [40M].

References

[1] Masini F, Ricci F, Fossati B, et al. Combination therapy with retinaldehyde (0.1%) glycolic acid (6%) and efectiose (0.1%) in mild to moderate acne vulgaris during the period of sun exposure—efficacy and skin tolerability. Eur Rev Med Pharmacol Sci. 2014;18(16):2283–6 [c].

[2] Faghihi G, Rakhshanpour M, Abtahi-Naeini B, et al. The efficacy of 5% dapsone gel plus oral isotretinoin versus oral isotretinoin alone in acne vulgaris: a randomized double-blind study. Adv Biomed Res. 2014;3:177 [C].

[3] El-Gohary M, van Zuuren EJ, Fedorowicz Z, et al. Topical antifungal treatments for tinea cruris and tinea corporis. Cochrane Database Syst Rev. 2014;4:8 [R].

[4] Gupta AK, Foley KA. 5% Minoxidil: treatment for female pattern hair loss. Skin Therapy Lett. 2014;19(6):5–7 [c].

[5] Ebrahimi B, Naeini FF. Topical tranexamic acid as a promising treatment for melasma. J Res Med Sci. 2014;19(8):753–7 [C].

[6] Gropper S, Albareda N, Chelius K, et al. Ozenoxacin 1% cream in the treatment of impetigo: a multicenter, randomized, placebo- and retapamulin-controlled clinical trial. Future Microbiol. 2014;9(9):1013–23 [C].

[7] Gropper S, Cepero AL, Santos B, et al. Systemic bioavailability and safety of twice-daily topical ozenoxacin 1% cream in adults and children with impetigo. Future Microbiol. 2014;9(8 Suppl):S33–S40 [C].

[8] Li W, Xin H, Ge L, et al. Induction of vitiligo after imiquimod treatment of condylomata acuminata. BMC Infect Dis. 2014;4:329 [A].

[9] Jariwala P, Kumar V, Kothari K, et al. Acute methotrexate toxicity: a fatal condition in two cases of psoriasis. Case Rep Dermatol Med. 2014;2014:946716 [A].

[10] Ito T, Furukawa F, Iwatsuki K, et al. Efficacious treatment of psoriasis with low-dose and intermittent cyclosporin microemulsion therapy. J Dermatol. 2014;41(5):377–81 [C].

[11] Ports WC, Khan S, Lan S, et al. A randomized phase 2a efficacy and safety trial of the topical Janus kinase inhibitor tofacitinib in the treatment of chronic plaque psoriasis. Br J Dermatol. 2013;69(1):137–45 [C].

[12] Kragballe K, van de Kerkhof P. Pooled safety analysis of calcipotriol plus betamethasone dipropionate gel for the treatment of psoriasis on the body and scalp. J Eur Acad Dermatol Venereol. 2014;28(Suppl 2):10–21 [M].

[13] Kim JT, Jeong HW, Choi KH, et al. Delayed hypersensitivity reaction resulting in maculopapular-type eruption due to entecavir in the treatment of chronic hepatitis B. World J Gastroenterol. 2014;20(42):15931–6 [A].

[14] Biesbroeck LK, Scott JD, Taraska C, et al. Direct-acting antiviral-associated dermatitis during chronic hepatitis C virus treatment. Am J Clin Dermatol. 2013;14(6):497–502 [A].

[15] Nishijima T, Gatanaga H, Teruya K, et al. Skin rash induced by ritonavir-boosted darunavir is common, but generally tolerable in an observational setting. J Infect Chemother. 2014;20(4):285–7 [c].

[16] Talpur R, Venkatarajan S, Duvic M. Mechlorethamine gel for the topical treatment of stage IA and IB mycosis fungoides-type cutaneous T-cell lymphoma. Expert Rev Clin Pharmacol. 2014;7(5):591–7 [C].

[17] Sahu J, Sepassi M, Nagao M, et al. Recent clinical evidence for topical mechlorethamine in mycosis fungoides. Clin Invest. 2014;4(8):745–61 [C].

[18] Larkin J, Del Vecchio M, Ascierto PA, et al. Vemurafenib in patients with BRAF(V600) mutated metastatic melanoma: an open-label, multicentre, safety study. Lancet Oncol. 2014;15(4):436–44 [C].

[19] Proctor AE, Thompson LA, O'Bryant CL. Vismodegib: an inhibitor of the Hedgehog signaling pathway in the treatment of basal cell carcinoma. Ann Pharmacother. 2014;48(1):99–106 [C].

[20] Censabella S, Claes S, Orlandini M, et al. Retrospective study of radiotherapy-induced skin reactions in breast cancer patients: reduced incidence of moist desquamation with a hydroactive colloid gel versus dexpanthenol. Eur J Oncol Nurs. 2014;18(5):499–504 [c].

[21] Bath-Hextall F, Ozolins M, Armstrong SJ, et al. Surgical excision versus imiquimod 5% cream for nodular and superficial basal-cell carcinoma (SINS): a multicentre, non-inferiority, randomised controlled trial. Lancet Oncol. 2014;15(1):96–105 [C].

[22] Jones RT, Evans W, Mersfelder TL, et al. Rare red rashes: a case report of levetiracetam-induced cutaneous reaction and review of the literature. Am J Ther. 2014. Case report: PDF only [A]. http://journals.lww.com/americantherapeutics/Abstract/publishahead/Rare_Red_Rashes___A_Case_Report_of.99214.aspx.

[23] Koubeissi MZ, Vismer M, Ehrlich A. Lacosamide-induced rash. Epileptic Disord. 2014;16(3):380–3 [A].

[24] Herstowska M, Komorowska O, Cubała WJ, et al. Severe skin complications in patients treated with antidepressants: a literature review. Postepy Dermatol Alergol. 2014;31(2):92–7 [R].

[25] Nguyen HP, Stiegel KR, Downing C, et al. Recent approval of Xerese in Canada: 5% acyclovir and 1% hydrocortisone topical cream in the treatment of herpes labialis. Skin Therapy Lett. 2014;19(3):5–8 [C].

[26] Wu ML, Deng JF. Toxic epidermal necrolysis after extensive dermal use of realgar-containing (arsenic sulfide) herbal ointment. Clin Toxicol (Phila). 2013;51(8):801–3 [A].

[27] Yin Z, Ma L, Xu J, et al. Pustular drug eruption due to Panax notoginseng saponins. Drug Des Devel Ther. 2014;16(8):957–61 [A].

[28] Alkhateeb H, Said S, Cooper CJ, et al. DRESS syndrome following ciprofloxacin exposure: an unusual association. Am J Case Rep. 2013;14:526–8 [A].

[29] Böckle BC, Jara D, Nindl W, et al. Adrenal insufficiency as a result of long-term misuse of topical corticosteroids. Dermatology. 2014;228(4):289–93 [A].

[30] Attaway A, Mersfelder TL, Vaishnav S, et al. Bullous pemphigoid associated with dipeptidyl peptidase IV inhibitors. A case report and review of literature. J Dermatol Case Rep. 2014;8(1):24–8 [A].

[31] Weinstein M, Laxer R, Debosz J, et al. Doxycycline-induced cutaneous inflammation with systemic symptoms in a patient with acne vulgaris. J Cutan Med Surg. 2013;17(4):283–6 [A].

[32] Beck LA, Thaçi D, Hamilton JD, et al. Dupilumab treatment in adults with moderate-to-severe atopic dermatitis. N Engl J Med. 2014;371(2):130–9 [C].

[33] Mahfouz A, Mahmoud AN, et al. A case report of hydralazine-induced skin reaction: probable toxic epidermal necrolysis (TEN). Am J Case Rep. 2014;15:135–8 [A].

[34] Franxman TJ, Howe LE, Baker Jr. JR. Infliximab for treatment of granulomatous disease in patients with common variable immunodeficiency. J Clin Immunol. 2014;34(7):820–7 [A].

[35] Bondalapati S, DR V, Rampure D, et al. Isoniazid induced cutaneous leukocytoclastic vasculitis in extra pulmonary tuberculosis (Pott's spine): a case report. J Clin Diagn Res. 2014;8(8):MD03–5 [A].

[36] Frances L, Guijarro J, Marin I, et al. Multiple eruptive keratoacanthomas associated with leflunomide. Dermatol Online J. 2013;19(7):18968 [A].

[37] Tsai MH, Yang JH, Kung SL, et al. Levamisole-induced myopathy and leukocytoclastic vasculitis: a case report and literature review. Dermatol Ther. 2013;26(6):476–80 [A].

[38] Belfonte CD, Shanmugam VK, Kieffer N, et al. Levamisole-induced occlusive necrotising vasculitis in cocaine abusers: an unusual cause of skin necrosis and neutropenia. Int Wound J. 2013;10(5):590–6 [A].

[39] Tran AN, Koo JY. Risk of systemic toxicity with topical lidocaine/prilocaine: a review. J Drugs Dermatol. 2014;13(9):1118–22 [M].

[40] Williams K, Mansh M, Chin-Hong P, et al. Voriconazole-associated cutaneous malignancy: a literature review on photocarcinogenesis in organ transplant recipients. Clin Infect Dis. 2014;58(7):997–1002 [M].

15

Antihistamines (H1 Receptor Antagonists)

Alan Polnariev[*],[†],[1]

[*]VA Healthcare System, East Orange, NJ, USA
[†]College of Pharmacy, University of Florida, Gainesville, FL, USA
[1]Corresponding author: apolnariev@gmail.com

GENERAL

Regarding their effects on the Central Nervous System (CNS), antihistamines can be classified into one of three categories. Those that markedly impair cognitive and psychomotor function by crossing the blood–brain barrier; those that despite crossing into the brain, do not cause significant impairment at low therapeutic doses; and those that do not cross into the brain and therefore, do not possess intrinsic potential for diminishing CNS function. The first-generation antihistamines have well-documented sedative, anticholinergic and dysrhythmogenic effects; there are also concerns regarding carry-over effects in terms of next-day somnolence and psychomotor responses following their use. These effects on movement dysfunction have been linked to altered neurotransmission in cholinergic and histaminergic pathways [1R]. One randomized, double-blind, crossover study was conducted to evaluate the effects of zolpidem (10 mg), diphenhydramine (50 mg), ketotifen (1 mg) or placebo on next-day sleepiness and psychomotor performance in 22 healthy male participants. The drugs were administered in four separate sessions before sleep with a greater than 1-week washout period. Participants were evaluated for subjective sleepiness, objective sleepiness and psychomotor performance, the morning and afternoon after administration. Ketotifen had the strongest carry-over effect followed by diphenhydramine, with no effect seen for zolpidem or placebo [2c]. The authors recommended that consideration be given to the risks associated with first-generation antihistamine use for the treatment of insomnia secondary to allergies.

In a double-blind, placebo-controlled, five-way cross-over study, 11 healthy subjects were examined at intervals of 1, 2 and 3 hours post-ingestion of first- and second-generation antihistamines with known anticholinergic effects to assess patients' levels of drowsiness, reaction time, and physiological tremor. It was found that promethazine (25 mg), desloratadine (5 mg) and fexofenadine (180 mg) caused drowsiness to varying degrees. Promethazine showed the greatest increase in simple and choice reaction time and reduced tremor. Desloratadine increased choice reaction time to a lesser extent, but was found to significantly increase tremor 1 hour after ingestion. Loratadine (10 mg) slowed simple and choice reaction time. Fexofenadine did not affect reaction time or tremor. The authors concluded that second-generation antihistamines offer patients a safer alternative to first-generation antihistamines because they generally lack the undesirable pharmacological effects of prolonged sedation and psychomotor effects [3c]. The efficacy and side effect profiles of two second-generation antihistamines, i.e., olopatadine (5 mg twice a day) and levocetirizine (5 mg once daily) were compared to a placebo in a double-blind, randomized, cross-over, placebo-controlled study of 12 healthy volunteers with a histamine-induced wheal and flare reaction. The histamine-induced wheal and flare model is a widely used, reproducible and standardized methodology. It gives an objective measure of the effectiveness of antihistamines in human subjects, and demonstrates any differences in onset and duration of action. Both antihistamines considerably suppressed the subjective itching and had no significant differences in reported drowsiness and objective cognitive function between drug- and placebo-treated subjects. [4c].

There are few reports that directly compare the antihistaminic efficacy and impairment of psychomotor functions of first-generation and second-generation drugs. A double-blind, placebo-controlled, crossover study in 24 healthy subjects compared promethazine, a first-generation antihistamine, with the second-generation antihistamines fexofenadine and olopatadine. The study

© 2015 Elsevier B.V. All rights reserved.

was done to measure their potency as peripheral inhibitors of histamine-induced wheal and flare together with examination of their sedative effects on the CNS using a battery of psychomotor tests. Compared with fexofenadine and promethazine, olopatadine showed the most rapid inhibitory effect on the histamine-induced wheal and flare test. In a battery of psychomotor assessments, promethazine significantly impaired psychomotor function while fexofenadine and olopatadine had no significant effect in any of the tests used. Promethazine, fexofenadine and olopatadine did not affect behavioral activity, as measured by wrist actigraphy. These results suggest that at therapeutic doses, olopatadine has greater inhibitory effect on the histamine-induced wheal and flare test compared with promethazine and that neither olopatadine nor fexofenadine cause significant cognitive or psychomotor impairment in healthy subjects [5c].

Two recent studies compared the sedative effects of first- and second-generation antihistamines, i.e., hydroxyzine and bilastine, respectively, under different conditions. The first study evaluated the psychomotor and subjective sedative effects of bilastine, hydroxyzine, and cetirizine, all in combination with alcohol in 24 volunteers. This randomized, double-blind, double-dummy, crossover, positive-controlled and placebo-controlled clinical trial assessed psychomotor performance tests (e.g., fine motor, finger tapping and simple reaction time) and subjective self-reports (drunkenness, drowsiness, and mental slowness) at 1-week intervals. Subjects received one of six regimens: (i) placebo, (ii) alcohol 0.8 g/kg alone (ALC), (iii) ALC in combination with: bilastine 20 mg (B20+A), (iv) bilastine 80 mg (B80+A), (v) cetirizine 10 mg (CET+A), and (vi) hydroxyzine 25 mg (HYD+A). The results showed that the most pronounced level of impairment was observed in the group receiving hydroxyzine 25 mg plus alcohol. In contrast, objective measures showed less impairment in groups that received bilastine 20 mg plus alcohol or alcohol alone, both to a similar extent. The authors concluded that concomitant administration of bilastine (at therapeutic dose) and alcohol does not induce central nervous system depressant effects greater than alcohol alone [6c]. The second study used positron emission tomography (PET) to determine histamine H1-receptor occupancy (H1RO), incidence of subjective sedation and objective psychomotor performance after a single oral dose of bilastine 20 mg, hydroxyzine 25 mg, or placebo. H1RO served as a marker of psychometric function since a level of H1RO greater than 50% has been clearly linked with a high rate of sleepiness and cognitive decline [7c]. While some subjects reported accounts of sleepiness and/or sedation with hydroxyzine, there were no such reported events with bilastine. It was therefore concluded that a single dose of bilastine 20 mg was not associated with subjective sedation or objective impairment of psychomotor performance and thus lacks clinically significant sedative side effects [7c].

SPECIAL REVIEW ON PHARMACOGENETICS

Pharmacogenetics is being used to develop personalized therapies tailored to a patient's distinct genetic composition of allele variations in the genes implicated with drug metabolizing processes, medication effectiveness, and clinical outcomes for conditions related to histamine pathways [8R,9R]. Several polymorphisms found in the genetic coding of enzymes such as CYP2D6 and CYP3A5 have been associated with the therapeutic efficacy and/or side effects of antihistamines. An individual's responsiveness to a medication can be affected by numerous genetic variations and is implicated in several pharmacokinetic stages of drug absorption, distribution, and metabolism [10M,11R]. Every pathway involved in drug metabolism has the potential to be affected by an individual's genetic makeup such as genes reflected in gender as well as different ethnic or racial groups. For example, the enzyme cytochrome P450 2D6 is involved in the metabolism of a number of antihistamines, including chlorpheniramine, promethazine and azelastine [12M]. As a therapeutic class, antihistamines undergo distinctive metabolic pathways and can be classified by their chemical structure into six categories: ethanolamines, alkylamines, ethylenediamines, piperazines, phenothiazines and piperidines. The former four categories undergo mainly cytochrome P450-mediated oxidative n-desalkylation and deamination whereas the aromatic rings of the latter two undergo P450-mediated oxidative hydroxylation and/or epoxide formation [13R,14R,15R]. Genetic differences are reflected in an individual's responsiveness to medications by a wide range of potential mechanisms.

Genetic polymorphisms in histamine-related genes, such as FCERI and HNMT, are theorized to influence mast cell activation and histamine metabolism. Mast cells are the major effector cell type that release histamine, cytokines and chemical mediators involved in the pathology of histamine-related conditions such as atopic dermatitis, chronic urticaria, and asthma [16c]. In a study conducted to better understand the association between HNMT polymorphisms and atopic dermatitis, researchers genotyped 763 Korean children for allelic determinants at four polymorphic sites in the HNMT gene. The researchers found that certain specific polymorphisms of the HNMT gene appear to incline susceptible individuals to develop non-atopic eczema and eczema (namely, HNMT 314C>T and 939A>G polymorphisms, respectively). This association between the 939A>G genotype and eczema is speculated to be related to raised serum IgE levels—a central element to the phenomenon of allergy and a diagnostic feature of atopic dermatitis [17c]. In another study examining histamine-related genes, researchers enrolled 93 children and adults to evaluate known single nucleotide polymorphisms (SNPs) in genes along the histamine biotransformation of the H1 receptor and the histamine response pathway. The researchers sought to determine how differences in the allele, genotype and haplotype frequency of subjects with and without asthma relate to HRH1 mRNA expression relative to genotype. While no differences in genetic expression and asthma were detected between subjects in the genotype/allele frequency for the SNPs, there were observed genetic differences relative to subjects' race and gender. Histamine pathway haplotype was associated with a diagnosis of asthma but genotype and allele were not [18c].

Pharmacogenetics is rapidly growing in its use to help researchers better understand the effects of genetic factors on clinical outcomes. Recent studies have shown how genetic polymorphisms can affect the gene expression of drug metabolizing enzymes, minimum effective drug dose and disease pathology. The following two studies examine how genetic polymorphisms can serve as pharmacodynamic predictors of antihistamine efficacy in patients with histamine-related conditions. In the first study, 384 patients with chronic urticaria (CU) were compared to 231 other patients as normal controls to assess the effect of the CRTH2 gene polymorphism. No significant differences were noted between the two groups in respect to the genotype and allele frequencies of the CRTH2 polymorphisms. Furthermore, no significant associations were observed within the clinical parameters examined by the researchers such as atopy status, serum total IgE, prevalence of autoantibodies and duration of CU. However, the patients with CU required higher doses of antihistamines to control their clinical symptoms than those in the control group. The authors concluded that although gene expression may not have had a direct observable effect on CU, it may have contributed to the required dose of the antihistamines needed to the treat the patients with the condition [19c]. In another study examining the polymorphisms of the C5AR1 −1330T/G gene and antihistamine therapy, 191 patients with chronic spontaneous urticaria (CSU) and 102 healthy controls were treated with various non-sedating antihistamines (i.e., desloratadine, mizolastine, and fexofenadine) as monotherapy for 4 weeks. In their research, the authors found for the first time that a genetic polymorphism of C5AR1 −1330GT could impact the therapeutic efficacy of desloratadine for a particular subset of patients with CSU. Specifically, it was observed that patients with −1330GT heterozygotes had the least clinical effect from desloratadine. To their surprise, the authors did not find a substantial clinical difference among −1330T/G genotypes when treated with mizolastine. The researchers concluded that the C5AR1 −1330T/G gene may serve as a useful pharmacodynamic predictor of the efficacy of non-sedating antihistamines in patients with chronic spontaneous urticaria [20C].

The significant inter-individual variations of genetic expression often cause differences in the pharmacokinetics, bioavailability and thus the therapeutic effect of antihistamines. In one study, researchers gave 12 healthy young males and 12 non-pregnant females a dose of combination doxylamine–pyridoxine which is indicated for treatment of nausea and vomiting in pregnancy. After a 21-day washout period, dose administration and blood samplings were repeated to measure the concentrations of doxylamine, pyridoxine and its metabolites. The differences between the two sexes were assessed and researchers found a higher maximum concentration for doxylamine in females and a higher maximum concentration for pyridoxal-5′-phosphate in males. The authors concluded that bioequivalence studies for drugs targeted for women should not be conducted in males because they poorly predict empirical treatment outcomes [21c]. Another study aimed to evaluate the effect on plasma concentrations of genetic polymorphisms, i.e., CYP3A5 and MDR1 after a single, oral dose of 10 mg rupatadine (RUP) was done using 36 healthy male Chinese volunteers as subjects. Researchers collected, assessed and compared rupatadine plasma concentrations and several pharmacokinetic parameters (e.g., Mean C_{max}, AUC $_{(0-t)}$ and AUC $_{(0-\infty)}$) among the various polymorphic alleles of CYP3A5 and MDR1. The results indicate statistically significant correlations between the varying polymorphisms of the alleles and their respective values observed. The authors speculate that CYP3A5 and MDR1 polymorphisms may be the main causative factor in explaining the pharmacokinetic differences and plasma concentrations of RUP. This study can therefore provide a rationale for the safe and effective use of the medication [22c].

OTHER ANTIHISTAMINES

Bilastine [SED-35; SEDA-36, 234]

Bilastine is a novel H1 receptor antagonist indicated for the treatment of seasonal or perennial allergic rhinitis and symptomatic chronic urticaria with little or no interactions with H2, H3 receptors, α1-adrenoceptors, β2-adrenoceptors, 5HT, bradykinin, leukotriene D4 or muscarinic M3 receptors. Its metabolism is unaffected by age, gender or renal function but may be affected by the co-administration of p-glycoprotein inhibitors [23r]. A recent review concluded that it is at least as effective as cetirizine or desloratadine with a documented lack of significant adverse CNS effects, drug–drug interactions or cardiac repolarization effects in the recommended doses [24r]. In terms of the latter, a comprehensive cross-over study in 30 healthy volunteers examined the effects of placebo, moxifloxacin 400 mg, bilastine at therapeutic and supratherapeutic doses (20 and 100 mg) and bilastine 20 mg co-administered with ketoconazole 400 mg on clinically relevant repolarization effects. Bilastine was found to have no significant effects on the morphology combination score or the heart rate QT interval providing further evidence for a very good safety profile for this drug with regard to cardiac repolarization. In another study involving 12 healthy volunteers, a randomized, single-dose, open-label, controlled two-arm crossover study design was used to examine the total oral bioavailability of bilastine. A single 20-mg oral tablet and a 10-mg intravenous formulation of bilastine were administered with a minimum 14-day washout period between the two single doses. The maximum bilastine concentration was achieved at 1.31 hours with a moderate bioavailability after oral administration in healthy subjects. No adverse events related to study medication were reported [25c].

Cetirizine [SEDA-34, 272; SEDA-35; SEDA-36, 235]

A 52-year-old woman with a 10-year history of chronic spontaneous urticaria (usually managed with mizolastine) developed generalized pruritus, erythema, facial and peripheral angioedema, vomiting, dyspnea, diaphoresis and severe abdominal cramping with pain. Because of the abdominal symptoms, paramedics administered intravenous morphine followed by intravenous chlorphenamine and oral prednisolone 3 hours later. Her acute tryptase level, a commonly used indicator to confirm a diagnosis of anaphylaxis, was 16.9 ng/ml (upper limit 11.4 ng/ml). Two months later, she developed severe abdominal pain, tachycardia, generalized urticaria, facial angioedema, erythema, and wheezing. Paramedics administered intravenous chlorphenamine and hydrocortisone. This time, the acute tryptase level was 15.8 ng/ml. The patient strongly believed cetirizine was the root cause of her reactions because she had taken cetirizine, instead of mizolastine, 30 minutes before both episodes. Consequently, a drug provocation test (DPT) was conducted with undiluted cetirizine oral solution and the results were initially negative. However, 20 minutes later, she developed acute rhinitis; generalized pruritus; erythema; angioedema of the face, hands, and feet, tachycardia (129 beats/min), and bronchospasm with a decrease in peak expiratory flow rate from 450 to 290 l/min. The patient's baseline tryptase level of 6.2 ng/ml spiked to 11.7 ng/ml. Oral chlorphenamine, prednisolone, and fluticasone propionate with salbutamol were administered. She recovered within an hour. DPT confirmed the patient's suspicion and she was advised to avoid cetirizine, its R-enantiomer levocetirizine and hydroxyzine, whose active metabolite is cetirizine. As of 6 months later, the patient's chronic condition was maintained with mizolastine and no further episodes of anaphylaxis were reported [26A].

A 63-year-old man with a 22-year history of urticaria pigmentosa for which he had been taking cetirizine 10 mg daily for 5 years, presented with a 9-month history of lethargy, thirst and nocturia [27a]. Investigations revealed raised urea and creatinine together with a heavy lymphocytic and plasma cell infiltrate seen within the interstitium of a renal biopsy. A diagnosis of acute interstitial nephritis (AIN) was made with an allergic etiology. Cetirizine was immediately discontinued and treatment commenced with oral prednisolone 60 mg. Although the patient quickly improved, only about 30% of normal renal function remained most likely as a result of the prolonged drug exposure and severity of nephritis. Second-generation antihistamines are widely used in the treatment of chronic urticaria, and serious complications arising from their use are very rare [28r]. AIN is a common form of acute kidney injury that can be allergic, infectious, autoimmune, systemic or idiopathic but 60–70% of cases are drug induced [29r]. The authors focused on cetirizine as the cause of AIN in this case as the biopsy was typical of a hypersensitivity reaction and the patient was receiving no other medication. They acknowledged this to be an extremely rare reaction and recommend renal function monitoring in those patients receiving long-term treatment with cetirizine or related products. However, given the wide availability and high degree of use of cetirizine, this would be a very difficult recommendation to realistically pursue.

An 18-year-old woman with no psychiatric history presented as an emergency with delusional thinking and passive suicidal ideations [30a]. These began 3 months prior to admission on commencing 10 mg cetirizine daily for 1 week to treat allergic rhinitis. A physical examination and all laboratory tests were normal and there was no evidence of substance abuse or a family history of mental disorders. The cetirizine was stopped and within 4 days the patient no longer experienced intrusive or paranoid thoughts and was discharged as an outpatient after 8 days. The authors speculate that cetirizine was the cause of delusional thinking and depression in this patient but this could not be confirmed by a subsequent challenge with cetirizine.

Chlorphenamine [SEDA-33, 345; SEDA-34, 272; SEDA-36, 235]

A report on two cases of elderly persons who suffered accidental fatalities in a home setting subsequently identified chlorphenamine overdose as a potential contributory factor following autopsy and toxicological analysis [31a]. In both cases, common cold medicines containing chlorphenamine were subsequently found at the scene of death. The authors suggested the fatalities might have been caused by the well-documented sedative effects of first-generation antihistamines such as chlorphenamine. This report was the subject of a letter to the editor to the same journal in which it was pointed out that serotonin syndrome following high doses of chlorphenamine may have been a possible contributory factor to the reported accidental fatalities [32a].

Diphenhydramine [SEDA-34, 272; SEDA-35; SEDA-36, 235]

Miss C, a 49-year-old retired nurse with a history of recurrent episodes of major depressive disorder and a history of alcohol dependence, is the subject of the first reported case of intramuscular diphenhydramine (IM DPH) usage. This led to drug dependence and complications of induced concurrent myonecrosis and prolonged QT interval. Six months prior to the incident, the patient received treatment for severe urticaria with a single, 30 mg dose of intramuscular diphenhydramine. After DPH use, she described feeling "good, relaxed, calm and slept better." Miss C began purchasing DPH and syringes at several pharmacies. She initially injected 30 mg DPH at night for her insomnia but increased the quantity and use of the drug every few days. She administered her first injection soon after waking up and the injection frequency increased to every 1–2 hours. Miss C's cravings for IM DPH increased to upwards of 450 mg per day and experienced withdrawal symptoms including anxiety, irritability and rebounding insomnia within hours of missing a dose. All of these aforementioned symptoms developed over the course of 4 months. Miss C had attempted to discontinue use of DPH injections but to no avail; she was admitted for detoxification, physical evaluation and depressive mood management when she could no longer maintain basic self-care. Physical examinations revealed multifocal myonecrosis of both thighs and buttocks and initial laboratory findings showed a prolonged QT interval of 420 ms with corrected QT interval of 503 ms. Miss C experienced signs/symptoms of withdrawal (similar to those stated above) upon abstinence of DPH and they resolved after initiating lorazepam. The patient's condition gradually improved and she was discharged 6 weeks later. The authors note that in their literature review, they found six case reports of DPH abuse involving daily oral DPH dosages ranging from 480 to 3000 mg and the subjects taking months to years to seek treatment. Miss C had been taking a lower dosage and for a shorter period of time compared to the other cases. The authors speculate that this patient's nursing experience might have inclined her to parenteral use of DPH and her history of major depressive disorder and/or alcohol dependence might have contributed to the development of drug dependence [33A].

A 37-year-old female was admitted to the emergency room in an unconscious state following an apparent suicide attempt with an overdose of acetaminophen and diphenhydramine. On arrival, the patient was profoundly hypothermic with a core rectal temperature of 17 °C with a Glasgow Coma Score of 10 which rose to 15 after rewarming/resuscitation and normalizing her temperature. The reported ingestion of 50 g of acetaminophen and 2.5 g of diphenhydramine was potentially hepatotoxic leading to administration of N-acetylcysteine therapy. The authors speculated that the lack of hepatotoxicity in this setting was likely due to intravenous infusion of N-acetylcysteine during warming therapy and that the patient's hypothermic state may have influenced the attenuated toxicity [34A].

Doxylamine [SEDA-32, 307; SEDA-34, 273; SEDA-36, 235]

Doxylamine succinate, an oral first-generation H1-antihistamine drug is commonly used in sleep-inducing OTC mediations. A 69-year-old woman was admitted to an emergency department with a 1-day history of worsening drowsiness and confusion following ingestion of 16 tablets of 25 mg of doxylamine 48 hours previously due to her recently exacerbated insomnia (recommended dose, 25 mg once daily). A diagnosis of acute severe hyponatremia in the setting of a syndrome of inappropriate antidiuresis (SIAD) was made [35A]. This appears to be a new adverse effect linked to doxylamine overdose. Following treatment, the patient was discharged as asymptomatic on day 8. The authors speculated that the doxylamine-induced hyponatremia was attributable to a SIAD originating from eutopic, non-osmotic release of antidiuretic hormone such as it has been described for antipsychotics and selective serotonin-reuptake inhibitors [36A]. They recommend that clinicians should be aware of this potential adverse effect of doxylamine overdose for those patients presenting with acute hyponatremia if no other causes are evident.

A fatal complication in a 1-year-old girl arose when she was prescribed an over-the-counter sleep remedy containing 250 mg doxylamine succinate per 100 ml for insomnia associated with teething. This previously healthy child died following aspiration of stomach contents after having received 3.5 ml of Sedaplus® Saft, which is within the manufacturer's recommended dose range for this age-group. A doxylamine blood level of 0.16 mg/l was found at toxicological examination and this was within the upper therapeutic range for adults. The authors suggest that extreme caution should be exercised when using over-the-counter sedatives in very young children and that there is a case for discontinuing their use in this age-group [37A].

Fexofenadine [SEDA-36, 236]

A 69-year-old man with a 10-month history of pruritic papules on his face and scalp was diagnosed as having allergic contact dermatitis that was treated with levocetirizine for 1 week with no improvement [38A]. He experienced episodes of itchy hives over his body approximately 2 hours after receiving 180 mg of fexofenadine in addition to 5 mg of levocetirizine. After ceasing fexofenadine for 2 days, the symptoms disappeared. Re-challenge with the same drugs the next day resulted in a recurrence of symptoms. Oral corticosteroid treatment for 3 days with subsequent levocetirizine given to control allergic contact dermatitis resulted in no further wheals being observed. Skin prick tests were performed 3 months later with fexofenadine dilutions of 0.01%, 0.05% and 0.1%. The latter concentration resulted in wheal development within 10 minutes. Oral provocation tests confirmed the diagnosis with urticarial eruptions observed over the body 1 hour after ingestion of a 180 mg dose of fexofenadine. The precise mechanism of urticaria induced by antihistamines was not elucidated in this study, but the findings emphasize that drugs of this class can act as causative agents.

Hydroxyzine [SEDA-36, 236]

A 47-year-old woman developed shortness of breath and generalized pruritus after taking a 25 mg tablet of hydroxyzine which necessitated treatment in the emergency department. Her physical examination was unremarkable except for mild eczema on her arms and hands and nasal mucosal edema. Her total IgE was 271 IU/ml and complete blood count showed eosinophilia of 910/μl. When subjected to a blinded oral challenge to hydroxyzine, the placebo (5 ml of water sweetened with sugar) caused no reaction. However, within 3 minutes after ingesting the hydroxyzine syrup the patient developed generalized pruritus and severe bronchospasm with little air movement on chest auscultation. She was treated with 0.3 mg of intramuscular epinephrine and required oxygen at 5 l by nasal cannula to bring her O_2 saturation to 95%. She was subsequently treated with nebulized albuterol. Within 30 minutes, her acute condition markedly improved. She was instructed to avoid hydroxyzine and its derivatives, cetirizine, and levocetirizine. She was prescribed fexofenadine for treatment of her allergic rhinitis and doxepin

for itching from eczema, both of which she tolerated well in the past. At another visit, a skin prick test (SPT) was performed with diphenhydramine (12.5 mg/5 ml), hydroxyzine (10 mg/ml), cetirizine (1 mg/ml), levocetirizine (2.5 mg/ml), fexofenadine (30 mg/ml), doxepin (10 mg/ml), and loratadine (5 mg/ml). A few minutes later the patient complained of pruritus, shortness of breath, and developed severe repetitive cough. Her vital signs showed blood pressure of 141/60 mmHg, heart rate of 96/min, and O_2 saturation of 100% on room air. Her oropharynx appeared normal, lungs were clear, and skin was clear except for marks of severe scratching. Because of the severity of her cough, she was given 0.3 mg of intramuscular epinephrine and 30 mg of fexofenadine for itching. Her symptoms significantly improved within 20 minutes [39A].

A 54-year-old female with acute severe headache had been taking hydroxyzine pamoate for several days as a treatment for skin eruptions. Neurological examination and computed tomography (CT) images of her brain revealed no abnormalities. A more detailed investigation was done on day 3 with 1.0 T magnetic resonance angiography. It revealed multiple segmental cerebral vasoconstrictive lesions in the bilateral anterior, middle and posterior cerebral arteries with subarachnoid hemorrhage (SAH) predominantly in the right frontal area on fluid-attenuated inversion recovery (FLAIR) images. Examination of cerebrospinal fluid revealed 5400 red blood cells per microlitre and a diagnosis of reversible cerebral vasoconstriction syndrome (RCVS) was made. Intravenous nicardipine therapy (2 mg/h) was started and the patient improved over the next 3 days with subsequent discharge with no neurological defect [40A]. The authors report this as the first instance of RCVS associated with SAH implicating hydroxyzine pamoate treatment. Although they could not confirm that hydroxyzine pamoate was the causative agent, the authors speculated that H1-antagonism or the anticholinergic action of hydroxyzine pamoate may have caused RCVS in this case.

A 33-year-old female with a history of chronic stable asthma, chronic sinusitis and allergic rhinitis noticed a pruritic rash several days after application of topical neomycin. She subsequently developed small and painful papulovesicular eruptions on her hands, elbows, shoulders and feet. Following clinical evaluation, the neomycin was discontinued and a 5-day course of prednisone and daily hydroxyzine started. The lesions were localized and resolved initially after the short course of oral prednisone with concurrent use of hydroxyzine. On stopping prednisone, the patient experienced reappearance of the intense pruritic skin lesions which worsened over 2 months of taking oral hydroxyzine. Patch testing was performed while the patient was still taking hydroxyzine with positive reactions observed at 48 hours and 1 week for 20%

neomycin sulphate and 1% ethylenediamine dihydrochloride. Due to suspected cross-reactivity to hydroxyzine in the setting of ethylenediamine sensitivity, hydroxyzine was discontinued and the patient experienced rapid clinical improvement [41A]. Although the authors did not repeat patch testing once the hydroxyzine was stopped, they recommended that ethylenediamine-sensitive patients should be instructed to avoid systemic and topical exposures to antihistamines that have piperazine (diethylenediamine)-derived chemically related structures.

A 60-year-old man took meprobamate and hydroxyzine for anxiety having previously taken the latter drug without incident. After 2 days, a pruritic symmetrical erythema with few small pustules developed on both inner thighs, cubital fossae, axillae and the gluteal area. The patient denied any intake of other medications during the previous weeks and had no history of mercury exposure. Laboratory tests (complete blood cell count and C-reactive protein, blood and pustule cultures, pustule mycology) were unremarkable with the exception of an eosinophilia (800/ml). A skin biopsy showed a perivascular lymphohistiocytic infiltrate with eosinophils and some neutrophils present in the dermis. Symmetrical drug-related intertriginous and flexural exanthema or baboon-type drug reaction was suspected. Both drugs were discontinued and the lesions resolved within 4 days without treatment. Despite being warned not to do so, the patient took one tablet of hydroxyzine and within 2–3 hours developed an acute episode of baboon syndrome. Hydroxyzine was stopped and the lesions resolved within 1 week. One month after complete resolution, the patient was patch tested with European standard series, ethylenediamine dihydrochloride, hydroxyzine, cetirizine and levocetirizine. Only hydroxyzine gave positive results at days 2 and 3 with pustular formation observed at day 4. Oral provocation tests with cetirizine and levocetirizine were negative. However, when combined with the accidental oral provocation test with hydroxyzine, the tests confirmed a case of what appears to be the first case of hydroxyzine-induced baboon syndrome [42A].

Levocetirizine

A 73-year-old female presented with multiple, recurrent generalized itching, rash and multiple, well-demarcated dark pigmented lesions with desquamation at fixed sites after taking several medications for the "common cold". She took bepotastine besilate (Talion®) and levocetirizine (Xyzal®) as antihistamine in addition to acetaminophen, pseudoephedrine 60 mg/triprolidine 2.5 mg (Actifed®), dihydrocodeine bitartrate 5 mg/di-methylephedrine hydrochloride 17.5 mg/chlorpheniramine maleate 1.5 mg/guaifenesin 50 mg (Codening®) and aluminium hydroxide 200 mg/magnesium carbonate 120 mg

(Antad®) at the same time. A patch test was performed for several medications including: cetirizine, hydroxyzine, fexofenadine and loratadine. The results were positive for piperazine derivatives (cetirizine and hydroxyzine) and negative for piperidine derivatives (fexofenadine and loratadine). To confirm the safety of an alternative candidate drug, a subsequent oral challenge test of 120 mg fexofenadine was given daily for 3 days and was well tolerated by the patient. Based on the history of repeated adverse reactions after taking levocetirizine and the result of patch test, the authors conclude that this is a confirmed case of levocetirizine-induced fixed drug eruption, with cross-reactivity to other piperazine derivatives such as cetirizine and hydroxyzine [43A].

An otherwise healthy 8-year-old girl with a history of allergic rhinitis (maintained on levocetirizine and fluticasone nasal spray) began suffering short-lasting stabbing headache attacks. The headaches began 1 month before her hospitalization and were usually preceded by physical activity (e.g., dancing, running). The pain, which was located in the right supraorbital region, lasted for only one second but occurred several times throughout the day. Upon physical examination, no other associated symptoms were observed and her brain MRI was normal. Based on the patient's clinical course and laboratory results, the proposed diagnosis was primary headache. The patient was discharged and it was suggested that she keep a headache diary. During a follow-up visit, an association was made between the cessation of the headache attacks and the discontinuation of levocetirizine. Six months later, the girl remained headache free further signifying that the headaches were most likely drug induced [44A].

Olopatadine [SEDA-36, 237]

A 14-year-old boy presented with dark-brown patches localized on the lateral margins of both eyes and was prescribed topical olopatadine 0.1% ophthalmic solution for recurrent allergic conjunctivitis. On the second day of the treatment, a rash appeared in the periorbital areas characterized by violaceous, erythematous, itchy plaques with a diameter of 1–2 cm. The erythematous patches healed in 1 month without any treatment leaving a dark-brown residual hyperpigmentation. The patient had a negative history of skin reactions with no history of any other drug intake during this period. A general examination of the patient and routine laboratory tests were unremarkable. Dermatological examination revealed darkly hyperpigmented patches of size between 1 and 2 cm in diameter over the lateral margins of the periorbital skin. A skin biopsy obtained from the hyperpigmented lesional skin showed thinning of the stratum malpighii, loss of rete ridges, vacuolar degeneration of the basal layer, pigment incontinence with capillary proliferation and perivascular lymphocytic infiltration in the dermis. A diagnosis of fixed drug eruption to olopatadine was based on the clinical and histopathological findings but could not be confirmed as the patient did not consent to patch testing [45A].

Oxatomide [SEDA-36, 237]

A 3-year-old Caucasian male who was treated for 2 days for conjunctivitis with oxatomide drops 2.5% developed abdominal pains, pallor and trouble speaking. These symptoms were followed by a serious bout of impaired consciousness and muscular hypotonia. The child was also suffering from concomitant acute gastroenteritis. After emergency admission, oxatomide was withdrawn but the state of impaired consciousness persisted with very low response to pain stimulation tests with a Glasgow Coma Score of 4. On admission to the pediatric emergency section, a CT scan was negative with normal deep tendon reflexes. Normal results were seen for blood gas analysis, serum electrolyte levels, hepatic and renal tests with unremarkable findings on analysis of urine or cerebrospinal fluid. Elevated leucocytes with decreased neutrophil numbers (39.5%) were present with a C-reactive protein (CRP) value of 0.47 mg/dl (physiologic range <0.25 mg/dl). This was compatible with a clinical picture of inflammation due to the concurrent gastroenteritis. Forty-eight hours after oxatomide withdrawal, the patient returned to normal and although asthenia and headache persisted, these afflictions remitted completely within days. A diagnosis of acute encephalitis was excluded and the symptoms attributed to an oxatomide adverse effect. The patient was screened for the main allelic variants of CYP3A4 but no polymorphisms were detected [46A]. The authors speculated that the release of pro-inflammatory molecules associated with concomitant gastroenteritis in this patient may have decreased CYP activities eventually leading to increased plasma oxatomide concentrations, thus contributing to the observed neurological symptoms. There is only one previously published article of a long-lasting impaired consciousness after therapeutic oxatomide treatment [47A]. This study reported six cases of acute dystonic reactions and long-lasting impaired consciousness in children 30–60 hours after the start of oxatomide treatment. Altered consciousness varied from lethargy and somnolence to frank encephalitis. The causes for those episodes of acute toxicity to oxatomide were not known.

Promethazine [SEDA-36, 237]

Many medical textbooks recommend the use of parenteral H1 and H2 antagonists in anaphylaxis, particularly in those hypotensive patients who are resistant to adrenaline [48R]. However, a systematic review did not identify any studies to support antihistamine administration as a first-line therapy for anaphylaxis [49R]. In this regard, an epidemiological study of 490 patients with anaphylaxis reported in a sub-study that three patients with anaphylaxis intravenously treated with promethazine 25 mg subsequently developed hypotension [50A]. All were then successfully treated with adrenalin. Although the authors accept that these observations do not prove causality, they do demonstrate the potential risk of using parenteral antihistamines in patients with anaphylaxis.

A 65-year-old woman who had undergone laparoscopic pancreatic surgery 10 days prior to admission and prescribed promethazine 25 mg for nausea on discharge was admitted with abnormal uncontrolled movements. Within 2–3 days of commencing promethazine, she experienced pain in her right calf, which then spread to both legs with a 'pins-and-needles' sensation that subsequently spread to her arms. She continued the promethazine for nausea and the uncontrolled movements became more serious. She was diagnosed with acute dystonic reaction due to promethazine and given intravenous diphenhydramine. This resulted in significant worsening of the abnormal movements that led to ICU admission. Routine laboratory blood parameters were within normal limits and magnetic resonance imaging of the brain and a neurological examination showed no abnormalities. Her uncontrollable movements in the lower extremities were proximal more than distal with minimal involvement of the upper extremities and the trunk and without orofacial involvement. These symptoms completely abated after intravenous administration of 2 mg of morphine. The patient did admit to having experienced mild RLS symptoms in previous years that were not reported to her physician. She was therefore diagnosed with severe exacerbation of restless leg syndrome and discharged on ropinirole with symptom control evident for over 2 years [51A]. The authors pointed out that drugs such as dopamine-blocking agents, some antidepressants, and antihistamines when used in patients with restless leg syndrome may have a synergistic effect in worsening their symptoms. They further speculated that the anesthetics used during surgery, diphenhydramine and promethazine may also have contributed in this case.

References

[1] Uesawa Y, Hishinuma S, Shoji M. Molecular determinants responsible for sedative and non-sedative properties of histamine H_1-receptor antagonists. J Pharmacol Sci. 2014;124(2):160–8 [R].
[2] Katayose Y, Aritake S, Kitamura S, et al. Carry over effect on next-day sleepiness and psychomotor performance of night time

administered antihistaminic drugs: a randomized controlled trial. Hum Psychopharmacol Clin Exp. 2012;27:428–36 [c].

[3] Naicker P, Anoopkumar-Dukie S, Grant GD, et al. The effects of antihistamines with varying anticholinergic properties on voluntary and involuntary movement. Clin Neurophysiol. 2013;124(9):1840–5 [c].

[4] Takeo T, Kasugai C, Tanaka R, et al. Evaluation of the antihistamine effects of olopatadine and levocetirizine during a 24-h period: a double-blind, randomized, cross-over, placebo-controlled comparison in skin responses induced by histamine iontophoresis. J Dermatol. 2013;40(12):987–92 [c].

[5] Kamei H, Isaji A, Noda Y, et al. Effects of single therapeutic doses of promethazine, fexofenadine and olopatadine on psychomotor function and histamine-induced wheal- and flare-responses: a randomized double-blind, placebo-controlled study in healthy volunteers. Arch Dermatol Res. 2012;304:263–72 [c].

[6] García-Gea C, Martínez J, Ballester MR, et al. Psychomotor and subjective effects of bilastine, hydroxyzine, and cetirizine, in combination with alcohol: a randomized, double-blind, crossover, and positive-controlled and placebo-controlled Phase I clinical trials. Hum Psychopharmacol. 2014;29(2):120–32 [c].

[7] Farré M, Pérez-Mañá C, Papaseit E, et al. Bilastine vs. hydroxyzine: occupation of brain histamine H1-receptors evaluated by positron emission tomography in healthy volunteers. Br J Clin Pharmacol. 2014;78(5):970–80 [c].

[8] Szalai C, Tölgyesi G, Nagy A, et al. Pharmacogenomics of asthma: present and perspective. Orv Hetil. 2006;147(4):159–69 [Review. Hungarian] [R].

[9] Losol P, Yoo HS, Park HS. Molecular genetic mechanisms of chronic urticaria. Allergy Asthma Immunol Res. 2014;6:13–21 [R].

[10] Cordova-Sintjago TC, Fang L, Bruysters M, et al. Molecular determinants of ligand binding at the human histamine H_1 receptor: site-directed mutagenesis results analyzed with ligand docking and molecular dynamics studies at H_1 homology and crystal structure models. J Chem Pharm Res. 2012;4(6):2937–51 [M].

[11] Saruwatari J, Matsunaga M, Ikeda K, et al. Impact of CYP2D6*10 on H1-antihistamine-induced hypersomnia. Eur J Clin Pharmacol. 2006;62(12):995–1001 [R].

[12] Morris AP, Zeggini E. An evaluation of statistical approaches to rare variant analysis in genetic association studies. Genet Epidemiol. 2010;34:188–93 [M].

[13] Hlavica P. N-oxidative transformation of free and N-substituted amine functions by cytochrome P450 as means of bioactivation and detoxication. Drug Metab Rev. 2002;34(3):451–77 [R].

[14] Hishinuma S, Sugawara K, Uesawa Y, et al. Differential thermodynamic driving force of first- and second-generation antihistamines to determine their binding affinity for human H1 receptors. Biochem Pharmacol. 2014;91(2):231–41 [R].

[15] Xu M, Ju W, Hao H, et al. Cytochrome P450 2J2: distribution, function, regulation, genetic polymorphisms and clinical significance. Drug Metab Rev. 2013;45(3):311–52 [R].

[16] Luquin E, Ap Kaplan, Ferrer M. Increased responsiveness of basophils of patients with chronic urticaria to sera but hypo-responsiveness to other stimuli. Clin Exp Allergy. 2005;35:456–60 [c].

[17] Lee HS, Kim SH, Kim KW, et al. Involvement of human histamine N-methyltransferase gene polymorphisms in susceptibility to atopic dermatitis in Korean children. Allergy Asthma Immunol Res. 2012;4(1):31–6 [c].

[18] Raje N, Vyhlidal CA, Dai H, et al. Genetic variation within the histamine pathway among patients with asthma—a pilot study. J Asthma. 2015;52:353–62 [c].

[19] Palikhe NS Kim SH, Ye YM, Hur GY, et al. Association of CRTH2 gene polymorphisms with the required dose of antihistamines in patients with chronic urticaria. Pharmacogenomics. 2009;10(3):375–83 [c].

[20] Yan S, Chen W, Wen S, et al. Influence of component 5a receptor 1 (C5AR1)-1330T/G polymorphism on nonsedating H1-antihistamines therapy in Chinese patients with chronic spontaneous urticaria. J Dermatol Sci. 2014;76(3):240–5 [C].

[21] Koren G, Vranderick M, Gill S, et al. Sex differences in pharmacokinetics of doxylamine-pyridoxine combination: implications for pregnancy. Obstet Gynecol. 2014;123(Suppl 1): 151S [c].

[22] Xiong Y, Yuan Z, Yang J, et al. CYP3A5*3 and MDR1 C3435T are influencing factors of inter-subject variability in rupatadine pharmacokinetics in healthy Chinese volunteers. Eur J Drug Metab Pharmacokinet. 2014; 1–8 [c].

[23] Corcóstegui R, Labeaga L, Innerárity A, et al. Preclinical pharmacology of bilastine, a new selective histamine H1 receptor antagonist: receptor selectivity and in vitro antihistaminic activity. Drugs R&D. 2005;6(6):371–84 [r].

[24] Scaglione F. Safety profile of bilastine: 2nd generation h1-antihistamines. Eur Rev Med Pharmacol Sci. 2012;16:1999–2005 [r].

[25] Sadaba B, Gomez-Guiu A, Azanza JR, et al. Oral availability of bilastine. Clin Drug Investig. 2013;33:375–81 [c].

[26] Rutkowski K, Wagner A. Cetirizine anaphylaxis. Ann Allergy Asthma Immunol. 2014;113(3):247–9 [A].

[27] Raghavendran R, Shipman AR, Langman G, et al. Acute interstitial nephritis secondary to long-term use of cetirizine for the treatment of urticaria pigmentosa. Clin Exp Dermatol. 2012;38:89–101 [a].

[28] Kavosh ER, Khan DA. Second generation H1 antihistamines in chronic urticaria, an evidence based review. Am J Clin Dermatol. 2011;12:361–76 [r].

[29] Praga M, Gonzalez E. Acute interstitial nephritis. Kidney Int. 2010;77:956–61 [r].

[30] Garden BC, Francois F. Cetirizine-associated delusions and depression in an 18-year old woman. Clin Neuropharmacol. 2013;36:96–7 [a].

[31] Karamanakos PN, Suzuki H, Shigeta A, et al. Accidental death of elderly persons under the influence of chlorpheniramine. Leg Med. 2013;15:253–5 [a].

[32] Karamanakos PN. Comment on: accidental death of elderly persons under the influence of chlorpheniramine. Leg Med. 2014;16:60 [a].

[33] Chen TY, Yeh YW, Kuo SC, et al. Diphenhydramine dependence through deep intramuscular injection resulting in myonecrosis and prolonged QT interval. J Clin Pharm Ther. 2014;39(3):325–7 [A].

[34] Rollstin AD, Seifert SA. Acetaminophen/diphenhydramine overdose in profound hypothermia. Clin Toxicol (Phila). 2013;51(1):50–3 [A].

[35] Carrascosa MF, Caviedes J-S, Lucena MI, et al. Syndrome of inappropriate antidiuresis in doxylamine overdose. BMJ Case Rep. 2012;http://dx.doi.org/10.1136/bcr-2012-007428 pii: bcr-2012-007428 [A].

[36] Covyeou JA, Jackson CW. Hyponatremia associated with escitalopram. N Engl J Med. 2007;356:94–5 [A].

[37] Turk EE, Ewald A. A fatal complication of doxylamine in a 1-year-old girl. Int J Leg Med. 2012;126:447–9 [A].

[38] Lee SW, Byun JY, Choi YW, et al. Fexofenadine-induced urticaria. Ann Dermatol. 2011;23:S329–32 [A].

[39] Shakouri AA, Bahna SL. Hypersensitivity to antihistamines. Allergy Asthma Proc. 2013;34(6):488–96 [A].

[40] Matano F, Murai Y, Adachi K, et al. Reversible cerebral vasoconstriction syndrome associated with subarachnoid hemorrhage triggered by hydroxyzine pamoate. Clin Neurol Neurosurg. 2013;115:2189–91 [A].

[41] Reid N, Jariwala S, Hudes G, et al. Worsening of contact dermatitis by oral hydroxyzine: a case report. Dermatol Online J. 2013;19:4 [A].

[42] Akkari H, Belhadjali H, Youssef M, et al. Baboon syndrome induced by hydroxyzine. Indian J Dermatol. 2013;58:244 [A].

[43] Kim MY, Jo EJ, Chang YS, et al. A case of levocetirizine-induced fixed drug eruption and cross-reaction with piperazine derivatives. Asia Pac Allergy. 2013;3(4):281–4 [A].

[44] Biedroł A, Kaciłski M, Skowronek-Bała B. Stabbing headache in an 8-year-old girl: primary or drug induced headache? Pediatrics. 2014;133(4):1068–71 [A].

[45] Bilgili SG, Karadag AS, Aradag R, et al. Fixed drug eruption induced by topical olopatadine ophthalmic solution. Hum Exp Toxicol. 2012;31(12):1292–4 [A].

[46] Antoniazzi S, Cattaneo D, Perrone V, et al. Inflammation and neurological adverse drugs reactions: a case of long lasting impaired consciousness after oxatomide administration in a patient with gastroenteritis. Ital J Pediatr. 2012;38:11 [A].

[47] Casteels-Van Daele M, Eggermont E, Caser P, et al. acute dystonic reactions and long-lasting impaired consciousness associated with oxatomide in children. Lancet. 1986;327:1204–5 [A].

[48] Tintinalli J, Stapczynski J, John Ma O, et al., Tintinalli's Emergency Medicine: A Comprehensive Study Guide. 7th ed. New York: McGraw Hill; 2013. ISBN-13: 978–0071484800 [R].

[49] Sheikh A, Ten Broek V, Brown SG, et al. H1-antihistamines for the treatment of anaphylaxis:cochrane systematic review. Allergy. 2007;62(8):830–7 [R].

[50] Ellis BC, Brown SG. Parenteral antihistamines cause hypotension in anaphylaxis. Emerg Med Australas. 2013;25(1):92–3 [A].

[51] Mehta SH, Dees DD, Morganand JC, et al. Severe exacerbation of undiagnosed restless legs syndrome presenting as a movement disorder emergency. Eur J Neurol. 2013;20:e35 [A].

16

Drugs that Act on the Respiratory Tract

Jayan George, Shehnoor Tarique, Gwyneth A. Davies[1]

Swansea University Medical School, Swansea, United Kingdom
[1]Corresponding author: gwyneth.davies@swansea.ac.uk

Inhaled Glucocorticoids [SEDA-32, 311; SEDA-33, 353; SEDA-34, 277; SEDA-35, 309; SEDA-36, 241]

Inhaled Corticosteroids and Risk of Pneumonia

Inhaled corticosteroids (ICS) are used in both asthma and Chronic Obstructive Pulmonary Disease (COPD) due to their anti-inflammatory effect. However, their effectiveness in COPD remains controversial. In recent years, studies have looked at the association between use of ICS and risk of developing pneumonia in COPD patients. Landmark studies from which such data were examined were TORCH (Towards a Revolution in COPD Health) study published in 2007 [1C] and INSPIRE (Investigating New Standards for Prophylaxis in Reducing Exacerbations) study published in 2008 [2C]. Both of these studies showed an increased risk of developing pneumonia and infective exacerbation in patients using inhaled corticosteroids. However, this remains a controversial area with many unanswered questions. The EIDOS and DoTS description of this adverse event (AE) is shown in Figure 1 as described in SEDA-36, [pxix].

A recent Cochrane review of 43 studies (26 studies for fluticasone $n = 21\,247$ and 17 studies for budesonide $n = 10\,150$) has found that use of fluticasone increased the risk of non-fatal serious pneumonia (requiring hospital admission) (Odds ratio (OR) = 1.78, 95% CI 1.50, 2.12). Budesonide use also resulted in an increased risk of non-fatal serious pneumonia event (OR = 1.62, 95% CI 1.00, 2.62) but less than fluticasone. However, no difference was noted in overall mortality rates between either of the ICS but no conclusion could be drawn as few such events were reported [3M].

A Canadian study looked at a cohort of 163 514 patients on ICS of which 20 344 had a serious pneumonia event (pneumonia needing hospitalization or resulting in death) during the 5.4 years of follow-up. All the patients were ≥65 years of age. It was found that current use of inhaled corticosteroid was associated with a 69% increase in the rate of serious pneumonia (Relative Risk (RR) = 1.69, 95% CI 1.63, 1.75). The risk of serious pneumonia was higher with fluticasone (RR = 2.01; 95% CI 1.93, 2.10) compared to budesonide (RR = 1.17, 95% CI 1.09, 1.26). They also found that the risk of serious pneumonia doubled at a higher dose of fluticasone (1000 µg/day). The risk was sustained with long-term use and declined gradually after stopping ICS use, disappearing after 6 months (RR = 1.08, 95% CI 0.99, 1.17) [4R].

A population-based, nested, case–control study of 653 cases of recurrent pneumonia (community acquired pneumonia ≥30 days of initial pneumonia) matched with 6244 controls showed a twofold increase in risk (5% absolute risk increase) of recurrent pneumonia in patients with current use of ICS. However, no relationship was found between the use of ICS in the past and recurrent pneumonias [5C].

Little is known about the causal factors for this adverse event. It has been speculated that impaired macrophage function, reduced bacterial adherence in the large airways, and alteration of the pulmonary microbiome might be responsible [6R]. The variable response to different ICS might be due to difference in their physiochemical properties [7E]. In summary, long-term use of ICS is associated with an increased risk of pneumonia and recurrent pneumonias especially in the elderly population. Clinicians are advised to consider this potential AE when prescribing long-term inhaled corticosteroid to patients with COPD.

SUSCEPTIBILITY FACTORS

Age

Effects on Growth

The effects of inhaled glucocorticoids on growth were reviewed in SEDA-36, [p244] identifying there may be less pronounced height loss with intermittent ICS use as opposed to long-term use in children. New

© 2015 Elsevier B.V. All rights reserved.

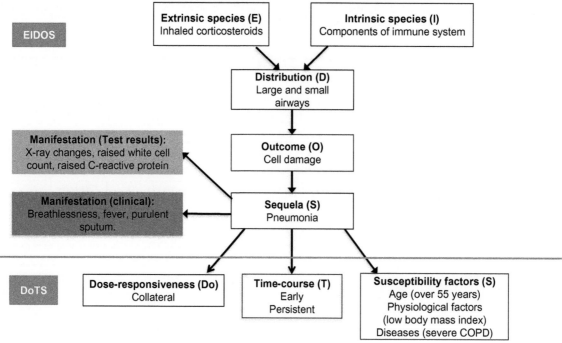

FIGURE 1   EIDOS and DoTS description of pneumonia with ICS.

information has arisen from a Cochrane meta-analysis focusing on ICS in children with asthma and effects on growth [8M]. Twenty-five trials included 8471 patients ($n = 5128$ ICS and $n = 3343$ control) over a period of 6 months to 6 years. Growth reduction appears to be maximal in the first year and less in subsequent years.

One Year

Linear growth velocity at or about 1 year of all dose ICS was assessed in 14 trials and showed a measured difference (MD) -0.47 cm/y (95% CI -0.66, -0.27, $p < 0.00001$) which is statistically significant but with significant heterogeneity between studies $I^2 = 60\%$. Further subset analysis at 1 year or nearly 1 year for different ICS is as follows: beclometasone 400 µg included three trials: MD -0.91 cm/y (95% CI -1.26, 0.55, $p = 0.33$), budesonide 100–400 µg included three trials: MD -0.59 cm/y (95% CI -0.73, -0.45, $p = 0.91$), ciclesonide 50–200 µg included one trial: MD -0.08 cm/y (95% CI -0.27, 0.11, $p = 0.41$), flunisolide 400 µg included two trials MD -0.22 cm/y (95% CI -0.63, 0.18, $p = 0.28$), fluticasone 100–200 µg included five trials MD -0.39 cm/y (95% CI -0.63, -0.15, $p = 0.34$), mometasone 100–200 µg included one trial MD -0.47 cm/y (95% CI -0.97, 0.03, $p = 0.07$).

Two Years

Linear growth velocity at 2 years of all dose treatments was assessed in five trials and the total results showed a MD -0.19 cm/y (95% CI -0.48, 0.11, $p = 0.22$). This was not deemed statistically significant and there was heterogeneity between the subgroups.

Three Years

One paper was deemed suitable for analysis of linear growth velocity at 3 years, which examined budesonide and placebo: MD -0.33 cm/y (95% CI -0.52, -0.14, $p = 0.0005$). Whilst this finding was statistically significant, there needs to be more research on the effect of ICS on height in children between 2 and 3 years of treatment and beyond.

Psychiatric

Previous studies describing neuropsychiatric symptoms were reviewed in SEDA-36, [p243]. ICS induced delirium has since been described in an elderly man. The symptoms started a week after initiating budesonide/formoterol and resolved once the medication was stopped. He was put back on the same combination later in the month and the symptoms resumed and resolved following discontinuation. The paper concluded that this was due to systemic absorption of glucocorticoids and should be noted in patients who have predisposing risk factors for delirium especially in the elderly population [9A].

Endocrine

Previous studies were examined in SEDA-36 [p243]. A Canadian nested case–control study examined the relationship between ICS and adrenal insufficiency. 392 patients were identified over a 15-year period and the study showed that the rate of adrenal insufficiency was not higher among all the users of ICS but that the risk was greater with those individuals on higher doses (OR 1.84, 95% CI 1.16–2.90) [10c].

INTERACTIONS

Drug–Drug Interactions

The interaction of cytochrome (CYP) P450 3A4 inhibitors, such as anti-fungals like ketoconazole or protein inhibitors such as ritonavir, in combination with fluticasone or budesonide where patients have developed Cushingoid features have been described in SEDA-36, [p245] and SEDA-35, [p314]. Three cases have subsequently been described with budesonide. A middle-aged female with common-variable immunodeficiency associated with autoimmunity developed an iatrogenic Cushing's Syndrome having been on long-term Fluticasone and 12 months of Posaconazole [11A]. The second case was an elderly gentleman on inhaled budesonide which had increased over a 6-month period whilst taking itraconozole for pulmonary aspergillosis. It is not clear whether these cases are due to underlying immune deficiency and ICS or ICS alone [12A]. A further report of a middle-aged female with a diagnosis of HIV treated with budesonide developed Cushingoid symptoms following the initiation of ritonavir [12A].

LONG ACTING BETA₂-ADRENOCEPTOR AGONISTS [SEDA-32, 314; SEDA-33, 357; SEDA-34, 280; SEDA 35, 315; SEDA-36, 245]

Combination Therapy

Asthma guidelines recommend adding long acting beta₂-adrenoceptor agonists (LABAs) to inhaled glucocorticoids at step 3 in adults and adolescents before increasing the dose of beclometasone or other glucocorticoids above 400 µg equivalents and certainly before increasing above 800 micrograms [13S]. They should not be used in isolation in asthma but as add-on therapy to inhaled glucocorticoids [14S]. The safety of LABAs has been examined in previous annuals and further findings are updated here.

Formoterol

An updated meta-analysis examined a total dataset of 149 trials; 75 026 were randomized to formoterol, 21 853 to non-LABA treatments, 4474 to salmeterol and 4394 to conventional best practice (CBP) [15M].

All-cause **mortality** was similar between patients randomized to formoterol and non-LABA for 1.5 and 1.6 per thousand treatment years (TTY), respectively (RR = 0.94, 95% CI 0.52, 1.80). There were 55 (0.07%) deaths in the formoterol group: 9 (0.01%) were asthma-related, 18 (0.02%) were cardiac-related and 28 (0.04%) other deaths. There were 3 (0.07%) deaths in the salmeterol group: 0 were asthma-related, 1 (0.02%) was cardiac-related, 2 (0.04%) were other deaths. There were 3 (0.07%) deaths in the CBP group: 0 were asthma-related, 3 (0.07%) were cardiac related. There were 16 (0.07%) deaths in the non-LABA randomized patients: 2 (0.01%) were asthma-related, 9 (0.04%) were cardiac-related and 5 (0.02%) were other deaths.

Asthma-related **serious adverse events** (SAE) occurred in 495 (0.66%) of the formoterol group, 38 (0.85%) of the salmeterol group, 25 (0.57%) of the CBP group and 213 (0.97%) of the non-LABA group. **Cardiac-related SAEs** occurred in 141 (0.19%) of the formoterol group, 12 (0.27%) of the salmeterol group, 3 (0.07%) of the CBP group and 47 (0.22%) of the non-LABA group. The analysis did not give a further breakdown of serious SAEs to comment further on.

Formoterol Versus Salmeterol

Two meta-analyses compared the safety profiles of formoterol versus salmeterol. A Cochrane meta-analysis included 23 trials comprising of 33 952 patients [16M]. 13 trials comprising 4824 adults looked at formoterol: Two deaths occurred in the formoterol group and none in the placebo group. The pooled mortality OR was 4.49 (95% CI 0.24, 84.80). The reviewers used a GRADE system for the quality of evidence and considered this low confidence. 10 trials comprised of 29 128 adults: 44/14 648 deaths occurred in the salmeterol group and 33/14 480 in the placebo group. The pooled OR was 1.33 (95% CI 0.85, 2.08), representing an absolute increase of 8 per 10 000 treated for 27 weeks (95% CI 3 less, 25 more). The GRADE of evidence was rated moderate. As few deaths occurred in the formoterol trials there was not enough evidence to compare mortality with salmeterol. One asthma-related death was reported in the formoterol group and none on placebo. The pooled OR was 4.54 (95% CI 0.07, 285.25). In the salmeterol treatment group 13 deaths were reported and three on placebo. The pooled OR was 3.49 (95% CI 1.31, 9.31). No reviews found a significant increase in death of any cause, nor could they rule out the possibility of a twofold increase in mortality on regular formoterol or salmeterol. Adults with non-fatal SAEs reported on salmeterol monotherapy were 587 (OR = 1.14, 95% CI 1.01, 1.28, I^2 = 0%). Non-fatal SAEs reported in the formoterol monotherapy group were 48 (OR = 1.26 95% CI 0.78, 2.04, I^2 = 15%). There was no statistical difference between the risks of non-fatal SAEs between these groups.

A systematic review examining the effects of asthma drugs in children (age range 0.5–17 years) included 12 studies, comprising of 2018 children completing the intervention [17R]. Groups included salmeterol ($n=212$), formoterol ($n=157$), and budesonide/formoterol ($n=139$) with the others being non-LABA drugs. The duration of treatment was up to 22 months. There were no reported deaths. Common adverse drug reactions (ADR) included asthma exacerbations, bronchitis, upper respiratory tract infections (URTI) and headache. 47 patients on salmeterol had an asthma exacerbation compared with 40 in the placebo group. 20 patients on formoterol had an asthma exacerbation compared to 17 in the placebo group. The trials included in the analysis had little information regarding the description of the severity of the AEs.

Indacaterol

Indacaterol is an ultra-long acting beta$_2$-adrenoceptor agonist used in the treatment of COPD. Safety has been reviewed in SEDA-36, [p246] and indacaterol has been found to have a generally acceptable AE profile. A meta-analysis assessing the use of indacaterol in the treatment of COPD patients comprised 12 RCTs [18M]. One death was related to the use of indacaterol 300 μg but the cause of death was not described. Patients on indacaterol were significantly more likely to experience nasopharyngitis compared to those on placebo (RR$=1.22$, 95% CI 1.01, 1.47, $I^2=15\%$). This result was statistically significant only at dosages >150 μg (RR$=1.27$, 95% CI 1.04, 1.54, $I^2=0\%$), doses ≤150 μg (RR$=1.24$, 95% CI 0.80, 1.91).

Vilanterol

Vilanterol is an ultra-long acting beta$_2$-adrenoceptor agonist which has been previously evaluated in SEDA-36, [p247]. New RCTs have been published evaluating its safety independently and in combination with other treatments.

An RCT examined once daily fluticasone furoate/vilanterol 200/100–500/100 μg preparations versus fluticasone propionate 200 μg on the risk of severe asthma exacerbations in patients aged over 12 [19C]. A total of 2019 patients were randomized and followed between ≥24 and 78 weeks. Severe asthma exacerbations leading to hospital admissions were seen in 9 ($<1\%$) of the fluticasone propionate group and 8 (1%) in the fluticasone furoate/vilanterol group. Treatment related AEs were the same, at 7% in each treatment group. Treatment related SAEs were 1% and 3% in the fluticasone furoate/vilanterol and fluticasone propionate group,

respectively. Headache, nasopharyngitis and upper respiratory tract infections (URTI) were the most common AE. Three fatalities occurred in the fluticasone propionate group and one in the fluticasone furoate/vilanterol group but these were not deemed to be treatment related. Reduction in diastolic blood pressure at week 44 (-0.8 mmHg, $p=0.022$) and at week 76/end of study (-0.7 mmHg, $p=0.032$) were statistically significant but these were deemed not to be clinically significant.

Vilanterol Versus Umeclidinium

An RCT examined umeclidinium/vilanterol combination (62.5/25 μg), umeclidinium 62.5 μg, vilanterol 25 μg and placebo in COPD patients. A total of 1536 patients were randomized over 24 weeks [20C]. AEs whilst on treatment were noted in 48% in the vilanterol group, 46% in the placebo group, 52% in the umeclidinium group, and 51% in the umeclidinium/vilanterol group. The most common treatment related AEs were headache, nasopharyngitis, URTI and cough amongst all groups. Fatal AEs were noted in all three treatment groups: 3 in the vilanterol group (sudden death, COPD exacerbation, COPD exacerbation/renal failure), 3 in the umeclidinium/vilanterol group (COPD exacerbation/respiratory failure, myocardial infarction (MI), unknown cause) and 3 in the umeclidinium group (COPD/acute respiratory failure, sudden death, cholecystitis and peritonitis). There were no deaths in the placebo group. No clinically meaningful changes were observed in vital signs, 12-lead ECG and 24-hour Holter monitoring in any of the groups compared with the placebo.

Anticholinergic Drugs [SEDA-32, 318; SEDA-33, 363; SEDA-34, 282; SEDA-35, 318; SEDA-36, 247]

There have been updates in relation to trials examining the safety of anticholinergic drugs and comparisons between the sub-classes.

A Cochrane meta-analysis assessed the use of combined inhaled short-acting anticholinergics (ipratropium bromide 120–500 μg and one trial used atropine sulfate 0.05–1 mg/kg) and short acting beta$_2$-adrenoceptor agonists (SABA) versus SABA monotherapy for initial acute asthma treatment in children. 9 trials were reviewed comprising of 524 patients [21M]. Tremor was less likely to occur in the combined anticholinergic/SABA group than in the SABA monotherapy group (RR$=0.69$, 95% CI 0.51, 0.93) which was statistically significant. 7 trials were reviewed comprising of 757 patients. Nausea was less likely to occur in the combined anticholinergic/SABA group than with the SABA monotherapy group

(RR = 0.60, 95% CI 0.38, 0.95) which was statistically significant. Anticholinergic/SABA was associated with a 39% reduced risk of tremor and 30% reduced risk of nausea. 8 trials were reviewed comprising of 1230 patients. There was no statistical difference between each group for vomiting (RR = 0.88, 95% CI 0.49, 1.56).

Glycopyrronium Bromide Versus Indacaterol

Glycopyrronium bromide in COPD airWays clinical study (GLOW) is a series of trials assessing the efficacy and safety of glycopyrronium bromide. The GLOW6 double-blind RCT of moderate–severe COPD patients compared combination of indacaterol and glycopyrronium versus indacaterol alone in a 12-week study [22C]. The regimes included were: Indacaterol 150 μg and glycopyrronium 50 μg or indacaterol 150 μg and placebo both delivered via separate breezhaler devices. A total of 449 patients were randomized: 226 to indacaterol and glycopyrronium and 223 to indacaterol and placebo.

Cardiovascular

SAEs occurred in 2.2% in the indacaterol and glycopyrronium group versus 2.3% in the indacaterol and placebo group. No deaths were reported. Incidence of Cardio/Cerebral events was 1.3% in the group on indacaterol and glycopyrronium and 2.3% in the indacaterol and placebo group. Newly diagnosed clinically relevant worsening QT interval with Fridericia's correction (QTcF) was 3.8% in the indacaterol and placebo groups and 2.8% in the indacaterol and glycopyrronium group.

Respiratory

Worsening of COPD was reported in 14.6% of the indacaterol and glycopyrronium group versus 12.7% in the indacaterol and placebo groups. AEs were present in 37.6% of the indacaterol and glycopyrronium group and 33.9% in the indacaterol and placebo groups. Common occurring AEs include nasopharyngitis, lower respiratory tract infection, cough, and upper respiratory tract infection in both groups.

Glycopyrronium Bromide Versus Tiotropium

GLOW5 is a blinded double-dummy parallel trial investigating once daily glycopyrronium 50 μg and once daily tiotropium 18 μg over 12 weeks for the treatment of moderate–severe COPD [23C]. A total of 657 patients were randomized: 327 to glycopyrronium and 330 to tiotropium. SAEs were 3.4% in the glycopyrronium group and 3.9% in the tiotropium group. Infections and infestation accounted for most of these.

Respiratory

AEs occurred in 40.4% of the glycopyrronium group and 40.6% of the tiotropium group. The most frequent AE was worsening of COPD, 15.3% in the glycopyrronium group and 17.6% in the tiotropium group.

Cardiovascular

Cardio/Cerebrovascular events were 0.6% in both groups. Two patients in the tiotropium group had a non-fatal stroke and two patients in the glycopyrronium group had a non-major cardiovascular adverse event. Clinically worsening clinically notable QTcF values were slightly higher with tiotropium than glycopyrronium 3.9–3.4%, respectively. Two patients in the glycopyrronium group had QTcF values >480 ms and none in the tiotropium group. The percentage increase of 30–60 ms from baseline in QTcF was similar in both the glycopyrronium and tiotropium groups at 3.4% and 3%, respectively. No new onset of atrial flutter was noted in either group. No deaths were reported in the study.

Ipratropium Bromide

Nervous System

Anisocoria has been reported in a child in SEDA 36, [p247]. A similar presentation has been reported in a young female with asthma who developed anisocoria due the systemic effects of using a metered dose inhaler of ipratropium bromide for 2 months at a dose of 20 micrograms per puff, 16 puffs a day. The anisocoria resolved a week after discontinuation. A re-challenge with ipratropium was performed and the patient again developed anisocoria which resolved following discontinuation [24A].

Tiotropium Versus Aclidinium Bromide

A double-blind RCT evaluated the efficacy of aclidinium bromide over placebo versus tiotropium over a 6-week period in mild–moderate COPD patients [25C]. Patients received 400 μg aclidinium bromide twice daily versus 18 μg tiotropium once daily. A total of 414 patients were randomized: 171 to aclidinium bromide, 158 to tiotropium and 85 to placebo: AEs were experienced in 25.9%, 27.5% and 29.7% of the respective groups. Headache occurred more frequently in the aclidinium bromide group than the tiotropium group in 7.0% versus 3.8%, respectively versus 3.5% for the placebo group. Nasopharyngitis occurred more frequently in the aclidinium bromide group than the tiotropium group; 5.8% and 5.7% versus 2.4% in the placebo group. No deaths were reported. There were few SAEs reported in the trial (1.7%) but these were not elaborated on.

Tiotropium Versus Ipratropium Bromide

A Cochrane meta-analysis compared the two drugs for treatment of patients with COPD [26M]. This included two studies with a total of 1073 patients. There were fewer people experiencing one or more non-fatal SAEs on tiotropium compared to ipratropium (OR = 0.5, 95% CI 0.34, 0.73). This was deemed to be high quality evidence. This represents an absolute reduction in risk from 176 to 97 per 1000 people over three to 12 months. Disease specific events were reported in one trial comprising of 535 patients. The tiotropium group were less likely to experience a COPD-related serious adverse event when compared to ipratropium bromide (OR 0.59, 95% CI 0.41, 0.85). This was deemed to be moderate quality evidence. There was no significant statistical difference in all-cause mortality between tiotropium and ipratropium groups (OR 1.39, 95% CI 0.44, 4.39, moderate quality evidence).

Umeclidinium Bromide

Umeclidinium is a relatively new long acting muscarinic antagonist (LAMA). Like most LAMAs it binds to muscarinic receptor subtypes M_1 and M_3 which are localized in the airway smooth muscle and block the bronchoconstrictor response to cholinergic nerve stimulation. It has been mainly developed for use in COPD patients [27E,28H]. An RCT examining different doses of umeclidinium over a 14-day period included 350 patients that were randomized to doses 15.6, 31.25, 62.5, 125, or 250 µg once daily preparations and 15.6 or 31.25 µg twice daily versus placebo [29C]. AEs were experienced in 9–21% in the umeclidinium groups and 12% of the placebo group. Headache was most frequently reported in the umeclidinium groups (2–5% versus 2% in the placebo group). Dysgeusia was reported in the umeclidinium groups (0–4% versus 0% in the placebo group). Non-fatal SAEs were not deemed to be due to the study treatment. No deaths were reported in the study.

These results were further supported in another RCT which also examined different doses of umeclidinium in COPD patients over a 7-day period [30C]. A total of 163 patients were randomized to different treatments. AEs across all groups ranged from 4–18%. Headache was most frequently reported in the umeclidinium group (2–5% and 3% in the placebo group). Dysgeusia was reported in the umeclidinium groups (2–3% versus 0% in the placebo group).

Cardiovascular

The mean change in diastolic blood pressure from baseline was −2.1 mmHg in the placebo group whereas in the umeclidinium treatment groups it was less (−0.8 to 0.6 mmHg) [29C]. The differences were statistically significant for all groups apart from the once daily dose of 31.25 µg of umeclidinium. Doses of umeclidinium 15.6 µg twice daily showed a change of 1.7–2.7 mmHg, $p \leq 0.030$. ECG changes post treatment occurred in 30–38% of patients in the umcelidinium groups and 30% in placebo group. The most common of these were repolarisation/depolarisation (frequent ventricular premature depolarisation) occurring in 15–20% of umeclidinium groups and 17% of the placebo group. There was no indication that this was treatment related.

Respiratory

Nasopharyngitis was reported in the umeclidinium groups (3–4%) and 2% in the placebo group [29C]. Pharyngitis was reported in the umeclidinium groups (0–4% versus <1% in the placebo group). Nasopharyngitis was reported in the umeclidinium groups (2% versus 0% in the placebo group). Sinusitis was reported in 3% of the umeclidinium 125 µg group but not in any of the other groups including placebo [30C].

Leukotriene Modifiers [SEDA-32, 319; SEDA-33, 366; SEDA-34, 283; SEDA-35, 320; SEDA-36, 251]

Montelukast

A Cochrane meta-analysis included an evaluation of the use of montelukast in the treatment of symptomatic cough in whooping cough [31M]. A total of 137 patients were randomized to montelukast and 139 to placebo. AEs in the montelukast group were 21 (15.3%) and 31 (22.3%) in the placebo group. Common AEs were increased mucus production; 6 in the montelukast group and 2 in the placebo group; and headache, 2 in the montelukast group and 6 in the placebo group.

INTERACTIONS

Drug Interactions

A possible drug interaction between montelukast and efavirenz was reported relating to neuropsychiatric symptoms. A middle-aged female with HIV who had been on long-term treatment with efavirenz for 5 years developed symptoms of confusion, irritability, disturbed sleep, concentration difficulties and vivid dream shortly after starting montelukast. These resolved 1 month after montelukast was withdrawn. Efavirenz inhibits CYP 2C9, 2C19 and 3A4 isoenzymes and CYP 3A4, 2C9 and 2C8 are involved in the metabolism of montelukast. [32A].

PHOSPHODIESTERASE INHIBITORS
[SEDA-32, 321; SEDA-33, 367; SEDA-34, 284; SEDA-35, 321; SEDA-36, 252]

A Cochrane meta-analysis looked at the safety and efficacy of the phosphodiesterase 4 inhibitors roflumilast and cilomilast in the management of stable COPD over a period of 6 weeks to a year [33M]. 15 trials comprising of 12 654 patients examined roflumilast and 14 trials comprising 6457 patients examined cilomilast. These included moderate to severe COPD patients. AEs were higher in patients on the phosphodiesterase 4 inhibitors compared to placebo (OR = 1.27, 95% CI 1.19, 1.36). There was no significant effect on non-fatal serious events between the two medications and placebo (OR = 1.01, 95% CI 0.91, 1.11) or on mortality (OR = 0.92, 95% CI 0.69, 1.22).

Cilomilast

The Cochrane meta-analysis included further information on the safety of cilomilast [33M]. There was an increased risk of suffering an AE on cilomilast (OR = 1.21, 95% CI 1.08, 1.36).

Respiratory

There was no significant increased risk of patients developing an upper respiratory tract infection (OR = 0.92, 95% CI 0.75, 1.13) or influenza type symptoms (OR = 0.88, 95% CI 0.44, 1.75).

Gastro-Intestinal

Diarrhoea was more common in treated groups than in controls (OR = 2.47, 95% CI 2.05, 2.98), as was nausea (OR = 4.37, 95% CI 3.49, 5.47), vomiting (OR = 4.06, 95% CI 2.83, 5.82), abdominal pain (OR = 1.97, 95% CI 1.55, 2.49) and dyspepsia (OR = 3.13, 95% CI 2.30, 4.27).

Roflumilast

Gastro-Intestinal

Diarrhoea was more common in treated groups than in controls (OR = 3.96, 95% CI 3.20, 4.89), as was nausea (OR = 3.54, 95%CI 2.63, 4.78) and vomiting (OR = 1.52, 95% CI 0.06, 37.37) [33M]. Weight loss was more likely in the treatment groups in the four roflumilast trials (OR = 3.94, 95% CI 3.11, 5.00). The lower dose of roflumilast (250 μg) was associated with fewer adverse effects than the 500 μg dose but this was only assessed in 3 trials.

Psychiatric

15 trials included data on psychiatric AEs. Events included depression, depressed mood, depressive symptoms or major depression. There was a higher risk in the roflumilast 500 μg group versus placebo of experiencing psychiatric AEs (OR = 2.13, 95% CI 1.79, 2.54). This included an increased risk of patients experiencing insomnia or sleep disorders (OR = 2.88, 95% CI 2.15, 3.86), symptoms of anxiety (OR = 1.81, 95% CI 1.26, 2.62) or depression (OR = 1.59; 95% CI 1.11, 2.27) in the roflumilast group compared with the placebo. For the 250 μg roflumilast group, there was no statistical difference compared with placebo as the confidence intervals crossed the midline. Review of the COPD roflumilast safety database revealed 2 suicide attempts and 3 completed suicides compared to none in the placebo group.

Cardiovascular

A systematic review looked at the incidence of major adverse cardiovascular events (MACE) in COPD patients with roflumilast versus placebo [34R]. 14 studies were assessed which examined roflumilast 250 or 500 μg orally daily versus placebo over a period of 12–52 weeks. 91 deaths occurred in the roflumilast group of which 52 were non-cardiovascular related versus 86 deaths in the placebo group of which 40 were non-cardiovascular related. 52 MACE events occurred in the roflumilast group including 35 cardiovascular deaths, 6 non-fatal strokes and 17 non-fatal MIs versus 77 MACE events in the placebo group including 22 non-fatal MIs, 43 cardiovascular deaths and 12 non-fatal strokes. Cardiovascular events were higher in the subgroup of patients with pre-existing cardiac risk factors. A greater statistical reduction in MACE was seen in the subgroup of patients without baseline cardiac risk factors treated with roflumilast versus placebo. The difference in MACE events was deemed statistically significant (hazard ratio 0.65, 95% CI, 0.45, 0.93, $p = 0.019$). Correcting for exposure to treatment, the adjudicated roflumilast event rate was 14.3 per 1000 patient-years compared with a placebo rate of 22.3 per 1000 patient-years. This analysis does not include the incidence of atrial fibrillation which was reviewed in SEDA-36 as increased in roflumilast patients. More information is required to investigate the cardiovascular safety of roflumilast.

Omalizumab (Xolair©)

Omalizumab is a monoclonal anti-IgE antibody which decreases circulating free IgE levels by the formation of trimeric and hexameric complexes. These complexes are cleared by the reiculoendothelial system and therefore there is no activation of the complement system [35c]. Omalizumab is mainly used in the treatment of patients with severe atopic asthma as it inhibits early and late phase bronchoconstriction induced by allergens [36c]. Trials on the use of omalizumab in chronic idiopathic/spontaneous urticaria are not included in this chapter on respiratory drugs.

A Cochrane meta-analysis examined omalizumab for adults and children (aged over 6 years) with asthma [37M]. 9 studies comprising of 4245 patients showed no significant difference in mortality reported between subcutaneous omalizumab and placebo (OR = 0.19, 95% CI 0.02, 1.67). Four deaths were reported, all in the placebo group. No deaths were asthma-related and three of the four deaths occurred in the severe asthma sub-group. SAEs were assessed in 15 studies comprising of 5713 patients. Few SAEs occurred in patients assigned to omalizumab compared to those in the placebo groups (OR = 0.72, 95% CI 0.57, 0.91). Heterogeneity was 7% and was deemed as low. This represents an absolute reduction in SAEs from 6% in those receiving placebo compared to 4% taking omalizumab. The breakdown of these events was not published in the analysis.

Endocrine

Omalizumab may have an association with hyperglycaemia. Two cases of middle-aged men with type 2 Diabetes Mellitus and allergic asthma, who were on omalizumab 375 and 300 mg, respectively, developed hyperglycaemia, on week 42 and on week 45 of treatment. Postprandial blood glucose readings were 13.9–16.7 mmol/L despite large decreases in carbohydrate. This increase only occurred during the first 6 hours of administering omalizumab [38A].

References

[1] Calverley PM, Anderson JA, Celli B, et al. Salmeterol and fluticasone propionate and survival in chronic obstructive pulmonary disease. N Engl J Med. 2007;356(8):775–89 [C].

[2] Wedzicha JA, Calverley PM, Seemungal TA, et al. The prevention of chronic obstructive pulmonary disease exacerbations by salmeterol/fluticasone propionate or tiotropium bromide. Am J Respir Crit Care Med. 2008;177(1):19–26 [C].

[3] Kew KM, Seniukovich A. Inhaled steroids and risk of pneumonia for chronic obstructive pulmonary disease. Cochrane Database Syst Rev. 2014;3:CD010115 [M].

[4] Suissa S, Patenaude V, Lapi F, et al. Inhaled corticosteroids in COPD and the risk of serious pneumonia. Thorax. 2013;68(11):1029–36 [R].

[5] Eurich DT, Lee C, Marrie TJ, et al. Inhaled corticosteroids and risk of recurrent pneumonia: a population-based, nested case-control study. Clin Infect Dis. 2013;57(8):1138–44 [C].

[6] Finney L, Berry M, Singanayagam A, et al. Inhaled corticosteroids and pneumonia in chronic obstructive pulmonary disease. Lancet Respir Med. 2014;2(11):919–32 [R].

[7] Lexmuller K, Gullstrand H, Axelsson BO, et al. Differences in endogenous esterification and retention in the rat trachea between budesonide and ciclesonide active metabolite. Drug Metab Dispos. 2007;35(10):1788–96 [E].

[8] Zhang L, Prietsch SO, Ducharme FM. Inhaled corticosteroids in children with persistent asthma: effects on growth. Evid Based Child Health. 2014;9(4):829–930 [M].

[9] Moss JM, Kemp DW, Brown JN. Combination of inhaled corticosteroid and bronchodilator-induced delirium in an elderly patient with lung disease. J Pharm Pract. 2014;27(1):79–83 [A].

[10] Lapi F, Kezouh A, Suissa S, et al. The use of inhaled corticosteroids and the risk of adrenal insufficiency. Eur Respir J. 2013;42(1):79–86 [c].

[11] Pilmis B, Coignard-Biehler H, Jullien V, et al. Iatrogenic Cushing's syndrome induced by posaconazole. Antimicrob Agents Chemother. 2013;57(11):5727–8 [A].

[12] Blondin MC, Beauregard H, Serri O. Iatrogenic Cushing syndrome in patients receiving inhaled budesonide and itraconazole or ritonavir: two cases and literature review. Endocr Pract. 2013;19(6):e138–e141 [A].

[13] SIGN/BTS. British Guideline on the Management of Asthma, Available from: https://www.brit-thoracic.org.uk/document-library/clinical-information/asthma/btssign-asthma-guideline-2014/ [S].

[14] Bacharier LB, Boner A, Carlsen KH, et al. Diagnosis and treatment of asthma in childhood: a PRACTALL consensus report. Allergy. 2008;63(1):5–34 [S].

[15] Sears MR, Radner F. Safety of formoterol in asthma clinical trials: an update. Eur Respir J. 2014;43(1):103–14 [M].

[16] Cates CJ, Wieland LS, Oleszczuk M, et al. Safety of regular formoterol or salmeterol in adults with asthma: an overview of Cochrane reviews. Cochrane Database Syst Rev. 2014;2:CD010314 [M].

[17] Aagaard L, Hansen EH. Adverse drug reactions associated with asthma medications in children: systematic review of clinical trials. Int J Clin Pharm. 2014;36(2):243–52 [R].

[18] Chung VC, Ma PH, Hui DS, et al. Indacaterol for chronic obstructive pulmonary disease: systematic review and meta-analysis. PLoS One. 2013;8(8):e70784 [M].

[19] Bateman ED, PM O'Byrne, Busse WW, et al. Once-daily fluticasone furoate (FF)/vilanterol reduces risk of severe exacerbations in asthma versus FF alone. Thorax. 2014;69(4):312–9 [C].

[20] Donohue JF, Maleki-Yazdi MR, Kilbride S, et al. Efficacy and safety of once-daily umeclidinium/vilanterol 62.5/25 mcg in COPD. Respir Med. 2013;107(10):1538–46 [C].

[21] Griffiths B, Ducharme FM. Combined inhaled anticholinergics and short-acting beta2-agonists for initial treatment of acute asthma in children. Cochrane Database Syst Rev. 2013;8:CD000060 [M].

[22] Vincken W, Aumann J, Chen H, et al. Efficacy and safety of coadministration of once-daily indacaterol and glycopyrronium versus indacaterol alone in COPD patients: the GLOW6 study. Int J Chron Obstruct Pulmon Dis. 2014;9:215–28 [C].

[23] Chapman KR, Beeh KM, Beier J, et al. A blinded evaluation of the efficacy and safety of glycopyrronium, a once-daily long-acting muscarinic antagonist, versus tiotropium, in patients with COPD: the GLOW5 study. BMC Pulm Med. 2014;14:4 [C].

[24] Alotaibi MA, Wali SO. Anisocoria with high dose ipratropium bromide inhaler. Saudi Med J. 2014;35(5):508–9 [A].

[25] Beier J, Kirsten AM, Mroz R, et al. Efficacy and safety of aclidinium bromide compared with placebo and tiotropium in patients with moderate-to-severe chronic obstructive pulmonary disease: results from a 6-week, randomized, controlled Phase IIIb study. COPD. 2013;10(4):511–22 [C].

[26] Cheyne L, Irvin-Sellers MJ, White J. Tiotropium versus ipratropium bromide for chronic obstructive pulmonary disease. Cochrane Database Syst Rev. 2013;9:CD009552 [M].

[27] Roffel AF, Elzinga CR, Zaagsma J. Muscarinic M3 receptors mediate contraction of human central and peripheral airway smooth muscle. Pulm Pharmacol. 1990;3(1):47–51 [E].

[28] Brusasco V. Reducing cholinergic constriction: the major reversible mechanism in COPD. Eur Respir Rev. 2006;15:32–6 [H].

[29] Lee LA, Briggs A, Edwards LD, et al. A randomized, three-period crossover study of umeclidinium as monotherapy in adult patients with asthma. Respir Med. 2015;109(1):63–73 [C].

[30] Church A, Beerahee M, Brooks J, et al. Dose response of umeclidinium administered once or twice daily in patients with COPD: a randomised cross-over study. BMC Pulm Med. 2014;14:2 [C].

[31] Wang K, Bettiol S, Thompson MJ, et al. Symptomatic treatment of the cough in whooping cough. Cochrane Database Syst Rev. 2014;9:CD003257 [M].

[32] Ibarra-Barrueta O, Palacios-Zabalza I, Mora-Atorrasagasti O, et al. Effect of concomitant use of montelukast and efavirenz on neuropsychiatric adverse events. Ann Pharmacother. 2014;48(1):145–8 [A].

[33] Chong J, Leung B, Poole P. Phosphodiesterase 4 inhibitors for chronic obstructive pulmonary disease. Cochrane Database Syst Rev. 2013;11:CD002309 [M].

[34] White WB, Cooke GE, Kowey PR, et al. Cardiovascular safety in patients receiving roflumilast for the treatment of COPD. Chest. 2013;144(3):758–65 [R].

[35] Corne J, Djukanovic R, Thomas L, et al. The effect of intravenous administration of a chimeric anti-IgE antibody on serum IgE levels in atopic subjects: efficacy, safety, and pharmacokinetics. J Clin Invest. 1997;99(5):879–87 [c].

[36] Fahy JV, Fleming HE, Wong HH, et al. The effect of an anti-IgE monoclonal antibody on the early- and late-phase responses to allergen inhalation in asthmatic subjects. Am J Respir Crit Care Med. 1997;155(6):1828–34 [c].

[37] Normansell R, Walker S, Milan SJ, et al. Omalizumab for asthma in adults and children. Cochrane Database Syst Rev. 2014;1: CD003559 [M].

[38] Yalcin AD, Gorczynski RM, Cilli A, et al. Omalizumab (anti-IgE) therapy increases blood glucose levels in severe persistent allergic asthma patients with diabetes mellitus: 18 month follow-up. Clin Lab. 2014;60(9):1561–4 [A].

17

Positive Inotropic Drugs and Drugs Used in Dysrhythmias

Cassandra Maynard[1], Jingyang Fan

SIUE School of Pharmacy, Edwardsville, IL, USA

[1]Corresponding author: cmaynar@siue.edu

CARDIAC GLYCOSIDES [SED-15, 648; SEDA-34, 287; SEDA-35, 327; SEDA-36, 257]

Digoxin is a cardiac glycoside which possesses a narrow therapeutic index. Caution must be exercised when using this medication as it has many drug interactions which can further increase the likelihood of adverse events.

Drug–Drug Interaction

P-glycoprotein (P-gp) is an efflux pump that has been detected in the luminal portion of the intestine, hepatocytes and renal tubule cells. Digoxin is a known substrate of P-glycoprotein and, as such, medications known to interfere with this efflux pump should be used with caution in combination with digoxin.

CIPROFLOXACIN

In addition to using P-glycoprotein inhibitors and inducers with caution in combination with digoxin, there is also the possibility of other P-gp substrates interfering with the absorption and clearance of digoxin. Ciprofloxacin, a P-gp substrate, has the potential to impede digoxin clearance through competitive inhibition.

- A 27-year-old female on digoxin 0.25 mg daily for arrhythmias associated with congenital heart disease was prescribed ciprofloxacin 500 mg by mouth daily as suppressive therapy for a sternal wound infection. A few days after starting ciprofloxacin, the patient complained of nausea and anorexia. These symptoms would occur 2–3 hours after taking her morning medications, which included ciprofloxacin and digoxin, and would dissipate as the day progressed. The symptoms resolved within 48 hours of

discontinuing the patient's digoxin. Digoxin was later restarted at 0.125 mg daily with no further symptoms [1A].

DRONEDARONE

Dronedarone has been identified as a P-glycoprotein inhibitor. In September 2012, the prescribing information for dronedarone was revised to include a recommendation that prescribers consider discontinuing digoxin when patients are receiving dronedarone. This expanded on prior recommendations for the digoxin dose to simply be reduced by one-half, along with close monitoring, when dronedarone was started [2S].

- An 82-year-old female was prescribed dronedarone and metoprolol during a hospital stay for newly diagnosed paroxysmal atrial fibrillation (AF). Following placement of drug-eluting stents for severe stenosis of the right coronary artery, the patient was started on a loading dose of digoxin due to continued AF. Following the third 0.25 mg oral dose of digoxin (0.75 mg total), an EKG revealed junctional bradycardia. A digoxin level was obtained which was found to be greater than 5 ng/mL (0.5–2 ng/mL), and the patient was given digoxin-specific antibody fragments. Additional lab results included a potassium level of 5 mEq/L, magnesium 1.8 mg/dL and SCr 0.6 mg/dL. All medications were discontinued and the patient's condition improved. Dronedarone and metoprolol were later re-instated without further adverse event [3A].
- A 77-year-old male was initiated on dronedarone 400 mg twice daily for the management of AF. He had already been receiving digoxin 0.25 mg daily, atenolol, hydrochlorothiazide/lisinopril, omeprazole,

© 2015 Elsevier B.V. All rights reserved.

sucralfate, trazodone and warfarin. Three weeks later, the patient presented to the emergency department with complaints of weakness, diarrhea, abdominal pain and weight loss. Laboratory findings included a potassium level of 2.4 mEq/L, digoxin level of 2.8 ng/mL and normal renal function. Digoxin and dronedarone were held during the hospital stay. The patient's electrolytes were replaced and the digoxin was later reduced to 0.125 mg/day. One week after discharge from the hospital, the patient continued to experience mild gastrointestinal symptoms. Given that the patient remained in atrial fibrillation, it was opted to discontinue the dronedarone [4A].

These cases illustrated various ways in which drone-darone can lead to increased digoxin levels and the potential for toxicity. The use of digoxin with medications which are P-glycoprotein inhibitors warrants caution. One must also be aware of the possibility of gastrointestinal complaints (e.g. diarrhea) leading to hypokalemia and dehydration as these conditions can also potentiate digoxin toxicity.

SPECIAL REVIEW—DIGOXIN USE AND MORTALITY IN ATRIAL FIBRILLATION

Despite the wide use of digoxin in AF, especially in those with heart failure (HF), and endorsement by various AF guidelines, no randomized studies have been conduct to evaluate the efficacy and safety of digoxin in the AF population. Since the publication of the landmark AFFIRM trial, where rate controlled strategy was compared to rhythm control, a few observational studies have called the safety of digoxin in AF into question. A sub-group analysis of the AFFIRM trial suggested that digoxin may increase the risk of mortality [5C]. A prospective cohort study, utilizing Swedish registry data, showed a higher mortality rate in patients taking digoxin for AF without HF [6C]. Another study evaluated the SPORTIF III and V trials and found increased vascular-related death with digoxin use [7C]. A subsequent Swedish study, however, failed to demonstrate an association between digoxin use and mortality in AF patients after multivariate adjustment and propensity score matching [8C] More studies have been published in the recent years in an attempt to explore the association between digoxin and mortality in AF and to elucidate whether the greater risk, if one indeed exists, is due to the inherent digoxin toxicity or due to confounding variables such as concomitant diseases and medications.

In addition to the sub-group analysis of the AFFIRM trials published in 2004 [5C], three *post hoc* analyses were recently published. The first analysis by Whitbeck et al. found that digoxin was associated with increased all-cause mortality, cardiovascular mortality, and arrhythmic

deaths, after controlling for multiple covariates. These increased risks were consistent whether patients had HF or not [9C]. Another *post hoc* analysis by Gheorghiade et al., which was published in the same issue based on the same AFFIRM data, focused only on patients who received digoxin as an initial therapy at baseline. This analysis showed that all-cause mortality was similar in those receiving and not receiving digoxin as an initial therapy in a propensity score matched cohort. When evaluating all patients without matching, all-cause mortality was still not significantly different between digoxin user and non-digoxin user, after adjustment for propensity scores [10C]. The third *post hoc* analysis was conducted by Patel et al. and specifically focused on patients with a left ventricular ejection fraction (LVEF) <30% from the AFFIRM trial. Interestingly, they found that digoxin use in patients with LVEF <30% was associated with decreased mortality [11c]. It should be noted that the number of patients with LVEF <30% in the AFFIRM trial was relatively small.

The TREAT-AF study, which is a retrospective cohort study conducted in the U.S. Veterans Affairs healthcare system, showed that digoxin was independently associated with a higher all-cause mortality rate in newly diagnosed AF, after adjusting for clinical covariates and matching for propensity scores [12C]. A population-based cohort study in Canada evaluated patients ≥65 years old who were admitted to a hospital with a primary or secondary diagnosis of AF. In the propensity-matched patients with concomitant AF and HF, digoxin use was associated with a higher risk of all-cause mortality. This increased risk of mortality was also seen in the propensity-matched patients with only AF without HF [13C]. Another population-based cohort study in Taiwan found similar results, in which patients with newly diagnosed AF but did not receive stroke thromboprophylaxis had a higher risk of ischemic stroke and all-cause mortality with digoxin use. The higher risk of clinical events was evident in patients without heart failure, but not in those with coexistence of heart failure. The authors noted that digoxin has been reported to increase platelet activity which may explain the increased risk of ischemic stroke seen in this study [14C]. The risk of stroke associated with digoxin was seen in another Taiwanese population-based cohort study where only 24% of patients taking digoxin were also taking warfarin [15C]. Furthermore, a prospective observational study in Italy found that digoxin use was associated with a significant increased rate of total mortality and cardiovascular (CV) death, in AF patients who were adequately anticoagulated with a vitamin K antagonist. The increase risk of CV death was consistent in patients with and without HF [16M]. Another retrospective cohort study, conducted in a U.S. managed care consortium, demonstrated that digoxin use was independently associated with a higher risk of death and a higher risk of hospitalization in patients with new diagnosis of AF without history of HF [17C]. Lastly, a meta-analysis of 11 studies showed that digoxin use was associated with an increased pooled risk of mortality using both Cox regression survival models and propensity score matching. Additional analysis showed that both AF patients with and without HF had an increased mortality with digoxin use. No significant publication bias was seen in the meta-analysis [18M].

Although a high quality randomized trial is needed to truly assess the effect of digoxin on mortality, literature suggests an association between digoxin and greater risk of mortality in AF patients. The analyses in patients with both AF and HF resulted in conflicting data; however, the risk of mortality with digoxin use was consistent in patients with only AF without HF. Therefore, digoxin should be reserved for AF patients who cannot achieve adequate rate control with other rate limiting agents and be used with caution especially in patients without concomitant HF.

OTHER POSITIVE INOTROPES

Milrinone [SED-15, 2346; SEDA-34, 290; SEDA-35, 329]

Electrolyte Balance

Vasodilator therapy is recommended for nonocclusive mesenteric ischemia. However, a rare case of hyperkalemia following milrinone infusion was recently reported.

- A 76-year-old woman presented with septic shock, which was later attributed to nonocclusive mesenteric ischemia based on CT and laparotomy. She had an elevated serum creatinine (2.23 mg/dL) but normal serum potassium (4.4 mmol/L) on admission. Patient was started on high dose norepinephrine (>0.3 mcg/kg/min) and vasopressin (0.05 units/kg/h) for her shock, until bowel resection was performed. In order to restore mesenteric blood flow to the remaining bowel, milrinone 0.05 mcg/kg/min was added to norepinephrine but vasopressin was stopped at that time. Serum creatinine was 1.7 mg/dL and potassium was 4.77 mmol/L at the time of milrinone initiation. Despite treatment with insulin and IV sodium bicarbonate, her potassium continued to rise. Within 60 minutes of milrinone initiation, patient developed hyperkalemia (7.18 mmol/L) and subsequent ventricular fibrillation which responded to defibrillation. Serum potassium was above 8 mmol/L when continuous hemodiafiltration (CHDF) was started. Although potassium decreased with CHDF, the last level reported was still elevated (>6 mmol/L) around 5 hours after milrinone initiation. No additional information was reported, except that the

patient died 21 days after surgery presumably owing to multiple-organ failure [19A].

This case suggested that hyperkalemia could have resulted from restoration of local blood flow by milrinone to an extensively ischemic bowel which led to a rapid washout of ischemic metabolites. This theory was supported by previous reports of hyperkalemia following revascularization for acute mesenteric ischemia. This unusual pathophysiology for reperfusion hyperkalemia should be kept in mind when vasodilators are used in nonocclusive mesenteric ischemia [20M].

Death

A previous meta-analysis of 13 trials in 2012 suggested that milrinone was associated with increased perioperative mortality in patients undergoing cardiac surgery, primarily driven by studies where milrinone was compared to an active inotrope [20M]. An updated meta-analysis by the same authors was conducted due to publication of new studies, inclusion of pediatric studies, and availability of mortality data from trials after contacting authors. This updated meta-analysis of 20 trials showed no difference in mortality in patients undergoing cardiac surgery when they received milrinone (2.2%) vs. control (2.1%), relative risk=1.15 (95% CI 0.55–2.43, $p=0.7$). The same holds true for both adult studies and pediatric studies. Sensitivity analyses were performed with 7 high quality studies, which showed a trend toward an increased mortality when using milrinone compared to any control [21M].

ANTIDYSRHYTHMIC DRUGS

Ajmaline [SED-15, 45; SEDA-34, 292; SEDA-35, 332; SEDA-36, 258]

Liver

Previous case studies reported liver injury associated primarily with chronic ajmaline administration. A second case in which cholestatic jaundice occurred after a single administration of ajmaline was recently reported [22A].

A 33-year-old Libyan man underwent an ajmaline (80 mg; 1 mg/kg) provocation test for pre-syncope. The test was negative with no complications. Three weeks after the test, he presented with jaundice and pruritus. He has no personal or family history of hepatic disease and took no medications, alcohol, recreational drugs, or herbal therapies. Examination showed no hepatomegaly or features of chronic liver disease. Workup was negative for biliary dilatation, gallstones, and other organ dysfunctions. Ten weeks after the ajmaline test, the patient's jaundice and pruritus had worsened, necessitating hospitalization.

Hepatitis serology, auto-antibody profile, a repeated ultrasound were all negative. A liver biopsy revealed features consistent with cholestatic drug reaction. His symptoms started to improve 9 days after the hospitalization and he eventually recovered 1 year after ajmaline exposure [22A].

In this patient case, a thorough workup had been conducted to rule out other possible etiologies; MRI and biopsy had confirmed drug induced liver injury. It was proposed that this patient's susceptibility may be due to a particular HLA subtype and non-functional allele of the CYP2Dy enzyme which is responsible for metabolism of ajmaline [22A].

Susceptibility Factor: Age

A sub-group analysis was conducted in patients who were diagnosed with Brugada syndrome by using ajmaline challenge between 1992 and 2013. Ajmaline-induced sustained ventricular arrhythmias (sVAs) occurred more frequently in the 40 pediatric patients (≤12 years of age) than the remaining 465 adult patients (10% vs. 1.3%, $p = 0.005$). Of the 4 pediatric patients who developed sVAs, 3 (7%) experienced an episode of ventricular fibrillation requiring defibrillation, whereas 1 (3%) had a polymorphic ventricular tachycardia that responded to high dose isoproterenol infusion. Furthermore, 3 of these pediatric patients who developed sVAs after ajmaline challenge presented initially with syncope (30% of symptomatic children), compared with 1 who was initially asymptomatic (3.3% of children presented for family screening), $p = 0.04$ [23c]. In a previous study, individuals ≤18 years were more likely to have ajmaline-induced intraventricular conduction delay and prolongation of ventricular repolarization, however, the risk of VA was similar to those ≥18 years old [24c]. This could be due to fewer number of symptomatic children (7%) in the previous study [24c] compared with those in the recent analysis (25%) [23c]. This analysis highlighted a higher risk of ajmaline-induced sVAs in children compared with adults, especially in those with history of syncope [23c].

Amiodarone [SED-15, 148; SEDA-34, 292; SEDA-35, 332; SEDA-36, 259]

Respiratory

Pulmonary toxicity is a well-known adverse effect of amiodarone which necessitates close monitoring.

- A 74-year-old male was prescribed amiodarone and acenocoumarol for AF. One month after starting amiodarone, the patient experienced hemoptysis and trepopnea (dyspnea in the left hemithorax) and a chest X-ray revealed an interstitial pattern. The patient received a cumulative dose of 6 grams when Amiodarone was discontinued and the patient's symptoms improved. Amiodarone was then restarted after 1 month. Three months later (and a total of 24 grams of amiodarone) the patient presented to the hospital with hemoptysis, worsening dyspnea and orthopnea. He was found to have a hemoglobin of 6.8 g/dL, an INR of 7.7 and prominent infiltrates on a chest X-ray. His hemoptysis, infiltrates and trepopnea continued for 8 days wherein a bronchoscopy revealed exudative hemorrhagic alveolar damage. Treatment involved discontinuation of amiodarone and initiation of prednisone 30 mg daily. Complete recovery was noted after 3 months [25A].

- An 80-year-old male developed AF following lung resection surgery for the treatment of Stage 1b adenocarcinoma. He was treated with IV amiodarone 0.5 mg/min and after 4 days amiodarone was transitioned to 400 mg orally three times a day. After receiving a total of 12.5 grams of amiodarone over 12 days, the patient developed severe dyspnea, a dry cough, diffuse dry crackles and syncope. Amiodarone was discontinued due to suspicion of pulmonary toxicity and prednisone was started. Other potential causes of dyspnea were excluded (e.g. pulmonary embolism, infection, etc.). The patient expired 112 days after his surgery [26A].

While often presenting after chronic use of amiodarone, there is literature to suggest that lung toxicity can occur in the acute setting—particularly in patients who receive large doses early on in therapy.

Psychiatric

Ataxia and tremor are documented adverse neurologic effects of amiodarone with delirium also being reported in the literature. It is possible that amiodarone may contribute to other neuropsychiatric effects as well.

- A 62-year-old male was receiving amiodarone 100 mg daily for AF. Six weeks after taking amiodarone, the patient developed a variety of psychiatric symptoms including somnolence, irritability, confusion and paranoia. After seeing no improvement with antipsychotics, cessation of steroids and reduction in opiate usage, amiodarone was discontinued as the patient was also experiencing QT-interval prolongation. Days later the patient's symptoms began to resolve [27A].

Musculoskeletal

Several case reports of back pain following IV infusion of amiodarone have been reported.

- A 39-year-old man with a history of AF, hypertension, obesity, sleep apnea and alcohol use was found to have

100% occlusion of the left anterior descending artery requiring CABG surgery. On the day of surgery the patient's AF was treated with amiodarone 150 mg IV over 10 minutes followed by a 2-hour infusion of 1 mg/min and then 0.5 mg/min for 13 hours without incidence. The patient was then prescribed amiodarone 400 mg twice a day for 2 days followed by 200 mg twice a day for 2 days. Due to uncontrolled AF the oral dose of amiodarone was increased back to 400 mg twice a day and the patient also received two 150 mg IV amiodarone doses, one each on post-operative day (POD) 5 and 6, respectively. During the infusion on POD 6, the patient experienced severe low back pain which radiated to the chest and arms. His symptoms resolved within 1 minute of stopping the infusion. Other possible causes of the pain, aortic dissection and pulmonary embolism, were ruled out in this patient [28A].

The mechanism of intravenous amiodarone causing musculoskeletal pain is unknown at this time. In most published cases the reaction has occurred with the first dose and can last up to 15 minutes. However, as noted in this case, it may also occur with subsequent doses.

Immunologic

Amiodarone-induced lupus is a rare adverse event with only a few cases found in the literature. Drug-induced lupus can take many years to develop.

- A 68-year-old female was diagnosed with drug-induced lupus after taking amiodarone 200 mg daily for 5 years. Upon presentation, she was noted to have a malar rash and joint pain which impaired her ability to walk. Laboratory findings supported a diagnosis of lupus in addition to a positive skin biopsy result. The patient's symptoms resolved completely following discontinuation of amiodarone and a course of steroids [29A].

Dofetilide [SED-15, 1173; SEDA-35, 338]

Cardiovascular

A retrospective cohort study evaluated the frequency of cardiac toxicity in 99 patients with symptomatic persistent AF who were loaded on dofetilide prior to cardioversion. In the 46 patients who cardioverted chemically, significant QT prolongation or torsades de pointes occurred in 8 patients (17%) that resulted in discontinuation of dofetilide (all converted after 1 dose of dofetilide); compared to 1 in 53 patients (2%) who required electrical cardioversion ($p=0.02$). Interestingly, of the 21 patients who chemically cardioverted after only 1 dose of dofetilide, 15 (71%) required dose adjustment or discontinuation due to QT prolongation. This study suggested that

patients who responded well to dofetilide were also more sensitive to its cardiac toxicity. Patients who are chemically cardioverted with dofetilide may require closer monitoring for proarrhythmia, especially if they respond after the first dose [30c].

Dronedarone [SEDA-34, 296; SEDA-35, 338; SEDA-36, 262]

Following the approval of dronedarone in 2009, there has been increased concern regarding its use in clinical practice. Studies have identified an increased risk of mortality in permanent AF [31C] and severe congestive heart failure (HF) [32C]. There have also been reports of severe liver damage prompting a warning to be issued by the FDA that providers should consider checking liver function tests during the first 6 months of therapy [33S].

OBSERVATIONAL STUDIES

A prospective study followed 191 patients, who were prescribed dronedarone 400 mg twice daily. Over the approximate 14 month follow-up period, 137 patients discontinued therapy, 95 due to lack of efficacy and 42 because of adverse effects. Side effects well-known to dronedarone, exercise intolerance and GI symptoms, occurred in 15 and 17 patients, respectively. There were no cases of torsades-de-pointes, however, five patients did experience major QT-interval prolongation. Three patients developed premature ventricular contractions which may have been due to their underlying coronary artery disease. One patient developed asystole following their second dosage of dronedarone. No deaths occurred during the study period. With respect to liver-related adverse effects, three patients required discontinuation of dronedarone secondary to markedly increased hepatic enzymes [34c].

Analysis of the Swedish Patient and Drug Registries was done to compare real-world usage of dronedarone to other antiarrhythmics. A total of 174 995 patients were identified of which 4856 received dronedarone. In contrast to other randomized controlled trials, patients exposed to dronedarone saw a reduced mortality rate when compared to the use of other agents including Class Ic antiarrhythmics. HF patients also demonstrated reduced mortality when exposed to dronedarone. Additionally, there were fewer cases of liver disease in those receiving dronedarone. While confounders were used to adjust for disparities between groups, those in the dronedarone group were significantly younger and healthier. Given that this was an observational study, it is unknown if those who filled a prescription actually ingested the medication. It is difficult to form a clinical decision regarding an impact on patient care from this study particularly in light of the contrasting results compared to previously published clinical trials [35c].

Cardiovascular

Dronedarone has been implicated in a number of adverse cardiac events, from QT-prolongation to atrial flutter with 1:1 atrioventricular (A-V) conduction.

- A 50-year-old male was prescribed dronedarone for atrial fibrillation/flutter. The patient experienced palpitations, shortness of breath and nausea 6 months after starting treatment. Dronedarone was determined to have caused atrial flutter cycle length slowing to produce 1:1 conduction [36A].

The package insert for dronedarone was revised in March 2013 to include atrial flutter with 1:1 A-V conduction as an adverse reaction that has been identified in post-marketing [2S].

- A 66-year-old male developed malaise, fatigue and rare palpitations 3 months after being prescribed dronedarone 400 mg BID for newly diagnosed paroxysmal AF. Cardiac monitoring revealed a prolonged QT-interval (>700 ms) and ventricular ectopy. Dronedarone was discontinued and follow-up monitoring revealed improvement in QT-prolongation (453 ms) and a reduction in ventricular ectopy along with the patient's symptomatic complaints [37A].

Sensory Systems

As dronedarone exposure increases, there appear to be more similarities to amiodarone's toxicity than once thought. Optic neuropathy is a well-known side effect of amiodarone, but had not been identified as an issue with dronedarone.

- A 74-year-old male patient with no known history of ocular disease was prescribed dronedarone 400 mg twice a day for lone AF. His only other medical history included remote migraines. Two months into treatment, the patient noted pain over his right eye and 5 months later, developed floaters and flashing lights in the same eye. An ophthalmology exam noted vision in the right eye to be 20/30 with a normal optic disc. The patient's symptoms progressed to include colored spots and decreasing visual acuity. Eleven months after starting dronedarone, the patient was found to have 16/200 vision in the right eye and optic atrophy. Once dronedarone was discontinued, the patient's eye pain ceased within 1 week. Visual acuity did not improve over the following 2 years [38A].

Like amiodarone, early recognition of vision complications and discontinuation of dronedarone is critical and may prevent permanent vision loss.

Hematologic

- A 71-year-old white male patient was prescribed dronedarone 400 mg twice a day for paroxysmal AF. Thirteen days after dronedarone was initiated, the patient presented to an emergency department with a burning, blistering lower extremity rash. A skin biopsy was obtained which revealed, along with clinical exam, leukocytoclastic vasculitis [39A].

Skin manifestations are a potential adverse effect of most medications, including dronedarone. It is important to monitor for a rash but also to be aware that it may be an indicator of a deeper issue.

Urinary Tract

From initial clinical trials, dronedarone was noted to increase serum creatinine levels. It is suspected that dronedarone inhibits the tubular secretion of creatinine, thereby resulting in an increase in serum creatinine but not necessarily a decline in glomerular filtration rate.

- A 71-year-old man required hemodialysis for acute kidney failure 7 days after being prescribed dronedarone 400 mg BID for AF. Six days prior to starting dronedarone, the patient was transitioned from sotalol to bisoprolol while remaining on his other anti-hypertensive medications. The day after dronedarone was initiated the patient experienced GI distress, bradycardia and hypotension. The patient's symptoms progressed to include oliguria, edema and hyperkalemia requiring hospitalization. Once the dronedarone was discontinued and hemodialysis was administered, he appeared to have resolution of his acute renal failure [40A].

A number of reports citing dronedarone as a possible cause of renal dysfunction have been submitted to a national reporting system, the Italian Medicines Agency, with each submission being outlined in a review. A total of nine reports implicating dronedarone were identified. Six cases involved renal failure while three reported an increased serum creatinine. Eight of the nine cases reported that recovery occurred once dronedarone was discontinued [41c].

Susceptibility Factors: Age and Concurrent Illness

There have been several reports implicating dronedarone as a possible cause of renal failure in patients. No direct nephrotoxic effect from dronedarone has been elicited at this time. It is likely that patients may experience such significant gastrointestinal symptoms that they developed dehydration, hypotension and ultimately renal hypoperfusion leading to renal injury. Those most at risk of renal impairment secondary to dronedarone appear to be older individuals and those with a concurrent illness. These individuals may be more prone to dehydration and hypotension thereby leading to acute kidney injury. Such patients should have their renal function monitored more closely.

Mexiletine [SED-15, 1370; SEDA-34, 298; SEDA-35, 341]

Immunologic

A drug-induced hypersensitivity syndrome (DIHS) has been reported with mexiletine [42A].

- A 71-year-old Japanese female developed a generalized maculopapular rash and periorbital/facial edema, along with intermittent fever, edema and general fatigue, 24 days after initiation of mexiletine. This was further complicated by hyperglycemia (466 mg/dL) with normal hemoglobin A1C, low C-peptide levels and negative diabetes-related antibodies. Twenty-eight days after the onset of rash, the patient also developed Hashimoto's thyroiditis. There was also an activation of both cytomegalovirus and human herpes virus 6. A patch test with mexiletine was positive. The patient responded to discontinuation of mexiletine, initiation of systemic prednisolone, insulin and levothyroxine.

The mechanism of mexiletine-induced hypersensitivity syndrome has not been fully elucidated, though it appears that the hypersensitivity tends to induce autoimmune diseases. Previously, several cases of mexiletine-induced hypersensitivity reactions with hepatic, pulmonary, or endocrine involvement have been reported, but interestingly in Asians primarily. Given the predominance of DIHS with mexiletine in this population, the HLA-B*1502 variant likely plays a role in the genetic predisposition to this adverse event.

Propafenone [SED-15, 2939; SEDA-34, 298; SEDA-35, 342; SEDA-36, 263]

Drug–Drug Interaction

Propafenone is metabolized by the CYP2D6 enzyme system, in which considerable polymorphism results in different rate of metabolism.

- A 69-year-old Caucasian male had been taking propafenone 325 mg twice daily chronically for paroxysmal AF. He developed new onset of seizures, symptomatic bradycardia with prolonged QTc, and hypotension, about 12 hours after he took just one dose of mirtazapine 15 mg. Blood work, CT and MRI were all negative, except EEG showed moderate diffuse encephalopathy. The patient responded to discontinuation of both propafenone and mirtazapine, as well as supportive care [43A].

It was proposed that the patient was a poor metabolizer of propafenone. Mirtazapine resulted in competitive inhibition of CYP2D6, which further increased the level of propafenone and its toxicity. Cautious clinical use and judicious dose titration are essential, especially in situations where concomitant medications are substrates for or inhibit CYP2D6.

Sotalol [SED-15, 3170]

Sotalol is a Class III antiarrhythmic agent that also possesses non-cardioselective beta-adrenergic effect. The most notable adverse effect of sotalol is QT interval prolongation which predisposes patients to *torsade de pointes*, sustained ventricular tachycardia, and cardiac arrest.

Cardiovascular

Due to its beta-adrenergic effect, sotalol is contraindicated in uncontrolled HF and must be used with caution and frequent monitoring in patients with compensated HF.

- A 73-year-old man was started on sotalol 40 mg twice daily and warfarin for atrial flutter. Echocardiogram at the time of diagnosis showed normal left ventricular (LV) size and mild to moderate systolic dysfunction. Two weeks after initiation of sotalol, the dose was increased to 80 mg twice daily. Patient only took one dose of sotalol 80 mg, before he developed cardiogenic shock with a prolonged QTc of 510 ms that was unresponsive to fluid resuscitation and high dose catecholamines vasopressors. His QT prolongation and hypotension responded to IV calcium and glucagon treatment. His echocardiogram showed normal LV function 2 months after the event [44r].

Previously cardiogenic shock had been reported with sotalol in combination with other negative inotropes, e.g., diltiazem or verapamil. However, this case patient was not taking any other cardiac medication that could affect rhythm or contractility. Literature has also shown that patients with severe hyperthyroidism are susceptible to beta-blockers' negative inotropic effect. This patient's thyroid function was not reported. In addition, renal function was not available to assess whether the sotalol dose was too high in this patient.

Susceptibility Factors: Age and Renal Disease

Elderly patients are at risk for hyperkalemia due to decreased renal function. Hyperkalemia, along with reduced renal clearance of sotalol, can lead to cardiac arrhythmias.

- An 85-year-old female developed hypotension and bradycardia, with an EKG that revealed junctional rhythm, left bundle-branch block, broad QRS complexes and peaked T-wave, after she had experienced diarrhea for 48 hours. She had been taking sotalol, valsartan, spironolactone chronically, and was recently started on trimethoprim–sulfamethoxazole. She was found to have a serum potassium level of 10.1 mmol/L, increased BUN and serum creatinine, and metabolic acidosis. Patient fully recovered after receiving hemodialysis and supportive care. The contributing factors included her drug combination, diarrhea that likely contributed to dehydration and acute kidney injury, and metabolic acidosis [45A].

This case illustrates the importance of avoiding polypharmacy that could lead to hyperkalemia and for close monitoring of serum potassium and renal function in elderly population.

References

[1] Moffett BS, Valdes SO, Kim JJ. Possible digoxin toxicity associated with concomitant ciprofloxacin therapy. Int J Clin Pharm. 2013;35(5):673–6 [A].

[2] U.S. Food and Drug Administration. Multaq (dronedarone hydrochloride) tablets: detailed view: safety labeling changes approved by FDA center for drug evaluation and research (CDER). Silver Springs, MD: U.S. Food and Drug Administration; 2014. Available at: http://www.fda.gov/Safety/MedWatch/SafetyInformation/ucm243762.htm. Accessed Feb 20, 2015 [S].

[3] Vallakati A, Chandra PA, Pednekar M, et al. Dronedarone-induced digoxin toxicity: new drug, new interactions. Am J Ther. 2013;20(6): e717–9 [A].

[4] Smith H, Battjes E, Yan S, et al. Chronic digoxin toxicity precipitated by dronedarone. Ann Pharmacother. 2014;48(7):923–7 [A].

[5] Corley SD, Epstein AE, DiMarco JP, et al. Relationships between sinus rhythm, treatment, and survival in the Atrial Fibrillation Follow-Up Investigation of Rhythm Management (AFFIRM) study. Circulation. 2004;109(12):1509–13 [C].

[6] Hallberg P, Lindback J, Lindahl B. Digoxin and mortality in atrial fibrillation: a prospective cohort study. Eur J Clin Pharmacol. 2007;63(1):959–71 [C].

[7] Gjesdal K, Feyzi J, Olsson SB. Digitalis: a dangerous drug in atrial fibrillation? An analysis of the SPORTIF III and V data. Heart. 2008;94(2):191–6 [C].

[8] Friberg L, Hammar N, Rosengvist M. Digoxin in atrial fibrillation: report from the Stockholm Cohort study of Atrial Fibrillation (SCAF). Heart. 2010;96(4):275–80 [C].

[9] Whitbeck MG, Charnigo RJ, Khairy P, et al. Increased mortality among patients taking digoxin—analysis from the AFFIRM study. Eur Heart J. 2013;34(20):1481–8 [C].

[10] Gheorghiade M, Fonarow GC, van Veldhuisen DJ, et al. Lack of evidence of increased mortality among patients with atrial fibrillation taking digoxin: findings from post hoc propensity-matched analysis of the AFFIRM trial. Eur Heart J. 2013;34(20):1489–97 [C].

[11] Patel NJ, Hoosien M, Deshmukh A, et al. Digoxin significantly improves all-cause mortality in atrial fibrillation patients with severely reduced left ventricular systolic function. Int J Cardiol. 2013;169(5):e84–6 [c].

[12] Turakhia MP, Santangeli P, Winkelmayer WC, et al. Increased mortality associated with digoxin in contemporary patients with atrial fibrillation: findings from the TREAT-AF study. J Am Coll Cardiol. 2014;64(7):660–8 [C].

[13] Shah M, Avgil Tsadok M, Jackevicius CA, et al. Relation of digoxin use in atrial fibrillation and the risk of all-cause mortality in patients ≥65 years of age with versus without heart failure. Am J Cardiol. 2014;114(3):401–6 [C].

[14] Chao TF, Liu CJ, Chen SJ, et al. Does digoxin increase the risk of ischemic stroke and mortality in atrial fibrillation? A nationwide population-based cohort study. Can J Cardiol. 2014;30(10):1190–5 [C].

[15] Chang SS, Chang KC, Wang YC, et al. Digoxin use is associated with increased risk of stroke in patients with non-valvular atrial fibrillation—a nationwide population-based cohort study. Int J Cardiol. 2013;169(2):e26–7 [C].

[16] Pastori D, Farcomeni A, Bucci T, et al. Digoxin treatment is associated with increased total and cardiovascular mortality in anticoagulated patients with atrial fibrillation. Int J Cardiol. 2015;180:1–5 [C].

[17] Freeman JV, Reynolds K, Fang M, et al. Digoxin and risk of death in adults with atrial fibrillation: the ATRIA-CVRN study. Circ Arrhythm Electrophysiol. 2015;8(1):49–58 [C].

[18] Ouyang AJ, Lv YN, Zhong HL, et al. Meta-analysis of digoxin use and risk of mortality in patients with atrial fibrillation. Am J Cardiol. 2015;115(7):901–6 [Epub ahead of print] [M].

[19] Miyashita K, Yasumura R, Yamazaki H, et al. Fatal hyperkalemia after vasodilator therapy for nonocclusive mesenteric ischemia. Am J Emerg Med. 2014;32(8):949. e3-4 [A].

[20] Zangrillo A, Biondi-Zoccai G, Ponschab M, et al. Milrinone and mortality in adult cardiac surgery: a meta-analysis. J Cardiothorac Vasc Anesth. 2012;26(1):70–7 [M].

[21] Majure DT, Greco T, Greco M, et al. Meta-analysis of randomized trials of effect of milrinone on mortality in cardiac surgery: an update. J Cardiothorac Vasc Anesth. 2013;27(2):220–9 [M].

[22] Mullish BH, Fofaria RK, Smith BC, et al. Severe cholestatic jaundice after a single administration of ajmaline; a case report and review of the literature. BMC Gastroenterol. 2014;14:60 [A].

[23] Conte G, Dewals W, Sieira J, et al. Drug-induced brugada syndrome in children. J Am Coll Cardiol. 2014;63(21):2272–9 [c].

[24] Sorgente A, Sarkozy A, De Asmundis C, et al. Ajmaline challenge in young individuals with suspected Brugada syndrome. Pacing Clin Electrophysiol. 2011;34(6):736–41 [c].

[25] Blasco LM. Trepopnea due to amiodarone-induced diffuse alveolar hemorrhage. Respir Care. 2013;58(2):e11–3 [A].

[26] Fadahunsi O, Krol R. Acute amiodarone pulmonary toxicity following lung resection. Int J Biomed Sci. 2014;10(3):217–20 [A].

[27] Yuppa DP, Nichols S. Amiodarone-induced delirium in advanced cancer: a case report. Psychosomatics. 2013;54(3):294–6 [A].

[28] Adams ML, Kujawski SZ, Bollinger J, et al. Low back pain induced by i.v. amiodarone. Am J Health Syst Pharm. 2014;71(10):782–4 [A].

[29] Fernandez Gonzalez F, Miranda S, Santiago Casiano M. An unexpected side-effect of a commonly used drug. Bol Asoc Med P R. 2013;105(3):50–2 [A].

[30] Brumberg G, Gera N, Pray C, et al. Frequency of toxicity with chemical conversion of atrial fibrillation with dofetilide. Am J Cardiol. 2013;112(4):505–8 [c].

[31] Connolly SJ, Camm AJ, Halperin JL, et al. Dronedarone in high-risk permanent atrial fibrillation. N Engl J Med. 2011;365(24):2268–76 [C].

[32] Kober L, Torp-Pederson C, McMurray JJ, et al. Increased mortality after dronedarone therapy for severe heart failure. N Engl J Med. 2008;358(25):2678–87 [C].

[33] U.S. Food and Drug Administration. FDA drug safety communication: severe liver injury associated with the use of dronedarone (marketed as multaq). Silver Springs, MD: U.S. Food and Drug Administration; 2011. Available at: http://www.fda.gov/Drugs/DrugSafety/ucm240011.htm. Accessed Feb 20, 2015 [S].

[34] Said SM, Esperer HD, Kluba K, et al. Efficacy and safety profile of dronedarone in clinical practice. Results of the Magdeburg Dronedarone Registry (MADRE study). Int J Cardiol. 2013;167(6):2600–4 [c].

[35] Friberg L. Safety of dronedarone in routine clinical practice. J Am Coll Cardiol. 2014;63(22):2376–84 [c].

[36] Rosman J, Hoffmeister P, Reynolds M, et al. Possible proarrhythmia with dronedarone. J Cardiovasc Electrophysiol. 2013;24(1):103–4 [A].

[37] Gonzalez JE, Sauer WH, Krantz MJ. Ventricular ectopy and QTc-interval prolongation associated with dronedarone therapy. Pharmacotherapy. 2013;33(10):e179–81 [A].

[38] Selvaraj V, Johnson KG. Dronedarone-induced optic neuropathy. Int J Cardiol. 2013;167(1):e8–9 [A].

[39] Smith SM, Al-Bataineh M, Lorfido SB, et al. A case report: Multaq-induced leukocytoclastic vasculitis. Am J Ther. 2014;21(3): e69–70 [A].

[40] Young C, Maruthappu M, Wayne RP, et al. Reversible acute kidney injury requiring haemodialysis five days after starting dronedarone in a stable 71-year-old man at risk of cardiovascular polypharmacy. J R Coll Physicians Edinb. 2013;43(2):122–5 [A].

[41] Biagi C, Venegoni M, Melis M, et al. Dronedarone-associated acute renal failure: evidence coming from the Italian spontaneous ADR reporting database. Br J Clin Pharmacol. 2013;75(5):1351–5 [c].

[42] Minegaki Y, Higashida Y, Ogawa M, et al. Drug-induced hypersensitivity syndrome complicated with concurrent fulminant type 1 diabetes mellitus and Hashimoto's thyroiditis. Int J Dermatol. 2013;52(3):355–7 [A].

[43] Rajpurohit N, Aryal SR, Khan MA, et al. Propafenone associated severe central nervous system and cardiovascular toxicity due to mirtazapine: a case of severe drug interaction. S D Med. 2014;67(4):137–9 [A].

[44] Leslie SD. Sotalol-associated cardiogenic shock in a patient with asymptomatic transient rate-related cardiomyopathy. Med J Aust. 2013;199(10):658–9 [r].

[45] Juvet T, Gourineni VC, Ravi S, et al. Life-threatening hyperkalemia: a potentially lethal drug combination. Conn Med. 2013;77(8):491–3 [A].

18

Beta-Adrenoceptor Antagonists and Antianginal Drugs

A. Nobili[*,1], *L. Pasina**, *R. Latini*[†]

*Department of Neuroscience, IRCCS-Istituto di Ricerche Farmacologiche Mario Negri, Milan, Italy
[†]Department of Cardiovascular Research, IRCCS-Istituto di Ricerche Farmacologiche Mario Negri, Milan, Italy
[1]Corresponding author: alessandro.nobili@marionegri.it

BETA-ADRENOCEPTOR ANTAGONISTS [SED-15, 452; SEDA-32, 363; SEDA-33, 397; SEDA-34, 303; SEDA-35, 351; SEDA-36, 267]

Beta-Blockers

Pulmonary

BETA-BLOCKERS ARE ASSOCIATED WITH A LOWER FORCED EXPIRATORY VOLUME IN 1 SECOND (FEV₁) AND FORCED VITAL CAPACITY FVC

A population-based cohort study investigated the effects of beta-blockers on pulmonary function. The population consisted of 1880 men (43.5%) and 2444 women (56.5%). Current use of non-cardioselective beta-blockers was significantly associated with a lower forced expiratory volume in 1 second (FEV_1) of −198 mL (95% CI −301, −96), with a lower forced vital capacity (FVC) of −223 mL (95% CI −367, −79) and with a decreased FEV_1:FVC of −1.38% (95% CI −2.74, −0.13%). Current use of cardioselective beta-blockers was significantly associated with a lower FEV_1 of −118 mL (95% CI −157, −78) and with a lower FVC of −167 mL (95% CI −222, −111), but did not affect FEV_1:FVC. The effects of cardioselective beta-blockers remained significant for FEV_1 (−142 mL [95% CI −189, −96]) and for FVC (−176 mL [95% CI −236, −117]) also after exclusion of patients with COPD, asthma and heart failure [1C].

Pulmonary

SELECTIVE BETA-BLOCKERS ARE BETTER TOLERATED BUT NOT COMPLETELY RISK-FREE

This systematic review and meta-analysis were performed to identify all randomized, blinded, placebo-controlled clinical trials evaluating acute beta-blocker exposure in asthma. Acute selective beta-blocker in the doses given caused a mean change in FEV_1 of −6.9% (95% CI, −8.5 to −5.2), a fall in FEV_1 of ≥20% in one in eight patients (P = 0.03), symptoms affecting one in 33 patients (P = 0.18), and attenuation of concomitant β2-agonist response of −10.2% (95% CI, −14.0 to −6.4). Corresponding values for acute nonselective beta-blockers in the doses given were −10.2% (95% CI, −14.7 to −5.6), one in nine patients (P = 0.02), one in 13 patients (P = 0.14), and −20.0% (95% CI, −29.4 to −10.7). Following investigation of heterogeneity, clear differences were found for celiprolol and labetalol. A dose–response relationship was demonstrated for selective beta-blockers. Selective beta-blockers are better tolerated but not completely risk-free. Risk from acute exposure may be mitigated using the smallest dose possible and beta-blockers with greater β1-selectivity. Beta-blocker-induced bronchospasm responded partially to β2-agonists in the doses given with response blunted more by non-selective beta-blockers than selective beta-blockers [2M].

Liver

Hepatorenal Syndrome

HEPATORENAL SYNDROME AND DEATH IN PATIENTS WITH CIRRHOSIS AND SPONTANEOUS BACTERIAL PERITONITIS TREATED WITH NON-SELECTIVE BETA-BLOCKERS (BBs)

A retrospective analysis of data from 607 consecutive patients with cirrhosis showed that among patients with spontaneous bacterial peritonitis, the use of non-selective BBs increased the proportion of hepatorenal syndrome (24% vs 11% of those not taking non-selective BBs,

ISSN: 0378-6080
http://dx.doi.org/10.1016/bs.seda.2015.08.011

© 2015 Elsevier B.V. All rights reserved.

$P=0.027$) and grade C acute kidney injury (20% vs 8% of those not taking NSBBs, $P=0.021$). Moreover, in patients with spontaneous bacterial peritonitis, non-selective BBs reduced the transplant-free survival (hazard ratio = 1.58; 95% CI: 1.098–2.274; $P=0.014$) and increased days of non-elective hospitalization (29.6 days/person-year in patients on non-selective BBs vs 23.7 days/person-year in those not taking non-selective BBs) [3C]. This study provides observational evidence on the detrimental effect of non-selective BB treatment after development of spontaneous bacterial peritonitis and it supports the hypothesis that indicates SBP as a clinical event that closes the therapeutic window for non-selective SS treatment. It remains unresolved whether the therapeutic window for non-selective SS treatment reopens after resolving an episode of spontaneous bacterial peritonitis.

Second Generation Effects

Pregnancy

In a historical cohort of pregnancies complicated by maternal heart disease, treatment with beta-blockers was found to be independently associated with an increased risk of delivering small for gestational age (SGA) infants. A cohort study on 175 women with heart disease, grouped according to beta-blocker treatment, and 627 women from background population matched on seven birth weight-determining factors was conducted to investigate the effect on fetal growth of treatment with oral beta-blockers during pregnancy in women with congenital or acquired heart disease. More of the infants exposed to beta-blockers were SGA compared with non-exposed infants (29.4% versus 15.3%; $P<0.05$). After adjustment for birth weight-determining factors, beta-blocker treatment and maternal body mass index (BMI) were the only factors independently associated with SGA. After adjustment for BMI, beta-blocker treatment was associated with an increased risk of SGA (OR 2.65; 95% CI 1.15–6.10; $P=0.02$). Beta-blocker treatment was the only independent predictor of SGA, adjusting for several factors influencing fetal growth (the relative difference in expected birth weight was −12.2%; 95% CI −19.9 to −3.9%; $P=0.001$) [4C].

Pregnancy

Treatment with beta-blockers was found to be associated with an increased risk of different adverse perinatal outcomes. An observational retrospective cohort study compared infant outcomes between mothers with hypertension treated by beta-blockers alone ($n=416$) with those receiving only methyldopa ($n=1000$) during pregnancy. The study found that beta-blockers appear to have a strong effect on adverse perinatal outcomes, with

an adjusted odds ratio of 1.95 (95% CI 1.21–3.14) for SGA < 10th percentile, 2.17 (95% CI 1.06–4.44) for SGA < 3rd percentile, and 2.17 (95% CI 1.09–4.34) for hospitalisation for respiratory distress syndrome, sepsis, and seizures during infancy, as compared with methyldopa, in pregnant women with chronic hypertension [5C].

Esmolol

Psychiatric

A first case of a probable association between excipient toxicity of esmolol and delirium has been reported. A 15-year-old boy with hypertrophic cardiomyopathy received in the pediatric intensive care unit high doses of continuous intravenous esmolol (range = 20–40 µg/kg/min) for cardiac rhythm control. After a few days he developed a delirium not responding to high doses of antipsychotics or discontinuation of benzodiazepines. It was realized that IV esmolol formulation contained high doses of propylene glycol and ethanol, which may accumulate after prolonged infusion causing intoxication. The Naranjo adverse reaction probability scale suggested a probable relationship (score = 6) between propylene glycol infusion and delirium [6A].

Levobunolol

Cardiovascular

BRADYARRHYTHMIAS WERE ASSOCIATED TO TOPICAL SOLUTION OF LEVOBUNOLOL

An 88-year-old man was admitted to the hospital with abdominal pain. His past history included coronary heart disease for which he underwent percutaneous coronary interventional treatment. He complained of fatigue, dizziness, and heart palpitations, and an electrocardiogram (ECG) demonstrated sinus bradycardia at a rate of 39 bpm (the day of hospitalization). Holter was taken the second day after being admitted to the hospital, which showed sinus bradycardia, atrioventricular block (first degree), and sinus arrest. The average heart rate was 54 bpm and the range of heart rate varied from 25 to 79 bpm. There were 265 episodes of sinus arrest lasting longer than 2 seconds and six arrests longer than 3 seconds. Serum electrolyte test, complete blood count, thyroid function test, and cardiac marker panel were all within normal limits. One hour prior to the onset of symptoms, he received levobunolol hydrochloride solution topically, which he had been using, one to two drops to each eye, two to three times per day for several years. Because of the clear relationship between onset of symptomatic bradycardia and the instillation of eyedrops, levobunolol hydrochloride solution was discontinued and replaced with latanoprost eyedrops and the bradycardia resolved. Intermittent sinus bradycardia and sinus arrest has been attributed to the topical application of beta-blocker [7A].

Nebivolol

Cardiovascular

EXTREME BRADYCARDIA HAS BEEN ASSOCIATED WITH NEBIVOLOL

A 56-year-old female patient diagnosed with hypertension has been admitted with nodal rhythm on the third day of 5 mg/day nebivolol treatment. From her medical history, 3 days prior to admission, nebivolol 5 mg/day was started due to hypertension and palpitations. Normal sinus rhythm (61/min) was seen during the electrocardiogram (ECG) test. She was also taking levothyroxine because of hypothyroidism and thyroid hormone levels were normal. Physical examination was unremarkable except bradycardia. Additionally, blood pressure was 130/60 mmHg. On electrocardiography test, nodal rhythm (31/min) was detected. The patient was transferred to the coronary care unit for rhythm monitoring and nebivolol treatment was discontinued. However, temporary pacemaker implantation was not performed to a patient with good general condition and normal blood pressure. On transthoracic echocardiographic examination and in laboratory parameters were not observed any pathologic findings. Eventually, 24 hours later, without any medication, the patient's sinus rhythm returned. At the end of the 3-day follow-up, the patient without arrhythmic finding was discharged to receive ramipril 5 mg/day and levothyroxine therapy [8r].

Metabolism and Electrolyte Imbalance

HYPOGLYCEMIA, POLYCYTHEMIA AND HYPONATREMIA HAVE BEEN ASSOCIATED TO NEBIVOLOL USE DURING PREGNANCY

An infant has been admitted about 24 hours after birth for a persistent severe hypoglycemia (blood glucose = 30 mg/dL) and jaundice (total bilirubin = 12.5 mg/dL, indirect bilirubin 11.75 mg/dL). He was born by spontaneous delivery after a normal term pregnancy and the birth weight was 3040 g. The mother reported taking nebivolol 5 mg/day for unspecified tachycardia in the last 4 months of pregnancy. Clinical and instrumental investigations carried out during hospitalization did not reveal any congenital or perinatal abnormalities. Because of jaundice and hypoglycemia, the infant immediately underwent phototherapy and intravenous administration of 10% glucose solution. The laboratory tests carried out at admission revealed polycythemia with hematocrit 63.7%, red blood cells count of 6 230 000/mm³, mild hyponatremia (132 mEq/L) and mild thrombocytopenia (platelets = 99 000/mm³). Tests during hospitalization showed blood glucose level within normal limits, despite treatment with intravenous glucose solution; coagulation remained deranged without overt clinical manifestations and hyponatremia became more pronounced. Urinary electrolytes were below normal; hence fluid intake was reduced, and the administration of sodium chloride increased. After treatment for metabolic and electrolyte imbalance, the infant was discharged on the 10th day of hospitalization, in good clinical condition and with normalization of clinical and laboratory parameters [9A].

Propranolol

Dermatological

A case of allergic contact dermatitis caused by propranolol hydrochloride topically applied for the treatment of a superficial haemangioma. A 5-month-old girl with a superficial haemangioma of the right hand and treated with topical propranolol 1% (lipid cream base) reported after 2 months a worsening of the haemangioma associated with pruritus. Scaling was evident on the haemangioma, and, at its periphery, there were vesicles and scratch marks. Propranolol was immediately stopped and corticosteroids were started. One month after the complete resolution of dermatitis, the patient was patch tested with propranolol 1% pet., propranolol 1% aq., and timolol 0.5% aq. Patch tests were applied on the back, and left in occlusion for 2 days. The test readings were performed after 48 and 96 hours. The reactions were classified according to ICDRG guidelines. Readings showed positive reactions only to propranolol 1% petroleum jelly (or Vaseline) and propranolol 1% aqueous. Ten healthy volunteers were patch tested with the same substances, and the results were negative [10A].

Susceptibility Factors

Age

According to this literature review propranolol has a favorable safety profile for the treatment of infantile hemangioma. In a recent meta-analysis of 85 IH articles 56% of patients had no reported complications. In the patients who did experience significant complications during propranolol use, the most frequently noted were asymptomatic hypotension, followed by pulmonary symptoms (bronchoconstriction or wheezing), hypoglycemia, and asymptomatic bradycardia. The most common non-serious adverse events reported were nightmares, somnolence, cool or mottled extremities, diarrhea, and gastroesophageal reflux. Another meta-analysis of more than 41 studies described an adverse event rate of 31%, with sleep disturbances and acrocyanosis as the most common, accounting for 11% and 5%, respectively. The authors suggest that monitoring for heart rate, blood pressure and symptoms of hypoglycemia should be performed. Blood pressure can be difficult to measure in infants and bradycardia may be a more easily obtained and reliable marker of adverse effects of the medication. Children with clinically significant abnormal vital signs are at higher risk of propranolol toxicity and in these patients, dose de-escalation should be considered. Hypoglycemia can be unpredictable and does not appear to be dose related. Patients who are most at risk are low birth weight infants, and those under 1 year of age [11R].

Metabolism and Electrolyte Imbalance

A 2-year-old male patient with intestinal haemangiomatosis and receiving propranolol was hospitalized for a severe hyperkalaemia. Propranolol was discontinued. 3000 cc/m^2 of body surface area/day, alkalinisation, furosemide 2 mg/kg/day and 0.15 mg/kg/dose 6 doses day inhaler salbutamol were started on the first day of hospitalization. He was monitored for cardiac effects of hyperkalaemia and was restricted for potassium containing diet. Sufficient dieresis was achieved and there were no ECG changes. At the second week of hospitalization, potassium was found to be 3.85 mmol/L and propranolol was started at a dose of 0.5 mg/kg/day. During a further 2 weeks propranolol was gradually increased to a dose of 2 mg/kg/day and a stepwise cessation of salbutamol, furosemide and hydration was managed. The patients had not had any symptoms [12A].

Timolol

Central Nervous System

Light-headedness has been reported as a side effect of intranasal administration ophthalmic timolol used for the treatment of epistaxis associated with hereditary haemorrhagic telangiectasia (HHT). A 59-year-old man presented to the emergency department with light-headedness. He had started intranasal administration of ophthalmic timolol for the prevention of epistaxis associated with HHT approximately 3 weeks earlier with excellent response. His heart rate was about half its normal rate, an ECG revealed sinus bradycardia and it was determined that he had significant cardiac issues in his family history. All other tests were normal. The discontinuation of the intranasal use of timolol resolved any further episodes of light-headedness and bradycardia. It has been found that the patient was an intermediate metaboliser of CYP2D6, the main enzyme contributing to the metabolism of timolol [13A].

INTERACTIONS

Drug–Drug Interactions

Propranolol

LACK OF PHARMACOKINETIC INTERACTION BETWEEN TOPIRAMATE AND PROPRANOL

Three phase-1 open-label studies in healthy subjects investigated the potential for drug–drug interactions between topiramate and diltiazem, hydrochlorothiazide of propranolol. The mean topiramate pharmacokinetic parameters when administered alone or in combination with propranolol at either 40 or 80 mg q12h dose appeared similar, and steady state C_{max} and AUC12 fell within 80–125% limits demonstrating equivalence of topiramate parameters in the presence or absence of propranolol. The authors conclude that plasma topiramate concentrations were increased by coadministration of hydrochlorothiazide, but were unaffected by diltiazem and propranolol. Moreover, topiramate coadministration resulted in a modest reduction in systemic exposure of diltiazem and one of its metabolites (desacetyl diltiazem), but did not affect hydrochlorothiazide of propranolol pharmacokinetics. Overall, no safety concern emerged when topiramate was administered with diltiazem, hydrochlorothiazide or propranolol [14c].

LONG-TERM EFFECTS

Drug Misuse

MEDICATION ERROR ASSOCIATE WITH THE USE OF BETA-BLOCKERS

A retrospective data analysis in Pakistan outpatient beta-blocker users identified 1627 medication errors in 450 prescriptions. During the study period (June 2011–June 2012) the 450 prescription containing beta-blockers were analyzed for the essential elements to be mentioned in prescription. Drug–drug interaction was analyzed by the Micromedex 2.0 DRUG-REAX Database and severity of medication errors by NCCMERP Index. Among the 1627 medication errors identified, the most frequent errors were lack of patient's weight (95%), missing of diagnosis (79.4%) and drug–drug interactions (69.5%). There was an association with number of drug prescriptions and in prescription written in outpatient setting of various hospitals and clinics. Significant differences were reported for those prescription orders having more than five drugs with beta-blockers. The involvement of pharmacists in the health care team could play a role in avoiding these types of medication errors [15c].

POTASSIUM CHANNEL ACTIVATORS

Nicorandil [SED-15, 2505; SEDA-32, 365; SEDA-33, 400; SEDA-34, 305; SEDA-35, 353; SEDA-36, 270]

Hematologic

Methaemoglobinaemia has been attributed to nicorandil in an elderly patient with chronic stable angina. A 75-year-old male patient on treatment with nicorandil at therapeutic dosage for chronic stable angina consulted his physician because he noticed that his fingernails had developed a bluish tinge. Following an accurate diagnostic and pharmacological assessment, and the exclusion of a cardiorespiratory causation of the cyanosis, the possibility of methaemoglobinaemia was considered (co-oximetry test = 8.7%) and nicorandil was theorized as being the potential cause. No specific therapy was undertaken, but nicorandil was omitted from the drug regime. Six weeks later the methaemoglobinaemia had decreased to 3.7% and the bluish discoloration was not perceptible. As methaemoglobinaemia can occur several years after administration of nitrates, regular checks for pseudocyanosis are prudent [16A].

Sensory System

A 78-year-old man experienced corneal ulceration at a second cataract surgery (right eye) while being treated with nicorandil for 3 years. Four years before, she had had an uneventful first cataract intervention (left eye). The lesion was not explained by mechanical, inflammatory infectious or local causes. No pathogen was found and corneal scraping for direct examination and culture was negative. Nicorandil was suspended and the patient underwent weekly medical supervision. After 6 weeks of a complete healing, disappearance of symptoms and improved visual acuity (20/40) was obtained. Nicorandil was not reintroduced. While the pathogenesis of nicorandil ulcerations is not yet clear, a recent hypothesis suggested that chemical ulceration is based on the effects of nicotinamide coupled with the direct ulcerating effects of nicotinic acid [17A].

CALCIUM CHANNEL BLOCKERS [SED-15, 598; SEDA-32, 366; SEDA-33, 401; SEDA-34, 306; SEDA-35, 354; SEDA-36, 270]

Cardiovascular

FLUSHING, PERIPHERAL EDEMA, HEADACHE

A surveillance program showed in 11 918 Japanese patients that vasodilation-related symptoms occurred significantly more frequently with dihydropyridines in females than in males (OR 1.28 [1.28–2.71]) and in particular females younger than 50 years complained symptoms more frequently (OR 2.39 [1.02–5.59]) than other age classes [18c].

Breasts

BREAST CANCER

The hypothesis that long-term use of calcium channel blockers increases the risk of breast cancer was revived by a recent case–control study (1900 cases and 856 controls) which showed a 2.4-fold increase in patients taking calcium channel blockers for more than 10 years. Biological mechanisms through which calcium channel blockers could influence breast cancer risk are unknown, though inhibition of apoptosis through increasing intracellular calcium levels has been suggested [18C]. Since the issue is still unsettled, in the presence of controversial results, a meta-analysis including 11 studies has performed: all were retrospective, observational studies. There was no evidence of an association between calcium channel blocker use and increased risk of breast cancer [19R].

Mouth and Teeth

GINGIVAL OVERGROWTH

Calcium channel blockers have been found to be responsible for a benign adverse reaction, gingival enlargement or overgrowth; reports on almost all types of calcium channel blockers can be found in the literature. The adverse reaction that can be serious can be managed by withdrawal of the drug and substitution with other classes of antihypertensive agents. Changing from one calcium channel blocker to another at lower risk may not be as effective, while in other cases lesions can be managed by nonsurgical or surgical methods, which provide usually short-term relief [20R].

Amlodipine [SED-15, 175; SEDA-32, 367; SEDA-33, 401; SEDA-34, 307; SEDA-35, 354; SEDA-36, 270]

Cardiovascular

PURPURA

A 60-year-old woman developed multiple petechiae and purpura on her right arm upon use of a tourniquet for blood drawing; she was receiving amlodipine 5 mg/day for hypertension. Purpura gradually disappeared within a week after amlodipine was substituted by enalapril and dihydrochlorothiazide [21c].

Hypertension

Allogeneic hematopoietic stem cell transplant requires chemotherapy with tacrolimus and cyclosporine A which can lead to worsening or *de novo* hypertension.

A 34-year-old patient, transplanted for acute myelogenous leukemia, was admitted for gastrointestinal symptoms attributable to graph versus host disease; the reaction was treated with 60 mg/8 hours of IV methylprednisolone and symptoms regressed in 5 days. Meanwhile, his blood pressure increased from 116/68 to 156/104 mmHg, and he was given amlodipine 5 mg/day orally. Starting from 2 days after first dose of amlodipine, ALT and AST progressively increased, after diagnostic exams which included liver biopsy, drug toxicity was suspected and after reviewing patient's therapy, amlodipine was suspended and carvedilol started. Liver enzymes normalized rapidly and the patient was discharged from hospital with normal liver function [22c].

Drug Administration

Drug Overdose

An 18-year-old girl was referred to the hospital after ingestion of 17 tables of a fixed dose combination of amlodipine 5 mg and atenolol 50 mg; heart rate was 130 bpm and pressure 70/50 mmHg, serum creatinine 1.9 mg/dL, arterial pH 7.31. No overt signs of beta-blocker toxicity such as conduction blocks or bradycardia were observed. After gastric lavage, norepinephrine and calcium gluconate were infused IV and oxygen was supplemented. The patient recovered completely 8 days later [23A].

Nicardipine [SED-15, 2502; SEDA-32, 367; SEDA-33, 402; SEDA-34, 308; SEDA-35, 355; SEDA-36, 271]

Respiratory
PULMONARY EDEMA

Nicardipine is used sometimes to delay preterm labor, given the reports of calcium channel blockers associated to pulmonary edema in mothers treated for preterm delivery, the French pharmacovigilance database was searched and 217 reports on IV nicardipine were reviewed. Pulmonary edema was reported in 23 women: all recovered after discontinuation of nicardipine and symptomatic treatment [24R].

Nifedipine [SED-15, 2516; SEDA-33, 402; SEDA-34, 308; SEDA-35, 355; SEDA-36, 271]

Cardiovascular
INTESTINAL OBSTRUCTION

Nifedipine is a widely used drug which has a short elimination half-life and for this reason is marketed as sustained-release formulation, among them the so-called GITS (gastrointestinal therapeutic system), for which cases of intestinal occlusion have been reported.

A retrospective population-based Canadian study in 103 657 patients newly treated with extended release nifedipine could not show any difference in risk of bowel obstruction with the group treated with amlodipine (0.6% vs 0.6%) [25C].

SEVERE HYPOTENSION

Nifedipine is widely used as a tocolytic, since it is well tolerated and inexpensive, nonetheless it should be considered that it can cause severe hypotension. A 18-year-old woman presented with risk of preterm delivery at 24 weeks of gestation; she was given a loading dose of 10 mg of oral nifedipine every 15 minutes, four times. After 2.5 hours her heart rate was 135 bpm and pressure 88/43 mmHg. The hypotension and tachycardia worsened constantly up to 7 hours after the first dose of nifedipine, when emergency caesarean section for delivery was performed, with rapid complete resolution of the clinical condition [26C].

Respiratory
PULMONARY EDEMA

Pulmonary edema during tocolysis with β2-agonists has been reported, but it appears to be less frequent with calcium channel blockers. A 38-year-old mother with 27-week twin pregnancy received 20 mg/6 hours and betamethasone 12 mg/day IV to improve fetal organ maturity. She was also infused 1 L of dextrose/saline solution. On the second day she developed tachycardia and hypotension (90/50 mmHg) and breathlessness; at chest X-ray pulmonary edema was diagnosed, which resolved in a few hours upon appropriate treatment [27A]. Although the course of the patient is suggestive of a role of nifedipine, the development of acute diastolic dysfunction as a consequence of volume overload may have contributed.

Verapamil [SED-15, 3618; SEDA-32, 367; SEDA-33, 403; SEDA-34, 308; SEDA-35, 356; SEDA-36, 272]

Drug Administration
DRUG OVERDOSE

A Case of Hypocalcemia Following Overdose of Verapamil and a Review Published A 37-year-old woman presented to Emergency Department with a chief compliant of chest pain 12 hours after ingesting five tablets of an unknown dose of verapamil. Her initial serum electrolytes were notable for a creatinine of 1.24 mg/dL (previously 1.0 mg/dL) and a calcium of 9.3 mg/dL (range of normal value = 8.6–10.5 mg/dL). After admission to cardiology ward, morning laboratory results 48 hours after verapamil overdose ingestion showed calcium of 5.5 mg/dL. A verapamil level was not obtained because the laboratory did not have this capability. The serum calcium concentration returned in the normal rage 56 hours after verapamil overdose ingestion and after 3750 mg of calcium gluconate. After the case description, a literature review of calcium channel blockers overdose effects has been reported. Although the most common severe symptoms include bradycardia and hypotension, and calcium channel blockers overdose pose a risk of significant morbidity and mortality, serum calcium should be closely monitored in these patients [28c].

NON-CARDIOGENIC PULMONARY EDEMA AND LIFE-THREATENING SHOCK

A case of massive intentional overdose of multiple medications including sustained-release verapamil has been reported. The patient developed a severe acute respiratory distress syndrome related to non-cardiogenic pulmonary edema and aspiration pneumonia. He was resistant to conventional support including fluid replacement, vasopressor and inotropic agent, and required mechanical ventilation, hyperinsulinemia–euglycemia, glucagon, intravenous calcium and bicarbonate, activate charcoal and intravenous lipid therapy. The mechanism of the non-cardiogenic pulmonary edema is not well known, but a possible mechanism is pre-capillary transudation. The reported case was successfully treated with lung-protective mechanical ventilation and was liberated from ventilator in 7 days [29C]. Furthermore, the authors provide a review of the mechanism and treatment of calcium channel blockers overdose.

PERIPORTAL EDEMA

A 41-year-old man with a history of diabetes mellitus and hypertension was admitted to Emergency Department with changes in consciousness, with a heart rate of 22 beats/min, a weak carotid pulse, respiration of 8 breaths/min and a Glasgow coma score of 3. Soon after arrival pulseless electrical activity cardiac arrest occurred. Circulation was restored after 2 minutes of cardiopulmonary resuscitation and one bolus dose of 1 mg IV adrenaline. After abdominal CT was evidenced a hypodense area around the portal veins of both lobes of the liver, compatible with periportal edema, dilated inferior vena cava, minimal ascites and marked submucosal edema of gallbladder wall. It was ascertained that the patient attempted suicide and claimed to have ingested 15 sustained-release tablets containing 240 mg of verapamil hydrochloride. The patient attained a complete recovery. Periportal edema is a compensatory increased flow of hepatic lymph due to hepatic lymphatic obstruction or fluid overload. It has rarely been reported after cardiac arrest. In this case, the increase in mediastinal pressure during cardiopulmonary resuscitation,

centralization of blood volume secondary to shock and vigorous IV fluid resuscitation may be the pathophysiological mechanism that caused periportal edema [30A].

References

[1] Loth DW, Brusselle GG, Lahousse L, et al. β-adrenoceptor blockers and pulmonary function in the general population: the Rotterdam Study. Br J Clin Pharmacol. 2014;77(1):190–200 [C].

[2] Morales DR, Jackson C, Lipworth BJ, et al. Adverse respiratory effect of acute β-blocker exposure in asthma: a systematic review and meta-analysis of randomized controlled trials. Chest. 2014;145(4):779–86 [M].

[3] Kapitein B, Biesmans RCG, van der Sijs H, et al. Propylene glycol-related delirium after esmolol infusion. Ann Pharmacother. 2014;48(7):940–2 [c].

[4] Ersbøll AS, Hedegaard M, Søndergaard L, et al. Treatment with oral beta-blockers during pregnancy complicated by maternal heart disease increases the risk of fetal growth restriction. BJOG. 2014;121(5):618–26 [C].

[5] Xie RH, Guo Y, Krewski D, et al. Beta-blockers increase the risk of being born small for gestational age or of being institutionalised during infancy. BJOG. 2014;121(9):1090–6 [C].

[6] Mandorfer M, Bota S, Schwabl P, et al. Non selective beta blockers increase risk for hepatorenal syndrome and death in patients with cirrhosis and spontaneous bacterial peritonitis. Gastroenterology. 2014;146(7):1680–90 [A].

[7] Lin L, Wang Y, Chen Y, et al. Bradyarrhythmias secondary to topical levobunolol hydrochloride solution. Clin Interv Aging. 2014;9:1741–5 [A].

[8] Bayar N, Arslan Ş, Çağırcı G, et al. Extreme bradycardia associated with nebivolol therapy. Int J Cardiol. 2014;177(1):e29–31 [r].

[9] Sullo MG, Perri D, Sibilio M, et al. Hypoglycemia, polycythemia and hyponatremia in a newborn exposed to nebivolol during pregnancy. J Pharmacol Pharmacother. 2015;6(1):45–8. [A].

[10] Bonifazi E, Milano A, Foti C. Allergic contact dermatitis caused by topical propranolol in a 5-month-old baby. Contact Dermatitis. 2014;71(4):250–1. [A].

[11] Admani S, Feldstein S, Gonzalez EM, et al. Beta blockers: an innovation in the treatment of infantile hemangiomas. J Clin Aesthet Dermatol. 2014;7(7):37–45 [R].

[12] Belen B, Oguz A, Okur A, et al. A complication to be aware of: hyperkalaemia following propranolol therapy for an infant with intestinal haemangiomatosis. BMJ Case Rep. 2014; http://dx.doi.org/10.1136/bcr-2014-203746 [A].

[13] Epperla N, Brilliant MH, Vidaillet H. Topical timolol for treatment of epistaxis in hereditary haemorrhagic telangiectasia associated with bradycardia: a look at CYP2D6 metabolising variants. BMJ Case Rep. 2014 Feb 11;2014. pii: bcr2013203056. http://dx.doi.org/10.1136/bcr-2013-203056 [A].

[14] Nesar S, Shoaib MH, Yousuf RI, et al. Incidence of medication error associated with the use of beta-blockers in Pakistan. Pak J Pharm Sci. 2014;27(3):531–6 [c].

[15] Manitpisitkul P, Curtin CR, Shalayda K, et al. Pharmacokinetic interaction between topiramate and diltiazem, hydrochlorothiazide, or propranolol. Clin Pharmacol Drug Dev. 2014;3(5):378–87 [c].

[16] Trechot F, Batta B, Petitpain N, et al. A case of nicorandil-induced unilateral corneal ulceration. Int Wound J. 2013;11(3):238–9 [A].

[17] Ekanayaka RAI. A case of pseudocyanosis. BMJ Case Rep. 2014; http://dx.doi.org/10.1136/bcr-2013-201915 [A].

[18] Kajiwara A, Saruwatari J, Kita A, et al. Younger females are at greater risk of vasodilation-related adverse symptoms

caused by dihydropyridine calcium channel blockers: results of a study of 11,918 Japanese patients. Clin Drug Investig. 2014;34(6):431–5 [c].

[19] Chen Q, Zhang Q, Zhong F, et al. Association between calcium channel blockers and breast cancer: a meta-analysis of observational studies. Pharmacoepidemiol Drug Saf. 2014;23(7):711–8 [R].

[20] Livada R, Shiloah J. Calcium channel blocker-induced gingival enlargement. J Hum Hypertens. 2014;28(1):10–4 [R].

[21] Balamurugesan K, Viswanathan S. Rumpel-leede phenomenon in a hypertensive lady on amlodipine. J Clin Diagn Res. 2014;8(4): YD01–2 [c].

[22] Hammerstrom AE. Possible amlodipine-induced hepatotoxicity after stem cell transplant. Ann Pharmacother. 2015;49(1):135–9 [c].

[23] Naha K, Suryanarayana J, Aziz RA, et al. Amlodipine poisoning revisited: acidosis, acute kidney injury and acute respiratory distress syndrome. Indian J Crit Care Med. 2014;18(7):467–9 [A].

[24] Nicardipine and preterm labour: pulmonary oedema. Prescrire Int. 2014;23(146):44 [r].

[25] Juurlink DN, Hellings C, Gomes T, et al. Extended-release nifedipine and the risk of intestinal obstruction: a population-based study. BMJ Open. 2014;4:e005377. http://dx.doi.org/10.1136/bmjopen-2014-005377 [C].

[26] Koo F, Mathur M. Severe resistant maternal hypotension following tocolysis with nifedipine. BMJ Case Rep. 2014; http://dx.doi.org/10.1136/bcr-2014-208059 [c].

[27] Girwalkar-Bagle A, Deshpande S, John J. Nifedipine induced pulmonary edema. Anaesth Pain & Intensive Care. 2014;18: 207–8 [A].

[28] Price D, Radke J, Albertson T. Hypocalcaemia after an occult calcium channel blocker overdose: a case report and literature review. Basic Clin Pharmacol Toxicol. 2014;114:217–21 [c].

[29] Siddiqi TA, Hill J, Uckleberry Y, et al. Non-cardiogenic pulmonary edema and life-threatening shock due to calcium channel blocker overdose: a case report and clinical review. Respir Care. 2014;59: e15–21 [c].

[30] Lu HC, Chen JD, How CH. Periportal edema after cardiac arrest due to calcium channel blocker overdose. J Formos Med Assoc. 2014;113:266–7 [A].

19

Drugs Acting on the Cerebral and Peripheral Circulations

Arduino A. Mangoni[1]

Department of Clinical Pharmacology, School of Medicine, Flinders University and Flinders Medical Centre,
Bedford Park, SA, Australia
[1]Corresponding author: arduino.mangoni@flinders.edu.au

DRUGS USED IN THE TREATMENT OF ARTERIAL DISORDERS OF THE BRAIN AND LIMBS AND IN THE TREATMENT OF MIGRAINE

Ergotamine [SEDA-36, 276] and Triptans [SEDA-36, 277]

Cardiovascular and Nervous System

A systematic review assessed the risk of serious cardiovascular events associated with use of either ergotamine or triptans in patients with migraine in observational studies [1M]. From a total of 3370 citations, only 4 studies met the inclusion criteria: cohort or case–control studies investigating the risk of any serious cardiovascular outcome in patients with migraine exposed to at least a triptan or an ergotamine compound. These studies investigated either the intensity (number of prescribed/dispensed doses) or the recency of exposure. When assessing intensity of exposure, the pooled odds ratio (OR) of serious ischaemic events was 2.28 (95% CI 1.18–4.41) for ergotamine and 0.86 (95% CI 0.52–1.43) for triptans. When assessing recency of exposure, only one, non-significant, study was identified for ergotamine. Two studies investigating triptans and risk of stroke reported ORs of 0.90 (95% CI 0.64–1.26) and 2.51 (95% CI 1.10–5.71), respectively. However, the high degree of heterogeneity precluded a pooled analysis [1M]. A systematic review assessed the incidence and type of adverse events associated with the use of triptans in patients with acute cluster headache [2M]. Four studies comparing sumatriptan or zolmitriptan vs. placebo were identified. The incidence of any adverse event was 27–37% with zolmitriptan vs. 15% with placebo, and

34–45% with sumatriptan vs. 16–19% with placebo. Most adverse events were rated as mild or moderate in intensity, largely consisting of localised reactions around the injection site with subcutaneous sumatriptan [2M]. There is no available evidence to support the potential role of pharmacogenetic factors on the reported associations between ergotamine and triptans and these adverse events.

Case

A 35-year-old female, heavy smoker, presented with a two-day history of worsening left foot pain and pallor [3A]. She had received a single 1 g dose of azithromycin 4 days earlier because of a genital infection. Doppler ultrasound was suggestive of acute arterial embolism. After heparin infusion was started the patient underwent emergency arterial embolectomy. During the procedure there was evidence of diffuse narrowing of the femoral artery, however, no thromboemboli were detected. Following further discussion with the patient it emerged that she was a long-term ergotamine user for migraine. Ergotamine treatment was stopped, and clinical findings and the vasospasm resolved after 5 days [3A].

Urinary Tract

A 22-year-old female on long-term treatment with ergotamine 2–4 mg daily because of chronic intermittent headache presented with severe headache, nausea and vomiting [4A]. She had a family history of hypertension but no other significant medical history apart from a ruptured ovarian cyst. Physical examination was unremarkable apart from high temperature and blood pressure 240/140 mmHg in both arms. Laboratory tests showed

© 2015 Elsevier B.V. All rights reserved.

serum creatinine 3.8 mg/dL (0.8 mg/dL 2 months earlier), urea 32 mg/dL, leukocytes 17 300/mm^3, haemoglobin 10.8 mg/dL and erythrocyte sedimentation rate 40 mm/h. Urinalysis showed 15 leukocytes/mm^3, four red blood cells/mm^3 and no proteinuria. Further blood tests and abdominal imaging did not reveal any significant abnormality. However, a renal biopsy demonstrated acute tubulointerstitial nephritis with glomerular ischaemic changes and vascular changes suggestive of nephrosclerosis [4A]. Symptoms, blood pressure and renal function progressively improved with blood pressure lowering agents and prednisolone 60 mg/day. Serum creatinine was 2.2 mg/dL after 6 weeks and 1.6 mg/dL after 6 months, respectively. It is unclear, however, whether ergotamine was continued or stopped after the histological diagnosis of acute tubulointerstitial nephritis.

SECOND GENERATION EFFECTS

Pregnancy and Teratogenicity

Using national databases, associations were investigated between prescribing of four triptans (sumatriptan, rizatriptan, eletriptan and zolmitriptan) and the incidence of congenital malformations and adverse pregnancy outcomes in Norway between 2004 and 2007 [5C]. The Norwegian prescription database was linked to the Medical Birth Registry of Norway. The latter provides information on pregnancy, delivery and maternal and neonatal health outcomes, based on the International Classification of Diseases, 10th Revision. Of the 181 125 women identified, 1465 (0.8%) redeemed treatment with triptans during pregnancy, 1095 (0.6%) before pregnancy only (disease comparison group), whereas the remaining 178 565 represented the population comparison. No significant associations were observed between triptan redemption during pregnancy and congenital malformations. However, there was an association between redemption in the second trimester and post-partum haemorrhage (adjusted OR 1.57, 95% CI 1.10–2.07). Further associations were observed in the disease comparison group with major congenital malformations (adjusted OR 1.48, 95% CI 1.11–1.97), low birth weight (adjusted OR 1.39, 95% CI 1.08–1.81) and pre-term birth (adjusted OR 1.30, 95% CI 1.06–1.60) [5C]. It remains to be established whether the reported associations are primarily related to the use of triptans, migraine severity, or pharmacogenetic factors.

Ginkgo biloba [SEDA-36, 276]

Tumorigenicity

Mutations, alterations in pathways associated with cancer development and global gene expression were investigated in hepatocellular carcinoma cells (B6C3F1 mice) treated with Ginkgo biloba leaf extract vs. spontaneous liver tumour cells [6E]. Two-year exposure of male and female B6C3F1 mice to 200, 600 and 2000 mg/kg Ginkgo biloba leaf extract 5 days/week resulted in dose-related hepatocellular hypertrophy, focal necrosis and increased incidence of hepatocellular adenomas and carcinomas. Compared to spontaneous hepatocellular carcinoma cells, treatment with Ginkgo biloba leaf extract was associated with alterations in H-ras and Ctnnb1 mutation spectra and dysregulation of the WNT signalling pathway. Furthermore, treatment with Ginkgo biloba leaf extract induced alterations of gene expression associated with oncogenesis, development of hepatocellular carcinoma and chronic xenobiotic and oxidative stress [6E].

Cytotoxicity and Mutagenicity

The toxic effects of three ginkgolic acids with different alkyl or alkenyl groups (13:0, 15:1, 17:1) were assessed in male Chinese hamster lung fibroblasts (V79 cells) and in Salmonella typhimurium strains (TA97a, TA98, TA100 and TA102) [7E]. Statistically significant reductions in V79 cell survival were observed with 13:0 (starting at a concentration of 25 µM), 15:1 (50 µM) and 17:1 (100 µM). However, no significant mutagenic effects were observed [7E].

Genotoxicity

The in vitro genotoxicity of Ginkgo biloba leaf extract (0.2–1.2 mg/mL) and its eight constituents (quercetin, quercetin-3-β-D-glucoside, kaempferol, isorhamnetin, ginkgolide A, ginkgolide B, ginkgolide C and bilobalide) was investigated in two cell assays, mouse lymphoma L5178Y cells and Comet [8E]. Ginkgo biloba leaf extract, and two of its constituents (quercetin and kaempferol), increased mutant frequency and DNA double-strand breaks in a dose-dependent fashion. This was associated with increased expression of γ-H2AX and phosphorylated Chk2 and Chk1. Ginkgo biloba leaf extract also stimulated the production of reactive oxygen species and reduced glutathione concentrations in L5178Y cells. There was evidence of extensive chromosomal damage with Ginkgo biloba leaf extract, quercetin or kaempferol [8E].

Hematologic

A 55-year old Chinese hypertensive woman presented with a 2-day history of jaundice, epigastric pain, general malaise and headache [9A]. Regular medications included nifedipine 60 mg/day, telmisartan 80 mg/day and atenolol 50 mg/day. Family history included a sister and a niece with glucose-6-phosphate dehydrogenase deficiency; however, she had not been tested for this. Three days before admission, she had received a single injection of Ginkgo biloba leaf extract 17.5 mg in a local dementia clinic for memory enhancement. She did not eat fava beans or take aspirin in the days prior to admission. Laboratory tests revealed acute haemolytic anaemia with haemoglobin 5.5 g/dL (normal range 11.3–15.3 g/dL), glucose-6-phosphate dehydrogenase deficiency, increased lactate dehydrogenase, decreased haptoglobin and increased total bilirubin concentrations. Both symptoms and laboratory abnormalities improved with volume repletion and supportive measures, while continuing her antihypertensive drugs, and she was discharged after 5 days. On follow-up 2 weeks later, she was asymptomatic with haemoglobin of 10.1 g/dL [9A]. Previous studies have suggested that *Ginkgo biloba* extracts might induce red blood cell damage *in vitro* by increasing cell fragility and by inducing glutathione depletion and methaemoglobin formation, particularly at high concentrations ($\geq$25 µg/mL) [10E]. The potential contribution of genetic factors remains unknown.

DRUGS USED IN THE TREATMENT OF VENOUS DISORDERS

Benzbromarone [SEDA-36, 276]

Liver

A study investigated the molecular mechanisms responsible for benzbromarone hepatocellular toxicity [11E]. Benzbromarone 25–50 µM for 24–48 h caused a reduction in ATP concentrations in HepG2 cells and primary human hepatocytes. Higher doses, 100 µM, induced both apoptosis and necrosis. In HepG2 cells, benzbromarone 50 µM decreased the mitochondrial membrane potential, induced mitochondrial uncoupling and decreased ATP turnover and maximal respiration. These effects were associated with a concomitant increase in lactate concentrations, suggesting enhanced glycolysis to compensate for ATP reduction, and increased reactive oxygen species. In HepG2 cells and isolated mitochondria, benzbromarone also reduced the metabolism of palmitic acid by inhibiting the long-chain acyl-CoA synthetase [11E].

Diosmin

Cardiovascular

A 55-year-old Caucasian woman with history of hypertension presented with leg oedema [12A]. Regular medications included amiloride 5 mg/day and hydrochlorothiazide 50 mg/day. Venous Doppler documented right ostial saphenofemoral incompetence and she was started on diosmin 450 mg twice daily. After 5 days of treatment with diosmin, she started to complain of worsening leg pain and myalgia. On day 7, she stopped diosmin and her myalgias disappeared after further 3 days. At day 29, she decided to restart treatment with diosmin at the same dose. Her myalgias reappeared, and she stopped treatment 2 days later. After further 3 days, laboratory tests documented raised serum creatine kinase concentrations (1500 IU/L, normal range 39–308 IU/L). There was no report of strenuous exercise over this period. Electrocardiogram and echocardiogram were both normal. She was not taking other medicines or herbal supplements. Two months after stopping diosmin serum creatine kinase concentrations returned within the normal range (180 IU/L) [12A]. A 77-year-old Caucasian man with history of hypertension was prescribed diosmin 900 mg three times daily, topical nifedipine 0.3 g and lidocaine hydrochloride 1.5 g for haemorrhoids. The only regular medication was amlodipine 10 mg/day. Although haemorrhoid-related symptoms disappeared after 10 days of treatment, the patient continued treatment with diosmin for further 21 days. Routine blood tests, performed shortly thereafter, documented increased lactate dehydrogenase concentrations (1100 IU/L, normal range 240–480 IU/L). The latter returned within normal range (265 IU/L) after 1 month [12A]. Previous reports have shown that diosmetin, diosmin's active metabolite, inhibits amine reuptake at the peripheral sympathetic nerve terminals, potentially leading to vasoconstriction [13E]. Moreover, diosmin has also been shown to inhibit catechol-O-methyltransferase activity in the venous wall, with reduced metabolism of noradrenaline. The authors speculate that the combination of arterial and venous vasoconstriction might lead to ischaemic muscle damage, with consequent increase in creatine kinase and lactate dehydrogenase concentrations [12A]. The potential role of genetic predisposition remains to be established.

OTHER PERIPHERAL VASODILATORS

Phosphodiesterase Type 5 Inhibitors [SEDA-36, 277]

Sensory Systems

A 37-year-old African American woman with sickle cell anaemia, pulmonary arterial hypertension, multiple pulmonary embolisms, type 2 diabetes and hypertension presented with a diagnosis of acute chest syndrome [15A]. One day later, she complained of sudden bilateral loss of vision. She had been on tadalafil 40 mg daily for the last 4 weeks for the treatment of pulmonary arterial hypertension, resulting from multiple sickle cell vaso-occlusive crises. Fundi examination revealed a cherry-red spot at the macula of each eye, indicative of central retinal artery occlusion. Fluorescein angiography showed delayed transit time with areas of blocked fluorescence secondary to retinal oedema. Furthermore, spectral-domain optical coherence tomography demonstrated inner retinal oedema in the macula [15A]. Although the patient was started on tadalafil 4 weeks before this complication, she had other risk factors for central retinal artery occlusion, i.e., sickle cell disease, hypertension and type 2 diabetes.

Liver

The effects of tadalafil on hepatic glucose homeostasis and output were investigated in the isolated perfused rat liver [14E]. Tadalafil concentrations up to 10 µM did not exert any significant effect on oxygen consumption, glucose release and synthesis of either lactate or pyruvate. However, when cAMP was administered at 10 min perfusion time, tadalafil 2.5–10 µM at 30 min led to a progressive reduction in glucose output. At 50 min perfusion time, i.e., after 20 min tadalafil infusion, the cAMP-induced glucose release was nearly abolished. Notably, the inhibitory effects on glucose release persisted 20 min after cessation of tadalafil infusion. Co-administration of glucagone 1 nM did not have any impact on the negative effects of tadalafil on glucose output. The concentrations of tadalafil causing half-maximal inhibition of cAMP- and glucagon-stimulated glucose release, 0.46 ± 0.04 and 1.07 ± 0.16 µM, respectively, are similar to plasma peak concentrations in humans following a 20 mg oral dose. Furthermore, tadalafil reduced glycogen phosphorylase activity and increased glucose-6-phosphatase, glucokinase, pyruvate kinase and glucose-6-phosphate dehydrogenase activities [14E]. The authors speculate that, even in the presence of phosphodiesterase inhibition, tadalafil-induced reduction in glucose output is the result of altered glycogen phosphorylase activity and/or increased futile cycling of glucose-6-phosphate and glucose with concomitant increased flow of hexose units in cellular metabolic pathways.

Immunologic

A 30-year-old male presented with recurrent red spots on the skin and genitalia over a period of 6 months [16A]. The only associated symptom was mild pruritus. Clinical examination revealed an isolated erythematous patch on the penile shaft. The lesion disappeared with a short-term treatment with topical steroids. Further disseminated patches on the penis, forearm and periorbital region also responded with topical steroids, but were also associated with the new onset of erosions in the buccal mucosa and the hard palate. Thorough medical history revealed that the onset of the recurring skin and mucosal lesions was always preceded by recreational use of tadalafil. The patient history is suggestive of tadalafil-induced fixed drug eruptions [16A]. The potential role of pharmacogenetic factors remains to be established.

References

[1] Roberto G, Raschi E, Piccinni C, et al. Adverse cardiovascular events associated with triptans and ergotamines for treatment of migraine: systematic review of observational studies. Cephalalgia. 2015;35(2):118–31 [M].

[2] Law S, Derry S, Moore RA. Triptans for acute cluster headache. Cochrane Database Syst Rev. 2013;7:CD008042 [M].

[3] Adam G, Kurt T, Cinar C, et al. Ergotamine-induced vasospastic ischemia mimicking arterial embolism: unusual case. Ulus Travma Acil Cerrahi Derg. 2014;20(4):291–4 [A].

[4] Pakfetrat M, Rasekhi A, Eftekhari F, et al. Ergotamine-induced acute tubulo-interstitial nephritis. Saudi J Kidney Dis Transpl. 2013;24(5):981–3 [A].

[5] Nezvalova-Henriksen K, Spigset O, Nordeng H. Triptan safety during pregnancy: a Norwegian population registry study. Eur J Epidemiol. 2013;28(9):759–69 [C].

[6] Hoenerhoff MJ, Pandiri AR, Snyder SA, et al. Hepatocellular carcinomas in B6C3F1 mice treated with Ginkgo biloba extract for two years differ from spontaneous liver tumors in cancer gene mutations and genomic pathways. Toxicol Pathol. 2013;41(6):826–41 [E].

[7] Berg K, Braun C, Krug I, et al. Evaluation of the cytotoxic and mutagenic potential of three ginkgolic acids. Toxicology. 2015;327:47–52 [E].

[8] Lin H, Guo X, Zhang S, et al. Mechanistic evaluation of Ginkgo biloba leaf extract-induced genotoxicity in L5178Y cells. Toxicol Sci. 2014;139(2):338–49 [E].

[9] Lai SW, Chen JH, Kao WY. Acute hemolytic anemia in glucose-6-phosphate dehydrogenase deficiency complicated by Ginkgo biloba. Acta Haematol. 2013;130(4):288–90 [A].

[10] He J, Lin J, Li J, et al. Dual effects of Ginkgo biloba leaf extract on human red blood cells. Basic Clin Pharmacol Toxicol. 2009;104(2):138–44 [E].

[11] Felser A, Lindinger PW, Schnell D, et al. Hepatocellular toxicity of benzbromarone: effects on mitochondrial function and structure. Toxicology. 2014;324:136–46 [E].

[12] Milano G, Leone S, Fucile C, et al. Uncommon serum creatine phosphokinase and lactic dehydrogenase increase during diosmin therapy: two case reports. J Med Case Rep. 2014;8:194 [A].

[13] Sher E, Codignola A, Biancardi E, et al. Amine uptake inhibition by diosmin and diosmetin in human neuronal and neuroendocrine cell lines. Pharmacol Res. 1992;26(4):395–402 [E].

[14] Vilela VR, de Oliveira AL, Comar JF, et al. Tadalafil inhibits the cAMP stimulated glucose output in the rat liver. Chem Biol Interact. 2014;220:1–11 [E].

[15] Murthy RK, Perez L, Priluck JC, et al. Acute, bilateral, concurrent central retinal artery occlusion in sickle cell disease after use of tadalafil (Cialis). JAMA Ophthalmol. 2013;131(11):1471–3 [E].

[16] Bjekic M, Markovic M, Sipetic S. Fixed drug eruption caused by tadalafil—case report. An Bras Dermatol. 2013;88(4):617–9 [A].

20

Antihypertensive Drugs

Nazeer Ahmed[1], Ashley Martinelli, Catherine Kiruthi

Department of Pharmacy, Johns Hopkins Bayview Medical Center, Baltimore, MD, USA
[1]Corresponding author: nahmed3@jhmi.edu

ANGIOTENSIN-CONVERTING ENZYME INHIBITORS [SED-15, 226; SEDA-33, 416; SEDA-34, 321; SEDA-35,364, SEDA-36, 282]

General Information

Angiotensin-converting enzyme inhibitors (ACEIs) have been shown to possess chemoprotective properties in a majority of the studies. An elevated risk of cancer has been noted patients taking Angiotensin II Receptor Blockers (ARBs) in meta-analysis of trials but these trials were not designed to assess cancer risk. A retrospective cohort study investigated the relationship between ACEIs, ARBs and cancer risk in patients with high drug compliance (over 80%). The results indicate that patients on ACEIs had an overall lower risk of developing cancer. ACEIs are thought to exert their protective effect by reducing the degradation of angiotensin I to angiotensin II. ARBs block type I angiotensin II receptor which is anticarcinogenic [1c].

Cardiovascular

A 51-year-old female was admitted with swollen tongue from taking an ACEI to which she had a reaction of angioedema about 5 months prior. She was advised never to take an ACEI again but later resumed the medication despite medical advice. She was intubated due to vocal cord and arytenoid edema. Her temperature was 36.7 °C, pulse rate was 80 beats per minute, blood pressure was 171/84 mmHg and oxygen saturation was 98% in room air. Her electrocardiogram showed deep T-wave inversion in the anterolateral leads and had a peak troponin-I level of 0.24 ng/mL leading to the diagnosis of non-ST segment elevation myocardial infarction. Her past medical history included diabetes mellitus, hypertension and tobacco use. She did not have a history of coronary artery disease or cardiomyopathy. Allergic myocardial infarction (Kounis syndrome) was included in her differential diagnosis. She had normal coronaries in her cardiac catheterization. She recovered in 1 week, and was discharged. Many drugs have been implicated as culprits in Kounis syndrome, however, none reported an ACEI. The name of the ACEI was not identified in this report [2A].

Delapril

General Information

Delapril is an ACEI that has been around since late 1980s and is available in a number of European and Asian countries. It has an indanylglycine moiety, differentiating it from captopril or enalapril, making it more lipophilic and thus more effective on ACE inhibition. It has less of an effect on bradykinin potentiation. It is metabolized in the liver into active and inactive metabolites. It has an elimination half-life of up to 3.4 hours with active metabolites and is renally excreted. The incidence of cough with delapril was 5% in one study. The antihypertensive effect of delapril is similar that the obtained with other ACEIs and has reno-protective and cardioprotective actions, with the potential to increase insulin sensitivity in hypertensive type 2 diabetic patients [3R].

Lisinopril [SED-15, 2071; SEDA-33, 418; SEDA-34,324; SEDA-35, 367, SEDA-36, 282]

Mouth and Teeth

Lisinopril contains a thiol group which has been reported to be involved in drug-induced pemphigus. Previously reported cases include the skin changes without mucosal involvement. Oral bullous eruption was reported with lisinopril in a case report in which a 78-year-old female suffered blisters and ulcers in vestibular, buccal, upper and lower jaw mucosa 3 weeks after taking

© 2015 Elsevier B.V. All rights reserved.

lisinopril. She had been taking amlodipine for a year without any complications. The oral lesions resolved in a month with topical therapy and withdrawal of lisinopril [4A].

Drug Interactions

A 58-year-old female suffered angioedema while undergoing treatment for metastatic clear-cell renal cell cancer with everolimus. She had also been on lisinopril for hypertension for a year prior to starting everolimus. With increasing use of everolimus in oncologic treatment, using alternative antihypertensives other than ACEI may be warranted [5A].

ANGIOTENSIN RECEPTOR BLOCKERS/ ANGIOTENSIN II RECEPTOR ANTAGONISTS [SEDA-15, 2071; SEDA-34, 324; SEDA-35; SEDA-36, 282]

General Information

Acute toxicity from exposure to ARBs was assessed in an observational case series. The ARBs reported in 206 cases included candesartan, eprosartan, irbesartan, losartan, olmesartan, telmisartan and valsartan. Out of the acute toxicities reported in 150 children, only one required intervention for a blood pressure of 60/40 mmHg for a 2.5 year old who ingested an 8.75-fold maximum daily dose based on weight. The authors reported that 16.7% of patients experienced mild symptoms including hypotension, fatigue, dizziness, nausea, vomiting and somnolence. Moderate to severe symptoms were reported in 8.9% of patients including syncope, coma and/or pronounced hypotension. There were no reports of acute toxicities of less than fivefold of the maximum daily dose based on weight. The study concluded that patients with accidental overdose must be evaluated thoroughly. Since ingestion of less than a fivefold of the maximum daily dose (MDD) yielded no severe symptoms, only symptomatic patients and those who have ingested a greater than fivefold of the MDD should be referred for medical assessment [6c].

Drug–Drug Interactions

A French pharmacovigilance study assessed the reported adverse drug reactions (ADRs) associated with concomitant use of nonsteroidal anti-inflammatory drugs (NSAIDs) with antihypertensive agents. Of the 81 084 ADRs reviewed by the authors of the study, 517 reports involved NSAIDS and of those, 125 (24.2%) were related to a drug–drug interaction with an antihypertensive agent. Cardiovascular ADRs such as heart failure, stroke, myocardial infarction, or increased blood pressure were found in 15 (2.9%) of reports, whereas acute

renal failure, hyponatremia, and hyperkalemia was reported in 116 (28.1%) of cases. Acute renal failure occurred in 105 cases (25.4%), and had increasing frequency when used in combination with ACEI/ARB/ diuretics. Nearly half of the cases (43/105) could not be connected to another cause. No particular NSAID was associated more frequently in adverse events. Women were found to be more likely to be exposed to concomitant use of both NSAIDs and antihypertensive agents. The authors advise caution, especially in women, to limit the use of NSAIDs in combination with ACEI/ARB/ diuretics due to an increased risk of renal failure [7c].

Fimasartan [SEDA-36, 283]

Comparative Study

The safety and efficacy of fimasartan were compared to valsartan in a Korean population. While both fimasartan and valsartan significantly decreased blood pressure, fimasartan 60 mg daily reduced diastolic blood pressure more significantly than valsartan 80 mg daily. Fimasartan was well tolerated with the most common side effect being headache in 5% of the patients. Other side effects included dizziness, insomnia, nasopharyngitis, chest pain, diarrhea and elevated alanine aminotransferase. At a higher dose of fimasartan, 120 mg daily, 6.7% of patients experienced a transient increase in alanine aminotransferase [8c].

Irbesartan [SED-15, 1908; SEDA-32, 386; SEDA-36, 371]

Skin

A 52-year-old female presented with asymptomatic diffuse purpuric eruption which had been present for 2 years. Affected areas included the intergluteal, axillary and inguinal folds. Irbesartan and hydrochlorothiazide combination product had been initiated 7 years prior to presentation. The product was discontinued with complete resolution in 9 weeks. The same medication combination was used in another patient, a 78-year-old female, who developed itching and a rash in the gluteal region, which cleared after stopping the drug. The drug was reinitiated 9 months after resolution with no relapse of the rash [9A].

Losartan [SED-15, 2168; SEDA-32, 387; SEDA-33, 419; SEDA-36, 371]

Genetic Factors

Most safety and efficacy studies conducted with losartan were in caucasian populations who may have distinct genetic variations from Asians. The effects of losartan in several Asian populations were recently evaluated in multiple studies involving the use of losartan in various Asian populations. In one study, researchers reported mild adverse reactions (5.8% of cases) in Indian patients. In another study, 11% of Japanese patients developed adverse effects. Chinese patients on losartan exhibited a significant decrease in serum urate levels. That authors suggest that Asian patients may have a genetic predisposition to experience dry cough with ACEI and therefore ARBs may be safer alternative antihypertensive agents [10R].

Olmesartan

Gastrointestinal

Several recent case reports with enteropathy adverse events have been reported recently with olmesartan. In one, a 78-year-old female prescribed and taking olmesartan for 4 years for hypertension presented with severe watery diarrhea over the past 4 months. Her biopsies showed mild villous blunting in the proximal small intestine with intraepithelial lymphocytosis and lamina propria inflammation, thickening of the subepithelial basement membrane, intraepithelial lymphocytosis and lamina propria chronic inflammation with eosinophil infiltration in the terminal ileum. She was diagnosed with celiac-like enteropathy, collagenous ileitis and collagenous colitis. Olmesartan was discontinued as the likely culprit along with atorvastatin and the diarrhea subsequently resolved. Upon re-challenge with olmesartan only, diarrhea returned. Ramipril was then substituted for olmesartan, which provided resolution of diarrhea. A repeat colonoscopy 4 months after initial findings revealed complete resolution of enteropathy-like changes. Given the long time course on olmesartan before presentation, this suggests a cell-mediated reaction [11A].

A 70-year-old female taking olmesartan for 2 years presented with worsening diarrhea, epigastric pain, and a 30 pound weight loss. Celiac tests were negative, computed tomography showed diffuse wall edema and thickening of the jejunum and ileum. After discontinuation of the drug, symptoms improved. Previous cases suggest sprue-like enteropathy with a likely cell-mediated immune response. This is the first case report to describe villous atrophy on push enteroscopy and capsule endoscopy due to olmesartan-induced enteropathy [12A].

A 62-year-old female presented with similar symptoms including abdominal pain, weight loss, and nausea despite following a gluten-free diet. The patient's biopsy findings revealed persistent villous blunting with epithelial lymphocytosis. Olmesartan was discontinued and within 2 months, the patient's symptoms resolved. Olmesartan may have been the reason for development of collagenous sprue [13A].

Sprue-like enteropathy associated with olmesartan use was subsequently found in a 57-year-old woman who initially presented with 3 weeks of nausea, vomiting, and diarrhea. Histological findings of diffuse villous blunting and increased intraepithelial lymphocytes determined this to be consistent with celiac disease or another sprue-like process. The patient's symptoms improved significantly after not receiving olmesartan due to formulary restrictions at a care facility. The symptoms completely resolved within 2 weeks of discharge [14A].

Drug Interactions

Recombinant tissue plasminogen activator (rt-PA) is known to increase the risk of angioedema especially in those using ACEIs. ARBs are generally not thought to carry the same risk of angioedema, however, several cases have been reported. One recent case is the first known case of its kind to showcase angioedema from use of an ARB and rt-PA therapy. A 80-year-old Asian female presented with left-sided weakness and was given rt-PA with improvement in symptoms. The patient started developing difficulty breathing, throat pain, dysarthria and an odd sensation in her mouth 6 minutes after the end of infusion. Angioedema of the tongue, uvula, and lips was diagnosed and steroids started for treatment with presentation attributed to rt-PA. Olmesartan was initiated at 20 mg daily for hypertension after angioedema developed. Angioedema did not fully recover until olmesartan was also discontinued, suggesting potentiation by olmesartan in persistent angioedema symptoms [15A].

Valsartan [SEDA-36, 383]

Dermatological

A 58-year-old woman treated with valsartan and hydrochlorothiazide combination for 7 days presented with asymptomatic purpuric eruption of the palms spreading to the forearms. After discontinuation of the drug, the rash resolved in 2 months. In a case with a 64-year-old male, a cutaneous eruption on the lower limbs and buttocks present for 3 months, started 3 months after a dose increase of valsartan 160 mg from 40 mg which was initially started 2 years prior. The rash completely resolved within 2 months of discontinuation of therapy. A possible mechanism for this type of cutaneous reaction could be due to reduction of collagen content in the arterial intima through inhibition of AT-receptors [11A].

Observational Study

The safety and efficacy of valsartan were studied in a population with ages ranging from 6 months to 5 years in a randomized, double-blind study for 8 weeks followed by an 18-week open label continuation. The dosing of valsartan was low: 0.25 mg/kg ($n=30$), medium: 1 mg/kg ($n=15$) or high: 4 mg/kg ($n=30$) once daily. No differences in adverse events were noted between the three different dosing strategies. Upper respiratory tract infections (8.1%) and abdominal pain (6.8%) were the most common adverse reactions reported. In regards to electrolytes and renal function, there were four patients who developed potassium levels >5.5 mmol/L all within the high dose regimen, although all had a history of renal conditions. One case resulted in discontinuation of therapy, but none were deemed serious by the researchers. Creatinine increases of more than 50% from baseline were observed in three patients in medium and high dose groups, however, there were no increases of more than 100% from baseline. A few patients had a decrease of more than 25% in glomerular filtration rate. In the extension study, the most reported adverse reactions by 57.6% of patients were fever (16.7%) and nasopharyngitis (10.6%). The adverse effects thought to be drug related were reported in 4.5% of patients included anorexia ($n=1$), hyperkalemia ($n=1$) and erythema ($n=1$). Adverse reactions of valsartan are generally mild to moderate in children aged 6 months to 5 years [16c].

CALCIUM CHANNEL BLOCKERS

Tumorigenicity

A population based study enrolled 880 women with invasive ductal breast cancer (IDC), 1027 with invasive lobular breast cancer (ILC) and 856 controls assessed the potential link between antihypertensive medication use and diagnosis of breast cancer. Patient interviews, past medical histories of hypertension, heart disease, use of antihypertensive agents such as: ACE inhibitors, angiotensin receptor blockers, β-blockers, calcium-channel blockers, diuretics, and combination therapies were collected at the time of use. There were no differences found between the three groups at baseline and 44% of the women in each group had a history of hypertension. While current, former, and short-term use of antihypertensive agents were not associated with risk of IDC or ILC, an increased risk was found in current users of calcium channel blockers for at least 10 years. This trend was found for both IDC (OR, 2.4; 95% CI, 1.2–4.9) ($P=0.04$ trend) and for ILC (OR 2.6; 95% CI, 1.3–5.3) ($P=0.01$ trend). Current use of short-acting formulations had a 3.7-fold increased risk for IDC (95% CI, 1.2–11.8) and 3.6-fold increased risk for ILC (95% CI, 1.2–11.4). Long-acting formulations did not have the same risk, however, use greater than 10 years did have increased risk (IDC: OR, 2.7; 95% CI, 1.2–5.7; ILC: OR, 2.5; 95% CI, 1.2–5.5). Current use of dihydropyridines for greater than 10 years also had an elevated risk of both ILC and IDC. The

associations did not vary based on the ER status of the breast cancer. This is the first study to examine duration of therapy for greater than 5 years. All associations with an increased risk of ILC and IDC occurred at more than 10 years. This was a population observational study and thus results must be validated in clinical trials before discontinuation of calcium channel blockers can be recommended [17C].

DIRECT RENIN INHIBITORS [SEDA-33, 420; SEDA-34, 328; SEDA-35, 373; SEDA-36, 283]

Aliskiren

Liver

A 61-year-old woman undergoing routine liver function monitoring in conjunction with long-term antiepileptic therapy was noted to have a drug-induced liver injury manifested as an asymptomatic acute hepatic cytolysis 1 month after the initiation of aliskiren therapy. Upon discontinuation of aliskiren use, the patient experienced rapid biological improvement, including normalization of serum AST and a sharp decline in serum ALT within 1 week [18A].

Kidney

A prospective, open-label study of 67 patients with CKD who were already being treated with other antihypertensives was conducted to assess the reno-protective effects of Aliskiren. Significant decreases in eGFR after 4 weeks of aliskiren treatment were noted and patients returned to a pretreatment level within 12 weeks of treatment initiation [19c].

A case reported of patient developed acute renal failure after the addition of aliskiren to the patient's regimen including a: diuretic, angiotensin-converting enzyme inhibitor and aldosterone antagonist. This case highlights the point that acute renal failure can occur as an adverse effect of aliskiren. Little to no conclusive evidence exists about the safety of aliskiren when used in combination with multiple drugs that inhibit renin angiotensin aldosterone system, therefore caution should be exercised [20A].

Drug–Drug Interaction

The authors review the most relevant information available, reported from the last 5 years, pertaining to the most important clinical trials on renin–angiotensin system blockers. Data reviewed include the trials of aliskiren, telmisartan, olmesartan and azilsartan and the possible risk of cancer associated with ARBs. The results of ASPIRE and ALTITUDE trials suggest that concomitant use of aliskiren with either ARBs or angiotensin converting enzyme inhibitors should be avoided. Olmesartan is an effective and safe antihypertensive agent but high-risk patients, such as those with coronary disease, should be carefully monitored for adverse events to avoid an excessive reduction in blood pressure [21R].

ACT-077825 (MK8151)

General Information

A study was conducted in healthy male subjects to evaluate the multiple-dose tolerability, pharmacokinetics, and pharmacodynamics of ACT-077825, a novel direct renin inhibitor [22c].

In this single-center, double-blind, placebo-controlled, active-controlled with 20 mg of enalapril, randomized multiple-ascending dose study, researchers found: adverse events, diarrhea, headache, and postural dizziness to be the most frequently cited side effects. The incidence of diarrhea was greater in the 1000 mg group and a dose of 500 mg of ACT-077825 was identified as the maximum tolerated dose [19c].

DIRECT VASODILATORS [SEDA-36, 284]

Hydralazine [SEDA-33, 427; SEDA-34, 331; SEDA-35, 379; SEDA-36, 284]

Immunologic

A 48-year-old woman with end-stage renal disease receiving continuous ambulatory peritoneal dialysis presented with polyarthritis. Painless cloudy peritoneal dialysis effluent was also noted. Analyses of the effluent dialysate showed an increased leukocyte count with a predominance of lymphocytes. The turbidity of effluent dialysate was still increased after 1 week of antibiotic treatment. Laboratory tests showed significant antinuclear antibody positivity. The patient had been taking hydralazine for 3 months prior to the event. Because drug-induced lupus was suspected, hydralazine was discontinued and low-dose steroids were initiated. Clinical symptoms and cloudy dialysate rapidly abated afterwards [23A].

A 68-year-old female presented with dyspnea on exertion and pleuritic chest pain of 1 week duration. Associated symptoms included low grade fever but no joint pain or rash. She had been maintained on warfarin for her paroxysmal atrial fibrillation and hypertension was managed with hydralazine 100 mg three times daily. Serology revealed anti-nuclear antibody anti-chromatin antibodies and anti-histone antibodies. A diagnosis of hydralazine-induced lupus syndrome was established, and the patient was started on high-dose prednisone after stopping hydralazine. The patient recovered with resolution of effusion on repeat echocardiograms [24A].

A case series reported four caucasian female patients who presented to a large, mid-western academic medical center on chronic hydralazine therapy with acute kidney injury, nephritic urine sediment on urine microscopy and had evidence of pauci-immune glomerulonephritis on kidney biopsy. This case series is of particular interest to rheumatologists due to the possibility of pauci-immune glomerulonephritis in patients taking hydralazine. It also highlights the presence of multiple antibodies in such cases and questions the long-term use of hydralazine especially in the elderly female population [25c].

DOPAMINE BETA-HYDROXYLASE INHIBITOR

Etamicastat

General Information

Etamicastat (also known as BIA 5–453) is a new generation, reversible, dopamine beta-hydroxylase inhibitor for hypertension. In a phase II study of males aged 18–65 years with mild to moderate hypertension, etamicastat 50, 100 and 200 mg daily showed dose-dependent decreases in both systolic and diastolic blood pressure after 10 days. However, the dose-dependent blood pressure effects were not clearly seen between doses 100 and 200 mg. The most common side effects experienced were dermatological, specifically maculopapular rash, pruritus, eczema and dry skin. This is could be a promising novel drug therapy that works by reducing the synthesis of norepinephrine [26C].

DRUGS THAT ACT ON THE SYMPATHETIC NERVOUS SYSTEM [SEDA-33, 424; SEDA-34, 329; SEDA-35, 376; SEDA-36, 286]

Guanfacine

Drug Overdose

A 12-year-old boy with attention-deficit/hyperactivity disorder and Tourette syndrome, presented 18 hours after ingesting three times his usual dose of extended-release guanfacine. On presentation, he was lethargic, bradycardic, and hypertensive with an otherwise nonfocal neurological examination. He remained hypertensive due to paradoxical initial stimulation of post synaptic receptors causing vasoconstriction, until administration of an intravenous antihypertensive agent, nicardipine, 24 hours after ingestion. Bradycardia may be a reflex response to hypertension. After cessation of the calcium-channel blocker, he continued to have intermittent episodes of symptomatic hypotension for the next 2.5 days. This hypotensive effect is due to stimulation of central nervous system alpha two receptors. This particular case report is unique in that hypertension followed by prolonged symptomatic hypotension is rare with ingestions of centrally acting α2-adrenergic agonists [27A].

Methyldopa [SED-15, 2291; SEDA-33, 424; SEDA-34, 330; SEDA-35, 377; SEDA-36, 286]

Drug Overdose

A 50-year-old woman developed sinus bradycardia, prolonged profound hypotension, and drowsiness after ingesting over 300 tablets (>75 g) of methyldopa. Upon presentation, her blood pressure was 59/27 mmHg, heart rate 49 beats/minute, and Glasgow Coma Scale Score of 14. Severe methyldopa overdose can be complicated by prolonged profound hypotension. The management of these patients should include close monitoring of vital functions and administration of intravenous fluids, colloids, and vasopressor agents [28A].

DIURETICS

Chlorthalidone

Renal Disease

Adverse events were assessed following chlorthalidone administration in moderate to advanced chronic kidney disease. An interventional pilot study evaluated adding chlorthalidone to existing medications in a dose of 25 mg/day, and the dose doubled every 4 weeks if the blood pressure remained elevated. The following adverse events were reported in seven subjects. Hypokalemia, hyperuricemia, hyponatremia, transient creatinine changes, dizziness, hyperglycemia, and constipation. One subject reportedly had an ischemic stroke during the study. Chlorthalidone may significantly reduce BP via volume contraction in moderate to advanced CKD with poorly controlled hypertension. The authors conclude that adverse events may take weeks to appear after initiation of therapy and patients should be carefully monitored [29c].

Drug–Drug Interactions

An 85-year-old African-American female with atrial arrhythmias, maintained on dofetilide therapy, presented to an ambulatory cardiology clinic with hypotension. A pharmacist identified a potential major drug–drug interaction between dofetilide and chlorthalidone causing increased risk for hypotension. After discontinuation of chlorthalidone, the patient's systolic BP was maintained between 140 and 145 mmHg with low-dose amlodipine and lisinopril. This case highlights the importance of proper prescribing and monitoring of patients on dofetilide [30A].

Hydrochlorothiazide

Eyes

A case of hydrochlorothiazide (HCTZ)-induced retinal detachment has been reported in a 48-year-old man that presented with a 3-week history of a painless loss of peripheral vision in his left eye. An afferent pupillary defect was present; the patient had recently started a combination medication for his hypertension that included hydrochlorothiazide. The use of HCTZ, a sulfa-derivative, in this patient predisposed to uveal effusion (short eye, thick sclera) caused ciliochoroidal effusion syndrome, severe exudative phenomena of peripheral serous pigment epithelial detachment (SPED), and serous retinal detachment (SRD). A positive challenge test was withheld due to ethical reasons, however, the patient improved with atropine eye drops twice daily and discontinuation of HCTZ [31A].

Electrolyte Balance

A cohort study evaluated risk and predictors of adverse events in older adults with multiple morbidities. The primary outcome was a composite of metabolic adverse events (AE) defined as sodium less than 135 mEq/L, potassium less than 3.5 mEq/L, or a decrease in the estimated glomerular filtration rate (eGFR) of more than 25% from the baseline rate. Secondary outcomes included severe AEs (sodium <130 mEq/L, potassium <3.0 mEq/L, or a decrease in eGFR of more than 50%). Over the course of 9 months of follow-up, low-to-normal and unmeasured baseline sodium and potassium values were among the strongest predictors of hyponatremia and hypokalemia, respectively. Of the patients treated with thiazides, 42% had laboratory monitoring within 90 days after treatment had begun. Greater attention should be paid to potential complications and closer laboratory monitoring before and after initiation of thiazides [32C].

A longitudinal retrospective cohort study in kidney transplant patients assessed safety and efficacy of thiazides in kidney transplantation. Safety and efficacy comparisons were measured using changes in blood pressure between thiazide recipients and control patients. After controlling for baseline differences, safety analysis revealed thiazide recipients were at higher risk to develop hyperkalemia or hypokalemia. Based on long-term outcomes, thiazides appear to be safe and effective antihypertensives; however, in the short-term, thiazides may increase the risk of developing potassium disturbances [33c].

Skin

While bullous pemphigoid, a common subepidermal blistering disorder, typically occurs in the elderly without any obvious inciting event, a recent episode involving a

32-year-old male was reported. A case study documents a patient's experience of generalized bullous pemphigoid induced by HCTZ [34A].

Tumerogenicity

Hydrochlorothiazide was examined as a putative chronic antigen in a cohort of prospectively staged patients after patients were observed with HCTZ-associated common cutaneous T cell lymphomas (CTCL). Patients with hypertensive CTCL were divided into two groups based on whether they were treated with HCTZ or not. Association between HCTZ use and CTCL was analyzed and about 30% of patients experienced complete remission after discontinuing HCTZ. Three patients were rechallenged and developed lesions that resolved or improved with discontinuation of the medication. HCTZ is commonly prescribed and may be a putative antigen in a small subset of patients with mycosis fungoides [35c].

Genetic Factors

A study finds a novel mechanism HCTZ-induced adverse metabolic effect in African-American population. A genome-wide association study and meta-analysis of the change in fasting plasma glucose and triglycerides were reported in response to HCTZ in two separate clinical trials. Two single-nucleotide polymorphisms achieved genome-wide significance for association with a change in fasting plasma triglycerides in African Americans, whereby each variant allele was associated with a marked increase in triglyceride levels. Two single-nucleotide polymorphisms (rs 12279250 and rs 4319515 9r(2) = 0.730) located at 11p15.1in the NELL1 encodes a cytoplasmic protein that contains epidermal growth factor-like repeats and has been shown to repress adipogenic differentiation. A novel mechanism underlying adverse, HCTZ-induced, metabolic effects can be inferred from these findings [36M].

A genome-wide association study evaluated uric acid (UA) and hyperuricemia associated with HCTZ therapy. Single-nucleotide polymorphisms (SNP) were replicated in caucasians and African Americans treated with HCTZ add-on therapy in the PEAR study [8c]. Replicated regions were followed up through expression and pathway analysis. Five unique gene regions were identified in African Americans and one region was identified in caucasians. Increases in UA were observed following HCTZ therapy in individuals homozygous for risk alleles. Several risk alleles were also associated with an increased risk of HCTZ-induced clinical hyperuricemia. Several novel gene regions were associated with HCTZ-induced UA elevations in African Americans and one such region was associated with in caucasians [37c].

Indapamide

Eyes

A case is reported of indapamide-induced, transient myopia with ciliary body edema and supraciliary effusion. A 39-year-old caucasian female patient presented with a chief complaint of headache and sudden bilateral loss of distant vision. Neurological assessment and cranial CT scans were unremarkable. For the patient's hypertension, twice a day bisoprolol 2.5 mg and once a day indapamide 1.5 mg tablets were prescribed several days before. Two days after the patient stopped taking indapamide, the ciliary body edema and detachment disappeared [38A].

Triamterene

Kidney

Triamterene crystalline nephropathy has rarely been reported and its histologic characteristics are not well characterized. The authors of the article describe two cases of triamterene crystalline nephropathy, one of which initially was misdiagnosed as 2,8-dihydroxyadenine crystalline nephropathy [39A].

ENDOTHELIAN RECEPTOR ANTAGONISTS

Ambrisentan [SEDA-33, 421; SEDA-34, 328; SEDA-35, 374; SEDA-36, 284]

Eyes

A 29-year-old woman presented with bilateral painless blurred vision with a duration of 1 week and began after initial treatment of daily ambrisentan 5 mg for her recently diagnosed idiopathic pulmonary arterial hypertension. Her past medical history was notable for hypertension for which her medication regimen consisted of aspirin 81 mg daily, amlodipine 5 mg daily, and lisinopril 40 mg daily. On the day of presentation, her blood pressure was 132/90 mmHg. On dilated fundus examination, multiple cotton wool spots were noted in both eyes, along with several small nerve fiber layer hemorrhages. No early perfusion defect was found, but fluorescein angiography demonstrated focal areas of late hyperfluorescence and leakage in the cotton wool spots. A laboratory workup was unremarkable and ambrisentan was discontinued due to the correlation between initiation of therapy and symptoms. At a 2-week follow-up appointment, resolution of cotton wool spots were observed on dilated fundus examination and blood pressure remained stable at 140/85 mmHg. Tadalafil 40 mg daily was initiated as an alternative therapy for the patient and she experienced no further visual changes or cotton wool spots [40A].

PROSTACYCLIN ANALOG

Treprostinil Diolamine

Hepatic Disease

The pharmacokinetics and safety of oral treprostinil diolamine was studied following a single-dose administration in 30 patients with mild, moderate, and severe hepatic impairment based on Child-Pugh classification. Mean plasma concentrations increased and clearance decreased by 89% with increasing severity of hepatic disease. The most frequently cited side effects were headache, nausea, diarrhea, and dizziness; 36 adverse events were reported in 12 (40%) of the 30 patients. The study ended enrollment for the severe group (Child-Pugh score >10) due to the severity of headache caused by treprostinil diolamine. Based on the results of this study, the authors suggest dose adjustments for Child-Pugh Class A with initial dose 0.125 mg twice daily and dose escalation every 3–4 days. Child-Pugh Class-B patients should start 0.125 mg twice daily with dose titration every 5 days. Treprostinil diolamine is contraindicated in patients with severe hepatic impairment [41c].

Infection Risk

A 14-year-old boy diagnosed with World Health Organization Group I idiopathic pulmonary arterial hypertension with an estimated ejection fraction of 30% was being treated with furosemide and bosentan when he began intravenous treprostinil continuous infusion. Two years later the patient presented with fatigue, muscle cramping, and fever and was subsequently treated for sepsis caused by a Gram-negative bacilli, Chryseomonas luteola, which was susceptible to ceftriaxone. The patient was treated with meropenem, amikacin, and ultimately ceftriaxone and was discharged with a 14-day course of ceftriaxone. Other studies have demonstrated a decrease in bacterial infections when treprostinil is prepared using epoprostenol diluent due to the more alkaline pH. The patient was later changed to the epoprostenol diluent without further infections. The authors advise consideration of this more alkaline diluent to prevent bacterial infections in patients on continuous intravenous treprostinil therapy [42A].

PULMONARY VASODILATORS [SEDA-33, 421; SEDA-34, 328; SEDA-35, 374; SEDA-36, 284]

Observational Study

A retrospective observational study was conducted to evaluate the safety and tolerability of treatment options for pulmonary hypertensive vascular disease (PVHD) in 63 children and to analyze the incidence and type of ADRs. As many as 90 different treatments were used between all the patients in the study, both monotherapy and combination therapy, with any of the following agents: sildenafil, bosentan, iloprost, treprostinil, epoprostenol, ambrisentan, and sitaxentan. The median age at therapy initiation was 3.4 years. NYHA functional class I–IV was 1.6%, 22.2%, 39.7%, and 36.5%, respectively. 39 patients (61.9%) were categorized as Group I pulmonary arterial hypertension, followed by 33 patients (52.4%) categorized as having congenital heart disease. Over the 12-month study period, a total of 90 episodes were recorded including 34 patients (54%) having ADRs and 37 events occurred with monotherapy, while 53 events occurred with combination therapy to give an incidence rate of 1.02 ADRs/patient/year. Most common events included gastrointestinal symptoms and spontaneous erection in male patients. The majority of reported events were considered mild (42, 46.7%) or moderate (39, 43.4%) versus severe (9, 10%). Headaches were found to have increased with patients greater than 8 years old, and gastrointestinal symptoms were more common for patients less than 2 years old. Gastrointestinal symptoms occurred in patients on sildenafil, which is likely due to relaxation of the esophageal sphincter and smooth muscle relaxant effect in patients who lack developed muscle tone. The ADR frequency was different than that of adults treated with these agents. More erections were noted in the pediatric population (12% versus unknown); however, less pediatric patients reported limb pain as compared to the reported adult ADR rate (2% versus ≥10%) while on sildenafil therapy. Pediatric patients also experienced higher rates of flushing and hypotension while on bosentan compared to reported adult rates (20% versus 1–10%). Increased transaminases are found in ≥10% of adult patients on bosentan, but the pediatric patients reported a lower rate of 4%. Patients receiving inhaled iloprost experienced higher frequencies of respiratory ADRs such as coughing, secretions, and bronchospasms as well as an increase in hypotension and vasodilation when compared to the adult population. This may be due to the developing airways of the pediatric patients which as more reactive and smaller in size. Treprostinil continuous infusion was well tolerated with 10% of the pediatric patients having local reactions causing discontinuation [43c].

In the United States, the Food and Drug Administration (FDA) recommends against the use of sildenafil in children. This is based on the results of the STARTS-2 trial which demonstrated decreased survival of children receiving high doses of sildenafil monotherapy. The STARTS-2 study followed the European Medicines Agency recommendations of 10 mg/8 h for patient

<20 kg, and 20 mg/8 h for patients >20 kg. Mean ADRs per treatment were higher for patients exceeding recommended dosing (1.47, IQR 0.78–2.16) compared to those receiving the recommended dosing regimen (0.68, IQR 0.36–1). Therefore, dosing in pediatric patients should not exceed the recommended dosing. This study was the largest report of ADRs for the pediatric population and demonstrated that these treatment options can be safely used in pediatric patients with PVHD [43c].

ANTIHYPERTENSIVES IN PREGNANCY

Observational Study

A cohort study found that women with chronic hypertension who were prescribed labetalol had infants that were more likely to require hospitalization for respiratory distress syndrome, seizures and sepsis than infants born to women who were prescribed methyldopa. More neonatal adverse effects have been reported in literature with beta-blockers than methyldopa and are most likely due to effects of fetal circulation. Another population based cohort study revealed the increased risk for low birth weight in infants was more likely in pregnant women who used vasodilators for hypertension. Beta-blockers and calcium channel blockers were, however, found to be relatively safe as antihypertensive agents [44c].

Genetic Factors

The bioavailability of several antihypertensive agents is lower in pregnant women than in non-pregnant women. There has been considerable research devoted to applying pharmacogenetics to assisting in individualized dosing in pregnancy. Polymorphisms in the eNOS gene are associated with variations in the pharmacological response to atenolol. Patients with a G498A polymorphism in the eNOS gene have a better blood pressure response to atenolol. A NAT enzyme associated with a polymorphism can lead to reduced enzymatic activity of hydralazine resulting in higher concentrations of hydralazine hence pronounced side effects such as hypotension. Nifedipine is metabolized by CYP3A family and polymorphisms in CYP3A5 can affect the maternal blood concentration of nifedipine [45R].

References

[1] Chiang YY, Chen KB, Tsai TH, et al. Lowered cancer risk with ACE inhibitors/ARBs: a population-based cohort study. J Clin Hypertens (Greenwich). 2014;16(1):27–33 [c].

[2] Movva R, Figueredo VM, Lynn Morris D. Kounis syndrome due to angiotensin converting enzyme inhibitor. Clin Res Cardiol. 2013;102(2):163–4 [A].

[3] Gonzalez-Juanatey JR, Cordero A. Benefits of delapril in hypertensive patients along the cardiovascular continuum. Expert Rev Cardiovasc Ther. 2013;11(3):271–81 [R].

[4] Baricevic M, Mravak Stipetic M, et al. Oral bullous eruption after taking lisinopril—case report and literature review. Wien Klin Wochenschr. 2013;125(13–14):408–11 [A].

[5] Rothermundt C, Gillessen S. Angioedema in a patient with renal cell cancer treated with everolimus in combination with an angiotensin-converting enzyme inhibitor. J Clin Oncol. 2013;31(5):e57–8 [A].

[6] Prasa D, Hoffmann-Walbeck P, Barth S, et al. Angiotensin II antagonists—an assessment of their acute toxicity. Clin Toxicol (Phila). 2013;51(5):429–34 [c].

[7] Fournier JP, Sommet A, Durrieu G, et al. Drug interactions between antihypertensive drugs and non-steroidal anti-inflammatory agents: a descriptive study using the French Pharmacovigilance database. Fundam Clin Pharmacol. 2014;28:230–5 [c].

[8] Lee H, Kim KS, Chae SC, et al. Ambulatory blood pressure response to once-daily fimasartan: an 8-week, multicenter, randomized, double-blind, active-comparator, parallel-group study in Korean patients with mild to moderate essential hypertension. Clin Ther. 2013;35(9):1337–49 [c].

[9] Foti C, Carbonara AM, Guida S, et al. Frictional purpuric eruption associated with angiotensin II receptor blockers. Dermatol Ther. 2014;27(2):97–100 [A].

[10] Cheung TT, Cheung BM. Managing blood pressure control in Asian patients: safety and efficacy of losartan. Clin Interv Aging. 2014;9:443–50 [R].

[11] Gallivan C, Brown I. Olmesartan induced enterocolitis. Pathology. 2014;46(4):360–1 [A].

[12] Khan AS, Peter S, Wilcox CM. Olmesartan-induced enteropathy resembling celiac disease. Endoscopy. 2014;46(Suppl 1 UCTN):E97–8 [A].

[13] Nielsen JA, Steephen A, Lewin M. Angiotensin-II inhibitor (olmesartan)-induced collagenous sprue with resolution following discontinuation of drug. World J Gastroenterol. 2013;19(40):6928–30 [A].

[14] Stanich PP, Yearsley M, Meyer MM. Olmesartan-associated sprue-like enteropathy. J Clin Gastroenterol. 2013;47(10):894–5 [A].

[15] Wang S, Bi X, Shan L, et al. Orolingual angioedema associated with olmesartan use after recombinant tissue plasminogen activator treatment of acute stroke. Ann Allergy Asthma Immunol. 2014;112(2):177–8 [A].

[16] Schaefer F, Coppo R, Bagga A, et al. Efficacy and safety of valsartan in hypertensive children 6 months to 5 years of age. J Hypertens. 2013;31(5):993–1000 [c].

[17] Li CI, Dalilng JR, Mei-Tzu CT, et al. Use of antihypertensive medications and breast cancer risk among women aged 55 to 74 years. JAMA Intern Med. 2013;173(17):1629–37 [C].

[18] Crepin S, Godet B, Carrier P, et al. Probable drug-induced liver injury associated with aliskiren: case report and review of adverse event reports from pharmacovigilance databases. Am J Health Syst Pharm. 2014;71(8):643–7 [A].

[19] Abe M, Suzuki H, Okada K, et al. Efficacy analysis of the renoprotective effects of aliskiren in hypertensive patients with chronic kidney disease. Heart Vessels. 2013;28(4):442–52 [c].

[20] Vallakati A, Chandra PA, Hollander G, et al. Direct renin inhibitor induced renal failure. Am J Ther. 2014;21(2):e53–5 [A].

[21] Escobar C, Barrios V. An evaluation of the latest evidence relating to renin-angiotensin system inhibitors. Expert Opin Drug Metab Toxicol. 2013;9(7):847–58 [R].

[22] Nicolas LB, Gutierrez M, Binkert C, et al. Pharmacokinetics, pharmacodynamics, and tolerability of ACT-077825, a new direct renin inhibitor after multiple-ascending doses in healthy subjects. J Cardiovasc Pharmacol. 2013;61(1):42–50 [c].

[23] Wen YK, Wen KI. An unusual cause of non-infectious peritonitis in a peritoneal dialysis patient. Int Urol Nephrol. 2014;46(1):265–8 [A].

[24] Chamsi-Pasha MA, Bassiouny M, Kim ES. Hydralazine-induced lupus syndrome presenting with large pericardial effusion. QJM. 2014;107(4):305–7 [A].

[25] Suneja M, Baiswar S, Vogelgesang SA. Hydralazine associated pauci-immune glomerulonephritis. J Clin Rheumatol. 2014;20(2):99–102 [c].

[26] Almeida L, Nunes T, Costa R, et al. Etamicastat, a novel dopamine beta-hydroxylase inhibitor: tolerability, pharmacokinetics, and pharmacodynamics in patients with hypertension. Clin Ther. 2013;35(12):1983–96 [C].

[27] Fein DM, Hafeez ZF, Cavagnaro C. An overdose of extended-release guanfacine. Pediatr Emerg Care. 2013;29(8):929–31 [A].

[28] Chan TY, Joynt GM. Prolonged profound hypotension complicating severe methyldopa overdose. Int J Clin Pharmacol Ther. 2014;52(7):628–30 [A].

[29] Agarwal R, Sinha AD, Pappas MK, et al. Chlorthalidone for poorly controlled hypertension in chronic kidney disease: an interventional pilot study. Am J Nephrol. 2014;39(2):171–82 [c].

[30] Crist LW, Dixon DL. Considerations for dofetilide use in the elderly. Consult Pharm. 2014;29(4):270–4 [A].

[31] Casparis H, Guex-Crosier Y, Wolfensberger TJ, et al. Peripheral serous pigment epithelial detachment and retinal detachment presumably associated with hydrochlorothiazide use. Klin Monbl Augenheilkd. 2013;230(4):437–9 [A].

[32] Makam AN, Boscardin WJ, Miao Y, et al. Risk of thiazide-induced metabolic adverse events in older adults. J Am Geriatr Soc. 2014;62(6):1039–45 [C].

[33] Taber DJ, Srinivas TM, Pilch NA, et al. Are thiazide diuretics safe and effective antihypertensive therapy in kidney transplant recipients? Am J Nephrol. 2013;38(4):285–91 [c].

[34] Warner C, Kwak Y, Glover MH, et al. Bullous pemphigoid induced by hydrochlorothiazide therapy. J Drugs Dermatol. 2014;13(3):360–2 [A].

[35] Jahan-Tigh RR, Huen AO, Lee GL, et al. Hydrochlorothiazide and cutaneous T cell lymphoma: prospective analysis and case series. Cancer. 2013;119(4):825–31 [c].

[36] Del-Aguila JL, Beitelshees AL, Cooper-Dehoff RM, et al. Genome-wide association analyses suggest NELL1 influences adverse metabolic response to HCTZ in African Americans. Pharmacogenomics J. 2014;14(1):35–40 [M].

[37] Vandell AG, McDonough CW, Gong Y, et al. Hydrochlorothiazide-induced hyperuricaemia in the pharmacogenomic evaluation of antihypertensive responses study. J Intern Med. 2014;276(5):486–97 [c].

[38] Vegh M, Hari-Kovacs A, Rez K, et al. Indapamide-induced transient myopia with supraciliary effusion: case report. BMC Ophthalmol. 2013;13:58. http://dx.doi.org/10.1186/1471-2415-13-58 [A].

[39] Nasr SH, Milliner DS, Wooldridge TD, et al. Triamterene crystalline nephropathy. Am J Kidney Dis. 2014;63(1):148–52 [A].

[40] Khan MA, Pitcher JD, Kawut SM, et al. Bilateral cotton wool spots after use of an endothelin receptor antagonist. Ophthalmic Surg Lasers Imaging Retina. 2014;45:156–9 [A].

[41] Peterson D, Marbury T, Marier J, et al. An evaluation of the pharmacokinetics of treprostinil diolamine in subjects with hepatic impairment. J Clin Pharm Ther. 2013;38:518–23 [c].

[42] Wen AY, Weiss IK, Kelly RB. Chryseomonas luteola bloodstream infection in a pediatric patient with pulmonary arterial hypertension receiving intravenous treprostinil therapy. Infection. 2013;41:719–22 [A].

[43] Roldan T, Deiros L, Romero JA, et al. Safety and tolerability of targeted therapies for pulmonary hypertension in children. Pediatr Cardiol. 2014;35:490–8 [c].

[44] Xie RH, Guo Y, Krewski D, et al. Association between labetalol use for hypertension in pregnancy and adverse infant outcomes. Eur J Obstet Gynecol Reprod Biol. 2014;175:124–8 [c].

[45] Haas DM. Pharmacogenetics and individualizing drug treatment during pregnancy. Pharmacogenomics. 2014;15(1):69–78 [R].

21

Diuretics

Yekaterina Opsha*,†,1

*Rutgers the State University of New Jersey, Piscataway, NJ, USA
†Saint Barnabas Medical Center, Livingston, NJ, USA
1Corresponding author: kate.opsha@pharmacy.rutgers.edu

CARBONIC ANHYDRASE INHIBITORS [SEDA-15, 643; SEDA-34, 339; SEDA-35, 387, SEDA-36, 289]

Acetazolamide

Eyes

Therapeutic use of acetazolamide post eye surgery may cause acetazolamide-induced bilateral choroidal effusion. A case report describing this effect in a 28-year-old patient was recently published discussing the uneventful surgery for hyperopia. However, 24 hours after surgery, the patient presented with bilateral shallow anterior chamber in both eyes. Ultrasound showed choroidal thickening in both eyes, which was consistent with choroidal effusion syndrome. When the drug was stopped, the condition improved slowly and resolved completely within 1 week [1A].

Dermatology

Cutaneous adverse drug reactions (CADR) to oral acetazolamide have been previously reported in the literature; however, skin tests have rarely been studied. Jachiet and colleagues sought to retrospectively evaluate acetalozamide CADR skin tests in nine patients and 12 controls. According to the authors, "seven patients developed maculopapular exanthema and four had acute generalized exanthematous pustulosis and patch tests were positive for 8/9 patients." This small study demonstrated the importance of skin tests in patients presenting with new onset dermatological reactions after initiation of oral acetazolamide therapy [2A]. Another similar reaction was reported in a second study of acute generalized exanthematous pustulosis due to oral acetazolamide administration. The reaction was initially negative on patch testing and confirmed by delayed-reading intradermal testing [3A].

Respiratory

Shock and transient non-cardiogenic pulmonary edema was identified in one patient after receiving a single oral dose of acetazolamide after eye surgery [4A].

LOOP DIURETICS [SEDA-15, 567, 1454; SEDA-34, 342; SEDA- 35, 390; SEDA-36, 290]

Azosemide

Urinary System

A single center study of 11 patients with type 2 diabetic kidney disease (DKD) and diuretic-resistant edema sought to evaluate the safety and efficacy of thiazide diuretic, hydrochlorothiazide (HCTZ) in addition to loop diuretics (azosemide or furosemide) and examine the clinical parameters of blood pressure (BP) control, proteinuria, and eGFR before and after addition of HCTZ. Each of the 11 patients had an estimated glomerular filtration rate (eGFR) <30 mL/min/1.73 m^2 and were suffering from severe edema even with loop diuretics. Patients were receiving either azosemide (60–120 mg/day) or furosemide (80 mg/day). In addition, patients were receiving a 13.6 ± 3.8 mg/day dose of HCTZ. After the addition of HCTZ therapy, systolic blood pressure (SBP) and diastolic blood pressures (DBP), as well as proteinuria significantly decreased (SBP: at 12 months, $p < 0.01$, DBP: at 12 months, $p < 0.05$, proteinuria: at 12 months, $p < 0.01$). The annual change in eGFR was not significantly different before and after HCTZ therapy. These findings suggest that the combination of HCTZ and loop diuretics (specifically azosemide and furosemide) may improve SBP and

© 2015 Elsevier B.V. All rights reserved.

DBP levels and decreases proteinuria even in advanced stage type 2 DKD patients with severe edema in whom previously HCTZ was thought to be less beneficial [5c].

Bumetanide

Urinary System

A retrospective single center study which analyzed 242 patient records with acute heart failure who received either continuous infusion of bumetanide or continuous infusion of furosemide alone or in combination with metolazone sought to evaluate the difference in these three regimens based on outcomes of urine output (UO) and incidence of worsening renal function. Compared to baseline, all regimens increased mean hourly urine output ($p < 0.0001$ for all). Incidence of worsening renal function was not different between regimens. The incidence of hyponatremia was higher with the combination therapy and bumetanide group versus furosemide alone [6c].

Ethacrynic Acid

Ethacrynic acid has been used in clinical practice for several decades, particularly in patients who require loop diuretics but have a true sulfa allergy as all other loop diuretics contain a sulfa moiety. This is currently the only sulfonamide-free loop diuretic. However, this agent is not a very potent diuretic and should only be reserved for those patients who cannot tolerate or have failed other diuretic therapies. Ethacrynic acid is also rarely used because of its increased incidence of ototoxicity as compared to the other loop diuretics. Amongst other expected diuretic side effects, this agent is known to cause: skin rash, Henoch–Schönlein purpura (IgA vasculitis), hematuria, agranulocytosis, severe neutropenia, thrombocytopenia, and vertigo [7S].

Electrolyte

A retrospective-cross-sectional study evaluated children (<18 years of age) who received ethacrynic acid as a continuous infusion in order to determined the mean/median effective dose as well as efficacy and safety markers. No significant differences were noted with magnesium and potassium levels. Five out of nine children (55%) developed metabolic alkalosis [8c].

Pharmacodynamics

The aim of this prospective study was to evaluate the effect of several cardiovascular agents (including ACE inhibitors, ARB's, HCTZ and ethacrynic acid) on the anticonvulsant activity of levetiracetam (LEV) in mice. The combinations of these agents with LEV were tested for adverse effects. The study found that ethacrynic acid at doses of 100 mg/kg did not affect the anticonvulsant activity of levetiracetam [9E].

Furosemide

Thrombocytopenia

Thrombocytopenia is a rare but serious concern with furosemide use because this agent is typically used on a chronic basis in the heart failure patient population.

- This is a report of an 84-year-old male with chronic symptomatic thrombocytopenia as a probable case of drug-induced side effect from long standing furosemide use. A dose-dependent change in platelet count was observed in association with the furosemide dose. The platelet count increased on discontinuation of furosemide and beginning of torsemide. Several months after discontinuation of furosemide, his platelet count increased to a 9-year high of $206 \times 10^3/mm^3$ from a low of $36 \times 10^3/mm^3$ while receiving furosemide therapy. Based on these observations, and other prior reports, clinicians should consider furosemide as a potential cause of thrombocytopenia [10A].

Urinary System

It is common knowledge among practitioner who treats patients with loop diuretics that renal function can become compromised. In this study by Triposkiadis and colleagues, the investigators sought to evaluate the effect of high-dose furosemide (20 mg/hour) in comparison to low-dose furosemide (5 mg/hour) and low-dose dopamine ($5 \mu g\,kg^{-1}min^{-1}$) or low-dose furosemide alone (5 mg/hour) in 161 patients presenting with acute decompensated heart failure (ADHF). Amongst several outcomes, the authors wanted to evaluate dyspnea relief (based on Borg index) and renal function based on serum creatinine (Scr) in each group. Worsening renal function was higher in the high-dose furosemide arm than in low-dose furosemide plus low-dose dopamine arm and low-dose furosemide groups at day 1, respectively (24% vs. 11% vs. 7%, $p < 0.0001$) but not at Scr peak (44% vs. 38% vs. 29%, $p = 0.27$). No significant differences were observed in dyspnea relief and no other significant differences in adverse events were noted [11C].

Another study looked at similar outcomes and wanted to evaluate the safety and efficacy of continuous infusion versus bolus injection of intravenous loop diuretics for the treatment of acute decompensated heart failure by performing a systematic review and meta-analysis of available randomized controlled trials. Ten randomized controlled trials with over 500 patients were identified. Continuous infusion of diuretics were associated with a significantly greater weight loss (weighted mean difference, 0.78; 95% confidence interval, 0.03–1.54) compared with bolus administration. Meta-analysis of the existing limited studies did not confirm any significant differences in the safety and efficacy with continuous administration of loop diuretic, compared with bolus injection in this patient population [12R].

Electrolytes

The EIDOS and DoTS descriptions of electrolyte disturbances due to loop diuretics, thiazide and thiazide-like diuretics have been described previously in [SEDA-35, 389].

Torsemide

Contrast-Induced Acute Kidney Injury

A review article on the use of torsemide for possible prevention of contrast-induced acute kidney injury (CI-AKI) was recently published. The authors speculated that based on observations and experiments of previous trials that RAAS (renin–angiotensin–aldosterone system) is potentially responsible for the development of CI-AKI through abnormalities of renal perfusion and other mechanisms and that torsemide could inhibit RAAS through its antialdosteronergic and diuretic functions. This review article provides some insight into the use of torsemide as an efficient, feasible and cost-effective strategy for the prevention of CI-AKI in combination with adequate hydration [13H].

THIAZIDE AND THIAZIDE-LIKE DIURETICS [SEDA-15, 3375; SEDA-34, 340; SEDA-35, 388; SEDA-36, 292]

Chlorothiazide

Metabolic

In a single center retrospective review of 82 patients hospitalized for heart failure, the authors sought to evaluate the safety and efficacy of oral hydrochlorothiazide (HCTZ) or intravenous chlorothiazide added to intravenous loop diuretic therapy (furosemide at total daily doses of >160 mg). After treatment, 24-hour urine output increased in both groups. Hypokalemia occurred frequently in both groups: 71.4% and 83.3% in the oral hydrochlorothiazide and intravenous chlorothiazide groups, respectively but was not statistically significantly different ($p = 0.21$) [14c]. This study suggests that both diuretic strategies are comparable but cost is a great consideration when making a decision regarding this type of therapy. Intravenous chlorothiazide costs over 50 times more than po hydrochlorothiazide in most countries.

Chlorthalidone

Hemodynamics

A retrospective self-controlled study of 40 patients who received HCTZ or chlorthalidone for blood pressure management evaluated the "within-patient clinic blood pressure readings, serum electrolyte levels, and renal function markers before and after a medication change from HCTZ to chlorthalidone." Both mean systolic and diastolic blood pressures showed statistically and clinically significant reductions after the medication change. A statistically significant decrease in sodium (-1.1 mmol/L [95% CI, 0.4–1.9], $p = 0.003$) and an increase in serum creatinine (0.06 mg/dL [95% CI, -0.09 to -0.02], $p = 0.002$) was observed after the patients were changed from HCTZ to chlorthalidone. However, it is up to the practitioner to decipher if these changed are deemed clinically significant [15c].

Hydrochlorothiazide

Electrolyte Balance—Hyponatremia

Hydrochlorothiazide (HCTZ) is frequently recommended as a first line antihypertensive agent. Some of the commonly known side effects of this agent are hypokalaemia and hyponatremia. A study involving 202 elderly patients (>65 years of age) evaluated the use of HCTZ to determine the frequency of hyponatremia as a potential side effect of this therapy. The reported incidence of hyponatremia was 24.87% (49 patients) in the whole group, and patients over the age of 75 were more likely to develop hyponatremia [16c].

Another similar study wanted to evaluate the rates of hyponatremia with the use of HCTZ versus chlorthalidone. The selected patients were over 18 years of age with a serum sodium levels of <130 mmol/L or hospitalized due to hyponatremic symptoms. Hyponatremia was more common with chlorthalidone than with hydrochlorothiazide at equal dose per day: adjusted odds ratio was 2.09 (95% confidence interval [CI], 1.13–3.88) for 12.5 mg/day and 1.72 (95% CI, 1.15–2.57) for 25 mg/day [17c].

Electrolyte Balance—Hypercalcemia

Due to its pharmacological mechanism of action, HCTZ has an effective capability to decreases urinary calcium excretion causing hypercalcemia. In this study, the authors assessed the frequency of hypercalcemia in 328 black patients who were receiving HCTZ for blood pressure control. At 3 months of therapy, the patients had higher calcium levels (0.2 mg/dL, $p < .001$) than nonhydrochlorothiazide participants, but only one participant in the hydrochlorothiazide group had hypercalcemia. These findings, although statistically significant, were not deemed to be clinically significant by the authors [18C].

Pharmacogenomics

Hyperuricaemia is a commonly observed side effect secondary to treatment with HCTZ. The authors of this study sought to identify a novel single nucleotide polymorphisms (SNPs) associated with HCTZ-induced elevations in uric acid (UA) and hyperuricaemia. Suggestive SNPs were replicated in Caucasians and African Americans patients from a prior study who were treated with HCTZ add-on therapy. The results indicated that there are at least "five unique gene regions identified in African Americans (LUC7L2, ANKRD17/COX18, FTO, PADI4 and PARD3B), and one gene region identified in Caucasians (GRIN3A)." Increases in uric acid levels of up to 1.8 mg/dL were observed following HCTZ therapy in patients who were homozygous for the above identified risk alleles [19C]. This may be a clinical concern in patients with underlying hyperuricaemia or a history of gout.

Metabolic

In a meta-analysis of 10 randomized controlled clinical trials, the investigators evaluated the metabolic profile (fasting plasma glucose and serum potassium) of low-dose thiazide diuretics. The cumulative mean change of fasting plasma glucose was +0.20 mmol/L for the diuretic arm versus +0.12 mmol/L ($p < 0.01$) for the comparator arm. The cumulative mean change of serum potassium was −0.22 mmol/L for the diuretic arm versus +0.05 mmol/L ($p < 0.01$) for the comparator arm. The change in glucose levels does not appear to place patients at a clinically significant risk of hyperglycemia. However, the observed change in potassium levels may be clinically significant especially in patients with underlying cardiovascular disease in whom maintaining an adequate potassium level is crucial [20M].

Skin

One case report of a 32-year-old male describes a subepidermal blistering disorder called bullous pemphigoid induced by losartan-HCTZ which was prescribed for hypertensive therapy in this patient. The patient presented with the typical flu-like prodromal symptoms and a nonspecific urticarial dermatitis primarily around the neck, trunk and both upper and lower extremities. The patient was transferred to a burn center where he was treated with oral steroids and successfully underwent several debridements of his lesions [21A].

Indapamide

Eyes

A case report of a 39-year-old female presenting with sudden headaches and bilateral loss of distant vision potentially due to indapamide 1.5 mg tablets which was prescribed several days prior to presentation is addressed below. Neurological exams and radiographic scans were unremarkable. After discontinuation of the offending agent (indapamide), the patient slowly regained her eye sight in both eyes. This is the third case in the available literature which describes indapamide-induced transient myopia. Currently, this side effect is not mentioned in indapamides package insert [22A].

ALDOSTERONE RECEPTOR ANTAGONISTS

Eplerenone [SEDA-15, 1227; SEDA-34, 344; SEDA-35, 391; SEDA-36, 293]

Electrolyte Balance

The EMPHASIS-HF study sought to evaluate the safety and efficacy of eplerenone in patients who are at a high risk for worsening renal function or high risk of hyperkalemia while receiving treatment of eplerenone for heart failure. The baseline glomerular filtration rate (eGFR) 30–60 mL/min/1.73 m^2 and serum potassium <5.0 mmol/L. Patients at high risk of hyperkalemia or worsening renal function were defined as patients >75 years of age, history of diabetes, and eGFR <60 mL/min/1.73 m^2. The results indicated that in all high-risk subgroups, patients treated with eplerenone had an increased risk of potassium >5.5 mmol/L but not of potassium >6.0 mmol/L. Eplerenone was both efficacious and safe when carefully monitored [23C].

Drug–Drug Interactions

In May of 2013, safety labeling changes approved by the U.S. Food and Drug administration indicated that there is an increased risk of hyperkalemia when eplerenone is used with other agents which may increase potassium levels (such as ACE inhibitors and ARB's). The FDA put out a warning that close monitoring of serum potassium and renal function is highly recommended. This side effect increases in patients who have baseline impaired renal function and the elderly [24S].

Spironolactone [SEDA-15, 3176; SEDA-34, 345; SEDA-35, 392; SEDA-36, 292]

Urinary System

The effects of spironolactone were studied in the TOP-CAT trial which evaluated mineralocorticoid-receptor antagonists and their effect on the improvement of prognosis in heart failure patients. In this trial, the authors enrolled 3445 patients with symptomatic heart failure who received either spironolactone (15–45 mg) or placebo in addition to optimal heart failure therapy. Of the multiple components in the primary outcomes, the only one that proved to be statistically significant was the incidence of hospitalization rates which were decreased in the spironolactone arm versus the placebo arm ($p = 0.04$). However, treatment with spironolactone was associated with increased serum creatinine and doubling of the rate of hyperkalemia. The authors concluded that with frequent monitoring, there was no significant difference in the incidence of serious adverse events [25C].

Gynecomastia

It is well known that gynecomastia is a potential side effect in patients being treated with spironolactone. In a small 12-week randomized, placebo-controlled trial of 82 dialysis patients with refractory hypertension this side effect was observed. Several adverse events led four patients to discontinue therapy with spironolactone. Gynecomastia was observed in one patient in the spironolactone arm who discontinued therapy. Two patients discontinued therapy due to hyperkalemia and one due to severe nausea [26C].

Gynecological Cancers

Investigators of the following study sought to evaluate the risk of gynecological and other cancers in a large Danish cohort population of female patient's ages >20-years old on spironolactone therapy. Based on a prescription drug registry, they were able to identify 2.3 million women who received spironolactone for at least 1 year of continuous therapy. Among these women, the risk of breast, uterus, ovary, and cervical cancers were generally increased about 10–30%. In the first year of drug exposure, incidences were increased, especially for ovarian cancers. With respect to breast, uterus, and cervical cancer, there was no evidence of increased risk with spironolactone use. Considering the nature of this study, it is difficult to decipher if the use of sprinolocatone alone lead to the increased risk of ovarian cancers or were there other underlying risk factors. However, prescribers need to be cognizant of this potentially dangerous side effect of spironolactone, especially in young patients who may be on this therapy for a prolonged period of time [27M].

OSMOTIC DIURETICS

Mannitol [SEDA-15, 2203; SEDA-34, 346; SEDA-35, 393; SEDA-36, 294]

Urinary System

In a retrospective study of 153 adult patients presenting with intracranial hemorrhage (ICH) receiving mannitol infusions, the investigators evaluated the impact of mannitol on the incidence of acute kidney injury (AKI) from the use of this agent. The overall incidence of AKI among the study participants was 10.5% ($n = 16$). The incidence also seemed to correlate with the dose of mannitol (infusion rates ≥1.34 g/kg/day), patient age ≥70 years, diastolic blood pressure (DBP) ≥110 mmHg, and an established renal dysfunction before starting mannitol therapy were associated with development of AKI (GFR < 60 mL/min/1.73 m^2). Knowing these risk factors, it is important to weight the risk versus benefit when initiating this agent at higher doses [28c].

Respiratory System

Inhaled mannitol is approved to be used in the European Union as a mucolytic agent in adult patients with cystic fibrosis which can be a life-threatening genetic disease characterized by the accumulation of viscous secretions in the airways, making it extremely difficult for patients to adequately breathe. Several studies have evaluated this agent in its inhaled form for the use in cystic fibrosis patients. The clinical results were primarily positive however, inhaled mannitol increased the risk of bronchospasm and haemoptysis. The authors concluded that due to these adverse effects, it is probably best to avoid inhaled mannitol in patients with cystic fibrosis [29c]. Another similar trial was performed in patients with non-cystic fibrosis bronchiectasis and the use of inhaled dry powder mannitol. This study showed that there was no difference between inhaled mannitol and inhaled placebo when it came to reported side effects. Both placebo and mannitol were well tolerated and similar proportion of patients reported side effects at rates of 80.4% versus 82.0%, respectively [30C].

References

[1] Rojas V, González-López F, Baviera J. Acetazolamide-induced bilateral choroidal effusion following insertion of a phakic implantable collamer lens. J Refract Surg. 2013;29(8):570–2 [A].

[2] Jachiet M, Bellon N, Assier H, et al. Cutaneous adverse drug reaction to oral acetazolamide and skin tests. Dermatology. 2013;226(4):347–52 [A].

[3] Benamara-Levy M, Haccard F, Jonville Bera AP, et al. Acute generalized exanthematous pustulosis due to acetazolamide: negative on patch testing and confirmed by delayed-reading intradermal testing. Clin Exp Dermatol. 2014;39(2):220–2 [A].

[4] Zimmermann S, Achenbach S, Wolf M, et al. Recurrent shock and pulmonary edema due to acetazolamide medication after cataract surgery. Heart Lung. 2014;43(2):124–6 [A].

[5] Hoshino T, Ookawara S, Miyazawa H, et al. Renoprotective effects of thiazides combined with loop diuretics in patients with type 2 diabetic kidney disease. Clin Exp Nephrol. 2014;1–2:247–53 [c].

[6] Ng TM, Konopka E, Hyderi AF, et al. Comparison of bumetanide- and metolazone-based diuretic regimens to furosemide in acute heart failure. J Cardiovasc Pharmacol Ther. 2013;18(4):345–53 [c].

[7] Edecrin® ethacrynic acid [package insert]. Bridgewater, NJ: Aton pharma, division of Valeant Pharmaceuticals North; 2011 [S].

[8] Miller JL, Schaefer J, Tam M, et al. Ethacrynic acid continuous infusions in critically Ill pediatric patients. J Pediatr Pharmacol Ther. 2014;19(1):49–55 [c].

[9] Lukawski K, Raszewski G, Czuczwar SJ. Interactions between levetiracetam and cardiovascular drugs against electroconvulsions in mice. Pharmacol Rep. 2014;66(6):1100–5 [E].

[10] Ochoa PS1, Fisher T. A 7-year case of furosemide-induced immune thrombocytopenia. Pharmacotherapy. 2013;33(7):e162–5 [A].

[11] Triposkiadis FK, Butler J, Karayannis G, et al. Efficacy and safety of high dose versus low dose furosemide with or without dopamine infusion: the dopamine in acute decompensated heart failure II (DAD-HF II) trial. Int J Cardiol. 2014;172(1):115–21 [C].

[12] Wu MY, Chang NC, Su CL, et al. Loop diuretic strategies in patients with acute decompensated heart failure: a meta-analysis of randomized controlled trials. J Crit Care. 2014;29(1):2–9 [R].

[13] Li XM, Jin DX, Cong HL. Could torsemide be a prophylactic agent of contrast induced acute kidney injury? A review about this field. Eur Rev Med Pharmacol Sci. 2013;17:1845–9 [H].

[14] Kissling KT, Pickworth KK. Comparison of the effects of combination diuretic therapy with oral hydrochlorothiazide or intravenous chlorothiazide in patients receiving intravenous furosemide therapy for the treatment of heart failure. Pharmacotherapy. 2014;34(8):882–7 [c].

[15] Matthews KA, Brenner MJ, Brenner AC. Evaluation of the efficacy and safety of a hydrochlorothiazide to chlorthalidone medication change in veterans with hypertension. Clin Ther. 2013;35(9):1423–30 [c].

[16] Diaconu CC, Balaceanu A, Bartos D. Diuretics, first-line antihypertensive agents: are they always safe in the elderly? Rom J Intern Med. 2014;52(2):87–90 [c].

[17] Van Blijderveen JC, Straus SM, Rodenburg EM, et al. Risk of hyponatremia with diuretics: chlorthalidone versus hydrochlorothiazide. Am J Med. 2014;127(8):763–71 [c].

[18] Chandler PD, Scott JB, Drake BF, et al. Risk of hypercalcemia in blacks taking hydrochlorothiazide and vitamin D. Am J Med. 2014;127(8):772–8 [C].

[19] Vandell AG, McDonough CW, Gong Y, et al. Hydrochlorothiazide-induced hyperuricaemia in the pharmacogenomic evaluation of antihypertensive responses study. J Intern Med. 2014;276(5):486–97 [C].

[20] Mukete BN, Rosendorff C2. Effects of low-dose thiazide diuretics on fasting plasma glucose and serum potassium—a meta-analysis. J Am Soc Hypertens. 2013;7(6):454–66 [M].

[21] Warner C, Kwak Y, Glover MH, et al. Bullous pemphigoid induced by hydrochlorothiazide therapy. J Drugs Dermatol. 2014;13(3):360–2 [A].

[22] Végh M, Hári-Kovásc A, Réz K, et al. Indapamide-induced transient myopia with supraciliary effusion: case report. BMC Ophthalmol. 2013;13(58):1–4 [A].

[23] Eschalier R, McMurray J, Swedberg K, et al. Safety and efficacy of eplerenone in patients at high risk for hyperkalemia and/or worsening renal function. J Am Coll Cardiol. 2013;62:1585–93 [C].

[24] U.S. Food and Drug administration. Inspra (eplerenone) tablets. Safety labeling changes approved by the FDA. Last revised: 6/13. http://www.fda.gov/Safety/MedWatch/SafetyInformation/Safety-RelatedDrugLabelingChanges/ucm119305.htm [S].

[25] Pitt B, Pfeffer M, Assmann S, et al. Spironolactone for heart failure with preserved ejection fraction. N Engl J Med. 2014;370:1383–92 [C].

[26] Ni Z, Zhang J, Zhang P, et al. Effects of spironolactone on dialysis patients with refractory hypertension: a randomized controlled study. J Clin Hypertens. 2014;16(9):658–63 [C].

[27] Biggar RJ, Andersen EW, Wohlfahrt J, et al. Spironolactone use and the risk of breast and gynecologic cancers. Cancer Epidemiol. 2013;37(6):870–5 [M].

[28] Kim MY, Park JH, Kang NR, et al. Increased risk of acute kidney injury associated with higher infusion rate of mannitol in patients with intracranial hemorrhage. J Neurosurg. 2014;120(6):1340–8 [c].

[29] Inhaled mannitol and cystic fibrosis. Unnecessary bronchial irritation. Prescrire Int. 2014;23(148):89–91 [c].

[30] Bilton D, Daviskas E, Anderson S, et al. Phase 3 randomized study of the efficacy and safety of inhaled dry powder mannitol for the symptomatic treatment of non-cystic fibrosis bronchiectasis. Chest. 2013;144(1):215–25 [C].

22

Metals

Swaran J.S. Flora[1], Vidhu Pachauri

Drug Discovery and Regulatory Toxicology Division, Defence Research and Development Establishment, Gwalior, India
[1]Corresponding author: sjsflora@drde.drdo.in

ALUMINIUM [SED-15, 97; SEDA-32, 413; SEDA-33, 447; SEDA-34, 349; SEDA-35, 397; SEDA-36, 297]

Aluminium (Al) is a ubiquitous metal that is encountered both naturally and intentionally due to its use in water, foods, pharmaceuticals, and vaccines. Small intake of aluminium is essential to human health, but some investigations suggest that toxicity occurs even with a minor change in daily dietary aluminium intake. An assessment of dietary aluminium exposure of the Chinese suggested that even with three decades of rapid development, residents in Shenzhen still face high dietary aluminium exposure, especially children. High dietary aluminium exposure thus still remains a great public health challenge in Shenzhen, China [1C]. It is also present in ambient and occupational airborne particulates. The toxicity of different chemical forms of aluminium depends largely on their physical behaviour and relative solubility in water [2R]. Exposure to aluminium has a negative influence on newborn babies and pregnant women [3H,4R]. Also, neonatal and paediatric parenteral nutrition (PN) contaminated with aluminium can impair bone mineralization and *delay neurological development*. Metallic forms of aluminium and common salts have not been shown to be genotoxic or carcinogenic [5R]. Hepatotoxicity due to aluminum trichloride was suggested in the rat model due to disorders of bile acid secretion inducing hepatocyte apoptosis [6E].

Biological Monitoring

A case–control analysis of population of U.S. aluminium production workers in 8 smelters and 43 other plants was recently done. Ninety-seven cases of acoustic neuroma (AN) were identified between 1996 and 2009 by using insurance claims data, and compared with four controls. Covariates included participation in a hearing conservation programme (HCP), working in an aluminium smelter, working in an electrical job, and hearing loss. Results suggest the incidental detection of previously *undiagnosed tumours* in workers who participated in the company-sponsored HCP. The increased medical surveillance among this population of workers most likely introduced detection bias, leading to the identification of AN cases that would have otherwise remained undetected [7C]. Another trace metals survey in 566 waterworks in the Norwegian population reported high incidences of hip fractures from hospitals throughout the country. This study investigated the relationship between cadmium, lead, and aluminium contamination of municipality drinking water and the incidence of hip fractures. A relatively high concentration of cadmium, lead and aluminium in drinking water increased the risk of hip fractures, and was also affected by gender, age, and urbanization degree. This study elucidated the complex effects on bone health by risk factors found in the environment [8c].

Management of Adverse Reactions

Aluminium salts have been successfully used as depot-adjuvants in essential prophylactic vaccinations with a convincing positive benefit-risk assessment. However, aluminium accumulation needs to be accurately measured for the entire treatment period. Currently, silica-enriched water is being used to measure aluminium accumulation in humans via non-invasive means and ascertain more accurate indications of an individual's body burden of aluminium. This may open up the possibility of providing an effective means of measurement in patients undergoing long-term subcutaneous immunotherapy (SCIT) treatment, as well as reducing the aluminium body burden [9c].

© 2015 Elsevier B.V. All rights reserved.

http://dx.doi.org/10.1016/bs.seda.2015.08.005

Another study investigated the exposure of nursing children to dietary aluminum (in breast milk and/or infant formulas) and through aluminum-adjuvanted vaccines (AAVs). This study analyzed the total hair-Al concentration of nursing children that had been immunized with hepatitis B, DTP, and meningococcal vaccines. Thirty-seven young children between ages 26 and 824 days were exposed to cumulative doses of Al ranging from 0.63 to 6.88 mg from AAVs. Results suggest median hair-Al was 47.7 μg g^{-1} (ranging from 12.2 to 221.9 μg g^{-1}). There was no statistically significant correlation between hair-Al concentration and age of the child and total exposure from vaccine or the time elapsed after the last AAVs [9c].

Nervous System

In a recent study aluminium neurotoxicity was examined in humans and animals in various conditions following different routes of administration which provided an overview of the various associated diseases with it. This study demonstrated that aluminium exposure in adults led to age-related *neurological deficits* resembling *Alzheimer's* and also linked to the Guamanian variant, ALS-PDC. Similar results were found in animal models and in young children [10R,11c]. A recent study demonstrated that apoptosis was the cause of aluminium-induced (3 mg/mL aluminium sulfate, daily for 2 weeks) neuronal death in the hippocampus of rats [12E]. Injection of aluminum adjuvants in an attempt to model Gulf War syndrome and associated neurological deficits led to an ALS phenotype in young male mice. Also, in young children, a highly significant correlation exists between the number of pediatric aluminum-adjuvanted vaccines administered and the rate of autism spectrum disorders [13M].

Cardiovascular System

Three cases of severe aluminium phosphide toxicity have been reported in humans. One case succumbed to intractable *ventricular arrhythmias* complicated by multiorgan failure before she died, while the other two cases required invasive hemodynamic support and eventually improved over the course of 10–14 days. Aluminium phosphide led to cardio-toxicity, resulting in a severe decrease in both ventricular heart functions [14A].

ARSENIC [SED-15, 339; SEDA-32, 414; SEDA-33, 448; SEDA-34, 351; SEDA-35, 399; SEDA-36, 298]

Genotoxicity

A well-known DNA damage marker, 8-hydroxydeoxyguanosine (8-OHdG) demonstrated a strong correlation with arsenic-induced genotoxicity. A study aimed to assess arsenic exposure and its effect on oxidative DNA damage and repair in young children exposed *in utero* and who continued to live in arsenic-contaminated areas. The study concluded that exposed children had a significant reduction in arsenic methylation capacity indicated by decreased primary methylation index and secondary methylation index in both urine and saliva samples. The study also found a defect in hOGG1 that resulted in ineffective cleavage of 8-OHdG. Multiple regression analysis showed that levels of inorganic arsenic (iAs) in saliva and urine had a significant positive association with salivary 8-OHdG and a significant negative association with salivary hOGG1 expression [15c].

Another important cytogenetic marker, the urothelial micronucleus assay (MN), is extensively used to monitor the arsenic-exposed population. 145 arsenic-exposed and 60 unexposed individuals were surveyed of which 128 exposed individuals and 54 unexposed controls could be followed up with in 2010–2011. In 2004–2005, the extent of arsenic content in the drinking water was 348.23 ± 102.67 μg/L, which was significantly lower at 5.60 ± 10.83 μg/L in 2010–2011. Comparison of the data generated between the years 2004–2005 and 2010–2011, a significant decline in the MN frequency was noticed. This study concluded that the urothelial MN assay is a good biomarker in detecting recovery from toxicity caused by low doses of arsenic in drinking water [16c].

Another case–control study in Europeans was performed to assess the impact of XRCC1 R399Q and XRCC3 T241M polymorphisms on the risk of non-melanoma skin cancer (NMSC) associated with sunlight and arsenic exposure. The study included 618 new cases of NMSC and 527 hospital-based controls. Criteria included frequency based on age, sex, and country of residence from non-melanoma skin cancer. Results indicated an increased risk of squamous cell carcinoma (SCC) for the homozygous variant genotype of XRCC1 R399Q and a protective effect against basal cell carcinoma (BCC) for the homozygous variant genotype of XRCC3 T241M. The study concluded that polymorphisms in XRCC genes may modify the associations between skin cancer risk and exposure to sunlight or arsenic [17c].

Systematic Reviews and Studies

This systematic review describes the association of low-level iAs exposure (i.e., <100–150 μg/L arsenic water concentration) and cardiovascular disease (CVD) in human populations. Thirteen cohort and case–control studies from the United States, Taiwan, Bangladesh, and China were identified and critically examined for evidence for derivation of a reference dose for assessing potential non-cancer health risks of arsenic exposure [18M].

Pregnancy

Arsenic, a common groundwater pollutant, is associated with adverse reproductive health but few studies have examined its effect on maternal health. A retrospective study was reported in which 795 women suffering from following symptoms during pregnancy: cold/flu/infection, nausea/vomiting, abdominal cramping, headache, vaginal bleeding, and/or swollen ankles. A positive trend was observed for abdominal cramping and a marginal negative association was observed between arsenic quartiles and the odds of self-reported cold/flu/infection. The study concluded that moderate exposure to arsenic contaminated drinking water early in pregnancy was associated with increased odds of experiencing nausea/vomiting and abdominal cramping. Preventing exposure to arsenic contaminated drinking water during pregnancy could improve maternal health [19c].

Nervous System

Arsenic exposure is associated with *neurodevelopment problems* in children [20c,21c,22M]. Studies in Bangladesh and elsewhere reveal that arsenic (As) exposure via drinking water is negatively associated with performance-related aspects of child intelligence (e.g., Perceptual Reasoning, Working Memory) after adjustment for social factors. The magnitude of the association between Arsenic exposure via drinking water (WAs) and negative trends in child IQ raises the possibility that levels of WAs $\geq 5\,\mu g/L$ pose a threat to child development [23c].

Skin

Arsenic-induced skin lesions have been found to be associated with aberrant DNA methylation in some studies. A follow-up study of 900 skin lesion cases and 900 controls identified 10 people who developed skin lesions since a baseline survey in 2001–2003. Drinking water and blood samples of these 10 subjects were collected from those diagnosed with a *skin lesion* by the physician. The study investigated epigenome-wide changes of DNA methylation in arsenic-induced skin lesions cases. Results concluded that examined DNA methylation changes were associated with the development of arsenic-induced *skin lesions* over time [24C].

Cardiovascular System

Arsenic exposure is a risk factor for atherosclerosis in adults and an early risk biomarker for atherosclerosis in children. Carotid intima-media thickness (cIMT) is an indicator of subclinical atherosclerotic burden that has been associated with plasma asymmetric dimethylarginine (ADMA), a predictor of *cardiovascular disease* risk. A cross-sectional study was conducted in 199 children 3–14 years of age in the residents of Zimapan, México. Urine samples were analyzed for ADMA, sICAM-1, and sVCAM-1 by ELISA, and measured the concentrations of total speciated arsenic (tAs) using hydride generation cryotrapping atomic absorption spectrometry. The study concluded that arsenic exposure and plasma ADMA levels were positively associated with cIMT in a population of Mexican children with environmental arsenic exposure through drinking water [25c].

Biomonitoring

Arsenic (As) exposure has been associated with both *urologic malignancy* and *renal dysfunction* [26C]. Several studies were conducted monitoring ground water arsenic across the globe thus confirming the respective population being exposed to arsenic concentrations above the permissible limits. These studies reported a good correlation of arsenic concentrations in ground water with arsenic found in human samples like urine and hair [27E,28c,29R,30c,31H,32M]. One of the studies measured the concentration of arsenic and other trace elements in the urine of urban school children and rural working children in Lahore. A cross-sectional study included 339 children aged 8–12 years (mean age 9.9 years, SD 1.4; 47% girls) from two elementary schools in Lahore—one situated in a high air pollution area ($n = 100$), one situated in an area with lower air pollution ($n = 79$), one from near the carpet weaving industry ($n = 80$), and one from near the brick industry ($n = 80$). A spot urine sample was collected and concentrations of 20 metals and metalloids were measured by inductively coupled plasma-mass spectrometry (ICP-MS). Concentrations of As were especially elevated in children working in the brick making industry and were also higher among urban school children than other metals.

Susceptibility

Diet and toenail arsenic concentrations were measured in a New Hampshire population with arsenic-containing water. The association between diet and toenail arsenic concentrations was evaluated for individuals with measured household tap water arsenic. This study did not find a correlation between arsenic-containing tap water and measured arsenic in toenails, suggesting that diet can be an important contributor to total arsenic exposure in U.S. populations regardless of arsenic concentrations in drinking water. Thus, dietary exposure to arsenic in the U.S. warrants consideration as a potential health risk [33A].

Another New Hampshire Birth Cohort Study investigated whether *in utero* exposure to arsenic enhanced infection susceptibility risks in infants. Information was obtained on 4-month-old infants ($n = 214$) using a parental telephone survey on infant infections and symptoms, including *respiratory infections, diarrhoea and specific illnesses*, as well as the duration and severity of infections. Results from the study provide initial evidence that *in utero* As exposure may be related to infant infection and infection severity [34c].

Another study evaluated the interaction between single nucleotide polymorphisms (SNPs) in genes associated with diabetes and arsenic exposure in drinking water and the risk of developing type 2 diabetes mellitus (T2DM). Findings from this study suggest that genetic variation in NOTCH2 increased susceptibility to T2DM among people exposed to inorganic arsenic. Additionally, genetic variants in ADAMTS9 may increase the risk of T2DM [35C]. A second report also suggested that epigenetic modifications may be an important pathway underlying arsenic toxicity. Analyzed samples from 400 participants found associations between arsenic exposure and gene-specific differential white blood cell DNA methylation, also identifying specific differentially methylated loci [36c].

Cancer

Arsenic is a known human carcinogen that has been associated with adverse health outcomes, including cancer. A study examined the association between arsenic exposure from food and incidence of cancer in a Japanese population (men and women aged 45–74 years). The study concluded that a significant dose–response trend was seen in the association of arsenic and inorganic intake with *lung cancer risk* in currently smoking men [37C,38c]. Investigating the mechanism, a recent study established critical roles of miR-199a-5p and its downstream targets HIF-1/COX-2 in arsenic-induced tumor growth and angiogenesis. The study utilized human lung epithelial BEAS-2B cells that were transformed through long-term arsenic exposure *in vitro*, and a human xenograft tumor model was established to assess tumor angiogenesis and tumor growth *in vivo* [39E].

ANTIMONY AND ANTIMONIALS [SED-15, 316; SEDA-32, 414; SEDA-33, 448; SEDA-34, 350; SEDA-35, 398; SEDA-36, 298]

Nervous System

A study was conducted based on a population-based birth cohort established in Sabadell (Catalonia, Spain) as part of the INMA [Environment and Childhood] Project. The aim of this study was to evaluate the potential neurotoxic effects of prenatal exposure to seven metals (cobalt, copper, arsenic, cadmium, antimony, thallium and lead) during the first and third trimester of pregnancy on child neuropsychological development at 4 years of age. Metals were analysed in the 485 urine samples collected from mothers during the first and third trimester of pregnancy. Results obtained negative coefficients for the exposure to cadmium first trimester, cadmium third trimester and lead third trimester on the general cognitive score of McCarthy Scales of Children's Abilities (MSCA). Results suggest that prenatal exposure to current low-levels of metals does not *impair children's cognitive development* during preschool years [40c].

Observational Study

A study was conducted in 55 recycling workers and 10 office workers at three formal e-waste recycling plants in Sweden. The purpose of this study was to evaluate workers' exposure to 20 potentially toxic metals, using biomarkers of exposure in combination with monitoring of personal air exposure. Metal concentration was measured in whole blood, plasma, urine, and air filters. Results showed significantly higher concentrations of chromium, cobalt, indium, lead, and mercury in blood, urine, and/or plasma of the recycling workers, compared with the office workers. Also, concentrations of antimony, indium, lead, mercury, and vanadium showed close to linear associations between the inhalable particle fraction and blood, plasma, or urine. The study concluded that workers performing recycling tasks for electronic wastes are exposed to multiple toxic metals [41c]. In an independent study analysing 205 human hair samples from Guiyu, e-waste recycling workers had higher hair antimony concentrations ($P < 0.001$). There was no significant difference of hair antimony concentrations among different occupation types in e-waste recycling [42c]. Use of antimony trioxide in food contact material and household plastics has been a point of concern with emphasis on risk assessment and investigations for its potential as a carcinogen and endocrine disruptor [43M].

BERYLLIUM [SEDA-34, 353; SEDA-35, 400; SEDA-36, 301]

Beryllium is commonly used in the dental industry. A study was conducted which investigated the association between particle size and shape in induced sputum (IS) upon beryllium exposure and oxidative stress in 83 dental technicians. Heme oxygenase-1 (HO1) gene expression in IS was evaluated by quantitative polymerase chain reaction. Results shown that high content of particles (92%) in IS >5 μ in size is correlated to a positive BeLPT risk (odds ratio [OR] = 3.4, 95% confidence interval [CI]: 0.9–13). These results suggested that parameters of size and shape of particles in IS are sensitive to workplace hygiene, affect the level of oxidative stress and also may be potential markers for monitoring hazardous dust exposures [44c].

CALCIUM SALTS [SED-15, 610; SEDA-33, 449; SEDA-34, 354; SEDA-35, 400; SEDA-36, 301]

Systematic Reviews and Studies

An observational study was performed in humans to evaluate the reported effects of treatments for calcium blocker poisoning [45E,46R,47c]. The primary outcomes of the study were *mortality* and *hemodynamic parameter* whereas secondary outcomes included length of stay in hospital, length of stay in an intensive care unit, duration of vasopressor use, functional outcomes, and serum calcium channel blocker concentrations. The results showed that humans examined for high-dose insulin and extracorporeal life support are associated with improved hemodynamic parameters and lower mortality. Extracorporeal life support was associated with improved survival in patients with *severe shock* or *cardiac arrest* at the cost of limb ischemia, thrombosis, and bleeding.

Observational Study

An observational study reported the role of Ca supplements in vascular risk elevation, suggesting that these supplements may also be associated with the occurrence of *brain lesions* in older adults [48c]. This cross-sectional clinical observational study investigated the association between Ca-containing dietary supplement use and lesion volumes in a sample of 227 older adults (60 years and above). The study concluded that use of Ca-containing dietary supplements, even low-dose supplements, by older adults may be associated with greater lesion volumes.

Cancer

A randomized clinical trial in patients was done to investigate whether the addition of a neutral, super-saturated, calcium phosphate mouth rinse benefits the severity and duration of *acute mucositis* in head and neck cancer patients treated with chemoradiation (chemotherapeutics followed by radiation) [49c]. 60 patients with malignant *neoplasms* of the head and neck receiving (chemo) radiation were included in this study. Patients were assessed twice in a week for oral mucositis and dysphagia using the National Cancer Institute

common toxicity criteria scale version 3, and oral pain was scored with a visual analogue scale. No significant difference in grade III *mucositis and dysphagia* was observed between the study group as compared to the control group. Therefore, there is currently no evidence that the use of calcium phosphate mouth rinse is useful for preventing acute mucositis in cancer patients.

Pregnancy

A study reported the effects of low levels of maternal calcium intake on postnatal growth. Epidemiological data link low dietary calcium with pre-eclampsia [50c,51r]. A prospective birth cohort study of 1150 pregnant women and their subsequent offspring used multivariable regression analysis to estimate the effects of prenatal maternal blood lead levels and low calcium intake on growth at each follow-up. Prenatal lead exposure (<5.0 μg/dL) adversely affected postnatal growth and low calcium intake aggravated the effect. It indicated that significant control of lead and sufficient intake of calcium is necessary to help children's health.

CHROMIUM [SED-15, 737; SEDA-32, 414; SEDA-33, 450; SEDA-34, 354; SEDA-35, 401; SEDA-36, 303]

Chromium (Cr) is an established environmental pollutant which is also classified as a carcinogen in humans. In case of chromium exposure in patients undergoing revision total hip arthroplasty (THA), sometimes adverse local tissue reactions occurring in metal-on-metal total hip arthroplasty (MoM THA) could potentially lead to secondary failure modes such as dislocation or infection [52c,53S,54c,55c].

Cancer

High concentrations of hexavalent chromium [Cr(VI)] in drinking water induce villous cytotoxicity and compensatory crypt hyperplasia in the small intestines of mice but not in rats. Exposure to such cytotoxic concentrations increases lifetime intestinal neoplasms in mice, suggesting that the mode of action for Cr(VI)-induced *intestinal tumors* involves chronic wounding and compensatory cell proliferation of the intestine [56E].

Exposure to hexavalent chromium [Cr(VI)] through the inhalation route is associated with increased lung cancer risk among workers in several industries, particularly in chromate production workers exposed to high concentrations of Cr(VI) (≥100 μg/m(3)) in which clear exposure–response relationships and respiratory irritation and tissue damage have been reported. This study provides data that was used to assess *lung cancer risk* associated with environmental and current occupational exposures, occurring at concentrations that are significantly lower. Mode of action (MOA) analysis was conducted for Cr(VI)-induced lung cancer evaluating toxicokinetic and toxicological data in humans and rodents [57E]. This MOA supports the use of non-linear approaches when extrapolating lung cancer risk occurring at high concentration occupational exposures.

Undertaking mechanistic investigations, a study assessed the impact of a mild Cr(VI) exposure on critical bioenergetic parameters (lactate production, oxygen consumption and intracellular ATP levels). A cell line derived from normal human bronchial epithelium (BEAS-2B), the main *in vivo* target of Cr(VI) carcinogenicity was used and exposed to 1 μM Cr(VI). A shift to a more fermentative metabolism resulting from the simultaneous inhibition of respiration and stimulation of glycolysis was reported [58E]. Another independent study suggested a new aspect of carcinogenic mechanism of Cr(VI). The study described that acute Cr(VI) resulted in a robust DNA double strand break and repair response, but that longer exposure to particulate zinc chromate induced concentration-dependent increases in DNA double strand breaks. Furthermore, acute (24 h) exposure induced DNA double strand break repair signaling by inducing Mre11 foci formation, ATM phosphorylation and phosphorylated ATM foci formation, Rad51 protein levels and Rad51 foci formation. However, longer exposures reduced the Rad51 response [59E].

Systematic Reviews and Studies

A systematic review on exposure–risk relationship for occupational chromium (VI) exposure and *lung cancer* was performed in order to establish exposure limits. Studies included in this review provided data for more than one level of occupational chromium exposure and also considered the confounders smoking and adequate methodological quality. Five studies of two cohorts of chromium production workers in Baltimore, Maryland, and Painesville, Ohio, were also included. On the basis of different estimates for the exposure effect, the absolute excess risk was found to be "acceptable" at a Cr(VI) concentration of $0.1 \mu g/m^3$, and became "intolerable" beyond a Cr(VI) concentration of $1 \mu g/m^3$. It concluded that occupational exposure limits for Cr(VI) based on excess absolute risks can be derived from published data identified by a systematic literature review [60M].

Genotoxicity

A pilot risk assessment study was carried out in painters exposed to strontium chromate ($SrCrO_4$) employed in the aeronautical industry. An analysis of chromium metal was done in blood and plasma. Genetic damage in workers was evaluated using the cytokinesis-block micronucleus assay (CBMN) and serum 8-hydroxyguanine (8-OHdG) ELISA assay. A significant association between blood Cr level and plasma miR-3940-5p level was found. Under high Cr exposure, a non-linear relationship with micronuclei frequency in CBMN and serum 8-OHdG level with micronuclei frequency was found. Study demonstrated that XRCC2 and BRCC3 protein levels were associated with miR-3940-5p level, respectively. Further, high Cr(VI) may not always aggravate genetic damage, this damage may instead be due to the regulation of miRNA on DNA repair genes responsive to high Cr(VI) exposure [61c,62c].

COBALT [SED-15, 847; SEDA-32, 415; SEDA-33, 450; SEDA-34, 354; SEDA-35, 402; SEDA-36, 303]

Systematic Reviews

Systematic reviews identified various published reports of toxicity related to metals such as cobalt and chromium which are released from hip implants. Medline (from 1950) and Embase (from 1980) were searched to 28 February 2014. These searches identified 281 unique references of which 23 contained original case data. Some cases associated with systemic toxicity were reported. Toxicity was first manifested months and often several years after placement of the metal-containing joint. Reported systemic features fell into three main categories: neuro-ocular toxicity (14 patients), cardiotoxicity (11 patients) and thyroid toxicity (9 patients). Neurotoxicity manifested as peripheral neuropathy (8 cases), sensorineural hearing loss (7) and cognitive decline (5); ocular toxicity presented as visual impairment (6). Analysis of blood or serum metal concentrations was reported in several studies ($n = 17$ for cobalt and $n = 14$ for chromium), and the median cobalt concentration was 398 μg/L (range, 13.6–6521) and the median chromium concentration in whole blood was 48 μg/L (range, 4.1–221 μg/L including serum and blood values). The report concluded that patients exposed to high circulating concentrations of cobalt from failed hip replacements resulted in *neurological damage, hypothyroidism and/or cardiomyopathy*. The major risk of systemic cobalt toxicity seems to result from accelerated wear of a cobalt-containing revision of a failed ceramic prosthesis, rather than from primary failure of a metal-on-metal prosthesis [63M,64M].

Multiorgan Dysfunctions

Various studies evaluating prosthetic hip-associated cobalt toxicity (PHACT) in animals and humans indicated that elevated serum or whole blood cobalt levels in humans are associated with local and systemic effects and induce *hypersensitivity reactions* [65c,66M,67c,68c].

In a study, 219 hips in 192 patients aged between 18 and 65 years were randomised to 28-mm metal-on-metal uncemented total hip replacements (THRs, 107 hips) or hybrid hip resurfacing (HR, 112 hips). Results shown that *Osteolysis* was found in 30 of 81 THR patients (37.4%), mostly in the proximal femur, compared with two of 83 HR patients (2.4%) ($P < 0.001$). Also, at 5 years the mean metal ion levels were $<2.5\ \mu g/L$ for cobalt and chromium in both groups [69c].

A single-center cross-sectional prospective cohort study of all patients who received a Birmingham Hip Resurfacing (BHR) prosthesis from 2005 to 2010 in Martini Hospital, Groningen, The Netherlands was conducted. Data were collected on patient and surgical characteristics, clinical hip outcome scores (Harris hip score and Oxford score), serum metal ion levels (cobalt and chromium), and radiographs. This study found that *pseudotumor* formation occurred in 28% of hips after an average follow-up of 41 months. Most pseudotumors (72.5%) were asymptomatic. Larger pseudotumors were associated with more complaints [70c].

Another independent study investigated the role of cobalt–chromium wear debris and Co ion in affecting lymphocytes contributing in metal-on-metal (MoM) implant failure. The study showed that prolonged exposure to metal debris induces lymphocyte proliferation, suggesting that activation of resting lymphocytes occurred. Cobalt toxicity may modulate IL-2 secretion, and even Co ion concentrations below the MHRA guideline levels (7 ppb) may contribute to the impairment of immune regulation *in vivo* in patients with MoM implants [71E].

COPPER [SED-15, 901; SEDA-32, 415; SEDA-33, 450; SEDA-34, 355; SEDA-35, 402; SEDA-36, 304]

Occupational exposure to copper leads to risks for developing occupational pathology. 358 Kola Transpolar copper–nickel miners who were diagnosed with 722 cases of occupational diseases in the years 1990–2013 were studied. Tunnellers (OR=12, 8) and operators of drilling rigs (OR=10, 4) were found to have the highest risk for developing occupational diseases, which are dominated by musculoskeletal disorders. A significant increase in the risk of occupational diseases was established in miners with 11–15 years of service and over 25 years of service [72c].

Cytotoxicity

A prospective study was conducted to compare the impact of copper-containing and levenorgestrel-releasing intrauterine contraceptives before and after insertion on cervicovaginal cytology and microbiological flora [73E]. In this study 108 Cu-IUDs and 42 LNG-IUSs were placed. Cervical cytological and vaginal microbiological findings before insertion and after 12 months were recorded. Non-specific inflammatory changes in cervical cytology became more frequent after 1 year of use of a Cu-IUD whereas no such changes were reported in women fitted with a LNG-IUS. Also, mycoplasma infections were diagnosed significantly more in Cu-IUD fitted devices women after 1 year of use. The study concluded that use of a Cu-IUD—but not that of a LNG-IUS—was associated with an alteration of the vaginal flora and showed a higher frequency of *nonspecific inflammatory changes* affecting cervical cytology.

Nervous System

Occupational exposure to copper is common through various sources including copper smelter plants. Workers employed in copper smelter plant underwent neuropsychological tests. Early subclinical effects of the exposure of the nervous system in copper smelters were detected [74c].

Numerous evidences robustly support the involvement of excess Cu-induced neurotoxicity in hepatocerebral (Wilson's disease) and neurodegenerative disorders (especially Alzheimer's disease and Parkinson's disease). But the ideal Cu neurotoxicity biomarker/s for early prognosis remains elusive. Non-ceruloplasmin bound Cu is a biological marker of Wilson's disease and recent studies have shown that its levels are also increased in Alzheimer's disease [75H,76H].

GOLD AND GOLD SALTS [SED-15, 1520; SEDA-32, 416; SEDA-33, 451; SEDA-34, 355; SEDA-35, 402; SEDA-36, 305]

A poisoning with gold potassium cyanide and other metallic cyanides in a jeweller has been reported [77c]. A cross-sectional study was conducted using a convenience sample of 340 pregnant women, ranging in age from 15–49 years, in six governmental antenatal clinics in the Geita District, Tanzania. The aim of the study was to examine geophagy practices of pregnant women in a gold mining area of the Geita District in northwestern Tanzania, and also examined the potential for exposure to chemical elements by testing soil samples. The study concluded that pregnant women who eat soil in Geita District are exposed to potentially high levels of chemical elements, depending upon the frequency of consumption, the daily amount consumed and the source location of the soil eaten [78R].

LANTHANUM CARBONATE [SEDA-32, 417; SEDA-33, 451; SEDA-34, 356; SEDA-35, 404; SEDA-36, 306]

Lanthanum carbonate (LC) is an effective non-calcium phosphate binder is widely used to manage *hyperphosphatemia* in patients with chronic kidney disease (CKD) on dialysis. Its safety and efficacy was confirmed by several studies reported [79M,80M].

A multicentre, randomized, double-blind, placebo-controlled trial was performed to investigate the efficacy and safety of LC in Japanese hyperphosphatemic stage in 4–5 CKD patients not on dialysis. Results showed that LC produced a significant reduction in serum phosphate level compared to placebo after 8 weeks of treatment. It also caused a significant decrease in serum Ca × P product and urinary phosphate excretion compared with placebo. The safety profile of LC was similar to that of placebo. This study demonstrated the effectiveness of LC to control hyperphosphatemia in pre-dialysis CKD patients [81c].

Another study evaluated the efficacy and tolerability of lanthanum carbonate (LC) in the treatment of hyperphosphatemia in dialysis patients. 950 patients in seven placebo-controlled RCTs were included. Results showed that LC could effectively control hyperphosphatemia compared with placebo. It was well tolerated and more effective than placebo during short-term trials in the treatment of hyperphosphatemia in dialysis patients. LC is an ideal choice for second-line treatment of hyperphosphatemia after therapy failure or other contraindication for calcium agents [82M].

LEAD [SED-15, 2013; SEDA-28, 247; SEDA-35, 404; SEDA-36, 307]

Lead (Pb) is a toxic element which is widely distributed throughout the environment. Children are more susceptible to lead exposure because of their higher absorption rate and the greater susceptibility of the developing nervous system. Furthermore, the combination of lead with other toxic metals like mercury and cadmium may aggravate the adverse effects of lead [83c,84C].

Fetotoxicity

A study conducted using event-related potentials (ERPs) for assessing the effects of low-level prenatal lead exposure on auditory recognition memory in 2-month-old infants. Infants were divided into four groups according to cord-blood lead concentration. The first group showed the normally expected differences in P2, P750, and late slow wave (LSW) amplitudes elicited

by mothers' and strangers' voices. These differences were not observed for one or more ERP components in the other groups. Thus, there was electrophysiological evidence of *poorer auditory recognition memory* at 2 months with cord-blood lead ≥2.00 µg/dL [85A].

Monitoring Therapy

The National Health and Nutrition Examination Survey (2003–2010) analyzed the environmental lead exposure in the United States for association of blood pressure and hypertension with blood lead. In this study 12 725 participants included 21.1% black, 20.5% Hispanic, 58.4% Caucasian, and 48.7% women. In multivariable analyses of all participants, doubling of blood lead was associated with higher ($P \leq 0.0007$) systolic and diastolic pressure but not with the odds of hypertension. Associations with blood lead were nonsignificant for systolic pressure in women and for diastolic pressure in non-whites. Systolic pressure increased with blood lead with effect sizes associated with blood lead doubling ranging from +0.65 mm Hg in whites to +1.61 mm Hg in blacks. Small and inconsistent effect sizes in the associations of blood pressure with blood lead likely exclude current environmental lead exposure as a major *hypertension* cause in the United States [86M].

Reproductive System

In this study occupational exposures and sperm morphology were tested to establish whether exposures affected motile sperm concentration. Men attending 14 fertility clinics across the UK gave semen samples that were analysed after the men completed questionnaires about their employment and lifestyle. Results associated with sperm morphology were available for 1861/2011 employed at the time of recruitment. Of these 1861, 296 (15.9%) had poor morphology; of the 2011, 453 (22.5%) had low MSC; 654/1981 (33.0%) had both conditions. Poor morphology was associated with self-reported lifetime exposure to lead [87A].

IRON SALTS [SED-15, 1911; SEDA-32, 417; SEDA-33, 451; SEDA-34, 355; SEDA-35, 402; SEDA-36, 305]

GI Tract

Oral iron supplementation is often associated with rapid onset of gastrointestinal side effects. A double-blind placebo-controlled study was planned to develop and test a short, simple questionnaire to capture these early side effects and to determine which symptoms are more discriminating. Subjects were randomized into two treatment groups ($n = 10$/group) to receive either ferrous sulphate (200 mg capsules containing 65 mg of iron) or placebo, both to be taken at mealtimes twice daily during the treatment period. Subjects completed the questionnaires daily for 14 days. The questionnaire included gastrointestinal symptoms commonly reported to be associated with the oral intake of ferrous iron salts (i.e. nausea, vomiting, heartburn, abdominal pain, diarrhoea, and constipation). Results obtained 75% of participants reporting the presence of one or more symptoms in the first week of the study were in the ferrous sulphate group. In the second week of the study (i.e. wash-out), 67% of the participants reporting one or more symptom(s) were in the ferrous sulphate group [88R].

Case Study

A first case was reported regarding the occurrence of widespread oral ulceration in an 87-year-old woman with Alzheimer's disease. The ulceration extended from the side of the tongue to the floor of the mouth. No clear explanation was found and various local treatments were ineffective. Once it was realized that the ferrous sulfate tablets (given as an iron supplement) were crushed prior to administration (due to the patient's deglutition disorder), withdrawal of this treatment led to rapid resolution of the ulceration. Nine other cases of oral ulcerations associated with ferrous sulfate were identified in the French National Pharmacovigilance Database. All patients were over 80 years of age and the youngest patient (a 54 years old) had dysphagia associated with facial paralysis [89A].

MAGNESIUM SALTS [SED-15, 2196; SEDA-32, 417; SEDA-33, 452; SEDA-34, 356; SEDA-35, 406; SEDA-36, 309]

Magnesium deficiency is associated with poor physical performance. A parallel-group, randomized controlled trial of 139 healthy elderly women (mean ± SD age: 71.5 ± 5.2 years) attending a mild fitness program were randomly allocated to a treatment group (300 mg Mg/days; $n = 62$) or a control group (no placebo or intervention; $n = 77$) by using a computer-generated randomization sequence. The study investigated whether 3 months of oral magnesium supplementation can improve physical performance in healthy elderly women. Magnesium supplementation may prevent or delay the age-related decline in physical performance [90c].

Case Study

A 35-year-old pregnant female with systemic lupus erythematosus and lupus nephritis underwent emergency cesarean section at 24 weeks of gestation under general anesthesia. The patient had received magnesium sulfate with a diagnosis of pregnancy-induced hypertension since 20 weeks of gestation. Anesthesia was induced with

thiopental 3.5 mg × kg⁻¹ and tracheal intubation was facilitated by administration of rocuronium 1.0 mg × kg⁻¹. No additional rocuronium was needed during operation. After operation, no twitch was noted on the ulnar nerve TOF monitor. When rocuronium is used to facilitate general endotracheal anesthesia in a patient for emergency cesarean delivery, it is important to recognize that magnesium may prolong neuromuscular block significantly [91A].

MERCURY AND MERCURIAL SALTS [SED-15, 2259; SEDA-32, 419; SEDA-33, 453; SEDA-34, 358; SEDA-35, 407; SEDA-36, 311]

Prenatal exposure to methylmercury leads to various health complications reported in children [83c,92c,93R,94C,95c,96M].

Nervous System

Chronic mercury intoxication leads to various severities of cognitive disorders. A discrimination analysis of neuropsychologic and neurophysiologic research data was performed comparing workers exposed to mercury during a long length of service with patients with early and marked stages of chronic mercurial intoxication. These authors observed cognitive disorders in chronic mercurial intoxication with three severity degrees; in the light degree, patients demonstrate lower amplitude of cognitive evoked potentials, poor long-term memory and associative thinking. Moderate cognitive disorders were characterized by decreased vision, long-term memory and concentration of attention, poor optic and spatial gnosis. Others marked cognitive disorders with chronic mercurial intoxication included a more decreased *long-term, short-term, picturesque memory, poor intellect, optic and spatial gnosis* and associative thinking [97C].

Case Study

A relationship between neurological effects and mercury/ methylmercury concentrations in various biomarkers, including meconium, hair, fingernail, and toenail was investigated. It was assumed that high fish consumption might be a critical risk factor for methylmercury levels in children and may cause a lower expressive language score. Three-year-old children in Taiwan were evaluating for the cognitive, language, and motor development calculated and validated. The geometric mean of the total mercury concentration in meconium was 89.6 ng g⁻¹ and in hair, fingernail, and toenail samples were 1.96, 0.64, and 0.55 μg g⁻¹, respectively. Seventy percent of children had hair methylmercury concentrations exceeding the U.S. environmental protection agency (EPA) reference of 1 μg g⁻¹. A significantly positive correlation was obtained between methylmercury levels in hair, fingernail, and toenail. These methylmercury levels were also significantly positively correlated with the children's fish intake and negatively correlated with a Bayley-III scale score of expressive language. High fish consumption appears to be a critical risk factor for methylmercury levels in children and may cause a lower expressive language score [98M].

Cardiovascular System

Exposure to methylmercury through maternal fish consumption leads to childhood blood pressure (BP) which is an important determinant of adult cardiovascular disease. It has been reported to increase the BP of children years later. A prospective cohort study conducted in Massachusetts included mother–child pairs from Project Viva.

In this study, erythrocyte mercury concentration and Systolic BP in children were measured up to five times per visit in early and mid-childhood (median ages 3.2 and 7.7 years). Among 1103 mother–child pairs, mean (SD) second trimester total erythrocyte mercury concentration was 4.0 (3.9) ng/g among mothers whose children were assessed in early childhood and 4.0 (4.0) ng/g for children assessed in mid-childhood. Mean (SD) offspring systolic BP was 92.1 (10.4) mm Hg in early childhood and 94.3 (8.4) mm Hg in mid-childhood [99C].

NICKEL [SED-15, 2502; SEDA-32, 419; SEDA-33, 453; SEDA-34, 358; SEDA-35, 409; SEDA-36, 313]

Genotoxicity

A study was conducted among 231 workers exposed to nickel in a stainless steel production enterprise and another 75 water pump workers in that enterprise were recruited as control group. The objective of the study was to analyse the excision repair capacity of human 8-oxoguanine DNA *N*-glycosylase 1 (hOGG1) for 8-OHdG and the oxidative DNA damage among workers exposed to nickel in stainless steel production environment. Results from the study concluded that exposure to nickel increases oxidative DNA damage among steel workers, and hOGG1 shows active excision repair capacity for 8-OHdG [100C].

Respiratory System

Nickel (Ni) is present in ambient air predominantly in the form of oxides and sulfates, with various sizes of Ni between the fine (particle aerodynamic diameter <2.5 μm; PM2.5) and coarser (2.5–10 μm) size-selected aerosol fractions of PM10 dependent on the aerosol's origin. It has been recommended that when a long-term health protective reference concentration for Ni in ambient air, the respiratory toxicity and carcinogenicity effects of the predominant Ni compounds is derived, its concentration in ambient air must be considered [101c].

Skin

Exposure to iPad tablet computers, a potential source of nickel exposure, leads to *Allergic contact dermatitis* in children [102c]. Also, another case of razor-associated *dermatitis* highlights a potential source of nickel exposure in allergic patients [103c].

Immunologic

Nickel is a strong immunological sensitizer and may induce contact hypersensitivity. Case reports of allergic reactions to intraoral nickel and these allergic reactions are generally of a delayed type (type IV). A case of a nickel allergic patient displaying frequent *laryngeal edema attacks* which required treatment with epinephrine injections followed by parenteral corticosteroid doses was reported [104H].

A prospective study was conducted in 60 young adults in which gum irritation and cytotoxicity caused by nickel–chromium (Ni–Cr) alloy porcelain, by interleukin-8 (IL-8), interleukin-6 (IL-6) and gingival crevicular fluid (GCF) volumes at different time points peri-crown restoration 30 male and 30 female subjects, aged 20–35 years old were enrolled in which total amount and concentrations of IL-8 and IL-6 per site, GCF volumes increased after nickel–chromium (Ni–Cr) alloy-porcelain crown restoration. It reached its peak at the third month as the GCF volume increased by 52.20%, the total amount and concentrations of IL-8 increased by 112.11% and 22.75%; the total amount and concentrations of IL-6 increased by 77.66% and 17.17% when compared to baseline. Results show that increase in the total amount and the concentrations of IL-8 and IL-6 and GCF volume may be related to the cytotoxicity induced by Ni–Cr alloy [105c].

Biological Monitoring

A study was conducted to assess whether occupational exposure to low doses of nickel (Ni) present in urban air could cause alterations in the concentration of plasma testosterone in workers of the Municipal Police of a large Italian city assigned to different types of outdoor tasks. In this study, 359 male subjects were included and divided on the basis of job, age, length of service and smoking habits. The dosage of whole blood Ni and of the plasma testosterone was carried out. The total sample was subjected to the independent-samples T-test and the Mann–Whitney U test for variables with 2 modes (smokers versus nonsmokers) and the ANOVA test and the Kruskal–Wallis test for variables with more than 2 modes (age, length of service and job function). Results were confirmed by multiple linear regressions, which indicated that Ni was the only important variable that can contribute to the alterations of testosterone. Occupational exposure to low doses of Ni present in the urban environment is able to influence some lines of the hypothalamic–pituitary–gonadal axis in exposed workers [106A].

POTASSIUM SALTS [SED-15, 2905; SEDA-31, 392; SEDA-35, 409; SEDA-36, 314]

Observational Study

Sodium–potassium intake imbalance leads to implications for dietetic practice [107c,108C]. In chronic kidney disease (CKD) patients, there is a deficient elimination of potassium. A study was performed in 477 stage-5 CKD patients referred for dialysis to The Dialysis Centre of the Emergency County Hospital Timişoara. 260 males and 217 females of average age of the patients was 57.41 ± 14.26 years were included. All were stage-5 CKD with GFR < 15 mL/min/1.73 m^2, with a group average value of eGFR of 5.72 ± 2.81 mL/min/1.73 m^2. This investigation showed *hypokalemia* in 14 patients (2.93%) and *hyperkalemia* was found in 179 patients [109c].

Diagnosis of Adverse Effects of Drugs

Sodium polystyrene sulfonate (Kayexalate) and calcium polystyrene sulfonate (CPS, Kalimate), may lead to significant obstruction of the gastrointestinal tract in some groups of patients [110A].

STRONTIUM SALTS [SEDA-32, 420; SEDA-33, 455; SEDA-34, 359; SEDA-35, 410; SEDA-36, 315]

Strontium ranelate is a relatively new medication with good safety profile for the treatment of postmenopausal osteoporosis [111c,112M,113C,114M].

Case Study

Severe cutaneous adverse drug reactions have been reported with strontium ranelate, such as drug rash with *eosinophilia* and systemic symptoms (DRESS), Stevens–Johnson syndrome (SJS), and toxic epidermal necrolysis (TEN). *A 70-year-old woman was reported to develop multiple itching erythematous macules and plaques*

about 1 month after beginning strontium ranelate medication. Cutaneous lesions progressed over the entire body with severe oral and ocular mucosa involvement whereas mild SJS was diagnosed and strontium ranelate was discontinued immediately [109c].

Cardiovascular System

A recent pooled analysis of randomised trials found an increased risk of myocardial infarction with use of the antiosteoporotic drug strontium ranelate. A cohort study in Denmark, 2005–2011, investigated the risk of *acute coronary syndrome* among postmenopausal women treated with strontium ranelate. Data obtained from this study of antiosteoporotic drug users do not support a significant association between use of strontium ranelate and acute coronary syndrome [115C].

SILVER SALTS AND DERIVATIVES [SED-15, 3140; SEDA-32, 420; SEDA-33, 454; SEDA-34, 359; SEDA-35, 409; SEDA-36, 314]

Case Study

Silver salt exposure leads to bluish-gray macules on hands at a workplace. *A 34-year-old man presented with asymptomatic bluish-gray macules on his hands. It developed over the previous 2 years, but otherwise the patient was healthy and was on no regular medication. A detailed clinical history and histologic examination allowed the diagnosis. Histopathologic examination illustrated deposits of aggregated granules of black pigment in the dermis, localized preferentially around the sweat glands. This was consistent with the deposition of silver salts. These deposits remain indefinitely in the skin and are characterized by a bluish-gray color, more prominent in the photo-exposed areas. The lesions remain unchanged after 1 year of follow-up. This exposure is usually occupational, iatrogenic, or accidental [116A].*

TITANIUM [SED-15, 3434; SEDA-32, 420; SEDA-33, 456; SEDA-34, 360; SEDA-35, 410; SEDA-36, 315]

Systematic Reviews

The use of metal-on-metal (MoM) total hip arthroplasty (THA) has increased in the last decades. A Systematic review of clinical trials (RCTs) and epidemiological studies with assessment of metal ion levels (cobalt, chromium, titanium, nickel, molybdenum) in body fluids after implantation of metalliferous hip replacements was published. The review suggested that the highest metal ion concentrations were observed after treatment with stemmed large-head MoM-implants and hip resurfacing arthroplasty [117c].

ZINC [SED-15, 3717; SEDA-32, 420; SEDA-33, 458; SEDA-34, 360; SEDA-35, 410; SEDA-36, 315]

Observational Study

Zinc phosphide-poisoned patients who were referred to Loghman-Hakim Hospital between March 2011 and September 2013 were retrospectively reviewed. Data reported in patients' records regarding demographic characteristics, characteristics of the poisoning, abdominal radiography results, and patients' outcome were recorded. Results shown that in 102 patients the most common signs/symptoms were *nausea and vomiting* (60%). Out of which four patients died and another seven had developed complications during their hospitalization (*metabolic acidosis, liver abnormalities, or acute renal failure*). Nineteen patients had radio-opaque abdominal radiographs, nine of whom had died or developed complications. Plain abdominal radiography had the sensitivity and specificity in predicting the patients' death or further development of complications [118].

Respiratory Effect

Zinc (Zn^{2+}) is a ubiquitous respiratory toxicant that has been associated with PM health effects. Zn^{2+} leads to multiple oxidative effects that are exerted through H_2O_2-dependent and independent mechanisms. Human airway epithelial cell (BEAS-2B) expressing the redox-sensitive fluorogenic sensors HyPer (H_2O_2) or roGFP2 (EGSH) in the cytosol or mitochondria were exposed to 50 μM Zn^{2+} for 5 min in the presence of 1 μM of the zinc ionophore pyrithione. Results showed that both cytosolic catalase overexpression and *ectopic catalase expression* in mitochondria were effective in ablating Zn^{2+}-induced elevations in H_2O_2. Compartment-directed catalase expression blunted Zn^{2+}-induced elevations in cytosolic EGSH and the increased expression of HO-1 mRNA levels [119E]. On the other hand utility of zinc as *panacea for common cold* in the form of intranasal (IN) zinc gluconate gel. Previous evidence has shown that IN zinc sulfate ($ZnSO_4$) solutions can cause *anosmia* in humans as well as significant damage to the olfactory epithelium in rodents. However, an *in vitro* (olfactory neuron model) study suggested Zn toxicity is not mediated through an acidification of intracellular pH in olfactory neurons [120E].

References

[1] Yang M, Jiang L, Huang H, et al. Dietary exposure to aluminium and health risk assessment in the residents of Shenzhen, China. PLoS One. 2014;9(3):e89715 [C].

[2] Krewski D, Yokel RA, Nieboer E, et al. Human health risk assessment for aluminium, aluminium oxide, and aluminium hydroxide. J Toxicol Environ Health B Crit Rev. 2007;10(Suppl 1):1–269 [R].

[3] Kuzmin DV. Hygienic evaluation of environment, morbidity among pregnant women and newborns within social hygienic monitoring system. Med Tr Prom Ekol. 2014;6:4–8 [H].

[4] Fanni D, Ambu R, Gerosa C, et al. Aluminum exposure and toxicity in neonates: a practical guide to halt aluminum overload in the prenatal and perinatal periods. World J Pediatr. 2014;10(2):101–7 [R].

[5] Willhite CC, Karyakina NA, Yokel RA, et al. Systematic review of potential health risks posed by pharmaceutical, occupational and consumer exposures to metallic and nanoscale aluminum, aluminum oxides, aluminum hydroxide and its soluble salts. Crit Rev Toxicol. 2014;44(Suppl 4):1–80 [R].

[6] She Y, Zhao H, Zhu Y, et al. Aluminum trichloride disorders bile acid secretion and induces hepatocyte apoptosis in rats. Cell Biochem Biophys. 2015;71(3):1569–77 [Epub ahead of print] [E].

[7] Taiwo O, Galusha D, Tessier-Sherman B, et al. Acoustic neuroma: potential risk factors and audiometric surveillance in the aluminium industry. Occup Environ Med. 2014;71(9):624–8 [C].

[8] Dahl C, Søgaard AJ, Tell GS, et al. Do cadmium, lead, and aluminum in drinking water increase the risk of hip fractures? A NOREPOS study. Biol Trace Elem Res. 2014;157(1):14–23 [c].

[9] Kramer MF, Heath MD. Aluminium in allergen-specific subcutaneous immunotherapy—a German perspective. Vaccine. 2014;32(33):4140–8 [c].

[10] Shaw CA, Tomljenovic L. Aluminum in the central nervous system (CNS): toxicity in humans and animals, vaccine adjuvants, and autoimmunity. Immunol Res. 2013;56(2–3):304–16 [R].

[11] Bohrer D, Schmidt M, Marques RC, et al. Distribution of aluminium in hair of Brazilian infants and correlation to aluminum-adjuvanted vaccine exposure. J Expo Sci Environ Epidemiol. 2013;23(5):474–80 [c].

[12] Çabuş N, Oğuz EO, Tufan AÇ, et al. A histological study of toxic effects of aluminium sulfate on rat hippocampus. Biotech Histochem. 2015;90(2):132–9 [E].

[13] Shaw CA, Tomljenovic L. Aluminum in the central nervous system (CNS): toxicity in humans and animals, vaccine adjuvants, and autoimmunity. Immunol Res. 2013;56(2–3):304–16 [M].

[14] Elabbassi W, Chowdhury MA, Fachtartz AA. Severe reversible myocardial injury associated with aluminium phosphide toxicity: a case report and review of literature. J Saudi Heart Assoc. 2014;26(4):216–21 [A].

[15] Hinhumpatch P, Navasumrit P, Chaisatra K, et al. Oxidative DNA damage and repair in children exposed to low levels of arsenic in utero and during early childhood: application of salivary and urinary biomarkers. Toxicol Appl Pharmacol. 2013;273(3):569–79 [c].

[16] Paul S, Bhattacharjee P, Mishra PK, et al. Human urothelial micronucleus assay to assess genotoxic recovery by reduction of arsenic in drinking water: a cohort study in West Bengal, India. Biometals. 2013;26(5):855–62 [c].

[17] Surdu S, Fitzgerald EF, Bloom MS, et al. Polymorphisms in DNA repair genes XRCC1 and XRCC3, occupational exposure to arsenic and sunlight, and the risk of non-melanoma skin cancer in a European case–control study. Environ Res. 2014;134:382–9 [c].

[18] Tsuji JS, Perez V, Garry MR, et al. Association of low-level arsenic exposure in drinking water with cardiovascular disease: a

systematic review and risk assessment. Toxicology. 2014;323:78–94 [M].

[19] Kile ML, Rodrigues EG, Mazumdar M, et al. A prospective cohort study of the association between drinking water arsenic exposure and self-reported maternal health symptoms during pregnancy in Bangladesh. Environ Health. 2014;13(1):29 [c].

[20] Hsieh RL, Huang YL, Shiue HS, et al. Arsenic methylation capacity and developmental delay in preschool children in Taiwan. Int J Hyg Environ Health. 2014;217(6):678–86 [c].

[21] Edwards M, Hall J, Gong G, et al. Arsenic exposure, AS3MT polymorphism, and neuropsychological functioning among rural dwelling adults and elders: a cross-sectional study. Environ Health. 2014;13(1):15 [c].

[22] Nahar MN, Inaoka T, Fujimura M, et al. Arsenic contamination in groundwater and its effects on adolescent intelligence and social competence in Bangladesh with special reference to daily drinking/cooking water intake. Environ Health Prev Med. 2014;19(2):159 [M].

[23] Wasserman GA, Liu X, Loiacono NJ, et al. A cross-sectional study of well water arsenic and child IQ in Maine school children. Environ Health. 2014;13(1):23 [c].

[24] Seow WJ, Kile ML, Baccarelli AA, et al. Epigenome-wide DNA methylation changes with development of arsenic-induced skin lesions in Bangladesh: a case–control follow-up study. Environ Mol Mutagen. 2014;55(6):449–56 [C].

[25] Osorio-Yáñez C, Ayllon-Vergara JC, Aguilar-Madrid G, et al. Carotid intima-media thickness and plasma asymmetric dimethylarginine in Mexican children exposed to inorganic arsenic. Environ Health Perspect. 2013;121(9):1090–6 [c].

[26] McClintock TR, Chen Y, Parvez F, et al. Association between arsenic exposure from drinking water and hematuria: results from the Health Effects of Arsenic Longitudinal Study. Toxicol Appl Pharmacol. 2014;276(1):21–7 [C].

[27] Ferreccio C, Smith AH, Durán V, et al. Case–control study of arsenic in drinking water and kidney cancer in uniquely exposed Northern Chile. Am J Epidemiol. 2013;178(5):813–8 [E].

[28] Dauphiné DC, Smith AH, Yuan Y, et al. Case–control study of arsenic in drinking water and lung cancer in California and Nevada. Int J Environ Res Public Health. 2013;10(8):3310–24 [c].

[29] Zhang Q, Rodriguez-Lado L, Liu J, et al. Coupling predicted model of arsenic in groundwater with endemic arsenism occurrence in Shanxi Province, Northern China. J Hazard Mater. 2013;262:1147–53 [R].

[30] Kalman DA, Dills RL, Steinmaus C, et al. Occurrence of trivalent monomethyl arsenic and other urinary arsenic species in a highly exposed juvenile population in Bangladesh. J Expo Sci Environ Epidemiol. 2014;24(2):113–20 [c].

[31] Shen H, Xu W, Zhang J, et al. Urinary metabolic biomarkers link oxidative stress indicators associated with general arsenic exposure to male infertility in a han chinese population. Environ Sci Technol. 2013;47(15):8843–51 [H].

[32] Agusa T, Trang PT, Lan VM, et al. Human exposure to arsenic from drinking water in Vietnam. Sci Total Environ. 2014;488–489:562–9 [M].

[33] Cottingham KL, Karimi R, Gruber JF, et al. Diet and toenail arsenic concentrations in a New Hampshire population with arsenic-containing water. Nutr J. 2013;12:149 [A].

[34] Farzan SF, Korrick S, Li Z, et al. In utero arsenic exposure and infant infection in a United States cohort: a prospective study. Environ Res. 2013;126:24–30 [c].

[35] Pan WC, Kile ML, Seow WJ, et al. Genetic susceptible locus in NOTCH2 interacts with arsenic in drinking water on risk of type 2 diabetes. PLoS One. 2013;8(8):e70792 [C].

[36] Argos M, Chen L, Jasmine F, et al. Gene-specific differential DNA methylation and chronic arsenic exposure in an epigenome-wide association study of adults in Bangladesh. Environ Health Perspect. 2015;123(1):64–71 [c].

[37] Sawada N, Iwasaki M, Inoue M, et al. Dietary arsenic intake and subsequent risk of cancer: the Japan Public Health Center-based (JPHC) Prospective Study. Cancer Causes Control. 2013;24(7):1403–15 [C].

[38] Melak D, Ferreccio C, Kalman D, et al. Arsenic methylation and lung and bladder cancer in a case–control study in northern Chile. Toxicol Appl Pharmacol. 2014;274(2):225–31 [C].

[39] He J, Wang M, Jiang Y, et al. Chronic arsenic exposure and angiogenesis in human bronchial epithelial cells via the ROS/miR-199a-5p/HIF-1α/COX-2 pathway. Environ Health Perspect. 2014;122(3):255–61 [E].

[40] Forns J, Fort M, Casas M, et al. Exposure to metals during pregnancy and neuropsychological development at the age of 4 years. Neurotoxicology. 2014;40:16–22 [c].

[41] Julander A, Lundgren L, Skare L, et al. Formal recycling of e-waste leads to increased exposure to toxic metals: an occupational exposure study from Sweden. Environ Int. 2014;73:243–51 [c].

[42] Huang Y, Ni W, Chen Y, et al. Levels and risk factors of antimony contamination in human hair from an electronic waste recycling area, Guiyu, China. Environ Sci Pollut Res Int. 2015;22(9):7112–9 [Epub ahead of print] [c].

[43] Snedeker SM, editor. Toxicants in food packaging and household plastics. Molecular and integrative toxicology, vol. 1. London: Springer-Verlag; 2014. p. 205–30.

[44] Stark M, Lerman Y, Kapel A, et al. Biological exposure metrics of beryllium-exposed dental technicians. Arch Environ Occup Health. 2014;69(2):89–99 [c].

[45] Thakrar R, Shulman R, Bellingan G, et al. Management of a mixed overdose of calcium channel blockers, β-blockers and statins. BMJ Case Rep. 2014. pii: bcr2014204732 [E].

[46] St-Onge M, Dubé PA, Gosselin S, et al. Treatment for calcium channel blocker poisoning: a systematic review. Clin Toxicol (Phila). 2014;52(9):926–44 [R].

[47] Kajiwara A, Saruwatari J, Kita A, et al. Younger females are at greater risk of vasodilation-related adverse symptoms caused by dihydropyridine calcium channel blockers: results of a study of 11,918 Japanese patients. Clin Drug Investig. 2014;34(6):431–5 [C].

[48] Payne ME, McQuoid DR, Steffens DC, et al. Elevated brain lesion volumes in older adults who use calcium supplements: a cross-sectional clinical observational study. Br J Nutr. 2014;112(2):220–7 [c].

[49] Lambrecht M, Mercier C, Geussens Y, et al. The effect of a supersaturated calcium phosphate mouth rinse on the development of oral mucositis in head and neck cancer patients treated with (chemo)radiation: a single-center, randomized, prospective study of a calcium phosphate mouth rinse + standard of care versus standard of care. Support Care Cancer. 2013;21(10):2663–70 [c].

[50] Hong YC, Kulkarni SS, Lim YH, et al. Postnatal growth following prenatal lead exposure and calcium intake. Pediatrics. 2014;134(6):1151–9 [c].

[51] Hofmeyr GJ, Belizán JM, von Dadelszen P. Low-dose calcium supplementation for preventing pre-eclampsia: a systematic review and commentary. BJOG. 2014;121(8):951–7 [r].

[52] Prieto HA, Berbari EF, Sierra RJ. Acute delayed infection: increased risk in failed metal on metal total hip arthroplasty. J Arthroplasty. 2014;29(9):1808–12 [c].

[53] Engh CA, MacDonald SJ, Sritulanondha S, et al. Metal ion levels after metal-on-metal total hip arthroplasty: a five-year, prospective randomized trial. J Bone Joint Surg Am. 2014;96(6):448–55 [S].

[54] Maezawa K, Yuasa T, Aritomi K, et al. Chromium level of salvaged blood in patients undergoing revision hip arthroplasty. J Orthop Surg (Hong Kong). 2013;21(2):195–8 [c].

[55] Fehring TK, Odum S, Sproul R, et al. High frequency of adverse local tissue reactions in asymptomatic patients with metal-on-metal THA. Clin Orthop Relat Res. 2014;472(2):517–22 [c].

[56] Thompson CM, Kirman CR, Proctor DM, et al. A chronic oral reference dose for hexavalent chromium-induced intestinal cancer. J Appl Toxicol. 2014;34(5):525–36 [E].

[57] Proctor DM, Suh M, Campleman SL, et al. Assessment of the mode of action for hexavalent chromium-induced lung cancer following inhalation exposures. Toxicology. 2014;325:160–79 [E].

[58] Cerveira JF, Sánchez-Aragó M, Urbano AM, et al. Short-term exposure of nontumorigenic human bronchial epithelial cells to carcinogenic chromium(VI) compromises their respiratory capacity and alters their bioenergetic signature. FEBS Open Bio. 2014;4:594–601 [E].

[59] Qin Q, Xie H, Wise SS, et al. Homologous recombination repair signaling in chemical carcinogenesis: prolonged particulate hexavalent chromium exposure suppresses the Rad51 response in human lung cells. Toxicol Sci. 2014;142(1):117–25 [E].

[60] Seidler A, Jähnichen S, Hegewald J, et al. Systematic review and quantification of respiratory cancer risk for occupational exposure to hexavalent chromium. Int Arch Occup Environ Health. 2013;86(8):943–55 [M].

[61] Li Y, Li P, Yu S, et al. Jia G.miR-3940-5p associated with genetic damage in workers exposed to hexavalent chromium. Toxicol Lett. 2014;229(1):319–26 [c].

[62] Lovreglio P, D'Errico MN, Basso A, et al. A pilot risk assessment study of strontium chromate among painters in the aeronautical industry. Med Lav. 2013;104(6):448–59 [c].

[63] Bradberry SM, Wilkinson JM, Ferner RE. Systemic toxicity related to metal hip prostheses. Clin Toxicol (Phila). 2014;52(8):837–47 [M].

[64] Devlin JJ, Pomerleau AC, Brent J, et al. Clinical features, testing, and management of patients with suspected prosthetic hip-associated cobalt toxicity: a systematic review of cases. J Med Toxicol. 2013;9(4):405–15 [M].

[65] Pizon AF, Abesamis M, King AM, et al. Prosthetic hip-associated cobalt toxicity. J Med Toxicol. 2013;9(4):416–7 [c].

[66] Hartmann A, Hannemann F, Lützner J, et al. Metal ion concentrations in body fluids after implantation of hip replacements with metal-on-metal bearing—systematic review of clinical and epidemiological studies. PLoS One. 2013;8(8):e70359 [M].

[67] Lutzner J, Hartmann A, Dinnebier G, et al. Metal hypersensitivity and metal ion levels in patients with coated or uncoated total knee arthroplasty: a randomised controlled study. Int Orthop. 2013;37(10):1925–31 [c].

[68] Smith JS, Shaffrey E, Klineberg E, et al. Prospective multicenter assessment of risk factors for rod fracture following surgery for adult spinal deformity. J Neurosurg Spine. 2014;21(6):994–1003 [c].

[69] Vendittoli PA, Rivière C, Roy AG, et al. Metal-on-metal hip resurfacing compared with 28-mm diameter metal-on-metal total hip replacement: a randomised study with six to nine years' follow-up. Bone Joint J. 2013;95-B(11):1464–73 [c].

[70] Bisschop R, Boomsma MF, Van Raay JJ, et al. High prevalence of pseudotumors in patients with a Birmingham Hip Resurfacing prosthesis: a prospective cohort study of one hundred and twenty-nine patients. J Bone Joint Surg Am. 2013;95(17):1554–60 [c].

[71] Posada OM, Tate RJ, Grant MH. Toxicity of cobalt-chromium nanoparticles released from a resurfacing hip implant and cobalt ions on primary human lymphocytes in vitro. J Appl Toxicol. 2015;35(6):614–22 [Epub ahead of print] [E].

[72] Siurin SA, Shilov VV. Occupational morbidity among miners engaged into contemporary method of extracting copper-nickel ores in Kola Transpolar regions. Med Tr Prom Ekol. 2014;9:26–31 [c].

[73] Erol O, Simavlı S, Derbent AU, et al. The impact of copper-containing and levonorgestrel-releasing intrauterine contraceptives on cervicovaginal cytology and microbiological flora: a prospective study. Eur J Contracept Reprod Health Care. 2014;19(3):187–93 [E].

[74] Halatek T, Sinczuk-Walczak H, Janasik B, et al. Health effects and arsenic species in urine of copper smelter workers. J Environ Sci Health A Tox Hazard Subst Environ Eng. 2014;49(7):787–97 [c].

[75] Pal A. Copper toxicity induced hepatocerebral and neurodegenerative diseases: an urgent need for prognostic biomarkers. Neurotoxicology. 2014;40:97–101 [H].

[76] Brewer GJ. Alzheimer's disease causation by copper toxicity and treatment with zinc. Front Aging Neurosci. 2014;6:92 [H].

[77] Prochalska C, Megarbane B, El Balkhi S, et al. Poisoning with gold potassium cyanide and other metallic cyanides in a jeweler. Clin Toxicol (Phila). 2014;52(8):907–8 [c].

[78] Nyanza EC, Joseph M, Premji SS, et al. Geophagy practices and the content of chemical elements in the soil eaten by pregnant women in artisanal and small scale gold mining communities in Tanzania. BMC Pregnancy Childbirth. 2014;14:144 [R].

[79] Zhang C, Wen J, Li Z, et al. Efficacy and safety of lanthanum carbonate on chronic kidney disease-mineral and bone disorder in dialysis patients: a systematic review. BMC Nephrol. 2013;14:226 [M].

[80] Guo H, Zhang X, Tang S, et al. Effects and safety of lanthanum carbonate in end stage renal disease patients with hyperphosphatemia: a meta-analysis—system review of lanthanum carbonate. Ren Fail. 2013;35(10):1455–64 [M].

[81] Takahara Y, Matsuda Y, Takahashi S, et al. Efficacy and safety of lanthanum carbonate in pre-dialysis CKD patients with hyperphosphatemia: a randomized trial. Clin Nephrol. 2014;82(3):181–90 [c].

[82] Huang W, Liu J, Tang Y, et al. Efficacy and tolerability of lanthanum carbonate in treatment of hyperphosphatemia patients receiving dialysis—a systematic review and meta-analysis of randomized controlled trials. Curr Med Res Opin. 2014;30(1):99–108 [M].

[83] Kim S, Arora M, Fernandez C, et al. Lead, mercury, and cadmium exposure and attention deficit hyperactivity disorder in children. Environ Res. 2013;126:105–10 [c].

[84] Kaufman AS, Zhou X, Reynolds MR, et al. The possible societal impact of the decrease in U.S. blood lead levels on adult IQ. Environ Res. 2014;132:413–20 [C].

[85] Geng F, Mai X, Zhan J, et al. Low-level prenatal lead exposure alters auditory recognition memory in 2-month-old infants: an event-related potentials (ERPs) study. Dev Neuropsychol. 2014;39(7):516–28 [A].

[86] Hara A, Thijs L, Asayama K, et al. Blood pressure in relation to environmental lead exposure in the national health and nutrition examination survey 2003 to 2010. Hypertension. 2015;65(1):62–9 [M].

[87] Cherry N, Povey AC, McNamee R, et al. Occupation exposures and sperm morphology: a case-referent analysis of a multi-centre study. Occup Environ Med. 2014;71(9):598–604 [A].

[88] Pereira DI, Couto Irving SS, Lomer MC, et al. A rapid, simple questionnaire to assess gastrointestinal symptoms after oral ferrous sulphate supplementation. BMC Gastroenterol. 2014;14:103 [R].

[89] Liabeuf S, Gras V, Moragny J, et al. Ulceration of the oral mucosa following direct contact with ferrous sulfate in elderly patients: a case report and a review of the French National Pharmacovigilance Database. Clin Interv Aging. 2014;9:737–40 [A].

[90] Veronese N, Berton L, Carraro S, et al. Effect of oral magnesium supplementation on physical performance in healthy elderly women involved in a weekly exercise program: a randomized controlled trial. Am J Clin Nutr. 2014;100(3):974–81 [c].

[91] Habe K, Kawasaki T, Sata T. A case of prolongation of rocuronium neuromuscular blockade in a pregnant patient receiving magnesium. Masui. 2014;63(7):817–9 [A].

[92] Valent F, Mariuz M, Bin M, et al. Associations of prenatal mercury exposure from maternal fish consumption and polyunsaturated fatty acids with child neurodevelopment: a prospective cohort study in Italy. J Epidemiol. 2013;23(5):360–70 [c].

[93] Morisset T, Ramirez-Martinez A, Wesolek N, et al. Probabilistic mercury multimedia exposure assessment in small children and risk assessment. Environ Int. 2013;59:431–41 [R].

[94] Croes K, De Coster S, De Galan S, et al. Health effects in the Flemish population in relation to low levels of mercury exposure: from organ to transcriptome level. Int J Hyg Environ Health. 2014;217(2–3):239–47 [C].

[95] Ohlander J, Huber SM, Schomaker M, et al. Risk factors for mercury exposure of children in a rural mining town in northern Chile. PLoS One. 2013;8(11):e79756 [c].

[96] Watson GE, van Wijngaarden E, Love TM, et al. Neurodevelopmental outcomes at 5 years in children exposed prenatally to maternal dental amalgam: the Seychelles Child Development Nutrition Study. Neurotoxicol Teratol. 2013;39:57–62 [M].

[97] Katamanova EV, Shevchenko OI, Lakhman OL, et al. Cognitive disorders in patients with chronic mercury intoxication. Med Tr Prom Ekol. 2014;4:7–12 [C].

[98] Hsi HC, Jiang CB, Yang TH, et al. The neurological effects of prenatal and postnatal mercury/methylmercury exposure on three-year-old children in Taiwan. Chemosphere. 2014;100:71–6 [M].

[99] Kalish BT, Rifas-Shiman SL, Wright RO, et al. Associations of prenatal maternal blood mercury concentrations with early and mid-childhood blood pressure: a prospective study. Environ Res. 2014;133:327–33 [C].

[100] Li Y, Sun J, Shang H. Effect of hOGG1 expression level on oxidative DNA damage among workers exposed to nickel in stainless steel production environment. Zhonghua Lao Dong Wei Sheng Zhi Ye Bing Za Zhi. 2014;32(8):578–81 [C].

[101] Oller AR, Oberdörster G, Seilkop SK. Derivation of PM10 size-selected human equivalent concentrations of inhaled nickel based on cancer and non-cancer effects on the respiratory tract. Inhal Toxicol. 2014;26(9):559–78 [c].

[102] Jacob SE, Admani S. iPad—increasing nickel exposure in children. Pediatrics. 2014;134(2):e580–e582 [c].

[103] Admani S, Matiz C, Jacob SE. Nickel allergy—a potential cause of razor dermatitis. Pediatr Dermatol. 2014;31(3):392–3 [c].

[104] Buyukozturk S, Gelincik A, Demirtürk M, et al. Nickel dental alloys can induce laryngeal edema attacks: a case report. J Dermatol. 2013;40(9):740–2 [H].

[105] Yu L, Su J, Zou D, et al. The concentrations of IL-8 and IL-6 in gingival crevicular fluid during nickel-chromium alloy porcelain crown restoration. J Mater Sci Mater Med. 2013;24(7):1717–22 [c].

[106] Sancini A, De Sio S, Gioffrè PA, et al. Correlation between urinary nickel and testosterone plasma values in workers occupationally exposed to urban stressors. Ann Ig. 2014;26(3):237–54 [A].

[107] Levings JL, Gunn JP. The imbalance of sodium and potassium intake: implications for dietetic practice. J Acad Nutr Diet. 2014;114(6):838–41 [c].

[108] O'Donnell M, Mente A, Rangarajan S, et al. Urinary sodium and potassium excretion, mortality, and cardiovascular events. N Engl J Med. 2014;371(7):612–23 [C].

[109] Gluhovschi G, Mateş A, Gluhovschi C, et al. Serum potassium in stage 5 CKD patients on their first presentation in a dialysis service of a county hospital in western Romania. Rom J Intern Med. 2014;52(1):30–8 [c].

[110] Tongyoo A, Sriussadaporn E, Limpavitayaporn P, et al. Acute intestinal obstruction due to Kalimate, a potassium-lowering agent: a case report and literature review. J Med Assoc Thai. 2013;96(12):1617–20 [A].

[111] Yang CY, Chen CH, Wang HY, et al. Strontium ranelate related Stevens-Johnson syndrome: a case report. Osteoporos Int. 2014;25(6):1813–6 [c].

[112] Fuksa L, Vytrisalova M, Hendrychova T, et al. Consumption of osteoanabolic drugs and strontium ranelate in the treatment of osteoporosis in the Czech Republic in 2005–2011. Acta Pol Pharm. 2014;71(2):329–35 [M].

[113] Audran M, Jakob FJ, Palacios S, et al. A large prospective European cohort study of patients treated with strontium ranelate and followed up over 3 years. Rheumatol Int. 2013;33(9):2231–9 [C].

[114] Reginster JY. Cardiac concerns associated with strontium ranelate. Expert Opin Drug Saf. 2014;13(9):1209–13 [M].

[115] Svanstrom H, Pasternak B, Hviid A. Use of strontium ranelate and risk of acute coronary syndrome: cohort study. Ann Rheum Dis. 2014;73(6):1037–43 [C].

[116] Pinto-Almeida T, Lobo I, Selores M. Unknown: Bluish-gray macules on the hands of a healthy 34 year-old man. Dermatol Online J. 2013;19(7):18964 [A].

[117] Hartmann A, Hannemann F, Lützner J, et al. Ion concentrations in body fluids after implantation of hip replacements with metal-on-metal bearing—systematic review of clinical and epidemiological studies. PLoS One. 2013;8(8): e70359 [c].

[118] Hassanian-Moghaddam H, Shahnazi M, Zamani N, et al. Plain abdominal radiography: a powerful tool to prognosticate outcome in patients with zinc phosphide poisoning. Clin Radiol. 2014;69(10):1062–5 [c].

[119] Wages PA, Silbajoris R, Speen A, et al. Role of H_2O_2 in the oxidative effects of zinc exposure in human airway epithelial cells. Redox Biol. 2014;3:47–55 [E].

[120] Hsieh H, Amlal H, Genter MB. Evaluation of the toxicity of zinc in the rat olfactory neuronal cell line, Odora. Hum Exp Toxicol. 2015;34(3):308–14 [E].

23

Metal Antagonists

Joshua P. Gray[*,1], *Sidhartha D. Ray*[†]

*Department of Science, United States Coast Guard Academy, New London, CT, USA
†Department of Pharmaceutical Sciences, Manchester University College of Pharmacy, Fort Wayne, IN, USA
[1]Corresponding author: joshua.p.gray@uscga.edu

INTRODUCTION

In patients with β-thalassemia and other disorders requiring frequent transfusions, iron overload develops due to the relatively slow excretion rate of 1 mg/day. Orally bioavailable chelation therapy accomplishes a faster rate of excretion either through the feces (deferasirox) or urine (deferiprone). Deferoxamine is a third option, although it must be administered intravenously.

Due to side effects that develop from each of these drugs, chelation therapy is sometimes halted which reverses most side effects, and patients are later returned to therapy. Combinations of metal chelators are increasingly being tested for safety and efficacy. The American Heart Association has concluded that deferiprone is superior in efficacy to deferoxamine, that combined deferiprone with deferoxamine is superior to deferoxamine alone, and that deferasirox is equivalent to deferoxamine [1S]. A meta-analysis of 16 randomized controlled trials evaluated side effects associated with metal chelators alone or in combination [2M] (Tables 1 and 2). A review details treatment options for iron overload in children, covering deferoxamine, deferiprone, and deferasirox [3R].

DEFERASIROX [SEDA-32, 426; SEDA-33, 466; SEDA-34, 368; SEDA-35, 420; SEDA-36, 323]

The most common side effects of deferasirox are non-progressive change in serum creatinine, gastrointestinal disturbances, and skin rash [33R]. Potential uses for deferasirox in the treatment of other diseases continue to grow. Several reports have suggested the use of deferasirox for the treatment of non-neoplastic cancers. One report states that chelators have not been translated into clinical practice for cancers due to side effects in preclinical model systems [34R]. Another review suggests iron chelation for use in multiple sclerosis [35R]. A phase IV open-label study is investigating the use of deferasirox for allogenic stem cell therapy [36c].

A critical review reports 4113 fatalities in patients treated with deferasirox. The author argues that ~500 of those fatalities were for individuals with normal iron stores being treated for cancer, leukemia, cardiovascular, and neurological diseases. The author also argues that these deaths were due to "indiscriminate and uncontrollable use of deferasirox" and that safer generic drugs deferiprone and deferoxamine be used in the treatment of thalassemia and other iron loading conditions [37R,38R]. A response by an employee of Novartis argues that several flaws exist in cited reports [39r]. Several reviews discuss deferasirox indications and adverse effects [33R,40R,41R,42R,43c,44c].

A cost-utility analysis comparing deferasirox and deferoxamine in Iran concluded that deferasirox was more cost-effective for the treatment of β-thalassemia [45r].

Organs and Systems

Cardiovascular

A consensus statement from the American Heart Association regarding the treatment of siderosis in β-thalassemia major concludes that deferasirox is equivalent in efficacy to deferoxamine [1S].

Respiratory

Upper respiratory tract infection (17.7%) was observed in a 1-year extension of the THALASSA clinical trial of 130 patients assessing deferasirox for non-transfusion-dependent thalassemia [46c].

© 2015 Elsevier B.V. All rights reserved.

TABLE 1 Adverse Effects of the Comparison of Deferiprone (DFP) Plus Deferoxamine (DFO) Versus DFO Treatment Group

Study or subgroup	DFX Events	DFX Total	DFO Events	DFO Total	Weight (%)	Risk ratio M-H, random, 95% CI
7.3.1 GASTROINTESTINAL SYMPTOMS						
[4C]	7	30	0	30	1.1	15.00 [0.89, 251.42]
[5c]	5	11	0	14	1.0	13.75 [0.84, 224.71]
[6c]	12	32	8	33	17.5	1.55 [0.73, 3.28]
Subtotal (95% CI)		73		77	19.6	2.92 [1.48, 5.77]
Total events	24		8			
Heterogeneity: Chi^2=5.23, df=2 (P=0.07); I^2=62%						
Test for overall effect: Z=3.09 (P=0.002)						
7.3.2 ARTHROPATHY						
[7c]	6	22	1	23	2.2	6.27 [0.82, 47.99]
[5c]	3	11	0	14	1.0	8.75 [0.50, 153.45]
[6c]	3	32	6	33	13.2	0.52 [0.14, 1.89]
Subtotal (95% CI)		65		70	16.3	1.78 [0.76, 4.17]
Heterogeneity: Chi^2=6.16, df=2 (P=0.05); I^2=68%						
Test for overall effect: Z=1.33 (P=0.18)						
7.3.3 NEUTROPENIA						
[8c]	1	8	3	12	5.3	0.5 [0.06, 4.00]
[7c]	1	22	1	23	2.2	1.05 [0.07, 15.70]
[4C]	0	30	1	30	3.3	0.33 [0.01, 7.87]
[6c]	2	32	0	33	1.1	5.15 [0.26, 103.30]
Subtotal (95% CI)		92		98	12.0	0.98 [0.30, 3.15]
Total events	4		5			
Heterogeneity: Chi^2=2.03, df=3 (P=0.57); I^2=0%						
Test for overall effect: Z=0.03 (P=0.97)						
7.3.4 AGRANULOCYTOSIS						
Subtotal (95% CI)		0		0		Not estimable
Total events	0		0			
Heterogeneity: Not applicable						
Test for overall effect: Not applicable						
7.3.5 OTHERS (HEADACHE, SKIN RASH, ETC.)						
[7c]	19	22	8	23	17.4	2.48 [1.39, 4.45]
[4C]	0	30	2	30	5.6	0.20 [0.01, 4.00]
[5c]	0	11	12	14	24.7	0.05 [0.00, 0.76]
[6c]	1	32	2	33	4.4	0.52 [0.05, 5.41]
Subtotal (95% CI)		95		100	52.1	0.92 [0.56, 1.50]
Total events	20		24			
Heterogeneity: Chi^2=16.77, df=3 (P=0.0008); I^2=82%						
Test for overall effect Z=0.34 (P=0.73)						
Total (95% CI)		325		345	100.0	1.46 [1.04, 2.04]
Total events	60		44			
Heterogeneity: Chi^2=25.18, df=13 (P=0.02); I^2=48%						
Test for overall effect: Z=2.21 (P=0.03)						

Reproduced with Permission from Ref. [2M], figure 12.

TABLE 2 Adverse Effects of the Comparison of Deferasirox (DFX) Versus Deferoxamine (DFO)

| Study or subgroup | DFX | | DFO | | Weight (%) | Risk ratio |
	Events	Total	Events	Total		M-H, random, 95% CI
7.4.1 GASTROINTESTINAL SYMPTOMS						
[9C]	31	303	0	197	16.3	61.15 [3.77, 992.42]
[4C]	31	47	8	21	31.4	1.73 [0.97, 3.10]
Subtotal (95% CI)		250		218	47.8	9.08 [0.05, 1521.87]
Total Events	62		8			
Heterogeneity: Tau^2 = 12.67, Chi^2 = 13.01, df = 1 (P = 0.0003); I^2 = 92%						
Test for overall effect: Z = 0.84 (P = 0.40)						
7.4.2 ARTHROPATHY						
[4C]	6	47	3	21	27.0	0.89 [0.25, 3.24]
Subtotal (95% CI)		47		21	27.0	0.89 [0.25, 3.24]
Total events	6		3			
Heterogeneity: Not applicable						
Test for overall effect: Z = 0.17 (P = 0.86)						
7.4.3 OTHERS						
[9C]	2	203	9	197	25.2	0.22 [0.05, 0.99]
Subtotal (95% CI)		203		197	25.2	0.22 [0.05, 0.99]
Total events	2		9			
Heterogeneity: Not applicable						
Test for overall effect: Z = 1.98 (P = 0.05)						
Total (95% CI)		500		436	100.0	1.53 [0.31, 7.49]
Total events	70		20			
Heterogeneity: Tau^2 = 2.00; Chi^2 = 17.28, df = 3 (P = 0.0006), I^2 = 83%						
Test for overall effect: Z = 0.53 (P = 0.60)						

A major review discussed the major side effects of the three major iron chelation therapy drugs, deferasirox, deferoxamine, and deferirpone [10r]. Side effects are listed in Table 3.
Reproduced from figure 13 of Ref. [2M] in accordance with the Creative Commons Attribution License.

Nervous System

Headache (n = 8) was observed in a 24-month trial of deferasirox in myelodysplastic patients (n = 55) [47c].

Sensory Systems

- Reversible retinopathy was observed in a 17-year-old girl with sickle cell anemia following change from deferoxamine to deferasirox for 2 years [48A].

Metabolism

- Hyperchloremic metabolic acidosis was reported in a 17-year-old patient with β-thalassemia on deferasirox 30 mg/kg daily, which resolved following withdrawal [49A].

Hematologic

- Acute pure red cell aplasia developed in 55-year-old and 68-year-old men with myelodysplastic syndrome refractory anemia treated with deferasirox [50A]. Removal of deferasirox caused reversal of the anemia.

Gastrointestinal

Palatability of deferasirox was improved in patients when taken with soft food at breakfast [51c]. Diarrhea (14.6%), gastroenteritis (6.1%), and upper abdominal pain (1.5%) were observed in a 1-year extension of the THA-LASSA clinical trial of 130 patients assessing deferasirox for non-transfusion-dependent thalassemia [46c]. Diarrhea (10.4% of 135) and nausea (5.2% of 135) were observed in sickle cell patients on deferasirox for up to

TABLE 3 Major Side Effects for Deferoxamine, Deferiprone, and Deferasirox [10R]

Drug	Adverse effects	Management	Recommendations
DFO	Local side effects at the subcutaneous injection site	Verify correct positioning of needle; hydrocortisone infused with DFO.	Adjust dose to serum ferritin levels. Monitor weight, height, and growth velocity every 3 months in children. Visual acuity tests, slit-lamp examination, and fundoscopy annually. Audiometry annually. Monitor renal function periodically.
	Stunted growth and bone changes (e.g., metaphyseal dysplasia) [11c,12c]	Reduce dose or change chelator.	
	Hypersensitivity reactions and systemic allergic reactions	Change treatment drug or desensitization [13c,14R].	
	High-frequency sensorineural hearing loss or visual disturbance [15A,16c,17A]	Rare if dosage guidelines followed and dose adjusted when ferritin declines; if abnormal tests or symptoms, discontinue treatment.	
	Increased serum creatinine, acute renal failure, and renal tubular disorders [18A,19c]	Reduce dose or discontinue treatment.	
	Increased susceptibility to *Yersinia entercolitica* and pseudotuberculosis and *Klebsiella pneumonia* infections [20R,21R]	Discontinue treatment if suspected signs and symptoms. Initiate antibiotic therapy.	
DFP	Nausea, abdominal pain, vomiting, diarrhea.	Usually transient without need to modify treatment; otherwise reduce dose and then increase gradually; as an alternative, switch to oral solution.	Weekly neutrophil count. Monitor hepatic and renal functions periodically. Monitor weight and body mass index. Avoid use of other neutropenia-inducing drugs.
	Neutropenia (neutrophils 0.5–1.5×10^9/L) [22c]	Discontinue DFP and repeat neutrophil count daily until normalization; rechallenge with caution.	
	Agranulocytosis (neutrophils $<0.5 \times 10^9$/L on two consecutive tests) [22c]	Immediately discontinue DFP; if signs/symptoms of infection, perform cultures and begin antibiotic treatment; granulocyte colony stimulating factor may be indicated.	
	Increased liver enzymes [22c,23R]	Usually asymptomatic and transient without need to modify treatment but may require lowering dose and gradually raising again	
	Increased appetite	Dietary measures.	
	Zinc deficiency [24c]	Oral zinc supplementation.	
	Arthralgia and arthropathy [25c,26A]	Mild arthralgia is usually transient; if more severe disease, reduce dose or discontinue treatment.	
	Neurologic disorders	Described in children taking long-term 2.5 times maximum recommended dose, often in absence of systemic iron overload; discontinue DFP.	
DFX	Nausea, vomiting, and abdominal pain [27c,28c]	Usually transient; if needed reduce dose or discontinue treatment.	Monitor serum creatinine, creatinine clearance, and/or plasma cystatin. C twice before initiation, weekly in the first month after initiation, or modification of therapy and then monthly. Monthly urinalysis for proteinuria. Monthly renal tubular function as needed. Monitor serum transaminases, bilirubin, and alkaline phosphatase before initiation of treatment, every 2 weeks. during the first month, and then monthly Auditory and ophthalmic testing annually.
	Diarrhea (may be due to coexistent lactose intolerance)	Consider administration with lactase-containing products.	
	Rash	Discontinue DFX; reintroduce at a lower dose after resolution (if necessary add short course of corticosteroids).	
	Increased serum creatinine, proteinuria, acute renal failure, renal tubulopathy, Fanconi syndrome [27c,29A,30A, 31A]	Reduce dose by 10 mg/kg if increase in serum creatinine by >33% above pretreatment average and if estimated creatinine clearance decreases below the lower limit of normal at two consecutive visits or if abnormalities of tubular markers; if no improvement, change chelator. For more severe changes, consider discontinuing DFX.	
	Increase liver enzymes, hepatic failure [9C,27c]	If persistent and progressive increase in serum transaminases, interrupt treatment; once normalized, cautious reinitiation at a lower dose.	

TABLE 3 Major Side Effects for Deferoxamine, Deferiprone, and Deferasirox [10R]—cont'd

Drug	Adverse effects	Management	Recommendations
	Upper gastrointestinal ulceration and hemorrhage	Observe carefully in patients in treatment with other potentially ulcerogenic drugs; discontinue treatment if signs or symptoms.	
	Auditory (decreased hearing) and ocular (lens opacities) disturbances.	Reduce dose or discontinue treatment.	
	Cytopenias [32A].	Discontinue treatment.	

Reproduced with permission from Elsevier.

2 years [51c]. Diarrhea ($n = 15$) and nausea ($n = 12$) were observed in a 24-month trial of deferasirox in myelodysplastic patients ($n = 55$) [47c]. Increased diarrhea (6.3% versus 1.1%) was observed in a 1-year randomized controlled trial of 197 beta-thalassemia patients comparing deferasirox versus deferoxamine for myocardial iron removal [52c]. In a study of first-time users of deferasirox between 2005 and 2008 in Taiwan's National Health Insurance Database, deferasirox users were found to have higher incidence of GI bleeding (2.03 per 10 000 patient-days) compared with other iron chelator users [53M]. Nausea and diarrhea similar to previous reports were also identified in a clinical trial [54c]. Lactose intolerance was not found to be linked to gastrointestinal adverse effects in beta thalassemia patients treated with deferasirox [55c].

Liver

Liver iron overload failed to resolve in all 30 patients of a small clinical trial of Indian thalassemia patients [56c]. Hepatitis severity grade 3 was observed in a 1-year extension of the THALASSA clinical trial of 130 patients assessing deferasirox for non-transfusion-dependent thalassemia [46c]. Increased ALT (6.3% versus 1.1%) and increased aspartate aminotransferase (6.3% versus 1.1%) were observed in a 1-year randomized controlled trial of 197 beta-thalassemia patients comparing deferasirox versus deferoxamine for myocardial iron removal [52c]. In a study of first-time users of deferasirox between 2005 and 2008 in Taiwan's National Health Insurance Database, deferasirox users were found to have higher incidence of acute liver necrosis (0.26 per 10 000 patient-days) compared with other iron chelator users [53M]. Alanine aminotransferase at 10-fold greater than normal which subsequently resolved was observed in two patients with active graft-versus-host disease in a study of deferasirox for the treatment of iron overload following allogenic stem cell transplantation [36c].

Urinary Tract

A review on pharmacological causes of Fanconi syndrome discussed the role of deferasirox [57R]. A review article discussed nephrotoxicity due to deferasirox [58R]. A phase 1, open-label study in beta-thalassemia patients receiving deferasirox concluded that negative impacts of deferasirox on renal hemodynamics were mild and reversible for up to 2 years of treatment, with no progressive worsening of renal function over time [59R].

Tubular dysfunction in a trial of 30 pediatric patients with β-thalassemia was observed. A significant increase in serum creatinine after 6 months of treatment (from 0.54 to 0.67), a decrease in estimate glomerular filtration rate (from 104.36 to 86.00), increase in mean serum potassium level, and decrease in serum calcium, magnesium, and uric acid levels were observed [60c]. Increased blood creatinine (8.3% versus 2.2%) and increased proteinuria (7.3% versus 3.3%) was observed in a 1-year randomized controlled trial of 197 beta-thalassemia patients comparing deferasirox versus deferoxamine for myocardial iron removal [52c]. In a study of first-time users of deferasirox between 2005 and 2008 in Taiwan's National Health Insurance Database, deferasirox users were found to have higher incidence of acute renal failure (1.45 per 10 000 patient-days) compared with other iron chelator users [53M]. Increased serum creatinine was observed in 12 patients in a study of deferasirox for the treatment of iron overload following allogenic stem cell transplantation [36c].

A 21-year-old male developed progressive decline in renal function and Fanconi syndrome after being prescribed deferasirox for iron overload. The patient continued to have hypokalemia, hypophosphatemia, proteinuria, and glucosuria 4 months after halting deferasirox treatment [61A].

Skin

Rash ($n = 8$) was observed in a 24-month trial of deferasirox in myelodysplastic patients ($n = 55$) [47c]. Maculopapular-type eruption was observed in a

75-year-old Japanese woman with acute myeloid leukemia and frequent drug transfusions. Within 4 hours of treatment with deferasirox (500 mg once a day), an eruption over her body and discomfort of the pharynx, high temperature, hypotension, tachycardia, and low blood oxygen saturation levels were observed. Removal of all medications caused symptoms to improve within 5 days [62A].

Immunologic

Immunologic abnormalities were observed in 17 patients with beta-thalassemia (12 females, media age 26) receiving deferasirox for a median duration of 27 months. Effects included increased total B- and T-lymphocytes ($n=14$ each), increased CD4+ ($n=13$), CD8+ ($n=12$), NK cells ($n=11$), and absolute counts for lymphocyte subsets [63c].

Body Temperature

Pyrexia was observed in a 1-year extension of the THALASSA clinical trial of 130 patients assessing deferasirox for non-transfusion-dependent thalassemia [46c].

Long-Term Effects

Genotoxicity

Genotoxicity was observed in rat bone marrow, which displayed increased mutageneity-related polymorphic band count in random amplification of polymorphic DNA [64E].

Susceptibility Factors

Age

Renal tubular dysfunction occurred with a very high incidence in a small cohort of transfusion-dependent mostly Chinese (94.4%) pediatric thalassemic patients on deferasirox treatment [65c]. Elevated urine beta-2 microglobulin, low serum calcium, phosphate, and potassium were identified in 100% of patients ($n=18$), most occurring within 100 months. The cumulative incidence of renal tubular dysfunction reach 90% by 6 years of deferasirox therapy, with a third of the patients developing dysfunction at 11 months in a retrospective analysis of beta-thalassemia patients from 2.6 to 23.8 years-of-age [65c].

Pediatric cancer patients ($n=13$) treated with deferasirox for iron overload due to transfusion displayed skin rash ($n=2$), gastrointestinal disturbance ($n=1$), and reversible acute renal failure ($n=1$) [66c].

DEFERIPRONE [SEDA-15, 1054; SEDA-32, 427; SEDA-33, 468; SEDA-34, 370; SEDA-35, 422, SEDA-36, 327]

A cost-utility analysis concluded that deferiprone was the most cost-effective treatment for management of chronic iron overload in beta-thalassemia patients [67H].

Organs and Systems

Cardiovascular

Reduced neutrophil count which may progress to agranulocytosis is a well-known side effect of deferiprone therapy, affecting 6% of patients with thalassemia [68c]. However, neutropenia was found to resolve within 4–7 days despite continued therapy with deferiprone in four patients in a study of 100 children investigating oral liquid deferiprone. One patient did progress to agranulocytosis and was halted. The authors suggest that deferiprone may not be responsible for the induction of neutropenia in patients with thalassemia [68c]. Agranulocytosis is a risk associated with deferiprone treatment, and the product label recommends halting treatment upon detection of an absolute neutrophil count less than $1.5 \times 10/L$. However, a study of 294 patients, nine of whom developed neutropenia and one of whom developed agranulocytosis found that the mean time to resolution of agranulocytosis was similar regardless of whether patients halted treatment or not [69r]. Reversible agranulocytosis was noted in a review discussing the use of deferiprone for Friedreich's ataxia [70r]. It was also noted in the treatment of superficial siderosis [71A]. Low ferritin levels were observed in four of 13 patients enrolled in a study investigating the use of deferiprone, idebenone, and riboflavin for the treatment of Friedreich's ataxia [72c].

Nervous System

Two generalized tonic–clonic seizures occurred in a patient with beta-thalassemia major 2 months after initiating treatment with deferiprone (75 mg/kg/day) [73A]. After halting for 2 months and returning to deferiprone treatment, the patient experienced another generalized tonic–clonic seizure. Since that time, the patient has not experienced any further seizures. Joint pain was more frequently noted in patients receiving deferiprone than desferrioxamine in a meta-analysis of 17 trials ($n=1061$ participants) comparing iron chelators [74M].

Neuromuscular Function

A review discussed the use of deferiprone for Friedreich's ataxia, stating that the disease can be worsened by higher doses of the drug, due to the fact that the disease is "more a condition of iron deficiency than of iron overload" [70r]. Doses higher than 20 mg/kg/day were concluded to worsen ataxia in a 6-month randomized controlled trial [75c].

Musculoskeletal

Bony dysplasia, deformation and impaired growth of ulnar epiphyses, metaphyses, and physes were hypothesized to be caused by deferiprone-related arthopathy in children with thalassemia major [76c].

Susceptibility Factors

Age

Ototoxicity was analyzed in a retrospective study of clinical records from January 1997 to December 2010 in patients receiving deferiprone. Three patients out of 100 experienced sensorineural hearing loss [77c]. Cytopenia ($n = 1$), neutropenia ($n = 2$), thrombocytopenia ($n = 2$), elevated alanine aminotransferase ($n = 5$), elevated serum creatinine ($n = 1$), proteinuria ($n = 1$), and gastrointestinal discomfort ($n = 4$) were observed in a study of 42 pediatric patients being treated with deferiprone and desferrioxamine for thalassemia major [78c]. Transient elevation of ALT was observed in 3 of 67 patients receiving deferiprone for 1 year [79c].

DEFEROXAMINE/DESFERRIOXAMINE
[SEDA-15, 1058; SEDA-32, 429; SEDA-33, 471; SEDA-34, 371, SEDA-35, 423]

Organs and Systems

Sensory Systems

Sudden bilateral visual loss and dyschromatopsia was observed in two patients with acute myelocytic leukemia and severe aplastic anemia being treated with intravenous deferoxamine for 1 month [80A]. Drug discontinuation allowed resolution of serous detachment. Decreased vision occurred in a 53-year-old man with beta-thalassemia 1 month after initiation of deferoxamine [81A]. Nyctalopia and decreased vision occurred in a 34-year-old man treated with high-dose intravenous deferoxamine [82A]. A retrospective review studied 20 patients with deferoxamine-induced retinopathy after a minimum of 10 years of deferoxamine treatment [83c].

Urinary Tract

Urine color changed to red-orange in a 21-year-old woman treated with deferoxamine (15 mg/kg/24 h) for ingestion of 5100 mg of ferrous sulfate (110 mg/kg) for a suicide attempt [84A].

Immunologic

Type 1 hypersensitivity was observed in a 13-year-old boy with beta-thalassemia [85A]. Desensitization was later successful.

Infection Risk

Mice administered deferoxamine mesylate had higher bacterial burden in liver and kidney following challenge with community-associated methicillin-resistant *Staphylococcus aureus* [86E].

Long-Term Effects
TUMORIGENICITY

Increased epithelial–mesenchymal transition and metastasis was observed in deferoxamine-treated colorectal cells [87E].

Susceptibility Factors

Age

Dysplasia-like skeletal abnormalities, mostly around the knees, were detected in 22 of 59 Egyptian children with thalassemia major and generalized arthralgia treated who were treated with deferoxamine [88c]. Mild, moderate, and severe dysplasia-like changes were observed in 4, 11, and 7 children, respectively.

EDETIC ACID (EDTA) [SED-15, 1300; SEDA-31, 405; SEDA-32, 431; SEDA-33, 474; SEDA-35, 372]

No kidney dysfunction was found in a meta-analysis investigating the use of EDTA for lead chelation therapy [89R]. A review discussed the decreasing popularity of edetic acid due to inconvenience of parenteral administration and neurotoxicity [90R].

HQK-1001 (2,2-DIMETHYLBUTYRATE)

HQK-1001 is an oral fetal globin inducer. A dose-escalation study in 52 subjects with hemoglobin SS or S/β(0) thalassemia was performed for 26 weeks, alone or in the presence of hydroxyurea. Adverse effects in the patients ($n = 41$) included gastrointestinal effects (79%), sickle cell disease-related adverse effects (75%), and neurologic effects (50%). The authors reported that the following adverse effects were attributed to the study drug: nausea (44%), vomiting (29%), somnolence (25%), headache and upper abdominal pain (17%), diarrhea (13%), and gastritis and abdominal pain (12%). HQK-1001 daily dose was subsequently limited to 30 mg/kg in all subjects and oral iron was no longer administered. Other adverse effects possibly related to the drug included one case each of pancreatitis, somnolence, and fatigue at the 50 mg/kg dose and one case each of epigastric pain and pancreatitis at 30 mg/kg dose [91c].

HYDROXYUREA [SEDA-36, 330]

Hydroxyurea is used to stimulate fetal hemoglobin production, which may be of use for the treatment of thalassemias and sickle cell disease. More recently, hydroxyurea is being considered as a substitute for regular blood transfusion [92c].

A systematic review of more than 500 articles found a modest but significant increase in hemoglobin in non-transfusion-dependent β-thalassemia major and transfusion-dependent beta-thalassemia major [130R]. A review article discussed side effects of hydroxyurea therapy for sickle cell disease, including neutropenia, bone marrow suppression, elevation of hepatic enzymes, anorexia, nausea, vomiting, and infertility [93R].

A review of the use of hydroxyurea for the treatment of non-transfusion-dependent beta-thalassemia major at a center that treats 1856 patients/year concluded that hydroxyurea is safe and effective [94R]. A single-arm clinical trial testing the efficacy and safety of hydroxyurea for the treatment of transfusion-dependent beta-thalassemia did not detect any adverse effects [95c]. A cross-sectional study with simple random sampling was performed on 56 patients with either sickle cell anemia ($n = 28$) or intermediate or major beta-thalassemia ($n = 28$) of a median age of 17.5 ± 8.55 years (range 4–52 years) who had received hydroxyurea therapy an average of 2.6 years. Side effects included neurologic (headache (13), vertigo (2), drowsiness (1), seizure (1)), dermatologic (hair loss (19), hyperpigmentation (6), skin ulcer (1), skin rash (2), nail hyperpigmentation (1)), gastrointestinal (abdominal pain (5), nausea and vomiting (3), constipation (1), anorexia (2)), hematologic (decreased PLT (2), decreased HB (2), neutropenia (2)), increased AST/ALT (4), weight gain (2), and edema (1) [96c].

Hydroxyurea was found to be effective in a mouse study wherein 70 BALB/c mice received intraperitonial injections of iron-sucrose [97E]. Hydroxyurea (500 mg/kg/day) decreased body weight gain, decreased circulating leukocytes, erythrocytes, and platelets, decreased cellularity of thymus, lymph nodes, and bone marrow, and caused epithelial degeneration and/or dysplasia of the stomach and small intestines in rats [98E]. Dogs receiving 50 mg/kg/day for 1 month had decreased circulating leukocytes, erythrocytes, and platelets; increased bone marrow cellularity with decreasing maturing granulocytes; increased creatinine kinase

activity; and increased iron pigment in bone marrow and hepatic sinusoidal cells [98E]. Increased diastolic blood pressure, heart rate, and change in blood pressure over time were observed in telemetered dogs receiving doses of 15 mg/kg or more [98E].

A combination therapy trial of hydroxyurea with deferasirox did not show any change in the efficacy, safety (including liver and kidney function), and pharmacokinetic properties of deferasirox [51c].

Organs and Systems

Endocrine

The incidence of hypothyroidism was not significantly affected in a small ($n = 31$) clinical trial investigating the use of hydroxyurea (8–15 mg/kg/day) in beta-thalassemia intermedia patients [99c].

Hematologic

Transient myelotoxicity was found in 4.8% of 203 patients administered hydroxyurea 10 mg/kg/day [100c]. Microparticles were increased in the serum of patients with sickle cell anemia receiving hydroxyurea treatment ($n = 10$) compared with control patients ($n = 13$) 25472687c. HUSOFT trial participants on continued hydroxyurea therapy for 15 years exhibited neutropenia causing temporary drug discontinuation 10 times in 4 of 28 patients [101c].

Gastrointestinal

Colonic ulcers were attributed to hydroxyurea therapy for the treatment of transfusion-dependent hemoglobin E/beta-thalassemia disease in a 37-year-old man. After beginning treatment in 2007, the patient suffered hematochezia, mucous diarrhea and epigastric pain intermittently between 2008 and April of 2010. Colonoscopies showed ulcerative lesions from the terminal ileum to the ascending colon and subsequently ulcerative lesions at the pharynx. The ulcerative lesions resolved within a month of discontinuation of hydroxyurea [102A].

Skin

A comprehensive review discussed hydroxyurea-induced skin ulcers [103R].

Reproductive System

A report discussed the adverse effects of long-term hydroxyurea treatment on sperm production and teratogenic effects [104r]. A systematic review evaluated evidence that hydroxyurea is associated with further decreasing fertility in men with sickle cell disease [105R].

Immunologic

Hydroxyurea did not affect immune function in patients with sickle cell disease [106c].

D-PENICILLAMINE [SEDA-15, 2729; SEDA-32, 430; SEDA-33, 472; SEDA-34, 372; SEDA-35, 424; SEDA-36, 330]

D-Penicillamine is an alpha-amino acid metabolite of penicillin with no antibiotic properties, primarily used to treat Wilson disease, a disorder of copper metabolism and elimination. D-penicillamine is associated with adverse effects in 20–40% of patients receiving treatment.

Patients with neurologic Wilson disease ($n=59$) and asymptomatic siblings ($n=4$) were prospectively evaluated. 30.2% of patients worsened following penicillamine treatment, especially those with chronic liver disease, leukpoenia, and thrombocytopenia [107c]. A comparison of D-penicillamine versus zinc sulfate as a first-line therapy for Wilson disease performed on 143 consecutive patients showed that adverse events were more common in penicillamine-treated patients (15% versus 3%) [108C]. A commentary discussed switching from penicillamine to zinc therapy to prevent penicillamine-induced elastosis perforans [109R].

Organs and Systems

Respiratory

A 47-year-old man with Wilson disease (diagnosed 20 years ago), initially treated with zinc and for past 2 years with penicillamine exhibited dyspnea on exertion. A lung function study showed irreversible obstructive changes, air trapping, and reduced carbon monoxide diffusing capacity. CT scan showed discrete bronchiectasis and diffuse bronchiolectasis. The authors reported an uncommon histological pattern for constrictive bronchiolitis obliterans characterized by changes in the bronchiolar wall caused by inflammation and fibrosis [110A].

Nervous System

A 38-year-old woman with severe pharmacoresistant depression for 3 years experienced a grandmal epileptic seizure 1 day following permanent decoppering therapy with 150 mg D-penicillamine per day [111A].

Gastrointestinal

Coadministration of penicillamine with food decreased plasma drug concentrations in dogs [112E].

Liver

Granulomatous hepatitis was observed in 63% of brown Norway rats treated with D-penicillamine (20 mg/day). Importantly, D-penicillamine inhibits the ALT assay, which may result in an under-diagnosis of liver injury resulting from D-penicillamine exposure [113E].

Urinary Tract (Kidney)

The first case of severe bilateral cystic kidney disease was observed in a patient with systemic toxicity from long-term penicillamine use [114A]. Membranous nephropathy was observed in a 26-year-old woman 18 months after receiving D-penicillamine for the treatment of Wilson Disease. Upon withdrawal of D-penicillamine, proteinuria disappeared within 7 months [115A].

Skin

Cutix laxa and elastosis perforans serpiginosa were observed in a patient with systemic toxicity resulting from long-term penicillamine use [114A]. Superficial pemphigus was observed in a 59-year-old male 1 year after starting D-penicillamine treatment for scleroderma [116E]. Penicillamine was detected in skin lesions in a case of elastosis perforans serpiginosa and pseudo-pseudoxanthoma elasticum in a patient who had received penicillamine for 25 years [117A]. Elastosis perforans serpiginosa was diagnosed in an elderly man (60s) who had been treated with penicillamine (1.0–1.5 g/day) for more than 40 years [118A]. Epiermolysis bullosa acquisita was observed in two family-related cases of individuals diagnosed 10 years earlier with Wilson disease. The authors concluded that D-penicillamine induced anticollagen VII autoimmunity [119A].

TRIENTINE (TRIETHYLENETETRAMINE) [SEDA-15, 3508; SEDA-32, 431, SEDA-33, 474; SEDA-34, 373; SEDA-35, 427; SEDA-36, 333]

Trientine is a chelating agent, primarily used to chelate copper in patients with Wilson's disease, particularly in patients with adverse effects resulting from D-penicillamine treatment.

A retrospective analysis of 380 patients with Wilson disease who had received either D-penicillamine ($n=326$) or trientine ($n=141$) showed liver transplants in patients receiving D-penicillamine ($n=3$) or trientine ($n=3$). Adverse effects were more frequent in those receiving D-penicillamine ($P=0.039$) [120M]. A prospective pilot study ($n=8$) of a single daily dosage trientine for 12 months for the treatment of Wilson disease showed ALT and AST fluctuation treatment in some patients but no change in liver function [121C].

A commentary discussed the problem that 20–40% of Wilson disease patients cannot be maintained on D-penicillamine due to severe side effects, including immediate hypersensitivity reactions, nephrotic syndrome, bone marrow toxicity, and neurological deterioration. Although trientine is well recognized as an alternative treatment, the author reports that the increase in cost from $800 to $11 000 per 100 tablets has made the drug inaccessible to most patients [122r].

TIOPRONIN [SED-15, 3430; SEDA-35, 373]

Tiopronin is a thiol used to prevent cystine precipitation and excretion and cystinuria.

Organs and Systems

Urinary Tract (Kidney)

Membranous nephropathy accompanied by uniformly thickened glomerular and rigid basement membrane and immunoglobulin and complement C3 deposited along the glomerular capillary wall was found in a 65-year-old Chinese man on long-term tiopronin treatment [123A].

POLYSTYRENE SULPHONATES [SEDA-15, 2894; SEDA-32, 433; SEDA-33, 474; SEDA-34, 373; SEDA-35, 427; SEDA-36, 333]

Sodium Polystyrene Sulfonate (Kayexalate)

Sodium polystyrene sulfonate is a potassium chelator used for the treatment of hyperkalemia. It is associated with intestinal necrosis. A review article details drug-induced injury of the GI-tract, covering sodium polystyrene sulfonate in contrast with other agents including colchicine, mycophenolate mofetil, olmesartan, paclitaxel, and tetracycline [124r].

A brief letter recommended sodium polystyrene sulfonate be considered a drug of last resort for the treatment of hyperkalemia, suggesting that insulin-glucose, calcium gluconate, sodium bicarbonate, diuretics, nebulized albuterol, and emergent dialysis be considered first [125r].

Organs and Systems

Gastrointestinal

A 66-year-old woman kidney transplant recipient with a history of hemodialysis and hypertension was admitted for a 3-month history of severe weight loss, fever, night sweats, and abdominal pain in the lower right quadrant. Laparotomy showed a thickened and inflamed ileocecal region with large lymph nodes and lightly basophilic and purple polygonal crystals were observed on a hematoxylin-eosin-saffron stain. Upon halting SPS administration, symptoms reversed and the patient regained weight [126A].

A calcium polystyrene sulfonate resin-associated bezoar was diagnosed in an 86-year-old man admitted for transarterial chemoembolization of a hepatoma who later developed fever and acute renal failure following the procedure. A video showing endoscopic fragmentation accompanies the publication [127A]. Complete intestinal obstruction occurred in a 52-year-old man treated with calcium polystyrene sulfonate for elevated serum potassium [128A]. Colonic perforation due to calcium polystyrene sulfonate administration was diagnosed in a 90-year-old woman complaining of severe upper abdominal pain [129A].

References

[1] Pennell DJ, Udelson JE, Arai AE, et al. Cardiovascular function and treatment in beta-thalassemia major: a consensus statement from the American Heart Association. Circulation. 2013;128(3):281–308 [S].

[2] Xia S, Zhang W, Huang L, et al. Comparative efficacy and safety of deferoxamine, deferiprone and deferasirox on severe thalassemia: a meta-analysis of 16 randomized controlled trials. PLoS One. 2013;8(12):e82662 [M].

[3] Ware HM, Kwiatkowski JL. Evaluation and treatment of transfusional iron overload in children. Pediatr Clin North Am. 2013;60(6):1393–406 [R].

[4] Piga A, Galanello R, Forni GL, et al. Randomized phase II trial of deferasirox (Exjade, ICL670), a once-daily, orally-administered iron chelator, in comparison to deferoxamine in thalassemia patients with transfusional iron overload. Haematologica. 2006;91(7):873–80 [C].

[5] Mourad FH, Hoffbrand AV, Sheikh-Taha M, et al. Comparison between desferrioxamine and combined therapy with desferrioxamine and deferiprone in iron overloaded thalassaemia patients. Br J Haematol. 2003;121(1):187–9 [c].

[6] Tanner MA, Galanello R, Dessi C, et al. A randomized, placebo-controlled, double-blind trial of the effect of combined therapy with deferoxamine and deferiprone on myocardial iron in thalassemia major using cardiovascular magnetic resonance. Circulation. 2007;115(14):1876–84 [c].

[7] El-Beshlawy A, Manz C, Naja M, et al. Iron chelation in thalassemia: combined or monotherapy? The Egyptian experience. Ann Hematol. 2008;87(7):545–50 [c].

[8] Aydinok Y, Ulger Z, Nart D, et al. A randomized controlled 1-year study of daily deferiprone plus twice weekly desferrioxamine compared with daily deferiprone monotherapy in patients with thalassemia major. Haematologica. 2007;92(12):1599–606 [c].

[9] Cappellini MD, Cohen A, Piga A, et al. A phase 3 study of deferasirox (ICL670), a once-daily oral iron chelator, in patients with beta-thalassemia. Blood. 2006;107(9):3455–62 [C].

[10] Marsella M, Borgna-Pignatti C. Transfusional iron overload and iron chelation therapy in thalassemia major and sickle cell disease. Hematol Oncol Clin North Am. 2014;28(4):703–27. vi R].

[11] Olivieri NF, Koren G, Harris J, et al. Growth failure and bony changes induced by deferoxamine. Am J Pediatr Hematol Oncol. 1992;14(1):48–56 [c].

[12] De Virgiliis S, Congia M, Frau F, et al. Deferoxamine-induced growth retardation in patients with thalassemia major. J Pediatr. 1988;113(4):661–9 [c].

[13] Cianciulli P, Sorrentino F, Maffei L, et al. Continuous low-dose subcutaneous desferrioxamine (DFO) to prevent allergic manifestations in patients with iron overload. Ann Hematol. 1996;73(6):279–81 [c].

[14] Bousquet J, Navarro M, Robert G, et al. Rapid desensitisation for desferrioxamine anaphylactoid reaction. Lancet. 1983;2(8354):859–60 [R].

[15] Olivieri NF, Buncic JR, Chew E, et al. Visual and auditory neurotoxicity in patients receiving subcutaneous deferoxamine infusions. N Engl J Med. 1986;314(14):869–73 [A].

[16] Gallant T, Boyden MH, Gallant LA, et al. Serial studies of auditory neurotoxicity in patients receiving deferoxamine therapy. Am J Med. 1987;83(6):1085–90 [c].

[17] Borgna-Pignatti C, De Stefano P, Broglia AM. Visual loss in patient on high-dose subcutaneous desferrioxamine. Lancet. 1984;1(8378):681 [A].

[18] Koren G, Bentur Y, Strong D, et al. Acute changes in renal function associated with deferoxamine therapy. Am J Dis Child. 1989;143(9):1077–80 [A].

[19] Koren G, Kochavi-Atiya Y, Bentur Y, et al. The effects of subcutaneous deferoxamine administration on renal function in thalassemia major. Int J Hematol. 1991;54(5):371–5 [c].

[20] Robins-Browne RM, Prpic JK, Stuart SJ. Yersiniae and iron. A study in host-parasite relationships. Contrib Microbiol Immunol. 1987;9:254–8 [R].

[21] Chan GC, Chan S, Ho PL, et al. Effects of chelators (deferoxamine, deferiprone and deferasirox) on the growth of Klebsiella pneumoniae and Aeromonas hydrophila isolated from transfusion-dependent thalassemia patients. Hemoglobin. 2009;33(5):352–60 [R].

[22] Cohen AR, Galanello R, Piga A, et al. Safety and effectiveness of long-term therapy with the oral iron chelator deferiprone. Blood. 2003;102(5):1583–7 [c].

[23] al-Refaie FN, Hershko C, Hoffbrand AV, et al. Results of long-term deferiprone (L1) therapy: a report by the International Study Group on Oral Iron Chelators. Br J Haematol. 1995;91(1):224–9 [C].

[24] al-Refaie FN, Wonke B, Wickens DG, et al. Zinc concentration in patients with iron overload receiving oral iron chelator 1,2-dimethyl-3-hydroxypyrid-4-one or desferrioxamine. J Clin Pathol. 1994;47(7):657–60 [c].

[25] Berkovitch M, Laxer RM, Inman R, et al. Arthropathy in thalassaemia patients receiving deferiprone. Lancet. 1994;343(8911):1471–2 [c].

[26] Chand G, Chowdhury V, Manchanda A, et al. Deferiprone-induced arthropathy in thalassemia: MRI findings in a case. Indian J Radiol Imaging. 2009;19(2):155–7 [A].

[27] Cappellini MD, Bejaoui M, Agaoglu L, et al. Iron chelation with deferasirox in adult and pediatric patients with thalassemia major: efficacy and safety during 5 years' follow-up. Blood. 2011;118(4):884–93 [c].

[28] Vichinsky E, Onyekwere O, Porter J, et al. A randomised comparison of deferasirox versus deferoxamine for the treatment of transfusional iron overload in sickle cell disease. Br J Haematol. 2007;136(3):501–8 [c].

[29] Rafat C, Fakhouri F, Ribeil JA, et al. Fanconi syndrome due to deferasirox. Am J Kidney Dis. 2009;54(5):931–4 [A].

[30] Rheault MN, Bechtel H, Neglia JP, et al. Reversible Fanconi syndrome in a pediatric patient on deferasirox. Pediatr Blood Cancer. 2011;56(4):674–6 [A].

[31] Wei HY, Yang CP, Cheng CH, et al. Fanconi syndrome in a patient with beta-thalassemia major after using deferasirox for 27 months. Transfusion. 2011;51(5):949–54 [A].

[32] Grandvuillemin A, Audia S, Leguy-Seguin V, et al. Severe thrombocytopenia and mild leucopenia associated with deferasirox therapy. Therapie. 2009;64(6):405–7 [A].

[33] Breccia M, Alimena G. Efficacy and safety of deferasirox in myelodysplastic syndromes. Ann Hematol. 2013;92(7): 863–70 [r].

[34] Bedford MR, Ford SJ, Horniblow RD, et al. Iron chelation in the treatment of cancer: a new role for deferasirox? J Clin Pharmacol. 2013;53(9):885–91 [R].

[35] Weigel KJ, Lynch SG, LeVine SM. Iron chelation and multiple sclerosis. ASN Neuro. 2014;6(1):e00136 [R].

[36] Vallejo C, Batlle M, Vazquez L, et al. Phase IV open-label study of the efficacy and safety of deferasirox after allogeneic stem cell transplantation. Haematologica. 2014;99(10):1632–7 [c].

[37] Kontoghiorghes GJ. A record number of fatalities in many categories of patients treated with deferasirox: loopholes in regulatory and marketing procedures undermine patient safety and misguide public funds? Expert Opin Drug Saf. 2013 Sep;12(5):605–9 [R].

[38] Kontoghiorghes GJ. A record number of fatalities in many categories of patients treated with deferasirox: loopholes in regulatory and marketing procedures undermine patient safety and misguide public funds? Author's response. Expert Opin Drug Saf. 2013;12(5):794–5 [r].

[39] Riva A. A record number of fatalities in many categories of patients treated with deferasirox: loopholes in regulatory and marketing procedures undermine patient safety and misguide public funds? Expert Opin Drug Saf. 2013;12(5):793–4 [r].

[40] Chaudhary P, Pullarkat V. Deferasirox: appraisal of safety and efficacy in long-term therapy. J Blood Med. 2013;4:101–10 [R].

[41] Shirley M, Plosker GL. Deferasirox: a review of its use for chronic iron overload in patients with non-transfusion-dependent thalassaemia. Drugs. 2014;74(9):1017–27 [R].

[42] Tanaka C. Clinical pharmacology of deferasirox. Clin Pharmacokinet. 2014;53(8):679–94 [R].

[43] Chen CH, Shu KH, Yang Y. Long-term effects of an oral iron chelator, deferasirox, in hemodialysis patients with iron overload. Hematology. 2015;20(5):304–10 [c].

[44] Baksi AJ, Pennell DJ. Randomized controlled trials of iron chelators for the treatment of cardiac siderosis in thalassaemia major. Front Pharmacol. 2014;5:217 [c].

[45] Keshtkaran A, Javanbakht M, Salavati S, et al. Cost-utility analysis of oral deferasirox versus infusional deferoxamine in transfusion-dependent beta-thalassemia patients. Transfusion. 2013;53(8):1722–9 [r].

[46] Taher AT, Porter JB, Viprakasit V, et al. Deferasirox effectively reduces iron overload in non-transfusion-dependent thalassemia (NTDT) patients: 1-year extension results from the THALASSA study. Ann Hematol. 2013;92(11):1485–93 [c].

[47] Improta S, Villa MR, Volpe A, et al. Transfusion-dependent low-risk myelodysplastic patients receiving deferasirox: long-term follow-up. Oncol Lett. 2013;6(6):1774–8 [c].

[48] Walia HS, Yan J. Reversible retinopathy associated with oral deferasirox therapy. BMJ Case Rep. 2013; published online July 17, 2013. [A].

[49] Dell'Orto VG, Bianchetti MG, Brazzola P. Hyperchloraemic metabolic acidosis induced by the iron chelator deferasirox: a case report and review of the literature. J Clin Pharm Ther. 2013;38(6):526–7 [A].

[50] Hayakawa F, Tomita A, Naoe T. Development of acute pure red cell aplasia after deferasirox administration in two cases of myelodysplastic syndrome. Rinsho Ketsueki. 2014;55(4):445–9 [A].

[51] Vichinsky E, Torres M, Minniti CP, et al. Efficacy and safety of deferasirox compared with deferoxamine in sickle cell disease: two-year results including pharmacokinetics and concomitant hydroxyurea. Am J Hematol. 2013;88(12):1068–73 [c].

[52] Pennell DJ, Porter JB, Piga A, et al. A 1-year randomized controlled trial of deferasirox vs deferoxamine for myocardial iron removal in beta-thalassemia major (CORDELIA). Blood. 2014;123(10):1447–54 [c].

[53] Huang WF, Chou HC, Tsai YW, et al. Safety of deferasirox: a retrospective cohort study on the risks of gastrointestinal, liver and renal events. Pharmacoepidemiol Drug Saf. 2014;23(11):1176–82 [M].

[54] Meerpohl JJ, Schell LK, Rucker G, et al. Deferasirox for managing transfusional iron overload in people with sickle cell disease. Cochrane Database Syst Rev. 2014 May 27;5:CD007477 [c].

[55] Pazgal I, Brown M, Perets TT, et al. Lactose intolerance is not the cause of gastrointestinal adverse effects in beta thalassemia patients treated with deferasirox. Am J Hematol. 2014;89(9):938–9 [c].

[56] Ahmed J, Ahmad N, Jankharia B, et al. Effect of deferasirox chelation on liver iron and total body iron concentration. Indian J Pediatr. 2013;80(8):655–8 [c].

[57] Hall AM, Bass P, Unwin RJ. Drug-induced renal Fanconi syndrome. QJM. 2014;107(4):261–9 [R].

[58] Diaz-Garcia JD, Gallegos-Villalobos A, Gonzalez-Espinoza L, et al. Deferasirox nephrotoxicity—the knowns and unknowns. Nat Rev Nephrol. 2014;10(10):574–86 [R].

[59] Piga A, Fracchia S, Lai ME, et al. Deferasirox effect on renal haemodynamic parameters in patients with transfusion-dependent beta thalassaemia. Br J Haematol. 2015;168(6):882–90 [R].

[60] Naderi M, Sadeghi-Bojd S, Valeshabad AK, et al. A prospective study of tubular dysfunction in pediatric patients with beta thalassemia major receiving deferasirox. Pediatr Hematol Oncol. 2013;30(8):748–54 [c].

[61] Murphy N, Elramah M, Vats H, et al. A case report of deferasirox-induced kidney injury and Fanconi syndrome. WMJ. 2013;112(4):177–80 [A].

[62] Ohshita A, Nakai N, Katoh N, et al. A maculopapular-type eruption associated with deferasirox administration. J Am Acad Dermatol. 2013;69(5):e265–7 [A].

[63] Aleem A, Shakoor Z, Alsaleh K, et al. Immunological evaluation of beta-thalassemia major patients receiving oral iron chelator deferasirox. J Coll Physicians Surg Pak. 2014;24(7):467–71 [c].

[64] Ila HB, Topaktas M, Arslan M, et al. Signs of deferasirox genotoxicity. Cytotechnology. 2014;66(4):647–54 [E].

[65] Dee CM, Cheuk DK, Ha SY, et al. Incidence of deferasirox-associated renal tubular dysfunction in children and young adults with beta-thalassaemia. Br J Haematol. 2014;167(3):434–6 [c].

[66] Ktena YP, Athanasiadou A, Lambrou G, et al. Iron chelation with deferasirox for the treatment of secondary hemosiderosis in pediatric oncology patients: a single-center experience. J Pediatr Hematol Oncol. 2013;35(6):447–50 [c].

[67] Bentley A, Gillard S, Spino M, et al. Cost-utility analysis of deferiprone for the treatment of beta-thalassaemia patients with chronic iron overload: a UK perspective. Pharmacoeconomics. 2013;31(9):807–22 [H].

[68] El-Beshlawy AM, El-Alfy MS, Sari TT, et al. Continuation of deferiprone therapy in patients with mild neutropenia may not lead to a more severe drop in neutrophil count. Eur J Haematol. 2014;92(4):337–40 [c].

[69] Elalfy M, Wali YA, Qari M, et al. Deviating from safety guidelines during deferiprone therapy in clinical practice may not be associated with higher risk of agranulocytosis. Pediatr Blood Cancer. 2014;61(5):879–84 [c].

[70] Pandolfo M, Hausmann L. Deferiprone for the treatment of Friedreich's ataxia. J Neurochem. 2013;126(Suppl 1):142–6 [r].

[71] Huprikar N, Gossweiler M, Callaghan M, et al. Agranulocytosis with deferiprone treatment of superficial siderosis. BMJ Case Rep. 2013; published online August 7, 2013 [A].

[72] Arpa J, Sanz-Gallego I, Rodriguez-de-Rivera FJ, et al. Triple therapy with deferiprone, idebenone and riboflavin in Friedreich's ataxia—open-label trial. Acta Neurol Scand. 2014;129(1):32–40 [c].

[73] Mallat NS, Beydoun A, Musallam KM, et al. Deferiprone-induced seizures in a patient with beta-thalassemia major. Blood Cells Mol Dis. 2013;51(2):94–5 [A].

[74] Fisher SA, Brunskill SJ, Doree C, et al. Oral deferiprone for iron chelation in people with thalassaemia. Cochrane Database Syst Rev. 2013;8:CD004839 [M].

[75] Pandolfo M, Arpa J, Delatycki MB, et al. Deferiprone in Friedreich ataxia: a 6-month randomized controlled trial. Ann Neurol. 2014;76(4):509–21 [c].

[76] Sharma R, Anand R, Chandra J, et al. Distal ulnar changes in children with thalassemia and deferiprone related arthropathy. Pediatr Blood Cancer. 2013;60(12):1957–62 [c].

[77] Tanphaichitr A, Kusuwan T, Limviriyakul S, et al. Incidence of ototoxicity in pediatric patients with transfusion-dependent thalassemia who are less well-chelated by mono- and combined therapy of iron chelating agents. Hemoglobin. 2014;38(5):345–50 [c].

[78] Songdej D, Sirachainan N, Wongwerawattanakoon P, et al. Combined chelation therapy with daily oral deferiprone and twice-weekly subcutaneous infusion of desferrioxamine in children with beta-thalassemia: 3-year experience. Acta Haematol. 2015;133(2):226–36 [c].

[79] Waheed N, Ali S, Butt MA. Comparison of deferiprone and deferrioxamine for the treatment of transfusional iron overload in children with beta thalassemia major. J Ayub Med Coll Abbottabad. 2014;26(3):297–300 [c].

[80] Van Bol L, Alami A, Benghiat FS, et al. Spectral domain optical coherence tomography findings in early deferoxamine maculopathy: report of two cases. Retin Cases Brief Rep. 2014;8(2):97–102 [A].

[81] Gelman R, Kiss S, Tsang SH. Multimodal imaging in a case of deferoxamine-induced maculopathy. Retin Cases Brief Rep. 2014;8(4):306–9 [A].

[82] Wu CH, Yang CP, Lai CC, et al. Deferoxamine retinopathy: spectral domain-optical coherence tomography findings. BMC Ophthalmol. 2014;14:88 [A].

[83] Viola F, Barteselli G, Dell'Arti L, et al. Multimodal imaging in deferoxamine retinopathy. Retina. 2014;34(7):1428–38 [c].

[84] Fernandez S, Castro P, Nogue S, et al. Acute iron intoxication: change in urine color during chelation therapy with deferoxamine. Intensive Care Med. 2014;40(1):104 [A].

[85] Surapolchai P, Poachanukoon O, Satayasai W, et al. Modified desensitization protocols for a pediatric patient with anaphylactic reaction to deferoxamine. J Med Assoc Thai. 2014;97(Suppl 8):S217–22 [A].

[86] Arifin AJ, Hannauer M, Welch I, et al. Deferoxamine mesylate enhances virulence of community-associated methicillin resistant Staphylococcus aureus. Microbes Infect. 2014;16(11):967–72 [E].

[87] Zhang W, Wu Y, Yan Q, et al. Deferoxamine enhances cell migration and invasion through promotion of HIF-1alpha expression and epithelial-mesenchymal transition in colorectal cancer. Oncol Rep. 2014;31(1):111–6 [E].

[88] Seif El Dien HM, Esmail RI, Magdy RE, et al. Deferoxamine-induced dysplasia-like skeletal abnormalities at radiography and MRI. Pediatr Radiol. 2013;43(9):1159–65 [c].

[89] Yang SK, Xiao L, Song PA, et al. Is lead chelation therapy effective for chronic kidney disease? A meta-analysis. Nephrology (Carlton). 2014;19(1):56–9 [R].

[90] Aaseth J, Skaug MA, Cao Y, et al. Chelation in metal intoxication—principles and paradigms. J Trace Elem Med Biol. 2015;31:260–6 [R].

[91] Kutlar A, Reid ME, Inati A, et al. A dose-escalation phase IIa study of 2,2-dimethylbutyrate (HQK-1001), an oral fetal globin inducer, in sickle cell disease. Am J Hematol. 2013;88(11):E255–60 [c].

[92] Karimi M, Cohan N, Pishdad P. Hydroxyurea as a first-line treatment of extramedullary hematopoiesis in patients with beta thalassemia: four case reports. Hematology. 2015;20(1):53–7 [c].

[93] Agrawal RK, Patel RK, Shah V, et al. Hydroxyurea in sickle cell disease: drug review. Indian J Hematol Blood Transfus. 2014;30(2):91–6 [R].

[94] Kosaryan M, Karami H, Zafari M, et al. Report on patients with non transfusion-dependent beta-thalassemia major being treated with hydroxyurea attending the Thalassemia Research Center, Sari, Mazandaran Province, Islamic Republic of Iran in 2013. Hemoglobin. 2014;38(2):115–8 [R].

[95] Bordbar MR, Silavizadeh S, Haghpanah S, et al. Hydroxyurea treatment in transfusion-dependent beta-thalassemia patients. Iran Red Crescent Med J. 2014;16(6):e18028 [c].

[96] Ghasemi A, Keikhaei B, Ghodsi R. Side effects of hydroxyurea in patients with Thalassemia major and thalassemia intermedia and sickle cell anemia. Iran J Ped Hematol Oncol. 2014;4(3):114–7 [c].

[97] Italia K, Colah R, Ghosh K. Hydroxyurea could be a good clinically relevant iron chelator. PLoS One. 2013;8(12):e82928 [E].

[98] Morton D, Reed L, Huang W, et al. Toxicity of hydroxyurea in rats and dogs. Toxicol Pathol. 2015;43(4):498–512 [E].

[99] Zekavat OR, Makarem AR, Haghpanah S, et al. Hypothyroidism in beta-Thalassemia Intermedia patients with and without hydroxyurea. Iran J Med Sci. 2014;39(1):60–3 [c].

[100] Dehury S, Purohit P, Patel S, et al. Low and fixed dose of hydroxyurea is effective and safe in patients with HbSbeta(+) thalassemia with IVS1-5(G–>C) mutation. Pediatr Blood Cancer. 2015;62(6):1017–23 [c].

[101] Hankins JS, Aygun B, Nottage K, et al. From infancy to adolescence: fifteen years of continuous treatment with hydroxyurea in sickle cell anemia. Medicine (Baltimore). 2014;93(28):e215 [c].

[102] Boonyawat K, Wongwaisayawan S, Nitiyanant P, et al. Hydroxyurea and colonic ulcers: a case report. BMC Gastroenterol. 2014;14:134 [A].

[103] Quattrone F, Dini V, Barbanera S, et al. Cutaneous ulcers associated with hydroxyurea therapy. J Tissue Viability. 2013;22(4):112–21 [R].

[104] Smith-Whitley K. Reproductive issues in sickle cell disease. Blood. 2014;124(24):3538–43 [r].

[105] DeBaun MR. Hydroxyurea therapy contributes to infertility in adult men with sickle cell disease: a review. Expert Rev Hematol. 2014;7(6):767–73 [R].

[106] Lederman HM, Connolly MA, Kalpatthi R, et al. Immunologic effects of hydroxyurea in sickle cell anemia. Pediatrics. 2014;134(4):686–95 [c].

[107] Kalita J, Kumar V, Chandra S, et al. Worsening of Wilson disease following penicillamine therapy. Eur Neurol. 2014;71(3–4):126–31 [c].

[108] Czlonkowska A, Litwin T, Karlinski M, et al. D-penicillamine versus zinc sulfate as first-line therapy for Wilson's disease. Eur J Neurol. 2014;21(4):599–606 [C].

[109] Ranucci G, Di Dato F, Leone F, et al. Penicillamine-induced elastosis perforans serpiginosa in Wilson's disease: is useful switching to zinc? J Pediatr Gastroenterol Nutr. 2014; Epub ahead of print. [R].

[110] Bruguera-Avila N, Sanchez-Martinez E, Garcia-Olive I, et al. Obliterating bronchiolitis in a patient treated with (D)-penicillamine. Arch Bronconeumol. 2013;49(9):411–2 [A].

[111] Berger B, Mader I, Damjanovic K, et al. Epileptic status immediately after initiation of D-penicillamine therapy in a patient with Wilson's disease. Clin Neurol Neurosurg. 2014;127:122–4 [A].

[112] Langlois DK, Lehner AF, Buchweitz JP, et al. Pharmacokinetics and relative bioavailability of D-penicillamine in fasted and nonfasted dogs. J Vet Intern Med. 2013;27(5):1071–6 [E].

[113] Metushi IG, Zhu X, Uetrecht J. D-penicillamine-induced granulomatous hepatitis in brown Norway rats. Mol Cell Biochem. 2014;393(1–2):229–35 [E].

[114] Koraishy FM, Cohen RA, Israel GM, et al. Cystic kidney disease in a patient with systemic toxicity from long-term D-penicillamine use. Am J Kidney Dis. 2013;62(4):806–9 [A].

[115] Kumar RP, Prasad ND, Tirumavalavan S, et al. D-penicillamine-induced membranous nephropathy. Indian J Nephrol. 2014;24(3):195–6 [A].

[116] Khashoggi M, Machet L, Perrinaud A, et al. D-penicillamine-induced pemphigus: changes in anti-32-2B immunostaining patterns. Ann Dermatol Venereol. 2013;140(8–9):531–4 [A].

[117] Neri I, Gurioli C, Raggi MA, et al. Detection of D-penicillamine in skin lesions in a case of dermal elastosis after a previous long-term treatment for Wilson's disease. J Eur Acad Dermatol Venereol. 2015;29(2):383–6 [A].

[118] Hellriegel S, Bertsch HP, Emmert S, et al. Elastosis perforans serpiginosa: a case of a penicillamine-induced degenerative dermatosis. JAMA Dermatol. 2014;150(7):785–7 [A].

[119] Ingen-Housz-Oro S, Grootenboer-Mignot S, Ortonne N, et al. Epidermolysis bullosa acquisita-like eruption with anticollagen VII autoantibodies induced by D-penicillamine in Wilson disease. Br J Dermatol. 2014;171(6):1574–6 [A].

[120] Weiss KH, Thurik F, Gotthardt DN, et al. Efficacy and safety of oral chelators in treatment of patients with Wilson disease. Clin Gastroenterol Hepatol. 2013;11(8):1028–35. e1-2 [M].

[121] Ala A, Aliu E, Schilsky ML. Prospective pilot study of a single daily dosage of trientine for the treatment of Wilson disease. Dig Dis Sci. 2015;60(5):1433–9 [c].

[122] Chandok N, Roberts EA. The trientine crisis in Canada: a call to advocacy. Can J Gastroenterol Hepatol. 2014;28(4):184 [r].

[123] Zheng Z, Xue Y, Jia J, et al. Tiopronin-induced membranous nephropathy: a case report. Ren Fail. 2014;36(9):1455–60 [A].

[124] Panarelli NC. Drug-induced injury in the gastrointestinal tract. Semin Diagn Pathol. 2014;31(2):165–75 [r].

[125] Varriale P, Ngai L. Sodium polystyrene sulfonate use revisited. Am J Med. 2014;127(8):e37 [r].

[126] Zaidan M, Loupy A, Rouquette A, et al. A kidney transplant patient with ileocecal inflammation. Sodium polystyrene sulfonate-associated intestinal ulcer and foreign-body reaction. Kidney Int. 2013;84(5): 1057–9 [A].

[127] Lai TP, Yang CW, Siaop FY, et al. Calcium polystyrene sulfonate bezoar in the ileum: diagnosis and treatment with double-balloon endoscopy. Endoscopy. 2013;45(Suppl 2 UCTN): E378–9 [A].

[128] Tongyoo A, Sriussadaporn E, Limpavitayaporn P, et al. Acute intestinal obstruction due to Kalimate, a potassium-lowering agent: a case report and literature review. J Med Assoc Thai. 2013;96(12):1617–20 [A].

[129] Takeuchi N, Nomura Y, Meda T, et al. Development of colonic perforation during calcium polystyrene sulfonate administration: a case report. Case Rep Med. 2013;2013:102614 [A].

[130] Kosaryan M, Zafari M, Alipur A, et al. The effect and side effect of hydroxyurea therapy on patients with beta-thalassemia: a systematic review to December 2012. Hemoglobin. 2014;38(4):262–71 [R].

24

Antiseptic Drugs and Disinfectants

Dirk W. Lachenmeier[1]

Chemisches und Veterinäruntersuchungsamt (CVUA) Karlsruhe, Karlsruhe, Germany
[1]Corresponding author: lachenmeier@web.de

ALL COMMONLY USED ANTISEPTICS AND DISINFECTANTS

Infection Risk

The FDA has reported a series of side effects of contaminated antiseptic solutions, ranging from localised infection at an injection site to deep infections and even fatal septicaemia. The products included all commonly used antiseptic agents such as alcohols, iodophors, chlorhexidine, and quaternary ammonium compounds. The microorganisms were introduced into the antiseptic solutions by diluting them with contaminated water, by inappropriate handling, or by storing them under non-sterile conditions [1r,2r]. An outbreak of *Burkholderia cenocepacia* infection was reported from a hospital in Korea, due to inadequate preparation of chlorhexidine solutions diluted with contaminated water [3c]. The FDA has published guidelines for proper handling of antiseptics to avoid contamination [4S].

ALDEHYDES [SED-15, 1439, 1513; SEDA-31, 409; SEDA-32, 437; SEDA-33, 479; SEDA-34, 377; SEDA-36, 339]

Considering all disinfectants, aldehydes have a special status as they are able to pose occupational hazards even at very low concentrations in air (SEDA-36, 339). A survey in Germany 2006–2009 shows that the use of formaldehyde releasers in cosmetics is common in 8% of all products in a random sample ($n = 4680$) [5M].

Formaldehyde

Respiratory

Exposure to formaldehyde occurs in certain occupational settings associated with its use as a sterilizing agent, but exposure to formaldehyde-emitting products such as particle board, urea formaldehyde insulation, carpeting and furniture is more common. Whether non-occupational exposure to formaldehyde is related to *asthma* is still a subject of intense debate [SEDA-32, 437; SEDA-34, 377; SEDA-36, 339]. In a birth cohort study of 3840 healthy full-term babies, domestic formaldehyde exposure was found to increase the occurrence of dry cough at night, but only among babies without parental history of allergy (adjusted OR per $10 \, \mu g/m^3$ increase 1.45, 95% CI 1.08–1.96) [6C]. This finding was consistent with previous studies reporting about respiratory system disorders in both adults and children residentially exposed to formaldehyde [see SEDA-36, 339]. Recent trends in risk assessment of formaldehyde exposure from indoor air were reviewed by Nielsen et al. [7R]. The authors provided strengthened evidence for the validity of the World Health Organization guideline of $0.1 \, mg/m^3$.

Gastrointestinal

The use of 1% formalin during colonoscopy to ablate angiodysplasia caused severe colonic necrosis in a 68-year-old patient with diabetes mellitus and end-stage renal disease. The authors advise against formalin application in the gastrointestinal tract beyond the rectum [8A].

Tumorigenicity

According to an updated assessment of the International Agency for Research on Cancer (IARC), formaldehyde was confirmed as carcinogenic to humans (Group 1). Formaldehyde causes cancer of the nasopharynx and leukaemia [9S]. Also, a positive association has been observed between exposure to formaldehyde and sinonasal cancer [9S]. An update of the National Cancer Institute (NCI) cohort ($n = 25619$) confirmed the link between formaldehyde exposure and nasopharyngeal cancer (RR in the highest exposure category 7.66, 95% CI

© 2015 Elsevier B.V. All rights reserved.

0.94–62.34) [10C]. Another study in a cohort of British chemical workers ($n=14008$), however, did not support an increased risk in myeloid leukemia, nasopharyngeal carcinoma or other upper airway tumours [11C]. The IARC assessment and specifically the epidemiologic evidence on the association between formaldehyde exposure and risk of leukaemia and other lymphohaematopoietic malignancies have been previously discussed controversially [SEDA-36, 339]. While the potential mechanisms associated with formaldehyde-induced cancer are not completely understood, some new studies have strengthened the mechanistic evidence of its genotoxic carcinogenicity in humans. Formaldehyde-exposed workers ($n=51$ vs. $n=54$ non-exposed controls) in the furnishing industry producing pressed-wood and laminate products were found to have increased oxidative stress status, which was indicated by urinary $15\text{-}F_{2t}$ isoprostane levels [12c]. In a similar study in plywood workers ($n=178$), a dose–response relationship was detected between the current formaldehyde exposure levels and DNA strand breaks and between the duration of exposure and chromosome damage in the peripheral blood lymphocytes [13c]. In a study of children ($n=413$) in Italy, the ones living near (<2 km) the chipboard industry had the highest average exposure to formaldehyde, which was also associated with markers of genotoxicity in exfoliated buccal cells (as determined by the comet and micronucleus assays) [14c]. A cross-sectional study of formaldehyde-exposed workers in China ($n=43$ vs. $n=51$ controls) showed decreased counts of natural killer cells, regulatory T cells and CD8$^+$ effector memory T cells. These alterations were judged as potential cause for alterations in immune function and anti-tumor response. However, due to the small sample size, the authors judged the results as preliminary needing confirmation in larger studies [15c].

Immunologic

Formaldehyde was pointed out as leading allergen in the cleaning industry (3.4%, 95% CI 2.0–4.7); standard single-use gloves with a limited material thickness (<0.2 mm) were pointed out as not being protective [16r]. A case of a 28-year-old Japanese female was described. The patient had developed general urticaria 1 hour after application of a paraformaldehyde-containing root canal disinfectant. The urticaria resolved after taking an oral antihistamine. Repeated dental procedures involving local paraformaldehyde application were judged to have accounted for the patient's sensitization [17A]. It should be noted that deficiency in ALDH2, which is prevalent in Asia, may contribute to the allergenic potential of aldehydes [18r]. Contact dermatitis may be caused by formaldehyde-releasing textile items (from 180 items tested, 10 exceeded the acceptable limit in the US of 75 ppm). Some guidelines were suggested to avoid formaldehyde-related textile dermatitis [19r].

Glutaraldehyde (Glutaral)

Gastrointestinal

A case of glutaraldehyde-induced colitis in a 52-year-old woman was described. Symptoms of abdominal pain, watery diarrhea and per rectal bleed developed soon following a screening colonoscopy. The temporal trend was consistent with that of a proctosigmoiditis secondary to glutaraldehyde. The symptoms resolved within 2 weeks after diagnosis [20A]. It should be noted that the case report did not point out the concentration or type of used disinfectant, or the actual practices of disinfectant use. Most probably, the sterilized instrument was not adequately rinsed and dried prior to the colonoscopy.

Immunologic

Glutaraldehyde was pointed out as relevant allergen in the cleaning industry (2.8%, 95% CI 1.3–4.2); similar to formaldehyde, standard single-use gloves with a limited material thickness (<0.2 mm) were pointed out as not being protective [16r].

GUANIDINES

Chlorhexidine [SED-15, 714; SEDA-31, 410; SEDA-32, 439; SEDA-33, 480; SEDA-34, 378; SEDA-36, 340]

Drug Formulations

Chlorhexidine is used extensively in oral hygiene but can cause staining of the teeth and oral mucosa, adversely affect taste and rarely cause pain [SEDA-30, 278; SEDA-31, 416; SEDA-34, 378; SEDA-36, 340]. A survey in Germany 2006–2009 shows that chlorhexidine is not only used in medicinal products but also in cosmetics with a prevalence of about 0.2% of all cosmetic products in a random sample ($n=4680$) [5M].

Skin

In a systematic Cochrane review on vaginal chlorhexidine use during labor to prevent early-onset neonatal group B streptococcal infection, mild maternal side effects were reported (stinging or local irritation in three trials, 1066 women) as more common in women treated with chlorhexidine (RR 8.50, 95% CI 1.60–45.28) [21M].

Immunologic

The prevalence of chlorhexidine-related allergic contact dermatitis was reported from patch-testing performed in Melbourne, Australia. The rate of relevant chlorhexidine allergic contact dermatitis was 19/7890 (0.24%) in the total collective of non-occupational and occupational patients, while the rate in occupationally exposed health care workers was higher (10/541, 2%) [22c]. A study in 899 Thai nurses also showed that occupational chlorhexidine exposure may be associated with dermal allergic symptoms in connection with latex glove use (OR 2.09, 95% CI 1.23–3.54) [23c]. A case series of six patients that were exposed to chlorhexidine in gels, swabs and catheters during surgery leading to anaphylaxis was reported [24A]. Another unusual case of a patient that showed acute allergic reaction after intravenous saline injection was described. The cannula connector was swabbed in this case with a disinfectant containing 70% isopropyl alcohol and 2% chlorhexidine [25A]. Finally, another case of anaphylactic reaction to intraurethral chlorhexidine was reported [26A].

Polyhexamethylene Guanidine [SEDA-36, 341]

Polyhexamethylene guanidine (PHMG) has been used as an antiseptic, especially for the suppression of hospital infection in the Russian Federation and as a disinfectant for sterilization of household humidifiers in Korea [SEDA-36, 341]. Following safety concerns, manufacture and sale of disinfectants containing PHMG were suspended in the Russian Federation [27A] and Korea [28C].

Respiratory

Further evidence was gathered on the association of the disinfectants PHMG and oligo(2-(2-ethoxy)ethoxyethyl)-guanidinium-chloride (PGH) with lung disease (see SEDA-36, 341 for description of first cases). A large nationwide retrospective study in South Korea was conducted between 2006 and 2011 to investigate the relationship between humidifier disinfectants and children's interstitial lung disease. In total, 138 children were diagnosed with this disease, from which 80 children (58%) died. Two years after humidifier disinfectant-sale suspension, no more new cases were found. The study suggested the causal relationship between humidifier disinfectant inhalation and an idiopathic type of children's interstitial lung disease [28C]. Sub-collectives of this nationwide study were published with similar findings [29c,30c]. The exposure characteristics were appreciated in another study from Korea in more detail. Out of 10 patients with fatal lung disease, nine were found to have used PHMG [31c]. The plausibility of the association between PHMG and PGH in household humidifiers and lung disease has been confirmed by several mechanistic studies. It was shown that both compounds can be found in the air following humidifier use under household conditions. The resulting consumer exposure was judged as indicating a significant health risk [32E]. The toxicity of

PHMG was investigated in human alveolar epithelial A549 cells *in vitro*. Potent cytotoxicity with cell death evident as low as 5 µg/ml was found, which is conferred through the generation of intracellular reactive oxygen species and alteration of gene expression [33E]. The effect of PHMG phosphate was studied in mice by direct exposure of the lungs *in vivo*. A dose-dependent exacerbation of both inflammation and pulmonary fibrosis was detected on day 14. PHMG phosphate also caused thymic atrophy [34E].

Polyhexamethylene Biguanidine [SEDA-36, 341]

Polyhexamethylene biguanidine (PHMB) has been applied as a substitute for chlorhexidine in local anti-infective treatments, but is also used in different nonmedical fields (swimming pool sanitizer) [SEDA-36, 341]. The mode of action of PHMB was recently reviewed and it was remarked that the European Chemicals Agency classified PHMB as "fatal if inhaled," which would discourage its use for disinfection by fumigation or fogging [35R].

Immunologic

A case of allergic contact dermatitis in a 42-year-old man following the use of wet wipes containing PHMB was reported. Chronic and recurrent itchy dermatitis in the anogenital region was found to be caused by the frequent use of wet wipes for intimate hygiene containing PHMB [36A].

BENZALKONIUM COMPOUNDS [*SED-15, 421; SEDA-32, 440; SEDA-33, 481; SEDA-34, 379; SEDA-36, 341*]

Sensory Systems

Reviews about the effect of glaucoma therapy on ocular surface disease (OSD) and the specific adverse effects of benzalkonium chloride were provided by Anwar et al. [37R], Inoue [38R] and Rasmussen et al. [39R]. It is believed that eye drops containing benzalkonium chloride as preservative may contribute to OSD [see also SEDA-36, 341]. An observational, cross-sectional study of patients with topically treated glaucoma was conducted ($n = 233$). Multivariate analysis confirmed that benzalkonium chloride exposure was a risk factor for developing OSD ($p < 0.001$) [40c]. A prospective single masked cohort study was conducted in glaucoma patients exposed to benzalkonium chloride ($n = 23$) compared to unexposed patients ($n = 27$). A greater increase in basal layer epithelium cell density was observed in the benzalkonium chloride exposed cohort ($p < 0.05$)

[41c]. A retrospective review of 128 glaucoma patients detected that increased preoperative exposure to ophthalmic solutions preserved with benzalkonium chloride is a risk factor for earlier surgical trabeculectomy failure [42A]. A retrospective case series in patients with limbal stem cell (LSC) disease found that benzalkonium chloride toxicity may have caused the LSC disease in 2 eyes out of 22 eyes [43A]. A prospective, randomized, investigator-masked comparative study in patients ($n=44$) comparing preservative-free artificial tears, or benzalkonium chloride-preserved artificial tears suggested that short-term exposure can cause disruption of the blood-aqueous barriers, without altering the blood–retinal barriers, in pseudophakic eyes [44c]. *In vitro* research on fibrillation of corneal dystrophy-associated peptides suggested that benzalkonium chloride in eye drops may accelerate amyloid fibrillation and deteriorate corneal dystrophies [45E]. Long-term experiments in nonhuman primates were suggested as necessary and are currently ongoing [39R].

ETHYLENE OXIDE [SED-15, 1296; SEDA-29, 242; SEDA-34, 379; SEDA-36, 341]

Ethylene oxide is used directly in the gaseous form to sterilize drugs, hospital equipment, disposable and reusable medical items, packaging materials, foods and other items [*SEDA-36, 341*]. A large number of samples of herbs, spices and other dried vegetables imported to Italy contained more than 0.3 mg/kg of ethylene oxide (29% of 63 analysed samples) [46E].

Tumorigenicity

According to IARC, there is strong evidence that the carcinogenicity of ethylene oxide, a direct-acting alkylating agent, operates by a genotoxic mechanism. A dose-related increase in the frequency of ethylene oxide-derived haemoglobin adducts has been detected in exposed humans and rodents, and a dose-related increase in the frequency of ethylene oxide-derived DNA adducts has been demonstrated in exposed rodents. Ethylene oxide is carcinogenic to humans (IARC Group 1) [47S], [*SEDA-36, 341*]. Two new mechanistic studies provided confirmation of the mode of action of ethylene oxide. The first study was conducted in male mice exposed by inhalation for up to 12 weeks and lung DNA samples were analyzed for levels of 3K-ras codon 12 mutations. Ethylene oxide exposure caused nonmonotonic changes in K-ras mutant fractions and the changes were consistent with early amplification of preexisting K-ras mutations, rather than induction through genotoxicity at codon 12 [48E]. The second new mechanistic research measured the ethylene oxide concentrations in blood of exposed rats, mice and humans *in vivo*. There were good agreements between calculated ethylene oxide adduct levels

(based on published adduct levels) and the measured levels of adducts to hemoglobin in rats and humans and to DNA in rats and mice [49E].

TRICLOSAN [SEDA-34, 379, SEDA-36, 342]

A survey in Germany during the period 2006–2009 [random sample ($n=4680$)] shows that triclosan is used in cosmetics with a prevalence of about 1% of all cosmetic products [5M]. A first human biomonitoring study in the US for exposures occurring during pregnancy ($n=181$) found that triclosan was detected in 100% of urine and 51% of cord blood samples. The results suggested that triclosan exposure is ubiquitous in the US population, even in expecting mothers and their unborn children [50c]. Due to safety concerns of antimicrobial soaps containing triclosan or triclocarban, the FDA proposed a plan to require makers of such products to conduct safety studies or be prepared to remove their products from the market [51r]. The timeline of scientific evidence and regulatory actions in the US concerning triclosan were reviewed by Halden [52R].

Tumorigenicity

The evidence about the potential carcinogenicity of triclosan was reviewed by Dinwiddie et al. [53R]. Currently, epidemiological evidence about carcinogenicity of triclosan is completely lacking and some conflicting results from *in vitro* and animal studies are available [53R]. For example, triclosan may act as tumor promoter in mice, e.g., by accelerating hepatocellular carcinoma development initiated by diethylnitrosamine [54E], or cause liver tumors in mice by activation of peroxisome proliferator-activated receptor alpha (PPARα) [55E]. The relevancy of these mechanisms in humans is questionable [53R].

Fertility

An *in vivo* study on triclosan in male rats suggests that triclosan has an accumulation tendency in the epididymis. Rats treated with the highest dose (200 mg/kg) showed a significant decrease in sperm production, abnormal sperm morphology and epididymal histophathology [56E].

Endocrine

Triclosan has been associated with endocrine effects [*SEDA-36, 342*]. The effects were corroborated in a study in rats *in vivo*, which found that triclosan markedly lowered maternal T4 levels in rat dams during gestation and lactation, and 9 days of exposure resulted in a LOAEL of 75 mg/kg bw/day [57E]. A review financed by the personal care industry suggested that only little evidence exists for the risk of endocrine disruptive adverse effects from triclosan exposure through personal care products [58R].

Immunologic

A retrospective analysis (1993–2012) of data from patch test results from Germany, Switzerland and Austria ($n = 113162$) reported a positive reaction to triclosan in 363 tested patients (0.32%) with clinically relevant reactions in 180 of 331 positive cases (54.4%). No time trends or increase in sensitization was detected in this time period despite the increasing use of triclosan [59C]. A case of an adolescent patient was reported with multiple, asymptomatic ulcerated lesions—resembling aphthous ulcerations—located in the oral cavity. Due to a history of utilization of a dentifrice containing triclosan, triclosan-induced contact stomatitis was diagnosed [60A].

Respiratory

The toxicity of triclosan was researched in a 28-day inhalation study in rats. Histopathological changes were found in the nasal septum and larynx at 0.40 mg/L. The no-observed adverse effect concentration was 0.13 mg/L [61E].

HALOGENS

Sodium Hypochlorite [SED-15, 3157; SEDA-28, 262; SEDA-34, 380; SEDA-36, 342]

Teeth

Sodium hypochlorite is used to irrigate root canals in dentistry and can cause many adverse reactions [SEDA-34, 380; SEDA-36, 342]. A literature review concerning the etiology and management of complications during root canal irrigation was published [62R]. A sodium hypochlorite accident occurred in a pediatric patient (1 year, 10-month-old) who was treated for early childhood caries. Symptoms included swelling of the upper lip, moderate periorbital ecchymosis and edema of the right eye causing decreased palpebral fissure height. The swelling and intensity of bruising had intensified on the following day. After 6 weeks, the patient revealed complete resolution of the facial hematoma without any detectable residual discoloration or swelling [63A]. Two similar cases of sodium hypochlorite dental accidents with facial swelling in adolescent patients following root canal therapy were described by Goswami et al. [64A].

Skin

The topical use of sodium hypochlorite for the treatment of infected atopic eczema was reviewed [65R]. The authors warned that neither the safety nor the efficacy of this practice has been proven in clinical trials. Side effects may include dermatitis or exacerbation of asthma.

Urinary Tract

An unusual case of sodium hypochlorite-induced acute kidney injury was described. The 60-year-old male patient inadvertently received an injection of 1.75 mL of sodium hypochlorite, instead of lidocaine, into his right infraorbital tissue during a dental procedure. The immediate symptoms were local facial swelling, hemorrhage into tissue and necrosis along the gum line. Four days after exposure, the patient complained about dark urine and urinalysis showed hematuria with >200 red blood cells per high-powered field and urine microscopy showed granular casts. Follow up after 20 days showed renal recovery from tubular insult [66A].

IODOPHORS [SED-15, 1896; SEDA-31, 411; SEDA-32, 440; SEDA-33, 485; SEDA-34, 380; SEDA-36, 342]

Iodine

ENDOCRINE

A systematic review was conducted about thyroid dysfunction in preterm neonates exposed to topical iodine. The incidence of (transient) hypothyroidism/hyperthyrotropinaemia ranged from 12% to 33% in infants, whereas the incidence in non-exposed infants was 0%. The authors concluded that neonatal exposure to iodine-containing disinfectants causes thyroid dysfunction in infants born <32 weeks. No studies regarding the impact of exposure on neurodevelopment were available. Currently, it would seem prudent practice to restrict the exposure of iodine-containing skin disinfectants in preterm infants [67M]. A case of a 50-year-old female patient with Graves' disease (a common form of hyperthyroidism) was reported. The patient was treated by misunderstanding for an extended period of time (30 days) with iodine solution, generating the so-called Jod-Basedow effect, with exacerbation of thyrotoxicosis and risk of thyroid storm [68A].

Polyvinylpyrrolidone (Povidone) and Povidone-Iodine

Breasts

The FDA concerns on the use of povidone-iodine with breast implants due to potential adverse effect on shell integrity that could lead to implant deflation or rupture were criticized in a letter to the editor [69r]. The author also reported the observation of persistent seroma following irrigation of the pocket with full-strength povidone-iodine (7–10%), while this was not seen with a 50:50 dilution with normal saline [69r].

Musculoskeletal

A chondrotoxic effect on the superficial cartilage layer was detected *in vitro* when povidone-iodine was used for time periods longer than 1 min. Further research was suggested as necessary to confirm this effect in human cartilage tissue [70E].

Sensory Systems

During the treatment of presumed viral conjunctivitis with dexamethasone 0.1%/povidone-iodine 0.4%, 13 participants (22.4%) compared to 1 participant (1.9%) in the control group ($p = 0.001$) reported stinging sensation as adverse effect [71c].

Skin

A 43-year-old male was diagnosed with iododerma following topical povidone-iodine use. The patient was a worker in a dairy farm and had been fumigating the barn air with 10% povidone-iodine for 6 months. The lesions appeared on his arm 3 days after he had used a povidone-iodine-soaked gauze to disinfect abrasions on his arm. The lesions resolved in 10 days when exposure ended and systemic steroid treatment was given [72A].

Immunologic

Two cases of allergic contact dermatitis were described, which occurred 24 hours after the usage of povidone-iodine as pre-operative antiseptic to prepare (scrub) the lower third of the face before surgical removal of third molars [73A].

References

[1] Anon. Antiseptics: sometimes the cause of infection. Prescrire Int. 2014;23(149):129 [r].
[2] Chang CY, Furlong LA. Microbial stowaways in topical antiseptic products. N Engl J Med. 2012;367(23):2170–3 [r].
[3] Lee S, Han SW, Kim G, et al. An outbreak of *Burkholderia cenocepacia* associated with contaminated chlorhexidine solutions prepared in the hospital. Am J Infect Control. 2013;41(9):e93–6 [c].
[4] FDA. FDA Drug Safety Communication: FDA requests label changes and single-use packaging for some over-the-counter topical antiseptic products to decrease risk of infection. US Food and Drug Administration, Silver Spring, MD, USA. 2013; [S]
[5] Uter W, Yazar K, Kratz EM, et al. Coupled exposure to ingredients of cosmetic products: II. Preservatives. Contact Dermatitis. 2014;70(4):219–26 [M].
[6] Roda C, Guihenneuc-Jouyaux C, Momas I. Environmental triggers of nocturnal dry cough in infancy: new insights about chronic domestic exposure to formaldehyde in the PARIS birth cohort. Environ Res. 2013;123:46–51 [C].
[7] Nielsen GD, Larsen ST, Wolkoff P. Recent trend in risk assessment of formaldehyde exposures from indoor air. Arch Toxicol. 2013;87(1):73–98 [R].
[8] Sallapant S, Angsuwatcharakon P, Thiptanakit C, et al. Formalin-induced severe colonic necrosis. Endoscopy. 2013;45(Suppl 2):E363–E364 [A].
[9] IARC Working Group on the Evaluation of Carcinogenic Risks to Humans. Formaldehyde. IARC Monogr Eval Carcinog Risks Hum. 2012;100F:401–35 [S].
[10] Beane Freeman LE, Blair A, Lubin JH, et al. Mortality from solid tumors among workers in formaldehyde industries: an update of the NCI cohort. Am J Ind Med. 2013;56(9):1015–26 [C].
[11] Coggon D, Ntani G, Harris EC, et al. Upper airway cancer, myeloid leukemia, and other cancers in a cohort of British chemical workers exposed to formaldehyde. Am J Epidemiol. 2014;179(11):1301–11 [C].
[12] Romanazzi V, Pirro V, Bellisario V, et al. 15-F$_{2t}$ isoprostane as biomarker of oxidative stress induced by tobacco smoke and occupational exposure to formaldehyde in workers of plastic laminates. Sci Total Environ. 2013;442:20–5 [c].
[13] Lin D, Guo Y, Yi J, et al. Occupational exposure to formaldehyde and genetic damage in the peripheral blood lymphocytes of plywood workers. J Occup Health. 2013;55(4):284–91 [c].
[14] Marcon A, Fracasso ME, Marchetti P, et al. Outdoor formaldehyde and NO$_2$ exposures and markers of genotoxicity in children living near chipboard industries. Environ Health Perspect. 2014;122(6):639–45 [c].
[15] Hosgood HD, Zhang L, Tang X, et al. Occupational exposure to formaldehyde and alterations in lymphocyte subsets. Am J Ind Med. 2013;56(2):252–7 [c].
[16] Bauer A. Contact dermatitis in the cleaning industry. Curr Opin Allergy Clin Immunol. 2013;13(5):521–4 [R].
[17] Tanaka Y, Nakase Y, Yamaguchi M, et al. Allergy to formaldehyde: basophil histamine-release test is useful for diagnosis. Int Arch Allergy Immunol. 2014;164(1):27–9 [A].
[18] Löffler H, Kampf G, Lachenmeier D, et al. Allergic or irritant contact dermatitis after patch testing with alcohol—that is the point. Contact Dermatitis. 2012;67(6):386–7 [r].
[19] Kiracofe E, Zirwas MJ. Formaldehyde in textiles—what dermatologists need to know about the relationship to contact dermatitis: a review of the US Government Accountability Office's Report to Congressional Committees. J Am Acad Dermatol. 2012;67(2):313–4 [r].
[20] Mohamad MZ, Koh KS, Chong VH. Glutaraldehyde-induced colitis: a rare cause of lower gastrointestinal bleeding. Am J Emerg Med. 2014;32(6):685.e1–685.e2 [A].
[21] Ohlsson A, Shah VS, Stade BC. Vaginal chlorhexidine during labour to prevent early-onset neonatal group B streptococcal infection. Cochrane Database Syst Rev. 2014;12(12):CD003520 [M].
[22] Toholka R, Nixon R. Allergic contact dermatitis to chlorhexidine. Australas J Dermatol. 2013;54(4):303–6 [c].
[23] Supapvanich C, Povey AC, de Vocht F. Respiratory and dermal symptoms in Thai nurses using latex products. Occup Med (Lond). 2013;63(6):425–8 [c].
[24] Nakonechna A, Dore P, Dixon T, et al. Immediate hypersensitivity to chlorhexidine is increasingly recognised in the United Kingdom. Allergol Immunopathol (Madr). 2014;42(1):44–9 [A].
[25] Mushtaq U, Tan A, Tan JA, et al. Acute allergic reaction after intravenous saline injection: an unusual presentation of chlorhexidine allergy. Med J Aust. 2014;200(10):599–600 [A].
[26] Dyer JE, Nafie S, Mellon JK, et al. Anaphylactic reaction to intraurethral chlorhexidine: sensitisation following previous repeated uneventful administration. Ann R Coll Surg Engl. 2013;95(6):e105–6 [A].
[27] Solodun YV, Monakhova YB, Kuballa T, et al. Unrecorded alcohol consumption in Russia: toxic denaturants and disinfectants pose additional risks. Interdiscip Toxicol. 2011;4(4):198–205 [A].
[28] Kim KW, Ahn K, Yang HJ, et al. Humidifier disinfectant-associated children's interstitial lung disease. Am J Respir Crit Care Med. 2014;189(1):48–56 [C].

[29] Lee E, Seo JH, Kim HY, et al. Toxic inhalational injury-associated interstitial lung disease in children. J Korean Med Sci. 2013;28(6):915–23 [c].

[30] Yang HJ, Kim HJ, Yu J, et al. Inhalation toxicity of humidifier disinfectants as a risk factor of children's interstitial lung disease in Korea: a case-control study. PLoS One. 2013;8(6):e64430 [c].

[31] Park D, Leem J, Lee K, et al. Exposure characteristics of familial cases of lung injury associated with the use of humidifier disinfectants. Environ Health. 2014;13(1):70 [c].

[32] Lee J-H, Kang H-J, Seol H-S, et al. Refined exposure assessment for three active ingredients of humidifier disinfectants. Environ Eng Res. 2013;18(4):253–7 [E].

[33] Jung H-N, Zerin T, Podder B, et al. Cytotoxicity and gene expression profiling of polyhexamethylene guanidine hydrochloride in human alveolar A549 cells. Toxicol In Vitro. 2014;28(4):684–92 [E].

[34] Song JA, Park H-J, Yang M-J, et al. Polyhexamethyleneguanidine phosphate induces severe lung inflammation, fibrosis, and thymic atrophy. Food Chem Toxicol. 2014;69:267–75 [E].

[35] Wessels S, Ingmer H. Modes of action of three disinfectant active substances: a review. Regul Toxicol Pharmacol. 2013;67(3):456–67 [R].

[36] Leysen J, Goossens A, Lambert J, et al. Polyhexamethylene biguanide is a relevant sensitizer in wet wipes. Contact Dermatitis. 2014;70(5):323–5 [A].

[37] Anwar Z, Wellik SR, Galor A. Glaucoma therapy and ocular surface disease: current literature and recommendations. Curr Opin Ophthalmol. 2013;24(2):136–43 [R].

[38] Inoue K. Managing adverse effects of glaucoma medications. Clin Ophthalmol. 2014;8:903–13 [R].

[39] Rasmussen CA, Kaufman PL, Kiland JA. Benzalkonium chloride and glaucoma. J Ocul Pharmacol Ther. 2014;30(2–3):163–9 [R].

[40] Rossi GC, Pasinetti GM, Scudeller L, et al. Risk factors to develop ocular surface disease in treated glaucoma or ocular hypertension patients. Eur J Ophthalmol. 2013;23(3):296–302 [c].

[41] Fernández Jiménez-Ortiz H, Toledano Fernández N, Fernández Escamez CS, et al. The effects of ocular hypotensive drugs on the cornea: an in vivo analysis with confocal microscopy. Arch Soc Esp Oftalmol. 2013;88(11):423–32 [c].

[42] Boimer C, Birt CM. Preservative exposure and surgical outcomes in glaucoma patients: the PESO study. J Glaucoma. 2013;22(9):730–5 [A].

[43] Kim BY, Riaz KM, Bakhtiari P, et al. Medically reversible limbal stem cell disease: clinical features and management strategies. Ophthalmology. 2014;121(10):2053–8 [A].

[44] Abe RY, Zacchia RS, Santana PR, et al. Effects of benzalkonium chloride on the blood-aqueous and blood-retinal barriers of pseudophakic eyes. J Ocul Pharmacol Ther. 2014;30(5):413–8 [c].

[45] Kato Y, Yagi H, Kaji Y, et al. Benzalkonium chloride accelerates the formation of the amyloid fibrils of corneal dystrophy-associated peptides. J Biol Chem. 2013;288(35):25109–18 [E].

[46] Bononi M, Quaglia G, Tateo F. Identification of ethylene oxide in herbs, spices and other dried vegetables imported into Italy. Food Addit Contam Part A Chem Anal Control Expo Risk Assess. 2014;31(2):271–5 [E].

[47] IARC Working Group on the Evaluation of Carcinogenic Risks to Humans. Ethylene oxide. IARC Monogr Eval Carcinog Risks Hum. 2012;100F:379–400 [S].

[48] Parsons BL, Manjanatha MG, Myers MB, et al. Temporal changes in K-ras mutant fraction in lung tissue of big blue B6C3F$_1$ mice exposed to ethylene oxide. Toxicol Sci. 2013;136(1):26–38 [E].

[49] Filser JG, Kessler W, Artati A, et al. Ethylene oxide in blood of ethylene-exposed B6C3F1 mice, Fischer 344 rats, and humans. Toxicol Sci. 2013;136(2):344–58 [E].

[50] Pycke BFG, Geer LA, Dalloul M, et al. Human fetal exposure to triclosan and triclocarban in an urban population from Brooklyn, New York. Environ Sci Technol. 2014;48(15):8831–8 [c].

[51] Kuehn BM. FDA pushes makers of antimicrobial soap to prove safety and effectiveness. JAMA. 2014;311(3):234 [r].

[52] Halden RU. On the need and speed of regulating triclosan and triclocarban in the United States. Environ Sci Technol. 2014;48(7):3603–11 [R].

[53] Dinwiddie MT, Terry PD, Chen J. Recent evidence regarding triclosan and cancer risk. Int J Environ Res Public Health. 2014;11(2):2209–17 [R].

[54] Yueh MF, Taniguchi K, Chen S, et al. The commonly used antimicrobial additive triclosan is a liver tumor promoter. Proc Natl Acad Sci U S A. 2014;111(48):17200–5 [E].

[55] Wu Y, Wu Q, Beland FA, et al. Differential effects of triclosan on the activation of mouse and human peroxisome proliferator-activated receptor alpha. Toxicol Lett. 2014;231(1):17–28 [E].

[56] Lan Z, Hyung Kim T, Shun Bi K, et al. Triclosan exhibits a tendency to accumulate in the epididymis and shows sperm toxicity in male Sprague-Dawley rats. Environ Toxicol. 2015;30(1):83–91 [E].

[57] Axelstad M, Boberg J, Vinggaard AM, et al. Triclosan exposure reduces thyroxine levels in pregnant and lactating rat dams and in directly exposed offspring. Food Chem Toxicol. 2013;59:534–40 [E].

[58] Witorsch RJ. Critical analysis of endocrine disruptive activity of triclosan and its relevance to human exposure through the use of personal care products. Crit Rev Toxicol. 2014;44(6):535–55 [R].

[59] Buhl T, Fuchs T, Geier J. Contact hypersensitivity to triclosan. Ann Allergy Asthma Immunol. 2014;113(1):119–20 [C].

[60] Lawrence LM, Farquharson A, Brown RS, et al. Oral tissue irritants in toothpaste: a case report. J Clin Pediatr Dent. 2013;38(1):75–8 [A].

[61] Yang YS, Kwon JT, Shim I, et al. Evaluation of toxicity to triclosan in rats following 28 days of exposure to aerosol inhalation. Regul Toxicol Pharmacol. 2015;71(2):259–68 [61E].

[62] Kishor N. Oral tissue complications during endodontic irrigation: literature review. N Y State Dent J. 2013;79(3):37–42 [R].

[63] Klein U, Kleier DJ. Sodium hypochlorite accident in a pediatric patient. Pediatr Dent. 2013;35(7):534–8 [A].

[64] Goswami M, Chhabra N, Kumar G, et al. Sodium hypochlorite dental accidents. Paediatr Int Child Health. 2014;34(1):66–9 [A].

[65] Barnes TM, Greive K. Use of bleach baths for the treatment of infected atopic eczema. Australas J Dermatol. 2013;54(4):251–8 [R].

[66] Peck BW, Workeneh B, Kadikoy H, et al. Sodium hypochlorite-induced acute kidney injury. Saudi J Kidney Dis Transpl. 2014;25(2):381–4 [A].

[67] Aitken J, Williams FLR. A systematic review of thyroid dysfunction in preterm neonates exposed to topical iodine. Arch Dis Child Fetal Neonatal Ed. 2014;99(1):F21–8 [M].

[68] Leustean L, Preda C, Ungureanu MC, et al. Jod-Basedow effect due to prolonged use of lugol solution-case report. Rev Med Chir Soc Med Nat Iasi. 2014;118(4):1013–7 [A].

[69] Wiener TC. Betadine and breast implants: an update. Aesthet Surg J. 2013;33(4):615–7 [r].

[70] von Keudell A, Canseco J, Gomoll AH. Deleterious effects of diluted povidone-iodine on articular cartilage. J Arthroplasty. 2013;28(6):918–21 [E].

[71] Pinto RDP, Lira RPC, Abe RY, et al. Dexamethasone/povidone eye drops versus artificial tears for treatment of presumed viral conjunctivitis: a randomized clinical trial. Curr Eye Res. In press. [c]. http://dx.doi.org/10.3109/02713683.2014.964419.

[72] Aliagaoglu C, Turan H, Uslu E, et al. Iododerma following topical povidone-iodine application. Cutan Ocul Toxicol. 2013;32(4):339–40 [A].

[73] Reyazulla MA, Gopinath AL, Vaibhav N, et al. An unusual complication of late onset allergic contact dermatitis to povidone iodine in oral & maxillofacial surgery—a report of 2 cases. Eur Ann Allergy Clin Immunol. 2014;46(4):157–9 [A].

CHAPTER

25

Beta-Lactams and Tetracyclines

Michelle M. Peahota*[,1], Lucia Rose[†], Jason C. Gallagher[‡]

*Infectious Diseases, Thomas Jefferson University Hospital, Philadelphia, PA, USA
[†]Infectious Diseases, Cooper University Hospital, One Cooper Plaza, Camden, NJ, USA
[‡]Temple University, Philadelphia, PA, USA
[1]Corresponding author: michelle.peahota@jefferson.edu

CARBAPENEMS

Ertapenem

Organs and Systems

NERVOUS SYSTEM

Acute prolonged neurotoxicity associated with dose-adjusted ertapenem in patients with advanced renal failure has not been previously reported. A 78-year-old female with Stage 5 chronic kidney disease (CKD) developed incoherent speech, hyperexcitability, and progressive cognitive impairment after the fourth dose of ertapenem 500 mg once daily for cholecystitis. A 70-year-old female with Stage 5 CKD developed hallucinations, incoherent speech, and cognitive impairment after the fifth dose of ertapenem 500 mg once daily for an arteriovenous fistula. Despite discontinuation of ertapenem and emergent high-flux hemodialysis in both patients, their neurologic symptoms persisted for 14 days. It is important to note that both patients received the recommended dose of ertapenem for their renal function. Clinicians should be aware of ertapenem-induced neurotoxicity in patients with advanced renal failure [1c].

SKIN

A 47-year-old man received ertapenem for erysipelas of the right foot and lower leg. He was initially started on clindamycin because he reported a history of allergies to penicillin and cephalosporins. Clindamycin was changed to ertapenem when his infection did not improve. He developed fever and a generalized nonfollicular pustular rash on day 2 of ertapenem therapy. A skin biopsy, which showed intraepidermal and subcorneal spongiform pustules with papillary edema, supported a diagnosis of acute generalized exanthematous pustulosis (AGEP).

Ertapenem was discontinued and he was started on linezolid which resulted in cure of his cellulitis. He underwent allergy testing and was subsequently found to be skin patch test positive to penicillin, cephalothin, meropenem, and ertapenem (his patch test to clindamycin was negative). The patient recalled that his reaction to penicillin and cephalexin was manifested as similar characteristics, including fever and pustulosis. The authors propose that this case demonstrates AGEP to multiple beta-lactam antibiotics and further study into the rates of cross-reactivity of beta-lactams in AGEP is warranted [2c].

Meropenem

General Adverse Drug Reactions

A retrospective cohort study of 5566 infants (<120 days old) sought to evaluate the incidence of adverse effects in hospitalized infants who received either meropenem or imipenem/cilastatin. Adverse effects were more common with meropenem compared to imipenem/cilastatin (62.8/1000 infant days versus 40.7/1000 infant days; $p < 0.001$). Laboratory abnormalities also were more common in the infants exposed to meropenem, with the most common adverse effect being hyperbilirubinemia. There was no difference in seizures between the two groups; however, the incidence of death, as well as the combined outcome of death or seizure was lower with meropenem use compared with imipenem/cilastatin use. The authors acknowledge the retrospective nature of this study was a limitation. The authors support the use of meropenem over imipenem/cilastatin in infants <120 days old; however, this may come at the expense of more frequent lab abnormalities [3C].

Side Effects of Drugs Annual, Volume 37
ISSN: 0378-6080
http://dx.doi.org/10.1016/bs.seda.2015.07.003

© 2015 Elsevier B.V. All rights reserved.

Interactions

DRUG–DRUG INTERACTIONS

A 14-year-old girl with well-controlled generalized juvenile absence epilepsy received meropenem for a pulmonary infection. On admission, her home valproate dose was continued and a serum valproate concentration was 44.7 µg/mL. Two days later, the patient experienced eye fluttering and brief episodes of unresponsiveness. Her serum valproate trough and peak concentrations dropped to 4.9 and 13.8 µg/mL, respectively. Meropenem was discontinued due to potential contribution to the decrease in valproate levels, resulting in seizures. The authors commented that meropenem is associated with a clinically significant decrease in serum valproate concentrations and alternative antimicrobials should be considered in the setting of valproate therapy [4c].

CEPHALOSPORINS

General Information

An open, prospective randomized, parallel group comparative study was conducted evaluating the efficacy and safety of cefotaxime/sulbactam versus cefepime/tazobactam in patients with urinary tract infections. A total of 60 patients were included in the study. Injection site reactions, diarrhea, and headache were similar and uncommon among both groups. Both agents seemed to be well tolerated and safe since no withdrawals of therapy occurred due to side effects [6c].

Cefazolin

Organs and Systems

DRUG ADMINISTRATION

Elevated plasma albumin can affect free drug concentrations, particularly those that are highly protein bound. Cefazolin is approximately 80% protein bound and its antimicrobial efficacy is reliant on the concentration of unbound drug. Less is known about the effect that varying degrees of plasma albumin in different populations can have on cefazolin concentrations. A pooled analysis of four studies including 237 patients was conducted. This study evaluated cefazolin plasma protein binding and found that unbound cefazolin concentrations varied significantly between neonates, pregnant women, and non-pregnant adults. Pregnant women and neonates had higher median unbound cefazolin fractions (unbound cefazolin concentrations/total cefazolin concentrations). Although this was attributed partly to plasma albumin concentration (which also varied greatly), other patient specific factors also likely played a role. While this study was unable to provide recommendations on dosage

modifications based on the pooled data, obtaining a patient's albumin may be useful to predict a patient's estimated unbound cefazolin concentration [5r].

Cefepime

Organs and Systems

GASTROINTESTINAL

The use of any antibiotic has a risk of leading to *Clostridium difficile-associated diarrhea* (CDAD) although certain agents have been more commonly reported. Although the factors causing CDAD are rather complicated and beyond the scope of this review, stratifying antibiotics in terms of risk for CDAD can be useful, particularly if equally effective alternatives with less CDAD risk exist. A retrospective single center study done by Muldoon et al. found when the institution switched their empiric treatment of choice for febrile neutropenia from meropenem to cefepime, CDAD rates increased. Although the testing method also changed, the remainder of the institution did not face the same CDAD rate increase as the hematology/oncology ward. This study highlights previous reports, which show that cephalosporins likely have a higher association to causing CDAD compared to carbapenems [7A].

Nervous System

Cefepime-induced neurotoxicity has been previously reported, particularly in patients with renal dysfunction who may inadvertently be at risk of overdose due to lack of dosage adjustment. Reports range from delirium and encephalopathy to status epilepticus [40c, 41A, 42c]. Reversal methods of neurologic toxicities reported in the literature are inconsistent with a lag time in recovery. Although most cases illustrate withdrawal of cefepime and supportive care as primary methods of reversal, some data exists on the benefits of intermittent hemodialysis. Mani and colleagues describe a case of severe, life threatening, highly probable cefepime-induced neurologic symptoms in an 88-year-old female started on cefepime 2 g IV every 12 hours. Two sessions of hemodialysis were completed early in the patient's course and recovery was achieved within 48 hours, decreasing the time to recovery. In certain patients with life-threatening cephalosporin-induced neurotoxicity, early initiation of hemodialysis may be beneficial [8c].

Cefozopran

Organs and Systems

SKIN

Cephalosporins have been well documented as potential causes of severe skin reactions. Cefozopran, a fourth generation cephalosporin, was reported to cause toxic epidermal necrolysis (TEN) in a 71-year-old woman with a history of psoriasis diagnosed with pyelonephritis and septicemia. While this agent has been reported to cause cutaneous adverse effects, this is the first case of reported TEN. To note, this patient had been treated with UV-B light for psoriasis for 10 years. The reaction occurred 7 days after administration of cefozopran, which included fever and widespread skin eruption of over 70% of her body surface. This resulted in death of the patient. The authors concluded that although the mechanism for TEN is complicated and not well defined, it is likely immunologic. This patient's history of psoriasis may have partly attributed via Th17 cells, which have been reported both in TEN and in the pathogenesis of psoriasis [9c].

Ceftaroline

Organs and Systems

GASTROINTESTINAL

A review of ceftaroline clinical trials stated that the most commonly reported side effect was diarrhea (4–5%), although not significantly higher than the comparator group [10R].

HEMATOLOGIC

Agranulocytosis and neutropenia are known, uncommon class-wide adverse effects of cephalosporins. In clinical trials, ceftaroline was well tolerated and hematologic toxicities were not noted. A 90-year-old female received ceftaroline 600 mg IV every 12 hours for complicated methicillin-resistant *Staphylococcus aureus* (MRSA) infections pneumonia and bacteremia. She clinically improved and was discharged back to her nursing home. Twenty-five days after starting therapy, she developed severe neutropenia with an absolute neutrophil count (ANC) of 0/μL. Upon discontinuation of the agent, her ANC increased to 100/μL 5 days later, and normalized in an additional 3 days up to 2400/μL. Based on timing of the ceftaroline in relation to the neutropenia, the authors concluded that it was the most likely cause [11c].

In a case series of patients who received ceftaroline for MRSA, 7 of 12 patients discontinued ceftaroline due to hematologic toxicities. Three discontinued due to anemia, two due to neutropenia, and two due to neutropenia in combination with either anemia or thrombocytopenia. The neutropenia was classified as severe or very severe in three of the four patients that developed this toxicity. Hematologic toxicities resolved in these patients after an average of 7 days after discontinuation. Although these effects are rare, it can be potentially fatal, therefore a complete blood count (CBC) with differential should be performed periodically while completing therapy [12c].

LUNG

A 46-year-old male was started on ceftaroline 600 mg IV every 8 hours for an MRSA post-operative spinal infection and bacteremia. On the fifth week of therapy (day 39), he developed symptoms of respiratory compromise including a dry cough and chest imaging revealed diffuse bilateral infiltrates. A bronchoalveolar lavage (BAL) was performed, which showed eosinophilic predominance in the fluid. Eosinophilia was also found on laboratory analysis. Ceftaroline was discontinued and corticosteroids were initiated. The patient improved over the next week and his eosinophilia resolved [13c].

A 65-year-old female with a penicillin allergy was started on ceftaroline 600 mg IV every 12 hours for MRSA pneumonia. The patient developed respiratory failure on day 5 of therapy along with eosinophilia (40%). Chest imaging revealed bilateral infiltrates and BAL analysis revealed 13% eosinophils. Based on these findings and exclusion of other causative factors, eosinophilic pneumonia was diagnosed. Ceftaroline was discontinued and corticosteroids were initiated. The patient' eosinophilia normalized and her respiratory status improved. Although penicillin and later generation cephalosporins such as ceftaroline have a 1–2% cross-reaction rate, it can still occur. Eosinophilic pneumonia is known to have an allergic component and given the patient's history, this may have been the likely cause [14c]. Although eosinophilia is listed as a rare adverse effect of ceftaroline by the manufacturer, the agent is still relatively new. Patients on ceftaroline should be closely monitored for respiratory compromise and a work up for eosinophilic pneumonia may be prudent if clinically indicated.

RENAL

A 52-year-old male developed acute interstitial nephritis (AIN) associated with ceftaroline usage. The patient was started on a prolonged course due to MRSA pneumonia with bacteremia. He was re-admitted to the hospital approximately 3 weeks after completion of therapy and found have AIN as evidenced by renal biopsy. To note, he also had a rise in creatinine and urine eosinophils. Shortly after discontinuation, his renal function improved [15c].

SKIN

In the case series described previously, ceftaroline discontinuation occurred in 2 of the 12 patients due to severe rash, which was likely unattributed to other causes. As with any beta-lactam, allergy (including rash) is a potential risk [12c].

Ceftriaxone

Organs and Systems

DRUG ADMINISTRATION

A meta-analysis was performed to compare the efficacy and safety of ertapenem with ceftriaxone for complicated infections. Studies that incorporated ceftriaxone combination therapy were included. Overall safety and tolerability was similar in both groups. A subgroup analysis comparing ceftriaxone with metronidazole to ceftriaxone monotherapy showed higher rates of local reactions (pain, erythema, tenderness) in the ceftriaxone plus metronidazole group. This difference was not observed in the ceftriaxone monotherapy group, indicating that the causative agent may have been metronidazole [16M].

DRUG INTERACTIONS

A 7-year-old male diagnosed with refractory stage 4 neuroblastoma developed fulminant hepatic toxicity after receiving ceftriaxone, fenretinide, and acetaminophen within the same day. He was started on ceftriaxone and acetaminophen for a fever that he developed on day 4 of admission. Within 3 days, the patient decompensated and found to be in severe hepatic failure, followed by death. The patient had no laboratory abnormalities associated with live failure prior to the start of these agents. Liver toxicity from fenretinide alone is uncommon. The mechanism of the interaction was proposed to be biliary sludging from ceftriaxone leading to impaired elimination of fenretinide and acetaminophen. The authors recommend against using this specific combination together; alternatives include using ibuprofen for fever and a different antibiotic within 24–48 hours of fenretinide administration [17c].

GASTROINTESTINAL

A 47-year-old woman was started on ceftriaxone 2 g IV daily for colonic diverticulitis. A repeat CT scan was completed 8 days into hospitalization to evaluate improvement of underlying disease. While improvement of diverticulitis was shown, stones and sludge in the gallbladder were present which were not previously seen prior to ceftriaxone. Six days after stopping ceftriaxone, the stones and sludge were resolved. The treating physicians diagnosed her with pseudocholethiasis secondary to ceftriaxone therapy. While this toxicity is known in neonates and children, it is thought to be rare in adults [18c].

HEMATOLOGIC

A 60-year-old female developed immune hemolytic anemia after 24 hours of receiving ceftriaxone 1 g IV every 12 hours. Her hemoglobin worsened from 9.6 g/dL on day 1 of admission to 7.5 g/dL on day 2 and 5.5 g/dL on day 3. Bilirubin increased from 0.4 mg/dL on day 1 to 2 mg/dL on day 3. The patient required a blood transfusion. Although difficult to undoubtedly conclude that ceftriaxone was the cause, the patient's hemoglobin improved after discontinuation of the agent and blood transfusion administration [19c].

HYPERSENSITIVITY

A 7-year-old boy received ceftriaxone for a respiratory infection. Soon after an outpatient injection, he developed a fever, maculopapular rash, eye congestion, and tachypnea. Measles was in the differential but ruled out and ceftriaxone was then continued. The rash worsened and he developed pruritus. He was started on corticosteroids and antibiotics were modified to azithromycin. Prior to receiving ceftriaxone, the patient did not react to a test dose or a skin test and did not have eosinophilia during therapy. However, reactions can be delayed and therefore, a test dose may not show an immediate reaction. Likewise, skin testing is not highly sensitive. Patients should always be closely monitored for reactions while on any antimicrobials [20c].

NEUROLOGIC

Neurologic toxicities such as encephalopathies have been more commonly reported in patients with underlying renal dysfunction. A 37-year-old female with a history of end stage renal disease (ESRD) on peritoneal dialysis received ceftriaxone 2 g IV daily for peritonitis. Her clinical status improved over the following 3 days. However, after 3 days of therapy, she developed signs of encephalopathy including agitation, paranoia, and visual hallucinations. Other medication-related causes and underlying diseases were ruled out as potential causes. Upon withdrawal of ceftriaxone and transition to ciprofloxacin, her mental status returned to baseline. The neurologic effects secondary to cephalosporins have been associated with gamma-aminobutyric acid (GABA) inhibition. Patients with ESRD are at increased risk for drug accumulation and dose-related adverse effects such as neurologic toxicity [21c].

Hoigé syndrome, an acute psychosensorial toxicity mainly associated with procaine penicillin administration, occurred in a 59-year-old male subsequently following a ceftriaxone 2 g intravenous injection. Within seconds after the injection, the patient developed major anxiety, nausea, headache, and chest tightness. While the pathogenesis of this syndrome is unknown, its clinical manifestations are seen within seconds to minutes after drug administration. To note, it is not considered an allergic reaction and therefore, if a patient develops Hoigé syndrome, it does not prohibit continuation of the agent [22c].

RENAL

A prospective, single-center study evaluating the difference in rates of urinary calcium excretion between ceftriaxone, cephalothin, and ampicillin in adult patients with or without stones was conducted. Urinary calcium excretion can lead to urolithiasis which includes nephrolithiasis. In this study, 180 patients with urinary tract infections were included, half with stones and half without stones. The groups were then equally divided to receive one of three drugs for 5 days, all given a 1 g IV infusion every 12 hours. The authors found statistically significant increases in calcium excretion after therapy for groups receiving either ceftriaxone or cephalothin. The calcium/creatinine ratio, collected via a 24-hour urine specimen, in the cephalosporin groups were also significantly increased after therapy. These effects were not seen in the ampicillin group. Hydration is critical in patients on cephalosporins who are at risk or have a history of urolithiasis and/or receiving high doses [23C]. This rare side effect has been previously reported as a class effect [24c].

Cefuroxime

Organs and Systems

SENSORY SYSTEMS

There have been multiple reports of intracameral cefuroxime causing severe ocular adverse effects. This agent is often chosen for prophylaxis of endophthalmitis in patients undergoing cataract surgery. Due to limited options, intracameral cefuroxime has been widely used as a first line agent for prophylaxis. However, it has a relatively narrow spectrum and may not cover the most concerning pathogens (i.e. *Pseudomonas aeruginosa*, *Staphylococcus aureus*). Two case reports have described anaphylaxis following administration and there has been a case series describing retinal hemorrhage. Since the necessity of endophthalmitis prophylaxis is also controversial, ophthalmologists should weight the risk versus benefit prior to administering cefuroxime. Data on alternative options is warranted [25r].

A case series described four patients who received intracameral cefuroxime at doses higher than recommended which resulted in elevated intravitreal concentrations and ultimately structural damage to the eye. The first patient received 70 mg (1 mg/0.1 × 7 mL) of cefuroxime developed retinal hemorrhage in central and inferior regions as well as optic atrophy. The second case received 60 mg (1 mg/0.1 × 6 mL) developed retinal hemorrhage in the peripapillary and macular regions as well as optic atrophy. The third case received 50 mg (1 mg/0.1 × 5 mL) also developed retinal hemorrhage in the peripapillary and inferior retinal regions as well as macular pucker. The fourth patient received

60 mg (1 mg/0.1 × 6 mL) developed retinal hemorrhage in the peripapillary, macular, and inferior regions. The authors recommend complying with current dosing recommendations when administering cefuroxime intracamerally [26c].

A 64-year-old female with a history of a non-anaphylactic penicillin allergy underwent cataract surgery with no complications. Following surgery, she received an injection of cefuroxime 1 mg/0.1 mL into the anterior chamber. Five minutes following the injection, the patient noticed redness and pruritus on her arms. She quickly developed tongue swelling, became hypotensive, and had difficulty breathing. She was treated with corticosteroids and oxygen was administered prior to admitting her to the hospital. Resolution of symptoms occurred within hours and returned home with no sequelae. Although the amount of drug administered was small and local, it was sufficient to produce an anaphylactic reaction. Ophthalmologists performing these surgeries should be cautious of patients with penicillin allergies and use alternatives such as moxifloxacin in those cases [27c].

A case series described six patients who received intracameral cefuroxime following cataract surgery. All six patients developed macular edema thought to be secondary to cefuroxime overdose. A component of this reaction may be retinal tolerance and therefore difficult to predict. However, it is thought to be a dose dependent toxicity and while the concentration is standard (1 mg/0.1 mL), the number of dilutions administered seems variable. The authors describe a recently approved cefuroxime preparation (Aprokam®) for this indication that is intended to assist in standardization and overdose prevention [28A].

DEATH

A 64-year-old male developed a probable disulfiram reaction secondary to cefuroxime, which was prescribed for a respiratory infection. During the infusion on the third day of therapy, the patient developed facial flushing, sweating, and weakness, dyspnea and hypotension. This was followed by dyspnea, loss of consciousness and death. To note, he had consumed alcohol prior to coming to clinic for his infusion and on autopsy analysis, ethanol level was 2110 mg/L and acetaldehyde was 60 mg/L. These levels, particularly acetaldehyde, are well above the expected level even after alcohol consumption which is why cefuroxime may have contributed to an inhibition of ethanol metabolism. The authors felt that there was a temporal relationship between cefuroxime/alcohol and death. It should be noted that this patient had severe coronary artery disease, cardiomegaly, and other comorbidities, which also may have attributed to his sudden death [29A].

Cephalexin

Organs and Systems

IMMUNOLOGIC

Cephalexin and a few other cephalosporins have been infrequently associated with drug-induced liver injury (DILI), specifically elevated transaminases. However, cholestatic jaundice has been rarely reported among this class of antimicrobials. A 57-year-old male who was prescribed cephalexin for a neck abscess developed a rash and pruritus 6 days after initiating cephalexin. He was later found to have elevated transaminases and total bilirubin and diagnosed with cholestatic jaundice. The patient improved after discontinuation of cephalexin. This reaction was thought to be due to an immunologic hypersensitivity response rather than a direct effect, consistent with prior case reports. Although rare, this is a potentially serious side effect that has been reported previously [30c].

MONOBACTAMS

Aztreonam

Organs and Systems

HYPERSENSITIVITY

Two randomized, double-blind, placebo-controlled phase 3 trials evaluating the efficacy and safety of inhaled aztreonam in patients with non-cystic fibrosis bronchiectasis were conducted. The difference between the two studies was the mean change from baseline quality of life-bronchiectasis respiratory symptoms. Adverse effects in both studies were more common in the aztreonam groups, which also led to higher discontinuation rates. The most common adverse events included dyspnea, cough, and increased sputum production. In these two particular studies, clinical benefit was not observed and therefore, the risk of adverse events does not warrant its use in this patient population for this indication [31R].

A meta-analysis aimed to evaluate the safety and efficacy of inhaled antibiotics in patients with stable non-cystic fibrosis bronchiectasis was conducted. Eight randomized trials on 590 patients, who had received six different inhaled antibiotics, were included in the analysis. The evaluation did not compare individual agents and thus aztreonam specific data was not published. Nonetheless, overall data showed that bronchospasm rates were higher in the inhaled antibiotic groups (10%) compared to placebo (2.3%). Cough, hemoptysis, death as well as withdrawal due to adverse effects were similar between both groups [32M].

In an observational study conducted by Roehmel and colleagues, hypersensitivity to various antibiotics in patients with cystic fibrosis was assessed. Out of the one hundred patients included in the study, 60% had at least one hypersensitivity reaction to antibiotics. Of the 3205 antibiotic courses evaluated, aztreonam had one of the highest risks for anaphylactic reactions ($\sim$6% of all treatment courses). Piperacillin/tazobactam and aztreonam were found to have similar risk for any reaction. To note, all patients who developed a hypersensitivity reaction to aztreonam, previously received ceftazidime. Caution should be taken in starting aztreonam in patients who develop hypersensitivity reactions to ceftazidime [33c].

PENICILLINS

Amoxicillin

Organs and Systems

CARDIOLOGY

An 18-year-old female presented to an emergency room with nausea, vomiting, and shortness of breath and died 3 days after admission. Three weeks prior to her arrival, she had received amoxicillin for a traumatic finger wound and developed facial rash with edema and generalized pruritus on day 5 of treatment. Autopsy findings were notable for clear fluid present in the pleural cavities, pericardium, and peritoneum. In addition, her myocardium was edematous and exhibited a mottled appearance with white patches. Histological exam revealed extensive myocardial necrosis with severe infiltration by lymphocytes, eosinophils and giant cells. The authors speculate this likely represents a case of hypersensitivity myocarditis with giant cell transformation [34c].

Kounis syndrome is a type of vasospastic myocardial ischemia or infarction that is being increasingly reported as an adverse effect of beta-lactams. A 16-year-old male, diagnosed with myocarditis after suffering chest pain, presented for a follow-up evaluation 3 weeks after his initial diagnosis. His physical exam was normal, but an ECG showed T wave inversions and ST elevations supporting inferolateral ischemia. He revealed at the follow-up visit that he took amoxicillin/clavulanic acid for sore throat just before his chest pain. The authors hypothesized that the chest pain and ST segment changes possibly corresponded to coronary spasm, and the patient was diagnosed with Kounis syndrome. The authors recommend that Kounis syndrome be considered in patients with coronary spasms in order to prevent subsequent acute coronary syndromes [35A].

A 52-year-old female with a history of smoking, hypertension, and hyperlipidemia experienced ventricular fibrillation after taking a single dose of 875 mg of amoxicillin/clavulanic associated with a dental operation. She was admitted to a cardiac intensive care unit and work-up revealed an unremarkable physical exam, no ECG abnormalities, and normal echocardiography. Additionally, a coronary angiography found only mild atherosclerosis. She was monitored closely during her hospital stay and no arrhythmias were detected. The authors acknowledge that Kounis syndrome may be a possible cause; however, it is usually associated with coronary artery disease, which was not present in this case. The authors propose that this woman experienced an anaphylactic reaction causing hemodynamic instability, resulting in ventricular tachycardia [36c].

BILIARY TRACT

Amoxicillin/clavulanate has been described to cause drug-induced hepatitis [37A, 38A]. A 63-year-old male developed hyperbilirubinemia after being admitted to a hospital for jaundice, choluria, pruritus, and nausea. His imaging work-up consisted of an abdominal ultrasound that demonstrated only cholesterolosis of the biliary vesicles and constricted biliary vessels on nuclear magnetic resonance. Both his infectious and autoimmune evaluations were negative. The patient was discovered to have taken amoxicillin/clavulanate 500 mg three times a day for 21 days approximately 45 days prior to presentation for acute otitis. The authors believed he had developed drug-induced cholestatic hepatitis, which was confirmed by a liver biopsy [39c].

SKIN

Two episodes of burning bullous desquamative eruptions of the palms and soles 24 hours after initiation of amoxicillin and rifamycin were reported by a 12-year-old female. She also reported a mild eruption after 48 hours of treatment with cefpodoxime, which resolved spontaneously. An allergic work up, consisting of prick, intradermal, and patch tests, was performed 8 months after the reaction to amoxicillin. The skin tests provided negative responses to beta-lactams. A challenge test with increasing doses of oral amoxicillin and rifamycin resulted in relapses of the palm and sole eruptions. Notably, she tolerated challenges of penicillin V and cefpodoxime. The child was diagnosed with non-pigmenting fixed drug eruption to amoxicillin and rifamycins [40c].

IMMUNOLOGIC

There was a case of toxic epidermal necrolysis (TEN) associated with a pneumothorax, pneumomediastinum, and subcutaneous emphysema following receipt of amoxicillin for the treatment of suspected pharyngitis. Three days after receiving amoxicillin, a 10-year-old male presented with diffuse erythematous macules with purpuric centers, hemorrhagic erosions, and blisters scattered on his trunk, back, and extremities. Bullae and erosions with sloughing were present on his face and his oropharynx had erythema of the buccal mucosa and several small erosions. Chest imaging showed pneumothorax, pneumomediastinum, and subcutaneous emphysema which required chest tube placement and intubation. Amoxicillin was discontinued immediately. After 3 weeks, the air leak syndrome resolved and his chest tube was removed. The patient was discharged home after a 1-month hospital stay and he has ongoing gastrointestinal (elevated transaminases) and ophthalmology (punctate keratitis) sequelae [41c].

Penicillin

Organs and Systems

SENSORY SYSTEMS

Antibiotic therapies, mostly aminoglycosides, have been associated with bilateral vestibulopathy (BV), a peripheral failure of the vestibule-ocular reflex that causes gait disturbances with oscillopsia. A 71-year-old female developed severe gait unsteadiness with oscillopsia 2 weeks after receiving a 10-day course of amoxicillin/clavulanic acid 875/125 mg twice daily. In addition, she took aspirin 100 mg daily for at least 4 years as part of her medication regimen. A 68-year-old male had a 5-year history of gait unsteadiness with oscillopsia and dizziness. Prior to the start of his symptoms, he received flucloxacillin 1 g twice daily for 10 days for a urologic surgery infection. In addition, he took etoricoxib for several days postoperatively for pain. Both patients showed BV during or immediately following receipt of a penicillin antibiotic and a non-steroidal anti-inflammatory drug (NSAID). Although penicillin alone is not associated with BV, the authors conclude that its use, in combination with a NSAID, may cause BV. The authors also believe that a prospective study investigating the prevalence of BV with this drug combination is warranted [42c].

HEMATOLOGIC

A 62-year-old man received high-dose floxacillin (12 g daily) for methicillin-susceptible *Staphylococcus aureus* endocarditis. His medication regimen included amiodarone and aspirin. He developed bleeding (severe epistaxis and bleeding from the bronchial tree and sternotomy) which required blood product transfusions and inotropic support. Platelet function tests indicated severe platelet dysfunction. Both floxacillin and amiodarone were immediately discontinued due to association concerns with platelet dysfunction, and daptomycin was initiated. Amiodarone was restarted 10 days later due to the development of recurrent arrhythmias. Subsequent platelet function tests were normal and bleeding did not recur while the patient received daptomycin, amiodarone, and aspirin. Although inhibition of platelet aggregation by amiodarone cannot be excluded, the authors propose the severe bleeding and platelet dysfunction was caused by high-dose floxacillin [43A]. In another case, a 42-year-old man was prescribed piperacillin/tazobactam 4/0.5 g every 8 hours for a postoperative intracranial infection. At the time of antibiotic initiation, his peripheral blood showed a white blood cell (WBC) count of $12.3 \times 10^9/L$, neutrophils of $8.8 \times 10^9/L$, platelets of $223 \times 10^9/L$, and hemoglobin of $133 \times 10^9/L$, aspartate aminotransferase (AST) of 12 IU/L and alanine aminotransferase (ALT) of 20 IU/L. Throughout his piperacillin/tazobactam course, his WBC, neutrophil, and platelet counts decreased, he expressed fevers, and developed a rash on his chest and back. On day 17 of therapy, he complained of a sharp pain in his upper thorax and neck during piperacillin/tazobactam infusion. Laboratory data revealed severe bone barrow suppression (WBC $1 \times 10^9/L$, neutrophils $0.21 \times 10^9/L$, platelets $34 \times 10^9/L$, and hemoglobin $134 \times 10^9/L$) and hepatic dysfunction (ALT 450 IU/L and AST 594 IU/L). Piperacillin/tazobactam was discontinued as it was suspected to be the likely cause of the agranulocytosis, thrombocytopenia, hepatic dysfunction and rash. The patient's antimicrobial therapy was changed to ceftazidime and amikacin; the patient's blood counts and hepatic function tests returned to baseline [44A].

URINARY TRACT

The combination of piperacillin/tazobactam and vancomycin has been described in adults to be associated with an increased incidence of acute kidney injury (AKI) [45c, 46c]. However, this has not previously been shown to be a concern in children. A 15-year-old female with alveolar rhabdomyosarcoma experienced elevated serum creatinine to 1.61 mg/dL (baseline 0.74 mg/dL) 3 days after receiving piperacillin/tazobactam, metronidazole, and vancomycin for neutropenic fever. Her serum creatinine continued to increase despite vancomycin discontinuation. Piperacillin/tazobactam was discontinued and her serum creatinine returned to baseline 13 days later. A 17-year-old male with B-cell lymphoma, initially started on vancomycin and ceftazidime, developed an increase in serum creatinine to 1.61 mg/dL (baseline 1.25 mg/dL) 2 days after his antibiotics were changed to piperacillin/tazobactam monotherapy for neutropenic fever. His piperacillin/tazobactam was discontinued and his creatinine returned to baseline on day 11. A 16-year-old male with acute myeloid leukemia developed an increase in serum creatinine from 0.93 to 3.79 mg/dL after he received piperacillin/tazobactam, vancomycin, and voriconazole. Vancomycin was held due to an elevated trough of 23 mg/L, but was restarted and continued for an additional 11 days for coagulase-negative staphylococcal bacteremia. Piperacillin/tazobactam was discontinued on day 4. His serum creatinine peaked at 11.78 mg/dL on day 11 and required

hemodialysis. A renal biopsy on day 26 showed marked inflammatory infiltrate and tubular damage consistent with interstitial nephritis. A 14-year-old male with neuroblastoma developed AKI with acute interstitial injury after 5 days of piperacillin/tazobactam for fever. He also received 48 hours of empiric vancomycin within this time frame for worsening fever. His serum creatinine returned to baseline 23 days after discontinuing piperacillin/tazobactam. The authors acknowledge that pediatric oncology patients may be at higher risk for AKI given the risk for dehydration, sepsis, and exposure to nephrotoxic agents, such as chemotherapy. They acknowledge a temporal relationship between piperacillin/tazobactam and AKI and note that all patients received vancomycin near the time of piperacillin/tazobactam therapy. The authors recommend that clinicians should be aware of the nephrotoxic potential of piperacillin/tazobactam, especially when used with vancomycin, in the management of children with neutropenic fever [47A].

A 63-year-old female developed frequent urination, dysuria, hematuria and pyuria on day 24 of penicillin G 400 million units every 4 hours for *Streptococcus agalactiae* septic arthritis. Her urine cultures were negative, had an elevated CRP at 3.57 mg/dL, and peripheral blood eosinophils at 18%. She was diagnosed with hemorrhagic cystitis: her symptoms and laboratory results normalized within 8 days after discontinuing penicillin. The authors performed a literature search of all studies written in English which described penicillin-induced hemorrhagic cystitis and found three previously reported cases. In all three reports, peripheral eosinophilia was noted and symptoms resolved after discontinuing penicillin. Clinicians should be aware of hemorrhagic cystitis as an adverse reaction to penicillin [48r].

SKIN

A 44-year-old man developed a rash on his thighs 1 day after piperacillin/tazobactam therapy for post-cholangiopancreatography induced pancreatitis. Dermatological evaluation revealed annular erythematous lesions with dozens of tiny non-follicular pustules on his upper thighs. A biopsy, revealing a thickened epidermis and a highly edematous upper dermis with scattered lymphocytes, neutrophils, and eosinophils, was consistent with acute generalized exanthematous pustulosis [49A].

TETRACYCLINES AND GLYCYLCYCLINES

Doxycycline

Organs and Systems

NERVOUS SYSTEM

A 6-week-old female infant with respiratory distress from macrocystic lymphatic malformations (LM) developed silent aspirations and Horner's syndrome following doxycycline sclerotherapy. She received three treatments of doxycycline 80 mg (at a concentration of 10 mg/mL) via an indwelling pigtail catheter for 3 days. Her airway symptoms resolved on day 1 after treatment and she was extubated. One week following treatment, she displayed right-sided ptosis and miosis and was diagnosed with Horner's syndrome. A video fluoroscopic swallow study (VFSS) additionally revealed silent aspiration. A VFSS confirmed improvement in swallow function at 1 month and a 1-year follow-up appointment revealed only mild ptosis. The authors believe her silent aspirations and Horner's syndrome developed secondary to doxycycline sclerotherapy since these were not present prior to treatment. Although neuropathies following doxycycline sclerotherapy have previously been described, this has been the first documentation of aspiration attributed to therapy [50A].

PSYCHIATRIC

A case series described three cases of young patients with no previous history of mental illness that developed suicidality after treatment with doxycycline. A 19-year-old man with no history of mental disorder or substance abuse received doxycycline 50 mg twice daily for perioral dermatitis. He engaged in normal behavior with his friends and family following initiation of doxycycline. Six days following the start of treatment he committed suicide and an autopsy report did not detect any alcohol or illicit substances in his blood. A 33-year-old female with stable family relationships was prescribed doxycycline 200 mg stat and then 100 mg once daily for acne treatment. She discontinued doxycycline days after initiation due to mood instability and suicidal ideations. She claimed her mental state returned to baseline 10 days after discontinuing doxycycline. An 18-year-old male with no history of mental disorder or concomitant medications was prescribed doxycycline 50 mg daily for mild acne. He discontinued the medication after 1 year due to abnormal behavior and negative effects on his mood and his disposition returned to baseline. He restarted doxycycline 6 months later and committed suicide after 8 weeks of therapy. The authors proposed that doxycycline may have caused suicidality in these cases due to the temporal relationship between treatment initiation, suicidal ideation, and the absence of other identifiable risk factors [51A].

METABOLISM

An observational placebo-controlled trial that compared patients with Q fever endocarditis to healthy controls was completed to evaluate the effects of oral doxycycline and hydroxychloroquine (OHCQ) on weight gain and gut microbiota. Of the 82 individuals included, 48 patients were treated with doxycycline and OHCQ for Q fever endocarditis and 34 individuals served as the control population. The study observed that 11/48 (23%) of the treatment group showed abnormal weight gain corresponding to a 4–8% increase in body mass index (BMI), which was significantly different from the control population 0/34 (0%); $p = 0.001$. Additionally, fecal samples examined in the treatment group yielded with lower concentrations of *Bacteroidetes*, *Firmicutes*, and *Lactobacillus*. The authors propose that there may be a causal relationship between gut microbiota depletion and weight gain. As a result, they suggest that patients undergoing long-term treatment with doxycycline and OHCQ, which have shown to modify gut microbiota, may require specific nutritional care [52c].

GASTROINTESTINAL

Medlicott et al. reported two cases of gastric ulceration following doxycycline therapy. A 27-year-old female developed severe retrosternal chest pain 6 days after swallowing a doxycycline tablet that was prescribed for urinary tract infection. A 26-year-old male developed odynophagia 3 days after exposure to doxycycline. In both cases endoscopy revealed esophageal ulcers with distinct histologic changes including mucosal ulceration, perivascular edema, and vascular mural damage. The authors suggest that endoscopic findings similar to these cases should prompt the observer to consider doxycycline-induced esophagitis [53r].

SKIN

A 15-year-old female presented to the emergency room after a 1-month history of skin eruptions over the extremities, myalgias, fatigue, swelling on her extremities and face, headache, and mood changes. She had been taking doxycycline for 2 years as treatment for acne vulgaris and was not taking other medications. Diffuse eruptions of erythematous, tender plaques on her legs were noted on physical exam and a skin biopsy revealed perivascular lymphocytic infiltrate. All symptoms resolved after she discontinued doxycycline. She developed similar symptoms after 1 month of a doxycycline rechallenge. In addition to other common side effects, clinicians should be aware of the possibility of cutaneous inflammation with systemic symptoms associated with doxycycline [54A].

A 13-year-old boy who received doxycycline 20 mg daily for severe periodontal disease complained of pain on the tips of his fingers and toes 1 week after sun exposure. He had played pinball while at the beach and wore garments to shield his skin from sun exposure. This activity left his hands, mostly his thumbs, exposed to the sun. A physical exam revealed onycholysis and hemorrhages at the proximal part of his nails; the thumbs were notably more pigmented than the other fingers. Doxycycline was discontinued and within 4 weeks, his pain disappeared. His nails returned to normal color within 3 months.

Interesting aspects of this case include the fact that photo-onycholysis is rarely observed in children, and phototoxic cutaneous reactions to doxycycline are thought to be dose-related (this child received a low dose) [55A].

Minocycline

Organs and Systems

SENSORY SYSTEMS

A 59-year-old woman developed blue discoloration of the sclera and diffuse hyperpigmentation of her skin over a 3-year period. She had been taking oral minocycline daily for acne vulgaris for over 20 years. An exam revealed bilateral blue pigmentation of the sclera, intact visual function, and diffuse brownish skin pigmentation. Clinicians should recognize that scleral hyperpigmentation is frequently seen in combination with skin pigment changes as noted in this case [56A].

MOUTH AND TEETH

Minocycline-induced hyperpigmentation (MIH) is well documented in a wide array of anatomic locations, and usually involves hard tissues, such as alveolar bone, roots, and crowns of teeth. Instances of MIH of the oral soft tissues have been rarely documented. Additionally, MIH is thought to occur after long courses of minocycline. A 22-year-old woman reported dark spots on her lips, gums, tongue and on her bilateral knees after receiving 2 weeks of minocycline 100 mg twice daily for acne vulgaris. Hyperpigmented macules on the tip of the tongue, inside the gingiva, and on the lower lip were noted on exam. The patient was instructed to stop minocycline and given doxycycline; however, the patient was lost to follow-up. Although rare, clinicians should be aware the MIH might occur on oral soft tissues and after short courses of minocycline [57A].

IMMUNOLOGIC

Reports of minocycline-induced polyarteritis nodosa vasculitis have been described [58A]. A 19-year-old male presented with fever, weight loss, myalgia, and polyarthralgia. He was a healthy individual who took minocycline 100 mg twice daily for acne vulgaris for the previous 3 years. In addition, he had been diagnosed with orchitis 1 month prior to presentation. Upon exam, arthralgias and myalgias were present without signs of arthritis. The patient was noted to have acute kidney injury evidenced by laboratory tests. Immunologic testing showed a positive antinuclear antibody at 1:40, negative double-stranded DNA antibody, positive perinuclear antineutrophilic cytoplasmic antibodies at 1:80, and elevated myeloperoxidase antibody titers at 7.26 U/mL. His acute kidney injury and symptoms rapidly resolved after minocycline discontinuation. Based on the clinical scenario and rapid improvement after discontinuation of minocycline, the authors support the diagnosis of minocycline-induced polyarteritis nodosa-like vasculitis [59A].

A 47-year-old man presented with right testicular pain and swelling associated with fevers, night sweats, abdominal pain, myalgias, and extremity numbness. He took daily minocycline for 12 months for rosacea. A testicular ultrasound revealed an avascular hypoechoic intratesticular lesion that had developed into an infarct. In addition, immunologic testing revealed positive serum antineutrophil cytoplasmic antibody and negative testis tumor markers. He was subsequently diagnosed with minocycline-induced vasculitis and his symptoms improved after minocycline discontinuation. The authors suggest that drug-induced vasculitis should be considered in patients who present with an otherwise unexplained testicular infarct [60A].

Tetracycline

Organs and Systems

GASTROINTESTINAL

A 36-year-old woman presented with severe sudden onset odynophagia, dysphagia and retrosternal chest pain 2 days after being started on tetracycline for acne. Endoscopy revealed extensive serpiginous ulceration resembling carcinoma in the mid-esophagus. Histopathological analysis of the biopsy revealed dense inflammatory infiltrates with no neoplasia. Clinicians should be aware that esophageal damage induced by tetracycline may resemble carcinoma [61A].

Tigecycline

Organs and Systems

HEMATOLOGIC

Life threatening coagulopathy and hypofibrinogenemia was described in a 43-year-old female with autoimmune cirrhosis who had received tigecycline. She was admitted in an intensive care unit for the management of acute kidney injury secondary to hepatorenal syndrome. On day 17 of admission, she was initiated on tigecycline 100 mg once followed by 25 mg twice daily for *Stenotrophomonas maltophilia* bacteremia. After 5 days of tigecycline therapy, she developed worsening hyperbilirubinemia and coagulation parameters. On day 6 of therapy, she had multiple episodes of rectal bleeding and tigecycline was subsequently discontinued. On day 7, following the initiation of tigecycline, her coagulation parameters continued to worsen evidenced by an indeterminable prothrombin time (PT) and an undetectable fibrinogen. Following the discontinuation, her PT, activated partial thromboplastin time, and fibrinogen levels began to improve and returned to baseline. The authors acknowledge that sepsis may have contributed towards the development of abnormal coagulation. Due to the fact that her coagulation parameters worsened during tigecycline therapy and resolved after discontinuation, the authors hypothesize this was an adverse effect of tigecycline. The authors suggest a strict monitoring of coagulation parameters in patients with advanced cirrhosis who receive treatment with tigecycline [62c].

References

[1] Wen M-J, Sung C-C, Chau T, et al. Acute prolonged neurotoxicity associated with recommended doses of ertapenem in 2 patients with advanced renal failure. Clin Nephrol. 2013;80:474–8. http://dx.doi.org/10.5414/CN107247 [c].

[2] Fernando SL. Ertapenem-induced acute generalized exanthematous pustulosis with cross-reactivity to other beta-lactam antibiotics on patch testing. Ann Allergy Asthma Immunol Off Publ Am Coll Allergy Asthma Immunol. 2013;111:139–40. http://dx.doi.org/10.1016/j.anai.2013.05.015 [c].

[3] Hornik CP, Herring AH, Benjamin DK, et al. Adverse events associated with meropenem versus imipenem/cilastatin therapy in a large retrospective cohort of hospitalized infants. Pediatr Infect Dis J. 2013;32:748–53. http://dx.doi.org/10.1097/INF.0b013e31828be70b [c].

[4] Taha FA, Hammond DN, Sheth RD. Seizures from valproate-carbapenem interaction. Pediatr Neurol. 2013;49:279–81. http://dx.doi.org/10.1016/j.pediatrneurol.2013.03.022 [c].

[5] Smits A, Roberts JA, Vella-Brincat JWA, et al. Cefazolin plasma protein binding in different human populations: more than cefazolin-albumin interaction. Int J Antimicrob Agents. 2014;43: 199–200. http://dx.doi.org/10.1016/j.ijantimicag. 2013.10.008 [r].

[6] Kaur K, Gupta A, Sharma A, et al. Evaluation of efficacy and tolerability of cefotaxime and sulbactam versus cefepime and tazobactam in patients of urinary tract infection-a prospective comparative study. J Clin Diagn Res JCDR. 2014;8:HC05–HC08. http://dx.doi.org/10.7860/JCDR/2014/9742.5090 [c].

[7] Muldoon EG, Epstein L, Logvinenko T, et al. The impact of cefepime as first line therapy for neutropenic fever on Clostridium difficile rates among hematology and oncology patients. Anaerobe. 2013;24: 79–81. http://dx.doi.org/10.1016/j.anaerobe. 2013.10.001 [A].

[8] Mani L-Y, Kissling S, Viceic D, et al. Intermittent hemodialysis treatment in cefepime-induced neurotoxicity: case report, pharmacokinetic modeling, and review of the literature. Hemodial Int Symp Home Hemodial. 2014. http://dx.doi.org/10.1111/hdi.12198 [c].

[9] Sawada Y, Kabashima-Kubo R, Hino R, et al. Fatal case of toxic epidermal necrolysis caused by cefozopran and associated with psoriasis. Acta Derm Venereol. 2014;94:341–2. http://dx.doi.org/10.2340/00015555-1704 [c].

[10] Frampton JE. Ceftaroline fosamil: a review of its use in the treatment of complicated skin and soft tissue infections and community-acquired pneumonia. Drugs. 2013;73:1067–94. http://dx.doi.org/10.1007/s40265-013-0075-6 [R].

[11] Rimawi RH, Frenkel A, Cook PP. Ceftaroline—a cause for neutropenia. J Clin Pharm Ther. 2013;38:330–2. http://dx.doi.org/10.1111/jcpt.12062 [c].

[12] Jain R, Chan JD, Rogers L, et al. High incidence of discontinuations due to adverse events in patients treated with ceftaroline. Pharmacotherapy. 2014;34:758–63. http://dx.doi.org/10.1002/phar.1435 [c].

[13] Desai KR, Burdette SD, Polenakovik HM, et al. Ceftaroline-induced eosinophilic pneumonia. Pharmacotherapy. 2013;33:e166–e169. http://dx.doi.org/10.1002/phar.1286 [c].

[14] Griffiths CL, Gutierrez KC, Pitt RD, et al. Eosinophilic pneumonia induced by ceftaroline. Am J Health-Syst Pharm AJHP Off J Am Soc Health-Syst Pharm. 2014;71:403–6. http://dx.doi.org/10.2146/ajhp130441 [c].

[15] Sulaiman K, Locati J, Sidhu I, et al. Allergic interstitial nephritis due to ceftaroline. Am J Med Sci. 2014;348:354–5. http://dx.doi.org/10.1097/MAJ.0000000000000323 [c].

[16] Bai N, Sun C, Wang J, et al. Ertapenem versus ceftriaxone for the treatment of complicated infections: a meta-analysis of randomized controlled trials. Chin Med J (Engl). 2014;127:1118–25 [M].

[17] Kang MH, Villablanca JG, Glade Bender JL, et al. Probable fatal drug interaction between intravenous fenretinide, ceftriaxone, and acetaminophen: a case report from a New Approaches to Neuroblastoma (NANT) Phase I study. BMC Res Notes. 2014;7:256. http://dx.doi.org/10.1186/1756-0500-7-256 [c].

[18] Tomoda T, Ueki T, Saito S, et al. A case of ceftriaxone-associated pseudolithiasis in an adult patient that disappeared after the discontinuation of ceftriaxone. Nihon Shokakibyo Gakkai Zasshi Jpn J Gastro-Enterol. 2013;110:1481–6 [c].

[19] Guleria VS, Sharma N, Amitabh S, et al. Ceftriaxone-induced hemolysis. Indian J Pharmacol. 2013;45:530–1. http://dx.doi.org/10.4103/0253-7613.117758 [c].

[20] Arulraj R, Venkatesh C, Chhavi N, et al. Hypersensitivity due to ceftriaxone mimicking measles in a child. Indian J Pharmacol. 2013;45:528–9. http://dx.doi.org/10.4103/0253-7613. 117756 [c].

[21] Safadi S, Mao M, Dillon JJ. Ceftriaxone-induced acute encephalopathy in a peritoneal dialysis patient. Case Rep Nephrol. 2014;2014:108185. http://dx.doi.org/10.1155/2014/108185 [c].

[22] Landais A, Marty N, Bessis D, et al. Hoigne syndrome following an intravenous injection of ceftriaxone: a case report. Rev Médecine Interne Fondée Par Société Natl Francaise Médecine Interne. 2014;35:199–201. http://dx.doi.org/10.1016/j.revmed. 2013.02.027 [c].

[23] Otunctemur A, Ozbek E, Polat EC, et al. Increasing urinary calcium excretion after ceftriaxone and cephalothin therapy in adults: possible association with urolithiasis. Urolithiasis. 2014;42:105–8. http://dx.doi.org/10.1007/s00240-013-0627-y [c].

[24] Mazhari R, Kimmel PL. Hematuria: an algorithmic approach to finding the cause. Cleve Clin J Med. 2002;69:870. 872–874, 876 passim [c].

[25] Lim CHL, Williams SC, Yun STH, et al. Persistent concerns regarding intracameral cefuroxime. J Cataract Refract Surg. 2014;40:1236–7. http://dx.doi.org/10.1016/j.jcrs.2014.05.015 [r].

[26] Çiftçi S, Çiftçi L, Dağ U. Hemorrhagic retinal infarction due to inadvertent overdose of cefuroxime in cases of complicated cataract surgery: retrospective case series. Am J Ophthalmol. 2014;157: 421–425.e2. http://dx.doi.org/10.1016/j.ajo.2013. 10.018 [c].

[27] Moisseiev E, Levinger E. Anaphylactic reaction following intracameral cefuroxime injection during cataract surgery. J Cataract Refract Surg. 2013;39:1432–4. http://dx.doi.org/10.1016/j.jcrs.2013.06.008 [c].

[28] Le Dû B, Pierre-Kahn V. Early macular edema after phacoemulsification and suspected overdose of cefuroxime: report of six cases. J Fr Ophtalmol. 2014;37:202–10. http://dx.doi.org/10.1016/j.jfo.2013.06.007 [A].

[29] Dong H, Zhang J, Ren L, et al. Unexpected death due to cefuroxime-induced disulfiram-like reaction. Indian J Pharmacol. 2013;45:399–400. http://dx.doi.org/10.4103/0253-7613.114991 [A].

[30] Agrawal A, Rao M, Jasdanwala S, et al. Cephalexin induced cholestatic jaundice. Case Rep Gastrointest Med. 2014;2014:260743. http://dx.doi.org/10.1155/2014/260743 [c].

[31] Barker AF, O'Donnell AE, Flume P, et al. Aztreonam for inhalation solution in patients with non-cystic fibrosis bronchiectasis (AIR-BX1 and AIR-BX2): two randomised double-blind, placebo-controlled phase 3 trials. Lancet Respir Med. 2014;2:738–49. http://dx.doi.org/10.1016/S2213-2600(14)70165-1 [R].

[32] Brodt AM, Stovold E, Zhang L. Inhaled antibiotics for stable non-cystic fibrosis bronchiectasis: a systematic review. Eur Respir J. 2014;44:382–93. http://dx.doi.org/10.1183/09031936.00018414 [M].

[33] Roehmel JF, Schwarz C, Mehl A, et al. Hypersensitivity to antibiotics in patients with cystic fibrosis. J Cyst Fibros Off J Eur Cyst Fibros Soc. 2014;13:205–11. http://dx.doi.org/10.1016/j.jcf.2013.10.002 [c].

[34] Martinez S, Miranda E, Kim P, et al. Giant cell myocarditis associated with amoxicillin hypersensitivity reaction. Forensic Sci Med Pathol. 2013;9:403–6. http://dx.doi.org/10.1007/s12024-013-9418-6 [c].

[35] Ilhan E, Akbulut T, Gürsürer M. An underdiagnosed syndrome; Kounis syndrome secondary to amoxicillin/clavulanic acid use in a 16 year-old child. Int J Cardiol. 2013;167:e90–e91. http://dx.doi.org/10.1016/j.ijcard.2013.03.158 [A].

[36] Shahar E, Roguin A. Ventricular fibrillation after oral administration of amoxicillin and clavulanic acid. Ann Allergy Asthma Immunol Off Publ Am Coll Allergy Asthma Immunol. 2013;111:573–4. http://dx.doi.org/10.1016/j.anai.2013.09.020 [c].

[37] Dandakis D, Petrogiannopoulos C, Hartzoulakis G, et al. Cholestatic hepatitis associated with amoxicillin and clavulanic acid combination. A case report. Ann Gastroenterol. 2007;15(1):8789–92.

[38] Fontana RJ, Shakil AO, Greenson JK, et al. Acute liver failure due to amoxicillin and amoxicillin/clavulanate. Dig Dis Sci. 2005;50: 1785–90. http://dx.doi.org/10.1007/s10620-005-2938-5 [A].

[39] Beraldo DO, Melo JF, Bonfim AV, et al. Acute cholestatic hepatitis caused by amoxicillin/clavulanate. World J Gastroenterol WJG. 2013;19:8789–92. http://dx.doi.org/10.3748/wjg.v19.i46.8789 [c].

[40] Ponvert C, Rufin P, de Blic J. An unusual case of non-pigmenting fixed drug eruptions in a child. Pediatr Allergy Immunol Off Publ Eur Soc Pediatr Allergy Immunol. 2013;24:715–6. http://dx.doi.org/10.1111/pai.12116 [c].

[41] Ellenburg JT, Josey D. An atypical presentation of pulmonary air-leak syndrome and multisystem toxic epidermal necrolysis. Pediatr Pulmonol. 2014;49:E130–E134. http://dx.doi.org/10.1002/ppul.22908 [A].

[42] Hertel S, Schwaninger M, Helmchen C. Combined toxicity of penicillin and aspirin therapy may elicit bilateral vestibulopathy. Clin Neurol Neurosurg. 2013;115:1114–6. http://dx.doi.org/10.1016/j.clineuro.2012.08.033 [c].

[43] Rau J, Simon M, Sander M, et al. Severe bleeding as a result of platelet inhibition caused by floxacillin treatment for endocarditis. J Thorac Cardiovasc Surg. 2013;146:e63–e65. http://dx.doi.org/10.1016/j.jtcvs.2013.07.071 [A].

[44] He Z-F, Wu X-A, Wang Y-P. Severe bone marrow suppression and hepatic dysfunction caused by piperacillin/tazobactam. Scand J Infect Dis. 2013;45:885–7. http://dx.doi.org/10.3109/00365548.2013.805426 [A].

[45] Gomes DM, Smotherman C, Birch A, et al. Comparison of acute kidney injury during treatment with vancomycin in combination with piperacillin-tazobactam or cefepime. Pharmacotherapy. 2014;34:662–9. http://dx.doi.org/10.1002/phar.1428 [c].

[46] Burgess LD, Drew RH. Comparison of the incidence of vancomycin-induced nephrotoxicity in hospitalized patients with and without concomitant piperacillin-tazobactam.

[47] Pratt JA, Stricherz MK, Verghese PS, et al. Suspected piperacillin-tazobactam induced nephrotoxicity in the pediatric oncology population. Pediatr Blood Cancer. 2014;61:366–8. http://dx.doi.org/10.1002/pbc.24720 [A].

[48] Kim M-K, Kang CK, Kim MJ, et al. Penicillin G-induced hemorrhagic cystitis: a case and review of the literature. Korean J Intern Med. 2013;28:743–5. http://dx.doi.org/10.3904/kjim.2013.28.6.743 [r].

[49] Huilaja L, Kallioinen M, Soronen M, et al. Acute localized exanthematous pustulosis on inguinal area secondary to piperacillin/tazobactam. Acta Derm Venereol. 2014;94:106–7. http://dx.doi.org/10.2340/00015555-1629 [A].

[50] Wang KL, Chun RH, Kerschner JE, et al. Sympathetic neuropathy and dysphagia following doxycycline sclerotherapy. Int J Pediatr Otorhinolaryngol. 2013;77:1613–6. http://dx.doi.org/10.1016/j.ijporl.2013.07.005 [A].

[51] Atigari OV, Hogan C, Healy D. Doxycycline and suicidality. BMJ Case Rep. 2013;2013. http://dx.doi.org/10.1136/bcr-2013-200723 [A].

[52] Angelakis E, Million M, Kankoe S, et al. Abnormal weight gain and gut microbiota modifications are side effects of long-term doxycycline and hydroxychloroquine treatment. Antimicrob Agents Chemother. 2014;58:3342–7. http://dx.doi.org/10.1128/AAC.02437-14 [c].

[53] Medlicott SAC, Ma M, Misra T, et al. Vascular wall degeneration in doxycycline-related esophagitis. Am J Surg Pathol. 2013;37:1114–5. http://dx.doi.org/10.1097/PAS.0b013e31828f5a3f [r].

[54] Weinstein M, Laxer R, Debosz J, et al. Doxycycline-induced cutaneous inflammation with systemic symptoms in a patient with acne vulgaris. J Cutan Med Surg. 2013;17:283–6 [A].

[55] Pazzaglia M, Venturi M, Tosti A. Photo-onycholysis caused by an unusual beach game activity: a pediatric case of a side effect caused by doxycycline. Pediatr Dermatol. 2014;31:e26–e27. http://dx.doi.org/10.1111/pde.12223 [A].

[56] Bosma JW, Veenstra J. A brown-eyed woman with blue discoloration of the sclera. Minocycline-induced hyperpigmentation. Neth J Med. 2014;72:33. 37.

[57] Filitis DC, Graber EM. Minocycline-induced hyperpigmentation involving the oral mucosa after short-term minocycline use. Cutis. 2013;92:46–8 [A].

[58] Odhav A, Odhav C, Dayal NA. Rare adverse effect of treatment with minocycline. Minocycline-induced cutaneous polyarteritis nodosa. JAMA Pediatr. 2014;168:287–8. http://dx.doi.org/10.1001/jamapediatrics.2013.3763 [A].

[59] Agur T, Levy Y, Plotkin E, et al. Minocycline-induced polyarteritis nodosa-like vasculitis. Isr Med Assoc J IMAJ. 2014;16:322–3 [A].

[60] Lyon TD, Ferroni MC, Casella DP, et al. Segmental testicular infarction due to minocycline-induced antineutrophil cytoplasmic antibody-positive vasculitis. Urology. 2014;84:e1–e2. http://dx.doi.org/10.1016/j.urology.2014.03.011 [A].

[61] Karaahmet F, Coşkun Y, Erarslan E, et al. Extensive esophageal damage resembling carcinoma due to tetracycline intake. Endoscopy. 2013;45(Suppl 2):E258. http://dx.doi.org/10.1055/s-0033-1344560. UCTN:E258.

[62] Rossitto G, Piano S, Rosi S, et al. Life-threatening coagulopathy and hypofibrinogenaemia induced by tigecycline in a patient with advanced liver cirrhosis. Eur J Gastroenterol Hepatol. 2014;26:681–4. http://dx.doi.org/10.1097/MEG.0000000000000087 [c].

26

Miscellaneous Antibacterial Drugs

Saira B. Chaudhry[1]

Ernest Mario School of Pharmacy, Rutgers University, The State University of New Jersey, Piscataway,
New Jersey and Jersey Shore University Medical Center, Neptune, New Jersey
[1]Corresponding author: sairac@pharmacy.rutgers.edu

AMINOGLYCOSIDES [SED-15, 118; SEDA-32, 461; SEDA-33, 509; SEDA-34, 399; SEDA 35, 463; SEDA-36, 363]

A retrospective, observational study performed in a single intensive care unit (ICU) investigated the risk of aminoglycoside nephrotoxicity in patients with severe sepsis or septic shock. Nephrotoxicity was investigated in patients who were in the ICU for greater than 3 days. Patients who had renal failure before day 3 or with endocarditis were excluded from the study. A total of 317 patients were included, of which 198 patients received an aminoglycoside. Acute kidney injury (AKI) occurred in 16.3% of patients, in a median time of 6 days. After adjusting for the clinical course and exposure to other nephrotoxic drugs from days 1 to 3, the risk of AKI was not increased in those receiving aminoglycosides (adjusted relative risk = 0.75 [0.32–1.76]). Therefore, septic patients receiving aminoglycosides for less than 3 days do not have an increased risk of nephrotoxicity [1c].

The use of aminoglycosides in patients ≥75 years old and the association with nephrotoxicity was evaluated by Fraisse et al. This was a multi-center, retrospective, observational study that included patients ≥75 years old, hospitalized for >24 hours, and received at least one dose of an aminoglycoside. Nephrotoxicity was defined as an increase in serum creatinine level >25% between admission and the last level. A total of 184 patients were included with a mean age of 84.4 years. Sixty-nine percent of the patients received at least one concomitant nephrotoxic drug. The two aminoglycosides used were gentamicin (70%) and amikacin (30%) with 92% of the patients received once daily dosing. The average treatment duration was 2.75 days for amikacin and 4.4 days for gentamicin. The average dose of amikacin was 13.5 mg/kg/day and gentamicin was 3.5 mg/kg/day.

Forty patients (22%) had an increase in their serum creatinine level of >25% at the end of their hospitalization. A multivariate analysis found that risk factors for an increase in serum creatinine were due to treatment >3 days ($p = 0.003$, OR 5.25, 95% CI [2.16–12.74]) and concomitant nephrotoxic drugs ($p = 0.0085$, OR 5.79, 95% CI [1.57–21.38]) [2c].

A prospective, cohort study researched whether serum trough levels of gentamicin and amikacin were associated with cochlear toxicity in newborns with neonatal sepsis. A total of 21 neonates met inclusion. The neonates were administered either gentamicin 5 mg/kg or amikacin 7.5 mg/kg. The dosing interval varied according to the age and body weight for gentamicin and age of gestation for amikacin. The authors found no statistical difference between the serum trough levels of aminoglycosides and the deterioration of cochlear function [3c] However, there are many limitations to this study: the sample size of 21 patients is small; the trough concentration range was not defined; it was unclear which level was used in the final analysis; and the length of treatment was not specified. Therefore, more studies are needed investing the correlation of aminoglycoside trough concentrations and ototoxicity in neonates with neonatal sepsis [4r].

Pharmacogenomics

Mutations in the mitochondrial 12S rRNA gene, particularly the m.1555A>G have been associated with increased susceptibility to the ototoxic effects of aminoglycosides. In a prospective, single-center, observational study, 66 children (mainly Caucasian and between the ages of 3–16 years) with a diagnosis of cystic fibrosis were included. Patients needed to have a history or future exposure to aminoglycosides. Genetic testing for the m.1555A>G mutation and audiological assessments

© 2015 Elsevier B.V. All rights reserved.

were done on these patients. Two of the 59 patients included had the m.1555A>G mutation. Of the two patients, one had severe deafness. The second child, despite having the mutation and repeated exposure to aminoglycosides, had well preserved hearing. In conclusion, further studies are needed to determine the true penetrance of m.1555A>G gene [5c].

Amikacin [SED-15, 111; SEDA-32, 461; SEDA-33, 510; SEDA-34, 400; SEDA-35, 463; SEDA-36, 363]

Sensory Systems

Recent literature supports the use of N-acetylcysteine (NAC) to prevent ototoxicity in end stage renal disease. A prospective, randomized, controlled, and open-label study evaluated the effect of NAC against amikacin-induced ototoxicity in peritoneal dialysis (PD) patients with peritonitis. All patients empirically received a dose of amikacin 2 mg/kg daily plus cefazolin 15 mg/kg daily intraperitoneally, when the diagnosis of peritonitis was made. Patients randomly received either NAC 600 mg twice-daily or placebo (control group) for 2 weeks. Otoacoustic emissions (OAE) were completed before exposure as well as 1 and 4 weeks after amikacin exposure. Oxidative stress measurements were completed concurrently to assess the effectiveness of NAC. A total of 46 patients were enrolled in the study: 23 patients were in the NAC treated group and 23 patients were in the control group. The OAE testing demonstrated an improvement in outer hair cell function at all frequencies, especially higher frequencies, in the NAC group. Total oxidative capacity statistically increased by the fourth week ($p = 0.009$). NAC was shown to have an ototoxic protective effect in aminoglycoside treated PD patients [6c].

Urinary Tract

A quasi-randomized clinical trial with parallel intervention and historical control groups was conducted to compare moderate twice-daily dosing of amikacin (12.5 mg/kg every 12 hours) to high once daily dosing (25 mg/kg daily) and risk of nephrotoxicity in patients with sepsis. A total of 40 patients were enrolled and received amikacin doses for 7 days. There was no statistical difference between groups for estimated glomerular filtration rate (eGFR) percent and serum creatinine percent change from baseline. The serum neutrophil gelatinase-associated lipocalin (NGAL) level change from baseline was statistically significant in the high dose group than the moderate dose group on days 3 and 5 of treatment ($p = 0.001$ and $p = 0.002$, respectively). Overall, this study demonstrated that moderate dosing of amikacin in septic patients may be a viable option [7c].

Respiratory

The use of aerosolized amikacin has a potential for reduced toxicity. Records were queried from the mycobacterial natural history study at the National Institutes of Health (NIH) Clinical Center to identify patients who met the diagnostic criteria for pulmonary nontuberculous mycobacterial disease established by the American Thoracic Society (ATS) guidelines and received treatment with aerosolized amikacin. The dose of amikacin sulfate used was 250 mg/mL solution diluted with 3 mL of saline and placed in a jet nebulizer for inhalation. Patients were started at 250 mg once daily and titrated to twice daily after 2 weeks if no dysphonia was noted. Patients were then told to titrate towards 500 mg twice daily at 2-week intervals. If dysphonia was encountered, they were instructed to hold the dose and then resume at the prior tolerated dose. A total of 20 patients were identified. They received an average of 60 months of treatment. Eleven patients developed sensorineural hearing loss; one patient developed nephrotoxicity. This study demonstrated that toxicity is still common in aerosolized amikacin [8M].

Pediatric

In a retrospective, cohort study, children aged 1–18-years-old, with cancer and with amikacin exposure (to treat febrile neutropenia), were evaluated for the development of vestibular dysfunction. Twenty-three patients had significant amikacin exposure (>15 days). Hearing loss was detected in three subjects (13%). Four patients had vestibular dysfunction (17%). The hearing loss was associated with days on amikacin ($p = 0.02$), cumulative amikacin exposure ($p = 0.005$), and cumulative amikacin exposure by weight ($p = 0.012$). The authors concluded the prolonged use of aminoglycosides in this patient population would benefit from prospective hearing screenings [9c].

Gentamicin [SED-15, 1500; SEDA-32, 461; SEDA-33, 510; SEDA-34, 400; SEDA-35, 463; SEDA-36, 364]

Urinary Tract

A retrospective, cohort study in patients with nosocomial infections compared those who received once daily dosing (ODD) of gentamicin and tobramycin for risk of nephrotoxicity. The dose of gentamicin and tobramycin was 4–6 mg/kg once daily for ≥3 days. Nephrotoxicity was compared in 202 patients in the gentamicin group versus 180 patients in the tobramycin group. Nephrotoxicity was defined by the acronym RIFLE (risk, injury, failure, loss of kidney function and end stage kidney disease). Nephrotoxicity developed in 21.3% of patients in the gentamicin group versus 10.6% who were given tobramycin (OR 2.4, 95% CI 1.2–4.7, $p = 0.012$). The mean serum creatinine increase was 13.3 nmol/mL for gentamicin and 0.1 nmol/mL for tobramycin ($p = 0.02$). Further prospective, randomized studies are needed to confirm the results from this study [10c].

Gentamicin nephrotoxicity was observed in a retrospective study evaluating patients who received extended interval dosing (mostly 24 hours) over a 14-year period. About 4% of the patients had gentamicin-associated nephrotoxicity. Of the four percent, 25% had irreversible nephrotoxicity [11c].

Tobramycin [SED-15, 3437; SEDA-32, 463; SEDA-33, 513; SEDA-35, 464; SEDA-36, 365]

Pediatrics

Tobramycin solution for inhalation (TSI) (300 mg dose) was given twice daily to small infants after receiving a 2-week treatment course of IV tobramycin 10 mg/kg plus either ticarcillin/clavulanate (100 mg/kg three times a day) or ceftazidime (50 mg/kg three times a day). Of the 142 patients, no detectable renal toxicity or ototoxicity was observed with the use of TSI [12c].

FLUOROQUINOLONES [SEDA-15, 1396; SEDA-32, 464; SEDA-33, 514; SEDA-34, 401; SEDA-36, 464; SEDA-36, 365]

Endocrine

A population-based inception, cohort study looked at dysglycemia in diabetic patients, who received oral levofloxacin, ciprofloxacin, moxifloxacin, second generation cephalosporins, and macrolides. The absolute risk of hyperglycemia per 1000 persons was found to be 1.6 for macrolides, 2.1 for cephalosporins, 6.9 for moxifloxacin, 3.9 for levofloxacin, and 4.0 for ciprofloxacin. The absolute risk of hypoglycemia was 3.7 for macrolides, 3.2 for cephalosporins, 10 for moxifloxacin, 9.3 for levofloxacin, and 7.9 for ciprofloxacin. Fluoroquinolones had an increased risk of dysglycemia compared to macrolides, especially moxifloxacin. Adjusted OR for moxifloxacin for hyperglycemia was 2.48 (95% CI 1.50–4.12) and 2.13 (95% CI 1.44–3.14) for hypoglycemia. Overall, dysglycemia was found with fluoroquinolone use, more so with moxifloxacin [13c].

Nervous System

In a pharmacovigilance analysis, it was demonstrated that fluoroquinolones were associated with causing peripheral neuropathy (PN). Of the 45 257 adverse events reported between 1997 and 2012, 539 reported PN. Nine percent of PN reports indicated Guillain-Barré Syndrome [14c]. Another case-controlled study, in men, also found a strong risk in developing PN after fluoroquinolone use (RR 1.83; 95% CI 1.49–2.27). Current new users were found to have the highest risk (RR 2.07; 95% CI 1.56–2.74) [15c].

Liver

A retrospective, matched, case–control study assessed the risk of hepatotoxicity associated with fluoroquinolone (FQ) use (ciprofloxacin, moxifloxacin, and levofloxacin) in adult patients admitted to Veteran Affairs institutions. Patients with a myocardial infarction (MI) diagnosis were used as the control group in the study. FQ use was associated with a 20% increased hepatotoxicity risk compared to the control group (OR 1.20, 95% CI 1.04–1.38). Patients taking ciprofloxacin were 1.29 times more likely to develop hepatotoxicity (95% CI 1.05–1.59) [16c].

Sensory System

Recently, fluoroquinolones (FQ) have been found to be associated with retinal detachment. This could be due to the fact that FQ are well distributed in the vitrous cavity and can have harmful effects on the collagen or connective tissue. Kuo and colleagues conducted a retrospective, population-based cohort study with parallel groups treated with oral FQs and oral amoxicillin. In the FQ cohort, 96 patients (0.054%) developed rhegmatogenous retinal detachment (RDD) versus 46 (0.026%) in the amoxicillin cohort. The adjusted hazard ratio (HR) for FQ use and RDD was 2.07 (95% CI 1.45–2.96) [17c]. Conversely, five recently published cohort studies found no association with FQ use and retinal detachment [18–21,22c].

Ciprofloxacin [SED-15, 783; SEDA-32, 465; SEDA-33, 514; SEDA-34, 402; SEDA-35, 465; SEDA-36, 365]

Drug–Drug Interaction

A 27-year-old female with a history of congenital heart disease, cardiac surgery, heart failure, and arrhythmias received oral ciprofloxacin 500 mg daily for suppression of her *Pseudomonas* sternal wound infection (which she received IV ceftazidime treatment). She was also taking digoxin 250 mcg daily. A few days after taking the ciprofloxacin, she presented with nausea and anorexia. Symptoms occurred when taking ciprofloxacin and digoxin together; therefore, there was concern for digoxin toxicity. The digoxin was reduced by 50% and the patient continued the ciprofloxacin without symptoms [23A].

Electrolyte Balance

A 68-year-old Caucasian woman suffered from ciprofloxacin-induced syndrome of inappropriate anti-diuretic hormone (SIADH). The patient was prescribed ciprofloxacin 500 mg twice daily for a urinary tract infection (UTI) on two occasions. She became hyponatremic; however, once the ciprofloxacin was discontinued, her sodium levels returned to normal (on both occasions) [24A].

Autocoids

A 24-year-old Hispanic female was prescribed ciprofloxacin for a UTI and developed Drug Reaction with Eosinophilia and Systemic Symptoms (DRESS). Two days after initiating ciprofloxacin, she complained of fever, diffuse rash, swelling of her face, arms and flanks, watery diarrhea and muscular pain. Five days after the onset of her symptoms, laboratory results showed a WBC of 38 810 cells/µL and absolute eosinophilia count of 17 080 cells/µL. A skin biopsy revealed superficial perivascular lymphocytic infiltration with dermal edema. Ciprofloxacin was discontinued and the patient's symptoms improved [25A].

Musculoskeletal

Two case reports found patients developed Achilles tendonitis and rupture after taking ciprofloxacin. A 70-year-old male presented with bilateral Achilles tendon rupture 4 days after ciprofloxacin exposure [26A]. A 59-year-old female presented with Achilles tendonitis 3 days after initiating ciprofloxacin [27A]. In both cases, the symptoms resolved after removal of ciprofloxacin.

Psychiatric

A 64-year-old male was given ciprofloxacin for chronic obstructive pulmonary disease (COPD) exacerbation with possible bronchiectasis and infection. Four days after the initiation of ciprofloxacin, the patient became disoriented and confused; therefore, he developed ciprofloxacin-induced psychosis. His cognitive state returned to normal 24 hours after discontinuing ciprofloxacin [28A].

Sensory System

An 81-year-old female, with a past medical history of temporal lobe epilepsy-induced psychotic episodes was prescribed ciprofloxacin 0.3% eye drops four times a day for nasolacrimal duct obstruction of the left eye. The patient was also taking phenytoin. Six days later she experienced breakthrough seizures and her phenytoin serum levels were subtherapeutic. Once the ciprofloxacin eye drops were discontinued, her phenytoin levels returned to the therapeutic range [29A].

Levofloxacin [SED-15, 2047; SEDA-32, 467; SEDA-33, 516; SEDA-34, 403; SEDA-35, 465; SEDA-36, 366]

Pediatric

A 13-year-old female developed levofloxacin-induced delirium with psychotic episodes. The patient developed these symptoms 2 hours after receiving oral levofloxacin 500 mg. The patient fully recovered after 6 days [30A]. Another case report of a 17-year-old male, describes how he developed levofloxacin-induced delirium 10 minutes after receiving one dose of intravenous levofloxacin 500 mg [31A].

Endocrine

Four days after starting levofloxacin (500 mg/day orally), an 81-year-old woman became unresponsive and severely hypoglycemic (blood glucose level of 39 mg/dL). After receiving boluses of 30% glucose and continuous intravenous 10% glucose infusion, her glucose returned to the normal range [32A].

Nervous System

A 93-year-old woman received levofloxacin 500 mg IV daily for pneumonia. Seven hours after the infusion of the second dose of levofloxacin, she had a relapsing generalized, tonic–clonic seizure that was controlled with diazepam and phenobarbital. The patient had no prior history of seizures. Levofloxacin was discontinued with no further bouts of seizures. Unfortunately, on the third day, she later developed multi-organ failure and died [33A].

Musculoskeletal

A 53-year-old woman was prescribed levofloxacin for worsening cellulitis from a cat bite. A few days later she was found to have worsening pain and swelling in her Achilles tendon. She also developed an abscess and hematoma on her Achilles tendon. She underwent incision and drainage a few days later to repair her Achilles tendon. It was determined that she suffered from levofloxacin-mediated Achilles tendon rupture [34A].

Pharmacogenomics

A 45-year-old female developed levofloxacin-induced seizures, without any predisposing factors. A blood sample was collected for pharmacogenetic analysis of the single nucleotide polymorphisms (SNP) that affects the expression or function of blood brain barrier (BBB) transporters; this was to assess if the seizures were due to the abnormal accumulation of the drug in the brain. The patient was found to have polymorphisms in the transporter genes that allowed higher penetration of drug across the BBB. The patient had one variant allele for all three SNPs in ABCB1 (1236C>T, 2677G>TA, and

3435C>T). The patient also had functional polymorphisms affecting the expression of ABCG2. Therefore, the seizures were due to the higher levofloxacin levels in the brain because of the patient's genetically impaired activity of the efflux proteins in the BBB [35A].

Moxifloxacin [SED-15, 2392; SEDA-32, 468; SEDA-33, 518; SEDA-34, 404; SEDA-35, 466; SEDA-36, 367]

Sensory Systems

A case–control study with a cohort of men aged 40–85 was conducted to determine the association of uveitis with moxifloxacin use. For all the identified uveitis cases, current use of moxifloxacin, levofloxacin, or ciprofloxacin was compared to nonuse. A total of 13 313 uveitis cases were identified. Current, first time users of moxifloxacin demonstrated the highest risk of uveitis (adjusted rate ratio 2.98, 95% CI 1.80–4.94). Current first time users of ciprofloxacin (adjusted rate ratio 1.96; 95% CI 1.56–2.47) showed an increased risk of uveitis; levofloxacin first time users did not show an association with uveitis (adjusted rate ratio 1.26; 95% CI 0.90–1.77) [36c].

Pharmacogenomics

A 65-year-old male who was septic and on hemodialysis developed moxifloxacin-induced thrombocytopenia. Antibody testing was performed using flow cytometry to demonstrate an immunoglobulin G (IgG) positive anti-platelet antibody reaction that was exacerbated in the presence of moxifloxacin but negative for immunoglobulin M (IgM). The patient's platelet count normalized after the removal of moxifloxacin [37M].

Ofloxacin [SED-15, 2597; SEDA-34, 405; SEDA-35, 466; SEDA-36, 368]

Pediatric

In a prospective, cohort study, children <5 years old or HIV-positive children aged <15 years old, and exposed to multi-drug resistant tuberculosis, were given preventive therapy with ofloxacin, ethambutol, and high dose isoniazid for 6 months. Three children developed grade 3 adverse events (hallucinations and insomnia) due to inadvertent overdosing of ofloxacin [38c].

GLYCOPEPTIDES [SEDA-32, 469; SEDA-33, 519; SEDA-34, 405; SEDA-35, 466, SEDA-36, 368]

Dalbavancin

Dalbavancin is a lipoglycopeptide antibiotic with a mechanism of action that works by binding to the D-alanyl-D-alanine terminus of the stem pentapeptide in the bacterial cell wall peptidoglycan, which prevents cross linking, therefore, interfering with bacterial cell wall synthesis. The pharmacokinetic profile allows for once weekly dosing. Dalbavancin is indicated for the treatment of acute bacterial skin and skin structure infections (ABSSI) caused by gram positive organisms [39R].

Drug Studies

The DISCOVER-1 and DISCOVER-2 trials were pooled to analyze the adverse events of dalbavancin. Because both the DISCOVER-1 and DISCOVER-2 trials were double-blind, double-dummy, international, multi-center, randomized trials that studied the treatment of acute bacterial skin and skin structure infections (comparing dalbavacnin with vancomycin-linezold), the data could be pooled for analysis. The most common adverse events in the dalbavancin group were nausea (2.5%), diarrhea (0.8%) and pruritus (0.6%). Infusion site-related reactions were exhibited in nine patients (1.4%). Cellulitis and anaphylactoid reaction were each found in one patient in the dalbavancin arm [40c].

A Phase 1 study in pediatric patients analyzed the pharmacokinetics of dalbavancin drug exposure. Patients who weighed ≥60 kg were given a single 1000 mg dose of dalbavancin. Patients who weighed <60 kg were administered a single 15 mg/kg dose of dalbavancin. Common side effects experienced were headache, diarrhea, nausea, and vomiting [41c].

Oritavancin

Oritavancin is a lipoglycopeptide with a dose-dependent disruption of the cell membrane through alteration of permeability and inhibition of cell wall synthesis. Oritavancin is unique with a half-life of ~393 hours (>2 weeks). Due to its uniquely long half-life, oritavancin is given as a single dose to treat gram positive infections [42R].

Drug Studies

Two major randomized, double-blinded trials studied patients who were given either oritavancin 1200 mg IV as a single dose or 7–10 days of intravenous vancomycin (1 g or 15 mg/kg of body weight) twice daily for acute bacterial skin and skin structure infections (SOLO I and SOLO II trials). The most frequently reported adverse events in the SOLO I trial were nausea, headache, vomiting, and diarrhea. In the SOLO II study common adverse events included nausea, headache, vomiting, cellulitis, increased alanine aminotransferase and infusion site phlebitis [43,44C].

Teicoplanin [SED-15, 3305; SEDA-32, 469; SEDA-33, 519; SEDA-34, 405; SEDA-35, 467; SEDA, 368]

Drug Studies

A prospective, multi-centered, observational study compared the efficacy and safety of vancomycin versus teicoplanin in patients with healthcare-associated methicillin-resistant *staphylococcus aureus* (MRSA) bacteremia. The most common adverse events with teicoplanin were acute renal injury, hepatotoxicity, bone marrow toxicity, and fever [45c].

Skin

A 74-year-old male was treated with teicoplanin for endocarditis. The patient developed pruritus and a rash over his trunk and limbs. He was then switched to vancomycin. Later the patient was reintroduced to teicoplanin and developed Stevens-Johnson syndrome. The patient was found to be heterozygous for two variants (rs2844682 of MUC21 and rs750332 of BAG6) [46c].

Telavancin [SEDA-33, 520; SEDA-34, 405; SEDA-35, 467; SEDA, 369]

Drug Studies

Data from both Phase 3 trials for the Assessment of Telavancin for Treatment of Hospital-Acquired Pneumonia (ATTAIN) were pooled to analyze patients with non-ventilator associated pneumonia. Both studies were double-blind, randomized controlled trials that demonstrated non-inferiority of telavancin versus vancomycin. In the pooled analysis, the adverse events for telavancin were diarrhea, constipation, nausea, acute renal failure, renal insufficiency, hematuria, and oliguria [47c]. Another double-blind, Phase 2 trial randomized patients to receive either telavancin or vancomycin for uncomplicated *Staphylococcus aureus* bacteremia. The most common adverse events for the telavancin arm were pyrexia, headache, anemia, and rash [48c].

Vancomycin [SED-15, 3593; SEDA-32, 470; SEDA-33, 520; SEDA-34, 406; SEDA-35, 467; SEDA-36, 369]

Urinary Tract

A retrospective, cohort study found nephrotoxicity at a rate of 24% in patients who received vancomycin for >3 days. Renal dysfunction occurred significantly more in the vancomycin patients than linezolid patients ($p = 0.032$, OR 2.01, 95% CI 1.05–3.85). Those patients with troughs >20 µg/mL were significantly more likely to develop renal impairment during therapy compared to patients with a trough range of 10–20 µg/mL ($p = 0.014$) [49c].

In a case–control study completed in a pediatric cardiac ICU, the authors analyzed the contribution of vancomycin to acute kidney injury (AKI). Vancomycin-associated AKI occurred in 30 (7.2%) patients. Vancomycin-associated AKI patients were more likely to have undergone extracorporeal membrane oxygenation and had greater exposure to other nephrotoxic drugs [50c].

Hematologic

A 49-year-old male developed vancomycin-induced thrombocytopenia after 8 days of therapy. The patient suffered from a purpuric rash and excessive bleeding with bruising and hematoma formation. After vancomycin was discontinued the patient's platelet count returned to normal after 3 days [51A].

Immunologic

Three case reports described the development of DRESS, after initiating vancomycin. All three patients had suffered from eosinophilia, facial angioedema, rash on limbs, and abnormal liver function tests. In all three cases, symptoms resolved after discontinuing vancomycin [52A].

An unusual case of vancomycin-related systemic reaction accompanied with severe thrombocytopenia resembling pacemaker-related infective endocarditis was reported in a 54-year-old female. Two days after discontinuing the vancomycin, the patient's erythrocyte sedimentation rate and C-reactive protein levels decreased and the platelet count normalized [53A].

A single case report of an 11-year-old boy, with end stage renal disease secondary to posterior urethral valves, on continuous ambulatory peritoneal dialysis received intraperitoneal (IP) vancomycin for peritonitis and developed red man syndrome 45 minutes into the dwell. The vancomycin IP dose was 1000 mg/L in a 1400 mL long dwell (40 mL/kg dwell), equivalent to a dose of 37.5 mg/kg. The vancomycin level at the time of the red man syndrome occurrence was 38.8 mcg/mL. The patient improved with oral diphenhydramine and draining the PD fluid. The vancomycin dose was lowered to 15 mg/kg/dose every 3 days without further occurrence. This case report suggests that lowering the IP vancomycin dose and avoiding supra-therapeutic vancomycin levels, can prevent red man syndrome from occurring [54A].

A unique case of a 52-year-old male developed a bullous skin eruption caused by an immune-mediated delayed hypersensitivity and red man syndrome 10 minutes after infusion of vancomycin 1 g IV every 12 hours [55A].

KETOLIDES [SED-15, 1976; SEDA-32, 471; SEDA-33, 521; SEDA-34, 407; SEDA-35, 469; SEDA-36, 370]

Solithromycin [SEDA-35, 469; SEDA-36, 370]

A randomized, double-blind, placebo controlled trial comparing solithromycin (800 mg IV day 1 followed by an oral 400 mg daily for the 5 remaining days) with levofloxacin (750 mg daily for 5 days) was conducted. Sixty-four patients were randomized to receive solithromycin and 68 received levofloxacin. Adverse events were more prevalent in the levofloxacin group. Adverse effects in the solithromycin group included diarrhea (4.7%), elevated CPK (1.5%) and hyponatremia (1.5%) [56C].

Telithromycin [SEDA-35, 469; SEDA-36, 371]

A meta-analysis comparing telithromycin with clarithromycin reviewed data from five randomized controlled trials. Adverse events were similar in both groups. Common adverse events included diarrhea, nausea, vomiting, flatulence, dyspepsia and abdominal pain. Other events included headache, oral candidiasis, dizziness, dysgeusia, abnormal liver function tests and fatigue. Serious adverse events included allergic reactions, abnormal liver function tests as well as death (in three cases) [57M].

LINCOSAMIDES [SED-15, 2063; SEDA-32, 472; SEDA-33, 522; SEDA-34, 407; SEDA-35, 469; SEDA-36, 371]

Clindamycin

Urinary Tract

A retrospective, biopsy-based case series, investigated the occurrence of clindamycin-induced acute kidney injury (AKI). Twenty-four patients were found to have clindamycin-induced AKI. The dose of clindamycin given to the patients was 0.5–0.75 g IV twice daily. The average onset of clindamycin-induced AKI occurred 1 day after the first dose. Renal biopsies were performed which found acute tubular necrosis in all 24 patients [58M].

MACROLIDES [SED-15, 2183; SEDA-32, 472; SEDA-33, 522; SEDA-34, 408; SEDA-35, 469; SEDA-36, 371]

Azithromycin [SED-15, 389; SEDA-33, 522; SEDA-34, 408; SEDA-35, 469; SEDA-36, 371]

Cardiovascular

A retrospective, population-based study compared the risk of ventricular arrhythmia and cardiovascular death among patients prescribed oral azithromycin, clarithromycin, moxifloxacin, levofloxacin, ciprofloxacin or amoxicillin-clavulanate. Azithromycin and moxifloxacin had significant increases in ventricular arrhythmia and cardiovascular death. The adjusted OR for ventricular arrhythmia was 4.32 (95% CI 2.95–6.33) for azithromycin [59c]. Azithromycin also was found to have a significantly increased risk of cardiac arrhythmias (HR = 1.77; 95% CI 1.20–2.62) and death (HR = 1.48; 95% CI, 1.05–2.09) compared to amoxicillin in a retrospective, cohort study of U.S. veterans [60c]. Conversely, in another retrospective, multi-center, cohort study, authors found a significantly lower 90-day mortality with azithromycin use versus those who did not receive azithromycin in patients ≥65 years old (exposed 17.4% vs. non-exposed 22.3%; OR 0.73, 95% CI 0.71–0.76). This study, however, did find a slight increased risk of myocardial infarctions in patients given azithromycin versus those not exposed to azithromycin (5.1% vs. 4.4%) [61c]. A meta-analysis of 12 randomized controlled trials found no increased risk of cardiovascular events and mortality with azithromycin use compared to placebo [62M].

A single case report described a 65-year-old woman who developed QT prolongation and inverted T waves on an electrocardiogram after one dose of azithromycin 500 mg IV. After azithromycin was discontinued, the patient's QT prolongation decreased and the inverted T waves disappeared [63A].

Sensory Systems

In a cohort study, 12 patients received azithromycin eye drops for ocular rosacea. Mild burning after instilling azithromycin was reported [64c].

Clarithromycin [SED-15, 799; SEDA-32, 473; SEDA-33, 523; SEDA-34, 408; SEDA-35, 470; SEDA-36, 372]

Drug–Drug Interactions

A retrospective, population-based, cohort study was conducted to determine the risk of adverse events with concomitant use of statins and clarithromycin or azithromycin. The concomitant use of statins and clarithromycin had the highest risk of acute kidney injury (RR 1.46; 95% CI 1.16–1.84), hyperkalemia (RR 1.87; 95% CI 1.05–3.32), and all-cause mortality (RR 1.32; 95% CI 1.07–1.62) [65c].

An 83-year-old woman developed rhabdomyolysis due to a drug interaction between simvastatin and an increased clarithromycin dose. The patient initially was placed on 250 mg twice daily of clarithromycin, which was increased to 500 mg twice daily. The patient complained of diffuse muscle pain and bilateral leg weakness that left her bedridden for 3 days prior to admission. Symptoms resolved once the simvastatin was discontinued and the clarithromycin dose was decreased to 250 mg twice daily [66M].

Psychiatric

A 28-year-old male experienced depersonalization-anxiety syndrome secondary to clarithromycin use. The patient had no prior underlying psychiatric history. The patient received a 500 mg dose of clarithromycin [67M].

Cardiovascular

In a prospective, cohort study, the objective was to determine if there was an association with the use of clarithromycin and roxithromycin with cardiac death compared to patients who used penicillin. A total of 285 cardiac deaths were reported. Compared to penicillin, clarithromycin did have a statistically significant association with cardiac death (5.3 per 1000 person years; adjusted rate ratio 1.76; 95% CI 1.08–2.85) [68c]. Alternatively, a systemic review of case reports found no statistical relationship between clarithromycin dose and QTc interval duration [69M].

Psychiatric

Two case reports describe two males (44 and 78 years old) who experienced mania after taking clarithromycin. The 78-year-old patient was thought to be experiencing a drug interaction between his prednisone and clarithromycin [70,71M].

Gastrointestinal

A single case report described a 67-year-old female who experienced haemorrhagic colitis caused by klebsiella oxytoca after the use of clarithromycin. The patient's symptoms were muco-bloody diarrhea and abdominal pain [72M].

Erythromycin [SED-15, 1237; SEDA-32, 474; SEDA-33, 523; SEDA-34, 409; SEDA-35, 470; SEDA-36, 373]

Cardiovascular

A systemic review of case reports was conducted to analyze the risk of QTc interval prolongation and torsades de pointes associated with erythromycin use. A total of 29 cases were analyzed. The authors found no significant relationship between erythromycin dose and QTc interval prolongation. Major risk factors identified were: female sex (22 cases), heart disease (19 cases), and elderly (13 cases) [73c].

OXAZOLIDINONES [SED-15, 2645; SEDA-32, 474; SEDA-33, 525; SEDA-34, 409; SEDA-35, 471; SEDA-36, 373]

Linezolid [SEDA-35, 469; SEDA-36, 373]

Hematologic

A prospective, observational study was conducted to determine risk factors associated with linezolid-induced thrombocytopenia. Thirty patients were included in the analysis and treated with linezolid 600 mg twice daily. Seventeen of the 30 patients developed thrombocytopenia (16.7%). Trough levels of linezolid were significantly higher in patients who developed thrombocytopenia than those who did not (13.4 vs. 4.3 mg/L, $p < 0.001$). Thrombocytopenia occurred more frequently in patients with a trough linezolid concentration >7.5 mg/L (OR 90, $p < 0.001$) and renal impairment (OR 39, $p = 0.0002$) [74c]. Similarly, a retrospective, cohort study found that an increase in serum creatinine (OR 1.51, 95% CI 1.01–2.50) and daily per kilogram dose (OR 1.14, 95% CI 1.05–1.26) were associated with linezolid-induced thrombocytopenia [75c]. A case report in a 72-year-old woman, also, developed thrombocytopenia after 10 days of linezolid therapy. Her platelet count normalized 7 days after linezolid withdrawal [76c].

Drug–Drug Interactions

Two case reports describe the development of serotonin syndrome with linezolid and selective serotonin reuptake inhibitors, escitalopram and citalopram. The first case was a 65-year-old female with depressive disorder receiving treatment with escitalopram 10 mg daily. The patient was prescribed linezolid 600 mg intravenously twice daily for pneumonitis. Within 24 hours, the patient developed serotonin syndrome. The linezolid and escitalopram were discontinued with symptom resolution within a few hours [77A]. The second case was a 98-year-old male with a history of depression and atrial fibrillation, who was receiving 2.5 mg citalopram and 200 mg amiodarone for 6 months. He was prescribed linezolid 600 mg intravenously twice daily for pneumonia. Within 3 days, the patient developed serotonin syndrome, requiring linezolid withdrawal. It was suspected that serotonin syndrome developed due to a drug–drug interaction with citalopram, amiodarone, and linezolid [78A].

Acid Base Balance

In a prospective, cohort study, the use of linezolid versus teicoplanin was analyzed to determine the incidence of linezolid-induced lactic acidosis with a total of 72 patients in each group. Lactic acidosis occurred in 6.8% of the cases in the linezolid group versus none in the teicoplanin group. The median change in the anion gap was significantly higher in the linezolid group than in the teicoplanin arm ($p = 0.026$) [79c]. A pediatric, prospective, cohort study was conducted in 50 children treated with linezolid to determine the incidence of lactic acidosis. Eight patients developed acidosis and eight developed lactic acidemia without acidosis [80c]. To further emphasize this association, four case reports were documented and described the development of lactic acidosis after linezolid administration. Unfortunately, lactic acidosis was fatal in one patient [81,82,83A].

Endocrine

Fifteen cases identified linezolid-induced hypoglycemia in a systemic review of case reports from the FDA Adverse Event Reporting System [84M].

Sensory System

Two case reports (41- and 45-year-old patients) describe the development of optic neuropathy after prolonged use of linezolid (17 months and 6 months) for multi-drug resistant tuberculosis [85,86A].

Tedizolid

Tedizolid is an oxolidinone that prevents protein synthesis, by binding to the V-domain of the 23S rRNA component of the 50S ribosomal subunit. Tedizolid has activity against both methicillin-resistant *Staphylococcus aureus* (MRSA) and vancomycin-resistant *Enterococcus* spp. Tedizolid is administered once daily due to its favorable pharmacokinetic profile [87R].

Drug Studies

A Phase 3, randomized, double-blind, non-inferiority trial was conducted to determine the Efficacy and Safety of 6-day Oral Tedizolid in Acute Bacterial Skin and Skin Structure Infections vs. 10-day Oral Linezolid Therapy (ESTABLISH-1). In this trial the most common adverse effects reported with tedizolid were nausea, headache and diarrhea. The incidences of these adverse events in the tedizolid arm occurred less than those patients in the linezolid arm. Other adverse events with tedizolid included alanine aminotransferase elevations and abnormal platelet counts [88C]. In the ESTABLISH-2 trial, gastrointestinal disorders were less common in the tedizolid group vs. the linezolid group. Thrombocytopenia and lower neutrophil count were also observed in the tedizolid group [89C]. In a pooled analysis of platelet profiles from patients in ESTABLISH-1 and ESTABLISH-2 trials, the authors found a lower incidence of thrombocytopenia among patients who received tedizolid versus those who received linezolid [90M].

POLYMYXINS [SED-15, 2891; SEDA-32, 476; SEDA-33, 527; SEDA-34, 412; SEDA-35, 473; SEDA-36, 374]

Colistin [SEDA-35, 473; SEDA-36, 374]

Respiratory

A 31-year-old female was reported to have developed acute respiratory failure requiring intubation and mechanical ventilation for 6 days after initiation of colistimethate sodium 200 mg IV every 12 hours for a multi-drug resistant *Pseudomonas aeruginosa* sacral wound infection. The patient's serum creatinine peaked at 3.7 mg/dL. Authors believed colistimethate was the cause of her respiratory failure and renal failure [91A].

STREPTOGRAMINS [SED-15, 3182; SEDA-32, 528; SEDA-34, 413; SEDA-35, 473; SEDA-36, 375]

Pristinamycin [SEDA-34, 413; SEDA-35, 469; SEDA-36, 375]

A meta-analysis was conducted to evaluate patients treated with pristinamycin in osteoarticular infections. A total of five studies were identified and included 247 patients. The analysis found that 25.7% of the patients experienced adverse events, with the most common being gastrointestinal complaints and rash [92c].

TRIMETHOPRIM AND CO-TRIMOXAZOLE [SED-15, 3216, 3510; SEDA-32, 477; SEDA-33, 528; SEDA-34, 414; SEDA-35, 474; SEDA-36, 375]

Trimethoprim-Sulfamethoxazole [SEDA-35, 474; SEDA-36, 375]

Musculoskeletal

A single case of trimethoprim-sulfamethoxazole (TMP-SMX) induced rhabdomyolysis was reported in a 65-year-old male who self-medicated for a UTI with three tablets of TMP-SMX 40/800 mg daily for 2 weeks. The patient also took numerous non-steroidal anti-inflammatory medications (NSAIDS), which also could have potentiated the rhabdomyolysis [93A].

Electrolyte Balance

A retrospective chart review was conducted to determine the association of hyperkalemia and acute renal failure in patients receiving high dose TMP-SMX. A dose of TMP-SMX was considered high if patients received >5 mg/kg/day. A standard dose was considered

<5 mg/kg/day. More patients developed hyperkalemia ($p < 0.001$) as well as a higher incidence of acute renal failure ($p = 0.0001$) [94c].

A 76-year-old female developed hyperkalemia intraoperatively when treated with prophylactic TMP-SMX for a tympanomastoidectomy. The patient was also taking an angiotensin receptor blocker for 6 months. The patient developed hyperkalemia within 1 hour of the surgery with a potassium level of 6.54 mEq/L [95A].

A 28-year-old HIV-infected patient developed hyponatremia after 7 days while being treated for pneumocystis jiroveci pneumonia with a 15 mg/kg/day dose of TMP-SMX. The patient's sodium level decreased from 135 to 117 mEq/L. A diagnosis of hyponatremia secondary to the diuretic effects TMP was confirmed [96A].

Psychiatric

Two case reports describe patients who developed TMP-SXS-induced acute psychosis and hallucinations in both patients. A 42-year-old patient developed the acute psychosis after 8 days of receiving high dose TMP-SXS (15 mg/kg/dose of TMP every 8 hours) for possible *Pneumocystis jiroveci* pneumonia. The patient returned to normal mental status 48 hours after the discontinuation of TMP/SXS. An 86-year-old patient was receiving a dose of TMP-SXS (80 mg/400 mg) two tablets every 12 hours for a urinary tract infection. After 2 days of treatment, the patient developed acute psychosis with auditory and visual hallucinations. Two days after the TMP/SXS was stopped the patient returned to normal mental status [97,98A].

OTHER ANTIMICROBIAL DRUGS

Daptomycin [SED-15, 1053; SED-32, 478; SEDA-33, 529; SEDA-34, 416; SEDA-35, 474; SEDA-36, 375]

Musculoskeletal

A single case report describes a 46-year-old female developing rhabdomyolysis and acute hepatotoxicity after being prescribed daptomycin 6 mg/kg IV every 24 hours. The patient's creatine kinase levels were 16, 710 U/L. The patient had a serum creatinine level of 4.7 mg/L with significantly elevated liver enzymes [99A].

Immunologic

An 82-year-old male with COPD was reported to have developed daptomycin-induced pneumonitis 16 days after starting daptomycin 10 mg/kg/day [100A].

A 61-year-old woman developed daptomycin-induced acute eosinophilic pneumonia 7 days after initiation of daptomycin. The patient had a white blood cell count of 16 100 per μL with 15% eosinophils and a chest X-ray

revealed bilateral pulmonary infiltrates. Once the daptomycin was discontinued the patient's chest X-ray and eosinophilia resolved [101A].

A single case report describes a 69-year-old female treated with a 2-minute rapid IV infusion of daptomycin 6 mg/kg every 48 hours and experienced an infusion-related flushing in the face with erythema. These symptoms occurred about an hour after infusion. The daptomycin infusion was extended to 30 minutes and the patient did not experience any adverse reactions [102A].

Fosfomycin [SED-15, 1448; SEDA-34, 417; SEDA-35, 476; SEDA-36, 376]

A total of 356 patients were included in a prospective, uncontrolled, open-label study was conducted to evaluate the efficacy and safety of three doses of 3 g fosfomycin orally for lower urinary tract infections. The doses were given on days 1, 3, and 5. About 5% of the patients complained about diarrhea. One patient complained about fatigue and another reported a mild backache [103c].

Fusidic Acid [SED-15, 1460; SEDA-32, 479; SEDA-33, 530; SEDA-34, 417; SEDA-35, 475; SEDA-36, 376]

A retrospective study was conducted to assess and compare the efficacy and safety between fusidic acid and petrolatum for the post-procedure care of clean dermatologic infections. Patients were instructed to apply either fusidic acid ointment or petrolatum to the wound area, once or twice a day for 1–2 weeks. Three subjects in the fusidic acid group developed adverse events including erythema and itching [104c].

References

[1] Picard W, Bazin F, Clouzeau B, et al. Propensity-based study of aminoglycoside nephrotoxicity in patients with severe sepsis or septic shock. Antimicrob Agents Chemother. 2014;58(12):7468–74 [c].

[2] Fraisse T, Gras Aygon C, Paccalin M, et al. Aminoglycosides use in patients over 75 years old. Age Ageing. 2014;43(5):676–81 [c].

[3] Setiabudy R, Suwento R, Rundjan L, et al. Lack of a relationship between the serum concentration of aminoglycosides and ototoxicity in neonates. Int J Clin Pharmacol Ther. 2013;51(5):401–6 [c].

[4] Samiee-Zafarghandy S, van den Anker JN. Aminoglycosides and ototoxicity in neonates: is there a relation with serum concentrations? Int J Clin Pharmacol Ther. 2013;51(12):993–4 [r].

[5] Al-Malky G, Suri R, Sirimanna T, et al. Normal hearing in a child with the m.1555A > G mutation despite repeated exposure to aminoglycosides. Has the penetrance of this pharmacogenetic interaction been overestimated? Int J Pediatr Otorhinolaryngol. 2014;78(6):969–73 [c].

[6] Kocyigit I, Vural A, Unal A, et al. Preventing amikacin related ototoxicity with N-acetylcysteine in patients undergoing peritoneal dialysis. Eur Arch Otorhinolaryngol. 2014; [c].

[7] Najmeddin F, Ahmadi A, Mahmoudi L, et al. Administration of higher doses of amikacin in early stages of sepsis in critically ill patients. Acta Med Iran. 2014;52(9):703–9 [c].

[8] Olivier KN, Shaw PA, Glaser TS, et al. Inhaled amikacin for treatment of refractory pulmonary nontuberculous mycobacterial disease. Ann Am Thorac Soc. 2014;11(1):30–5 [M].

[9] Chen KS, Bach A, Shoup A, et al. Hearing loss and vestibular dysfunction among children with cancer after receiving aminoglycosides. Pediatr Blood Cancer. 2013;60(11):1772–7 [c].

[10] van Maarseveen E, van Buul-Gast MC, Abdoellakhan R, et al. Once-daily dosed gentamicin is more nephrotoxic than once-daily dosed tobramycin in clinically infected patients. J Antimicrob Chemother. 2014;69(9):2581–3 [c].

[11] Plajer SM, Chin PK, Vella-Brincat JW, et al. Gentamicin and renal function: lessons from 15 years' experience of a pharmacokinetic service for extended interval dosing of gentamicin. Ther Drug Monit. 2015;37(1):98–103 [c].

[12] Hennig S, McKay K, Vidmar S, et al. Safety of inhaled (Tobi(R)) and intravenous tobramycin in young children with cystic fibrosis. J Cyst Fibros. 2014;13(4):428–34 [c].

[13] Chou HW, Wang JL, Chang CH, et al. Risk of severe dysglycemia among diabetic patients receiving levofloxacin, ciprofloxacin, or moxifloxacin in Taiwan. Clin Infect Dis. 2013;57(7):971–80 [c].

[14] Ali AK. Peripheral neuropathy and Guillain-Barre syndrome risks associated with exposure to systemic fluoroquinolones: a pharmacovigilance analysis. Ann Epidemiol. 2014;24(4):279–85 [c].

[15] Etminan M, Brophy JM, Samii A. Oral fluoroquinolone use and risk of peripheral neuropathy: a pharmacoepidemiologic study. Neurology. 2014;83(14):1261–3 [c].

[16] Alshammari TM, Larrat EP, Morrill HJ, et al. Risk of hepatotoxicity associated with fluoroquinolones: a national case–control safety study. Am J Health Syst Pharm. 2014;71(1):37–43 [c].

[17] Kuo SC, Chen YT, Lee YT, et al. Association between recent use of fluoroquinolones and rhegmatogenous retinal detachment: a population-based cohort study. Clin Infect Dis. 2014;58(2):197–203 [c].

[18] Chui CS, Man KK, Cheng CL, et al. An investigation of the potential association between retinal detachment and oral fluoroquinolones: a self-controlled case series study. J Antimicrob Chemother. 2014;69(9):2563–7.

[19] Chui CS, Wong IC, Wong LY, et al. Association between oral fluoroquinolone use and the development of retinal detachment: a systematic review and meta-analysis of observational studies. J Antimicrob Chemother. 2015;70(4):971–8.

[20] Eftekhari K, Ghodasra DH, Haynes K, et al. Risk of retinal tear or detachment with oral fluoroquinolone use: a cohort study. Pharmacoepidemiol Drug Saf. 2014;23(7):745–52.

[21] Fife D, Zhu V, Voss E, et al. Exposure to oral fluoroquinolones and the risk of retinal detachment: retrospective analyses of two large healthcare databases. Drug Saf. 2014;37(3):171–82.

[22] Pasternak B, Svanstrom H, Melbye M, et al. Association between oral fluoroquinolone use and retinal detachment. JAMA. 2013;310(20):2184–90 [c].

[23] Moffett BS, Valdes SO, Kim JJ. Possible digoxin toxicity associated with concomitant ciprofloxacin therapy. Int J Clin Pharm. 2013;35(5):673–6 [A].

[24] Babar SM. SIADH associated with ciprofloxacin. Ann Pharmacother. 2013;47(10):1359–63 [A].

[25] Alkhateeb H, Said S, Cooper CJ, et al. DRESS syndrome following ciprofloxacin exposure: an unusual association. Am J Case Rep. 2013;14:526–8 [A].

[26] Kawtharani F, Masrouha KZ, Afeiche N. Bilateral achilles tendon ruptures associated with ciprofloxacin use in the setting of minimal change disease: case report and review of the literature. J Foot Ankle Surg. 2014; [A].

[27] Tam PK, Ho CT. Fluoroquinolone-induced Achilles tendinitis. Hong Kong medical journal = Xianggang yi xue za zhi / Hong Kong Academy of Medicine. 2014;20(6):545–7 [A].

[28] Ben-Chetrit E, Rothstein N, Munter G. Ciprofloxacin-induced psychosis. Antimicrob Agents Chemother. 2013;57(8):4079 [A].

[29] Malladi SS, Liew EK, Ng XT, et al. Ciprofloxacin eye drops-induced subtherapeutic serum phenytoin levels resulting in breakthrough seizures. Singap Med J. 2014;55(7):e114–5 [A].

[30] Raj V, Murthy TV. Levofloxacin induced delirium with psychotic features in a young patient. Med J Armed Forces India. 2013;69(4):404–5 [A].

[31] Ghoshal A, Damani A, Salins N, et al. Management of levofloxacin induced anaphylaxis and acute delirium in a palliative care setting. Indian J Palliat Care. 2015;21(1):76–8 [A].

[32] Fusco S, Reitano F, Gambadoro N, et al. Severe hypoglycemia associated with levofloxacin in a healthy older woman. J Am Geriatr Soc. 2013;61(9):1637–8 [A].

[33] Famularo G, Pizzicannella M, Gasbarrone L. Levofloxacin and seizures: what risk for elderly adults? J Am Geriatr Soc. 2014;62(10):2018–9 [A].

[34] Budny AM, Ley AN. Fluoroquinolone-mediated achilles rupture: a case report and review of the literature. J Foot Ankle Surg. 2014;54:494–6 [A].

[35] Gervasoni C, Cattaneo D, Falvella FS, et al. Levofloxacin-induced seizures in a patient without predisposing risk factors: the impact of pharmacogenetics. Eur J Clin Pharmacol. 2013;69(8):1611–3 [A].

[36] Eadie B, Etminan M, Mikelberg FS. Risk for uveitis with oral moxifloxacin: a comparative safety study. JAMA Ophthalmol. 2015;133(1):81–4 [c].

[37] Mailman JF, Stigant C, Martinusen D. Moxifloxacin-induced immune-mediated thrombocytopenia in a chronic kidney disease patient receiving hemodialysis. Ann Pharmacother. 2014;48(7):919–22 [M].

[38] Seddon JA, Hesseling AC, Finlayson H, et al. Preventive therapy for child contacts of multidrug-resistant tuberculosis: a prospective cohort study. Clin Infect Dis. 2013;57(12):1676–84 [c].

[39] Cada DJ, Ingram K, Baker DE. Dalbavancin. Hosp Pharm. 2014;49(9):851–61 [R].

[40] Boucher HW, Wilcox M, Talbot GH, et al. Once-weekly dalbavancin versus daily conventional therapy for skin infection. N Engl J Med. 2014;370(23):2169–79 [c].

[41] Bradley JS, Puttagunta S, Rubino CM, et al. Pharmacokinetics, safety and tolerability of single dose dalbavancin in children 12 through 17 years of age. Pediatr Infect Dis J. 2015;34(7):748–52 [c].

[42] Tice A. Oritavancin: a new opportunity for outpatient therapy of serious infections. Clin Infect Dis. 2012;54(Suppl 3):S239–43 [R].

[43] Corey GR, Kabler H, Mehra P, et al. Single-dose oritavancin in the treatment of acute bacterial skin infections. N Engl J Med. 2014;370(23):2180–90.

[44] Corey GR, Good S, Jiang H, et al. Single-dose oritavancin versus 7–10 days of vancomycin in the treatment of gram-positive acute bacterial skin and skin structure infections: the SOLO II noninferiority study. Clin Infect Dis. 2015;60(2):254–62 [C].

[45] Yoon YK, Park DW, Sohn JW, et al. Multicenter prospective observational study of the comparative efficacy and safety of vancomycin versus teicoplanin in patients with health care-associated methicillin-resistant Staphylococcus aureus bacteremia. Antimicrob Agents Chemother. 2014;58(1):317–24 [c].

[46] Yang LP, Zhang AL, Wang DD, et al. Stevens-Johnson syndrome induced by the cross-reactivity between teicoplanin and vancomycin. J Clin Pharm Ther. 2014;39(4):442–5 [c].

[47] Rubinstein E, Stryjewski ME, Barriere SL. Clinical utility of telavancin for treatment of hospital-acquired pneumonia: focus on non-ventilator-associated pneumonia. Infect Drug Resist. 2014;7:129–35 [c].

[48] Stryjewski ME, Lentnek A, O'Riordan W, et al. A randomized Phase 2 trial of telavancin versus standard therapy in patients with uncomplicated Staphylococcus aureus bacteremia: the ASSURE study. BMC Infect Dis. 2014;14:289 [c].

[49] Fujii S, Takahashi S, Makino S, et al. Impact of vancomycin or linezolid therapy on development of renal dysfunction and thrombocytopenia in Japanese patients. Chemotherapy. 2013;59(5):319–24 [c].

[50] Moffett BS, Hilvers PS, Dinh K, et al. Vancomycin-associated acute kidney injury in pediatric cardiac intensive care patients. Congenit Heart Dis. 2015;10(1):E6–E10 [c].

[51] Rowland SP, Rankin I, Sheth H. Vancomycin-induced thrombocytopaenia in a patient with severe pancreatitis. BMJ Case Rep. 2013;2013:1–3 [A].

[52] Young S, Ojaimi S, Dunckley H, et al. Vancomycin-associated drug reaction with eosinophilia and systemic symptoms syndrome. Intern Med J. 2014;44(7):694–6 [A].

[53] Candemir B, Aribuca A, Koca C, et al. An unusual case of vancomycin-related systemic reaction accompanied with severe thrombocytopenia mimicking pacemaker-related infective endocarditis: a case report and review of literature. J Interv Card Electrophysiol. 2013;38(2):143–5 [A].

[54] Domis MJ, Moritz ML. Red man syndrome following intraperitoneal vancomycin in a child with peritonitis. Front Pediatr. 2014;2:55 [A].

[55] Li Q, Chen J, Li R, et al. A unique case of bullous drug eruption related to vancomycin and cefoperazone. Eur J Dermatol. 2014;24(3):378–9 [A].

[56] Oldach D, Clark K, Schranz J, et al. Randomized, double-blind, multicenter phase 2 study comparing the efficacy and safety of oral solithromycin (CEM-101) to those of oral levofloxacin in the treatment of patients with community-acquired bacterial pneumonia. Antimicrob Agents Chemother. 2013;57(6):2526–34 [C].

[57] Li XM, Wang FC, Yang F, et al. Telithromycin versus clarithromycin for the treatment of community-acquired respiratory tract infections: a meta-analysis of randomized controlled trials. Chin Med J. 2013;126(11):2179–85 [M].

[58] Xie H, Chen H, Hu Y, et al. Clindamycin-induced acute kidney injury: large biopsy case series. Am J Nephrol. 2013;38(3):179–83 [M].

[59] Chou HW, Wang JL, Chang CH, et al. Risks of cardiac arrhythmia and mortality among patients using new-generation macrolides, fluoroquinolones, and beta-lactam/beta-lactamase inhibitors: a Taiwanese nationwide study. Clin Infect Dis. 2015;60(4):566–77 [c].

[60] Rao GA, Mann JR, Shoaibi A, et al. Azithromycin and levofloxacin use and increased risk of cardiac arrhythmia and death. Ann Fam Med. 2014;12(2):121–7 [c].

[61] Mortensen EM, Halm EA, Pugh MJ, et al. Association of azithromycin with mortality and cardiovascular events among older patients hospitalized with pneumonia. JAMA. 2014;311(21):2199–208 [c].

[62] Almalki ZS, Guo JJ. Cardiovascular events and safety outcomes associated with azithromycin therapy: a meta-analysis of randomized controlled trials. Am Health Drug Benefits. 2014;7(6):318–28 [M].

[63] Yu T, Niu T. Giant inverted T waves and substantial QT interval prolongation induced by azithromycin in an elderly woman with renal insufficiency. Canadian family physician Medecin de famille canadien. 2014;60(11):1012–5 [A].

[64] Mantelli F, Di Zazzo A, Sacchetti M, et al. Topical azithromycin as a novel treatment for ocular rosacea. Ocul Immunol Inflamm. 2013;21(5):371–7 [c].

[65] Li DQ, Kim R, McArthur E, et al. Risk of adverse events among older adults following co-prescription of clarithromycin and statins not metabolized by cytochrome P450 3A4. CMAJ:

Canadian Medical Association journal = journal de l'Association medicale canadienne. 2015;187(3):174–80 [c].

[66] Page SR, Yee KC. Rhabdomyolysis in association with simvastatin and dosage increment in clarithromycin. Intern Med J. 2014;44(7):690–3 [M].

[67] Negrin-Gonzalez J, Peralta Filpo G, Carrasco JL, et al. Psychiatric adverse reaction induced by clarithromycin. Eur Ann Allergy Clin Immunol. 2014;46(3):114–5 [M].

[68] Svanstrom H, Pasternak B, Hviid A. Use of clarithromycin and roxithromycin and risk of cardiac death: cohort study. BMJ. 2014;349:g4930 [c].

[69] Vieweg WV, Hancox JC, Hasnain M, et al. Clarithromycin, QTc interval prolongation and torsades de pointes: the need to study case reports. Ther Adv Infect Dis. 2013;1(4):121–38 [M].

[70] Khalili N. Sunny hypomania associated with clarithromycin: a case report. J Clin Psychopharmacol. 2014;34(3):416–7.

[71] Liu EY, Vasudev A. Mania induced by clarithromycin in a geriatric patient taking low-dose prednisone. Prim Care Companion CNS Disord. 2014;16(3) [M].

[72] Miyauchi R, Kinoshita K, Tokuda Y. Clarithromycin-induced haemorrhagic colitis. BMJ Case Rep. 2013;2013 [M].

[73] Hancox JC, Hasnain M, Vieweg WV, et al. Erythromycin, QTc interval prolongation, and torsade de pointes: case reports, major risk factors and illness severity. Ther Adv Infect Dis. 2014;2(2):47–59 [c].

[74] Nukui Y, Hatakeyama S, Okamoto K, et al. High plasma linezolid concentration and impaired renal function affect development of linezolid-induced thrombocytopenia. J Antimicrob Chemother. 2013;68(9):2128–33 [c].

[75] Natsumoto B, Yokota K, Omata F, et al. Risk factors for linezolid-associated thrombocytopenia in adult patients. Infection. 2014;42(6):1007–12 [c].

[76] Cossu AP, Musu M, Mura P, et al. Linezolid-induced thrombocytopenia in impaired renal function: is it time for a dose adjustment? A case report and review of literature. Eur J Clin Pharmacol. 2014;70(1):23–8 [c].

[77] Kulkarni RR, Kulkarni PR. Linezolid-induced near-fatal serotonin syndrome during escitalopram therapy: case report and review of literature. Indian J Psychol Med. 2013;35(4):413–6 [A].

[78] Ma J, Zhu P, Tu G, et al. Serotonin syndrome under combination of linezolid and low-dose citalopram with amiodarone. Psychiatry Clin Neurosci. 2013;67(6):457 [A].

[79] Im JH, Baek JH, Kwon HY, et al. Incidence and risk factors of linezolid-induced lactic acidosis. Int J Infect Dis. 2015;31:47–52 [c].

[80] Ozkaya-Parlakay A, Kara A, Celik M, et al. Early lactic acidosis associated with linezolid therapy in paediatric patients. Int J Antimicrob Agents. 2014;44(4):334–6 [c].

[81] Djibre M, Pham T, Denis M, et al. Fatal lactic acidosis associated with linezolid therapy. Infection. 2015;43(1):125–6.

[82] Del Pozo JL, Fernandez-Ros N, Saez E, et al. Linezolid-induced lactic acidosis in two liver transplant patients with the mitochondrial DNA A2706G polymorphism. Antimicrob Agents Chemother. 2014;58(7):4227–9.

[83] Sawyer AJ, Haley HL, Baty SR, et al. Linezolid-induced lactic acidosis corrected with sustained low-efficiency dialysis: a case report. Am J Kidney Dis. 2014;64(3):457–9 [A].

[84] Viswanathan P, Iarikov D, Wassel R, et al. Hypoglycemia in patients treated with linezolid. Clin Infect Dis. 2014;59(8): e93–5 [M].

[85] Han J, Lee K, Rhiu S, et al. Linezolid-associated optic neuropathy in a patient with drug-resistant tuberculosis. J Neuroophthalmol. 2013;33(3):316–8.

[86] Karuppannasamy D, Raghuram A, Sundar D. Linezolid-induced optic neuropathy. Indian J Ophthalmol. 2014;62(4):497–500 [A].

[87] Rybak JM, Roberts K. Tedizolid phosphate: a next-generation oxazolidinone. Infect Dis Ther. 2015;4:1–14 [R].

[88] Prokocimer P, De Anda C, Fang E, et al. Tedizolid phosphate vs linezolid for treatment of acute bacterial skin and skin structure infections: the ESTABLISH-1 randomized trial. JAMA. 2013;309(6):559–69 [C].

[89] Moran GJ, Fang E, Corey GR, et al. Tedizolid for 6 days versus linezolid for 10 days for acute bacterial skin and skin-structure infections (ESTABLISH-2): a randomised, double-blind, phase 3, non-inferiority trial. Lancet Infect Dis. 2014;14(8):696–705 [C].

[90] Lodise TP, Fang E, Minassian SL, et al. Platelet profile in patients with acute bacterial skin and skin structure infections receiving tedizolid or linezolid: findings from the Phase 3 ESTABLISH clinical trials. Antimicrob Agents Chemother. 2014;58(12):7198–204 [M].

[91] Shrestha A, Soriano SM, Song M, et al. Intravenous colistin-induced acute respiratory failure: a case report and a review of literature. Int J Crit Ill Inj Sci. 2014;4(3):266–70 [A].

[92] Cooper EC, Curtis N, Cranswick N, et al. Pristinamycin: old drug, new tricks? J Antimicrob Chemother. 2014;69(9):2319–25 [c].

[93] Petrov M, Yatsynovich Y, Lionte C. An unusual cause of rhabdomyolysis in emergency setting: challenges of diagnosis. Am J Emerg Med. 2015;33(1), 123 e1-3. [A].

[94] Gentry CA, Nguyen AT. An evaluation of hyperkalemia and serum creatinine elevation associated with different dosage levels of outpatient trimethoprim-sulfamethoxazole with and without concomitant medications. Ann Pharmacother. 2013;47(12):1618–26 [c].

[95] Lee SW, Park SW, Kang JM. Intraoperative hyperkalemia induced by administration of trimethoprim-sulfamethoxazole in a patient receiving angiotensin receptor blockers. J Clin Anesth. 2014;26(5):427–8 [A].

[96] Babayev R, Terner S, Chandra S, et al. Trimethoprim-associated hyponatremia. Am J Kidney Dis. 2013;62(6):1188–92 [A].

[97] Hsiao HH, Chu NS, Tsai YF, et al. Trimethoprim/sulfamethoxazole-related acute psychosis in the second course of treatment after a stem cell transplant: case report and literature review. Exp Clin Transplant. 2013;11(5):467–8.

[98] Stuhec M. Trimethoprim-sulfamethoxazole-related hallucinations. Gen Hosp Psychiatry. 2014;36(2), 230 e7-8. [A].

[99] King ST, Walker ED, Cannon CG, et al. Daptomycin-induced rhabdomyolysis and acute liver injury. Scand J Infect Dis. 2014;46(7):537–40 [A].

[100] Yamamoto K, Hayakawa K, Ohmagari N. Daptomycin-induced pneumonitis in a patient with chronic obstructive pulmonary disease (COPD). Intern Med. 2014;53(21):2559–60 [A].

[101] Patel JJ, Antony A, Herrera M, et al. Daptomycin-induced acute eosinophilic pneumonia. WMJ. 2014;113(5):199–201 [A].

[102] Caulder CR, Sloan A, Yasir A, et al. Infusion-related reaction following daptomycin two-minute rapid intravenous administration. Hosp Pharm. 2014;49(7):644–6 [A].

[103] Qiao LD, Zheng B, Chen S, et al. Evaluation of three-dose fosfomycin tromethamine in the treatment of patients with urinary tract infections: an uncontrolled, open-label, multicentre study. BMJ Open. 2013;3(12):e004157 [c].

[104] Lee DH, Kim DY, Yoon SY, et al. Retrospective clinical trial of fusidic acid versus petrolatum in the postprocedure care of clean dermatologic procedures. Ann Dermatol. 2015;27(1):15–20 [c].

27

Antifungal Drugs

Dayna S. McManus[1]

Department of Pharmacy Services, Inova Farifax Hospital, Falls Church, VA, USA
[1]Corresponding author: dayna.mcmanus@inova.org

ALLYLAMINES [SEDA-34, 427; SEDA-35,483; SEDA-36, 381]

Terbinafine [SEDA-34, 427; SEDA-35,483; SEDA-36, 381]

Immunology/Liver

A 30-year-old woman presented to the emergency department with a 3-week history of malaise, itching, nausea, decreased appetite, weight loss, dark orange urine and intermittent epigastric pain. The patient reported that 3 weeks prior to admission she had completed a 3-week course of oral terbinafine 250 mg tablets daily for treatment of tinea unguium, which had completely resolved upon presentation to the hospital. The patient denied any alcohol use and was only on paracetamol as needed for pain. A percutaneous liver biopsy revealed mild portal inflammation, interface hepatitis, lobular inflammation and Kuppfer cell hyperplasia. Moderate cholestasis was present without any steatosis. Because of the lack of other causes including viral etiologies the diagnosis was most likely chronic active hepatitis secondary to a drug reaction with the most likely drug being terbinafine. Three days into the admission, the patient developed a maculopapular pruritic rash over her arms, thighs and trunk that were also thought to be related to the terbinafine. The patient was discharged home and started on topical betamethasone valerate 0.1% cream and topical urea 5% cream by dermatology. Five days after the liver biopsy, the patient was re-admitted to the hospital due to discrete erythematous, papular and painful skin lesions over her shins. The appearance was consistent with erythema nodosum and the skin biopsy showed underlying inflammation and mild septal panniculitis without vasculitis and occasional mast cells. The patient was started on oral prednisolone 40 mg once daily for 7 days followed by 5 mg/week reductions until down to 0 mg. Extensive work up for erythema nodosum was preformed which reviewed inflammatory bowel disease, other medications, and tuberculosis as possible causes. When the work ups were all negative, there was concern terbinafine could have been the cause. Soon after initiating the steroids the patient's liver function tests normalized as well as her jaundice, pruritus, skin rash and erythema nodosum [1A].

A systematic review of literature from 1966 to 2012 on severe acute liver injury related to terbinafine use was published. Seventeen English and three Chinese case reports were included in the review. Fourteen articles were excluded because of lack of relation between acute liver injury and terbinafine in the cases. Based on this review, it was found that acute liver injury related to terbinafine was most likely to occur in patients over the age of 40. For patients who were on terbinafine for less than 2 weeks at the time of liver injury recovered, when terbinafine was stopped. Patients that were on terbinafine for over 3 weeks required medical treatment in addition to stopping terbinafine in order to have a good outcome. Two patients in all of the included literature required liver transplantation. One patient that required a transplant was on terbinafine for 3 months and the other took three other medications that can cause liver injury in addition to terbinafine. Acute liver injury related to terbinafine use is rare, however, it can be life threatening. Therefore, terbinafine should be discontinued if liver injury is suspected while taking this medication [2M].

Skin

A 27-year-old man presented to his outpatient clinic with a red inflamed rash that first started on the lateral sides of his trunk before quickly spreading throughout his body. Upon review of his past medical history, it

© 2015 Elsevier B.V. All rights reserved.

was discovered he was taking terbinafine for 14 days for treatment of onychomycosis. He had no family history consistent with psoriasis. Upon examination vital signs were normal except a temperature of 38.3 °C. Upon dermatologic examination he was found to have non-follicular pustules with erythematous, edematous and occasionally coalescing plaques of variable sizes. His oral mucosal membranes were tender with a reported burning sensation and were found to be erythematous with non-erosive mucositis that extended from the soft palate to the pharynx. All cultures of the pustules were negative and histologic examination revealed spongiform pustules filled with neutrophils in the subcorneal region, mild edema and perivascular mixed cellular infiltrate including eosinophils in the papillary dermis. Because of these findings the patient was given the diagnosis of acute generalized exanthematous pustulosis (AGEP) triggered by terbinafine. Terbinafine was stopped and he was started on methyl-prednisolone at a dose of 32 mg/day. On the 14th day of steroid treatment, the lesions completely resolved [3A].

A 25-year-old woman with no past medical history or drug allergies who took no medications except oral terbinafine for onychomycosis presented to the clinic due to erythematous, pruritic, burning skin eruptions that presented just minutes after sun exposure. The patient had no personal history or family history of autoimmune disease or photosensitivity. Phototesting was performed which revealed an UVB-sensitive urticarial reaction, confirming the diagnosis of solar urticaria. Terbinafine was discontinued at this time since it was her only medication and therefore thought to be the cause. After 4 months of sunscreen, antihistamines and sun avoidance the patient's reactions ceased in the presence of the sun. Because terbinafine has been shown to be present in the sebum and stratum corneum for up to 2 months and the half-life for redistribution from the sebum can be 14.5 ± 8.5 days, it is possible the terbinafine can be present for months after discontinuation. This timeline would coincide with the slow and gradual resolution of solar urticaria over 4 months that the patient experienced rather than abrupt resolution. This is the first potential case of terbinafine associated solar urticaria and although extremely rare it should be of concern in any patients presenting with similar symptoms while taking terbinafine [4A].

Drug–Drug Interactions

Metoprolol

A 63-year-old Caucasian man was admitted to the hospital from his nursing home due to confusion and multiple falls that were thought to be due to sinus bradycardia and worsening dementia. Forty-nine days prior to presentation the patient was started on terbinafine 250 mg/day for treatment of onychomycosis. Additional home medications that had not been changed in the last 90 days consisted of metoprolol tartrate 200 mg/day orally, acetylsalicylic acid 80 mg/day orally, clopidogrel 75 mg/day orally, trandolapril 2 mg/day orally, atorvastatin 80 mg/day orally, furosemide 40 mg/day orally, potassium chloride 24 meq/day orally, and domperidone 40 mg/day orally. After review of these medications, it was determined that terbinafine could have been inhibiting the metabolism of metoprolol, leading to the bradycardia that developed in this patient. The proposed mechanism behind this drug–drug interaction was thought to be mediated by CYP2D6. Terbinafine is a highly potent competitive inhibitor of CYP2D6 and 70–80% of metoprolol's metabolism has been shown to be through CYP2D6. Therefore, if terbinafine was competitively inhibiting CYP2D6, there could be greater concentrations of metoprolol due to decrease metabolism, which would result in the side effect of bradycardia. Based on the temporal relationship between the terbinafine and the development of bradycardia, this interaction was graded by the authors as a 7 on the Naranjo scale, which is indicative of a probable relationship between the side effect of bradycardia and the drug–drug interaction of metoprolol and terbinafine. The patient was changed to bisoprolol, which is not metabolized through CYP2D6, and the patient's bradycardia resolved. Therefore, β-blockers such as metoprolol, carvedilol, timolol, and propranolol should not be given with terbinafine since these β-blockers undergo extensive metabolism from CYP2D6 [5A].

Perhexiline

Perhexiline is approved in many countries world wide, except the United States, for treatment of chronic refractory angina. Hepatotoxicity and neurotoxicity have been associated with chronic use of perhexiline. Because of these side effects plasma perhexiline concentrations are typically monitored closely to ensure levels remain non-toxic (<0.6 mg/L). This case report described a 63-year-old man who was on perhexiline 200 mg daily with stable levels of <0.6 mg/L for 4 months until he was started on terbinafine 250 mg daily for onychomycosis. Terbinafine was the only medication change for the patient and it was started 4 weeks prior to a follow-up appointment in which the perhexiline level was found to be elevated at 1.39 mg/L. The patient only experienced intermittent nausea as a side effect. Perhexiline and terbinafine were held and the follow-up level from 3 weeks after stopping these medications was still detectable at 0.35 mg/L. Perhexiline was then re-started at 100 mg weekly and slowly increased to original 200 mg daily without supratherapeutic levels at follow up [6A].

Pharmacogenomics

The drug interactions in the cases presented above highlight the importance of pharmacogenomics in relation to terbinafine. Approximately 5–10% of Caucasians are categorized as "poor metabolisers" of drugs that are broken down by CYP2D6 due to a genetic polymorphism that results in a lack of functional CYP2D6 enzyme. Since terbinafine is an inhibitor of CYP2D6, it has the potential to cause significant drug–drug interactions especially when used in a patient who has a genetic polymorphism resulting in poor metabolism of drugs metabolized by CYP2D6. Consideration of pharmacogenetic testing for individuals who are on terbinafine in addition to other medications that undergo significant metabolized by CYP2D6 may be beneficial in preventing unwanted adverse effects [6A,7R].

AMPHOTERICIN [SEDA-33, 542; SEDA-34, 427; SEDA-35,483; SEDA-36, 382]

Adverse Event Comparison of Available Amphotericin Formulations

The electronic medical records of 327 patients who were treated with either liposomal amphotericin (L-AmB) (105 patients) or amphotericin lipid complex (ABLC) (222 patients) were compared retrospectively to determine the difference in incidents of nephrotoxicity and other adverse events among inpatients. Patients in this study were placed on one of these two forms of amphotericin due to intolerance to amphotericin B deoxycholate (CAB). Between the patient population that received L-AmB and those that received ABLC there were no significant differences in baseline serum creatinine, exposure to other nephrotoxic agents, and total exposure to amphotericin. In the patients available for pre- and post-analysis, nephrotoxicity developed in 10.6% (9/85) of patients treated with L-AmB and 22.6% (38/168) with ABLC ($p = 0.02$). Therefore, the odds of developing nephrotoxicity were 3.48 times higher for ABLC patients than L-AmB patients (OR = 3.48; 95% CI: 1.05–11.52; $p = 0.041$). Development of hypomagnesaemia (44.3% versus 28.1%, $p = 0.033$) and infusion-related reactions requiring treatment (23.9% versus 9.5%, $p = 0.002$) were also statistically significantly more common in the ABLC group versus L-AmB, respectively. The main limitations of this study were that the patients included were only those that could not tolerate CAB and therefore may not be a reflection of all patients that receive these medications and the study was retrospective and observational and although they tried to account for differences in patient populations this is still a possibility that can affect the results. Furthermore, there was heterogeneity of the patient populations, which may lead to confounding of the results. This study provides a good addition to the available literature related to the adverse event profiles between ABLC and L-AmB. However, further studies that also review efficacy in addition to toxicity along with economic considerations should be performed to fully understand how to select the optimal amphotericin B agent [8c].

Recently, a budget impact model was created to estimate the costs associated with using amphotericin lipid complex (ABLC) compared to liposomal amphotericin (L-AmB) for the treatment of adult patients with *Aspergillus*, *Candida* and *Cryptococcus* spp. infections who are admitted to the hospital. Hospital-related cost for the drugs as well as the drug-related adverse events (nephrotoxicity with and without dialysis, infusion-related reactions, anaphylaxis, and electrolyte abnormalities) were analyzed. The estimated per-patient costs per hospital episode were found to be US$ 14 563 for L-AMB and US$ 16 748 for ABLC. Cost of adverse events accounted for 85.4% of the costs for ABLC and 68.7% of the costs for L-AMB. Because of the difference in cost of not only the medications but also the treatment of adverse events, these findings, while worth considering, need to be further investigated within individual institutions [9H].

Amphotericin Lipid Complex (ABLC)

A retrospective observation review study compared the safety and efficacy of micafungin versus ABLC for prophylaxis in liver transplant patients at high risk of acquiring fungal infections. A total of 24 patients in the study received ABLC and 18 received micafungin. The median duration of prophylaxis was 20 days in the micafungin group and 27 in the ABLC group ($p = 0.157$). Serum creatinine was found to be significantly higher at day 14 in the ABLC group compared to the micafungin group ($p = 0.04$), however, there was no difference between the groups at day 28 ($p = 0.58$). There was no significant difference in total bilirubin between the micafungin and ABLC groups ($p = 0.61$). Overall, there was no statically significant difference in mortality at 90 days between the two groups [10c].

Respiratory

A retrospective review of 32 patients who received aerosolized amphotericin B lipid complex (ABLC) (50 mg in 10 mL of saline) twice daily for adjunctive treatment of fungal lung infections in patients with immunosuppression due to malignancy or hematopoietic stem cell transplant was reported. All patients were also given systemic antifungal treatment with either an echinocandin monotherapy (22%, 7/32 patients), an echinocandin in combination with a mold-active triazole (31%, 10/32 patients), an echinocandin in combination with liposomal amphotericin (28%, 9/32 patients), or a mold-active triazole (19%, 6/32 patients). Modest cough, transient chest pain, mild bronchospasm, nausea and vomiting occurred in 9% (3/32) of patients in the study, which resolved when the aerosolized ABLC was stopped. There appeared to be minimal absorption of the medication due to the fact that there were no systemic side effects such as nephrotoxicity or electrolyte abnormalities. The side effects seen in this study are much different than those seen when ABLC is given intravenously and it is therefore important to recognize the different side effects that patients may present with when using ABLC as an aerosolized product [11c].

Liposomal Amphotericin (L-AmB)

Sensory Systems

A 65-year-old male from India was admitted to the hospital and started on L-AmB 150 mg daily (3 mg/kg/day) for treatment of visceral *Leshmania donovani*. On the 5th day of therapy with L-AmB, the patient complained of some minor hearing loss in both ears. The L-AmB was stopped on the same day the patient noticed some hearing loss and by the 10th day since the L-AmB was started the patient had complete hearing loss in both ears. Based on otoscopic examination, there were no abnormalities found; however, a pure tone audiometry (PTA) was performed and revealed bilateral sensorineural deafness of profound grade. The patient's prior and current medications were thoroughly reviewed and there were no identifiable causes for the ototoxicity except for the L-AmB based on the temporal relationship. The patient was started on oral prednisone 30 mg/day which was tapered gradually over 4 weeks and L-AmB was never re-started. At follow-up 4 weeks after completing the prednisone taper the patient had a repeat PTA with an otolaryngologist. The results of the PTA showed the patient had normal hearing both clinically and audiometrically. Although many medications have been implicated as causes of ototoxicity, this is the first case of potential L-AmB associated ototoxicity. Because this patient had underlying renal insufficiency (creatinine at admission was 3.0 mg/dL) this effect may be related to elevated concentrations of L-AmB. Another potential mechanism for this reaction could be due to the inner ear tissues relation to kidney tissues. This relationship between ear and kidney tissue could explain that ototoxicity is a result of altering the ionic homeostasis of the inner ear which results in hearing loss just like altering of renal tubular ion-transport system causes reversible nephrotoxicity in the kidney. This relationship has been described and hypothesized with other medications that cause both nephrotoxicity and ototoxicity, such as the aminoglycosides [12A].

Cardiovascular

A case of a 9-month-old girl, ex-premature of 35 weeks, was treated with L-AmB (3 mg/kg/day) for *Candida*

parapsilosis of the blood. Two days after starting the L-AmB, the patient began having episodes of short-term bradycardia which would spontaneously return to normal sinus rhythm. Cardiac examination, laboratory work-up, and ECG were all normal and without evidence of myocarditis, myocardial infarction, or cardiomyopathy. 24-hour ECG monitoring was preformed and revealed a second degree atrioventricular block Mobitz type 1 alternating with Mobitz type 2. The patient was also on ganciclovir (day 15 of therapy) for CMV in addition to the L-AmB (day 3 of therapy). The L-AmB was stopped and changed to fluconazole, and slowly over the following 7 days the number of episodes of bradycardia decreased in frequency each day, stopping completely 8 days after stopping L-AmB. At the 6-month follow-up, the patient did not report any repeat episodes of bradycardia or cardiac abnormalities. Cardiac abnormalities including toxicity, ventricular arrhythmias, and bradycardia have been reported with CAB overdoses and with conventional doses. Due to the lack of other possible causes for this bradycardia and heart block it is likely that amphotericin may have caused this adverse event [13A].

Immunology

Two patients who were receiving treatment for visceral leishmaniasis with liposomal amphotericin B reported hypersensitivity reactions during therapy. The first patient was a 43-year-old male who was started on L-AmB of 5 mg/kg daily who developed shortness of breath with clear lungs and drop in blood pressure to 60/20 mmHg and tachycardia 10 minutes into the infusion. The patient was treated with 0.5 mL of IM adrenaline with IV diphenhydramine and hydrocortisone and the patient's symptoms resolved over the next 20 minutes. The next day a subsequent dose of L-AmB was given with diphenhydramine and hydrocortisone prophylaxis, but the patient developed the same reaction and L-AmB was not re-tried again. The second case reported in this publication was an 11-year-old girl who was given a test dose of L-AmB with plans to start the patient on daily therapy for visceral leishmaniasis. During administration of the test dose the patient experienced chills and rigors, facial flushing, puffiness, chest tightness and respiratory distress. For the reaction the patient was given IV antihistamines and hydrocortisone. Because liposomes and lipid excipient-based drugs are generally recognized by the immune system as foreign it may be the actual lipid component of the drug that patients have a hypersensitivity reaction to and not the amphotericin component, especially since the reactions occurred with the first dose. Based on these findings, it is important to closely monitor first doses of L-AmB due to the possibility of hypersensitivity reactions to either the amphotericin or the liposomal component [14A].

For metronidazole, see Chapter Antiprotozoal drugs by Thurston et al.

Adverse Event Comparison of Available Azole Antifungals

The safety and efficacy of posaconazole versus fluconazole for prophylaxis of invasive fungal infections in neutropenic patients with either AML or MDS was evaluated in a multicentre, randomized open-label study in China. The most common adverse event, with similar occurrence in both groups, was liver function abnormalities which occurred in 11 patients on posaconazole (8.8%) and 6 patients on fluconazole (5%) ($p = 0.221$) [15C].

A single center retrospective study reviewed 150 pediatric patients that underwent allogeneic hematopoietic stem cell transplantation and compared the safety and efficacy of voriconazole, posaconazole, and itraconazole for the prevention of invasive fungal infections. There were no statistical differences in occurrence of side effects between the three groups; however, voriconazole had the most potential drug related adverse events ($p = 0.62$). Adverse events related to the drug occurred in seven patients (14.0%) on voriconazole, six itraconazole patients (12.0%), and in four patients (8%) on posaconazole treatment. These adverse events were of severity grades I or II. Oral antifungal prophylaxis was stopped due to side effects in 3 of the 6 cases treated with itraconazole, in 4 of the 7 receiving voriconazole, and in 3 of the 4 receiving posaconazole [16c].

A population-based study looked at the use of oral antifungal agents from 2002 to 2008 using the Taiwan National Insurance Database to assess the risk of liver injury from oral antifungals in the Taiwanese population. Of the 90 847 patients that received an oral antifungal 52 (0.06%) of them experienced drug induced liver injury (DILI). The most common antifungals to cause DILI were ketoconazole, fluconazole, griseofulvin, itraconazole and terbinafine. The incidence rate of DILI per 10 000 persons was 31.6 for ketoconazole, 4.9 for fluconazole, and 4.3 for griseofulvin. With all oral antifungals, the duration of exposure significantly increased the risk of DILI. Six patients died as a complication of their DILI and all six were receiving fluconazole therapy and were of older age (>60 years of age). Overall incidence of DILI related to oral antifungals is rare; however, it can result in fatal outcomes especially in elder patients. Therefore the risks of DILI related to extended durations of therapy, patients' age and oral antifungal agent being used should be taken into account [17C].

Fluconazole [SEDA-33, 551; SEDA-34, 430; SEDA-35,485; SEDA-36, 382]

Skin

A 1580 g female baby born at 35 weeks gestation was started on fluconazole 10 mg/kg daily for treatment of a *Candida albicans/dubliensis* urinary tract infection. Five days into treatment with fluconazole, the patient broke out in blisters and bullae on her lower abdomen and perineal area which were draining clear fluid. Initially, these blisters and bullae were thought to be due to skin tension and edema, but 9 days into treatment with fluconazole the patient abruptly broke out in more widespread skin lesions which became extensive, coalesced and malodorous with green discharge. Fluconazole and deferoxamine were discontinued at that time due to concerns of a drug related reaction. The following day her skin and oral and laryngeal mucosa began sloughing off in the sheets. The patient had to be intubated and progressed further into multi-organ failure and died 2 days after discontinuing fluconazole. Post-mortem revealed greater then 90% of skin and oral mucosa were sloughed and dermatopathology was consistent with toxic epidermal necrolysis (TEN). Case reports of TEN most likely related to fluconazole in adults have been published in the literature before. In all the cases of potential fluconazole-related TEN, the timelines of developing TEN in relation to starting fluconazole were extremely similar to the case presented here. None of the other medications the patient was receiving have been associated with TEN and the temporal relationship of when those medications were started did not quite fit with the development of TEN. Although rare, TEN appears to be a potentially fatal adverse effect associated with fluconazole use in both adults and pediatrics. Therefore, providers should be aware of this rare and serious adverse effect of fluconazole so that early signs of TEN can be promptly identified and managed promptly [18A].

Itraconazole [SED-15, 1969; SEDA-33, 552; SEDA-34, 430; SEDA-35,485; SEDA-36, 383]

A total of 128 patients who had undergone allogeneic hematopoietic stem cell transplant were randomized to receive short-term (+30 days post-transplant) or long-term (+90 days post-transplant) prophylaxis with itraconazole for the prevention of invasive fungal infections. Patients in both groups were given a loading dose of itraconazole 400 mg/day for 2 days followed by 200 mg/day and adjusted based on trough concentrations. More patients withdrew from the study due to side effects in the long term treatment group (6.78%) compared with short term group (0%) ($p = 0.05$). Drug-related adverse events occurred in 19 patients (19/121, 15.7%), including 15 with gastrointestinal (GI) side effects (15/121, 12.4%), 2 with abnormal liver function (2/12, 1.65%), 1 with hypokalemia (1/121, 0.8%), and 1 with hydrothorax (1/121, 0.8%). There was no statistical difference in drug related adverse events in the 2 arms (11/59, 18.6% in the long-term arm vs. 8/62, 12.9% in the short-term arm, $p = 0.386$). Three cases of serious adverse events were documented in the long term arm and one in the short-term arm; only one case in the long-term arm (hydrothorax) was considered related to itraconazole [19C].

Cardiovascular

The US FDA AERS reporting database was used to assess if reported cases of congestive heart failure (CHF) events related to antifungal agents are a class effect or specific to a certain medication. In addition, this study sought to determine if, based on reported adverse events, development of CHF from antifungals was related to drug–drug interactions. Based on the review of this database, it appears that CHF is not a class effect of the azole antifungals but rather specific to itraconazole and it does not appear to be related to drug–drug interactions [20H].

A case of CHF associated with itraconazole use was reported in a 60-year-old man who was on itraconazole 200 mg daily for treatment of dermatomycosis of his right lower leg. The patient had a history of acute myocardial infarction that required urgent percutaneous coronary intervention and ICD implantation resulting in a left ventricular ejection fraction (LVEF) of 30%. The patient's heart condition was stable for 6 years on medication until 1.5 months into his therapy with itraconazole when the patient's dyspnea worsened causing an increase in NYHA class from I to IV and an increase in his diuretic requirements. The patient stopped the itraconazole on his own and within a month of stopping his symptoms resolved and he was back at his baseline NYHA class of I. Worsening of heart failure is a known side effect of intraconazole that continues to be reported and therefore it is important for providers to weigh the risks and benefits in starting this medication in someone with a history of cardiovascular disease and heart failure [21A].

A similar case of a 60-year-old female who had no history of cardiovascular disease or CHF presented to her doctor with shortness of breath, swelling of her legs and bilateral edema 5 days after starting itraconazole 200 mg/day for onchomycosis. The itraconazole was stopped and the patient's symptoms resolved within 1 week without any abnormalities on her cardiac work-up, which suggested this was all caused by itraconazole [22A].

Ketoconazole [SEDA-34, 430; SEDA-35, 486; SEDA-36, 383]

Hepatic

A meta-analysis was performed to evaluate the incidence of hepatotoxicity with ketoconazole use. A total

of 204 eligible studies were included in the analysis which showed the incidence of ketoconazole associated hepatotoxicity was 3.6–4.2%. There was an increased rate of hepatotoxicity in children and patients >60 years of age at 1.4% (95% CI: 0.5–4.2%) and 3.2% (95% CI: 1.1–8.7%), respectively. The incidence was also increased 5.7% (95% CI: 4.5–7.2%) in people who used doses higher then the FDA approved instructions. Caution, therefore, should be advised when using ketoconazole in children, people over the age of 60 and in higher off-label doses [23M].

Luliconazole

Luliconazole is an azole antifungal 1% cream available for the treatment of dermatophytoses. The structure and mechanism of action is similar to the other azole antifungals.

A meta-analysis of six published randomized controlled trials reviewed the safety and efficacy of luliconazole cream. Luliconazole was not found have any statistically significant differences in adverse events when compared to other topical antifungals. No patients in the luliconazole group withdrew from therapy due to side effects and most adverse events that were reported were likely not due to the drug. The adverse events that did occur were contact dermatitis, irritation and pruritus. These events were considered to be of mild severity [24M].

Posaconazole [SEDA-33, 553; SEDA-34, 430; SEDA-35, 486; SEDA-36, 383]

Information on posaconazole can be found in the drug interactions and the general comparison of azole adverse effects sections.

Voriconazole [SEDA-33, 554; SEDA-34, 431; SEDA-35, 486; SEDA-36, 384]

Hair/Nails

A total of 152 patients who received voriconazole for at least 1 month for probably or confirmed fungal infection were asked to complete a survey regarding any alopecia and/or nail changes that they noticed while on therapy. Of the 152 patients, 125 of them (82%) reported alopecia in the scalp (96%), arms and legs (42%), and eyebrows and eyelashes (38%). Nineteen of these patients (15%) reported the hair loss to be so extensive they needed to wear a wig or hat. The alopecia was found to develop, on average, about 75 days after starting voriconazole. In the 114 patients that were able to stop voriconazole for at least 3 months hair loss stopped for 94 patients (82%) and regrowth began for 79 of them (69%) including patients who were changed to either itraconazole or posaconazole. There were no changes in nails or loss of nails reported for 106 patients (70%). Although alopecia and nail changes were not side effects that were commonly reported with voriconazole it appears it is much more common than once thought especially in patients on therapy for at least 75 days [25c].

Sensory System

A single-center, double-blind, randomized, placebo-controlled, parallel-group study of 36 volunteers who received voriconazole 400 mg every 12 hours for 1 day then 300 mg every 12 hours for 27.5 days (18 patients) or placebo (18 patients). These patients were followed throughout this time period and monitored to see the incidence of voriconazole induced visual adverse effects. Fifteen patients (83.3%) in the voriconazole group experienced one or more treatment side visual side effects. None of the adverse effects experienced were severe and they ranged from enhanced visual perceptions, blurred vision, and color vision changes, to photophobia. None of these effects progressed and became worse in severity throughout the treatment course and they were all reversible when voriconazole was stopped. The proposed mechanism behind this effect is that voriconazole may have an effect on the rod and cone pathways in the eye which may reversibly put the retina in a more light-adapted stated which leads to increased sensitivity. However, this mechanism remains a hypothesis at this time [26c].

Cardiovascular System

Cases of bradycardia related to voriconazole continue to be reported. In one case report, two pediatric patients that developed severe bradycardia that were on 12 mg/kg/day of voriconazole were described. In both cases, the bradycardia resolved within 24 hours of decreasing the voriconazole dose to 10 mg/kg/day and remained within normal limits throughout hospital admission and at follow-up. Pediatric patients on doses of voriconazole of 12 mg/kg/day should be closely monitored for development of bradycardia which may result in the need for voriconazole dose reduction [27A].

Liver

A retrospective review of patient's trough levels and incidence of hepatotoxicity was published. Thirty-nine patients were separated into three different groups depending on three consecutive therapeutic levels for voriconazole. One group was individuals with two levels <4 µg/mL (25 patients), the second was one level <4 µg/mL and second was >4 µg/mL (8 patients) and the third group had both levels >4 µg/mL (6 patients). The incidence of hepatotoxicity was greatest in the group with two levels >4 µg/mL at 83.3%, the second highest was the group with one level <4 µg/mL and second

was >4 µg/mL at 25% and the last group with two levels <4 µg/mL had an incidence of 16%. These results suggest that high trough concentrations of voriconazole may increase the incidence of hepatotoxicity and therefore it is important to closely monitor trough levels and ensure they are therapeutic but potentially less the 4 µg/mL [28c].

Skin

A 45-year-old female who had a history of bilateral lung transplant was started on voriconazole 200 mg twice daily for 13 months for treatment of Aspergillus when she noted mild erythema on her forehead and cheeks along with dryness and scaling of forearms and dorsa of her hands. Her physician thought this was most likely due to a photosensitivity reaction. Two months later, severe skin squamous cell carcinoma (SCC) lesions were noted on the dorsa of her hands. Voriconazole was stopped at this time because her fungal infection had resolved. The following year the fungal infection returned and the patient was re-started on voriconazole twice daily when 3 months into treatment she noticed a photosensitivity rash on her lower legs and forearms. About a year later, while still on voriconazole, she was noted to have six skin SCC lesions on her forehead, left hand, chest and ankles. Voriconazole was stopped and 5 months later posaconazole prophylaxis was started and continued for 12 months when she was diagnosed with parotid gland metastasis from an SCC. The patient underwent parotidectomy as well as chemotherapy, but ultimately passed away from metastatic disease. There have been reports of SCC related to voriconazole in the past; however, it is unclear if the posaconazole also played a role since the patient developed the parotid gland metastasis and aggressive skin SCC lesions while on posaconazole prophylaxis. Previous reports have shown the SCC fading after changing from voriconazole to posaconazole or itraconazole; however that was not the case in this patient. Therefore, voriconazole remains a risk factor for development of SCC especially in areas of high sun exposure and more information is needed to survey the risk of other azole antifungals [29A].

A 37-year-old woman presented to the emergency department for evaluation of severely painful bullae of her feet. The patient had been started on voriconazole 1 week prior to admission for concern of fungal infection after partial gastrectomy procedure. The patient regularly used tanning beds and continued to do so after the initiation of voriconazole. The bullae were filled with straw colored fluid and skin biopsy showed vacuolar interface dermatitis compatible with phototoxic drug reaction. Voriconazole was stopped, she was given acetic acid wet dressing and triamcinolone 0.1% cream which improved the condition. This case highlights the importance of counselling patients to avoid sun and especially artificial sun like tanning beds while on voriconazole therapy [30A] (Figure 1).

Periostitis

Cases of voriconazole-induced periostitis continue to be reported. Voriconazole preparations contain fluoride and the mechanism of this adverse effect has been linked to the accumulation of fluoride which usually results in elevated levels in patients on therapy for at least 6 months. In most cases, the periostitis and fluoride accumulation ceases once voriconazole is stopped. The EIDOS and DoTS descriptions of this reaction are shown in Figure 2.

Fluoride integrates as fluorapatite into the bone crystal structure and promotes bone formation by stimulating osteoblasts. The integration of fluorapatite into bone causes alterations in bone crystal size and structure, making these more resistant to resorption. Ultimately, this increases bone density and leads to osteosclerosis associated with brittleness, exostoses, pain, decreased mechanical competence of bone and increased susceptibility to fractures [31C].

Fluoride intoxication resembles hypertrophic osteoarthropathy and periostitis deformans, and several common features have been observed in skeletal imaging. Symmetric diffuse periosteal reactions including osteosclerosis and hyperostotic periostitis have been described together with osteoporosis, ligamentous calcification and periarticular changes; these have been located in various parts of the skeleton. Contrary to hypertrophic osteoarthropathy, voriconazole-induced periostitis is strongly associated with an elevated alkaline phosphatase and shows characteristically no digital clubbing [31C,32H].

Several etiological explanations may be considered for voriconazole-associated fluorosis. Fluorine is organically bound in voriconazole and hepatic oxidative metabolism may increase unbound fluoride levels after extensive voriconazole administration. Pharmacogenomic variations, especially polymorphisms in CYP2C19 enzyme may further alleviate this phenomena. Secondly, renal insufficiency or failure may increase the risk for toxicity during fluorine exposure, since its renal clearance is dependent on the patients renal function [32H].

Periostitis: Cases

A case of voriconazole-induced periostitis was reported in a 52-year-old woman who was started on voriconazole 600 mg/day (trough levels of 3 g/mL), for treatment of possible pulmonary Aspergiollosis. Four weeks after starting the voriconazole, there was a rapid elevation of the alkaline phosphatase (ALP) and the patient presented with diffuse pain in the shoulders, humeri, scapulae along with hypochondriac and femoral regions. Two months later, a bone scintigraphy was performed which showed multiple areas of increase radio tracer uptake in the same areas in which the patient experienced pain. MRI results as well as bone biopsy were compatible with periostitis. The voriconazole was stopped and the patient was changed to itraconazole 200 mg/day. Three weeks after discontinuing voriconazole, the patient's bone pain resolved and ALP decreased [33A].

Another report of two cases of potential voriconazole related periostitis was reported. The first patient in this case presentation was a 60-year-old woman with a

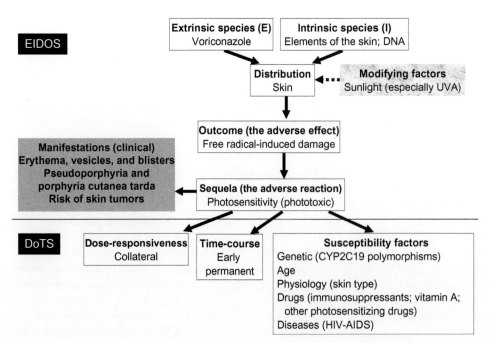

FIGURE 1 The EIDOS and DoTS descriptions of voriconazole-induced photosensitivity.

FIGURE 2   The EIDOS and DoTS descriptions of voriconazole-induced periostitis.

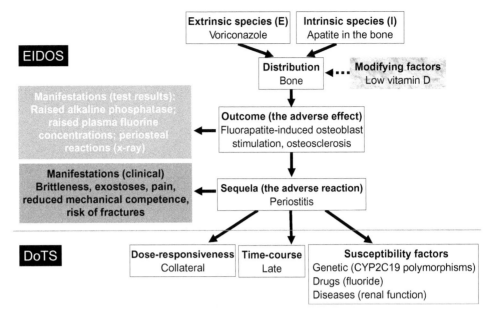

history of heart transplant who presented with a 2-week history of refractory polyarticular pain with fever and malaise. The patient had been started on voriconazole 5 months prior to presentation for prophylaxis after her heart transplant. Plain radiograph images showed periostitis of the proximal femoral shafts and humeral shafts. Voriconazole was thought to be the cause due to the time period of presentation and at 3- and 4-month follow-up after discontinuing voriconazole the patient's symptoms as well as imagining markedly improved. The second case presented within this publication was a 48-year-old man with acute lymphocytic leukemia who had undergone stem cell transplant and therefore started voriconazole prophylaxis 10 months prior to his presentation with joint pain in his elbows, ankles, knees and wrists. His bone marrow biopsy showed his leukemia was in remission and plain radiographs were again consistent with periostitis. Voriconazole was stopped given the concern it was the underlying cause of the periostitis and the patient's pain dramatically improved since stopping voriconazole [34A].

Drug–Drug Interactions and Pharmacogenomics of the Azoles Antifungals

Since many of the azole antifungals affect the hepatic cytochrome P450 system, there are a large number of drug–drug interactions with many of these agents. Because of the large number of drug–drug interactions associated with the azole antifungals, it is important to always review all medications, both prescription and over-the-counter, whenever starting a

patient on an azole antifungal. The chart below shows the extent of the interactions with cytochrome P450 system that are commonly associated with drug interactions and the different azole antifungals affect on those cytochromes.

The other important factor that affects the potential severity with these drug–drug interactions involved pharmacogenomics. As discussed briefly in the section on terbinafine, some individuals are classified as poor metabolizers or rapid metabolizers of certain cytochrome P450 enzyme systems. Depending on the patient's pharmacogenomics and therefore ability to metabolize certain medications through the CYP 450 system they may be at risk of being undertreated by a certain medication or potentially being over treated and therefore at risk for developing more side effects [35H,36R].

Voriconazole, in particular, has been one of the most difficult azoles to utilize effective dosing strategies because of the significant intra-patient variability in plasma concentrations due to nonlinear pharmacokinetics and patient characteristics such as age, sex, weight, liver disease, and genetic polymorphisms in the cytochrome P450 2C19 gene (CYP2C19) encoding for the CYP2C19 enzyme. The largest portion in variability in voriconazole dosing is the CYP2C19 polymorphisms and therefore it may be important, especially from an efficacy standpoint, to test CYP2C19 genotypes to help optimize the efficacy of voriconazole while decreasing the toxicity [36R].

A study done in pediatric patients in Japan highlight that there is a value to identifying these polymorphisms because they found there is an association between voriconazole plasma concentrations and the CYP2C19 phenotype. In this study 37 pediatric patients who had voriconazole plasma concentrations measured and were categorized as normal metabolizers, intermediate metabolizers, poor metabolizers, or hypermetabolizers based

	CYP3A4		CYP2C9		CYP2C19	
	Substrate	Inhibitor	Substrate	Inhibitor	Substrate	Inhibitor
Fluconazole		Moderate		Moderate		Strong
Itraconazole	Major	Strong				
Voriconazole	Minor	Strong	Major	Moderate	Major	Moderate
Posaconazole		Strong				
Ketoconazole	Major	Strong		Moderate		Moderate
Miconazole						

This figure highlights some of the most common cytochrome P450 enzymes that are affected by antifungals and therefore are important to be aware of for pharmacogenomics differences as well as drug-drug interactions [35H, 36R].

on genotype testing were retrospectively reviewed. Trough plasma concentrations of voriconazole were statistically significantly higher in the poor metabolizer and intermediate metabolizer groups compared with the normal metabolizer and hypermetabolizer groups ($p = 0.004$). Syndromes of inappropriate antidiuretic hormone secretion and cardiac toxicities were experienced by two patients in the high voriconazole concentration group. Dose adjustment based on CYP2C19 phenotype therefore may be useful during voriconazole therapy to improve efficacy and avoid toxicity. Japanese children, in particular, may benefit from this since they have a higher incidence of the poor metabolizer and intermediate metabolizer phenotypes as a group [37c].

Apixaban

A recent pharmacokinetic study was designed to determine the effect of ketoconazole, an inhibitor of both CYP3A4 and P-gp, on apixaban which is metabolized through both of these systems. 18 patients in the study were started on apixaban 10 mg daily and ketoconazole 400 mg daily. There was a twofold increase in apixaban exposure with co-administration of ketaconazole. Because of the bleeding risk associated with apixaban and the fact that many of the azoles inhibit CYP3A4 caution should be given when these medications are used in combination [38E].

Corticosteroids

A 48-year-old woman who was on oral budesonide 9 mg/day for treatment of Crohn's disease was started on oral voriconazole 200 mg every 12 hours for treatment of Candida albicans esophagitis that was resistant to fluconazole. Because the patient was still having symptoms after 3 weeks of voriconazole therapy, the decision was made to give her a second 3-week course. Seven weeks after initially starting voriconazole, she presented to her primary care clinic with lower extremity edema, weight gain, and elevated blood pressure. There was concern she was developing renal dysfunction so she was asked to follow-up with a nephrologist and she was given a prescription for a diuretic. Six weeks later, the patient again followed up with her primary care clinic due to further elevations in blood pressure and worsening lower extremity edema. On physical examination, by three different physicians, they all noted the patient had moon facies and posterior cervical fat pad predominance associated with Cushingoid. Voriconazole was discontinued due to the concern it was inhibiting budesonide's metabolism from inhibiting CYP3A4 and budesonide was continued at 9 mg/day. At follow-up 2 months after stopping the voriconazole the patient's physical examination as well as blood pressure and lower extremity edema were markedly improved. Although cases of iatrogenic Cushing syndrome have been described with other triazoles and corticosteroids, this is the first case with voriconazole [39A].

A 71-year-old male who was on inhaled budesonide for chronic obstructive pulmonary disease, which was recently increased to 400 µg/day, and itraconazole 400 mg/day for pulmonary Aspergillosis, rapidly developed Cushing syndrome with weight gain, increased blood pressure, moon face, buffalo hump, and suppressed cortisol levels. The dose of budesonide was lowered and hydrocortisone was started. Unfortunately, the patient passed away 4 days later from a massive myocardial infarction [40A].

A potentially similar interaction occurred in a patient on posaconazole for treatment of Aspergillus and inhaled fluticasone. The patient was a 51-year-old female with common-variable immunodeficiency and bronchiectasis who was on itraconazole for 7 years for treatment of Aspergillus fumigatus bronchial colonization. Prophylaxis was changed from itraconazole to posaconazole 200 mg three times daily after 7 years when a different species of Aspergillus was identified from her sputum. After 12 months of posaconazole treatment, she presented for follow-up due to weight gain, moon face, increase blood pressure and glucose. Because there were no other changes in her medications, it was thought that these changes were due to posaconazole and systemic corticosteroid therapy was required due to corticotrophin insufficiency [38E]. It is important to recognize and monitor for potential drug–drug interaction in patients on a triazole antifungal that inhibits CYP3A4 and corticosteroids as many of the azoles have been implicated in causing Cushing's syndrome in patients on this combination [39A,40A,41A].

Rivaroxaban

In this study, all available literature on P-glycoprotein (P-gp)-associated drug–drug interactions with the new oral anticoagulants is reviewed. Within this review, it was found that there are reports of fluconazole and ketoconazole interactions with rivaroxaban through P-gp that result in increased rivaroxaban concentrations. Because of the bleeding risk associated with rivaroxaban, providers should be extra cautious in monitoring for side effects of bleeding if this medication is used in combination with fluconazole or ketoconazole [42H].

Warfarin

INR results in patients taking warfarin and an azole antifungal were retrospectively reviewed to capture the severity of this drug–drug interaction. Of the 18 patients in the review taking the combination of fluconazole and warfarin, the mean INR increased from 1.40 to 2.94. Of the five patients taking the combination of voriconazole and warfarin, the mean INR increased from 1.95 to 2.89. The increases in INR seen in patients treated with fluconazole or voriconazole and warfarin occurred within a week of starting antifungal therapy. The six patients who were on itraconazole as well as warfarin had no observed change in INR. Based on these findings, it is important to closely monitor for elevations in INR when starting fluconazole or voriconazole with warfarin especially within the first week of therapy [43c].

Vincristine

An *in vitro* activity study of vincristine and fluconazole alone and in combination against *Candida* spp. has shown that the antifungal activity of fluconazole is enhanced in a synergistic fashion with used in combination with vincristine. This is a unique effect that may help to improve treatment of life threatening invasive infections due to *Candida* spp. However, further research on this topic is necessary since there is the potential risk of increased vincristine toxicity when this combination is given together has also been reported [44E].

PYRIMADINE ANALOGUES
[SEDA-36, 383]

Flucytosine

Flucytosine is a pyrimadine analogue that has activity against fungal species by interfering with purine and pyrimidine uptake and by deaminated to 5-fluorouracil (5-FU) and then converted to 5-fluorodeoxyuridylic acid monophosphate, a noncompetitive inhibitor of thymidylate synthetase which interferes with DNA synthesis. The most common side effects seen with flucytosine are abdominal pain, leukopenia, and myelosuppresssion. Because of these side effects, flucytosine use today is mainly limited to treatment of Cryptococcal meningitis in combination with amphotericin.

A case of possible flucytosine-induced colitis has been reported in a 52-year-old man with a history of HIV who was started on flucytosine for treatment of Cryptococcal meningitis. Ten days after starting flucytosine, the patient developed watery diarrhea. After extensive work-up and colonoscopy, the patient was found to have severe acute colitis of the colon without any infectious or autoimmune causes on biopsy. Since there was no cause for the diarrhea and colitis to be found the providers attributed to it to flucytosine and stopped the medication. Five days after stopping the flucytosine, the patient's diarrhea resolved [45A].

ECHINOCANDINS [SEDA-33,556; SEDA-34,434; SEDA-35,489; SEDA-36, 388]

Cardiac Effects of the Echinocandins

The first patient in this case series was an 81-year-old woman with a past medical history of hypertension and aortic valve stenosis who was admitted to the hospital after a motor vehicle crash. She was started on meropenem and caspofungin due to hypotension and concern for sepsis. After starting the loading dose of caspofungin, 70 mg, the patient's cardiac index dropped within 15 min from 3.2 to 2.7 L/m/m^2 and lasted for a few hours. The next day, when the second dose of caspofungin was given, this effect did not occur. The second case in this series was a 71-year-old man who had a history of chronic kidney disease, arterial hypertension and NYHA class III heart failure. He was admitted for resection of the right upper pulmonary lobe due to cavernous chronic infection. After the surgery, the patient's condition deteriorated and she was started on imipenem/cilastatin, linezolid and cotrimoxazole in addition to anidulafungin. During the administration of anidulafungin, his cardiac index dropped from 2.0 to 1.6 L/m/m^2 which required pressers and fluids to be given. This drop in cardiac index also occurred with the administration of third anidulafungin dose for this patient, but not with any subsequent doses. The third case was a 66-year-old male with ischemic cardiomyopathy resulting in NYHA class III heart failure who was admitted to the ICU for acute ischemia of his lower leg requiring amputation. A week after his amputation, he developed hemodynamic instability and was started on levofloxacin, vancomycin and anidulafungin. Fifteen minutes after starting the anidulafungin loading dose, the patient had a drop in cardiac index from 3.5 to 2.1 L/m/m². Further information in large scale trials or meta-analysis are needed to validate these effects; however, it is important to be aware of these reports to closely monitor patients who are started on echinocandins in the ICU with comorbid cardiac conditions [46A].

ANIDULAFUNGIN [SEDA-35,489; SEDA-36, 388]

Hair/Nails

A 34-year-old woman who was started on fluconazole 400 mg daily and anidulafungin 100 mg daily for treatment of *Candida albicans* that was isolated from the site of her chronic femoral osteomyelitis and peripatellar fistula. Initially, the patient was treated with fluconazole for about 3 months. However, her cultures continued to be positive for Candida, so she was started on the combination of fluconazole and anidulafungin. One month into this treatment regimen the patient complained of greater hair loss than usual. After 3 months on the combination therapy, the patient stopped taking anidulafungin because of the continued hair loss and alopecia plaques 1–2 cm in size. However, fluconazole was continued at 200 mg/day. After stopping the anidulafungin the hair loss slowed down, fragility had improved and the volume was re-establishing. Two months after stopping anidulafungin, the fistulas worsened and the patient was started on micafungin 100 mg daily in addition to the fluconazole 400 mg daily. After 90 days of micafungin and fluconazole, the patient was changed back to anidulafungin due to concerns of liver toxicity with the fluconazole being continued at the same dose. Within the first month of restarting anidulafungin, the patient did notice reactivation of the hair loss. However, over time it stabilized and then started to improve again. On the Naranjo scale, the alopecia was described as a probably relationship to the anidulafungin. Although alopecia has been reported with the azole antifungals, this is the first case related to anidulafungin treatment [47A].

CASPOFUNGIN [SEDA-33, 556; SEDA-34, 434; SEDA-35,490; SEDA-36, 389]

Eosinophilia

A 68-year-old Eurasian lady was admitted to the ICU for severe necrotizing pancreatitis and was started on empiric therapy with caspofungin for empiric fungal coverage during severe septic shock. In addition to the caspofungin, she was also started on piperacillin-tazobactam and vancomycin. Five days into therapy, the patient's absolute eosinophil count started to climb to a peak of 2.87×10^9/L. Two days after this peak eosinophil level, she developed respiratory distress with oxygen saturation of 88% along with wheezing on exam. She was started on oral prednisolone, but continued to have wheezing and low oxygen saturation. Caspofungin was stopped due to concerns of eosinophilia. After stopping the caspofungin, her eosinophil count began to slowly decrease. Two weeks later, she developed new fevers and was re-started on anti-fungal coverage with anidulafungin. Her antibiotic coverage was also changed at the time from piperacillin-tazobactam to meropenem for coverage of multi-drug resistant Gram-negative organisms. Six days after starting anidulafungin, the patient's eosinophils rose to 4.88×10^9/L and anidulafungin was therefore discontinued. Two weeks after stopping anidulafungin, the eosinophils returned to normal. Eosinophilia has been reported with caspofungin before; however, this is the first case in which another echinocandin may also have been implicated as the cause of eosinophilia. It is important for providers to stop the offending agent in a case of eosinophil to prevent accumulation in tissues which can lead to end-organ damage [48A].

References

[1] Kumar K, Gill A, Shafei R, et al. A curious case of cholestasis: oral terbinafine associated with cholestatic jaundice and subsequent erythema nodosum. BMJ Case Rep. 2014;1–3: [A].
[2] Yan J, Wang X, Chen S. Systematic review of severe acute liver injury caused by terbinafine. Int J Clin Pharm. 2014;36(4):679–83 [M].
[3] Turan H, Acer E, Erdem H, et al. Acute generalized exanthematous pustulosis associated with terbinafine: a case report. Cutan Ocul Toxicol. 2013;32(4):325–6 [A].
[4] Kuo S, Sivamani RK. UVB-sensitive solar urticara possibly associated with terbinafine. Dermatol Online J. 2014;20(3):1–8 [A].
[5] Bebawi E, Jouni SS, Tessier AA, et al. A metoprolol-terbinafine combination induced bradycardia. Eur J Drug Metab Pharmacokinet. 2014; Online, http://dx.doi.org/10.1007/s13318-014-0205-x [A].
[6] Sheikh AR, Westley I, Sallustio B, et al. Interaction of terbinafine (an anti-fungal agent) with perhexiline: a case report. Heart Lung Circ. 2014;23(6):e149–e151 [A].
[7] Meletiadis J, Chanock S, Walsh TJ. Defining targets for investigating the pharmacogenomics of adverse drug reactions to antifungal agents. Pharmacogenomics. 2008;9(5):561–84 [R].
[8] Wade RL, Chaudhari P, Natoli JL, et al. Nephrotoxicity and other adverse events among inpatients receiving liposomal amphotericin B or amphotericin B lipid complex. Diagn Microbiol Infect Dis. 2013;76(3):361–7 [c].
[9] Yang H, Chaudhari P, Zhou ZY, et al. Budget impact analysis of liposomal amphotericin B and amphotericin B lipid complex in the treatment of invasive fungal infections in the United States. Appl Health Econ Health Policy. 2014;12(1):85–93 [H].

[10] Sun HY, Cacciarelli TV, Singh N. Micafungin versus amphotericin B lipid complex for the prevention of invasive fungal infections in high-risk liver transplant recipients. Transplantation. 2013;96(6):573–8 [c].

[11] Safdar A, Rodriguez GH. Aerosolized amphotericin B lipid complex as adjunctive treatment for fungal infections in patients with cancer-related immunosuppression and recipients of hematopoietic stem cell transplantation. Pharmacotherapy. 2013;33(10):1035–43 [c].

[12] Das P, Kandel R, Sikka K, et al. Reversible ototoxicity: a rare adverse reaction of liposomal amphotericin-B used for the treatment of antimony-resistant visceral leishmaniasis in an elderly male. Clin Med Insights Case Rep. 2014;7:63–6 [A].

[13] Sanches BF, Nunes P, Almeida H, et al. Atrioventricular block related to liposomal amphotericin B. BMJ Case Rep. 2014;2014: [A].

[14] Nath P, Basher A, Harada M, et al. Immediate hypersensitivity reaction following liposomal amphotericin-B (AmBisome) infusion. Trop Doct. 2014;44(4):241–2 [A].

[15] Shen Y, Huang XJ, Wang JX. Posaconazole vs. fluconazole as invasive fungal infections prophylaxis in China: a multicenter, randomized, open-label study. Int J Clin Pharmacol Ther. 2013;51(9):738–45 [C].

[16] Doring M, Blume O, Haufe S, et al. Comparison of itraconazole, voriconazole and posaconazole as oral antifungal prophylaxis in pediatric patients following allogeneic hematopoietic stem cell transplant. Eur J Clin Microbiol Infect Dis. 2014;33(4):629–38 [c].

[17] Kao WY, Su CW, Huang YS, et al. Risk of oral antifungal agent-induced liver injury in Taiwanese. Br J Clin Pharmacol. 2014;77(1):180–9 [C].

[18] Islam S, Singer M, Kulhanjian JA. Toxic epidermal necrolysis in a neonate receiving fluconazole. J Perinatol. 2014;34(10):792–794 [A].

[19] Lin R, Xu X, Sun J, et al. Comparison of long-term and short-term administration of itraconazole for primary antifungal prophylaxis in recipients of allogeneic hematopoietic stem cell transplant: a multicenter, randomized, open-label trial. Transpl Infect Dis. 2014;16(2):286–94 [C].

[20] Hauben M, Hung EY. A quantitative analysis of the spontaneous reporting of congestive heart failure-related adverse events with systemic anti-fungal drugs. J Clin Pharmacol. 2013;53(7):762–72 [H].

[21] Vollenbroich R, Maeder MT, Weilenmann D. Congestive heart failure related to antifungal therapy with itraconazole. Int J Cardiol. 2014;172(1):e170–e171 [A].

[22] Okuyan H, Altin C. Heart failure induced by itraconazole. Indian J Pharmacol. 2013;45(5):524–5 [A].

[23] Yan JY, XI N, Tao QM, et al. Ketoconazole associated hepatotoxicity: a systematic review and emta anaylsis. Biomed Environ Sci. 2013;26(7):605–10 [M].

[24] Feng X, Xie J, Zhuang K, et al. Efficacy and tolerability of luliconazole cream 1% for dermatophytoses: a meta-analysis. J Dermatol. 2014;41(9):779–82 [M].

[25] Malani AN, Kerr L, Obear J, et al. Alopecia and nail changes associated with voriconazole therapy. Clin Infect Dis. 2014;59(3):e61–e65 [c].

[26] Zrenner E, Tomaszewski K, Hamlin J, et al. Effects of multiple doses of voriconazole on the vision of healthy volunteers: a double-blind, placebo-controlled study. Ophthalmic Res. 2014;52(1):43–52 [c].

[27] Uludag D, Ozdemir N, Tuysuz G, et al. Voriconazole induced bradycarida. Pediatr Hematol Oncol. 2013;30(7):674–6 [A].

[28] Suzuki Y, Tokimatsu I, Sato Y. Association of sustained high plasma trough concentrations of voriconazole with the incidence of hepatotoxicity. Clin Chim Acta. 2013;424:119–22 [c].

[29] Neoh CF, Snell GI, Levvey B. Lung transplant recipients receiving voriconazole and skin squamous cell carcinoma risk in Australia. Med J Aust. 2014;201(9):543–4 [A].

[30] Barbosa NS, Wetter DA. Bollous phototoxicity from voriconazole. J Emerg Med. 2014;46(3):e83–e84 [A].

[31] Lindsay R. Fluoride and bone—quantity versus quality. N Engl J Med. 1990;322(12):845–6 [C].

[32] Whitford GM. Intake and metabolism of fluoride. Adv Dent Res. 1994;8(1):5–14 [H].

[33] Hirota K, Yasoda A, Fujii T, et al. Voriconazole-induced periostitis in a patient with overlapping syndromes. BMJ Case Rep. 2014;2014: [A].

[34] Bucknor MD, Gross A, Link TM. Voriconazole-induced periostitis in two post-transplant patients. J Radiol Case Rep. 2013;7(8):10–7 [A].

[35] Ashbee HR, Gilleece MH. Has the era of individualized medicine arrived for antifungals? A review of antifungal pharmacogenomics. Bone Marrow Transplant. 2012;47(7):881–94 [H].

[36] Owusu Obeng A, Egelund EF, Alsultan A, et al. CYP2C19 polymorphisms and therapeutic drug monitoring of voriconazole: are we ready for the clinical implication of pharmacogenomics? Pharmacotherapy. 2014;34(7):703–18 [R].

[37] Narita A, Muramatsu H, Sakaguchi H. Correlation of CYP2C19 phenotype with voirconazole plasma concentration in children. J Pediatr Hematol Oncol. 2013;35(5):e219–e223 [c].

[38] Frost CE, Byon W, Song Y, et al. Effect of ketoconazole and diltiazem on the pharmacokinetics of apixaban, an oral direct factor Xa inhibitor. Br J Clin Pharmacol. 2015;79(5):838–46 [E].

[39] Jones W, Chastain CA, Wright PW. Iatrogenic cushing syndrome secondary to probable interaction between voriconazole and budesonide. Pharmacotherapy. 2014;34(7):e116–e119 [A].

[40] Blondin MC, Beauregard H, Serri O. Iatrogenic Cushing syndrome in patients receiving inhaled budesonide and intraconazole or ritonavir: two cases and literature review. Endocr Pract. 2013;19(6):e138–e141 [A].

[41] Pilmis B, Coignard-Biehler H, Jullien V, et al. Iatrogenic Cushing's syndrome induced by posaconazole. Antimicrob Agents Chemother. 2013;57(11):5727–8 [A].

[42] Stollberger C, Finsterer J. Relevance of P-glycoprotein in stroke prevention with dabigatran, rivaroxaban and apixaban. Herz. 2015;40(Suppl 2):140–5 [H].

[43] Yamamoto H, Habu Y, Yano I, et al. Comparison of the effects of azol antifungal agents on the anticoagulant activity of warfarin. Biol Pharm Bull. 2014;37(12):1990–3 [c].

[44] Kahn AA, Khurshid M, Tawfik AF. In vitro evaluation of vincristine and fluconazole combination against Candida. Pak J Pharm Sci. 2013;26(5):1037–40 [E].

[45] Sohail MA, Ikram U. Fluctosine-induced colitis. BMJ Case Rep. 2014;2014: [A].

[46] Lichtenstern C, Wolff M, Arens C, et al. Cardiac effects of echinocandin preparations—three case reports. J Clin Pharm Ther. 2013;38(5):429–31 [A].

[47] Ruiz-Ramos J, Salavert-Lleti M, Monte-Boquet E, et al. Anidulafungin-induced alopecia. Ann Pharmacother. 2014;48(5):660–2 [A].

[48] Chua NG, Zhou YP, Lingegowda PB, et al. Echinocandin-induced eosinophilia: a case report. Scand J Infect Dis. 2014;46(11):809–12 [A].

28

Antiprotozoal Drugs

Scott Thurston, Gary L. Hite, Alyssa N. Petry, Sidhartha D. Ray[1]

Department of Pharmaceutical Sciences, Manchester University College of Pharmacy, Fort Wayne, IN, USA
[1]Corresponding author: sdray@manchester.edu

INTRODUCTION

Chemotherapy for protozoal infections continues to cause adverse effects, some at doses in their normal therapeutic index. A literature search of >4300 PubMed articles was reviewed against already published data in online pharmaceutical databases to present the contents included in this year's chapter. The inclusion of the combination of trimethoprim–sulfamethoxazole and thiamine, which are non-antiprotozoal therapies, was required as these agents were used in two clinical trials treating protozoal infections. The use of combination therapies and the correlated increase in adverse events is a recurring theme this year as investigators make advances in the treatment of protozoal infections. Phase II results of fexinidazole are included in this chapter; however, it is not currently FDA approved in the United States.

ALBENDAZOLE

Methyl N-(6-propylsulfanyl-1H-benzimidazol-2-yl) carbamate

Albendazole is a benzimidazole and anthelmintic agent most commonly used in the treatment of echinococcosis (also known as Hydatid cysts) and neurocysticercosis [1,2]. It causes degenerative alterations to the tegument and intestine of worms; this leads to impaired uptake of glucose and causes a depletion of glycogen stores [2]. Albendazole ultimately causes a decrease in the production of ATP which causes immobilization and death of the worm.

Drug-Interaction

The investigators of a recent trial evaluated the effectiveness of combined therapy of praziquantel and albendazole (50 mg/kg/day and 15 mg/kg/day, respectively) in comparison to two different doses of just albendazole (15 or 22.5 mg/kg/day) in the treatment of neurocysticercosis [3C]. Praziquantel is also an anthelmintic that works by causing strong contractions within the parasite that causes paralysis and eventual dislodgment [4,5]. The purpose of the study was to determine if combining the two different mechanisms would be more effective than single agent therapy. It has also been noted in the past that praziquantel increases the serum concentration of the active metabolite of albendazole [2]. The side effects listed by the study were described as seizures, headache, pregnancy, drug-induced hepatitis, and "other" which included spontaneous abortion, urinary tract infection, motor vehicle accident, dizziness, fever, vomiting, and intracranial hypertension. While all of the side effect groups except for the drug-induced hepatitis were more common in the increased dose of albendazole or the combination therapy than in the standard albendazole therapy, the study found that the increased prevalence of adverse effects was not statistically significant. Currently, there is not a listed interaction between albendazole and praziquantel with the active ingredients of birth control.

ARTEMETHER–LUMEFANTRINE

(3R,5aS,6R,8aS,9R,10S,12R,12aR)-Decahydro-10-methoxy-3,6,9-trimethyl-3,12-epoxy-12H-pyrano[4,3-j]-1,2-benzodioxepin; 2,7-Dichloro-9-[(4-chlorophenyl)methylene]-α-[(dibutylamino)methyl]-9H-fluorene-4-methanol

Artemether is a semisynthetic derivative of artemisinin, a naturally occurring sesquiterpene lactone obtained from the Chinese herb Artemisia annua (qing hao) [6].

© 2015 Elsevier B.V. All rights reserved.

Lumefantrine is an antimalarial agent initially developed in China for treatment of *Plasmodium falciparum* mediated malaria. It is a synthetic racemic fluorene derivative (a dichlorobenzylidine) with broad schizontocidal activity, and conforms structurally, physiochemically, and mechanistically to the aryl amino alcohol group of antimalarial agents (e.g., halofantrine, mefloquine, quinine) [7]. In an open randomized controlled clinical trial comparing the efficacy and safety of three artemisinin-based combinations, the incidence of labial herpes of 3.37% occurred in the combination of artemether–lumefantrine in doses of 20 mg/120 mg respectively.

Labial herpes is also called fever blisters or cold sores. It is caused by herpes simplex virus type 1. The virus lies latent (dormant) in the body and is reawakened (reactivated) by factors such as stress, sunburn, or fever from a wide range of infectious diseases including colds [8S]. The median age of those affected was 13 years. It is thought that the adverse event reported is not due to the combination of artemether-lumefantrine; instead, it is transmitted when a child rubs their sores and then touches another person and/or through kissing [9C,10C].

DIHYDROARTEMISININ–PIPERAQUINE

Dihydroartemisinin

(3*R*,5a*S*,6*R*,8a*S*,9*R*,12*S*,12a*R*)-Decahydro-3,6,9-trimethyl-3,12-epoxy-12*H*-pyrano[4,3-*j*]-1,2-benzodioxepin-10-ol

Piperaquine

1,3-Bis[4-(7-chloroquinolin-4-yl)piperazin-1-yl] propane

Dihydroartemisinin–piperaquine is an antimalarial combination drug. In a meta-analysis including 27 studies comparing Dihydroartemisinin-piperaquine (DHA-P) and Artemisinin-based Combination Therapy (ACT) it was found that the DHA-P patients experience less side effects such as palpitations, sleeplessness, dizziness, vomiting, or nausea. However, there was low quality evidence indicating that DHA-P could have an association with higher frequency of QTc interval prolongation [11M].

FEXINIDAZOLE

1-Methyl-2-{[4-(methylsulfanyl)phenoxy]methyl}-5-nitro-1H-imidazole

Fexinidazole is a 5-nitroimidazole that may be useful in the treatment of both stages of human African Trypanosomiasis, or sleeping sickness, spread through the bite of the tsetse fly carrying either *Trypanosoma brucei gambiense* or *Trypanosoma brucei rhodesiense* [12C]. A study was completed in order to determine tolerability of a variety of different dosages and formulations. A total of 154 healthy males were used in the studies [12C,8S]. Headache was the most commonly reported adverse event followed by vomiting, nausea, and diarrhea. Other, less common adverse events include: gastro-esophageal reflux disease, abdominal pain, dizziness, flushing, increased transaminases, somnolence, regurgitation, fever, palpitations, sweating, insomnia, paresthesia, myalgia, keratitis, chest pain, dysuria, asthenia, anxiety, and dyspepsia.

FUMAGILLIN

4-(1,2-Epoxy-1,6-dimethylhex-4-enyl)-5-methoxy-1-oxaspiro[2.5]oct-6-yl hydrogen deca-2,4,6,8-tetraenedioate

Fumagillin is an antibiotic with activity in microsporidial infection and acts to inhibit RNA synthesis [13].

Microsporidia are obligate intracellular spore-forming protozoan parasites that are acquired by multiple pathways such as ingestion, inhalation, direct contact with the conjunctiva, animal contact, or person-to-person transmission and are heavily associated in individuals with human immunodeficiency virus [8S,14].

One review of fumagillin noted that significant bone marrow toxicity, not defined, had occurred in 4 patients receiving 60 mg orally daily for 2 weeks. These effects resolved within days of treatment cessation [15R,16A].

NITAZOXANIDE

[2-[(5-Nitro-1,3-thiazol-2-yl)carbamoyl]phenyl] ethanoate

Nitazoxanide is an antiprotozoal agent most commonly used in the treatment of diarrhea caused by *Cryptosporidium parvum* or *Giardia lamblia* but can also be used to treat *Clostridium difficile* infections. It is believed that nitazoxanide works through the interference of pyruvate:ferredoxin oxireductase (PFOR) enzyme-dependent electron transfer reaction which is essential to anaerobic metabolism [17,18]. Both *Clostridium* and *Giardia* can be found in almost all surface water and have been found to be extremely resistant to the disinfectants most commonly used to make water drinkable; in order to effectively protect a population from these organisms, filtration of drinking-water is required [8S]. Even in very small amounts, these organisms can cause infection.

It has also been shown that nitazoxanide may be effective in the treatment of some viruses including influenza, parainfluenza, coronavirus, and respiratory syncytial virus through the inhibition of viral replication [19C]. When used together with neuraminidase inhibitors in cells, nitazoxanide provides a synergistic effect.

A recent, randomized clinical trial examined the efficacy of nitazoxanide at two different doses in the treatment of acute uncomplicated influenza. Patients reported a variety of different adverse events throughout the course of treatment. Some of these adverse effects can likely be ruled out due to the fact that the patients were being treated for influenza; these include: rhinorrhea, nasal congestion, sore throat, cough, headache, myalgia, fatigue, pyrexia, and sweats/chills. Others, such as bronchitis, sinusitis, and otitis may be ruled out as complications of influenza; however, nitazoxanide can cause infection. Other adverse events reported by participants in the nitazoxanide group were uncommon (reported in <2% of participants) and included diarrhea, oropharyngeal pain, abdominal pain, vomiting, abnormal liver function tests, otitis media, constipation, dry mouth, and nasopharyngitis. Chromaturia was reported in 3% of patients receiving 300mg of nitazoxanide and 4% of patients receiving 600mg. These adverse events were more common in at least one of the nitazoxanide treatment groups when compared to placebo and are not commonly associated with influenza in adults.

OXANTEL PAMOATE–ALBENDAZOLE

Methyl [5-(propylthio)-1H-benzoimidazol-2-yl] carbamate

Although albendazole is the drug of choice against hookworm, it shows low efficacy at treating T. trichuria, a helminthes transmitted from the soil.

A clinical study involving 458 patients included an incident where one child who was receiving the combination of oxantel pamoate and albendazole had a case of fever and diarrhea within 24 hours of administration [20C]. While this case may be isolated, it was worth mentioning the rare, but possible, interaction.

POSACONAZOLE

4-(4-(4-(4-(((3R,5R)-5-(2,4-Difluorophenyl)-5-(1,2,4-triazol-1-ylmethyl)oxolan-3-yl)methoxy)phenyl)piperazin-1-yl)phenyl)-2-((2S,3S)-2-hydroxypentan-3-yl)-1,2,4-triazol-3-one

Posaconazole is an ergosterol inhibitor, triazole antifungal medication commonly used in Candida and Asperigillus, but it can also be used against Chaga's disease, also known as American Trypanosomiasis, which is caused by T. cruzi. This parasite can spread through both the lymphatic system and the vasculature and eventually accumulates in the muscle and ganglionic cells, most commonly infecting the heart [21C].

Posaconazole is known to cause inflammation of the mucosal tissue, called mucositis. While mucositis is often associated with chemotherapy, it can also result from the use of ergosterol inhibitors like posaconazole. An incidence was reported regarding the possibility of developing mucositis likely leading to dryness of the mucosal tissue. During a randomized trial testing the efficacy of posaconazole for the treatment of chronic Chaga's disease involving 26 patients in each study arm, the author's noted mucosal dryness in approximately 12% of the patients taking a high dose of posaconazole and 8% in patients taking a low dose [22C]. The authors found posaconazole to be ineffective in the treatment of Chaga's disease, but could potentially be used as a suppressive agent used as adjunct therapy for anti-trypanosomal treatment.

PRIMAQUINE

(RS)-N-(6-Methoxyquinolin-8-yl)pentane-1,4-diamine

Primaquine is an aminoquinoline used in the treatment of Plasmodium falciparum and P. vivax malaria and the prevention of relapse of P. vivax malaria [23,24C]. Its treatment works by eradicating the infection present in tissue; it prevents relapse by eliminating the parasite present in the blood. P. vivax is more resistant to other treatments than P. falciparum which is due to a variety of reasons including: P. vivax has a dormant liver stage that is difficult to kill, the earlier appearance of gametocytes during infection, and the tolerance of its sporogonic cycle to low temperatures [8S]. Currently, there are no other treatments other than primaquine that is effective in killing P. vivax while it is in its dormant stage. While this makes primaquine the best option for the treatment of P. vivax, it is not used often because of the risk of acute hemolytic anemia in patients that have glucose-6-phosphate dehydrogenase (G6PD) deficiency. A review article compiled information from four different studies dating from the late 1960s to 2000 in the mass distribution of primaquine in populations that have high prevalence of G6PD deficiency [25R]. Overall, it was found that primaquine was relatively well tolerated especially when taken with food. Around 2–4% of patients experienced side effects such as headache, epigastric pain, nausea/vomiting, dizziness, anorexia, chromaturia, and black urine (a possible symptom of hemolytic anemia). The study completed in Korea found that 0.1% of the treated population experienced black urine despite a higher prevalence of G6PD deficiency. The studies conducted in Azerbaijan and Afghanistan both reported <1% of patients that experienced changes in urine color. Many of the patients in Azerbaijan and Afghanistan have the Mediterranean variant of G6PD which is commonly associated with severe hemolytic reactions after receiving primaquine. The study conducted in Tajikistan did not report specific adverse effects, but stated that there were very few. Combined, the four studies treated millions of people and reported only a few cases of serious adverse effects, none of which resulted in hospitalization or death.

QUINACRINE

(RS)-N'-(6-Chloro-2-methoxy-acridin-9-yl)-N,N-diethylpentane-1,4-diamine

Prions are infectious proteinaceous particles that are thought to cause Creutzfeld–Jakob disease which is a transmissible spongiform encephalopathy [8S]. Quinacrine is an antiprotozoal drug that is also known for having inhibitory effects on prion formation. One study looked at this inhibitory effect on the prions for the treatment of Creutzfeld–Jakob disease. This study enrolled 54 patients and randomized them 1:1 comparing quinacrine vs placebo. The study found that quinacrine does not improve survival for patients with Creutzfeld-Jacob disease. Within the first two months, there was one case of severe gastrointestinal distress in a patient receiving quinacrine. Elevated liver function tests and gastrointestinal distress were the most commonly reported adverse events by patients in the quinacrine group after the initial two months of treatment [26C].

TAFENOQUINE–CHLOROQUINE

N-[2,6-Dimethoxy-4-methyl-5-[3-(trifluoromethyl)phenoxy]quinolin-8-yl]pentane-1,4-diamine
(RS)-N'-(7-Chloroquinolin-4-yl)-N,N-diethyl-pentane-1,4-diamine

Tafenoquine, an 8-aminoquinoline, is a synthetic analog of primaquine that has been around awhile but is just now entering phase III trials for the treatment and prevention of relapse in the case of Plasmodium vivax malaria. The DETECTIVE study, which evaluates use of tafenoquine used concurrently with chloroquine, and the GATHER study (anticipated), which compares tafenoquine versus primaquine, has been introduced to determine end points such as safety, efficacy, tolerability and incidence of hemolysis. Tafenoquine is not currently approved for use but has been granted breakthrough status with the FDA to expedite the process [27].

Like primaquine, tafenoquine can cause glucose-6-phosphate dehydrogenase (G6PD) deficient patients to experience an adverse effect of hemolysis [28R]. Testing for G6PD deficiencies is thus warranted prior to tafenoquine administration.

In a study of 58 healthy subjects, some common side effects include nausea (31%), vomiting (12%), diarrhea (17%), abdominal pain (9%), headache (29%), and dizziness (19%). One patient had an event that may indicate declination in visual acuity is a potential effect which spontaneously resolved. This study also indicated application site erosion (17%) where the EKG sticker was placed. This study also found the adverse effect of QTc prolongation to be clinically insignificant when administered in combination with chloroquine [24,29C].

The DETECTIVE Trial is a phase 2b study of the safety and tolerability of the combination of chloroquine and tafenoquine in a dose ranging from 50 to 600 mg for treating P. vivax [30C]. The study enrolled 329 patients where 69% reported adverse events. Notably, 3 patients in this study were G6PD deficient and none of which experienced hemolysis. While these results are positive, more studies would need to be considered before removing hemolysis as a potential threat in G6PD deficient patients on tafenoquine. Adverse events in the tafenoquine plus chloroquine groups (n=55) that differed from the chloroquine alone group (n=56) include headache (25% vs 37%), chills (29% vs 37%), pyrexia (33% vs 39%), nausea (13% vs 6%), asthenia (9% vs 0%), and dizziness (13% vs 9%). In the case of asthenia, it is thought that this reaction may not have been drug related. The investigators were not able to make an association with QTc prolongation and tafenoquine; however, they were defining QTc prolongation as more than 500 ms. While these adverse effects may be attributable to the use of the drug, some of them are also signs of the disease state being treated since malarial infections can cause headache, fever, as well as vomiting [27S, 8S].

THIAMINE HYDROCHLORIDE

N-(5-Acetoxy-3-acetylthiopent-2-en-2-yl)-N-(4-amino-2-methylpyrimidin-5-ylmethyl)formamide hydrochloride monohydrate

Thiamine hydrochloride is converted to the active coenzyme thiamine pyrophosphate by the enzyme thiamine diphosphokinase. Thiamine pyrophosphate functions in carbohydrate metabolism in decarboxylation of alpha-keto acids and in the hexose monophosphate shunt [31].

A randomized, double blind, parallel, placebo controlled trial for the treatment of falciparum malaria in southern Laos, utilized oral thiamine hydrochloride supplementation at 10mg daily for 7 days following the standard of anti-malarial care, then 5mg daily for an additional 35 days to determine if thiamine would decrease the number of adverse events experienced by patients receiving anti-malarial treatment. Of the 630 randomized participants, 27% of the subjects were considered biochemically thiamine deficient. Three percent of participants that received thiamine experienced diarrhea at some point during the 42 days of treatment with thiamine and 25% experienced dizziness on the first day of thiamine supplementation [32C].

TRIMETHOPRIM–SULFAMETHOXAZOLE

5-(3,4,5-Trimethoxybenzyl)pyrimidine-2,4-diamine; N1-(5-Methylisoxazol-3-yl)sulphanilamide

Doxycycline interferes with the third stage of bacterial protein synthesis. After amino acids are activated and attached to t-RNA (transfer RNA), the resulting amino acyl-t-RNA migrates to the bacterial ribosome for synthesis of proteins. Doxycycline binds to the 30S subunit on the ribosome and inhibits binding of the aminoacyl-t-RNA molecule [33,34].

Trimethoprim–sulfamethoxazole is used in the treatment of Pneumocystis carinii infection (called *Pneumocystis jirovecii* is a yeast-like fungus; was considered a protozoan in the past) that causes pulmonary disease in immunocompromised patients. It acts to inhibit folic acid synthesis [34].

Melioidosis, also known as Whitmore's disease, is an infection caused by the bacteria *Burkholderia pseudomallei*. This pathogen of the genus *Pseudomonas* is known to affect both humans and animals [8S].

Drug-Interaction

In a multicentered, double blinded, non-inferiority randomized clinical trial comparing trimethoprim–sulfamethoxazole to trimethoprim–sulfamethoxazole plus doxycycline for the treatment of melioidosis, three patients experienced nail bed changes as an adverse effect to combination therapy. Trimethoprim–sulfamethoxazole was administered via weight-based dosing along with doxycycline 100 mg for twenty weeks in five locations in northeast Thailand [35C]. *P. aeruginosa* paronychia has been correlated with frequent placement of the hands in water in these countries, where discoloration results from diffusion of pyocyanin into the nail bed, and therefore the interaction between trimethoprim-sulfamethoxazole in combination with doxycycline is not likely [8S].

ARTESUNATE

(3R,5aS,6R,8aS,9R,10S,12R,12aR)-Decahydro-3,6,9-trimetyl-3,12-epoxy-12H-pyrano[4,3-j]-1,2-benzodioxepin-10-ol, hydrogen succinate

Artesunate is a water soluble derivative of artemisinin. It is used to treat *Plasmodium falciparum* malaria and is considered first-line therapy [8s]. It is believed to work by creating free radicals from cleaving portions of the endoperoxide bridge and may also have other damaging effects on cATP and protein folding 36 (lexicomp). Artesunate is combined with other antimalarial drugs to avoid resistance from developing and is referred to as ACT (Artmisinin-based combination therapy). One such combination is artesunate–mefloquine therapy. Mefloquine works by destroying the asexual blood form of malaria.

In an open label, single-arm study the team of Valecha et al. evaluated the pharmacodynamics, safety and efficacy of artesunate–mefloquine combination therapy for uncomplicated malaria caused by *Plasmodium falciparum*. This was a small study with as few as 77 patients who ranged between ages 18 and 55 years old with a cure rate of nearly 100% (58/59 or 98.3; 95% CI 90.9–99.9%) [37C].

Valecha et al. reported potential adverse effects from taking a combination artesunate–mefloquine therapy including toothache, pallor, and anemia among other known adverse effects [37C]. Though these findings may seem new, the authors could not determine that this adverse effect was directly related to the drug combination and ruled it out stating that, of all the adverse events recorded, the only ones they could logically associate to the drug combination was gastritis and diarrhea. Overall, the combination therapy was well tolerated by the patient population.

MEFLOQUINE

[(R*,S*)-2,8-bis(trifluoromethyl)quinolin-4-yl]-(2-piperidyl)methanol

The indication for mefloquine hydrochloride is mefloquine-susceptible P. falciparum and P. vivax infections that may cause mild to moderate acute malaria. Malarial infections caused by P. falciparum and P. vivax may be prevented with the prophylactic use of mefloquine hydrochloride. Mefloquine hydrochloride has been linked to neurological side effects (dizziness, tinnitus, and balance problems) and psychiatric side effects (hallucinations, having the feeling of anxiousness, depression, or mistrustfulness). A five year study conducted in Denmark examined the psychiatric adverse events associated with the use of mefloquine [38R]. Patients that reported possible psychiatric side effects were assessed with SCL-90-R tool. Using the SCL-90-R, the study found clinical significance for anxiety, phobic anxiety, and depression for patients receiving mefloquine. The study found that women experienced hallucinations more often than men. The study also found that neurological side effects can become long term and sometimes even permanent side effects. As a result, the FDA has issued a black box warning about the neurological and psychiatric side effects. If a patient develops neurological or psychiatric symptoms while taking mefloquine for the prevention of malaria, the patient should discuss his symptoms with his physician and the physician should consider discontinuing the use of mefloquine and using an alternative drug [39S,40].

ACETAZOLAMIDE

N-(5-Sulfamoyl-1,3,4-thiadiazol-2-yl)acetamide

The study of Stienlauf et al. was designed to examine the interactions between chronic medications used in the treatment of pre-existing disease states and medications used for prophylaxis in patients traveling to developing countries. The study was a retrospective cohort that evaluated mefloquine, primaquine, doxycycline, atovaquone/proguanil, fluoroquinolone antibiotics, rifaximin, azithromycin, and acetazolamide to determine if there were interactions with chronic medications. This was a large study of over 16 000 individuals. Fluoroquinolones, as well as azithromycin, were shown to most commonly have drug–drug interactions with chronic medications. About 45% of study subjects were given a preventative medication that interacted with at least one of their chronic medications. Interactions identified in about 20% of the individuals were most commonly attributed to use of acetazolamide, primaquine and mefloquine. Also of note was the presence of drug allergies in patients taking acetazolamide where 8.1% of those in the study experienced a drug allergy. Further studies are needed to verify the results, but clinicians should be aware of such interactions between medicine used for travel with chronic conditions and/or maintenance medications [41r].

References

[1] Albendazole. Lexi-Drugs, Lexi-Comp Online, Hudson, OH: Lexi-Comp, Inc.; 2015. Available at: http://online.lexi.com/crlsql/servlet/crlonline Accessed Mar 14, 2015.

[2] Albendazole. DrugPoint Summary, Greenwood Village, CO: Truven Health Analytics, Inc.; 2015. Available at: http://www.micromedexsolutions.com. Accessed Mar 16, 2015.

[3] Garcia HH, Gonzales I, Lescano AG, et al. Efficacy of combined antiparasitic therapy with praziquantel and albendazole for neurocysticercosis: a double-blind, randomized controlled trial. Lancet Infect Dis. 2014;14(8):687–95 [C].

[4] Praziquantel. Lexi-Drugs, Lexi-Comp Online, Hudson, OH: Lexi-Comp, Inc.; 2015. Available at: http://online.lexi.com/crlsql/servlet/crlonline. Accessed Mar 14, 2015.

[5] Praziquantel. DrugPoint Summary. Greenwood Village, CO: Truven Health Analytics, Inc.; 2015. Available at: http://www.micromedexsolutions.com. Accessed Mar 16, 2015.

[6] Artemether. DrugPoint Summary. Greenwood Village, CO: Truven Health Analytics, Inc.; 2015. Available at: http://www.micromedexsolutions.com. Accessed Mar 14, 2015.

[7] Lumefantrine. DrugPoint Summary, Greenwood Village, CO: Truven Health Analytics, Inc.; 2015. Available at: http://www.micromedexsolutions.com. Accessed Mar 14, 2015.

[8] http://www.who.int/trypanosomiasis_african/en/ (http://www.who.int/water_sanitation_health/dwq/admicrob5.pdf) [S].

[9] Sowunmi A, Gbotosho GO, Adedeji AA, et al. Herpes simplex labialis in children with acute falciparum malaria. Acta Trop. 2008;106(1):68–71. Elsevier 2008-4. 0001-706X [C].

[10] Sylla K. Monitoring the efficacy and safety of three artemisinin based-combinations therapies in Senegal: results from two years surveillance. BMC Infect Dis. 2013;13:598. BioMed Central. 1471-2334 [C].

[11] Babalwa Z, Michael G, Donegan S, et al. Dihydroartemisinin-piperaquine for treating uncomplicated Plasmodium falciparum malaria, Cochrane database of systematic reviews, vol. 1. Chichester, West Sussex, Uk: John Wiley & Sons, Ltd; 2014. http://dx.doi.org/10.1002/14651858.CD010927. http://onlinelibrary.wiley.com/doi/10.1002/14651858.CD010927/abstract [M].

[12] Tarral A, Blesson S, Mordt OV, et al. Determination of an optimal dosing regimen for fexinidazole, a novel oral drug for the treatment of human African trypanosomiasis: first-in-human studies. Clin Pharmacokinet. 2014;53(6):565–80 [C].

[13] Fumagillin. DrugPoint Summary. Greenwood Village, CO: Truven Health Analytics, Inc.; 2015. Available at: http://www.micromedexsolutions.com. Accessed Mar 14, 2015.

[14] http://www.merckmanuals.com/professional/infectious_diseases/intestinal_protozoa/microsporidiosis.html.

[15] van den Heever Johan P. Fumagillin: an overview of recent scientific advances and their significance for apiculture. J Agric Food Chem. 2014;62(13):2728–37. American Chemical Society 2014-4-2. 0021-8561 [C].

[16] Desoubeaux G, Maakaroun-Vermesse Z, Lier C, et al. Successful treatment with fumagillin of the first pediatric case of digestive microsporidiosis in a liver-kidney transplant. Transpl Infect Dis. 2013;15(6):E250–9 [A].

[17] Nitazoxanide. Lexi-Drugs, Lexi-Comp Online, Hudson, OH: Lexi-Comp, Inc.; 2015. Available at: http://online.lexi.com/crlsql/servlet/crlonline. Accessed Mar 14, 2015.

[18] Nitazoxanide. DrugPoint Summary, Greenwood Village, CO: Truven Health Analytics, Inc.; 2015. Available at: http://www.micromedexsolutions.com. Accessed Mar 14, 2015.

[19] Haffizulla J, Hartman A, Hoppers M, et al. Effect of nitazoxanide in adults and adolescents with acute uncomplicated influenza: a double-blind, randomised, placebo-controlled, phase 2b/3 trial. Lancet Infect Dis. 2014;14(7):609–18 [C].

[20] Speich B. Oxantel pamoate-albendazole for Trichuris trichiura infection. N Engl J Med. 2014;370(7):610–20. 2014-2-13 0028-4793 [C].

[21] Kirchhoff LV, Rassi Jr. A. Chagas' disease and trypanosomiasis, In: Longo DL, Fauci AS, Kasper DL, et al., editors. Harrison's principles of internal medicine. 18th ed. New York: McGraw Hill; 2012. Retrieved March 14, 2015 from, http://accesspharmacy.mhmedical.com/content.aspx?bookid=331&Sectionid=40726978 chapter 213 [C].

[22] Molina I. Randomized trial of posaconazole and benznidazole for chronic Chagas' disease. N Engl J Med. 2014;370(20):1899–908 [C].

[23] Primaquine. Lexi-Drugs, Lexi-Comp Online, Hudson, OH: Lexi-Comp, Inc.; 2015. Available at: http://online.lexi.com/crlsql/servlet/crlonline. Accessed Mar 16, 2015.

[24] Primaquine. DrugPoint Summary, Greenwood Village, CO: Truven Health Analytics, Inc.; 2015. Available at: http://www.micromedexsolutions.com. Accessed Mar 16, 2015 [C].

[25] Kondrashin A, Baranova AM, Ashley EA, et al. Mass primaquine treatment to eliminate vivax malaria: lessons from the past. Malar J. 2014;13:51 [R].

[26] Geschwind Michael D, et al. Quinacrine treatment trial for sporadic Creutzfeldt-Jakob disease. Neurology. 2013;81(23):2015–23, PMC. Web [C].

[27] GSK and MMV announce start of phase III programe of tafenoquine for Plasmodium vivax malaria. Issued April 28, 2014. Accessed March 14, 2014 [C].

[28] Price RN, Nosten F. Single-dose radical cure of Plasmodium vivax: a step closer. Lancet. 2014;383(9922):1020–1 [R].

[29] Miller Ann K. Pharmacokinetic interactions and safety evaluations of coadministered tafenoquine and chloroquine in healthy subjects. Br J Clin Pharmacol. 2013;76(6):858–67. Blackwell Publishing Limited 2013-12 0306-5251 [C].

[30] Llanos-Cuentas A, Lacerda MV, Rueangweerayut R, et al. Tafenoquine plus chloroquine for the treatment and relapse prevention of Plasmodium vivax malaria (DETECTIVE): a multicentre, double-blind, randomised, phase 2b dose-selection study. Lancet. 2014;383(9922):1049–58 [C].

[31] Thiamine hydrochloride. DrugPoint Summary, Greenwood Village, CO: Truven Health Analytics, Inc.; 2015. Available at: http://www.micromedexsolutions.com. Accessed Mar 14, 2015.

[32] Mayfong M. Thiamin supplementation does not reduce the frequency of adverse events after anti-malarial therapy among patients with falciparum malaria in southern Laos. Malar J. 2014;13:275. BioMed Central 2014. 1475-2875 [C].

[33] Doxycycline. DrugPoint Summary, Greenwood Village, CO: Truven Health Analytics, Inc.; 2015. Available at: http://www.micromedexsolutions.com. Accessed Mar 14, 2015.

[34] Trimethoprim/sulfamethoxazole. DrugPoint Summary, Greenwood Village, CO: Truven Health Analytics, Inc.; 2015. Available at: http://www.micromedexsolutions.com. Accessed Mar 14, 2015.

[35] Ploenchan P, Chetchotisak D. Trimethoprim-sulfamethoxazole versus trimethoprim-sulfamethoxazole plus doxycycline as oral eradicative treatment for melioidosis (MERTH): a multicentre, double-blind, non-inferiority, randomised controlled trial. Lancet. 2014;383(9919):807–14. Elsevier 2014-3-1. 1474-54 [C].

[36] Artesunate. Lexi-Drugs. Lexi-Comp Online. Hudson, OH: Lexi-Comp, Inc. Available at: http://online.lexi.com/crlsql/servlet/crlonline [accessed Mar 14, 2015].

[37] Valecha N, et al. Safety, efficacy and population pharmacokinetics of fixed-dose combination of artesunate-mefloquine in the treatment of acute uncomplicated Plasmodium falciparum malaria in India. J Vector Borne Dis. 2013;50(4):258–64 [c].

[38] Ringqvist Å, Bech P, Glenthøj B, et al. Acute and long-term psychiatric side effects of mefloquine: a follow-up on Danish adverse event reports. Travel Med Infect Dis. 2015;13(1):80–8 [R].

[39] http://www.fda.gov/Safety/MedWatch/SafetyInformation/SafetyAlertsforHumanMedicalProducts/ucm362887.htm.

[40] Ritchie EC, Block J, Lee Nevin R. Psychiatric side effects of mefloquine: applications to forensic psychiatry. J Am Acad Psychiatry Law. 2013;41(2):224–35.

[41] Stienlauf S, Meltzer E, Kurnik D, et al. Potential drug interactions in travelers with chronic illnesses: a large retrospective cohort Study. Travel Med Infect Dis. 2014;12(5):499–504. http://dx.doi.org/10.1016/j.tmaid.2014.04.008. Epub 2014 May 5 [r].

29

Antiviral Drugs

Sreekumar Othumpangat*,1, John D. Noti*, Sidhartha D. Ray†

*Allergy and Clinical Immunology Branch, Health Effects Laboratory Division, National Institute for Occupational Safety and Health, Centers for Disease Control and Prevention, Morgantown, WV, USA
†Department of Pharmaceutical Sciences, Manchester University College of Pharmacy, Fort Wayne, IN USA
1Corresponding author: seo8@cdc.gov

Key to abbreviations and alternative names of some antiviral drugs

3TC	lamivudine (dideoxythiacytidine)
D4T	stavudine (didehydrodideoxythymidine)
TMC125	etravirine
AZT	zidovudine (azidothymidine)
DDI	didanosine (dideoxyinosine)
FTC	emtricitabine
SOF	sofosbuvir
TMC 278	rilpivirine
TDF	tenofovir
RBV	ribavirin

DRUGS ACTIVE AGAINST CYTOMEGALOVIRUS

Cidofovir [SED-15, 771; SEDA-32, 529; SEDA-33, 577; SEDA-34, 447, SEDA-35, 503; SEDA-36, 401]

Observational Studies

Topical cidofovir treatment in herpes simples virus infections resulted in irreversible acute kidney injury [1A]. A 58-year-old man underwent a matched unrelated donor (MUD) stem cell transplant for secondary myelodysplastic syndrome. His conditioning regimen consisted of busulfan, fludarabine, and antithymocyte globulin. The patient received oral valganciclovir during the peritransplantation phase at a dose of 900 mg twice daily for CMV prophylaxis, and prophylactic valacyclovir was initiated on day 1. The patient was readmitted within 2 weeks of his initial hospital discharge with neutropenic fever, worsening mucositis, and acute cutaneous graft-versus-host disease (GVHD). The patient was treated with intravenous (IV) acyclovir at 5 mg/kg followed by antiviral therapy containing 5% cidofovir administered as oral gel.

The patient's creatinine had increased to 1.8 mg/dL prior to the initiation of topical cidofvir. The frequency of administration of topical cidofvir was increased to three times daily, and the dose of IV acyclovir was adjusted to 5 mg/kg every 12 hours. Despite 8 days of therapy with both topical cidofvir and IV acyclovir, the oral lesions persisted; both agents were discontinued, and dose-adjusted foscarnet was initiated, and he developed progressive oliguric acute kidney injury (AKI). While receiving cidofvir therapy, the patient developed glucosuria (≥1000 mg/dL), proteinuria and hypouricemia, an indication of proximal tubule injury. Intermittent hemodialysis began approximately 2 weeks after initial treatment with high-dose acyclovir and topical cidofvir. His post transplantation course was complicated by grade IV acute cutaneous GVHD, multiple infections, acute liver injury, and persistent oral herpes simplex virus (HSV) infection. Based on the Naranjo adverse drug reaction (ADR) probability scale, it is possible that topical cidofvir was the cause of AKI in this patient.

A 52-year-old man with a history of small lymphocytic lymphoma underwent an MUD stem cell transplant. His conditioning regimen included fludarabine, cyclophosphamide, rituximab, and antithymocyte globulin. The patient had normal renal function before undergoing transplantation. He was given oral valganciclovir (900 mg) twice daily during the peritransplantation phase for CMV prophylaxis, and prophylactic valacyclovir was initiated on day 1. Patient was readmitted with perianal lesions that were positive for HSV, and the valacyclovir oral dose was increased to 1 g three times daily. Later valacyclovir was discontinued, and 44 mg/kg of foscarnet was administered IV every 8 hours and the patient had improved kidney functions. On the basis of these case reports, the authors recommend caution when

© 2015 Elsevier B.V. All rights reserved.

using topical cidofovir in patients who have the potential for high systemic absorption that could affect renal function.

A 67-year-old female was referred for ophthalmologic monitoring while receiving IV cidofovir treatment for extensive recurrent laryngotracheal papillomatosis. She underwent three laser excisions with intralesional injections of cidofovir (75 mg/mL). Due to the extension of the lesion, she was treated with IV cidofovir (dose: 4 mg/kg) every 2 weeks. The patient developed mild bilateral anterior uveitis without iridocapsular synechiae. The patient's vision decreased and the IV cidofovir was discontinued. The authors suspected that ocular hypotonia due to cidofovir was caused by lesion of the non-pigmented ciliary epithelium [2A].

The current therapy for the treatment of CMV retinitis including its limitation by drug toxicity and antiviral resistance has been reviewed [3r].

Respiratory papillomatosis patients were treated with 7.5 mg/mL of cidofovir in adjuvant therapy. Thirty one adult patients were treated with the drug and 26 (83.9%) patients showed good response and 19 cured of respiratory papillomatosis. Six patients developed dysplasia during the treatment with cidofovir [4c].

Dermatological Studies

Plantar warts are benign lesions produced by the human papillomavirus (HPV) [5c]. A retrospective observational study was reported in patients with plantar warts. Patients received treatment with cidofovir cream between July 2008 and July 2011. Patients used 1% or 3% cidofovir cream, with or without occlusion, and once or twice a day for 4–40 weeks. Study was conducted in 35 patients between the ages of 6 to 55 years. In 19 patients (54.3%), there was total disappearance of the lesions, in 9 (25.7%), the response was partial, with a reduction in the number and/or size of the warts but without complete disappearance, and seven patients showed no response. Only two patients (5.7%) reported local irritation.

A 55-year-old man with human immunodeficiency virus (HIV) and hepatitis C virus (HCV) coinfection presented with new lesions on his scrotum and perianal area. He was treated with darunavir (DRV), ritonavir (RTV), FTC/tenofovir (TDF), and trimethoprim-sulfamethoxazole. The patient was treated for HSV with a high-dose of oral acyclovir, valacyclovir, and famciclovir. However, the lesions increased, and a biopsy confirmed the original diagnosis of verrucous HSV. Given concern for acyclovir-resistant HSV, oral therapy was discontinued, and IV cidofovir treatment was started. Cidofovir (IV) caused elevations in serum creatinine levels and IV was discontinued. Intralesional cidofovir was administered every other week, and the patients lesions improved with 6 treatments [6A].

Foscarnet [SED-15 1447, SEDA-34 448, SEDA-35, 504, SEDA-36, 403]

Observational Study

A 42-year-old female solid organ transplant recipient underwent a double lung transplantation for cystic fibrosis. The recipient was CMV-seronegative and received a graft from a CMV-seropositive donor. Two months post-transplant, the patient developed CMV infection, while treatment with IV ganciclovir failed due to antiviral drug resistance, and her viral load increased. The treatment was then switched to foscarnet, followed by a second course of CMV-specific immune globulins. The viral load was reduced within 2 weeks of treatment. However, the patient developed side effect of hypokalemia, hypomagnesaemia, impaired renal function, weight gain occurred due to generalized edema, loss of appetite, nausea, and fever. Due to the severity of side effects, foscarnet was discontinued, and leflunomide administered. Consequently, symptoms and electrolyte disturbances disappeared and kidney function recovered [7A].

A case of foscarnet resistance arising from a UL54 mutation after a short duration of foscarnet exposure was reported [8A]. A 46-year-old Caucasian man with acute myelogenous leukemia, underwent conditioning chemotherapy with fludarabine and melphalan, followed by a MUD allogeneic hemaptopoetic stem cell transplantation (HSCT). Despite continued broad-spectrum antimicrobial therapy, the patient developed recurrent neutropenic fevers. He was later diagnosed with human herpes virus -6 (HHV) and antiviral therapy was initiated with foscarnet 90 mg/kg/day. During foscarnet treatment, the patient developed a diffuse, maculopapular skin rash as well as gastrointestinal symptoms, including bloating, diarrhea, and nausea.

Ganciclovir and Valganciclovir [SED-15, 1480; SEDA-34, 449, SEDA-35, 504, SEDA-36, 404]

Observational Study

18-year-old female, immune-compromised was diagnosed with lupus nephritis and treated with prednisolone and cellcept. After 7 months, she was re-admitted with acute renal failure and showed mild edema in her lower limb. Her laboratory investigations revealed hemoglobin: 9 g/dL, WBCs $3.6 \times 10/\mu$L [9], plate-let count $163 \times 109/\mu$L, serum creatinine 160 µmol/L and 24-hour urine protein 600 mg/day with normal serum aspartate aminotransferase (AST) and alanine aminotransferase (ALT) and serum albumin. Patient received 1 g methylprednisolone IV and cellcept orally. She was detected with CMV infection, and ganciclovir 200 mg IV infusion twice daily was administered, but, after 5 days, the patient developed acute liver injury. A chest radiograph showed right lower lobe consolidation and abdominal sonar revealed ascites. Ganciclovir was then stopped and liver function subsequently improved. The authors conclude from the study that ganciclovir may induce acute liver injury, thus it is important to monitor liver function while treating with ganciclovir.

A meta-analysis was conducted in patients, with lung or heart transplant recipients having CMV genotypic resistance. Patients infected with resistant CMV received valganciclovir for a median of seven months. Twelve percent (2/16) of patients were seen to be infected with ganciclovir-resistant virus upon their initial CMV infection. The other 87% (14/16) of patients were diagnosed with ganciclovir-resistant infections a median of 88 days. Ganciclovir resistance was diagnosed at a median of 8.5 months (range 5–21) post-transplant. The median duration of treatment with foscarnet-containing regimens was 38 days (range 17–210). Twenty-nine percent (4/14) of patients treated with a foscarnet-containing regimen failed to achieve serum virologic suppression. This group included three patients who died from CMV pneumonitis and one patient who recovered from pneumonitis but had persistent viremia for over seven months. The remaining 71% (10/14) of patients treated with a foscarnet-containing regimen achieved virologic suppression after a median of 23 days. Twenty percent (2/10) of patients who had virologic suppression subsequently died; one patient died of persistent CMV pneumonitis, and one patient died of allograft failure without evidence of active CMV infection. The other 80% (8/10) of patients who had virologic suppression suffered relapsing infections. Seventy-eight percent (11/14) of patients treated with foscarnet experienced toxicity, including renal injury (71%, 10/14), electrolyte abnormalities (71%, 10/14), and GI disturbances (28%, 3/14) (9 patients had multiple toxicities). One patient required hemodialysis. Foscarnet was discontinued due to toxicity in 36% (5/14) of patients. One patient treated with ganciclovir developed drug-related neutropenia that required treatment with granulocyte colony-stimulating factor [9c].

A 17-year-old boy diagnosed with CMV retinitis after chemotherapy for ALL had aggravated blurred vision, and CMV retinitis in both eyes. IV ganciclovir therapy (250 mg twice daily) was given, accompanied by intra-vitreous ganciclovir injection (0.1 mg twice weekly) and in 3 weeks the viral copies were reduced. Upon the completion of ganciclovir therapy, right retinal detachment developed, and surgery by vitrectomy and buckling with an encircling band procedure was performed. After surgery, the retinitis of the left eye improved without the retinal detachment [10A].

Neurological Studies

A 35-year-old woman infected with HIV received anti-retroviral therapy for 7 weeks and ganciclovir for 3 months. She developed CMV retinitis with varied neuro-logic complaints. Addition of corticosteroids to anti-CMV therapy improved neurological complications [11c].

A retrospective cohort study was reported in CMV retinitis patients without HIV. Ten patients with a mean age of 33.7 years were included in the study. The patients received intravitreal ganciclovir injection (2 mg/0.1 mL) alone until quiescence. Thirteen eyes with active lesions (mean best-corrected visual acuity (BCVA) of 0.51 ± 0.41) received 5.54 ± 3.36 intravitreal ganciclovir injections and were healed in 1.81 ± 1.25 months. Immune recovery uveitis was observed in six eyes (33.33%) and retinal detachment developed in one eye. One eye had recurrence of uveitis 1 month after stopping ganciclovir injections. The rest of the patients had no recurrence follow-up for 12 months [12c].

A retrospective monocentric study was performed in 547 patients undergone allogeneic stem cell transplantation [13R]. One hundred and ninety patients were presented with CMV reactivation (35%). Eighty of 160 (50%) patients presented Ganciclovir-related neutropenia, 39 patients had grade III neutropenia and 41 patients had grade IV neutropenia. The average time between the introduction of ganciclovir and the occurrence of neutropenia was 35 days (range 2–216 days). All patients with grade III–IV neutropenia (80 patients in all) received granulocyte colony-stimulating factor. Twenty-seven patients (14%) developed a CMV disease (18 had disseminated gastrointestinal colitis, two pneumonitis and seven disseminated gastrointestinal and lung disease). In those 80 patients with ganciclovir-related neutropenia, 20 patients (25%) developed concomitant bacterial infections, and 16 patients (20%) developed concomitant fungal infections. Antiviral therapy may become a potentially life-threatening complication in patients with neutropenia and CMV activation because of the risk of bacterial or fungal infections.

Combination Study

A 51-year-old woman diagnosed with HIV-1 infection was under antiretroviral therapy (ART) with TDF 300 mg, FTC 200 mg, and efavirenz 600 mg, once daily. Ganciclovir 250 mg and fluconazole 150 mg were given 14 days prior to ART for loss of appetite and dysphagia. The patient underwent left nephrectomy, for unknown reasons. She was found to have pallor, with no signs of icterus, cyanosis, lymphadenopathy, clubbing and pedal edema. A drug interaction occurred between TDF and ganciclovir. TDF concentration increased and that led to acute kidney injury. Ganciclovir was discontinued and the patient's renal function recovered. In conclusion, patients who are on TDF-based ART should avoid co-administration of ganciclovir or valganciclovir. In case ganciclovir or valganciclovir are indicated for treatment of the co-infection, then TDF may be substituted with any other appropriate antiretroviral drug, to preserve renal function [14c].

DRUGS ACTIVE AGAINST HERPES VIRUSES [SEDA-32, 530; SEDA-33, 577; SEDA-34, 450, SEDA-35, 507, SEDA-36, 407]

Acyclovir

Nervous System

A 69-year-old morbidly obese woman reported with mental status changes after she was treated with acyclovir for shingles. Acyclovir-induced acute renal injury induced her creatinine level to 7.4 mg/dL. Acyclovir was discontinued and the patient returned to the baseline [15A]. Neurotoxicity was reported in a 75-year-old lady on administration of acyclovir IV and on termination of acyclovir patient recovered from neurological abnormalities [16A].

Renal Function

A 45-year-old male with acute retinal necrosis treated with IV acyclovir developed nephrotoxicity. Switching to oral valacyclovir led to toxic hepatitis. Withdrawal of the drug resulted in return of renal and liver function to normal levels [17A].

A 58-year-old man with acquired immune deficiency syndrome on highly active antiretroviral therapy had severe thrombocytopenia when administered with acyclovir [18A].

Famciclovir

Renal Function

Efficacy and safety of famciclovir among herpes zoster patients with renal dysfunction has been reported [19c]. Fifty-three herpes zoster patients with a creatinine clearance (Ccr) of less than 90 mL/min, including nine patients treated with hemodialysis were included in the study. Famciclovir was administered to each individual according to their Ccr. No ADR were reported in the participants. Famciclovir did not alter the Ccr and did not have any AEs on renal function after herpes treatment.

Skin Lesions

Three cases of the use of famciclovir for recurrent herpes-associated erythema multiforme have been reported [20A]. A 50-year-old Caucasian woman with HSV 2 reported with herpes-associated erythema multiforme (HAEM). Mycophenolate mofetil, cyclosporine, methotrexate, adalimumab, IV immunoglobulin (IVIg), valacyclovir, acyclovir, doxycycline, hydroxychloroquine, oxycodone, hydroxyzine, and long-term

prednisone were tried, but were unsuccessful. She had red, targetoid, confluent plaques, some eroded, on her face, trunk, and extremities without mucosal involvement. The patient was given methylprednisolone 125 mg IV followed by prednisone 60 mg and famciclovir 500 mg three times daily. Patient completely recovered in 19 months.

Patient 2 was a 65-year-old Caucasian woman treated for erythematous targetoid lesions on her right lower extremity. She was treated with doxycycline 100 mg twice daily for 2 weeks, but had no effect. She failed to recover even after treating with valaciclovir 1 g daily and desoximetasone 0.25% ointment twice daily for 5 days. The patient was free of the lesions after switching to famciclovir 500 mg daily.

Patient 3, a 27-year-old Latina woman with serologically proven HSV 1 and 2 had targetoid macules and bullae of her hands and elbows and erosions of her hard palate. After valacyclovir treatment failed she was put on prednisone, but her lesions recurred. She was Cushingoid with erythematous targetoid lesions with central bullae on her fingers and erosions on her hard palate. Biopsy confirmed she had HAEM. Following treatment with famciclovir 500 mg orally twice daily, her palatal and cutaneous erosions resolved completely.

Neurological

A 67-year-old man's control of trigeminal neuralgia with botulinum toxin A injections was lost after herpes labialis and herpes zoster infection. Famciclovir treatment improved patient's trigeminal neuralgia [21].

Valaciclovir

Sixty HIV type 1 (HIV-1)/HSV-2-coinfected adults on suppressive ART were included in the study, had placebo, low-dose valaciclovir (500 mg twice daily), or high-dose valaciclovir (1 g twice daily). Valaciclovir did not decrease systemic immune activation or inflammatory biomarkers in HIV-1/HSV-2-coinfected adults on suppressive ART. One of the low dose valaciclovir administered patients showed nausea (1/20) and in high dose reported with 1 episode of nausea, headache and diarrhea. Eight patients had adverse events related to the study drug (5 placebo, 1 low-dose, 2 high-dose) [22c]. Maternal valaciclovir did not show any effect on infant CMV acquisition or breast milk CMV viral loads [23C].

Comparative Studies

A randomized trial was conducted to compare the efficiency of valganciclovir and valaciclovir prophylaxis for prevention of CMV in renal transplantation. One hundred nineteen recipients with renal transplants (recipient or donor CMV-seropositive) were randomly allocated (1:1) with valaciclovir (2 g, four times daily) or valganciclovir (900 mg daily) for 3 months. The incidence of CMV disease was 2% with valaciclovir and 5% with valganciclovir prophylaxis and more patients with valaciclovir prophylaxis developed biopsy-proven acute rejection of the renal transplant [24C].

Neurological

A 58-year-old female patient diagnosed with herpetic skin lesion treated with valaciclovir 500 mg daily. After 4 days she developed confusion, drowsiness, restless and talked irrelevantly. Electroencephalography (EEG) showed generalized slowing of brain wave activity but no epileptic discharges. Valaciclovir discontinued and she underwent dialysis. She regained normal sensorium on day 5 [25A].

Chronic fatigue syndrome presents with fatigue, low motivation, diminished mood, and reduced activity, with depression have been reported in a retrospective study in 15 adolescents and preteens treated with valaciclovir for viral disease [26c].

DRUGS ACTIVE AGAINST HEPATITIS VIRUSES

Adefovir [SED-15, 35; SEDA-32, 530; SEDA-33, 578; SEDA-34, 452; SEDA-35, 507; SEDA-36, 409]

A 64-year-old woman with chronic hepatitis B was given 3TC and adefovir, even-though her serum creatinine level was normal (<1.01 mg/dL). She developed bone pain due to Fanconi syndrome and osteomalacia and subsequently adefovir was discontinued. The patient medication was switched to entecavir, and she recovered from the syndrome [27c].

Urinary Tract

A 64-year-old man suffering polyarthralgia and bone pain had renal dysfunction, hypophosphatemia and increased levels of bone alkaline phosphatase. The patient was taking oral adefovir 10 mg/day and 3TC 100 mg/day. The patient's serum creatinine level had gradually increased after the initiation of adefovir dipivoxil administration for hepatitis B. An iliac bone biopsy revealed an abnormal increase in osteoid tissues. Reducing the dose of adefovir 10 mg to 5 mg and initiating the administration of eldecalcitol were effective for reducing proteinuria and glucosuria, and for ameliorated bone pain. This case reported to be a clinical course of hypophosphatemic osteomalacia caused by secondary Fanconi's syndrome for 8 years after administration of adefovir [28c].

A retrospective study was reported of 292 patients with Hepatitis B infection. Patients were on treatment with adefovir (10 mg/day) and 3TC (100 mg/day) for 6 months. During the duration of treatments, 28 (9.6%) patients developed renal impairment (defined as eGFR < 50 mL/min/1.73 m^2), and 73 (27.1%) developed hypophosphatemia, including 14 with persistent hypophosphatemia. Three of the 14 patients with persistent hypophosphatemia developed Fanconi's syndrome; their serum creatinine level was normal, but eGFR was lower. According to author's long-term treatment of hepatitis B with low-dose adefovir and 3TC could potentially cause renal impairment and hypophosphatemia [29c].

Adefovir dipivoxil and entecavir carry significant risks for the development of lactic acidosis and hepatic dysfunction, as discussed in this report [30A].

Antiviral therapy could lead to the emergence of mutant strains in chronic hepatitis B patients. In 147 patients, the antiviral resistance rate was 17% (25/147) for 3TC 5.44% (8/147) for adefovir, and 0.68% (1/147) for 3TC and adefovir. The change in nucleotide sequence in a particular (YMDD, YVDD, or YIDD) portion of the gene was responsible for the generation of resistant strains [31c].

Comparative Study

A phase 3, multicentred, randomized, double-blind, controlled trial compared the efficacy and safety of tenofovir disoproxil fumarate (TDF) with adefovir dipivoxil (ADV) in Chinese patients with chronic hepatitis B. A total of 509 patients, 202 hepatitis B e antigen (HBeAg) were received TDF 300 mg once daily with ADV 10 mg once daily for 48 weeks. The most common side effect reported was upper respiratory tract infection (8.2% in TDF group vs 6.7% in ADV group). Grade 3/4 ALT abnormalities were reported in TDF group (8.9%) compared with the ADV group (7.1%). The study is still continuing for 192 weeks with TDF 300 mg/daily to generate more safety data [32C].

A 50-year-old Chinese man with chronic hepatitis B and kidney transplantation received nucleos(t)ide analog therapy with sequential monotherapy and combination therapy. Patient received entecavir plus adefovir that resulted in decreased hepatitis B virus load, normal hepatic function, and stabilized CCr but resulted in multidrug resistance, subsequently the patient was administered with TDF plus entecavir for 8 weeks, which improved the hepatic function and Ccr. Compared with combination therapy with adefovir plus entecavir, TDF plus entecavir showed a potent antiviral effect for multidrug resistance and minimized renal injury [33A].

Nucleos(t)ide analogues in patients with chronic hepatitis B virus infection and chronic kidney disease have been reviewed [34R].

DIRECT-ACTING ANTIVIRAL PROTEASE INHIBITORS [SEDA-35, 508; SEDA-36, 409]

Boceprevir

Acute Pancreatitis

A 43-year-old white man with hepatitis was treated for 17 weeks with peg-interferon, ribavirin and 13 weeks on boceprevir. The patient was hospitalized with epigastric pain that radiated to his back, along with nausea, and vomiting. The patient's hemoglobin level was 14 g/L, hematocrit was 43, leukocytes were 5700 mm³, platelets 163000 mm³, amylase was 1209 IU/mL, lipase was 6462 IU/mL, aspartate aminotransferase was 34 IU/mL, alanine aminotransferase was 42 IU/mL, total Ca 9.0 mg/dL, ionized Ca 4.5 mg/dL, and triglycerides were 195 mg/dL. Peg-interferon, ribavirin and boceprevir were discontinued and the patient was placed under supportive care. In the author's opinion acute pancreatitis was associated with boceprevir [35c].

Patients with chronic hepatitis C when treated with boceprevir and telaprevir to peg-interferon α and ribavirin developed seizures [36c].

A case of red cell aplasia in a patient treated with ribavirin, peg-interferon alpha and telaprevir has been reported [37c].

HCV causing complexities in using boceprevir and other antiviral agents were also reviewed [38R].

Drug–Drug Interactions

A randomized, open-label study reported the pharmacokinetic interactions between boceprevir and RTV-boosted protease inhibitors (PI/r). The patients received boceprevir (800 mg, three times daily) for 6 days and then atazanavir (ATV) 300 mg once daily, lopinavir (LPV) 400 mg twice daily, or DRV 600 mg twice daily, each with RTV 100 mg on days 10–31, plus concomitant boceprevir on days 25–31. Boceprevir decreased the exposure of all RTV-boosted protease inhibitors with no unexpected AEs. The authors note that these drug–drug interactions may reduce the effectiveness of boceprevir co-administered with protease inhibitors [39c].

Telaprevir

Combination

Hepatitis C virus (HCV) reinfection occurs universally after liver transplantation, with accelerated cirrhosis rates of up to 30% within 5 years after liver transplantation. Dual antiviral therapy with pegylated interferon-2a (peg-IFN) and ribavirin (RBV) only reached sustained virological response rates of ∼30% after liver transplantation. Telaprevir (TVR), boceprevir, and simeprevir and the NS5B polymerase inhibitor SOF, combination therapy offers a new therapeutic option for HCV-infected patients. Three cases were reported of TVR-based triple antiviral therapy in HCV genotype 1 reinfected patients after liver transplantation, a 57-year-old Caucasian female and a 43-year-old Caucasian male were therapy naïve, whereas, a 49-year-old Caucasian male patient was pretreated ineffectively. TVR of 750 mg thrice daily were administered over 12 weeks. Initial peg-IFN and RBV doses ranged from 135–180 μg/week and 800–1200 mg/day depending on the patient's body weight. Doses of peg-IFN and RBV were adapted to 90–135 μg/week and 400–800 mg/day after 2–12 weeks of protease inhibitor therapy. Dual therapy was continued for 36 weeks with total treatment duration of 48 weeks in the therapy naïve patients. After 4 weeks of TVR based therapy, viral load decreased and became negative in naïve patients in 6–8 weeks. The pretreated patient showed a negative viral load in week 4. In the pretreated patient a breakthrough was detected in week 24 and therapy was discontinued. Side effects reported were dysgeusia and anemia leading to erythropoietin application and blood transfusions [40c].

Severe anemia occurred in one-third of patients who received telaprevir-based triple therapy. Risk was greater in patients with diabetes and advanced liver fibrosis [41C].

A 65-year-old man developed a *Mycobacterium abscessus* pulmonary infection during treatment with telaprevir, peginterferon and ribavirin [42c].

Liver Function

Three patients were treated with telaprevir 750 mg/daily for 12 weeks after liver transplantation. Side effects with telaprevir treatment reported included dysgeusia and anemia leading to erythropoietin application and blood transfusions [40c].

A 50-year-old woman was presented with diffuse, intensely pruritic pink-red combination therapy with papules on her trunk and extremities 3 weeks after starting ribavirin, telaprevir, and interferon. She also had cervical lymphadenopathy, fever, eosinophilia, and transaminitis consistent with a severe drug reaction to telaprevir. Severe cutaneous eruptions secondary to telaprevir have resulted in fatal skin reactions, including drug reaction with Eosinophilia and Systemic Symptoms (DRESS) and Stevens-Johnson syndrome (SJS), and toxic epidermal necrolysis (TEN) [43c].

Skin

A case study reported in a 50-year-old woman with diffuse, intensely pruritic pink-red papules on her trunk and extremities 3 weeks after combination therapy with ribavirin, telaprevir, and interferon [43c].

Dermatological side effects in hepatitis C infected patients treated with a triple regimen PEG-interferon, ribavirin and telaprevir have also been reported [44c].

Entecavir [SEDA-33, 578, SEDA-34, 452, SEDA-35 512; SEDA-36, 411]

Observational Study

A 44-year-old man presented with a 3-month history of myalgia and progressive weakness. He received entecavir for 5 years for hepatitis B. Serum creatine kinase levels were elevated and muscle histopathology showed abundant T-lymphocyte infiltration of muscle fibers, symptoms reduced after withdrawing entecavir [45A].

Ribavirin [SEDA-33, 578; SEDA-34, 452, SEDA-35, 512; SEDA-36, 412]

Anemia is a well-known ribavirin (RBV)-related event in HCV therapy which is exacerbated by the addition of telaprevir and boceprevir. This retrospective study evaluated and compared RBV exposure and parameters able to influence decreased hemoglobin in a large population of patients treated with dual or triple therapy. Patients on triple therapy had higher RBV concentrations (3460 ng/mL vs 1843 ng/mL). The proportion of patients with a >20 mL/min/1.73 m^2 decreased in eGFR at 12 weeks of treatment and was higher in patients on triple therapy, whereas it was 32%, 14%, and 5% for boceprevir, telaprevir, and dual therapy, respectively. There was no correlation between boceprevir and telaprevir concentrations and hemoglobin or eGFR decrease. Exacerbation of anemia in patients on triple therapy was related to higher RBV concentrations [46c].

Telbivudine [SEDA-33, 582; SEDA-34, 455; SEDA-35, 515; SEDA-36, 412]

Potential benefit of telbivudine on renal function as well as AEs were reviewed [47R].

A systematic review and meta-analysis showed that telbivudine was effective and safe for preventing intrauterine transmission of HBV [48R].

Neurological

Myopathy or neuropathy were associated with 3TC/telbivudine therapy in hepatitis B patients. A retrospective study was reported in six patients diagnosed with nucleotide analogues-associated myopathy or neuropathy and depletion of mitochondrial DNA that was responsible for the mitochondrial dysfunction in the 3TC/telbivudine-associated neuromyopathy [49c].

A long-term efficacy and safety study in a Chinese population showed that telbivudine as a monotherapy or as a combination therapy with adefovir dipivoxil in chronic hepatitis B patients had the same safety and efficacy [50C].

Faldaprevir

Faldaprevir, a first generation, second-wave protease inhibitor, in combination with a peg-interferon/RBV regimen, has been shown to increase treatment success and reduce the treatment duration [51R].

Sofosbuvir

The first global approval of SOF was granted by the US FDA on December 6, 2013 [52R]. SOF, is a potent first-in-class nucleoside inhibitor for treatment of HCV. The drug has low toxicity, a high resistance barrier, and minimal drug interactions with other HCV direct-acting antiviral agents, such as protease inhibitors or anti-NS5A agents. SOF is safe and can be used across different viral genotypes, disease stages, and special patient groups, such as those coinfected with HIV. When used in combination with ribavirin or another direct-acting antiviral agent, SOF has improved the HCV treatment spectrum for universal HCV antiviral therapy.

A multicenter, open-label, nonrandomized, uncontrolled phase 3 trial study was conducted in patients chronically infected with HCV receiving 400 mg of SOF administered orally once daily along with ribavirin orally twice daily for 24 weeks. Patients treated with SOF plus ribavirin had a rapid decrease in serum HCV within 2 weeks. Of the 223 patients who received at least 1 dose of the study drug, 7 (3%) discontinued treatment due to an adverse event. Fourteen patients (6%) experienced serious ADs. The grade 1 or 2 AEs were mostly fatigue, insomnia, nausea, and headache. Thirty-four patients (15%) had decreased hemoglobin less than 10 mg/dL with three patients reported with less than 8.5 mg/dL hemoglobin. Forty-three patients (19%) required dose reduction of ribavirin due to AEs. Overall, 32 patients (14%) experienced elevations of total bilirubin greater than 3.0 mg/dL [53C].

Simeprevir

A randomized, double-blind multicenter trial undertaken in 394 patients (aged ≥18 years) with chronic HCV genotype 1 infection and no history of HCV treatment, were randomly treated with simeprevir (150 mg once daily, orally) plus peg-interferon alpha-2a plus RBV for 12 weeks, followed by peg-interferon alfa-2a plus RBV (simeprevir group), or placebo orally plus peg-interferon alpha-2a plus ribavirin for 12 weeks, followed by peg-interferon alpha-2a plus RBV (placebo group). Treatment lasted for 24–48 weeks in the simeprevir group and 48 weeks in the placebo group. AEs in the first 12 weeks of treatment led to discontinuation of simeprevir in two (<1%) patients and one placebo patient discontinued. Fatigue and headache were the most common AEs reported in both groups. The prevalence of anemia (42 [16%] vs 14 [11%], respectively) and rash (72 [27%] vs 33 [25%]) were similar in the simeprevir and placebo groups [54C].

An open-label, phase 3 study conducted in 39 sites in 7 Europe and North America countries from September 20, 2011–August 28, 2013. One hundred and six patients with chronic HCV genotype 1 infection and documented HIV-1 co-infection were enrolled in the study. Patients received simeprevir (150 mg once daily) with peg-IFN/RBV (peg-IFN alfa-2a 180 μg/week plus RBV 1000 or 1200 mg/day depending on body weight) for 12 weeks. During the simeprevir plus peg-interferon/RBV treatment phase, 63.2% of the worst recorded AEs were grade 1/2, and 33.0% were grade 3/4. The most frequent AEs (>25% of patients) were fatigue, headache, and nausea. Six (5.7%) patients were reported with angina pectoris, increased aspartate aminotransferase, dyspnea, general physical health deterioration, hyperbilirubinemia, intervertebral disc protrusion, mental status changes, pneumothorax, and thoracic vertebral fracture. Four (3.8%) patients discontinued simeprevir due to AEs. Rash was reported in 16.0% of patients, photosensitivity reactions in 1.9%, and sunburn in 2.8%. Grade 3 hyperbilirubinemia was reported in two patients (1.9%). Grade 3 neutropenia was reported in 18 (17.0%), grade 4 neutropenia in 4 (3.8%) patients, and grade 3 anemia reported in 3 (2.8%) patients [55C].

DRUGS ACTIVE AGAINST HUMAN IMMUNODEFICIENCY VIRUS: COMBINATIONS

Fixed Dose Combination Antiretrovirals

Abacavir/Lamivudine

OBSERVATIONAL STUDY

A retrospective, multicenter, cohort study with ABC/3TC/NVP in 78 HIV-infected, ARV-naïve patients for 96 weeks were reported. One or more drugs of the regimen were discontinued in 33 (42.3%) patients. In 15 (19.2%) patients (13 NVP, 2 ABC/3TC), therapy was stopped due to toxicity. Eighty percent of them had rash/liver toxicity. Six (7.7%) patients discontinued ART due to virologic failure. The authors conclude that the toxicity was mostly associated with NVP [56c].

A retrospective, multicenter cohort study was conducted in 183 patients. Patients received 600 mg of ABC 300 mg of 3TC (fixed-dose combination) plus DRV/RTV; in >90% of patients, DRV/RTV was given in a once-daily dose of 900/100 mg for 48 weeks. After 48 weeks the regimen was DRV/RTV 800/100 mg. Of these, nine patients had dyslipidaemia, three had gastrointestinal symptoms, and two had suspected hypersensitivity due to ABC. One patient of each had the following conditions: renal failure, neutropenia, arthralgia, lipodystrophy and osteoporosis. Authors suggests that ABC/3TCplus DRV/RTV may be an effective and well-tolerated alternative regimen for naive and experienced HIV-1-infected patients [57C].

Abacavir/Lamivudine/ZDV

A systematic review and meta-analysis on virological efficacy of ABC has been reported [58R].

OBSERVATIONAL STUDY

An open-label, noninferiority study in ART-naïve patients treated with AZT/3TC and lopinavir/RTV for 96 weeks was reported. One hundred and twenty patients were randomized to receive ABC/3TC/ZDV ($n = 61$) or to continue the PI-based ART ($n = 59$). Switching to ABC/3TC/ZDV was not inferior compared with continuing the PI regimen; the difference in failure rate (ABC/3TC/ZDV) was −4.4% and +0.4% respectively. AEs leading to discontinuation of these drugs occurred in seven patients in the PI arm and in six patients in the ABC/3TC/ZDV arm. Five patients developed lipodystrophy or dyslipidemia, and one patient developed Hodgkin's lymphoma. In the ABC/3TC/ZDV arm two patients experienced hypersensitivity to ABC, one patient developed anemia, and one patient reported myopathy on ZDV, without any myocardial infarctions in either group [59C].

New Component Drugs

ELVITEGRAVIR (FORMERLY GS-9137)

6-[(3-chloro-2-fluorophenyl) methyl]-1-[(2S)-1-hydroxy-3-methylbutan-2-yl]-7-methoxy-4-oxoquinoline-3-carboxylic acid) is a potent inhibitor of HIV-1 integrase.

COBICISTAT (FORMERLY GS-9350)

Thiazol-5-ylmethyl N-[1-benzyl-4-[[2-[[(2-isopropylthiazol-4-yl) methyl-methyl-carbamoyl]amino]-4-morpholino-butanoyl]amino]-5-phenyl-pentyl]carbamate is an inhibitor of cytochrome P450 3A.

OBSERVATIONAL STUDY

A phase 3, non-comparative, open-label study was conducted in 73 patients to evaluate the efficacy and safety of switching RTV to COBI in patients with CCr 50–89 mL/min, who are virologically suppressed on a stable regimen containing RTV-boosted ATV or DRV. Serious AEs occurred in 7% patients treated with ATV or DRV and were discontinued in 10% of the patients. There were two cases of renal discontinuations and no cases of proximal renal tubulopathy reported [60c].

Elvitegravir

The pharmacokinetics (PK) and safety of COBI boosted elvitegravir (EVG/COBI) were evaluated in subjects with impaired liver function [61c]. A phase 1, open-label, parallel-group study evaluated the steady-state pharmacokinetics of EVG and COBI in HIV-infected subjects with moderate hepatic impairment versus control subjects with normal hepatic function. Twenty subjects were enrolled and 10 subjects received EVG (150 mg) plus COBI (150 mg) once daily for 10 days, followed by an 11-day follow-up period and 10 were the control group. Subjects in the hepatic impairment group reported three grade 1 AEs (mild) and one grade 2 AE (moderate), while subjects in the normal control group reported five grade 1 AEs. In summary, the study suggested no clinically relevant changes in EVG or COBI PK following multiple dose administration.

A review examined the safety data of the three FDA-approved INSTIs: RAL, EVG and DTG, and reported that the most common clinical AEs for these drugs were diarrhea, nausea and headache. DTG and COBI, a component of Stribild™, increase serum creatinine and decrease estimated CCr [62R].

The potential use of EVG for the treatment of HIV infection has been reviewed [63R].

Cobicistat

OBSERVATIONAL STUDIES

Pharmacokinetic [64R], and uses in combination with COBI [65H], have been reported.

Elvitegravir/Cobicistat/FTC/Tenofovir

A randomized double-blinded study compared the first integrase inhibitor–based single-tablet regimen combined EVG/COBI/FTC/TDF vs RTV-boosted ATV plus FTC/TDF showed AEs after 144 weeks of treatment. Twenty one subjects (5.9%) discontinued the study drug because of an AE with EVG/COBI/FTC/TDF and 30 subjects (8.5%) in ATV+RTV+FTC/TDF in 144 weeks of treatment. From weeks 96 to 144, 6 and 9 patients from

each group, respectively discontinued the study due to AE. Rates of study drug discontinuation because of renal events remained low through week 144 [5 (1.4%) vs 8 (2.3%)], including 2 subjects in EVG/COBI/FTC/TDF group and 6 subjects in the ATV+RTV+FTC/TDF group since week 96. There were no cases of PRT among EVG/COBI/FTC/TDF subjects and three cases among ATV+RTV+FTC/TDF subjects. Through 144 weeks, fractures occurred in 10 EVG/COBI/FTC/TDF subjects (2.8%) vs 19 ATV+RTV+FTC/TDF subjects (5.4%) [66r].

DRUGS ACTIVE AGAINST HUMAN IMMUNODEFICIENCY VIRUS: NUCLEOSIDE ANALOGUE REVERSE TRANSCRIPTASE INHIBITORS (NRTI)
[SED-15, 2586; SEDA-32, 534; SEDA-33, 585; SEDA-34, 456; SEDA-35, 516; SEDA-36, 415]

Abacavir [SED-15, 3; SEDA-32, 534; SEDA-33, 585; SEDA-34, 456; SEDA-35, 516; SEDA-36, 415]

An open-label, randomized study conducted for 96-week compared the safety and efficacy of ABC/3TC and TDF/FTC plus EFV in HLA-B 5701-negative antiretroviral-naive adults A total of 385 subjects were enrolled. AEs reported were decreased hip bone mineral density in both arms, with a greater decline with TDF/FTC (ABC/3TC 2.2% and TDF/FTC 3.5%; $p < 0.001$) at week 96. Patients in the ABC/3TC arm reported increased total cholesterol, high-density lipoprotein cholesterol, low-density lipoprotein cholesterol and triglycerides [67C].

Didanosine [SED-15, 1113; SEDA 32, 535; SEDA-33, 587; SEDA-35, 516; SEDA-36, 416]

A systematic review analyzed the diagnosis, pathogenesis, natural history, and management of nodular regenerative hyperplasia (NRH) in patients with HIV. The authors conclude that the NRH vary from patients being completely asymptomatic to the development of portal hypertension. There was a strong association between the occurrence of NRH and the use of antiviral therapies such as DDI [68R].

Emtricitabine [SEDA-35, 517; SEDA-36, 416]

A study conducted in 161 patients in Spain on the safety, efficacy, and persistence of emtricitabine/TDF versus other nucleoside analogues [69c]. Patients were in the age group of 50 to 55 years. One hundred and twelve patients were on emtricitabine and TDF and 49 with other nucleotide reverse transcriptase inhibitors. Followed-up for 19 months and 21.9% of subjects developed at least one laboratory adverse event of grade 3, 5.6% interrupted cART due to adverse events, and 19.3% had virologic failure. There was no significant differences between emtricitabine and TDF and nucleotide reverse transcriptase inhibitor users for any output except for longer persistence.

Lamivudine [SED-15, 1989; SEDA-32, 531; SEDA-33, 587; SEDA-34, 456; SEDA-35, 517; SEDA-36, 416]

Observational Studies

Safety and effectiveness of antiretrovirals (300 mg of 3TC and 600 mg of ABC) marketed in Japan was studied between January 2005 and March 2009 (final follow-up in December 2010). Six hundred and twenty four patients were enrolled in the study. Age group were 10–81 years, the adults (15≤ and ≤64 years) being 96.0% (599 cases) and the elderly patients (over 65 years) were 3.7% (23 cases). Two hundred and two of the 624 patients had ADRs 32.4% (202/624). The highest incidence of ADR was the metabolism and nutrition disorders (13.9%, 87/624 patients), followed by gastrointestinal disorders (4.3%, 27/624), skin and subcutaneous tissue disorders (4.0%, 25/624), hepatobiliary disorders (3.7%, 23/624), psychiatric disorders (1.3%, 8/624) and nervous system disorders (1.3%, 8/624). Serious AEs were reported on 19 patients (30 events), including two cases each of pancreatitis acute, fever, liver disorder and drug eruption. Of these serious AEs, two events (hepatic dysfunction and immune reconstitution inflammatory syndrome) reported in two patients were associated with 3TC/ABC interactions [70C].

A case report of a man with HIV infection and acquired immune deficiency syndrome was diagnosed with drug-induced pure red cell aplasia due to 3TC treatment [71A]. The patient had a hemoglobin level of 7.6 g/dL and a hematocrit proportion of 21.2%, with normal leukocyte and platelet counts. ART consist of 3TC (300 mg), EFV (600 mg) and ABC (600 mg). 3TC treatment was discontinued and D4T was added in the ART. Subsequently the patient's hemoglobin concentration and hematocrit level returned to normal. This case indicated that 3TC can induce severe anemia without the influence of AZT.

A meta-analysis of randomized trials comparing the efficacy of 3TC and FTC reported that the two drugs are clinically equivalent [72R].

Stavudine (D4T) [SED-15, 3180; SEDA-32, 535; SEDA-33, 587; SEDA-34, 456, SEDA-35, 517; SEDA-36, 417]

Metabolic complication [73R], and neurological and psychiatric AEs from D4T were reviewed [74R].

Observational Studies

In a cross sectional study, 203 HIV-infected Malawian adult patients on D4T-containing ART and 64 healthy controls, on standard first-line D4T containing ART, for at least 6 months, were recruited. The D4T related AEs reported were peripheral neuropathy in 21% (43/203), lipodystrophy in 18% (20/112) and elevated lactate level (>2.5 mmol/L) in 17% (19/113). They studied mitochondrial DNA as a biomarker for the toxicity of D4T, and suggested the use of peripheral blood mtDNA/nDNA ratio as a marker of mitochondrial toxicities of D4T [75c].

A cross sectional study in India was conducted on 80 HIV infected children aged 2–18 years of age who were on D4T based HAART (protease inhibitors, D4T and NVP) for ≥2 years. Lipodystrophy was observed in 33.7% of children followed by lipohypertrophy was the result of long duration HAART [76c].

Zidovudine [SED-15, 3713; SEDA-32, 536; SEDA-33, 588; SEDA-34, 458; SEDA-35, 517; SEDA-36, 417]

In an experimental study, AZT-induced oxidative stress selectively down regulated mitochondrial thymidine kinase 2 and deoxyguanosine kinase, leading to decreased mitochondrial DNA precursor pools. The authors suggests that these enzymes have significant implications for the regulation of mitochondrial nucleotide biosynthesis and antiviral therapy [77E].

A study in 195 HIV patients from China were switched from AZT/D4T+DDI+NVP to 3TC+TDF and LPV+RTV resulted in less multidrug resistant mutation [78c].

Anemia appeared to be marginally increased among children ($p = 0.05$) treated with AZT [79c].

DRUGS ACTIVE AGAINST HUMAN IMMUNODEFICIENCY VIRUS: NUCLEOTIDE ANALOGUE REVERSE TRANSCRIPTASE INHIBITORS

Tenofovir [SED-15, 3314; SEDA-32, 537; SEDA-33, 588; SEDA-34, 458; SEDA-35, 518; SEDA-36, 418]

A Phase 2, double-blind, double-dummy, multicenter, active-controlled study in antiretroviral naive adults with

HIV-1 (RNA 5000 copies per milliliter and a CD4 count 50 cells per microliter) were randomized, 2:1 to receive an STR of EVG/COBI/FTC/tenofovir alafenamide (EVG/COBI/FTC/TAF) or EVG/COBI/FTC/TDF, plus placebo for 48 weeks. Mild to moderate AEs reported in both treatments. Patients on EVG/COBI/FTC/TAF had higher increases in total cholesterol, low-density lipoprotein, and high-density lipoprotein [80c].

Over a 9-year period (2001–2010), a total of 407 category II Yellow Card reports (Medicines and Healthcare Products Regulatory Agency) of patients with suspected kidney related ADRs due to TDF were reviewed. Among the 106 reports analyzed, 53 (50%) had features of kidney tubular dysfunction, 35 (33%) had glomerular dysfunction and 18 (17%) had Fanconi syndrome. Of the 106 patients, 33 (31.4%) patients required hospitalization due to TDF-related kidney effects with a mortality of 18.2% (6 out of 33 patients) [81M].

Long-term kidney toxicity as a modest but significant risk for TDF-containing regimens [82R].

DRUGS ACTIVE AGAINST HUMAN IMMUNODEFICIENCY VIRUS: NON-NUCLEOSIDE REVERSE TRANSCRIPTASE INHIBITORS (NNRTI) [SED-15, 2553; SEDA-31, 486; SEDA-32, 537; SEDA-33, 590; SED-34, 459; SEDA-35, 519; SEDA-36, 420]

Efavirenz [SED-15, 1204; SEDA-32, 537; SEDA-33, 590; SEDA 34, 459; SEDA-35, 519; SEDA-36, 420]

Observational Studies

In a retrospective cohort study, 3089 adults received a fixed dose combination of D4T, 3TC and NVP. A total of 180 (5.8%) individuals discontinued efavirenz or NVP due to severe liver toxicity. The risk was highest in co-infected patients treated with NVP (11.3% for HBV and 15.2% for HCV), compared to 8.0% for HBV and 6.9% for HCV co-infected individuals treated with efavirenz. One hundred and eighty two patients discontinued ART due to skin rash [83C].

Genetic Variation

Inter-individual variability in plasma efavirenz concentrations has been reported in 800 patients from Ghana with confirmed HIV infection. Efavirenz was administered orally as a single fixed dose of 600 mg daily for 24 months. Five hundred and seventy-eight (72.3%) patients were on antiretroviral therapy, while 222 (27.8%) were antiretroviral therapy naive at the time of sampling. Genotyping for the allelic discrimination was done from the genomic DNA isolated from

patient's serum. Plasma concentration of efavirenz was depends on the variation in allele CYP2B6 gene. In conclusion, CYP2B6 and CYP2A6 SNPs were associated with higher plasma efavirenz concentrations due to reduction in major and minor phase I routes of elimination [84C].

A prospective study reported on the use of ART containing efavirenz in pregnant women in Rio de Janeiro, Brazil and the incidence of ADR were discussed [85C].

Etravirine [SEDA-33, 592; SEDA-34, 459; SEDA-35, 520; SEDA-36, 421]

A combination of TMC125 plus RAL treatment in 24 patients for 48 weeks did not cause any drug interactions and no liver toxicity [86c].

A 46-year-old HIV-positive patient with BEACOPP chemotherapy for advanced Hodgkin's lymphoma, switched from DRV, TDF and FTC to TMC125 (200 mg BID)+RAL (400 mg BID)+FTC (200 mg QD)+TDF (300 mg QD) showed less drug–drug interactions [87c].

Nevirapine [SEDA-33, 593; SEDA-34, 460; SEDA-35, 521; SEDA-36, 421]

Pharmacokinetics and pharmacodynamics of the antiviral drugs affecting the nervous system was discussed in this review [88R].

Comparative Study

A systematic review and meta-analysis on the use of nevirapine versus efavirenz for patients co-infected with HIV and tuberculosis has been reported [89R]. This meta-analysis compared five randomized clinical trials and four retrospective clinical trials. Eight hundred and thirty three patients received nevirapine, and 1424 received efavirenz, including patients co-infected with HIV and TB. NVP-based regimens showed higher AEs and were discontinued more frequently than efavirenz.

Observational Study

A longitudinal prospective cohort study was conducted in Rwandan children infected with HIV. HIV-infected 183 cART-naïve children below 15 years of age initiated cART between March 2008 and December 2009 were included in the study and monitored for 18 months. cART regimen was NVP, efavirenz, or protease-inhibitor based. The most common side effects reported were nausea and vomiting (14.8%), NVP-associated skin rash and hypersensitivity (13.2%), anemia

(7%), diarrhea (6%), and dizziness and fatigue (5%). Most of the symptoms were reversed after discontinuation of NVP [90C].

Rilpivirine [SEDA-35, 521; SEDA-36, 423]

The effectiveness and safety of TMC 278 in treatment-naive adults infected with HIV-1 has been reported. Randomized controlled trials from multiple databases on the effectiveness and safety of TMC 278 in treatment-naive adults infected with HIV-1 was collected. The data analysis included the four randomized controlled trials with a total of 2522 patients. TMC 278 demonstrated noninferior antiviral efficacy in viral load and baseline CD4 count. TMC 278 showed significantly higher difference in virological failure rates compared with the efavirenz group. The most commonly reported AEs were rash and neurological events, which were lower with TMC 278 than efavirenz (RR, 0.11; 95% CI, 0.03–0.33; RR, 0.52; 95% CI, 0.45–0.60, respectively) [91C].

Liver toxicity in HIV-infected patients receiving TMC125 and TMC 278 has been reported in this review [92R]. According to the authors both TMC125 and TMC 278 are safe to be used in patients with liver abnormalities.

DRUGS ACTIVE AGAINST HUMAN IMMUNODEFICIENCY VIRUS: PROTEASE INHIBITORS [SED-15, 2586; SEDA-32, 541; SEDA-33, 593; SEDA-34, 461, SEDA-35, 522; SEDA-36, 423]

Fosamprenavir/Amprenavir

An open-label study reported on the drug–drug interaction of fosamprenavir (FPV)-RTV on DTG PK parameters, in 12 healthy subjects with a mean age of 33.4 years. All patients received 50 mg DTG daily for 5 days and were on a regimen of 50 mg DTG every 24 hours in combination with 700/100 mg FPV-RTV every 12 hours for 10 days. No deaths or serious AEs occurred. Abnormal dreams were reported by 2 subjects. Rash was reported by 2 subjects (17%) who were receiving both DTG and FPV-RTV [93c].

Experimental Study

Chronic effects of antiretrovirals (3TC, D4T, delavirdine, nelfinavir, amprenavir and LPV/RTV) of 3 or 9 times doses were given to pregnant albino rats. D4T increased maternal weight ($p = 0.001$), while 3TC at 3 and 9-time doses reduced maternal weight. Higher rates of maternal death were reported with amprenavir at all of the doses, and LPV/RTV at 3- and 9-times doses. None of the antiretroviral drugs studied were harmful to the fetuses with regard to implantation, reabsorption, teratogenity and mortality. D4T at all doses reduced the litter weights ($p < 0.001$); however, 3TC, delavirdine, and amprenavir all at 3-times dose increased the litter weight [94E].

Atazanavir

A phase 3, randomized, open-label study reported the efficacy and tolerability of 3 non-nucleoside reverse transcriptase inhibitor-sparing antiretroviral regimens for treatment-naïve volunteers infected with HIV-1 in a 1:1:1 ratio. Follow-up were done for at least 96 weeks. Of the three inhibitor studies, RAL treatment was superior to the other two inhibitors [95c].

The efficacy of abacavir/3TC+ATV (ABC/3TC +ATV) to TDF/FTC+ATV/RTV in a population, HIV-1 infected patients over a period of 24 weeks were reported [96C]. After 24 weeks, ABC/3TC+ATV ($n = 199$) was found to be noninferior to TDF/FTC +ATV/RTV ($n = 97$) by both the primary analyses (87% in both groups) and all secondary efficacy analysis. Fasting HDL was increased from the baseline levels for the ABC/3TC+ATV group compared to the TDF/3TC +ATV/RTV group. Rates of AEs were of moderate or greater severity (grade 2–4) between the two groups (40% [79/199] for ABC/3TC+ATV and 37% [36/97] for TDF/FTC+ATV/RTV), with only upper respiratory tract infection observed in ≥5% of patients in either treatment group (4% [5/199] for ABC/3TC+ATV and 6% [6/97] for TDF/FTC+ATV/RTV). There were few grade 2–4 treatment-related AEs in either group (8% [16/199] for ABC/3TC+ATV and 5% [6/97] for TDF/ FTC+ATV/r). In the TDF/FTC+ATV/RTV group, one patient had grade 2 palpitations. In the ABC/3TC +ATV group, two patients had grade 2 cardiomyopathy, one patient had grade 2 coronary artery disease, and one patient had a grade 4 acute inferior myocardial infarction.

A drug interaction study showed that RTV was responsible for the adverse interactions that occurred when telaprevir and ATV were administered together [97A].

A systematic review suggests that RTV-boosted ATV appears to be a safe, effective and durable option for treatment-naive and early treatment-experienced HIV-1 patients, including non-pregnant and pregnant women [98R].

Another study indicates that some of the AEs associated with ARV use may be mediated through 'off-target' effects involving nuclear receptor activation. ARV drugs activate pregnane X receptors and constitutive androstane receptors, increasing the risk of drug interactions due to altered drug metabolism and disposition. The closely related liver X receptors (LXRα/β), estrogen receptors (ERα/β) and glucocorticoid receptor (GR) regulate many endogenous processes such as lipid/cholesterol homeostasis, cellular differentiation and inflammation. ATV and RTV activated LXRα/β, while tipranavir enhanced transcriptional activity of ERα. Direct ligand-binding domains interact with LXRα and/or LXRβ were confirmed in vitro studies for DRV, efavirenz, flavopiridol, maraviroc and tipranavir. Likewise, efavirenz was also predicted and confirmed as a ligand of ERα-LBD [99E].

Darunavir

In a randomized clinical trial, 178 patients received once-daily ATV/RTV ($n=90$) or DRV/RTV ($n=88$) plus TDF/FTC. After 24 weeks, the mean cholesterol levels had increased (7.26 and 11.47 mg/dL in the ATV/RTV and DRV/RTV arms). However, the ratio of total to HDL cholesterol decreased in patients treated with ATV/RTV compared to DRV/RTV [100C].

In another study, sixteen HIV-1-infected pregnant women were enrolled and received DRV/RTV 600/100 mg. The pharmacokinetic plasma concentration of total DRV during the second and third trimesters in the pregnant woman was 28% and 19% lower than the postpartum, and the total RTV plasma concentrations were higher during the postpartum period compared with the second and third trimesters of pregnancy. The most common AEs, were infections and infestations (44%), gastrointestinal disorders (25%) and premature labor (25%). Of 12 infants, four were born prematurely (at weeks 30, 36, 36 and 37) [101c].

The efficacy and safety of DRV/ritonavir compared with LPV/RTV in HIV-1-infected treatment-naïve patients has been reported [102]. Six hundred and eighty-nine patients were involved in the study. Patients received DRV/RTV 800/100 mg or LPV/r 800/200 mg total daily dose (either once or twice daily) plus TDF/FTC. In the DRV/RTV and LPV/RTV arms, 85/343 and 114/346, respectively, had discontinued by week 192. No protease inhibitor (PI) primary mutations developed and only low levels of nucleoside reverse transcriptase inhibitor resistance developed in virological failures in both groups. AEs reported were treatment-related diarrhea, increases in total cholesterol and triglyceride mostly in LPV/RTV group. DRV (once-daily) was found to be non-inferior and statistically superior in virological response to LPV/RTV.

A prospective, observational, multicenter, cohort study assessed the incidence of AEs in patients receiving DRV. Four hundred and twenty-nine patients were enrolled in the study and were given DVR once or twice daily. The authors were of the opinion that DRV

administrated both once daily or twice daily was safe and well tolerated [103C].

Nelfinavir

Drug–Drug Interactions

The interactions between nelfinavir and rifabutin have been reported in a case of bilateral uveitis associated with co-administration of rifabutin and nelfinavir. Uveitis did not subside until rifabutin was discontinued. The study showed that drug–drug interaction and AEs led to the discontinuation of rifabutin [104A].

Ritonavir

A retrospective study reported on HIV-infected patients treated with double-dose of lopinavir-ritonavir (LPV/RTV) based ART during concomitant rifampicin-containing antituberculosis treatment for 2 months. Optimal treatment for tuberculosis (TB) in HIV infected was treated with lopinavir-ritonavir (LPV/RTV 800 mg/200 mg) twice daily. During co-administration, gastrointestinal toxicity occurred in 9/25 patients and increased aspartate aminotransferase or alanine aminotransferase of any grade in three patients (12%). AEs reported were gastro-intestinal toxicity in 9/25 (36%) patients and diarrhea in 7 (28%) patients, and vomiting in five patients. Treatment discontinued in three patients due to AEs [105c].

Saquinavir

The Polish Observational Cohort of HIV/AIDS Patients (POLCA) study group assessed the efficacy and side effects of saquinavir in 259 naive patients, of these 56.1% continued the drug for 24 months. Twenty three percentage of patients discontinued saquinavir containing regimen due to gastrointestinal side effects. A gradual decrease in proteinuria (44.4–26%), and increase in HDL was also reported [106c].

DRUGS ACTIVE AGAINST HUMAN IMMUNODEFICIENCY VIRUS: INHIBITORS OF HIV FUSION [SEDA-33; 598; SEDA-34, 464; SEDA-35, 525; SEDA-36, 428]

Enfuvirtide

The effectiveness of Enfuvirtide (ENF) was studied in a cohort of 40 HIV-1-infected patients in Mexico. The median age was 44.8%, and 90% of the patients were men. Twenty-seven of those patients were followed through the 48-week analyses. Significant reduction in viral copy numbers were reported in 81% patients. Pain at the site of injection was the main adverse event in 100% of patients. Another AE was the presence of subcutaneous nodules at the injection site in 45.4% of the patients and 19% of patients developed instant side reactions, but none of the patients discontinued the treatment [107c].

Drugs Active Against Human Immunodeficiency Virus: Integrase Inhibitors [SEDA-33, 599, SEDA-34, 465, SEDA-35, 525; SEDA-36, 428]

Dolutegravir

A systematic review and meta-analysis on relative efficacy and safety of DTG are reported [108r], [109R].

DTG was reported to caused headache and insomnia [110R], [111R].

DTG administration showed hypersensitivity reactions in <1% of patients and elevations in liver transaminases were reported in patients co-infected with HBV and HCV [112r].

OBSERVATIONAL STUDIES

A 96-week, phase 3b, randomized, open-label, active-controlled, multicenter, parallel-group, non-inferiority study was conducted at 64 research centers with 484 patients. The patients were randomly assigned (1:1) to receive DTG 50 mg once daily or DRV 800 mg plus RTV 100 mg once daily. The most frequently reported AEs with grade 1 and grade 2 were diarrhea, nausea, headache, and nasopharyngitis. Serious AEs were reported in the DTG group (11%) than in the DRV plus RTV group (5%). Creatinine toxic effects were reported infrequently (DRV, 10 patients (4%); DRV plus RTV two patients (<1%); two (<1%) patients in the DTG group had grade 2 toxic effects [113C].

Raltegravir

OBSERVATIONAL STUDY

Extensive pulmonary involvement with RAL-induced DRESS syndrome in a postpartum woman with HIV was reported. An 18-year-old postpartum woman with HIV, was treated with 3TC–AZT, LPV–RTV and RAL, for 1-week had developed rash and fevers. She had high fever, respiratory distress, hypotension and tachycardia. She also had febrile (102°F) with cervical and submandibular lymphadenopathy, diffuse morbilliform rash, generalized pruritus, facial edema, and oedematous hands and feet. After discontinuing RAL and starting prednisone, her DRESS symptoms completely resolved [114c].

An open-label, randomized, multicenter study was reported in patients with 3 age groups in 4 cohorts.

Cohort I, ≥12 to <19 years and cohort IIA, ≥6 to <12 years, were assigned to receive film-coated tablets, as used in the adult formulation. In all, 126 subjects were treated with RAL of these, 96 received the final selected dose. AEs reported were rash and drug-induced liver injury [115C].

A 39-year-old man positive for HIV had CD4+ T-lymphocyte count 3 cells/μL, and HIV RNA was 4.5×106 copies/mL, but urine analysis showed a heavy proteinuria (3 g/day). He was treated for atypical mycobacteriosis with ethambutol, azytromycin, and rifabutin for a total of 6 months, and highly active antiretroviral therapy (AZT/3TC+DRV/RTV), along with cotrimoxazole prophylaxis. The patient developed a symptomatic muscular toxicity (creatine phosphokinase increased to 5000 UI/L, n.v. <186 UI/L) and AZT/3TC was replaced by RAL. The patient subsequently developed fever with an itchy rash on the limbs and scalp, and painful oral aphthae. The patient was then treated with prednisone (1 mg/kg), and the symptoms subsided [116A].

A non-randomized, Phase I, parallel-assignment, open-label pharmacokinetic study in HIV/HCV-coinfected patients with advanced liver cirrhosis (Child-Pugh C), were given RAL (400 mg twice daily) showed no AEs even with the highest dose of RAL [117c].

MUSCULOSKELETAL

A prospective, observational, multicenter study (Surveillance Cohort Long-Term Toxicity of Antiretrovirals) was reported in a cohort of HIV-infected patients receiving RAL-based ART. A total of 496 HIV-infected patients were included in the study [333 (67.1%) male]. The mean age at enrolment was 45.9 ± 9.3 years, the mean CD4 cell count was 386 ± 277 cells/μL and the mean HIV-RNA level was 2.99 ± 1.56 log10 copies/mL. Of these, 192 patients (38.7%) were positive for hepatitis C antibody, 196 (39.5%) had lipodystrophy and 29 patients (5.8%) were antiretroviral therapy naïve. A total of 26 patients (5.2%) reported muscle symptoms; 16 of them had muscle pain and 17 had muscle weakness (7 had both). Seven patients (1.4%) discontinued RAL because of muscular events (three for muscle pain/weakness and four for creatinine phosphokinase increases). No cases of rhabdomyolysis were reported. Authors suggest that monitoring of muscle symptoms and creatinine phosphokinase levels should be considered in patients receiving RAL co-administered with ATV and in those with CNS symptoms [118C].

A retrospective, cohort study in adult patients with HIV-1 infection were treated with RAL-containing antiretroviral therapy from May 2009 to May 2013. The study contained 155 subjects, 117 (75.5%) were men, 141 (91%) were white, and the mean (±SD) age was 49.2 (±9.2) years. The median duration of the RAL-containing regimen at the end of follow-up was 30.7 months. Other antiretroviral drugs taken in association with RAL, 84 (54.2%) patients received TDF/FTC, 39 (25.2%) ABC/3TC, 53 (34.2%) DRV/RTV, 32 (20.6%) lopinavir/RTV, and 14 (9%) efavirenz. AEs reported were skeletal muscle toxicity in 37 (23.9%) patients during the RAL-containing treatment. Creatinine kinase elevation was observed in 33 (21.3%) patients, diffuse myalgia without weakness in three (2%) patients, and proximal muscle weakness in one (0.6%) subject, while no cases of rhabdomyolysis were reported. A creatinine kinase elevation prior to RAL treatment was observed in 18 (48.6%) out of 37 patients with skeletal muscle toxicity. AZT was included in the previous antiretroviral regimen in 15 (40.5%) out of 37 patients who developed skeletal muscle toxicity. According to the authors, the major factors associated with skeletal muscle toxicity were previous use of AZT, higher baseline creatinine kinase levels, previous increase of the creatinine kinase levels, and a higher body mass index [119C].

A retrospective observational study reported on HIV-1-positive ART-experienced adults was switched to an RAL/ATV or RAL/ATV/RTV regimen between July 2008 and June 2013, in France. Twenty-seven patients (69%) experienced at least one adverse event. A total bilirubin elevation occurred in 64% of patients (grade 1, $n=13$; grade 2, $n=12$), and raised CPK in 13% of patients (grade 1, $n=5$). There was elevation in total bilirubin levels, with a mean increase of 18 μmol/L at week 24 (95% CI, 8–29, $p<0.005$). Other grade 1 AEs related or possibly related to dual therapy included: muscle pain ($n=8$), asthenia ($n=6$), scleral icterus ($n=6$), jaundice ($n=5$), nausea and diarrhea ($n=4$), pain ($n=3$), headache ($n=3$), sleep disturbances ($n=3$), raised alanine aminotransferase ($n=2$), and loss of libido ($n=1$) [120c].

The safety and efficacy of RAL as an alternative to efavirenz for patients co-infected with HIV and TB has also been reported [121C]. A multicentre, phase 2, non-comparative, open-label, randomised trial at eight sites in Brazil and France in patients co-infected with HIV and tuberculosis. Participants in the efavirenz group received 600 mg per day of efavirenz (one tablet), 300 mg per day of 3TC (one 300 mg tablet in France, two 150 mg tablets in Brazil), and 245 mg per day of TDF (one tablet). RAL 400 mg twice daily given as an alternative to efavirenz for the treatment of patients co-infected with HIV and TB. One patient in the RAL 800 mg group had liver failure, Serious AEs reported with efavirenz in 19 patients (37%) and 17 (33%) patients in RAL group. Hepatotoxicity was reported in two patients with RAL that lead to discontinuation of treatment. Cutaneous rash reported in one patient in each efavirenz and RAL group.

DRUGS ACTIVE AGAINST HUMAN IMMUNODEFICIENCY VIRUS: CHEMOKINE RECEPTOR CCR5 ANTAGONISTS [SEDA-33, 600; SEDA 34, 465; SEDA-35, 528; SEDA-36, 430]

Maraviroc

A long-term randomized, double-blind, multicenter phase IIb/III study (5 years) on the efficacy and safety of maraviroc (MVC) vs efavirenz in treatment-naive HIV-1 patients was reported. Naive patients with CCR5-tropic HIV-1 infection received MVC 300 mg twice daily or efavirenz 600 mg once daily, and AZT/3TC 300 mg/150 mg twice daily. Fewer patients on MVC vs efavirenz experienced treatment-related AEs (68.9% vs 81.7%) and discontinued on any adverse event (10.6 vs 21.3%). Nausea (MVC 38.6% vs EFV 36.6%) was the most common adverse event in both treatment arms observed. Other AEs (≥20% of patients, either arm) included dizziness (MVC 17.2% vs EFV 32.1%) and headache (MVC 30.3% vs EFV 29.1%). The other AEs (≥10% of patients, either arm) were nausea (MVC 30.8% vs EFV 28.5%), headache (MVC 19.4% vs EFV 18.0%), dizziness (MVC 11.9% vs EFV 28.0%), fatigue (MVC 10.6% vs EFV 9.1%), diarrhea (MVC 8.9% vs EFV 14.7%), vomiting (MVC 7.8% vs EFV 10.5%), and abnormal dreams (MVC 5.8% vs EFV 12.5%). Dizziness, rash and pregnancy each led to the discontinuation of eight patients (2.2%) in the EFV treatment arm [122c].

Selective and dual targeting of CCR2 and CCR5 receptors, including MVC for the treatment of HIV-1 infections, has been reviewed [123A].

An in vitro experimental study showed antagonistic effects with the combination of CCR5 inhibitors [124E].

The efficacy and safety of changes in highly active antiretroviral therapy regimens for HIV-infected patients has been evaluated [125c].

A retrospective cohort study was also conducted to evaluate the efficacy and safety of MVC plus RTV-boosted DRV-r once-daily in HIV-infected pretreated patients [126c]. Changing the treatment regimen reduced the AEs in 38 patients and improved viral clearance.

In an open-label, fixed-sequence, phase I study, 14 volunteers received MVC 150 mg BID (every 12 hours) for 5 days, followed by MVC 150 mg BID plus BOC 800 mg TID (every 8 hours) for 10 days, then MVC 150 mg BID plus TVR 750 mg TID (every 8 hours) for subsequent 10 days. AEs were higher with MVC+BOC and MVC+TVR versus MVC alone. Dysgeusia (50%) and pruritus (29%) occurred most commonly with MVC+BOC, and fatigue (46%) and headache (31%) with MVC+TVR. There were no serious AEs reported [127c].

Regulatory T cells play a key role in HIV-associated immunopathology, and the regulatory T cells in MVC-treated peripheral blood mononuclear cells (PBMCs) were reduced significantly [128E].

DRUGS ACTIVE AGAINST INFLUENZA VIRUSES: ION CHANNEL INHIBITORS
[SED-15, 105, 3051; SEDA-32, 544; SEDA-33, 269, 602; SEDA-34, 467; SEDA-35, 529; SEDA-36, 430]

Amantadine

Amantadine, at high dose (10 mg/kg), did not prevent dopamine depletion but exacerbated the behavioral manifestations of methamphetamine toxicity such as akinesia and catalepsy. Lower dose of amantadine (1 mg/kg) produced significant scavenging of the reactive oxygen species induced by methamphetamine. The authors suggests that amantadine should not be used concomitantly with methamphetamine as it may results in excessive neurotoxicity [129E].

DRUGS ACTIVE AGAINST INFLUENZA VIRUSES: NEURAMINIDASE INHIBITORS
[SED-15, 2436; SEDA-32, 544; SEDA-33, 601; SEDA-34, 466; SEDA-35, 528; SEDA-36, 431]

Oseltamivir (Tamiflu)

A meta-analysis by Dobson and colleagues was performed that includes all available data from randomized, double-masked, placebo-controlled adult trials, including trials that did not reach recruitment targets and had not been published (nine trials including 4328 patients). Oseltamivir treatment with 75 mg twice daily for 5 days resulted in a significant 21% (95% CI, 15–26) reduction, from 123 to 98 hours, in reported symptom duration in adult and adolescent patients with laboratory-confirmed influenza (the intention-to-treat infected with influenza group). The oseltamivir treatment resulted in an increased risk of nausea (6.2%) in the placebo group as compared with 9.9% and an increased risk of vomiting (3.3% vs 8.0%) [130M].

A retrospective analysis was reported of oseltamivir and zanamivir in 150 randomly-selected confirmed H1N1 patients between July 2009 and December 2009, where patients were in the age group of 18–65 years received oseltamivir alone or along with zanamivir. Oseltamivir alone treated patients (48%) developed gastrointestinal intolerance [131C].

OTHER DRUGS

Imiquimod [SED-15, 1718; SEDA-35, 530; SEDA-36, 431]

Dermatological Studies

In a multicenter, open label, randomized, phase 2 study, the feasibility of cidofovir and imiquimod for treatment of vulval intraepithelial neoplasia was reported. One hundred and eighty patients with vulval intraepithelial neoplasia grade 3 were included in the study. Eighty nine patients were treated with 1% cidofovir (supplied as a gel in a 10 g tube, to last 6 weeks) and 91 patients were treated with 5% imiquimod (one 250 mg sachet for every application), self-applied three times a week for a maximum of 24 weeks. A complete response was reported in 41 (46%; 90% CI, 37.0–55.3) patients allocated cidofovir and by 42 (46%; 37.2–55.3) patients assigned imiquimod. AEs of grade 3 or higher were reported in 31 (37%) of 84 patients allocated cidofovir and 39 (46%) of 84 patients assigned imiquimod. The most frequent grade 3 and 4 AEs were pain in the vulva, pruritus, fatigue, and headache [132C].

References

[1] Saunders IM, Lahoti A, Chemaly RF, et al. Topical cidofovir-induced acute kidney injury in two severely immunocompromised patients with refractory multidrug-resistant herpes simplex virus infections. J Oncol Pharm Pract. 2014; in press, http://dx.doi.org/10.1177/1078155214560921 [A].
[2] Orssaud C, Wermert D, Roux A, et al. Urrets-Zavalia syndrome as a complication of ocular hypotonia due to intravenous cidofovir treatment. Eye. 2014;28(6):776–7 [A].
[3] Dunn JP. An overview of current and future treatment options for patients with cytomegalovirus retinitis. Expert Opin Orphan Drugs. 2014;2(10):999–1013 [r].
[4] Grasso M, Remacle M, Bachy V, et al. Use of cidofovir in HPV patients with recurrent respiratory papillomatosis. Eur Arch Otorhinolaryngol. 2014;271(11):2983–90 [c].
[5] España LP, Del Boz J, Fernández Morano T, et al. Topical cidofovir for plantar warts. Dermatol Ther. 2014;27(2):89–93 [c].
[6] Wanat KA, Gormley RH, Rosenbach M, et al. Intralesional cidofovir for treating extensive genital verrucous herpes simplex virus infection. JAMA Dermatol. 2013;149(7):881–3 [A].
[7] Kneidinger N, Giessen C, vonWulffen W, et al. Trip to immunity: resistant cytomegalovirus infection in a lung transplant recipient. Int J Infect Dis. 2014;28:e140–2 [A].
[8] Gregg K, Hakki M, Kaul DR. UL54 foscarnet mutation in an hematopoietic stem cell transplant recipient with cytomegalovirus disease. Transpl Infect Dis. 2014;16(2):320–3 [A].
[9] Minces LR, Nguyen MH, Mitsani D, et al. Ganciclovir-resistant cytomegalovirus infections among lung transplant recipients are associated with poor outcomes despite treatment with foscarnet-containing regimens. Antimicrob Agents Chemother. 2014;58(1):128–35 [c].
[10] Han SB, Lee JH, Lee JW, et al. Cytomegalovirus retinitis diagnosed after completion of chemotherapy for acute lymphoblastic leukemia in an adolescent. J Pediatr Hematol Oncol. 2015;37(2):e128–30 [A].

[11] Kerkhoff AD, Reyes JA, Roberts AD, et al. A rare complication of cytomegalovirus infection: meningoventriculoencephalitis immune reconstitution inflammatory syndrome. Infect Dis Clin Pract. 2014;22(6):365–7 [c].

[12] Agarwal A, Kumari N, Trehan A, et al. Outcome of cytomegalovirus retinitis in immunocompromised patients without human immunodeficiency virus treated with intravitreal ganciclovir injection. Graefes Arch Clin Exp Ophthalmol. 2014;252(9):1393–401 [c].

[13] Venton G, Crocchiolo R, Fürst S, et al. Risk factors of Ganciclovir-related neutropenia after allogeneic stem cell transplantation: a retrospective monocentre study on 547 patients. Clin Microbiol Infect. 2014;20(2):160–6 [R].

[14] Soanker R, Udutha SJC, Subbalaxmi MVS, et al. Ganciclovir–tenofovir interaction leading to tenofovir-induced nephrotoxicity. J Pharmacol Pharmacother. 2014;5(4):265–7 [c].

[15] Sacchetti D, Alawadhi A, Albakour M, et al. Herpes zoster encephalopathy or acyclovir neurotoxicity: a management dilemma. BMJ Case Rep. 2014; http://dx.doi.org/10.1136/bcr-2013-201941 [A].

[16] Berry L, Venkatesan P. Aciclovir-induced neurotoxicity: utility of CSF and serum CMMG levels in diagnosis. J Clin Virol. 2014;61(4):608–10 [A].

[17] Guney E, Sezgin Akcay BI, Erdogan G, et al. Systemic side effects of antiviral therapy in a patient with acute retinal necrosis. Ocul Immunol Inflamm. 2014;22(3):233–5 [A].

[18] Kamboj J, Wu F, Kamboj R, et al. A rare case of acyclovir-induced thrombocytopenia. Am J Ther. 2014;21(5):e159–62 [A].

[19] Kusakari Y, Tanita M, Egawa T, et al. Efficacy and safety of famciclovir for the treatment of herpes zoster patients with renal dysfunction. Nishinihon J Dermatol. 2014;76(1):44–51 [c].

[20] Routt E, Levitt J. Famciclovir for recurrent herpes-associated erythema multiforme: a series of three cases. J Am Acad Dermatol. 2014;71(4):e146–7 [A].

[21] Emeriewen K, Macgregor C, Athanasiadis Y, et al. Neuropathic pain in multiple sclerosis improved with oral famciclovir: a case report. Ophthal Plast Reconstr Surg. 2014; in press, http://dx.doi.org/10.1097/IOP.0000000000000300 [A].

[22] Yi TJ, Walmsley S, Szadkowski L, et al. A randomized controlled pilot trial of valacyclovir for attenuating inflammation and immune activation in hiv/herpes simplex virus 2-coinfected adults on suppressive antiretroviral therapy. Clin Infect Dis. 2013;57(9):1331–8 [c].

[23] Roxby AC, Atkinson C, Ásbjörnsdóttir K, et al. Maternal valacyclovir and infant cytomegalovirus acquisition: a randomized controlled trial among HIV-infected women. PLoS One. 2014;9(2):e87855 [C].

[24] Reischig T, Kacer M, Jindra P, et al. Randomized trial of valganciclovir versus valacyclovir prophylaxis for prevention of cytomegalovirus in renal transplantation. Clin J Am Soc Nephrol. 2015;10(2):294–304 [C].

[25] Singh NP, Shah HR, Aggarwal N, et al. Valacyclovir associated neurotoxicity in a patient on dialysis. Indian J Nephrol. 2014;24(2):128–9 [A].

[26] Henderson TA. Valacyclovir treatment of chronic fatigue in adolescents. Adv Mind Body Med. 2014;28(1):4–14 [c].

[27] Iizuka Y, Sakai H, Kobayashi K, et al. A case of chronic hepatitis B managed with continued adefovir despite treatment-related Fanconi syndrome and osteomalacia. Nihon Shokakibyo Gakkai Zasshi. 2014;111(8):1618–23 [c].

[28] Terasaka T, Ueta E, Ebara H, et al. Long-term observation of osteomalacia caused by adefovir-induced Fanconi's syndrome. Acta Med Okayama. 2014;68(1):53–6 [c].

[29] Tanaka M, Suzuki F, Seko Y, et al. Renal dysfunction and hypophosphatemia during long-term lamivudine plus adefovir dipivoxil therapy in patients with chronic hepatitis B. J Gastroenterol. 2014;49(3):470–80 [c].

[30] Ahrens CL, Manno EM. Neurotoxicity of commonly used hepatic drugs. Handb Clin Neurol. 2014;120:675–82 [A].

[31] Özekinci T, Mese S, Ozbek E, et al. Lamivudine and Adefovir motif variants detected in chronic hepatitis B patients. Clin Ter. 2014;165(1):13–7 [c].

[32] Hou JL, Gao ZL, Xie Q, et al. Tenofovir disoproxil fumarate vs adefovir dipivoxil in Chinese patients with chronic hepatitis B after 48 weeks: a randomized controlled trial. J Viral Hepat. 2015;22(2):85–93 [C].

[33] Shan C, Yin GQ, Wu P. Efficacy and safety of tenofovir in a kidney transplant patient with chronic hepatitis B and nucleos(t)ide multidrug resistance: a case report. J Med Case Rep. 2014;8(1):281 [A].

[34] Pipili C, Cholongitas E, Papatheodoridis G. Review article: nucleos(t)ide analogues in patients with chronic hepatitis B virus infection and chronic kidney disease. Aliment Pharmacol Ther. 2014;39(1):35–46 [R].

[35] Bilar JM, Carvalho-Filho RJ, Mota CFMGP, et al. Acute pancreatitis associated with boceprevir: a case report. Braz J Infect Dis. 2014;18(4):454–6 [c].

[36] Milazzo L, Falvella FS, Magni C, et al. Seizures in patients with chronic hepatitis C treated with NS3/4A protease inhibitors: does pharmacological interaction play a role? Pharmacology. 2014;92(5–6):235–7 [c].

[37] Hernández Segurado M, Martín Gozalo EM, Bonilla Porras M, et al. Pure red cell aplasia in a patient treated with triple therapy for hepatitis C. Atencion Farmaceutica. 2014;16(4):289–92 [c].

[38] Rosenberg WM, Tanwar S, Trembling P. Complexities of HCV management in the new era of direct-acting antiviral agents. QJM. 2014;107(1):17–9 [R].

[39] Hulskotte EGJ, Feng HP, Xuan F, et al. Pharmacokinetic interactions between the hepatitis C virus protease inhibitor boceprevir and ritonavir-boosted HIV-1 protease inhibitors atazanavir, darunavir, and lopinavir. Clin Infect Dis. 2013;56(5):718–26 [c].

[40] Knapstein J, Grimm D, Wörns MA, et al. Triple antiviral therapy with telaprevir after liver transplantation: a case series. Transpl Res Risk Manag. 2014;6:73–8 [c].

[41] Crismale JF, Martel-Laferrière V, Bichoupan K, et al. Diabetes mellitus and advanced liver fibrosis are risk factors for severe anaemia during telaprevir-based triple therapy. Liver Int. 2014;34(7):1018–24 [C].

[42] Soza A, Labbé P, Arrese M, et al. Mycobacterium abscessus pulmonary infection during hepatitis C treatment with telaprevir, peginterferon and ribavirin. Ann Hepatol. 2015;14(1):132–6 [c].

[43] Shuster M, Do D, Nambudiri V. Severe cutaneous adverse reaction to telaprevir. Dermatol Online J. 2015;21(1) [c].

[44] Bernardeschi C, Valeyrie-Allanore L, Ortonne N, et al. Dermatological side-effects in hepatitis C infected patients under a triple regimen associating pegylated interferon, ribavirin and telaprevir. J Eur Acad Dermatol Venereol. 2014; Sep 3. http://dx.doi.org/10.1111/jdv.12635 [c].

[45] Yuan K, Guochun W, Huang Z, et al. Entecavir-associated myopathy: a case report and literature review. Muscle Nerve. 2014;49(4):610–4 [A].

[46] Bodeau S, Nguyen-Khac E, Solas C, et al. Patients treated with first-generation HCV protease inhibitors exhibit high ribavirin concentrations. J Clin Pharmacol. 2015;55(5):517–24 [c].

[47] Yapali S, Lok AS. Potential benefit of telbivudine on renal function does not outweigh its high rate of antiviral drug resistance and other AEs. Gastroenterology. 2014;146(1):15–9 [R].

[48] Lu YP, Liang XJ, Xiao XM, et al. Telbivudine during the second and third trimester of pregnancy interrupts HBV intrauterine

transmission: a systematic review and meta-analysis. Clin Lab. 2014;60(4):571–86 [R].

[49] Xu H, Wang Z, Zheng L, et al. Lamivudine/telbivudine-associated neuromyopathy: neurogenic damage, mitochondrial dysfunction and mitochondrial DNA depletion. J Clin Pathol. 2014;67(11):999–1005 [c].

[50] Liu Y, Liu L, Peng D, et al. Long-term efficacy and safety of telbivudine as monotherapy and as combination therapy with adefovir dipivoxil in HBeAg-positive chronic hepatitis B patients. Zhonghua Gan Zang Bing Za Zhi. 2014;22(3):181–4 [C].

[51] Agarwal K, Barnabas A. Faldaprevir for the treatment of genotype-1 hepatitis C virus. Expert Rev Gastroenterol Hepatol. 2015;9(3):277–88 [R].

[52] Keating GM, Vaidya A. Sofosbuvir: first global approval. Drugs. 2014;74(2):273–82 [R].

[53] Sulkowski MS, Naggie S, Lalezari J, et al. Sofosbuvir and ribavirin for hepatitis C in patients with HIV coinfection. JAMA. 2014;312(4):353–61 [C].

[54] Jacobson IM, Dore GJ, Foster GR, et al. Simeprevir with pegylated interferon alfa 2a plus ribavirin in treatment-naive patients with chronic hepatitis C virus genotype 1 infection (QUEST-1): a phase 3, randomised, double-blind, placebo-controlled trial. Lancet. 2014;384(9941):403–13 [C].

[55] Dieterich D, Rockstroh JK, Orkin C, et al. Simeprevir (TMC435) with pegylated interferon/ribavirin in patients coinfected with HCV genotype 1 and HIV-1: a phase 3 study. Clin Infect Dis. 2014;59(11):1579–87 [C].

[56] Podzamczer D, Rojas JF, Neves I, et al. Effectiveness and tolerability of abacavir-lamivudine-nevirapine (ABC/3TC/NVP) in a multicentre cohort of HIV-infected, ARV-naive patients. J Int AIDS Soc. 2014;17(4 Suppl 3):19773 [c].

[57] Podzamczer D, Imaz A, Perez I, et al. Abacavir/lamivudine plus darunavir/ritonavir in routine clinical practice: a multicentre experience in antiretroviral therapy-naive and -experienced patients. J Antimicrob Chemother. 2014;69(9):2536–40 [C].

[58] Cruciani M, Mengoli C, Malena M, et al. Virological efficacy of abacavir: systematic review and meta-analysis. J Antimicrob Chemother. 2014;69(12):3169–80 [R].

[59] Sprenger H, Langebeek N, Mulder P, et al. A randomized controlled trial of single-class maintenance therapy with abacavir/lamivudine/zidovudine after standard triple antiretroviral induction therapy: final 96-week results from the FREE study. HIV Med. 2015;16(2):122–31 [C].

[60] McDonald CK, Martorell C, Ramgopal M, et al. Cobicistat-boosted protease inhibitors in HIV-infected patients with mild to moderate renal impairment. HIV Clin Trials. 2014;15(6):269–73 [c].

[61] Custodio JM, Rhee M, Shen G, et al. Pharmacokinetics and safety of boosted elvitegravir in subjects with hepatic impairment. Antimicrob Agents Chemother. 2014;58(5):2564–9 [c].

[62] Del Mar Gutierrez M, Mateo MG, Vidal F, et al. Drug safety profile of integrase strand transfer inhibitors. Expert Opin Drug Saf. 2014;13(4):431–45 [R].

[63] Reviriego C. Elvitegravir for the treatment of HIV infection. Drugs Today. 2014;50(3):209–17 [R].

[64] Lyseng-Williamson KA, Deeks ED. Cobicistat: a guide to its use as a pharmacokinetic enhancer of atazanavir and darunavir in HIV-1 infection. Drugs Ther Perspect. 2014;30(9):309–15 [R].

[65] Lyseng-Williamson KA. Darunavir/cobicistat fixed-dose single tablet (Rezolsta™): a guide to its use in HIV-1 infection in adults in the EU. Drugs Ther Perspect. 2015;31(3):77–82 [H].

[66] Clumeck N, Molina JM, Henry K, et al. A randomized, double-blind comparison of single-tablet regimen elvitegravir/cobicistat/emtricitabine/tenofovir DF vs ritonavir-boosted atazanavir plus emtricitabine/tenofovir DF for initial treatment of HIV-1 infection: analysis of week 144 results. J Acquir Immune Defic Syndr. 2014;65(3):e121–4 [r].

[67] Moyle GJ, Stellbrink HJ, Compston J, et al. 96-Week results of abacavir/lamivudine versus tenofovir/emtricitabine, plus efavirenz, in antiretroviral-naive, HIV-1-infected adults: ASSERT study. Antivir Ther. 2013;18(7):905–13 [C].

[68] Sood A, Castrejón M, Saab S. Human immunodeficiency virus and nodular regenerative hyperplasia of liver: a systematic review. World J Hepatol. 2014;6(1):55–63 [R].

[69] Blanco J, Caro-Murillo A, Castaño M, et al. Safety, efficacy, and persistence of emtricitabine/tenofovir versus other nucleoside analogues in naive subjects aged 50 years or older in Spain: the TRIP study. HIV Clin Trials. 2013;14(5):204–15 [c].

[70] Kurita T, Kitaichi T, Nagao T, et al. Safety analysis of Epzicom® (lamivudine/abacavir sulfate) in post-marketing surveillance in Japan. Pharmacoepidemiol Drug Saf. 2014;23(4):372–81 [C].

[71] Nakamura K, Tateyama M, Tasato D, et al. Pure red cell aplasia induced by lamivudine without the influence of zidovudine in a patient infected with human immunodeficiency virus. Intern Med. 2014;53(15):1705–8 [A].

[72] Ford N, Shubber Z, Hill A, et al. Comparative efficacy of lamivudine and emtricitabine: a systematic review and meta-analysis of randomized trials. PLoS One. 2013;8(11):e79981 [R].

[73] Finkelstein JL, Gala P, Rochford R, et al. HIV/AIDS and lipodystrophy: implications for clinical management in resource-limited settings. J Int AIDS Soc. 2015;18(1):19033 [R].

[74] Abers MS, Shandera WX, Kass JS. Neurological and psychiatric adverse effects of antiretroviral drugs. CNS Drugs. 2014;28(2):131–45 [R].

[75] Kampira E, Dzobo K, Kumwenda J, et al. Peripheral blood mitochondrial DNA/nuclear DNA (mtDNA/nDNA) ratio as a marker of mitochondrial toxicities of stavudine containing antiretroviral therapy in HIV-infected Malawian patients. OMICS. 2014;18(7):438–45 [c].

[76] Bhutia E, Hemal A, Yadav TP, et al. Lipodystrophy syndrome among HIV infected children on highly active antiretroviral therapy in northern India. Afr Health Sci. 2014;14(2):408–13 [c].

[77] Sun R, Eriksson S, Wang L. Zidovudine induces downregulation of mitochondrial deoxynucleoside kinases: implications for mitochondrial toxicity of antiviral nucleoside analogs. Antimicrob Agents Chemother. 2014;58(11):6758–66 [E].

[78] Zhang M, Shang M, Yang W, et al. Treatment effect and drug-resistant mutations in Chinese AIDS patients switching to second-line antiretroviral therapy. PLoS One. 2014;9(10):e110259 [c].

[79] Jaganath D, Walker AS, Ssali F, et al. HIV-associated anemia after 96 weeks on therapy: determinants across age ranges in Uganda and Zimbabwe. AIDS Res Hum Retrovir. 2014;30(6):523–30 [c].

[80] Sax PE, Zolopa A, Brar I, et al. Tenofovir alafenamide vs. tenofovir disoproxil fumarate in single tablet regimens for initial HIV-1 therapy: a randomized phase 2 study. J Acquir Immune Defic Syndr. 2014;67(1):52–8 [c].

[81] Danjuma MI, Mohamad-Fadzillah NH, Khoo S. An investigation of the pattern of kidney injury in HIV-positive persons exposed to tenofovir disoproxil fumarate: an examination of a large population database (MHRA database). Int J STD AIDS. 2014;25(4):273–9 [M].

[82] Moss DM, Neary M, Owen A. The role of drug transporters in the kidney: lessons from tenofovir. Front Pharmacol. 2014;5:248 [R].

[83] Van Griensven J, Phirum L, Choun K, et al. Hepatitis B and C co-infection among HIV-infected adults while on antiretroviral treatment: long-term survival, CD4 cell count recovery and antiretroviral toxicity in Cambodia. PLoS One. 2014;9(2):e88552 [C].

[84] Sarfo FS, Zhang Y, Egan D, et al. Pharmacogenetic associations with plasma efavirenz concentrations and clinical correlates in a

retrospective cohort of Ghanaian HIV-infected patients. J Antimicrob Chemother. 2014;69(2):491–9 [C].

[85] Santini-Oliveira M, Friedman RK, Veloso VG, et al. Incidence of antiretroviral adverse drug reactions in pregnant women in two referral centers for HIV prevention of mother-to-child-transmission care and research in Rio de Janeiro, Brazil. Braz J Infect Dis. 2014;18(4):372–8 [C].

[86] Casado JL, Bañón S, Rodriguez MA, et al. Efficacy and pharmacokinetics of the combination of etravirine plus raltegravir as novel dual antiretroviral maintenance regimen in HIV-infected patients. Antivir Res. 2015;113:103–6 [c].

[87] Kurz M, Stoeckle M, Krasniqi F, et al. Etravirine: a good option for concomitant use with chemotherapy for Hodgkin's lymphoma. Int J STD AIDS. 2015;26(3):212–4 [c].

[88] Calcagno A, Di Perri G, Bonora S. Pharmacokinetics and pharmacodynamics of antiretrovirals in the central nervous system. Clin Pharmacokinet. 2014;53(10):891–906 [R].

[89] Jiang HY, Zhang MN, Chen HJ, et al. Nevirapine versus efavirenz for patients co-infected with HIV and tuberculosis: a systematic review and meta-analysis. Int J Infect Dis. 2014;25:e130–5 [R].

[90] Mutwa PR, Boer KR, Asiimwe-Kateera B, et al. Safety and effectiveness of combination antiretroviral therapy during the first year of treatment in HIV-1 infected Rwandan children: a prospective study. PLoS One. 2014;9(11):e111948 [C].

[91] Li SL, Xu P, Zhang L, et al. Effectiveness and safety of rilpivirine, a non-nucleoside reverse transcriptase inhibitor, in treatment-naive adults infected with HIV-1: a meta-analysis. HIV Clin Trials. 2014;15(6):261–8 [C].

[92] Casado JL. Liver toxicity in HIV-infected patients receiving novel second-generation nonnucleoside reverse transcriptase inhibitors etravirine and rilpivirine. AIDS Rev. 2013;15(3):139–45 [R].

[93] Song I, Borland J, Chen S, et al. Effect of fosamprenavir-ritonavir on the pharmacokinetics of dolutegravir in healthy subjects. Antimicrob Agents Chemother. 2014;58(11):6696–700 [c].

[94] Nakamura Jr. MU, Araujo Júnior E, Simões MJ, et al. Effect of six antiretroviral drugs (delavirdine, stavudine, lamivudine, nelfinavir, amprenavir and lopinavir/ritonavir in association) on albino pregnant rats (Rattus norvegicus albinus, Rodentia, Mammalia): biological assay. Ceska Gynekol. 2014;79(4):295–304 [E].

[95] Lennox JL, Landovitz RJ, Ribaudo HJ, et al. Efficacy and tolerability of 3 nonnucleoside reverse transcriptase inhibitor-sparing antiretroviral regimens for treatment-naïve volunteers infected with HIV-1: a randomized, controlled equivalence trial. Ann Intern Med. 2014;161(7):461–71 [c].

[96] Wohl DA, Bhatti L, Small CB, et al. Simplification to abacavir/lamivudine + atazanavir maintains viral suppression and improves bone and renal biomarkers in ASSURE, a randomized, open label, non-inferiority trial. PLoS One. 2014;9(5):e96187 [C].

[97] Gutierrez-Valencia A, Ruiz-Valderas R, Torres-Cornejo A, et al. Role of ritonavir in the drug interactions between telaprevir and ritonavir-boosted atazanavir. Clin Infect Dis. 2014;58(2):268–73 [A].

[98] Johnson M, Walmsley S, Haberl A. A systematic review of the use of atazanavir in women infected with HIV-1. Antivir Ther. 2014;19(3):293–307 [R].

[99] Svärd J, Blanco F, Nevin D, et al. Differential interactions of antiretroviral agents with LXR, ER and GR nuclear receptors: potential contributing factors to AEs. Br J Pharmacol. 2014;171(2):480–97 [E].

[100] Martinez E, Gonzalez-Cordon A, Ferrer E, et al. Early lipid changes with atazanavir/ritonavir or darunavir/ritonavir. HIV Med. 2014;15(6):330–8 [C].

[101] Zorrilla CD, Wright R, Osiyemi O, et al. Total and unbound darunavir pharmacokinetics in pregnant women infected with HIV-1: results of a study of darunavir/ritonavir 600/100mg administered twice daily. HIV Med. 2014;15(1):50–6 [c].

[102] Orkin C, Dejesus E, Khanlou H, et al. Final 192-week efficacy and safety of once-daily darunavir/ritonavir compared with lopinavir/ritonavir in HIV-1-infected treatment-naïve patients in the ARTEMIS trial. HIV Med. 2013;14(1):49–59.

[103] Menzaghi B, Ricci E, Carenzi L, et al. Safety and durability in a cohort of HIV-1 positive patients treated with once and twice daily darunavir-based therapy (SCOLTA Project). Biomed Pharmacother. 2013;67(4):293–8 [C].

[104] Cheng WH, Chang CH, Lu PL, et al. Bilateral uveitis associated with concurrent administration of rifabutin and nelfinavir. Taiwan J Ophthalmol. 2015; in press, http://dx.doi.org/10.1016/j.tjo.2014.08.004 [A].

[105] Sunpath H, Winternheimer P, Cohen S, et al. Double-dose lopinavir-ritonavir in combination with rifampicin-based anti-tuberculosis treatment in South Africa. Int J Tuberc Lung Dis. 2014;18(6):689–93 [c].

[106] Kubicka J, Ignatowska A, Kowalska JD, et al. Saquinavir/r containing initial antiretroviral therapy (ART)-long term evaluation in Polish Observational Cohort of HIV/AIDS patients (POLCA) Study Group. HIV AIDS Rev. 2014; in press [c].

[107] Huerta-García G, Chavez-García M, Mata-Marín JA, et al. Effectiveness of enfuvirtide in a cohort of highly antiretroviral-experienced HIV-1-infected patients in Mexico. AIDS Res Ther. 2014;11(1):323 [c].

[108] Wu G, Abraham T, Saad N. Dolutegravir for the treatment of adult patients with HIV-1 infection. Expert Rev Anti-Infect Ther. 2014;12(5):535–44 [r].

[109] Patel DA, Snedecor SJ, Tang WY, et al. 48-week efficacy and safety of dolutegravir relative to commonly used third agents in treatment-naive HIV-1-infected patients: a systematic review and network meta-analysis. PLoS One. 2014;9(9):e105653 [R].

[110] Osterholzer DA, Goldman M. Dolutegravir: a next-generation integrase inhibitor for treatment of HIV infection. Clin Infect Dis. 2014;59(2):265–71 [R].

[111] Rathbun RC, Lockhart SM, Miller MM, et al. Dolutegravir, a second-generation integrase inhibitor for the treatment of HIV-1 infection. Ann Pharmacother. 2014;48(3):395–403 [R].

[112] DOlutegravir (tivicay) for hiv. JAMA. 2014;312(4):428–9 [r].

[113] Clotet B, Feinberg J, Van Lunzen J, et al. Once-daily dolutegravir versus darunavir plus ritonavir in antiretroviral-naive adults with HIV-1 infection (FLAMINGO): 48 week results from the randomised open-label phase 3b study. Lancet. 2014;383(9936):2222–31 [C].

[114] Yee BE, Nguyen NH, Lee D. Extensive pulmonary involvement with raltegravir-induced DRESS syndrome in a postpartum woman with HIV. BMJ Case Rep. 2014; in press, http://dx.doi.org/10.1136/bcr-2013-201545 [c].

[115] Nachman S, Zheng N, Acosta EP, et al. Pharmacokinetics, safety, and 48-week efficacy of oral raltegravir in HIV-1-infected children aged 2 through 18 years. Clin Infect Dis. 2014;58(3):413–22 [C].

[116] Ripamonti D, Benatti SV, Di Filippo E, et al. Drug reaction with eosinophilia and systemic symptoms associated with raltegravir use: case report and review of the literature. AIDS. 2014;28(7):1077–9 [A].

[117] Hernández-Novoa B, Moreno A, Pérez-Elías MJ, et al. Raltegravir pharmacokinetics in HIV/HCV-coinfected patients with advanced liver cirrhosis (Child-Pugh C). J Antimicrob Chemother. 2014;69(2):471–5 [c].

[118] Madeddu G, De Socio GVL, Ricci E, et al. Muscle symptoms and creatine phosphokinase elevations in patients receiving raltegravir in clinical practice: results from the SCOLTA project long-term surveillance. Int J Antimicrob Agents. 2015;45(3):289–94 [C].

[119] Calza L, Danese I, Colangeli V, et al. Skeletal muscle toxicity in HIV-1-infected patients treated with a raltegravir-containing antiretroviral therapy: a cohort study. AIDS Res Hum Retrovir. 2014;30(12):1162–9 [C].

[120] Gantner P, Koeppel C, Partisani M, et al. Efficacy and safety of switching to raltegravir plus atazanavir dual therapy in pretreated HIV-1-infected patients over 144 weeks: a cohort study. Scand J Infect Dis. 2014;46(12):838–45 [c].

[121] Grinsztejn B, De Castro N, Arnold V, et al. Raltegravir for the treatment of patients co-infected with HIV and tuberculosis (ANRS 12 180 Reflate TB): a multicentre, phase 2, non-comparative, open-label, randomised trial. Lancet Infect Dis. 2014;14(6):459–67 [C].

[122] Cooper DA, Heera J, Ive P, et al. Efficacy and safety of Maraviroc vs. Efavirenz in treatment-naive patients with HIV-1: 5-year findings. AIDS. 2014;28(5):717–25 [c].

[123] Junker A, Kokornaczyk AK, Strunz AK, et al. Selective and dual targeting of CCR2 and CCR5 receptors: a current overview. Topics Med Chem. 2015;14:187–242 [A].

[124] Asin-Milan O, Sylla M, El-Far M, et al. Synergistic combinations of the CCR5 inhibitor VCH-286 with other classes of HIV-1 inhibitors. Antimicrob Agents Chemother. 2014;58(12):7565–9 [E].

[125] Tanaka H, Wada T, Takayama Y, et al. Evaluation of the efficacy and safety of changes in antiretroviral regimens for HIV-infected patients. J Pharm Pharm Sci. 2014;17(3):316–23 [c].

[126] Macías J, Recio E, Márquez M, et al. Efficacy and safety of once-daily maraviroc plus ritonavir-boosted darunavir in pretreated HIV-infected patients in a real-life setting. HIV Med. 2014;15(7):417–24 [c].

[127] Vourvahis M, Plotka A, Kantaridis C, et al. The effects of boceprevir and telaprevir on the pharmacokinetics of maraviroc: an open-label, fixed-sequence study in healthy volunteers. J Acquir Immune Defic Syndr. 2014;65(5):564–70 [c].

[128] Pozo-Balado MM, Martínez-Bonet M, Rosado I, et al. Maraviroc reduces the regulatory T-cell frequency in antiretroviral-naive HIV-infected subjects. J Infect Dis. 2014;210(6):890–8 [E].

[129] Thrash-Williams B, Ahuja M, Karuppagounder SS, et al. Assessment of therapeutic potential of amantadine in methamphetamine induced neurotoxicity. Neurochem Res. 2013;38(10):2084–94 [E].

[130] Dobson J, Whitley RJ, Pocock S, et al. Oseltamivir treatment for influenza in adults: a meta-analysis of randomised controlled trials. Lancet. 2015;385(9979):1729–37 [M].

[131] Arora HR, Singh KS, Ghongane BB. Retrospective analysis of Oseltamivir and Zanamivir in patients of H1N1 influenza in a tertiary care hospital in Western India. Int J Pharm Bio Sci. 2015;6(1):P672–8.

[132] Tristram A, Hurt CN, Madden T, et al. Activity, safety, and feasibility of cidofovir and imiquimod for treatment of vulval intraepithelial neoplasia (RT3VIN): a multicentre, open-label, randomised, phase 2 trial. Lancet Oncol. 2014;15(12):1361–8 [C].

30

Drugs Used in Tuberculosis and Leprosy

F.R. Tejada, A.R. Walk, M.K. Kharel[1]

School of Pharmacy and Health Professions, University of Maryland Eastern Shore, Princess Anne, MD, USA

[1]Corresponding author: mkkharel@umes.edu

RIFAMYCINS

Rifamycins, natural products-based antibiotics, have remained in the first-line antituberculosis (anti-TB) therapeutics since the launch of rifamycin SV as an antimycobacterial agent in the mid-1960s. Since then four other analogues of rifamycin SV, namely, rifampicin (RMP) in 1967, rifamixin in 1988, rifabutin in 1992, and rifapentine in 1998 have been approved by the U.S. FDA or equivalent organizations [1R].

Rifampicin

Multi-drug regimens including rifampicin (RMP), isoniazid (INH), ethambutol (EMB), pyrazinamide (PZA) are commonly prescribed to treat TB. Despite several therapeutic implications, anti-TB drugs possess significant cytotoxic and mutagenic potential, especially in combination therapy. A recent comparative study by Fatima et al. revealed RMP to possess the highest cytotoxic potential among INH, PZA and RMB. The results showed RMP to cause the strongest decline ($p < 0.001$) in cell numbers at the concentration of 250 µg/mL with LC_{50} at 325 µg/mL. Moreover, combination of RMP, INH, PZA and EMB (RIPE) demonstrated a significant reduction ($p < 0.01$) in cell number at the concentration of 25, 500, 500, and 500 µg/mL, respectively. The corresponding LC_{50} values were 60–1200–1200–1200 µg/mL. RMP was also proven to be highly mutagenic of all the tested drugs ($p < 0.01$) at 0.0525 µg/plate against *Salmonella* strain TA98 strain with S9 [2E].

Urinary Tract

TB is a common opportunistic infection in renal transplant patients. A retrospective study of patients who underwent a renal transplant and were diagnosed with TB has shown very high toxicity, high mortality, and considerable rates of rejection and graft loss [3c]. Of the 641 renal transplants, 12 cases had TB. Pulmonary (50%) and disseminated TB (33.3%) were the most frequent forms and required prolonged treatment. The first phase of treatment consisted of 3 months of HPRE (INH, PZA, RMP and EMB) in 75% of the cases and IPME (INH, PZA, moxifloxacin and EMB) in 25% of the cases. During the second phase of the treatment, 75% of the cases received INH and RMP, and 25% received INH and EMB. In 41.7% of patients, hepatotoxicity was associated with the beginning of anti-TB therapy. During a year-long follow-up, renal function remained stable, and the mortality rate was 16.7% [3c].

Although relatively uncommon, cases of RMP-induced acute kidney injury (AKI) have been reported. Moreover, little is known about the renal outcomes and prognostic factors, especially in an aging population. A retrospective study conducted at the National Taiwan University Hospital has shown that 7.1% (99 out of 1394) patients, with a median age of 68 years of old and predominantly male, on anti-TB treatment had AKI [4c]. Sixty-one percent developed AKI within 2 months of anti-TB treatment, including 11% with a prior history of RMP exposure. It is important to note that permanent renal impairment occurs in approximately one-third of the AKI patients [4c].

- A 47-year-old patient was diagnosed with pulmonary TB and was referred to the hospital for inpatient treatment. Following the initiation of treatment, which consisted of a daily regimen of RMP (450 mg), INH (300 mg), PZA (1.2 g) and EMB (750 mg), the patient's symptoms initially improved. On the 19th day, he developed AKI with a fever and chills. Renal biopsy specimens indicated tubulointerstitial nephritis. Suspecting RMP-induced AKI, RMP was discontinued and levofloxacin was administered. The patient's serum creatinine level subsequently gradually improved [5A].

ISSN: 0378-6080
http://dx.doi.org/10.1016/bs.seda.2015.06.009

© 2015 Elsevier B.V. All rights reserved.

Immunologic

Although RMP is often associated with drug interactions and has common serious side effects that include hepatic and immunologic events, it is generally considered a safe drug. The immunologic side effects range from flu-like syndrome to shock. Other immunologic side effects include thrombocytopenia, gastrointestinal symptoms, rash and cutaneous leukocytoclastic vasculitis. A rare case of anti-TB therapy-associated cutaneous leukocytoclastic vasculitis (CLV) has been reported [6A].

- A 14-year-old male diagnosed with disseminated TB developed purpuric lesions after 1.5 months of treatment. Histopathology was consistent with leukocytoclastic vasculitis. Skin lesions improved after cessation of RMP and PZA therapy and treatment with corticosteroids was initiated [6A].

    Thrombocytopenia induced by RMP in the absence of prior sensitization is remarkable, especially when it occurs in a patient without risk factors [7A].

- A 25-year-old patient with no past history of medical, surgical or knowledge of having taken RMP previously, was hospitalized for treatment of thrombocytopenic purpura occurring after the initiation of fixed combination quadruple therapy (INH, RMP, PZA and EMB) for pulmonary TB. On day 9 after initiation of treatment, the patient presented with thrombocytopenic purpura 30 000/mm^3. After 10 days of discontinuation of treatment, the platelet count returned to normal. A phased reintroduction of INH, EMB and PZA was conducted with no recurrence of the thrombocytopenia. However, RMP was not reintroduced given the strong likelihood that it was responsible for this complication. The patient tolerated the remainder of the treatment [7A].

    Although thrombocytopenia with RMP was first documented in 1970, thrombocytopenia with PZA is extremely rare and limited case reports are available. An even rarer adverse event is thrombocytopenia with oral mucosal ecchymosis followed by ulceration and petechiae on legs and forearms caused by both RMP and PZA [8A]. The following case emphasizes the importance of continuous supervision of patients on anti-TB drugs since patients are capable of causing thrombocytopenia at any time during the course of therapy.

- A 32-year-old male patient was diagnosed as having pulmonary TB and was placed on category II antitubercular regime (STR 750 g, INH 600 mg, RMP 450 mg, EMB 1200 mg, and PZA 1500 mg along with daily pyridoxine 10 mg at bed time) since he had a history of anti-TB treatment 10 years ago. After 20 days, patient presented with ulcers in mouth, and blood analysis confirmed thrombocytopenia. RMP-induced thrombocytopenia was suspected and

antitubercular treatment stopped. Upon re-exposure of the patient to the drugs one after the other, the platelet count decreased drastically and oral mucosal ecchymosis reappeared after re-exposure with PZA. Additionally, after re-exposure to RMP, the patient developed thrombocytopenia accompanied with petechiae on legs and forearms. However, re-exposure to INH, EMB, and STR was uneventful and thus was continued [8A].

In addition to the above-mentioned RMP associated side effects, an association between angioedema and RMP has never been reported. The following case study revealed an incidence of angioedema in a patient a month after starting RMP [9A].

- A 62-year-old woman was in close contact of a patient with active, sputum positive TB. She had a positive Quantiferon test and no evidence for active disease. She had never taken RMP before. She began RMP 600 mg daily. After 4 days of treatment, the patient developed mild itching that was unresponsive to diphenhydramine. After 23 days, her lips and eyelid swelled and she developed a generalized rash. She was admitted to the hospital for angioedema. No abnormality was found in routine laboratory tests. She recovered 2 days after stopping RMP. RMP-induced angioedema is a life threatening side effect and should not be readministered in this case [9A].

Hepatic

Although several randomized trials have been conducted to compare the efficacies of nevirapine (NVP) and efavirenz (EFV) based regimens in HIV-associated TB, the use of these drugs remains controversial. RMP, a key component of anti-TB therapy, is a potent inducer of the cytochrome P450 enzyme system; activation of this system leads to enhanced clearance of nevirapine or efavirenz [10c]. A comprehensive search of the literature has shown that EFV regimen for patients co-infected with HIV and TB is associated with more successful virological outcomes compared to the standard NVP regimen [11M].

Although it is known that INH, RMP, NVP, and EFV are all associated with hepatotoxicity, little is known about the relative rates of hepatotoxicity with either NVP or EFV in the setting of RMP-based TB treatment. Further, there is no information on rates of hepatotoxicity among HIV–TB co-infected patients treated with an intermittent (three times weekly) regimen.

- A prospective four arm observational study confirmed that TB–HIV co-infected patients receiving concomitant HIV and TB therapy are at a higher risk to develop severe drug-induced liver injury (DILI) than HIV patients receiving highly active antiretroviral treatment (HAART) alone or TB patients receiving anti-TB therapy alone. Of the 1060 patients enrolled into four treatment groups, 15% developed DILI with varying severity grades. Incidence of DILI was highest in TB–HIV co-infected patients with CD4 ≤ 200 cells/μL, receiving concomitant RMP based anti-TB and EFV-based HAART. Concomitant anti-TB–HIV therapy increased the risk of DILI by 10-fold than anti-TB alone ($p < 0.0001$) [12c]. Hepatotoxicity was not a major concern when HIV-infected TB patients, with normal baseline liver function, initiate once-daily NVP or EFV-based ART along with RMP-containing anti-TB treatment. HIV–TB patients treated with an intermittent anti-TB regimen and once-daily NNRTI-based ART regimen did not experience significant changes in liver function over 12 months [13c].

Drug–Drug Interactions

Given the need of multi-drug therapy for the treatment of TB, drug–drug interaction is always a major concern. A case of profound hypotension after anesthesia induction with propofol in a patient who was treated with two 600 mg doses of RMP for prophylaxis of infection before surgery was reported. A retrospective case–control study of 75 patients confirmed this potentially serious drug–drug interaction. The patient who received RMP experienced a significant and prolonged arterial blood pressure drop with propofol, but not thiopental [14A].

Rifabutin (RBT)

RBT, the semisynthetic derivative of rifamycin S, is routinely used to treat TB. This drug can be used as an alternative to rifapentine (RPT) in anti-TB regimens in the circumstances when the adverse effects of the latter are not tolerated. A recent study of 39 elderly patients (mean age was 69 years) who received RBT resulted in a good tolerance and patient compliance [15c]. However, 72% of the patients (28 patients) experienced treatment-related adverse effects including gastrointestinal complications (16 cases), liver dysfunction (7 cases), skin rashes (6 cases), renal dysfunction (1 case), and thrombocytopenia (1 case).

Drug–Drug Interactions

RMP and protease inhibitors are difficult to use concomitantly in patients with HIV-associated TB because of drug–drug interactions. Recently, some international guidelines have recommended a higher dose of RBT (150 mg daily) in combination with boosted lopinavir (LPV/r), than the previous dose of RBT (150 mg three times weekly) [16c]. An open-label, randomized, three-period, crossover drug interaction study was undertaken to assess the tolerability and safety of RBT and LPV/r. Sixteen patients with TB–HIV co-infection received RBT 300 mg QD in combination with TB chemotherapy (initially PZA, INH and EMB then only INH) and were then randomized to receive INH and LPV/r based ART with

RBT 150 mg thrice a week or RBT 150 mg daily. The RBT dose with ART was switched after 1 month. RBT was well tolerated at all doses and there were no grade 4 laboratory toxicities. One case of uveitis (grade 4), occurred in a patient taking RBT 300 mg daily prior to starting ART, and grade 3 neutropenia (asymptomatic) was reported in 4 patients. These events were not associated with increases in RBT or metabolite concentrations [17c].

Due to the drug–drug interactions associated with conventional RMP and protease inhibitors, the use of RBT is favored in patients receiving HAART. However, a recent case highlights the importance of considering the diagnosis of drug-induced lupus (DIL) in the setting of RBT treatment. To date, only 3 cases of RBT-induced lupus have been reported and none has been reported in blacks. Drug-induced lupus (DIL) is a rare adverse reaction to medications with features resembling idiopathic systemic lupus erythromatosis [18A].

- A 55-year-old woman with HIV presented with intermittent headache, weakness, and lightheadedness for 2 months. She had self-discontinued her antiretroviral (ARV) medications 3 months prior to presentation. Tuberculous skin test in the current admission was positive and she was started empirically on anti-TB medications using RBT, INH, PZA and EMB. RBT was used since she was planning to resume her HIV antiretroviral therapy. TB treatment was discontinued for 10 weeks due to INH hepatotoxicity. After 4 weeks of restarting treatment with RBT, EMB and PZA, she presented with severe generalized arthralgias which began in her knees and later progressed to her joints in the ankle, wrists, and hands. She also had recurrent oral ulcers but had no associated fever or rash. During this time, her antinuclear antibody (ANA) was 1:1280 homogenous patterns. Within 2 months of stopping RBT, her symptoms resolved while continuing other anti-TB medications and her ANA titer started to decrease [18A].

Latent TB Infection

In many countries with a low incidence of TB, many new cases emerge as a result of reactivation of latent TB infection (LTBI), which is often acquired in high-incidence areas or from recent exposure in occasional outbreaks. Therefore, promising new regimens that may be more effective in treating LTBI are being introduced. Because few regimens can be directly compared, using a network meta-analyses approach enables the indirect comparison of regimens and thus produces inferences of relative efficacy that would not otherwise be possible. Using this approach, a comparison study of 15 different regimens from 53 different studies has shown that INH for 6 months or 12 months or longer, RMP for 3–4 months and RMP–INH regimens for 3–4 months were efficacious compared with placebo within the network [19M]. Furthermore, RMP-only and RPT–INH regimens had lower rates of hepatotoxicity than an INH-only regimen of 6 or 9 months, or 9 or 12 to 72 months, respectively. RMP–INH regimens also potentially had lower hepatotoxicity compared to INH-only regimens. The analyses also revealed lower incidences of hepatotoxicity in 6 months of INH or 12 weeks of RPT–INH therapy compared to the regimens containing PZA. These results favored an improved efficacy and lower toxicity of the therapies containing rifamycin over INH [19M].

Rifapentine

Rifapentine (RPT), the semisynthetic analogue of RMP, is generally included in three- or four-drug regimens and is currently approved for intermittent dosing in the treatment of TB. Recent clinical studies revealed that a 6-month regimen that included a continuation phase of intermittent treatment with high-dose RPT (1200 mg) and moxifloxacin (400 mg) administered once weekly was equally effective compared to the 6-month control regimen that included daily administration of INH and RMP. Additionally, the 4-month regimen of RPT (900 mg) and moxifloxacin (400 mg) was not noninferior to the 6-month control regimen. Among 827 patients eligible for the safety analysis, there were a total of 45 grade 3 or 4 adverse events in treatment among 38 patients. These events were approximately equally distributed across the treatment groups. Additionally, there were a total of 25 deaths with a slightly increased number in the 4-month regimen. These results could facilitate the strategy of directly observed treatment and could be used as first-line treatment in certain settings, for instance patients with high rates of INH resistance [20c].

BEDAQUILINE

Bedaquiline (BDQ) possesses a unique mechanism of action that disrupts the activity of the mycobacterial adenosine triphosphate synthase [21R]. Clinical trials have been conducted evaluating the use of BDQ in combination with a background regimen for the treatment of adults with pulmonary multidrug-resistant TB (MDR-TB). However, its side effect profile limits its use against MDR-TB when no other effective regimen can be provided. BDQ carries Black Box warnings for increased risk of unexplained mortality and QT prolongation. BDQ is metabolized via the CYP3A4 isoenzyme and thus interacts with rifamycins and several antiretrovirals [22R]. BDQ has been associated with accelerated sputum-culture conversion in patients with MDR-TB, when added to a preferred background regimen for 8 weeks. In a phase 2b trial, 160 randomly assigned

patients with newly diagnosed, smear-positive MDR-TB received either 400 mg of BDQ once daily for 2 weeks, followed by 200 mg three times a week for 22 weeks, or placebo, both in combination with a preferred background regimen [23c]. The primary efficacy end point was the time to sputum-culture conversion in liquid broth. Patients were then followed for 120 weeks from baseline. Cure rates at 120 weeks were 58% in the BDQ group and 32% in the placebo group ($p = 0.003$). The overall incidence of adverse events was similar in the two groups. Overall, 10 of 79 patients (13%) in the BDQ group and 2 of 81 patients (2%) in the placebo group died ($p = 0.02$), with no causal pattern evident. The reason for higher mortality in the BDQ group compared to the placebo group is unclear [23c].

There have been a few reports of BDQ use in a non-trial setting from Europe. A study consisting of a series of five patients is the first series of drug-resistant TB (DR-TB) patients from India to receive BDQ. All five patients showed striking improvement, with microbiological conversion and an absence of notable adverse effects (e.g., prolonged QTcF), indicating the potential impact of this drug in such a population [24c].

LINEZOLID

Linezolid (LNZ) is the first member of a new synthetic class of antimicrobials known as oxazolidinones with activity against many important pathogens including multidrug-resistant tubercle *Bacillus*, methicillin-resistant *Staphylococcus* and *Streptococcus* [25E]. There is limited data available regarding the efficacy and safety of LNZ in MDR-TB since it is always administered as part of combination therapy. LNZ has been used for the treatment of MDR-TB in adults and pediatric population [26c]. There is mounting evidence on the utility of LNZ in managing extensively drug-resistant (XDR-TB) cases. Limitations of LNZ include high cost and toxicity (myelosuppression and neuropathy), which appears to be determined by dose (>600 mg daily) and duration.

Hematologic

It was found that LNZ is an effective medicine for pulmonary MDR-TB treatment with an acceptable side effect profile [27A].

- A 29-year-old refugee man was referred to the clinic for TB evaluation with positive tuberculin skin (PPD > 13 mm) and QuantiFERON-TB tests. He was living in a camp in Nepal for several years before moving to the United States. The patient underwent excisional biopsy of the cervical lymph nodes, which the pathological examination reported as chronic necrotizing granulomatosis inflammation consistent with TB. Anti-TB therapy was started empirically with a regimen including: INH, RMP, PZA, and EMB on direct observe therapy. Eight weeks later, the sputum and lymph node cultures reported *Mycobacterium TB* complex, and drug susceptibility test (DST) confirmed the presence of a multiple drug-resistant strain. The previous anti-TB regimen was modified to LNZ 300 mg/day, cycloserine 500 mg/day, levofloxacin 750 mg/day and capreomycin 1300 mg/week. Treatment was maintained for 18 months, and closely monitoring toxicities did not reveal evidence of any neurologic adverse effects. However, thrombocytopenia was seen after 2 years follow-up [27A].

Published data for LNZ in the treatment of pediatric DR-TB are limited. A structured review of existing literature identified 8 reports of 18 children receiving LNZ for difficult to treat DR-TB. Adverse events were reported in 9 of 18; a LNZ dose reduction was required in 5 of 18, and 2 of 18 permanently discontinued LNZ because of adverse events [28R].

Hematologic

Eosinophilia and severe neutropenia are rare adverse effects of LNZ. An incident of severe neutropenia was reported in a child during the course of LNZ therapy [29A].

- A 15-month-old boy who was recently diagnosed with TB was admitted for isolation and treatment. The patient had been vaccinated according to the Spanish schedule, which does not include the BCG vaccine. The child began anti-TB therapy with: moxifloxacin 100 mg/day orally administered, ethionamide 125 mg/12 h orally administered, cycloserine 125 mg/12 h orally administered, LNZ 60 mg/12 h orally administered, pyridoxine 25 mg/day orally administered, and capreomycin 175 mg/day by subcutaneous reservoir. The child was kept in strict respiratory isolation until 15 days of treatment were completed. One month later the patient was discharged, continuing outpatient treatment that was well tolerated without adverse effects. In the two subsequent analyses, the child showed moderate neutropenia, with an absolute neutrophil count (ANC) of 840 and 600/μL, respectively. The patient recovered spontaneously on both occasions, without modification or discontinuation of linezolid. The fluctuating course of neutropenia, even when LNZ was continued, was attributed by doctors to a recurrent virus infection. After 2 months, severe neutropenia was detected in the patient with an ANC of 200/μL. Finally, the patient was treated with granulocyte colony-stimulating factor, filgrastim. The child received only two subcutaneous doses of 65 μg of filgrastim (5 μg/kg), after which neutrophils count gradually improved [29A].

Sensory Systems

Although EMB is the most common anti-TB drug implicated to cause toxic optic neuropathy it is important to be aware that if withdrawal of one drug does not show visual recovery or there is further deterioration of vision, the possibility of toxicity due to other drugs should be investigated [30A].

- A 45-year-old male patient who was on treatment with multiple second-line anti-tuberculous drugs including LNZ and EMB for XDR-TB presented with painless progressive loss of vision in both eyes for the past 10 days. Medical history included XDR-TB on treatment with LNZ (600 mg/day), EMB (800 mg/day), moxifloxacin (400 mg/day), cycloserine (500 mg/day), ethionamide (500 mg/day), and kanamycin (750 mg/day) for the past 6 months. Color vision was defective and fundus examination revealed optic disc edema in both eyes. Deterioration of vision occurred despite withdrawal of EMB. Discontinuation of linezolid resulted in marked improvement of vision [30A].

ISONIAZID

Isoniazid (INH, pyridine-4-carboxy hydrazide), a hydrazide derivative of isonicotinic acid, has remained among the current first-line drugs to treat TB after its first clinical use half century ago [31R]. Excellent potency, a high target selectivity, and relatively predictable toxicity exhibited by this molecule favors this drug for the extensive treatment period needed to cure TB [32R]. Although the exact mechanism of its antibacterial action is not fully understood, literature reports support the production of reactive nitric oxide radicals and formation of $NAD^+/NADP^+$ adducts to be responsible for the antimycobacterial activity of the drug [31R]. Doses of INH and treatment period vary depending upon the stage of infection (latent vs active), patients' condition, and level of drug resistance. INH monotherapy (5 mg/kg daily dose for 6 months, maximum dose 300 mg daily) is preferred as a preventive therapy for persons with latent TB who are living with HIV positive individuals [33M,34R,35M]. INH and RMP are also given for 6 months to treat drug-susceptible TB whereas EMB and PZA are included in the regimen for the first 2 months of the 6-month regimen [34R]. In addition, a high dose (daily dose 16–20 mg/kg for 6 months) of INH has been considered as a treatment option for selected cases where other options are not feasible [34R,36R]. However, a number of side effects of INH therapy have been known to cause low patient adherence with the medication making the prevention and treatment of TB a challenging task. A plethora of side effects of INH observed during late 2013 and 2014 are briefly discussed under the following subsections.

Hepatotoxicity

INH is extensively metabolized in the liver and is responsible for the general hepatotoxicity in patients under INH-alone or INH-containing multi-drug therapy [37R]. Hepatic N-acetyltransferase 2 (NAT2) catalyzes the acetylation step of INH where the products undergo further modifications to yield hydrazine and acetylated hydrazine derivatives. Recent studies revealed that hepatotoxicity of INH mainly arise from hydrazine instead of acetylated derivatives of INH (Scheme 1). In the lack of sufficient acetylation activities, INH undergoes hydrolysis to produce the toxic metabolite hydrazine. As a consequence, slow acetylators have more than a twofold risk of developing hepatic diseases compared to fast acetylators [37R,38c]. Animal studies revealed a novel mechanism for liver injury where co-treatment of INH and RMP altered heme biosynthesis through pregnane X-receptor mediated pathway [39E]. A recent study also revealed previously unrecognized mechanisms such as INH-induced modulation of the adaptive and innate immune system, mitochondrial dysfunction and environmental factors [40R].

A retrospective study of 926 patients with non-multi drug resistance (non-MDR) pulmonary TB revealed an incidence rate of 0.59 for INH-treatment associated hepatotoxicity per 100 person-months (2% of total TB patients under study), where patients were treated with INH (4–6 mg/kg), RMP (RMP, 8–12 mg/kg), and pyrazinamide (PZA, 20–25 mg/kg) in a sequence for 4122.9 person-months as per TB-treatment guideline in Taiwan. INH evidently displayed the least toxicity among the three drugs and the cumulative incidences of hepatotoxicity were the highest among females over 67.5 years of age. During hepatotoxicity, patients experienced varieties of symptoms including malaise, poor appetite, nausea, vomiting and skin rash [41c]. A study involving 195 patients with active TB also revealed similar results where 1.02% of the INH-treated TB patients developed hepatotoxicity when single daily dose of INH (300 mg) was co-administered with RMP (450 mg), ethambutol (EMB, 800 mg) and PZA (1000 mg) to patients with body wt. ≤50 kg [42c]. The negative impact of INH on liver function was better demonstrated in the clinical study where 5 out of 100 patients who were prescribed INH (300 mg daily dose) alone for 9 months as a preventive therapy developed hepatitis [43c]. One patient who developed grade 3 or 4 hepatitis [peak level of bilirubin 100 μM/L and alanine transferase (ALT) 1268 IU/L]

did not have pre-existing liver function test abnormalities, and his liver function was restored following the cessation of INH therapy. INH-induced hepatitis has often been a key reason for discontinuation of the course of preventive therapy among people with LTBI. A retrospective study revealed that 8 out of 1587 adolescents and children receiving INH as a preventive therapy had to quit INH-therapy as a result of hepatitis and about 20% of the total follow-up visits were primarily due to the symptoms of adverse effects [44c]. A similar retrospective study of 1582 children who received INH as a preventive therapy for 9 months revealed higher incidences (13 patients, 0.8%) of hepatotoxicities [45c]. The majority of hepatotoxicities were noted within 6 months of therapy and the liver function restored to normal in all cases when INH therapy was stopped.

Genetic Susceptibility

N-acetyltransferase 2 (NAT-2) and glutathione S-transferases (GSTs) are involved in the metabolism/detoxification of INH and related metabolites. To explore the correlation between genetic polymorphism of the genes involved in INH metabolism and INH-mediated hepatotoxicity, Xiang and co-workers have conducted a study in over 2244 TB patients who were treated INH and pyrazinamide (PZA) [46C]. Genotype analysis of 89 patients (4%) who developed drug induced liver injury within 2 months of treatment revealed an association between NAT2*5 allele and the drug induced hepatotoxicity. The toxicity was more prevalent in people with the CT genotype compared to CC (prevalence ratio = 1.70, 95% CI = 1.10–2.70, $p = 0.0623$). The results also revealed twofold increased in toxicity among slow acetylators compared to the rapid acetylators. Similar results were found in a parallel study that involved 26 patients with INH-induced hepatotoxicity [47c]. However, conflicting results were reported for the association of polymorphisms of GSTs with INH-induced hepatotoxicity. Two independent pharmacogenomics studies conducted Chinese TB patients did not reveal any statistically significant association between drug-induced liver injury and null mutation genotypes GSTM1 and GSTM2 [46C,48c]. In contrast, Gupta and coworkers have reported a statistically significant association of drug induced hepatotoxicity with the null mutation in GSTM1 gene alone ($p < 0.02$) or with GHSTM1 and T1 genes ($p < 0.007$) among western Indian TB patients who received multi-drug therapy including INH (INH: 5 mg/kg, max. 300 mg/day; RMP: 10 mg/kg, max. 600 mg/day; pyrazinamide (PZA): 25 mg/kg, max. 2000 mg/day; ethambutol (EMB): 15–25 mg/kg, max. 1500 mg/day) [49c]. Since multiple drugs were included in the regimen, the exact correlation of the individual drugs to the hepatotoxicity and genetic variation could not be established.

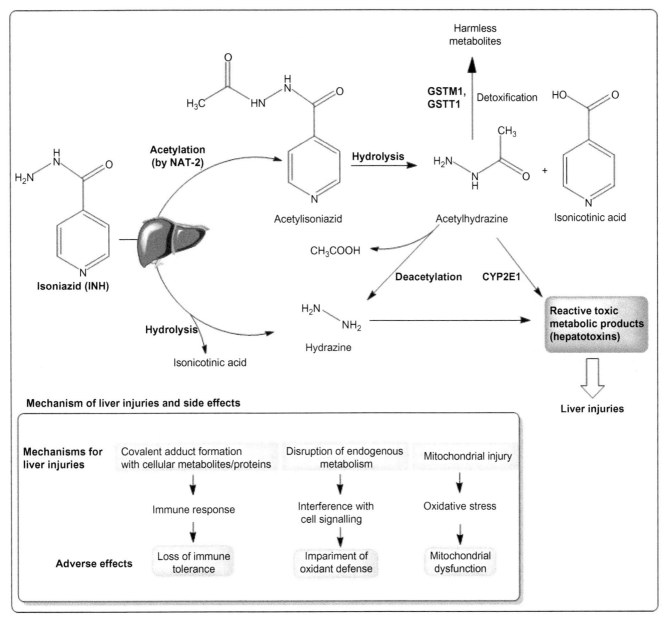

SCHEME 1 Mechanism of INH-induced hepatic injuries and adverse effects [40R]. NAT2: *N*-acetyltransferase 2; CYP2E1 (a CYP450 isoform); GSTM1 and GSTT1: glutathione *S*-transferases. INH is metabolized in the liver into hydrazine and acetylated hydrazine. Both products can further convert into reactive toxic metabolites. Hepatic glutathione *S*-transferases (GSTM1 and GSTT1) modify acetylated hydrazine and prevent them from converting into reactive species. Mechanism of injuries and associated adverse effects is summarized in a box.

Gastrointestinal and Dermatological

Gastrointestinal (GI) side effects are common for many medications and INH is not an exception. A prospective clinical study that involved INH alone (300 mg, single dose daily for 9 months) as a preventive therapy for 100 patients with LTBI revealed GI side effects in 21 patients [43c]. Although the majority of these adverse effects were observed at the beginning of the treatment period and resolved spontaneously, two patients were forced to quit the therapy due to the persistence and severity of the side effects. Dermatological manifestations occurred in 15 patients where 7 patients developed acneiform rashes, 7 patients developed generalized rashes, and one patient developed both. It is notable that one of the patients who had pre-existing acne developed a severe flare and required subsequent treatment with isotretinoin.

Neurotoxicity

Peripheral neuropathy is a known side effect of INH therapy. It is reported that 2% of the patients under isoniazid medication develop peripheral neuropathy due to the interference of INH in the metabolism of pyridoxine [36R,50R]. The level of toxicity is positively correlated to the dose of INH [51A]. Ophthalmic evaluation of 20 patients who were receiving INH and ETM treatment for pulmonary or extra-pulmonary TB displayed a significant thinning of retinal nerve fiber layer (RNFL) in both eyes compared to pre-treatment baseline levels (p values for right eye's average RNFL, superior quadrant RNFL, left eye's average RNFL, superior quadrant, and inferior quadrant RNFLs were 0.024, 0.006, 0.001, 0.008, and <0.001, respectively) [52c]. Although the results were indicative of INH and ETM induced optic neuropathy, the extent of individual drug's contribution to the development of this condition was not determined. Development of severe optic neuropathy was also reported in a case study where a 59-year-old Nigerian woman with multi-drug resistant TB was treated with INH and ETM. The patient recovered complete visual function after 10 months from the suspension of anti-TB therapy [53A]. Isolated Jarisch–Herxhemier reaction manifested by the anterior chamber inflammation, optic disc swelling, cystoid macular edema, periphlebitis in both eyes and abnormal visual acuity (20/200) was reported in a separate case report where a 7-year-old girl with positive tuberculin test was treated with INH [54A].

Denholm and co-workers reported 4 incidences of grade 1 neuropathy among 100 patients who were taking INH as a single drug preventive therapy [43c]. Three out of four episodes of neuropathy developed following the introduction of INH therapy. Furthermore, nine patients experienced perceived cognitive impairment and 7 patients reported lethargic effects. Numerous reports on high doses of INH-induced seizure are available in the literatures [55A]. Ingestion of high doses of INH is known to cause seizures ($\geq$30 mg/kg body wt.) or death ($\geq$80 mg/kg body wt.) [51A]. Although there are limited reports on induction of seizure caused by a therapeutic dose of INH, a recent report presented a case of convulsive seizures that was associated with the short-term administration of a therapeutic dose of INH [51A].

- An 86-year-old woman with tuberculous peritonitis and pulmonary TB was treated with INH (4.4 mg/kg, 200 mg daily), RMP (10 mg/kg, 450 mg daily) ethambutol (16.6 mg/kg, 750 mg daily). On the fifth day of the treatment, the patient complained of visual disturbances and auditory abnormalities. Disturbances on consciousness and tonic–clonic convulsions were developed after 2 days. No abnormality was found on physical exam, head CT or magnetic resonance imaging (MRI) scans, cerebrospinal fluid (CSF) examination, and in the culture of acid-fast bacterial strains and other culture tests. No specific cause for convulsions was identified through the test except the remarkably low serum vitamin B_6 level [pyridoxamine:

<0.2 ng/mL (normal level: <0.6 ng/mL), pyridoxal: <2.0 ng/mL (normal range: 4.0–19.0 ng/mL) and pyridoxine: <3.0 ng/mL (normal level: <3.0 ng/mL). Since no other medications that are known to cause low plasma level of vitamin B_6 were administered during the course of anti-TB therapy, the low level of vitamin B_6 was concluded to cause convulsion. The clonic convulsive seizure did not stop with the IV administration of diazepam (10 mg), phenobarbital (500 mg) and phenytoin (500 mg). This prompted the discontinuation of anti-TB drugs and administration of pyridoxal phosphate hydrate (60 mg per day). The intensity of seizure gradually decreased and disappeared completely in 3 days following the vitamin B_6 therapy [51A].

Psychiatry

Cognitive impairment and lethargy represent emerging side effects of INH therapy. Denholm and co-workers reported a transient psychosis in a patient following a month of INH therapy. Psychosis, obsessive–compulsive disorders, and mood alterations are well-documented side effects of INH [32R].

Autoimmune Disorders

The use of INH in relieving the symptoms of multiple sclerosis, particularly cerebellar tremors, dates back to early 1980s [56c]. INH is still a treatment option for relapsing-remitting multiple sclerosis (RRMS) [57R]. Nourbakhsh et al. reported a rare case concerning the development lupus erythematosus and multiple sclerosis (MS) by INH therapy [58A].

- A 39-year-old man with tuberculin skin test developed neurological symptoms following isoniazid (INH) as preventive therapy for TB. The patient developed multiple symptoms such as fatigue, a tremor of his neck and extremities, and heat sensitivity. Although he was first diagnosed with drug-induced lupus erythematosus (DILE), continuous progression of neurological disorders prompted for further diagnostic testing including magnetic resonance imaging (MRI) of his brain and spinal cord and cerebrospinal fluid (CSF) analyses. The results led to the diagnosis of primary progressive multiple sclerosis (PPMS). A chest X-ray was normal and the following laboratory tests were negative or within normal limits: thyroid stimulating hormone, anti-aquaporin-4 antibody, antinuclear antibodies, rheumatoid factor, hemoglobin A1C, human immunodeficiency virus 1 and 2, and a vitamin B_{12} level. The patient reported urinary incontinence, erectile dysfunction and was unable to ambulate. Neurological examinations revealed a bilateral intermittent gaze-associated pendular nystagmus, a 4–5-beat clonus over both ankles, intermittent irregular holding tremor of the hands, weakened strength in the lower extremities, and a bilateral intention tremor [58A].

Although the exact mechanism for INH-induced PRMS is not known, it is suggested that INH may facilitate the onset of demyelinating disease through the activation of central nervous system (CNS) autoantigen-reactive CD4+T cells [58A].

Tenosynovitis

Although infections of *Mycobacterium bovis* and other atypical mycobacterial species are recently known to cause recurrent tenosynovitis [59A]. This condition is rarely known as an adverse effect of INH therapy. Yamamoto and coworkers have reported two cases of such rare incidences [60A].

- A 49-year-old diabetic mellitus man with hypoesthesia experienced difficulty in grasping with his right hand after 1 month of anti-TB drug therapy (isoniazid, RMP, ethambutol, and pyrazinamide). He was diagnosed with tenosynovitis following the MRI imaging. Isoniazid was identified to be correlated to the tenosynovitis in the clinical course and isoniazid challenge test. The patient's symptoms gradually improved after discontinuation of isoniazid treatment [60A].
- A 78-year-old man with the history of gout developed edema and arthralgia on both hands 3 weeks after the surgery of rectal cancer. His TB was identified during preoperative screening tests for rectal cancer and he was given anti-TB therapy. Discontinuation of pyrazinamide did not improve the symptoms of gout. He was diagnosed with tenosynovitis based on MRI results. A slight improvement on his symptoms was observed at the end of 6-month anti-TB treatment [60A].

ETHAMBUTOL

Visual Impairment

The bacteriostatic drug ethambutol (EMB) is widely used to treat both tubercular and non-tubercular mycobacterial infections. EMB is a drug of choice for the treatment of infections caused by *Mycobacterium avium* complex (MAC). Although this drug is considered as the least toxic among the first-line anti-TB drugs, EMB-associated ocular toxicity is widely reported in the literatures [61c]. An analysis of 36 patients with drug-related visual impairment reported 12 (33.3%) cases with EMB (dose range 800 mg–1.2 g daily)-induced neuropathy where 7 patients experienced permanent vision loss

[62c]. EMB-induced optic neuropathy is often manifested by a decrease in visual acuity, deficit in color vision and cecocentral scotomas, and is related to dose and duration of treatment [53A,61c]. However, the latter was disputed in case reports where patients developed optic neuropathy with the treatment of renal function-adjusted doses of EMB in increased dosing intervals or even after cessation of EMB therapy [63E,64A,65A]. Abnormalities in optic chiasm are also reported in MRI images of patients with EMB-induced bitemporal hemianopia [66A]. Other rarely occurring adverse effects of EMB therapy include peripheral neuropathy, cutaneous reactions, thrombocytopenia, and hepatitis [67R].

The exact mechanism by which EMB exerts toxic effect is not fully known. EMB is proposed to cause cellular injuries by facilitating the production of reactive oxygen species which disrupts oxidative phosphorylation and mitochondrial function by interfering with iron-containing complex I and copper-containing complex IV [68M,69R]. Observation of notable damage of retinal ganglion cells with EMB-induced optic neuropathies in monkeys provides explanation for observation of temporal pallor in neuropathy patients where damage in mitochondria-rich ganglionic cells was apparent [69R]. Although a recent clinical study revealed a significant decrease of vitamin E and vitamin B levels among patients who developed EMB-induced toxic optic neuropathy, the exact of correlation between these factors and toxicity has not fully established [70c].

Association of EMB treatment with ocular toxicity was further investigated in a prospective cohort study, where 64 Indian TB patients were treated with combination drugs involving EMB [61c]. Patients were divided into two categories based on the treatment regimen (category I: treatment with RMP (450 mg), INH (600 mg), EMB (1200 mg), and PZA (1500 mg), thrice weekly for 2 months followed by 4 months of RMP and INH of the same dose; category II: treatment with streptomycin (STR, 750 mg), INH (600 mg), RMP (450 mg), EMB (1200 mg), and PZA (1500 mg) for 2 months followed by 1 month of the same regimen without STR, and an intensive phase of 5 months (thrice per week) of RMP, INH, and EMB. At the second month follow-up, a notable loss in visual acuity from the baseline, visual field defects, optic disc abnormalities and color vision abnormalities were observed in 9.4% eyes ($p=0.001$), 6.3% eyes ($p=0.0412$), 4.7% ($p=0.013$) and 12.6% eyes ($p=0.003$), respectively. Improvement on visual acuity was observed in 1–2 months after patients stopped taking EMB. However, discontinuation of EMB did not affect overall outcome of treatment.

Genetic Predisposition

Charcot–Marie–Tooth disease Type 2A2 (CMT2A2) is part of a group of genetic disorders and is associated with mutations in the mitofusin 2 (*MFN2*) gene that encodes a protein involved in mitochondrial fusion. A case study indicated EMB to accelerate the onset of numerous adverse effects including acceleration of weakness, vocal cord paralysis, and optic atrophy in a patient with pre-existing CMT2A2 and MFN2 mutations (T669G and F223L) [71A]. EMB is also known to cause a defect in mitochondrial coupling through the reduction of the activity of complex IV by 25% in fibroblasts of a person carrying mutations on functionally related optic atrophy 1 (*OPA1*) gene [72A]. The results taken together support a higher risk of EMB-induced ocular toxicity among patients with mutation on genes encoding proteins implicated in mitochondrial fusion.

Hypersensitivity Reactions

EMB-induced hypersensitivity reactions such as rash, dermatosis-like pigmentations, lichenoid eruptions, and drug fever are widely reported in the literatures. Despite the use of multiple drugs in anti-TB treatment regimen, multiple drug allergy (MDA) that occurs as result of simultaneous use of two or more chemically unrelated drugs is scarce. Özkaya reported such a rare case where 58-year-old TB patient who developed a generalized eczematous eruption after receiving a combination therapy involving INH, EMB, RMP and morphazinamide. Patch tests indicated INH and EMB to be responsible for the generalized hypersensitivity [73A].

EMB-induced drug reactions with eosinophilia and systemic symptoms (DRESS) are relatively rare. DRESS can lead to potentially life-threatening conditions that involve eruption of skin, hematologic abnormalities, lymphadenopathy, and damage of internal organs including kidney, lungs and liver [74R]. EMB was reported to induce DRESS in a Korean patient [75A].

- A 68-year-old woman, who was under multi-drug anti-TB therapy for the treatment of her tuberculous pericarditis for 7 weeks was admitted to the emergency department with rashes on her trunk and extremities along with painful erosions on her oral mucosa. Based on laboratory findings and physical examination, she was suspected of having Stevens–Johnson Syndrome (SJS). Therefore, anti-tuberculous medications were stopped and methylprednisolone (1 mg/kg/day) was administered systemically. A gradual improvement on her skin rash and oral mucosal lesions was observed. On the day 11, she developed maculopapular eruptions and painful cervical lymphadenopathy. Notable differences in her cutaneous manifestations such as development targetoid lesion or blister formation were observed at this time compared to the initial findings. Follow-up laboratory tests revealed leukocytosis (13020/mm³)

with hypereosinophilia (2734/mm³), atypical lymphocytosis (10%; normal <1%), acute renal dysfunction (serum creatinine 4.7 mg/dL) and elevated ALT (63 IU/L). Immunological tests were negative for cytomegalovirus and Epstein–Barr virus on day 12. Five days later, both AST/ALT and serum creatinine increased to peaks of 95/118 IU/L and 5.4 mg/dL, respectively. Based on the RegiSCAR scoring system, DRESS was diagnosed. Treatment of the patient with three courses of hemodialysis and a high-dose systemic corticosteroid facilitated recovery, and the patient was discharged after 1 month of hospitalization. An oral low dose of corticosteroid was maintained for an additional month. After 4 months, patch tests were conducted in petroleum ether using individual anti-TB drugs. EMB caused a grade 2 positive reaction at 48 h. Lymphocyte transformation test (LTT) was only positive for EMB with stimulation index of >2.5 [75A].

- A rare incidence of EMB-induced pulmonary eosinophilia was reported in an Indian patient who was under multi-drug anti-TB therapy (daily doses of RMP, INH, EMB and PZA) [76A]. Follow-up test and analysis revealed EMB to be the sole drug to cause eosinophilia. Such EMB-induced life threatening reactions necessitate a need of a desensitization procedure prior to beginning of treatment and a careful observation following the initiation of treatment with EMB [77A].

FLUOROQUINOLONES

The synthetic antibiotics fluoroquinolones are broadly active against both Gram-positive and -negative bacterial species. Bactericidal activity of fluoroquinolones arises from the inhibition of bacterial DNA gyrase and topoisomerase IV, which are necessary for bacterial DNA duplication [78R]. High potencies, broad-spectrum activities, and excellent oral bio-availabilities of fluoroquinolones made these drugs suitable to treat varieties of infectious diseases including TB. Members of fluoroquinolones such as levofloxacin, moxifloxacin and ofloxacin are generally considered as the second-line therapy due to the high incidences of drug resistance against these drugs. While many clinical studies reported a good toleration of fluoroquinolones among patients, numerous adverse effects associated with these drugs are noted in other studies [79M,80c,81c]. Dose- and duration-dependent cartilage injury of fluoroquinolones observed in animal studies raised a major safety concern for their use in treating infections in children. However, none of such adverse effect was observed in a randomized prospective clinical study where 124 children with acute otitis media and community-acquired pneumonia were treated with levofloxacin (L) and followed up for 5 years of post-treatment [82C]. Considering a longer duration of treatment needed in anti-TB therapy, further study is need to ascertain the safety of fluoroquinolones in treating TB in children. A randomized control trial involving 416 subjects compared the efficacy of gatifloxacin- and moxifloxacin-containing regimens (gatifloxacin, INH and RMP, and moxifloxacin, INH and RMP) to the control (INH, RMP, EMB, and PZA) group [83c]. The results revealed a significant increase of adverse effects associated with the former regimens. The incidences of anthralgia, cutaneous, dizziness, gastrointestinal, seizures were 1.2- to 5-fold higher among subjects who received fluoroquinolones compared to the control subjects. A separate study reported gastrointestinal adverse effects (nausea, vomiting and diarrhea) to be the primary cause for the discontinuation of moxifloxacin therapy [84c].

Although clinical studies assure safety of levofloxacin and moxifloxacin concerning hepatotoxicity [85c], sporadic incidences of other severe adverse effects such as sudden onset of hyperglycemia, generalized pruritus, seizure, myasthenic crisis and drug-induced hypersensitivity warrant a need for a closer look while treating patients with these drugs [86A,87A,88A,89A,90A].

- Pulmonary TB of a 27-year-old man was treated with INH, RMP, EMB, and PZA. Due to the development of hepatic dysfunction and visual impairment, a three-drug regimen including INH, RMP and levofloxacin was used to replace the initial four-drug regimen. At the ninth week of levofloxacin-containing therapy, the patient developed cervical lymphadenopathy, fever, systemic erythema, and hepatic dysfunction. Drug-induced hypersensitivity syndrome (DIHS) was diagnosed based on positive HHV-6 reactivation test. The symptoms gradually improved following the withdrawal of the anti-TB drugs and initiation of steroid therapy [90A].

PYRAZINAMIDE

Although pyrazinamide (PZA) is considered as an effective and well-tolerated first-line anti-TB drug, it is known to cause numerous adverse effects including hepatitis and hypersensitivity. A case study report revealed PZA-induced hepatitis and gastritis in a patient undergoing anti-TB therapy [91A]. Similarly, the other report revealed a rare incidence of PZA-induced olfactory disturbance in a patient [92A]. Similarly, PZA is reported to cause the retention of uric acid [93c]. PZA is metabolized by xanthine oxidase to produce pyrazinoic acid which is proposed to be responsible for the hyperuricemic effect [94A]. In handful of incidences PZA-associated hyperuricemia have been recently reported [95A,96A]. A prospective study of 39 Indian patients who were treated with PZA revealed an increase in serum uric acid level in 41.02% of the patients, but the data were not statistically significant to establish PZA as the cause [96R].

Photosensitivity

Photosensitivity reactions due to PZA rarely occur. A case report revealed such incidence in a patient [97A].

- A 40-year-old woman with TB was treated with an appropriate doses of multi-drug therapy including RMP, INH, EMB and PZA. After 3 weeks of drug therapy, mild pruritus with macular rash appeared on her face and arms after exposure to sunlight, and the condition worsened to blisters formation. PZA-induced photosensivity was suspected. Discontinuation of PZA and avoidance of exposure to sunlight led to the recovery of the patient in 4 months [97A].

Hematology

Hypersensitive reactions of PZA leading to hematological disorders such as DRESS and thrombocytopenia are relatively scarce. A direct role of antituberculosis therapy to induce thrombocytopenia has become apparent after several reports on antituberculosis drugs-induced thrombocytopenia in recent years [98A,99A,100R]. Recently, Bansal and co-workers identified both PZA and RMP to be responsible for causing thrombocytopenia. Authors have used discontinuation of one drug at a time approach to pinpoint the causative drug in a patient who under multi-drug therapy developed thrombocytopenia [101A]. Similarly, a separate study reported PZA to cause DRESS syndrome in a patient [102A].

- A 32-year-old male patient who received anti-TB treatment a decade ago developed tubercular pleural effusion and was treated with category II anti-TB treatment under DOTS (streptomycin 750 g, INH 600 mg, RMP 450 mg, EMB 1200 mg, and PZA 1500 mg for three times a week, and a daily dose of 10 mg pyridoxine). After about 20 days of treatment, he developed ulceration in the mouth. His hemogram were as follows: hemoglobin (Hb) 8.3 gm%, total leukocyte count (TLC) 9800 cells/mm^3, erythrocyte sedimentation rate (ESR) 45 mm/1 h, and platelet count 21 000/mm^3. Peripheral smear revealed a shift to the left with thrombocytopenia; prothrombin time Index (PTI) was 76.92%, and international normalized ratio (INR) was 1.43. Enzyme-linked immunosorbant assay (ELISA) test for human immunodeficiency virus (HIV) was negative and random blood sugar level and urinalysis results were normal. RMP was suspected to cause potential thrombocytopenia and all drugs were stopped. Ulcers were healed, platelet count and INR both increased to 472 000/mm^3, and 1.82, respectively. The RMP was removed from the original regimen and the therapy was resumed. The patient developed ulcers in the mouth the next day and the platelet count decreased to 10 000/mm^3. The treatment was stopped for a month that allowed the elevation of platelet count to 505 000/mm^3 and the patient was treated with one drug at a time. Treatment with INH (300 mg) went uneventful. When the patient was treated with 750 mg of PZA, the patient developed ecchymosis ulcers in the mouth within 24 h and the platelet count dropped to 23 000/mm^3. PZA was discontinued, but INH (300 mg) was continued. Patient recovered promptly. When the patient was retreated with RMP 150 mg along with INH 300 mg, petechiae on legs and forearms appeared within 6 h, the patient developed fever with chills and the platelet count decreased to 25 000/mm^3. The lesions subsided within 48 h of RMP withdrawal. Sequential treatment of the patient with EMB and STR went uneventful. The patient was then treated with isoniazid 300 mg, EMB 1000 mg, and STR 750 mg without any further lesions [101A].

- A 21-year-old female with tubercular cervical lymphadenitis began antituberculosis therapy with first-line drugs (RMP, INH, PZA and EMB). She developed fever (41 °C), pruritic maculopapular rash in limbs and face, facial edema, generalized weakness, hepatomegaly, and enlargement of inguinal lymph node. Lab investigation revealed leucocytosis (16 000 cells/mm^3), eosinophilia (3200 cells/mm^3), lymphocytosis (5500 cells/mm^3), thrombocytopenia (75 000 cells/mm^3), and an ESR of 130 mm/h Abnormal LFT findings were ALAT, 180 IU/L; ASAT, 140 IU/L; alkaline phosphatase, 780 IU/L. Blood and urine culture and bone marrow biopsy results were normal. Serological tests negative for hepatitis B and C virus and human immunodeficiency virus and no family history of such adverse reactions with these drugs were identified. Based on these findings, the patient was diagnosed with hypersensitivity to anti-TB drugs. The anti-TB therapy was stopped and steroids were prescribed to the patient for 3 weeks. The anti-TB drugs were then reintroduced one at a time basis. With the reintroduction of PZA, the symptoms reappeared within 1 week and disappeared after 4 weeks following the withdrawal of the drug and treatment with corticosteroids. PZA produced positive hypersensitivity reaction on a PATCH test when the patient was not taking any other drugs except vitamin supplements [102A].

CLOFAZIMINE

Clofazimine (CFZ), a fat-soluble riminophenazine dye, is used to treat leprosy worldwide. The drug has been proven in both pre-clinical and clinical studies to be effective to treat drug-resistant mycobacterial infections caused by *Mycobacterium avium*, *Mycobacterium kansasii* and *Mycobacterium avium* complex [103c]. Discoloration of skin, a well-known side effect of CFZ, was the most prominent adverse effect observed in a randomized control study of 105 subjects with multi drug resistance TB (MDR-TB). 94.3% of the patients (50 out of 53) who were treated with CFZ (45 patients, 100 mg daily dose for 21 months) developed skin discoloration whereas 47.2% of the patients experienced ichthyosis [103c]. Similarly, all of the leprosy patients who received CFZ treatment developed skin discoloration [104c]. Although it is becoming apparent that discoloration of skin is a temporary side effect and is reversible upon cessation of therapy, the adverse effect reportedly contributed to causing depression in patients [105c,106R]. A meta-analysis reviewed CFZ-containing treatment regimens in 3489 children and adults with either XDR-TB or MDR-TB. Mortality, treatment interruptions, adverse effects and defaults in CFZ-treated patients were comparable to the established therapies [107M]. Similarly, a separate report noted a 65% in favorable outcomes (cure or treatment completion, 95% CI 54–76) when CFZ-containing regimen was used in treating XDR- and MDR-TB [108M]. Gastrointestinal disturbances and skin pigmentation were the most common adverse effects of the therapy. It is important to note that CFZ was only a part of the therapeutic regimen. Therefore, the contribution of other drugs in causing these adverse effects cannot be ruled out.

Poor aqueous solubility of CFZ has been a concern for treating patients with a high oral dose (100 mg twice or thrice a day). The drug may crystallize in the GI tract to cause gastric enteropathy. Such adverse effect of CFZ has been reported in a recent case study [109A].

- A 19-year-old male leprosy patient who was receiving multi-drug therapy for the last 8 months presented with 1-week history of abdominal pain complained of periumbilical, intermittent and dull-aching pain lasting for hours. The patient described the experience of pain during the night and was not related to food intake. The pain was not relieved by a proton pump inhibitor or an antacid. Physical examination revealed few enlarged lymph nodes at the left cervical region and mild tenderness at the umbilical region without guarding or stiffness. Hepatosplenomegaly or enlargements of the superficial nerve were not detected. Serological test for HIV virus was negative. Other abnormal findings were eosinophilia, hypoalbuminemia, and mild hyperglobulinemia. No indication of malignant lymphoma was found in lymph node biopsy results. Endoscopic biopsies revealed a mild, chronic inflammation of the gastric and duodenal mucosa. Few crystal-storing (red colored) histiocytes were detected in the lamina propria of the duodenum, but several crystal-storing histiocytes were found in the lamina propria of the jejunum. Further investigation concluded these crystals to be of CFZ. The patient had lepra-2 reaction (Erythema Nodosum Leprosum (ENL)) during multi drug therapy course. Therefore, he was prescribed with a high dose of CFZ (100 mg thrice a day for 1 month followed by 100 mg twice a day for next 15 days with additional appropriate corticosteroid) that followed the continuation of regular multi-drug treatment. CFZ was then replaced with an appropriate alternative that facilitated gradual improvement of the patient's condition over about 2 months [109A].

CYCLOSERINE

The broad spectrum antibiotic cycloserine (CS) has been widely used to treat mycobacterial infections since its first introduction in 1954. However, frequent incidences of psychiatric and CNS-related side effects of CS restricted its use as a second-line anti-TB drug for MDR-TB. A recent meta-analysis reviewed 2164 patients covered in 27 studies revealed 9.1% (95% CI 6.4–11.7) incidences of adverse effects associated with CS therapy where psychiatric and CNS-related adverse effects accounted for 5.7% (95% CI 3.7–7.6) and 1.1% (95% CI 0.2–2.1), respectively [110M]. Although the study revealed manageable patients' compliance, the results also highlighted a need for educating patients and health care workers regarding the potential adverse effects of CS-containing regimens.

Psychiatric

A case of CS-induced acute psychosis in a young female during the treatment of tubercular meningitis was presented in the following case study [111A].

- A 20-year-old female, known case of tubercular meningitis on anti-tubercular treatment (ATT) for 8 months, presented with 10-days history of headache, vomiting, and photophobia. A provisional diagnosis of drug-resistant TB was made, and second-line ATT including CS (750 mg/day) and levofloxacin (750 mg/day) was added. Three days after the start of CS and levofloxacin, the patient developed psychosis with delusions and hallucinations. Since the patient was on several drugs with potential to cause psychotic

reaction, a provisional diagnosis of drug-induced acute psychosis was considered. Two days following CS withdrawal, the patient improved significantly, and on the third day, she was absolutely normal with disappearance of psychotic symptoms [111A].

DELAMANID

Delamanid is another very promising compound that has entered Phase III clinical trials. In a study reporting the effects of delamanid in combination with an optimized background regimen, a higher proportion of favorable outcomes was observed in the subset of patients with XDR-TB after extended treatment with delamanid (61.4%) compared with patients receiving the drug for shorter periods (50%). Notably, all 44 patients with XDR-TB who had received delamanid for at least 6 months survived [112c]. While clinical efficacy and safety of delamanid in small cohort-based studies look promising, further clinical studies in bigger subject populations are necessary to validate these initial findings.

DAPSONE

Dapsone (4,40-diaminodiphenylsulfone) has been widely used in the treatment of leprosy since its discovery in the 1940s, and some of its reported side effects include methemoglobinemia, hemolysis, agranulocytosis, and dapsone-induced hypersensitivity reactions (DIHRs). Correlation of genetic susceptibility and dapsone-related adverse effects have become more apparent in recent years.

Genetic Susceptibility

A case–control study from June 2009 to June 2012 was conducted in Southern China and screened 1058 cases of leprosy patients [113c]. Major histocompatibility complex (MHC) I region typing and gene polymorphisms of related metabolism enzymes were detected in 122 leprosy patients exposed to dapsone and 96 healthy controls. It was found that *HLA-B*1301* and *HLA-Cw*0304* were present in significantly higher frequencies in DIHR patients than in either dapsone-tolerant patients or healthy controls. This indicated that the presence of the human leukocyte antigens *HLA-B*1301* haplotype is strongly associated with DIHR development. DIHR mechanism appears to be immunologically related to HLA, but not to dapsone metabolism. However, a larger-scale prospective study is needed to verify the value of *HLA-B*1301* as a predictive biomarker for DIHR. Results of a genome-wide association analysis further shed light into the pathogenesis on this syndrome by showing that single-nucleotide polymorphisms (SNPs) rs2844573, located between the HLA-B and MICA loci, were significantly associated with the dapsone hypersensitivity syndrome among patients with leprosy (odds ratio, 6.18; $p = 3.84 \times 10^{-13}$) [114c]. *HLA-B*13:01* was confirmed to be a risk factor for the dapsone hypersensitivity syndrome (odds ratio, 20.53; $p = 6.84 \times 10^{-25}$) [114c].

- A 42-year-old Chinese woman with borderline lepromatous leprosy that included life-threatening hypersensitivity pneumonitis and fulminant hepatitis was tested after the fact and indeed was *HLA*B13:01* positive [115A].

STREPTOMYCIN

The use of streptomycin (STR) in treating TB is in a gradual decline in recent years. However, it still represents one of the most common injectable anti-TB medication. Ototoxicity is a common side effect of all aminoglycosides including STR regardless of route of their administration. STR is generally administered by deep intramuscular injection and inflammation at the injection site is a common side effect. A clinical study evaluated drug tolerance and safety of short-term (6–23 days) STR treatment in 27 TB patients where the drug was delivered through the intravenous (IV) route. In the study, standard treatment of RMP, INH and PZA was supplemented with IV administration of STR (15 mg/kg/24 h in 100 mL of saline over 45–60 min). While no incidences of vestibular or cochlear toxicity was observed, three patients developed circumoral paresthesia during or immediately after STR infusion highlighting a need for close monitoring of STR treatment [116c].

References

[1] Cragg GM, Grothaus PG, Newman DJ. New horizons for old drugs and drug leads. J Nat Prod. 2014;77(3):703–23 [R].

[2] Fatima R, Ashraf M, Ejaz S, et al. In vitro toxic action potential of anti tuberculosis drugs and their combinations. Environ Toxicol Pharmacol. 2013;36(2):501–13 [E].

[3] Higuita LM, Nieto-Rios JF, Daguer-Gonzalez S, et al. Tuberculosis in renal transplant patients: the experience of a single center in Medellin-Colombia, 2005–2013. J Bras Nefrol. 2014;36(4):512–8 [c].

[4] Chang CH, Chen YF, Wu VC, et al. Acute kidney injury due to anti-tuberculosis drugs: a five-year experience in an aging population. BMC Infect Dis. 2014;14:23 [c].

[5] Chiba S, Tsuchiya K, Sakashita H, et al. Rifampicin-induced acute kidney injury during the initial treatment for pulmonary tuberculosis: a case report and literature review. Intern Med. 2013;52(21):2457–60 [A].

[6] Bhatia V, Sibal A, Rajgarhia S. Antituberculosis therapy-associated cutaneous leukocytoclastic vasculitis. J Trop Pediatr. 2013;59(6):507–8 [A].

[7] Neino Mourtala Mohamed A, Tummino C, Gouitaa M, et al. Thrombocytopenia induced by rifampicin not previously sensitized: a case presentation. Rev Mal Respir. 2013;30(9):785–8 [A].

[8] Bansal R, Sharma PK, Sharma A. A case of thrombocytopenia caused by rifampicin and pyrazinamide. Indian J Pharmacol. 2013;45(4):405–7 [A].

[9] Mirsaeidi M, Schraufnagel D. Rifampin induced angioedema: a rare but serious side effect. Braz J Infect Dis. 2014;18(1):102–3 [A].

[10] Ramachandran G, Kumar AK, Ponnuraja C, et al. Lack of association between plasma levels of non-nucleoside reverse transcriptase inhibitors & virological outcomes during rifampicin co-administration in HIV-infected TB patients. Indian J Med Res. 2013;138:955–61 [c].

[11] Jiang HY, Zhang MN, Chen HJ, et al. Nevirapine versus efavirenz for patients co-infected with HIV and tuberculosis: a systematic review and meta-analysis. Int J Infect Dis. 2014;25:130–5 [M].

[12] Yimer G, Gry M, Amogne W, et al. Evaluation of patterns of liver toxicity in patients on antiretroviral and anti-tuberculosis drugs: a prospective four arm observational study in Ethiopian patients. PLoS One. 2014;9(4):e94271 [c].

[13] Padmapriyadarsini C, Bhavani P, Tang A, et al. Early changes in hepatic function among HIV–tuberculosis patients treated with nevirapine or efavirenz along with rifampin-based anti-tuberculosis therapy. Int J Infect Dis. 2013;17(12):e1154–e1159 [c].

[14] Mirzakhani H, Nozari A, Ehrenfeld JM, et al. Case report: profound hypotension after anesthetic induction with propofol in patients treated with rifampin. Anesth Analg. 2013;117(1):61–4 [A].

[15] Morimoto K, Yoshiyama T, Kuse M, et al. Clinical experience using rifabutin for treating infection with Mycobacterium tuberculosis in elderly Japanese patients. Kekkaku. 2013;88(8):625–8 [c].

[16] Reves R, Heilig CM, Tapy JM, et al. Intermittent tuberculosis treatment for patients with isoniazid intolerance or drug resistance. Int J Tuberc Lung Dis. 2014;18(5):571–80 [c].

[17] Naiker S, Connolly C, Wiesner L, et al. Randomized pharmacokinetic evaluation of different rifabutin doses in African HIV-infected tuberculosis patients on lopinavir/ritonavir-based antiretroviral therapy. BMC Pharmacol Toxicol. 2014;15(1):61 [c].

[18] Anyimadu H, Saadia N, Mannheimer S. Drug-induced lupus associated with rifabutin: a literature review. J Int Assoc Provid AIDS Care. 2013;12(3):166–8 [A].

[19] Stagg HR, Zenner D, Harris RJ, et al. Treatment of latent tuberculosis infection: a network meta-analysis. Ann Intern Med. 2014;161(6):419–28 [M].

[20] Jindani A, Harrison TS, Nunn AJ, et al. High-dose rifapentine with moxifloxacin for pulmonary tuberculosis. New Engl J Med. 2014;371(17):1599–608 [c].

[21] Patel RV, Riyaz SD, Park SW. Bedaquiline: a new hope to treat multi-drug resistant tuberculosis. Curr Top Med Chem. 2014;14(16):1866–74 [R].

[22] Chahine EB, Karaoui LR, Mansour H. Bedaquiline: a novel diarylquinoline for multidrug-resistant tuberculosis. Ann Pharmacother. 2014;48(1):107–15 [R].

[23] Diacon AH, Pym A, Grobusch MP, et al. Multidrug-resistant tuberculosis and culture conversion with bedaquiline. New Engl J Med. 2014;371(8):723–32 [c].

[24] Udwadia ZF, Amale RA, Mullerpattan JB. Initial experience of bedaquiline use in a series of drug-resistant tuberculosis patients from India. Int J Tuberc Lung Dis. 2014;18(11):1315–8 [c].

[25] De Vriese AS, Coster RV, Smet J, et al. Linezolid-induced inhibition of mitochondrial protein synthesis. Clin Infect Dis. 2006;42(8):1111–7 [E].

[26] Anger HA, Dworkin F, Sharma S, et al. Linezolid use for treatment of multidrug-resistant and extensively drug-resistant tuberculosis, New York city, 2000–06. J Antimicrob Chemother. 2010;65(4):775–83 [c].

[27] Farshidpour M, Ebrahimi G, Mirsaeidi M. Multidrug-resistant tuberculosis treatment with linezolid-containing regimen. Int J Mycobacteriol. 2013;2(4):233–6 [A].

[28] Garcia-Prats AJ, Rose PC, Hesseling AC, et al. Linezolid for the treatment of drug-resistant tuberculosis in children: a review and recommendations. Tuberculosis (Edinb). 2014;94(2):93–104 [R].

[29] Hernandez Segurado M, Arias Moya MA, Gomez Perez M, et al. Filgrastim therapy in a child with neutropenia induced by linezolid. Int J Clin Pharm. 2013;35(4):538–41 [A].

[30] Karuppannasamy D, Raghuram A, Sundar D. Linezolid-induced optic neuropathy. Indian J Ophthalmol. 2014;62(4):497–500 [A].

[31] Timmins GS, Deretic V. Mechanisms of action of isoniazid. Mol Microbiol. 2006;62(5):1220–7 [R].

[32] Padmapriyadarsini C, Jawahar M. Drugs used in tuberculosis and leprosy. Side effects of drugs annual. Kidlington, Oxford, UK: Elsevier; 2014, p. 445 [R].

[33] Adams LV, Talbot EA, Odato K, et al. Interventions to improve delivery of isoniazid preventive therapy: an overview of systematic reviews. BMC Infect Dis. 2014;14(1):281 [M].

[34] Lienhardt C, Vernon A, Raviglione MC. New drugs and new regimens for the treatment of tuberculosis: review of the drug development pipeline and implications for national programmes. Curr Opin Pulm Med. 2010;16(3):186–93 [R].

[35] Makanjuola T, Taddese HB, Booth A. Factors associated with adherence to treatment with isoniazid for the prevention of tuberculosis amongst people living with HIV/AIDS: a systematic review of qualitative data. PLoS One. 2014;9(2):e87166 [M].

[36] Norton BL, Holland DP. Current management options for latent tuberculosis: a review. Infect Drug Resist. 2012;5:163 [R].

[37] Tostmann A, Boeree MJ, Aarnoutse RE, et al. Antituberculosis drug-induced hepatotoxicity: concise up-to-date review. J Gastroenterol Hepatol. 2008;23(2):192–202 [R].

[38] Huang YS, Chern HD, Su WJ, et al. Polymorphism of the N-acetyltransferase 2 gene as a susceptibility risk factor for antituberculosis drug–induced hepatitis. Hepatology. 2002;35(4):883–9 [c].

[39] Li F, Lu J, Cheng J, et al. Human PXR modulates hepatotoxicity associated with rifampicin and isoniazid co-therapy. Nat Med. 2013;19(4):418–20 [E].

[40] Boelsterli UA, Lee KK. Mechanisms of isoniazid-induced idiosyncratic liver injury: emerging role of mitochondrial stress. J Gastroenterol Hepatol. 2014;29(4):678–87 [R].

[41] Shu C, Lee C, Lee M, et al. Hepatotoxicity due to first-line anti-tuberculosis drugs: a five-year experience in a Taiwan medical centre. Int J Tuberc Lung Dis. 2013;17(7):934–9 [c].

[42] Jeong I, Park J-S, Cho Y-J, et al. Drug-induced hepatotoxicity of anti-tuberculosis drugs and their serum levels. J Korean Med Sci. 2015;30(2):167–72 [c].

[43] Denholm JT, McBryde ES, Eisen DP, et al. Adverse effects of isoniazid preventative therapy for latent tuberculosis infection: a prospective cohort study. Drug Healthc Patient Saf. 2014;6:145 [c].

[44] Chang S-H, Eitzman SR, Nahid P, et al. Factors associated with failure to complete isoniazid therapy for latent tuberculosis infection in children and adolescents. J Infect Public Health. 2014;7(2):145–52 [c].

[45] Chang S-H, Nahid P, Eitzman SR. Hepatotoxicity in children receiving isoniazid therapy for latent tuberculosis infection. J Ped Infect Dis Soc. 2014;3:221–2277. pit089 [c].

[46] Xiang Y, Ma L, Wu W, et al. The incidence of liver injury in Uyghur patients treated for TB in Xinjiang Uyghur autonomous region, China, and its association with hepatic enzyme polymorphisms nat2, cyp2e1, gstm1 and gstt1. PLoS One. 2014;9(1):e85905 [C].

[47] Ng C-S, Hasnat A, Al Maruf A, et al. N-acetyltransferase 2 (NAT2) genotype as a risk factor for development of drug-induced liver injury relating to antituberculosis drug treatment in a mixed-ethnicity patient group. Eur J Clin Pharmacol. 2014;70(9):1079–86 [c].

[48] Liu F, Jiao A-X, Wu X-R, et al. Impact of glutathione S-transferase M1 and T1 on anti-tuberculosis drug-induced hepatotoxicity in Chinese pediatric patients. PLoS One. 2014;9(12): e115410 [c].

[49] Gupta VH, Singh M, Amarapurkar DN, et al. Association of GST null genotypes with anti-tuberculosis drug induced hepatotoxicity in Western Indian population. Ann Hepatol. 2013;12(6):959–65 [c].

[50] Ghavanini AA, Kimpinski K. Revisiting the evidence for neuropathy caused by pyridoxine deficiency and excess. J Clin Neuromuscul Dis. 2014;16(1):25–31 [R].

[51] Tsubouchi K, Ikematsu Y, Hashisako M, et al. Convulsive seizures with a therapeutic dose of isoniazid. Intern Med. 2014;53(3):239–42 [A].

[52] Gumus A, Oner V. Follow up of retinal nerve fiber layer thickness with optic coherence tomography in patients receiving anti-tubercular treatment may reveal early optic neuropathy. Cutan Ocul Toxicol. 2014;1–5 [c].

[53] Rodriguez-Marco NA, Solanas-Alava S, Ascaso FJ, et al. Severe and reversible optic neuropathy by ethambutol and isoniazid. An Sist Sanit Navar. 2014;37(2):287–91 [A].

[54] Neunhoffer H, Gold A, Hoerauf H, et al. Isolated ocular Jarisch-Herxheimer reaction after initiating tuberculostatic therapy in a child. Int Ophthalmol. 2014;34(3):675–7 [A].

[55] Skinner K, Saiao A, Mostafa A, et al. Isoniazid poisoning: pharmacokinetics and effect of hemodialysis in a massive ingestion. Hemodial Int. 2015. http://dx.doi.org/10.1111/hdi.12293 [A].

[56] Sabra A, Hallett M, Sudarsky L, et al. Treatment of action tremor in multiple sclerosis with isoniazid. Neurology. 1982;32(8):912–3 [c].

[57] Feinstein A, Freeman J, Lo AC. Treatment of progressive multiple sclerosis: what works, what does not, and what is needed. Lancet Neurol. 2015;14(2):194–207 [R].

[58] Nourbakhsh B, Stuve O. Isoniazid in autoimmunity—a trigger for multiple sclerosis? Ther Adv Neurol Disord. 2014;7(5):253–6. 1756285614540361 [A].

[59] Valença-Filipe R, Costa J, Martins A. Mycobacterium bovis: a rare cause of hand tenosynovitis. J Hand Surg Eur Vol. 2014;39(7):780–1 [A].

[60] Yamamoto K, Takasaki J, Morino E, et al. Tenosynovitis confirmed by MRI during anti-tuberculous treatment suspected due to isoniazid–2 case reports and literature review. Kekkaku. 2014;89(7):659–65 [A].

[61] Garg P, Garg R, Prasad R, et al. A prospective study of ocular toxicity in patients receiving ethambutol as a part of directly observed treatment strategy therapy. Lung India. 2015;32(1):16 [c].

[62] Cumberland PM, Russell-Eggitt I, Rahi JS. Active surveillance of visual impairment due to adverse drug reactions: findings from a national study in the United Kingdom. Pharmacol Res Perspect. 2015;3(1):1–9 [c].

[63] Scoville BA, De Lott LB, Trobe JD, et al. Ethambutol optic neuropathy in a hemodialysis patient receiving a guideline-recommended dose. J Neuroophthalmol. 2013;33(4):421–3 [E].

[64] Divya G, Ranganayakulu D. A rare case report on ethambutol induced optic neuritis. Int J Basic Clin Pharmacol. 2015;4(1):172–4 [A].

[65] Undrakonda V, Yashodhara B, Gonsalves S, et al. Bilateral retrobulbar neuritis following cessation of ethambutol. Int J Case Rep Image. 2015;6(2):76–80 [A].

[66] Osaguona VB, Sharpe JA, Awaji SA, et al. Optic chiasm involvement on MRI with ethambutol-induced bitemporal hemianopia. J Neuroophthalmol. 2014;34(2):155–8 [A].

[67] Chan R, Kwok A. Ocular toxicity of ethambutol. Hong Kong Med J. 2006;12(1):56 [R].

[68] Ezer N, Benedetti A, Darvish-Zargar M, et al. Incidence of ethambutol-related visual impairment during treatment of active tuberculosis. Int J Tuberc Lung Dis. 2013;17(4):447–55 [M].

[69] Wang MY, Sadun AA. Drug-related mitochondrial optic neuropathies. J Neuroophthalmol. 2013;33(2):172–8 [R].

[70] Rasool M, Malik A, Manan A, et al. Determination of potential role of antioxidative status and circulating biochemical markers in the pathogenesis of ethambutol induced toxic optic neuropathy among diabetic and non-diabetic patients. Saudi J Biol Sci. 2014 [c] http://dx.doi.org/10.1016/j.sjbs.2014.09.019.

[71] Fonkem E, Skordilis MA, Binkley EM, et al. Ethambutol toxicity exacerbating the phenotype of CMT2A2. Muscle Nerve. 2013;48(1):140–4 [A].

[72] Guillet V, Chevrollier A, Cassereau J, et al. Ethambutol-induced optic neuropathy linked to OPA1 mutation and mitochondrial toxicity. Mitochondrion. 2010;10(2):115–24 [A].

[73] Özkaya E. Eczematous-type multiple drug allergy from isoniazid and ethambutol with positive patch test results. Cutis. 2013;92:121–4 [A].

[74] Husain Z, Reddy BY, Schwartz RA. DRESS syndrome: part I. Clinical perspectives. J Am Acad Dermatol. 2013;68(5):693, e1-e14 [R].

[75] Kim J-Y, Sohn K-H, Song W-J, et al. A case of drug reaction with eosinophilia and systemic symptoms induced by ethambutol with early features resembling Stevens-Johnson syndrome. Acta Derm Venereol. 2013;93(6):753–4 [A].

[76] Saha K, Bandyopadhyay A, Sengupta A, et al. A rare case of ethambutol induced pulmonary eosinophilia. J Pharmacol Parmacother. 2013;4(4):300 [A].

[77] Cernadas JR, Santos N, Pinto C, et al. Hypersensitivity reaction and tolerance induction to ethambutol. Case Rep Med. 2013;2013:1 [A].

[78] Drlica K, Zhao X. DNA gyrase, topoisomerase IV, and the 4-quinolones. Microbiol Mol Biol Rev. 1997;61(3):377–92 [R].

[79] Ziganshina LE, Titarenko AF, Davies GR. Fluoroquinolones for treating tuberculosis (presumed drug-sensitive). Cochrane Database Syst Rev. 2013; http://dx.doi.org/10.1002/14651858. CD004795.pub4 [M].

[80] Seddon JA, Hesseling AC, Finlayson H, et al. Preventive therapy for child contacts of multidrug-resistant tuberculosis: a prospective cohort study. Clin Infect Dis. 2013;57:1676–84. cit655 [c].

[81] Adler-Shohet FC, Low J, Carson M, et al. Management of latent tuberculosis infection in child contacts of multidrug-resistant tuberculosis. Pediatr Infect Dis J. 2014;33(6):664–6 [c].

[82] Bradley JS, Kauffman RE, Balis DA, et al. Assessment of musculoskeletal toxicity 5 years after therapy with levofloxacin. Pediatrics. 2014;134(1):e146–53 [C].

[83] Jawahar MS, Banurekha VV, Paramasivan CN, et al. Randomized clinical trial of thrice-weekly 4-month moxifloxacin or gatifloxacin containing regimens in the treatment of new sputum positive pulmonary tuberculosis patients. PLoS One. 2013;8(7):e67030 [c].

[84] Trieu L, Proops DC, Ahuja SD. Moxifloxacin prophylaxis against MDR TB, New York, New York, USA. Emerg Infect Dis. 2015;21(3):500 [c].

[85] Alshammari TM, Larrat EP, Morrill HJ, et al. The risk of hepatotoxicity associated with fluoroquinolones: a national case-control safety study. Am J Health Syst Pharm. 2014;71(1):37–43 [c].

[86] Fusco S, Reitano F, Gambadoro N, et al. Severe hypoglycemia associated with levofloxacin in a healthy older woman. J Am Geriatr Soc. 2013;61(9):1637–8 [A].

[87] Dewachter P, Mouton-Faivre C. Anaphylaxis to levofloxacin. Allergol Immunopathol. 2013;41(6):418–9 [A].

[88] Gervasoni C, Cattaneo D, Falvella FS, et al. Levofloxacin-induced seizures in a patient without predisposing risk factors: the impact of pharmacogenetics. Eur J Clin Pharmacol. 2013;69(8):1611–3 [A].

[89] Gutiérrez-Gutiérrez G, Sereno M, García Vaquero C, et al. Levofloxacin-induced myasthenic crisis. J Emerg Med. 2013;45(2):260–1 [A].

[90] Katsube O, Anzai M, Nomura Y, et al. A case of drug-induced hypersensitivity syndrome caused by levofloxacin used for treating pulmonary tuberculosis. Kekkaku. 2014;89(2):51–6 [A].

[91] Sivakumar T. Pyrazinamide induced multiple adverse drug reactions: a case report. World J Pharmacy Pharm Sci. 2015;4(03):1317 [A].

[92] Tsou C-C, Chien J-Y. Olfactory disturbance related to pyrazinamide. QJM. 2014;107(3):217–8 [A].

[93] Gutman AB, Yü TF, Berger L. Renal function in gout: III. Estimation of tubular secretion and reabsorption of uric acid by use of pyrazinamide (pyrazinoic acid). Am J Med. 1969;47(4):575–92 [c].

[94] Pham AQ, Doan A, Andersen M. Pyrazinamide-induced hyperuricemia. Pharmacol Ther. 2014;39(10):695 [A].

[95] Gerdan V, Akkoc N, Ucan ES, et al. Paradoxical increase in uric acid level with allopurinol use in pyrazinamide-induced hyperuricaemia. Singapore Med J. 2013;54(6):e125–6 [A].

[96] Mahantesh A, Hanumantharayappa B, Reddy M, et al. Effect of pyrazinamide induced hyperuricemia on patient compliance undergoing DOTS therapy for tuberculosis. Res Rev J Pharmacol Toxicol Stud. 2014;2(2):12–7 [R].

[97] Al-Amiry MH. Pyrazinamide induced photosensitivity: a case report from Iraq. J Pharmacovigil. 2013;1:103 [A].

[98] Kant S, Verma SK, Gupta V, et al. Pyrazinamide induced thrombocytopenia. Indian J Pharmacol. 2010;42(2):108 [A].

[99] Verma AK, Singh A, Chandra A, et al. Rifampicin-induced thrombocytopenia. Indian J Pharmacol. 2010;42(4):240 [A].

[100] Kant S, Natu N, Mahajan V. Rifampicin ethambutol and pyrazinamide-induced thrombocytopenia. Int J Clin Pharmacol Ther. 2008;46(8):440–2 [R].

[101] Bansal R, Sharma PK, Sharma A. A case of thrombocytopenia caused by rifampicin and pyrazinamide. Indian J Pharmacol. 2013;45(4):405 [A].

[102] Patil V, Pattar R, Ichalkaranji R, et al. DRESS syndrome secondary to pyrazinamide—a rare case report. Int J Biomed Adv Res. 2014;5(6):322–3 [A].

[103] Tang S, Yao L, Hao X, et al. Clofazimine for the treatment of multidrug-resistant tuberculosis: prospective, multicenter, randomized controlled study in China. Clin Infect Dis. 2015;60(9):1361–7. civ027 [c].

[104] Maia MV, Cunha Mda G, Cunha CS. Adverse effects of alternative therapy (minocycline, ofloxacin, and clofazimine) in multibacillary leprosy patients in a recognized health care unit in Manaus, Amazonas, Brazil. An Bras Dermatol. 2013;88(2):205–10 [c].

[105] Xu HB, Jiang RH, Xiao HP. Clofazimine in the treatment of multidrug resistant tuberculosis. Clin Microbiol Infect. 2012;18:1104–10.

[106] Cholo MC, Steel HC, Fourie PB, et al. Clofazimine: current status and future prospects. J Antimicrob Chemother. 2012;67(2):290–8 [R].

[107] Dey T, Brigden G, Cox H, et al. Outcomes of clofazimine for the treatment of drug-resistant tuberculosis: a systematic review and meta-analysis. J Antimicrob Chemother. 2013;68(2):284–93 [M].

[108] Gopal M, Padayatchi N, Metcalfe JZ, et al. Systematic review of clofazimine for the treatment of drug-resistant tuberculosis. Int J Tuberc Lung Dis. 2013;17(8):1001–7 [M].

[109] Singh H, Azad K, Kaur K. Clofazimine-induced enteropathy in a patient of leprosy. Indian J Pharmacol. 2013;45(2):197–8 [A].

[110] Hwang TJ, Wares DF, Jafarov A, et al. Safety of cycloserine and terizidone for the treatment of drug-resistant tuberculosis: a meta-analysis. Int J Tuberc Lung Dis. 2013;17(10):1257–66 [M].

[111] Sharma B, Handa R, Nagpal K, et al. Cycloserine-induced psychosis in a young female with drug-resistant tuberculosis. Gen Hosp Psychiatry. 2014;36(4):451. e3-4 [A].

[112] Skripconoka V, Danilovits M, Pehme L, et al. Delamanid improves outcomes and reduces mortality in multidrug-resistant tuberculosis. Eur Respir J. 2013;41(6):1393–400 [c].

[113] Wang H, Yan L, Zhang G, et al. Association between HLA-B*1301 and dapsone-induced hypersensitivity reactions among leprosy patients in China. J Invest Dermatol. 2013;133(11):2642–4 [c].

[114] Zhang FR, Liu H, Irwanto A, et al. HLA-B*13:01 and the dapsone hypersensitivity syndrome. N Engl J Med. 2013;369(17):1620–8 [c].

[115] Markova A, Duquesnoy R, Levis W. T-cell plasticity of dapsone and DRESS. J Drugs Dermatol. 2014;13(1):12–3 [A].

[116] Perez Tanoira R, Sanchez-Patan F, Jimenez Giron A, et al. Tolerance and safety of intravenous streptomycin therapy in patients with tuberculosis. Infection. 2014;42(3):597–8 [c].

Antihelminthic Drugs

Igho J. Onakpoya[1]

Nuffield Department of Primary Care Health Sciences, Oxford, United Kingdom
[1]Corresponding author: igho.onakpoya@phc.ox.ac.uk

ALBENDAZOLE (SEDA-31, 508; SEDA-32, 572; SEDA-33, 647; SEDA-36, 458)

Observational Studies

In a long-term follow up study (61–210 months) of 101 patients to assess the effectiveness and safety of albendazole in the prevention of secondary hydatidosis and/or hydatid disease recurrence, no haematological abnormalities were observed [1c].

In a non-randomized study, the safety and effectiveness of a single oral dose of 400 mg albendazole in the treatment of infestation with *Ascaris*, *Trichuris* and hookworm in 298 school children was evaluated [2C]. Frequently observed side effects were *nausea, abdominal discomfort, headache* and *fatigue*. These effects were reported as mild and transient.

Comparative Studies

The safety and efficacy of single versus extended dose albendazole in the treatment of *Ascaris*, *Trichuris* and hookworm has been assessed in a randomized, controlled, assessor-blinded clinical trial involving 175 children [3c]. No clinically relevant adverse events were observed.

The safety and efficacy of albendazole or mebendazole administered randomly for 1 or 2 days has been examined in 385 school children with heavy intensity *Trichuris trichuria* infection [4C]. No adverse events were observed.

Drug Combination Studies

The safety of combination therapy with albendazole and praziquantel in the treatment of human hydatid disease has been assessed in a retrospective observational study including 57 patients [5c]. Adverse events were

reported in 14% of patients; the most common of which were diarrhea (5.2%) and *vomiting* (3.5%). These events were mild, and disappeared when treatment was stopped. No clinically relevant haematological changes were noted.

The safety and efficacy of combined albendazole and praziquantel for treatment of neurocysticercosis has been evaluated in a 6-month randomized, double-blind comparative trial including 118 patients: albendazole plus praziquantel (n = 39) versus standard albendazole (n = 41) versus albendazole (n = 38) [6c]. Serious adverse events reported included *seizures, headache*, and *drug-induced hepatitis*. There were no significant differences in the frequencies of severe adverse events between groups.

In a four-arm, randomized clinical trial (n = 431), the efficacy and safety of albendazole plus ivermectin, albendazole plus mebendazole, albendazole plus oxantel pamoate, and mebendazole alone against *Trichuris trichiura* and concomitant soil-transmitted helminth infections in children were compared [7C]. Adverse events were observed in 20% of children, the most common of which were *abdominal cramps* and *headache*. No serious adverse events were observed.

In a randomized double-blind, placebo-controlled four-arm trial (n = 458), the safety and efficacy of albendazole-oxantel pamoate combination in the treatment of *Trichuris trichuria* infection in children was compared with albendazole, oxantel pamoate or mebendazole alone [8C]. Adverse events were reported in 30% of participants; *abdominal cramps* and *headaches* were the most common. No serious adverse events occurred.

Placebo-Controlled Studies

In a randomized double-blind study (n = 140), the safety and effectiveness of albendazole (400 mg/day for 3 days) therapy in tuberculosis patients who were

© 2015 Elsevier B.V. All rights reserved.

co-infected with helminths was assessed. No adverse events were observed with albendazole [9c].

Liver

Case Study 1

INHIBITION OF MICROTUBULE-RELATED CELLULAR FUNCTIONS AFTER LONG-TERM HIGH DOSE EXPOSURE TO ALBENDAZOLE

A 26-year-old patient was diagnosed with a hydatid cyst in the liver. He underwent surgery and received a 3-month course of 500 mg daily albendazole as postoperative therapy. Two years later, he suffered a relapse with multiple new hydatid cysts in the liver and was treated with albendazole 800 mg daily. Liver enzymes at that time were within the normal ranges. One month later, the patient was admitted to the surgery department for upper right abdominal pain and jaundice. A physical examination was normal except for icteric sclerae. Laboratory investigations showed a hemoglobin level of 8.9 mg/dL, mean corpuscular volume (MCV) 89 fL, mean corpuscular hemoglobin (MCH) 29 pg, reticulocyte count 53 000 per mm^3, a white blood cell count of 5400/L, and a platelet count of 119×10^3/L. Serum levels of hepatic enzymes were as follows: alanine aminotransferase (ALT) 2454 IU/L, aspartate aminotransferase (AST) 1451 IU/L, and alkaline phosphatase 198 IU/L; total bilirubin was 341 mg/dL. The prothrombin index was 77% Hepatitis viral serology was negative, as were the results for auto-antibodies (anti-nuclear, anti-smooth muscle, anti-mitochondria, and anti-liver kidney microsomal). Liver ultrasound revealed multiple cystic images without alteration of the biliary ducts. This picture was thought to be related to the intake of albendazole, and therefore, the drug was withdrawn. Clinical symptoms resolved within 1 week and laboratory tests showed progressive improvement, with complete resolution of the hematologic and hepatic disorders at 4 and 15 days after drug withdrawal respectively. Authors postulate inhibition of microtubule-related cellular functions may be related to long-term high dose exposure to albendazole [10A].

Case Study 2

RECURRENT ACUTE HEPATITIS DUE TO SINGLE DOSE OF ALBENDAZOLE IN A CHILD

A 5-year-old male child presented with repeated episodes of acute-hepatitis, each episode occurring after 2–3 days of administering albendazole [11A]. He presented during the fourth episode with complaints of acute onset fever, anorexia and vomiting followed by yellowish discoloration of eyes and urine. Liver was palpable 3.5 cm below the right costal margin, soft and mildly tender. There were no signs of chronic liver disease. Serum

bilirubin on admission was 11.5 mg/dL (Direct: 9.5 and indirect: 2.0). Serum alanine transaminase (ALT), aspartate transaminase (AST), alkaline phosphatase (ALP) and gamma glutamyl transpeptidase (GGT) were 2720, 4100, 1247 and 26 IU/L, respectively. Albumin and globulin levels were 3.3 and 3.0 g/dL, respectively. Prothrombin time was 22 s (INR-1.6, control 12.6 s) and aPTT was 31.0 s (N-25–35 s). Ceruloplasmin level was 35.64 mg/dL. Hepatic viral serology, antinuclear antibodies, anti-LKM antibody and anti-smooth muscle antibody were negative. His condition improved within 2 weeks with subsidence of jaundice and hepatomegaly. On follow up, at 2 months, he was asymptomatic without hepatomegaly and with normal levels of bilirubin.

Case Study 3

RECURRENT ACUTE HEPATITIS DUE TO REPEATED INGESTION OF ALBENDAZOLE

A 7-year-old boy presented with his fourth episode of jaundice. During each episode, he had prodromal symptoms (nausea, anorexia, vomiting) starting 3–4 days prior to jaundice. There was no history of fever, pruritus, clay-coloured stools or abdominal pain in any of the episodes. Each episode of jaundice lasted for 7–10 days and then subsided spontaneously. There was no history of ascites, encephalopathy or gastrointestinal bleeding. Each onset of symptoms was within 7 days of taking albendazole 400 mg single dose prescribed by a pediatrician. On examination, icterus was absent. The liver was palpable 1 cm below the costal margin, soft in consistency, and had a smooth surface and regular margins. Gall bladder and spleen were not palpable. There was no family history of liver disease or ingestion of any other drug. Initial LFT showed elevated liver enzymes. Repeat LFT within 10 days of peak enzyme levels showed normal values. His prothrombin time, INR value, total protein and albumin levels were normal. Red and white blood cell counts were normal, and there was no eosinophilia. Abdominal ultrasound showed a mildly hypo-echoic liver with normal spleen and no evidence of ascites or portal hypertension. Hepatic viral serology was negative. His serum ceruloplasmin level was normal. ANA, ASMA, anti-LKM and AMA tests were negative [12A].

Case Study 4

GRANULOMATOUS HEPATITIS IN AN ADULT RESULTING FROM ALBENDAZOLE

A 25-year-old Hispanic woman, without significant past medical history, presented with progressive jaundice, associated with right upper quadrant pain, fatigue, weakness, dark urine, fever, and vomiting. On physical examination, she had icteric sclerae, no hepatomegaly and no stigmata of chronic liver disease. The results of ultrasonography of the liver and biliary tract were normal. Initial LFTs revealed AST of 933 U/L, ALT 1649 U/L, GGT 28 U/L and total bilirubin 13.75 mg/dL. Hepatic viral serology was negative. Based on the clinical and laboratory findings, a preliminary diagnosis of acute hepatitis of unknown aetiology was made. An ultrasound-guided percutaneous liver biopsy revealed portal inflammatory infiltrate of lymphocytes, plasma cells and neutrophils, with necrosis of the hepatocytes of the limiting plate, and macrophage infiltrate composed of epithelioid granulomas, forming a non-necrotizing aspect in the hepatic sinusoids. Special stains for tuberculosis and fungi were negative. Contrasted computed tomography of the chest and abdomen were normal. The patient had a favorable outcome, with gradual improvement of her liver biochemical profile, without any specific treatment. At this point, the possibility of drug-related granulomatous hepatitis was considered. Further questioning revealed that 2 weeks prior to the jaundice, the patient had received empirical treatment with albendazole, paracetamol and hyoscine butyl bromide for nonspecific gastrointestinal symptoms. The self-limiting condition, as well as the gradual normalization in her liver profile, supported the possibility of toxic hepatitis. Patient monitoring without any intervention was decided. The toxic granulomatous hepatitis spontaneously resolved [13A].

Case Study 5

TOXIC HEPATITIS IN AN ADULT INDUCED BY ALBENDZOLE

A 28-year-old male diagnosed with allergic dermatitis and bronchitis presented for follow-up at the clinic. Due to his increased complaints over the last year, a thoracic computed tomography (CT) scan was requested, which showed multiple cysts in the liver. He had no history of alcohol consumption, had taken minimal anti-allergic drugs and had no significant family history. His physical examination was normal. All dermatologic and other systemic examinations were normal. Results of the laboratory tests were as follows: alanine aminotransferase (ALT) 21 IU/L, alkaline phosphatase (ALP) 154 IU/L, lactate dehydrogenase (LDH) 400 IU/L (reference value: 240–480), white blood cell (WBC) 7430/μL, hemoglobin (Hb) 14.6 g/dL, platelets 339000/μL, hydatid cyst-specific immunoglobulin (Ig)E 0.76 (++), and indirect hemagglutination (IHA) test was positive at 1/512 titer. A diagnosis of hydatid cyst was made, 800 mg/day albendazole was administered, and surgery was planned. 20 days prior to surgery, preoperative control tests revealed: aspartate aminotransferase (AST) 659, ALT 968, ALP 209 IU/L, gamma glutamyl transpeptidase (GGT) 108 U/L, LDH 667 IU/L, prothrombin time (PT) 18.1 s (international normalized ratio [INR] 1.48),

activated partial thromboplastin time (aPTT) 41.3 s, WBC 15400/μL (eosinophils 33%), Hb 12.8 g/dL, and platelets 505000/μL. Hepatic viral serology was negative. Abdominal ultrasound showed hepatic enlargement and presence of multiple cysts. On CT scan, six cystic masses were found in the eighth hepatic segment. A diagnosis of drug toxicity was made and albendazole was stopped. All hepatic enzyme levels subsequently decreased and the patient had surgery. Cystotomy plus drainage were applied to five of the cysts. For the remaining cyst, a scolicidal solution was injected into the cyst under operative ultrasound, and albendazole was re-administered postoperatively. On the third day of the therapy, liver enzymes became elevated and albendazole administration was once again stopped. The patient was re-scheduled for follow-up without medical therapy. On follow-up tests, a decrease in liver enzyme levels to normal reference values was observed [14A].

Case Study 6

HEPATITIS IN AN ADULT CAUSED BY CONTINUOUS ALBENDAZOLE THERAPY

A 47-year-old male patient presented with a 2-month history of fever, generalized jaundice, and pain in the right abdomen associated to paresthesia on the ipsilateral lower limb. He was referred to a hepatology clinic. Upon admission, hepatic profile was total bilirubin 1.85 mg/dL, AST 22 U/L, ALT 30 U/L, GGT 393 U/L. Hepatic viral serology was negative. Carcinoembryonic antigen (CEA) and alpha-fetoprotein (AFP) were within normal limits. Magnetic resonance imaging (MRI) revealed two cystic lesions: one located between the middle hepatic vein and the right hepatic vein, with sub-capsular enhancement, without septa or nodules; the second lesion occupied the whole right lobe of liver with multiple enhancing septa. No ischemic liver damage was observed and the bile duct was normal. Based on these findings, a diagnosis of hepatic hydatidosis was made and treatment was commenced with 600 mg albendazole every 24 hours. After 5 months of uninterrupted treatment, the patient was again admitted and hospitalized because of jaundice. Physical exam revealed mild hepatomegaly and tenderness in the right hypochondrium, icterus in mucosa and dysesthesias in lower right limb. The patient denied consumption of other medications or nutritional supplements after discharge. It was decided to discontinue albendazole and continuously monitor the patient's hepatic function. Again, hepatic viral serology, CEA, and AFP were negative; additionally, a new MRI showed a mild decrease of cysts. After 4 days of hospitalization, improved hyperbilirubinemia was noted along with decreased transaminases. A diagnosis of albendazole-induced liver damage was made and after progressive clinical improvement, the patient was discharged. Three months later, the patient was asymptomatic and his hepatic profile was normal [15A].

Case Study 7

ACUTE HEPATITIS DUE TO REPEAT TREATMENT WITH ALBENDAZOLE IN A PATIENT WITH CHRONIC TOXOCARA CANIS INFECTION

A 15-year-old female presented to the clinic for routine check-up. She had a history of mild asthma treated with salbutamol. Prior to presentation, she had received four courses of treatment with albendazole (400 mg every 12 hours for 7 days) due to moderate asymptomatic eosinophilia associated with IgG *Toxocara* positive serology. She has been on monthly injectable hormonal contraceptives for 1 year. She denied use of other medication, herbs, alcohol and illicit drugs. She had no history of recent travel and had no pets. She denied a family history of liver disease. On routine check-up, moderate eosinophilia was detected, and she was again prescribed albendazole 400 mg 12 hourly for 7 days on suspicion of asymptomatic reactivation of toxocariasis. Twelve days after completing therapy, she presented in the emergency department with a 1-week history of progressive jaundice, dark urine, nausea, anorexia and epigastric discomfort. On physical examination, she was hemodynamically stable, afebrile, jaundiced, had no stigmata of chronic liver disease, and no evidence of bleeding. Laboratory results revealed hyperbilirubinemia with elevated direct bilirubin, elevated transaminases, coagulopathy and hypokalaemia. She was admitted to the intensive care unit for monitoring, and supportive treatment and intravenous vitamin K were instituted. Liver ultrasound showed a normal morphology with features suggestive of hepatic inflammatory gallbladder disease. Hepatitis viral serology was negative. Her clinical condition improved with rapid remission of symptoms without encephalopathy. The patient rejected a request for liver biopsy. She was discharged after 16 days of monitoring, and was advised to suspend further injections of contraceptives. She was monitored as an outpatient monthly, remained asymptomatic and showed evidence of normalization of liver function. The spontaneous improvement of liver function in the absence of the drug supported the diagnosis of albendazole-induced toxic hepatitis. To confirm the diagnosis, a quantitative level Council for International Organizations of Medical Sciences (CIOMS) scale was used to assess the causality relationship between albendazole and the observed hepatotoxicity. The patient had a CIOMS score of 6, indicating a probable association between consumption of albendazole and development of hepatitis Importance of monitoring liver function in patients on albendazole treatment is emphasized [16A].

Renal System

Acute Renal Failure due to Albendazole Therapy

A 72-year-old Caucasian woman presented to the hospital with a 3-week history of cramping abdominal pain, nausea, vomiting, diarrhea, fatigue, weight loss, dehydration, confusion with memory impairment and reported visual hallucinations. Exposure history revealed that she had intermittently consumed raw meat products. Pertinent medical history included IgG deficiency, diagnosed in the patient's fifth decade of life and requiring monthly intravenous immunoglobulin infusions, type 2 diabetes mellitus, coronary artery disease, sleep apnea, chronic obstructive pulmonary disease and stage 2 chronic kidney disease. She was a former tobacco smoker and denied history of alcohol consumption. Physical examination was normal. However, her short-term memory recall was impaired. Systemic examination revealed mild right upper quadrant tenderness, pupillary anisocoria (unequal pupil sizes) and chronic stasis dermatitis on bilateral lower extremities. The remainder of the systemic examination was normal. Her complete blood count showed leukocytosis and 30% peripheral eosinophilia with an absolute eosinophil count of 3.1×10^9/L. The complete metabolic profiles showed reduction in sodium, potassium, chloride and bicarbonate. Alkaline phosphatase (ALP) was elevated at 181 units/L. AST, ALT and bilirubin were within normal limits. Albumin was 3.2 g/dL and pre-albumin was 7 mg/dL. Creatine kinase was 15 units/L. C-reactive protein and sedimentation rate were elevated at 37.1 mg/L and 33 mm/L h, respectively. Lipase, serum lactate, serum osmolality, glycated hemoglobin and thyroid stimulating hormone were normal. Serology was positive for *Trichinella* antibody by ELISA. Serology for cysticercosis was negative. Testing for HIV, giardia, strongyloides, toxocara and stool ova and parasites were all negative. CT scan of the head was negative for any acute intracranial findings. Chest X-ray showed calcified and tortuous aorta and mild prominence of the central pulmonary arteries. ECG demonstrated normal sinus rhythm, left atrial enlargement, prolonged QTc interval, right bundle branch block and left anterior fascicular block. The patient was commenced on albendazole 400 mg orally twice daily. However, on day 2 of hospital stay, she was become febrile and her creatinine was noted to have risen to 1.9 mg/dL and blood urea nitrogen elevated to 25 mg/dL. Urinalysis with microscopy was significant for protein/osmolality ratio 1.32, white cell count 11–20/hpf, 1–3 transitional epithelial cells/hpf, 4–10 squamous epithelial cells/hpf and urine eosinophils 1–5%. A renal ultrasound showed no evidence of hydronephrosis or dilation of the collecting system for either kidney. The left and right kidneys had normal cortical thickness and parenchymal echogenicity. These findings were consistent with stage 2 acute kidney injury likely secondary to albendazole therapy. Albendazole was discontinued and oral prednisone therapy was initiated for treatment of possible hypersensitivity reaction or acute interstitial nephritis. Alternative treatment for trichinosis with pyrantel was considered. However, pyrantel is active only against worms in the gut and has no efficacy once the larvae have migrated outside of the intestine. As the patient's symptoms had been present for several weeks and her symptoms were most consistent with the systemic phase of disease, pyrantel was unlikely to be of benefit. The decision was made to proceed with observation as the patient did not tolerate the treatment. The patient received a total of 30 days of prednisone. Her serum creatinine slowly decreased after discontinuation of albendazole. She was seen in the outpatient clinic 3 weeks after discharge from the hospital for a follow-up visit. Her creatinine had improved to 1 mg/dL. Her absolute eosinophil count had normalised to $0.30 \times 10^9/L$. Her symptoms of confusion, memory impairment and visual hallucinations had completely resolved [17A].

IVERMECTIN (SEDA-31, 509; SEDA-32, 575; SEDA-33, 649; SEDA-36, 460)

Comparative Studies

In a randomized double-blind study including 127 adults, the safety and effectiveness of ivermectin and moxidectin in the treatment of *Onchocerca volvulus* infection were compared [18c]. All ivermectin-treated participants and 97–100% of moxidectin-treated participants experienced *Mazzotti reactions*. The frequencies of adverse drug reactions were significantly less with ivermectin compared with moxidectin for pruritus (56% vs 87%), rash (42% vs 63%), tachycardia (36% vs 61%), and reduction in mean arterial on standing still for 2 minutes after at least 5 minutes supine relative to pre-treatment (27% vs 61%).

Nervous System

Neurotoxicity with resulting death due to persistently elevated serum levels of ivermectin has been reported [19A].

- A 64-year-old man was admitted to intensive care unit for postoperative care after aortic valve replacement. His previous medical history was relevant for giant cell arteritis for which he was using prednisone. Three days postoperatively, severe sepsis with multiorgan failure developed. Sputum test results showed high numbers of mobile *Strongyloides stercoralis* larvae, and a diagnosis of *S. stercoralis* hyperinfection syndrome

with dissemination was made. Ivermectin therapy, first orally and later subcutaneously, was initiated. Although numbers of live *Strongyloides* decreased rapidly and his clinical condition improved, he remained in a persistent vegetative state and the patient died. Given the fact that other causes for a persistent coma were excluded, we suspected that neurotoxicity of ivermectin might have been responsible for the persistent coma. To analyze whether drug accumulation was present in our patient, we measured ivermectin levels in serum during and after treatment as well as in autopsy-derived brain tissue. A steady state of serum levels was reached after 5 days, but hereafter no reduction was observed even after ivermectin treatment had been discontinued for 11 days. In line with this, the ivermectin level in brain tissue was still markedly elevated (30 ng/g brain tissue) at the time of death, 14 days after the last ivermectin treatment. Such a markedly elevated concentration may have been attributed to severe neurotoxicity.

The authors cautioned against prescribing further dosages of ivermectin to patients after effective serum levels have been achieved, unless the infection was still uncontrolled and the serum levels of the drug has significantly reduced.

LEVAMISOLE (SEDA-31, 510; SEDA-32, 575; SEDA-33, 649; SEDA-36, 460)

Nervous System

- A 42-year-old man presented with subacute onset of right hemiparesis and mild cognitive impairment. Prior to presentation, he has taken 600 mg oral levamisole for ascariasis 30 days. Neuroimaging revealed two irregular lesions in the white matter of bilateral frontal lobes. The left larger lesion showed the shape of a concentric ring, and after Gd-DTPA administration, both lesions demonstrated prominent ring enhancement. The patient was diagnosed with levamisole-induced leukoencephalopathy, mimicking Baló disease, and treated with high-dose IV glucocorticoid therapy. Within 3 months, the patient's symptoms improved and a repeat MRI scan showed that the previous lesions had decreased in size [20A].

Levamisole-Contaminated Cocaine

Levamisole is used by South American drug cartels to increase cocaine bulk prior to shipment [21r]. Levamisole-contaminated cocaine was first detected by the FDA in 2003 [22r], and as at 2009, 69% of cocaine seized by the FDA in the US contained levamisole [23R]. There is also an increasing trend in the occurrence of levamisole-contaminated cocaine in Europe [24R]. Possible harms associated with abuse of levamisole-contaminated cocaine include neutropenia, agranulocytosis, arthralgias, retiform purpura, and skin necrosis [25R]. Several cases of unusual presentations secondary to abuse of levamisole-contaminated cocaine, such as kidney injury and fatal cardiovascular toxicity have also recently appeared in the literature, and these are described below.

CARDIOVASCULAR

Acute coronary syndrome with subsequent fatality due to levamisole abuse [26A].

A 25-year-old man, who was known to be a cocaine addict, died suddenly at home after complaining of retrosternal pain. The electrocardiogram performed by the rescue team showed ventricular fibrillation. A year prior to death the patient had presented to the emergency room with a Q-wave myocardial infarction. His blood lipid levels were normal. The patient refused coronarography and did not follow the prescribed treatment plan. He complained of pins and needles in the left arm, especially in the mornings, and of retrosternal pain after an effort. A complete post-mortem examination was performed the day after he died. There were signs of resuscitation attempts (sternal fracture, and defibrillator and injection marks). Native (unenhanced) CT scan and multi-phase post-mortem CT angiography (MPMCTA) were performed by a trained forensic. Peripheral blood, cerebrospinal and vitreous fluids, and hair samples for toxicological analysis were collected according to standard autopsy protocol prior to the injection of the contrast agent. Samples of bile and urine were obtained under CT-guidance. MPMCTA, was performed using a Virtangio® perfusion device and the oily contrast agent Angiofil® Radiological findings included pulmonary edema and pleural effusion, which was already visible in the unenhanced CT-scan. The arterial phase of MPMCTA revealed pathological enhancement of the myocardium of the left ventricle and septum, as well as a luminal stenosis of the proximal portion of the left anterior descending artery. The heart weighted 330 g (predicted heart weight for the local population 207.5–378 g). The ventricles were dilated; the left ventricle thickness was 1.4 cm and the cardiac valves were unremarkable. A small eroded plaque was found in the proximal portion of the left anterior descending artery (LAD). There were two fibrous scars of healed infarction in the left ventricular myocardium: a transmural scar in the anterolateral wall and a subendocardiac scar in the anterior part of the ventricular septum. Pleural effusion (250 mL on the right and 100 mL on the left) and pulmonary edema were present. The other organs were normal. Histological examinations were performed using standard H&E and trichrome staining. Myocardial examination revealed fibrous tissue in the anterolateral wall and in the anterior septum. A few contraction bands were observed in the anterior wall. There was no eosinophilic infiltration in the myocardium and the intramural coronary arteries were free from inflammation. Microscopic examination of the proximal portion of the LAD

artery showed fibrous thickening of the intima and an infiltration of numerous eosinophils into the adventitia and intima. A small amount of thrombotic material adhering to the eroded plaque was detected. Fibrinoid necrosis and granulomatous changes were not found in the inflammatory areas. The toxicological analyses of femoral blood obtained before radiological examination and performed by GC-MS revealed the presence of cocaine (340 μg/L) and its metabolites (benzoylecgonine 610 μg/L, methylecgonine 210 μg/L). Screening analyses detected levamisole in the urine and pericardial fluid, and phenacetin in the pericardial fluid. No alcohol was detected. Cocaine was detected in the hair samples (9 ng/mg). Post-mortem laboratory investigations demonstrated a normal CRP level, elevated levels of troponin I (0.28 μg/L; normal < 0.04) and NT-proBNP (211 ng/L; normal < 115 ng/L) and tryptase at its upper limit (12.1 μg/L, normal < 13.5 μg/L).

Skin

Case Study

PYODERMA GANGRENOSUM IN A COCAINE USER [27A]

A 51-year-old Caucasian female presented with a 2-month history of painful, expanding ulcerations on her forehead, torso and fingers. The patient reported a history of smoking crack cocaine 1 week prior to admission. Physical examination revealed 14 skin lesions, including a large ulcerated plaque with a pink firm border and central boggy ulceration on the forehead and temple. Round ulcers with friable gunmetal gray borders and fluid-filled necrotic centers were observed on the abdomen, back, thigh and pubis. The patient was admitted for further evaluation. Laboratory studies were positive for perinuclear anti-neutrophil cytoplasmic antibodies, antinuclear antibodies, lupus anticoagulant, anticardiolipin antibodies (IgM and IgA), and trace cryoglobulins. Hepatic viral serology was negative. Blood cultures and cutaneous cultures for bacteria, fungus, and mycobacterial cultures were negative. Serum electrophoresis with immunofixation was within normal limits. A skin biopsy of the left forehead lesion demonstrated dense dermal inflammatory infiltrate composed of neutrophils with scattered lymphocytes, plasma cells, and eosinophils without evidence of vasculitis. Colonoscopy, bone marrow biopsy, and a total body computed tomography scan were without remarkable findings. Clinical and histopathological findings were suggestive of pyoderma gangrenosum. No other underlying condition was identified other than illicit drug use. The patient was started on oral prednisone 60 mg daily and was encouraged to refrain from cocaine abuse. After 5 months of therapy and cocaine abstinence, the lesions had not recurred. The patient's non-compliance during drug cessation precluded repeat autoantibody testing. At the 12-month follow-up, most lesions had healed with cribriform scarring; however, she developed a new eruption with similar morphology involving the left dorsal wrist, abdomen, right breast, and right thigh.

The onset of these lesions coincided with cocaine use 1 week earlier. The authors concluded that physicians should have a higher index of suspicion for a wide variety of dermatological disorders in patients with a history of cocaine abuse [27A].

A 52-year-old male presented with complaints of a rash and pain in his perineal area for 4 days. The rash first appeared in his upper right thigh and was purpuric with a central black discoloration. He also complained of general malaise, fever of 103 °F and diarrhea for 4 days. His past history included chronic hepatitis C, alcoholism, liver cirrhosis and substance abuse. Laboratory studies revealed leukopenia (400 per mm^3) with an absolute neutrophil count (ANC) of zero. Differential diagnosis at this point included infection, autoimmune conditions and medications. Viral, Babesiosis and Lyme serologies were negative. Blood, urine and stool cultures were also negative. Biopsy of the perineal region showed skin and subcutaneous tissue with extensive necrosis. Wound cultures grew Escherichia coli, Streptococcus ludginous and Candida, which were treated with broad-spectrum antibiotics and antifungals. Autoimmune panel for p-ANCA, c-ANCA, anti-neutrophil antibody, complement levels and Jak2 v617F was also negative. A full review of his home medications did not indicate a cause of such a drastic neutropenia. A urine levamisole level and urine drugs of abuse screen were obtained (2 days after admission), and the patient was found to be positive for cocaine with a high levamisole level of 210 ng/dL. Subsequently, the patient was placed on filgastrim, which ultimately resulted in an increase in his WBC. His abscess was then drained and several weeks later the patient made a full recovery. The authors cautioned clinicians to suspect levamisole contamination in suspected drug abusers with very low neutrophil count and neutropenia [27A].

A 54-year-old man presented with bilateral axillary adenopathy and fatigue of 2 weeks' duration. His medical history was unremarkable. He had been performing light construction work in a rural environment but denied insect bites or toxic exposure. He was started trimethoprim-sulfamethoxazole followed by cephalexin without improvement. The enlarging axillary lymph nodes subsequently were lanced, and Serratia marcescens was cultured from the expressed material. Several days later, the axillary lymph nodes became ulcerated and the patient developed fever, night sweats, oral ulcers, and dysphagia. He was subsequently admitted to the hospital. On admission, the patient was noted to have bilateral axillary adenopathy with lymph nodes measuring up to 2 cm as well as oral ulcers involving the proximal tongue and left maxillary gum. A chest radiograph was normal. Complete blood analysis showed leukopenia with severe neutropenia, with a white blood cell count of $2.4 \times 10^3/\mu L$ (reference range, $4.5-11.0 \times 10^3/\mu L$) and an absolute neutrophil count of $0.12 \times 10^3/\mu L$ (reference range, $1.5-7.0 \times 10^3/\mu L$). Hemoglobin, haematocrit, platelet count and serum electrolytes were all within their respective reference ranges. He was started on granulocyte colony-stimulating factor and broad-spectrum antibiotics, and a bone marrow biopsy was performed to evaluate for hematopoietic malignancy. Shortly after admission to the hospital, the patient developed

rapid onset of progressive cutaneous violaceous ecchymosis, areas of purpura, and hemorrhagic bullae, most notably affecting the nasal tip, lips, and ears, which became ischemic and blackened. After several days, 40% of the skin surface was involved, including the extremities, trunk, and face, yielding second and third degree burn-like skin loss of approximately 30% and 10% of the skin surface area, respectively. Complete blood cell count revealed the onset of thrombocytopenia, with the platelet count dropping to $98 \times 10^3/\mu L$. A skin biopsy revealed numerous intravascular thrombi involving superficial and deep dermal vessels without vasculitis that were consistent with vascular occlusive disease, excluding Stevens–Johnson syndrome secondary to antibiotic therapy. Special stains for infectious organisms were negative. Laboratory data showed increased PT and aPTT, decreased fibrinogen, decreased antithrombin III antigen, and decreased serum complement levels. All infectious serologies were negative. A positive ANCA and weakly positive IgM antiphospholipid autoantibody were present. Additional patient history obtained at this time revealed recent cocaine use that started prior to the initial symptoms of fatigue and adenopathy. The bone marrow was negative for a hematologic malignancy but showed reactive myeloid hyperplasia. The possibility of purpura fulminans with disseminated intravascular coagulation secondary to bacterial lymphadenitis was considered, but given its rarity in adults and the lack of systemic changes such as hypotension generally seen with this entity in addition to the patient's history and clinical findings, it was determined that the disease process was consistent with exposure to levamisole-contaminated cocaine. The patient was administered anticoagulants, with appropriate skin and wound care. A follow-up skin biopsy 3 days later revealed intravascular thrombi. The patient developed respiratory distress requiring transfer to the intensive care unit; he subsequently was transferred to a local burn unit. He continued to deteriorate, with development of renal and hepatic failure, and he lapsed into a transient coma. The cutaneous lesions also progressed, with complete necrosis of the nose; substantial skin and soft tissue loss in the chest and extremities, requiring extensive skin grafts; and focal necrosis of lower extremity muscles and bone. He remained hospitalized with ongoing therapy at the time of this report [28A].

Case Study
LEG ULCERATION

A 48-year-old woman with a history of hypertension was admitted for evaluation of a skin rash, fever and a cough. She rapidly developed a red, pruritic and painful rash on her legs bilaterally few days after snorting cocaine. She also reported fever, chills, cough and a left-sided pleuritic chest pain. The physical examination was significant for large violaceous plaques and large flaccid bullae, involving bilateral lower extremities Complete blood count was remarkable for neutropenia with absolute neutrophil count of 0.64×10^9 cells/L and urine toxicology positive for cocaine. A chest X-ray showed left lower lobe infiltrate suggestive of pneumonia and the patient was started on antibiotics. Further serologies were performed including antinuclear antibody (ANA), anti-double-stranded DNA and perinuclear antineutrophil cytoplasmic antibody (p-ANCA) was positive by immunofluorescent assay and enzyme immunoassay that were positive. An extractable nuclear antigen panel was positive for antichromatin antibody. Cytoplasmic antineutrophil cytoplasmic antibody antihistone antibody and cryoglobulins were negative. A wound swab was negative for any bacterial or fungal culture and stain. A skin lesion biopsy showed thrombogenic vasculopathy with multiple microthrombi within the superficial vascular plexuses with no inflammatory infiltrates. Histopatholgical findings along with neutropoenia were most consistent with levamisole that is usually added to powdered cocaine to increase weight. Test for levamisole was positive. A few days after admission, the skin lesions improved and the patient was discharged home in stable condition. She was advised to stop misusing cocaine. Within 10 days of being discharged, she was readmitted again with new skin lesions and worsening necrotic ulcers from the old ones. The patient was confronted and she admitted for ingesting cocaine again from the same dealer [29A].

A 39-year-old female presented with diffuse non palpable retiform purpura on her breasts, trunk and extremities following a recent binge of "crack". She required hospital admission for progression of her retiform purpura to ecchymotic purpura and eventually skin necrosis. Her presentation was linked to levamisole with positive urine toxicology. Her tissue pathology showed microvascular thrombosis with leukocytoclastic vasculitis, a pattern attributable to levamisole-induced skin necrosis. Her lesions improved significantly in her periods of abstinence from cocaine, without residual scar or deformity. The patient suffered a number of relapses with varying degrees of purpura and ulceration. Approximately 2 years after initial presentation, a major binge of cocaine prompted admission for extensive purpura covering 40% body surface area, with accompanying skin necrosis including both of her legs, buttocks, breasts, and abdomen. She underwent debridement with split thickness skin grafting over multiple procedures. She developed necrosis of the left leg secondary to extensive scarring and ulceration consistent with late sequelae of thombosing vasculopathy, which necessitated amputation. The grafts healed well and the patient was discharged for rehabilitation [30A].

Case Study

FACIAL CUTANEOUS NECROSIS DUE TO LEVAMISOLE TOXICITY IN A COCAINE USER

A 29-year-old woman with a history of cocaine abuse presented with a several-hour history of painful and tender purpuric patches on her auricles bilaterally, hard palate, nose, and lips, as well as scattered purpuric patches on her right upper arm and left shoulder, and a 1-week history of epistaxis and generalized malaise. Otolaryngology was consulted, and her physical exam was significant for extensive violaceous purpura over both auricles, nose, upper and lower lips, both cheeks, as well as an eschar of her central hard palate. A large patch of retiform purpura was also found over her right lateral upper arm, and several small purpuric patches were evident on her left anterior and lateral shoulder. Laboratory data revealed a normal white blood cell count, normal D-dimer and fibrinogen levels, normal platelet count, mild microcytic anemia, moderate bandemia (excess immature white blood cells), anti-proteinase-3 (anti-PR3) ANCA positivity, negative anti-myeloperoxidase (anti-MPO) antibodies, and cocaine and opiates in her urine. An antiphospholipid antibody panel was positive for phosphatidyl glycerol IgG and phosphatidyl serine IgG, borderline positive for anticardiolipin IgG, and negative for anticardiolipin IgM. Punch biopsies of the cutaneous lesions revealed leukocytoclastic vasculitis with foci of fibrin microthrombi. She was treated with intravenous vancomycin and piperacillin-tazobactam and oral prednisone, but the cutaneous lesions demonstrated little improvement at discharge 9 days later. She was discharged with oral prednisone and sulfamylon 8.5% cream for her facial lesions and saline nasal spray for both nares, but unfortunately she did not return for follow-up.

The authors concluded that early recognition of the syndrome and cessation of use of cocaine-tainted levamisole remains a cornerstone in the treatment of this drug abuse complication [31A].

Hair

Case Study

DETECTION OF LEVAMISOLE IN HAIR SAMPLES OF A PATIENT WITH PANNICULITIS SECONDARY TO ABUSE OF LEVAMISOLE-CONTAMINATED COCAINE

A 39-year-old female cocaine addict consulted for recurrent (six stereotypic episodes per year) painful panniculitis with erythematous reticulated skin lesions of the lower limbs, polyarthralgia, myalgia and fever of 10 years duration, without obvious etiology. Biopsy of an erythematous reticulated lesion showed a septal panniculitis with leucocytoclastic vasculitis. Antineutrophil cytoplasm antibodies (ANCA) were present at 1/1280 with anti-myeloperoxydase (MPO) antibodies at 126 UI/mL (Elisa; Euroimmun). Oral prednisone (80 mg/day) and methotrexate (20 mg/week) were administered but adherence to treatment was poor. Hair samples were analyzed; levamisole and benzoylecgonine (a cocaine metabolite) were detected over the entire length of the hair (which measures 12 cm), proving that the patient had regularly consumed levamisole during the past 12 months. It was concluded levamisole abuse could be responsible for the observed clinical and immunological events. The patient was followed up and remained asymptomatic for the next 8 months. During the following 7 months, the symptoms recurred then persisted. A new 16-cm hair sample was collected to measure concentrations of levamisole and cocaine. Since hair growth is approximately 1 cm per month, this was consistent with retrospective analysis of more than an annual levamisole exposition. After pre-treatment, hair sample testing was positive for both levamisole and cocaine in the slightly modified previously published methods (UPLC-MS/MS and FPIA-AXSYM Abbott, respectively). The results showed that the recurrence of symptoms and consumption of levamisole were concomitant. The authors emphasized the importance of measuring levamisole in hair samples of patients with a history of cocaine abuse [32A].

Immune

Case Study

TOXICITY MIMICKING AUTOIMMUNE DISEASE

A 44-year-old woman was admitted with a diffuse painful skin eruption of 3 weeks duration. She regularly used heroin and intranasal cocaine, with last use 3 days prior to admission. Two weeks earlier, she had been treated for cocaine-induced vasculitis and abdominal-wall cellulitis with oral antibiotics. After that admission, she used cocaine again, noted progression of her skin lesions, and re-presented for medical evaluation. Physical examination revealed large, stellate, purpuric plaques on her trunk, arms, and earlobes, overlying flaccid blisters on her breasts, and livedo reticularis on her back, thighs, and forearms. A urine toxicology screen on admission was positive for cocaine, opioids, and acetaminophen. Skin biopsy specimens from the right forearm and back showed thrombotic vasculopathy and neutrophilic dermatitis. Laboratory studies demonstrated positive perinuclear-ANCA (p-ANCA), anti-myeloperoxidase, anti-double-stranded DNA (dsDNA), antic-ardiolipin (ACL), and antinuclear antibodies (ANA). She was started on systemic corticosteroids and cyclophosphamide for presumed severe systemic granulomatosis with polyangiitis, and anticoagulated with heparin and switched to warfarin before discharge. Her skin lesions improved over the course of the 7-day hospital stay. After discharge, she completed a 3-month course of cyclophosphamide and an extended predni-sone taper. She abstained from cocaine and heroin following hospitalization. Follow-up testing after treatment demon-strated negative dsDNA and ANA titres, and her p-ANCA titres and ACL antibodies normalized. Cyclophosphamide and prednisone were discontinued when her original cocaine supply was obtained from the police and subsequently tested positive for levamisole, confirming a suspicion of levamisole-induced vasculopathy. Her skin lesions healed with thick, scle-rotic scars over the upper aspect of her right arm and mid aspect of her back. She has demonstrated no systemic complications or recurrences of her condition [33A].

A 50-year-old woman with a history of heroin and cocaine abuse presented with pain and swelling of her hands and a skin eruption on her legs and ears. She reported a 6-month history of joint pain and swelling and stated that her flares were related to cocaine use. Her medical history included von Willebrand dis-ease and hepatitis C. She experienced a miscarriage 12 weeks prior while using cocaine and was found to have a positive

ANA and indeterminate dsDNA, resulting in a diagnosis of systemic lupus erythematosus. On examination, she had ten-der, purpuric, reticulated patches on her thighs and pinna bilat-erally and faint livedo reticularis on her arms and legs. A biopsy specimen of a lesion revealed thrombotic vasculopathy without evidence of vasculitis. Laboratory findings were also notable for an elevated p-ANCA, with positive myeloperoxi-dase and leukopenia. She was started on prednisone and hydroxychloroquine, but she self-discontinued the hydroxy-chloroquine, and her lesions resolved on prednisone alone. Her ANA normalized shortly after. One year later, she experi-enced episodic arthralgia despite reported abstinence from cocaine, but her p-ANCA continued to decline [33A].

A 48-year-old woman with a history of cocaine dependence and idiopathic neutropenia presented to the emergency depart-ment with the complaint of 4 days of fevers, cough, rhinorrhea, shortness of breath, and diffuse body aches. Her initial vital signs were as follows: temperature of 36.8 °C, heart rate of 69 beats per minute, blood pressure of 83/44 mm Hg. Initial labs were significant for a white blood cell count of 2300/μL with an absolute neutrophil count of 1000/μL consistent with her history of idiopathic neutropenia, negative blood cultures, chest X-ray with stable hilar adenopathy, and urine toxicology screen positive for cocaine. Her last use of cocaine was 6 days prior. She was admitted from the emergency department to the general medicine floor for observation, given her history of severe pneumonia, recent fevers at home, and neutropenia. On the night of admission, the patient became febrile and was started on broad spectrum antibiotics. She remained afe-brile for 36 hours and her antibiotics were tapered, but became febrile again with associated hypotension and tachycardia not responsive to intravenous fluid boluses. She was transferred to the medical intensive care unit for suspected sepsis where she required intubation for airway protection. Repeat infectious workup was notable for bilateral patchy infiltrates on CXR. Antibiotic coverage was broadened again with improvement in hemodynamics. On her initial exam in the medical ICU (hospital day 2), she was found to have large non-blanching purpuric patches on both forearms. Dermatology was con-sulted, and a punch biopsy demonstrated a vaso-occlusive vasculitis. Autoimmune workup was significant for positive perinuclear anti-neutrophil cytoplasmic antibodies (p-ANCA) at 1:1280, negative cytoplasmic antineutrophil cytoplasmic antibodies (c-ANCA), and negative anticardiolipin antibodies. The patient's ICU course was also complicated by anxiety and agitation, for which psychiatry was consulted, and she was started on quietapine 100 mg daily. She was hemodynamically stabilized, extubated, and transferred back to the general med-icine service, where she completed an 8-day course of meropen-em. Her violaceous patches developed into bullae on hospital day 3 and began to necrose and slough on hospital day 6. Once she completed the course of IV antibiotics, she requested and was granted a discharge against medical advice. On discharge, she was provided with a 3-week course of cephalexin due to lack of intact skin barrier. Her dermatologic findings were thought to be attributable to the levamisole-induced cutaneous vasculo-pathy. The authors concluded that adulteration of cocaine with levamisole and other substances is a worldwide phenomenon, and that public enlightenment about the potentially dangerous effects associated with such practices could be an important deterrent [34A].

A 40-year-old woman presented to the emergency department with a chief complaint of a painful rash. She had noticed lesions on her skin accompanied by burning pain that intensi-fied over a 24-hour period. The patient admitted to smoking "crack" cocaine 4 days prior to presentation. Her past medical history was significant for hepatitis C, anti-phospholipid anti-body syndrome, migraine headaches, and chronic lower back pain. She admitted smoking cigarettes and polysubstance abuse (marijuana, heroin, and daily cocaine use). The patient's exam was notable for retiform purpuric skin lesions with eschar on her left external pinnae, tongue, roof of her mouth, and bilater-ally on her upper and lower extremities. Pus was expressible on palpation of the tibial skin lesions. Laboratory evaluation revealed a white blood cell count of 3.1×109 cells/L and a pos-itive urine toxicology screen for cocaine. A biopsy obtained from her right thigh during a prior similar presentation showed luminally thrombosed fibrin-containing small vessels sur-rounded by neutrophils and nuclear dust. The adjacent dermis contained extravasated erythrocytes [35A].

Thrombotic vasculitis due to levamisole-contaminated cocaine has been described [36A].

A 49-year-old African-American presented with a 1-week history of a painful eruption consisting of retiform purpura of the trunk and extremities and necrotic palpable purpura of the earlobes, cheeks, and nasal tip. Two skin biopsies, one from each upper arm, revealed necrotizing vasculitis of the reticular dermal vessels with mural infiltration by neutrophils and lumi-nal occlusion with fibrinous material. Direct immunofluores-cence demonstrated granular deposition of immunoglobulin M (IgM), C3, and fibrin in the superficial reticular dermal vessel walls. Cytoplasmic (c-ANCA) and atypical perinuclear (p-ANCA) anti-neutrophil cytoplasmic antibodies were detected. Levels of antibodies to myeloperoxidase and proteinase-3 were 14.7 U/mL (normal range: 0–9 U/mL) and 82.5 U/mL (normal range: 0–3.5 U/mL), respectively. Lupus anticoagulant and anticardiolipin IgM and IgG antibodies were present. A urine toxicology screen was positive for cocaine. The patient experi-enced marked improvement with a short taper of oral prednisone and cessation of cocaine use.

A 33-year-old woman presented to the emergency depart-ment complaining of painful skin lesions on her cheeks, nose, back, and bilateral upper and lower extremities that had been developing for the past week. She admitted to recent heroin and cocaine use. She also reported fever, chills, nausea, decreased appetite, non-productive cough, chest tightness, and loose stools but denied chest pain, vomiting, trauma, and dysuria. Physical exam revealed ecchymotic lesions on the malar eminences and on the nasal tip, supratip, nasal ala, nasal sill, and columella. Nasal mucosa was erythematous and edematous with left septal deviation and left anterior septal mucosa excoriation without perforation. Purpuric and ecchy-motic lesions were also noted on the left scapular region, right triceps region, and bilateral lower extremities. The patient had a past medical history significant for previous episodes of levamisole-induced skin necrosis. She was started on 60-mg oral prednisone for her skin lesions before admission. Initial lab-oratory investigations revealed thrombocytopenia with a plate-let count of 125000 per mm^3 and a white blood cell count within normal limits. Absolute neutrophil count was 2600 per mm^3. Antinuclear antibodies were weakly positive with a titer of 1:80, and ANCA were positive with a titer of 1:1280. Antimyeloperoxidase antibodies (anti-MPO) were within nor-mal limits, and antiserine protease 3 antibodies (anti-PR3) were elevated at 31 (0–20). Hepatitis B core antibodies were positive, and HIV antibodies were negative. Gas chromatogra-phy mass spectrometry analysis was positive for cocaine, levamisole, and nicotine. Toxicology screen was positive for cocaine and opiates. Urinalysis was suggestive of a urinary tract infection, and blood culture was positive for Escherichia coli. On the second day of admission the patient was started on cefepime, had fevers with a max temperature of 38.7 °C, and was tachypneic. She also had an episode of hypotension and elevated lactic acid, which improved after a 2-L bolus of normal saline. Her skin lesions appeared lighter, except for lesions on the right triceps and nasal area, which appeared necrotic. She was continued on 50-mg oral prednisone. Over the course of the rest of her hospital stay, the patient developed additional necrotic lesions on the left helix, right anterior thigh, and left triceps region. Her platelet count decreased to 74000 per mm^3, and her white blood cell decreased to 3400 per mm^3. Her antibiotics were switched from cefepime to ceftriax-one once sensitivities were available. The patient was dis-charged on hospital day 5 on 20-mg oral prednisone for 10 days and oral ciprofloxacin after improvement of her skin lesions and multiple negative blood cultures. She returned to the emergency department 4 weeks later after continued cocaine use and auto amputation of the tip of her nose [37A].

Renal System

Case Study

CASES OF KIDNEY INJURY RESULTING FROM INGESTION OF LEVAMISOLE-CONTAMINATED COCAINE

A 36-year-old woman with a history of sarcoidosis presented to the emergency department with purple lesions over her face and limbs present for 3 days. She admitted to smoking cocaine on a regular basis but denied intravenous drug abuse. Her tem-perature was 101.4 °F, heart rate of 119 beats per minute, respiratory rate of 20 breaths per minute, and blood pressure of 120/65 mm Hg. Her skin was noted to be warm and dry, with violaceous lesions in a malar distribution over her face, hands, wrists, and a patchy distribution over her legs. She had significant perioral swelling and mucosal breakdown with serosanguineous drainage. Laboratory results were significant for sodium of 131 mEq/L, potassium of 3.1 mEq/L, bicarbonate of 13 mmol/L, creatinine of 2.8 mg/dL, glomerular filtration rate (GFR) of 24 mL/min/1.73 m^2, venous pH of 7.23, and lactate of 1.8 mmol/L. Complete blood cell count and liver function tests were within normal limits. Urine toxicology screen was positive for cocaine metabolites. She was admitted to the intensive care unit for intravenous fluids, antimicrobials, and further evaluation of her acute renal failure. Testing for syphilis, HIV, hepatitis panel, and complement were negative. Immunologic panel was negative for antinuclear antibody, centromere antibodies, rheumatoid factor, IgM cardiolipin antibodies, β-2 glycoprotein, perinuclear antineutrophil cytoplasmic antibodies (p-ANCA), and cytoplasmic antineutrophil cytoplasmic antibodies (c-ANCA). Quantitative titers for p-ANCA and c-ANCA were less than 1:10. Haptoglobin was found to be 320 mg/dL. Blood and urine cultures were all negative. Over the course of 3 days, she received 7 L of fluid, a sodium bicarbonate infusion, and her serum creatinine improved to 1.5 mg/dL (GFR, 48 mL/min/1.73 m^2). The patient's bicarbonate improved to 30 mmol/L. Nephrologists and other consultants involved in her care concluded that levamisole was the culprit. By day 18, her serum creatinine improved to a level of 0.8 mg/dL (GFR, 98 mL/min/1.73 m^2) [38A].

A 36-year-old Caucasian man with history of antibodies to hepatitis C infection, smoking, and intravenous use of cocaine and brown heroin, on treatment with methadone, presented to the hospital with purpuric skin lesions on extremities and earlobes. The patient had been admitted to the hospital 4 months earlier due to intravenous drug-induced cellulitis and abscess on his forearms and legs. He had received treatment with amoxicillin-clavulanic acid, and skin lesions had improved. A transthoracic echocardiogram had ruled out infectious endocarditis. One month before the current presentation, purpuric lesions on extremities and earlobes had appeared and a skin punch biopsy had been performed. The histopathologic findings were suggestive of mixed cryoglobulinemia. Blood tests showed polyclonal hypergammaglobulinemia and deterioration of renal function (serum creatinine 1.6 mg/dL, normal range of 0.9–1.3 mg/dL). On physical examination, the patient was afebrile. Skin examination revealed a purpuric and violaceous, non-blanching rash in a retiform pattern with areas of necrosis and infected ulcers, located on helix and earlobes and upper and lower extremities. There were no mucosal lesions or peripheral lymphadenopathy and no heart murmur or rub. Hepatosplenomegaly was present. Laboratory testing showed a white blood cell (WBC) count of 2720 per mm^3 (normal range of 4300–11000 per mm^3), hemoglobin 5.6 g/dL (normal range of 12.5–17.5 g/dL); hepatic function was normal; renal function test revealed serum creatinine 2.71 mg/dL, glomerular filtration rate (GFR) 28 mL/min/1.73 m^2; urinary sediment showed hematuria and 4750 mg of protein excretion in 24-hour urine collection. Erythrocyte sedimentation rate was 121 mm per hour and C-reactive protein was 200 mg/dL. Test

result for cryoglobulin was negative; anti-nuclear antibody (ANA) positive at 1:80 dilution with a homogeneous pattern; complement C3 89 and C4 14 mg/dL (normal range of 19–152 and 16–43 mg/dL, respectively); ELISA for antiproteinase 3 antineutrophil cytoplasmic antibodies (PR3-ANCA) was negative and for antimyeloperoxidase (MPO-ANCA) was positive at 145 AU/mL (normal 0–5 AU/mL). Anti-glomerular basement membrane antibodies were negative. Skin punch biopsy performed 1 month before the current admission (suggestive of mixed cryoglobulinemia) demonstrated pathologic findings consistent with leukocytoclastic vasculitis. An ultrasound scan showed slightly enlarged kidneys suggestive of nephrotic syndrome induced by probable glomerulonephritis. The patient provided a cocaine sample for personal use and an analysis was performed using mass spectrometry–gas chromatography. Levamisole was detected in the cocaine sample. The patient received a 3-week course of amoxicillin-clavulanic acid for infected skin ulcers. In addition, six packed red cell transfusions were required due to severe anemia. Considering signs of inflammation and end-organ damage (nephrotic syndrome induced by probable glomerulonephritis) in a toxic context, three boluses of intravenous methylprednisolone were administered, followed by oral prednisone 1 mg/kg per day. Sulfamethoxazole-trimethoprim was started for Nocardia and Pneumocystis jiroveci prophylaxis. An angiotensin-converting enzyme (ACE) inhibitor was added to decrease protein loss in the urine. The patient was discharged with tapering down of prednisone. Three months later, the patient denied cocaine use since last admission. On physical examination, he had gained weight and was fully active, skin lesions had disappeared, and he reported only migrating joint pains. WBC count had normalized. Renal function had improved, reaching serum creatinine of 1.83 mg/dL (GFR 45 mL/min/1.73 m^2) and 1915 mg of protein excretion in 24-hour urine collection. Complement C4 was normal and MPO-ANCA decreased to 83 AU/mL. Patient counselling to avoid cocaine use was provided [39A].

Hematologic: Agranulocytosis due to levamisole-contaminated cocaine has again been described [40A].

A 36-year-old man was referred to a specialty clinic because of an episode of high fever and infections on his hands, mouth and ears. Laboratory testing showed neutropenia. The infections were treated successfully with antibiotics. The neutropenia disappeared, but returned with recurrence of the infections. Upon presentation at the emergency care unit, the patient had signs of intoxication. This patient's urine contained metabolites of cocaine (benzoylecgonine and ecgonine methyl ester), whereupon additional testing showed levamisole to be present in serum. The patient discontinued cocaine use. Following treatment of the infections, the neutropenia fully resolved and did not recur.

The first case of agranulocytosis due to levamisole in a cocaine user has been reported in Argentina in a 36-year-old male with a 22-year smoking history and occasional use of ketamine, ecstasy, LSD and marijuana [41A].

A 50-year-old man presented with a 10 day history of fever, chills and profuse sweating, myalgia associated with polyarthritis, odynophagia with anorexia, and cough. He had a history of "snorting" cocaine up to 4 g per day. On admission, vital parameters were pulse rate 120 beats per minute, fever 39.3 °C and normal blood pressure. Physical examination revealed tender cervical lymphadenopathy. Ear, nose and throat (ENT) examination revealed bilateral earache without otorrhea and perforation of the right nasal septum. The remainder of the physical examination was normal. Laboratory analysis revealed agranulocytosis, moderate lymphopenia, normocystic aplastic anemia, normal platelet counts, and increased CRP. Bacteriological tests were negative. Thoraco-abdomino-pelvic CT scan did not reveal any abnormality. A myelogram showed a poor marrow without immature or abnormal cells. The patient was commenced on empirical antibiotic therapy with piperacillin/tazobactam. The ENT symptoms resolved gradually over 72 hours. His aplastic anemia resolved within 10 days of hospitalization after which antibiotic therapy was stopped. In the absence of regular drug intake, spontaneous improvement of neutropenia with the stoppage of drug abuse and the lack of hematologic etiology, a toxic cause related to high dose cocaine use was suspected. The HIV tests were negative but HBV and HCV serology suggested a history of a past infection. There was no sign of hemolysis. Anti-nuclear, anticardiolipin and anti-β2GP1 antibodies were negative, the complement was normal and cryoglobulinemia was positive. ANCA was very positive by indirect immunofluorescence with anti-Elisa myeloperoxidase specificity (67 U/mL), anti-proteinase 3 (228 U/mL) and anti-elastase. Testing for circulating lupus anticoagulant was positive. The direct Coombs test was positive for IgG. Intent on contributing to knowledge development, the patient provided two samples of cocaine that he had consumed just before hospitalization. The SINTES (national identification system and toxic substances) was contacted to collect and analyze the products. Analysis of the two samples showed the presence of levamisole, at a rate of 13% and 15% of the total weight, respectively. These results were returned to the patient, and used to support a specialized maintenance risk reduction based on the actual composition of drugs sold on the black market. The diagnosis was therefore that of immune-mediated agranulocytosis due to levamisole. After discharge, the patient resumed taking cocaine, "sniffed" at 1 g per day. He was hospitalized again a month later for recurrence of febrile agranulocytosis. He was again put under empiric antibiotic therapy, and a rapid improvement in clinical symptoms and laboratory results were noted after detoxification. Urinary levamisole assay carried out 3 days after the entry was negative, probably because of the short half-life of the molecule. He was subsequently transferred with his consent to a residential facility specializing in addiction to help maintain the prolonged withdrawal desired by the patient [42A].

DEATH

A case of death secondary to sepsis in a patient who consumed to levamisole-contaminated cocaine [43A].

A 22-year-old man, with a long history of cannabis (>10 years) and cocaine (>5 years) abuse, was admitted with headache, ataxia, and right-sided paresthesias of several days duration. He had no relevant medical history and had no recognized occupational exposures. Cerebrospinal fluid (CSF) analysis revealed a hyperproteinorrachia (excess protein in the CSF) at 2.49 g/L with low cellularity (15 cells/mm^3, mainly lymphocytes) and no CSF-specific IgG oligoclonal bands. Serological testing was negative for antinuclear antibody (ANA), antineutrophil cytoplasmic antibody (ANCA), and anticardiolipine antibodies. Complement was normal, as was the activity of antithrombin III, protein C and S. Comprehensive screening for infectious diseases was negative. Brain magnetic resonance imaging (MRI) revealed diffusely severe multiple sclerosis (MS)-like leukoencephalopathy with numerous small foci of T2-weighted hypersignal intensity throughout the supra- and infratentorial white matter. Multiple lesions were present within the corpus callosum (i.e., on the midline) raising a strong suspicion for Susac syndrome; they progressively evolved to necrotic, cystic lesions. Only a faint contrast enhancement was observed within a few lesions, thereby decreasing the probability of an acute disseminated encephalomyelitis (ADEM). Despite heavy steroid pulse therapy, the neurological status rapidly worsened, with altered consciousness, mutism and quadriparesis. The follow-up MR examination revealed a progression of the T2-weighted images. Occlusion of some branch retinal arteries was noted at fundoscopy performed by a neuro-ophthalmologist. Brainstem auditory evoked potentials were normal. Despite maximal immunosuppressive therapy, the patient remained in a minimally conscious state. He deteriorated with spasticity and dysautonomic symptoms. He died 3 months later from septic complications. In order to explore possible toxic etiologies, hair sampling was done from hair specimens collected 2 months after he was initially hospitalized. The analysis was performed using an ultra-performing liquid chromatography tandem mass spectrometry operating in positive electrospray mode (Quattro Premier, Waters, Milford, MA, USA). Analysis included investigation for cocaine, levamisole, opioids, and several amphetamines. Except for cocaine (C), benzoylecgonine (B), and levamisole (L), no other compounds were detected.

MEBENDAZOLE (SEDA-36, 461)

Comparative Studies

In a nonrandomized study of school children, the safety and efficacy of 1-day versus 2-day regimen of mebendazole in heavy intensity *Trichuris trichuria* infection was compared [4C]. There were no adverse events.

Drug Combination Studies

See albendazole.

PRAZIQUANTEL (SEDA-31, 511; SEDA-33, 650; SEDA-36, 461)

Observational Studies

The efficacy and safety of praziquantel for treating *S. mansoni* infection in school aged children has been evaluated in a nonrandomized study including 342 participants [44C]. *Abdominal cramps, fatigue, diarrhea* and *headache* were reported as the most frequent adverse effects.

In a prospective study to examine the safety and efficacy of praziquantel for the treatment of *S. haematobium* in 197 of 243 participants who tested positive to *S. haematobium* infection using urine dipsticks, the most common side effects reported post-treatment were *nausea, abdominal pain* and *headache* [45C].

Comparative Studies

The safety and efficacy of praziquantel alone for prophylaxis against *S. mansoni* infection has been compared with combination therapy (mefloquine–praziquantel or mefloquine–artesunate–praziquantel) in a randomized clinical trial including 71 children [46C]. 56% of children reported adverse events following praziquantel administration. *Abdominal pain, headache, vomiting* and *diarrhea* were the most common adverse events reported. The adverse events were mild, apart from abdominal pain which was reported to be moderate in severity. At 24 hours post-treatment, praziquantel and mefloquine-artesunate were significantly better tolerated than mefloquine ($P < 0.05$). There were no significant differences in cure rates.

Drug Combination Studies

In a cross-sectional survey of 752 school-age children, adverse events following co-administration of praziquantel and albendazole for prophylaxis against urogenital schistosomiasis and soil-transmitted helminthiasis were examined [47C]. Reported adverse events were described as mild, transient, and no worse in severity compared with monotherapy. The most common adverse events reported were *abdominal pain* (46.3%), *dizziness* (33.2%) and *nausea* (21.1%). Over 80% of the reported adverse events were self-resolving. The frequency of adverse events were significantly greater in girls than with boys ($P = 0.027$).

Systematic Reviews and Meta-Analyses

The relationship between praziquantel therapy for liver fluke (*Opisthorchis viverrini*) infestation, and the incidence of cholangiocarcinoma has been investigated in a systematic review and meta-analysis of three studies ($n = 637$) [48M]. There was no significant relationship in a pooled analysis of two studies with 237 participants (OR 1.8, 95% CI 0.81–4.16). The authors concluded that because of the significant methodological limitations in the review, further research into this relationship is warranted.

The safety of praziquantel therapy for intestinal and urinary schistosomiasis has been evaluated in a systematic review and meta-analysis of 40 comparative and non-comparative studies including a total of 12 435 subjects [49M]. The most common adverse events reported were gastrointestinal, dermatological and neurological. The incidence of adverse events ranged from 2.3% (*urticaria*) to 31.1% (*abdominal pain*). There was a significantly increased risk of experiencing adverse events with praziquantel, 56.9% (95% CI 47.4–69.0%).

The safety and efficacy of different dosages of praziquantel for treating *S. japonicum* infection has been systematically reviewed [50M]. Six studies were included in the meta-analysis, four of which had good methodological quality. There were no significant differences in the frequencies of adverse events for 30 versus 40 mg/kg (RR 0.97, 95% CI 0.68–1.38; $P = 0.87$), 40 versus with 60 mg/kg (RR 0.79, 95% CI 0.46–1.35; $P = 0.39$) and 50 versus with 60 mg/kg (RR 0.89, 95% CI 0.56–1.42; $P = 0.63$).

TRIBENDIMIDINE (SEDA 36, 462)

Comparative Studies

The safety and efficacy of two doses of tribendimidine (200 and 400 mg) in the treatment of co-infection with *Clonorchis sinensis* and other helminths has been compared with praziquantel in an open-label study including 156 patients [51c]. Adverse events reported included *vertigo, headache, fever, fatigue, nausean vomiting* and *anxiety*. The frequency of adverse events were significantly less in the two tribendimidine groups compared with praziquantel ($P = 0.034$ and $P = 0.0002$, respectively).

References

[1] Karabulut K, Ozbalci GS, Kesicioglu T, et al. Long-term outcomes of intraoperative and perioperative albendazole treatment in hepatic hydatidosis: single center experience. Ann Surg Treat Res. 2014;87(2):61–5 [c].

[2] Samuel F, Degarege A, Erko B. Efficacy and side effects of albendazole currently in use against Ascaris, Trichuris and hookworm among school children in Wondo Genet, southern Ethiopia. Parasitol Int. 2014;63(2):450–5 [C].

[3] Adegnika AA, Zinsou JF, Issifou S, et al. Randomized, controlled, assessor-blind clinical trial to assess the efficacy of single- versus repeated-dose albendazole to treat ascaris lumbricoides, trichuris trichiura, and hookworm infection. Antimicrob Agents Chemother. 2014;58(5):2535–40 [c].

[4] Mekonnen Z, Levecke B, Boulet G, et al. Efficacy of different albendazole and mebendazole regimens against heavy-intensity

Trichuris trichiura infections in school children, Jimma Town, Ethiopia. Pathog Glob Health. 2013;107(4):207–9 [C].

[5] Alvela-Suárez L, Velasco-Tirado V, Belhassen-Garcia M, et al. Safety of the combined use of praziquantel and albendazole in the treatment of human hydatid disease. Am J Trop Med Hyg. 2014;90(5):819–22 [c].

[6] Garcia HH, Gonzales I, Lescano AG, et al. Working Group in Peru. Efficacy of combined antiparasitic therapy with praziquantel and albendazole for neurocysticercosis: a double-blind, randomised controlled trial. Lancet Infect Dis. 2014;14(8):687–95 [c].

[7] Speich B, Ali SM, Ame SM, et al. Efficacy and safety of albendazole plus ivermectin, albendazole plus mebendazole, albendazole plus oxantel pamoate, and mebendazole alone against Trichuris trichiura and concomitant soil-transmitted helminth infections: a four-arm, randomized controlled trial. Lancet Infect Dis. 2015;15(3):277–84. pii: S1473-3099(14)71050-3 [C].

[8] Speich B, Ame SM, Ali SM, et al. Oxantel pamoate-albendazole for Trichuris trichiura infection. N Engl J Med. 2014;370(7):610–20 [C].

[9] Abate E, Elias D, Getachew A, et al. Effects of albendazole on the clinical outcome and immunological responses in helminth co-infected tuberculosis patients: a double blind randomised clinical trial. Int J Parasitol. 2015;45(2–3):133–40.

[10] Ben Fredj N, Chaabane A, Chadly Z, et al. Albendazole-induced associated acute hepatitis and bicytopenia. Scand J Infect Dis. 2014;46(2):149–51 [A].

[11] Nandi M, Sarkar S. Albendazole-induced recurrent hepatitis. Indian Pediatr. 2013;50(11):1064 [A].

[12] Shah C, Mahapatra A, Shukla A, et al. Recurrent acute hepatitis caused by albendazole. Trop Gastroenterol. 2013;34(1):38–9 [A].

[13] Marin Zuluaga JI, Marin Castro AE, Perez Cadavid JC, et al. Albendazole-induced granulomatous hepatitis: a case report. J Med Case Rep. 2013;7:201 [A].

[14] Gözüküçük R, Abci İ, Güçlü M. Albendazole-induced toxic hepatitis: a case report. Turk J Gastroenterol. 2013;24(1):82–4 [A].

[15] Ríos D, Restrepo JC. Albendazole-induced liver injury: a case report. Colomb Med (Cali). 2013;44(2):118–20 [A].

[16] Verdugo Thomas F, Tapia Mingo A, Ramírez Montes D, et al. Albendazole-induced toxic hepatitis [Article in Spanish]. Gastroenterol Hepatol. 2014. pii: S0210-5705(14)00224-6 [A].

[17] Batzlaff CM, Pupaibool J, Sohail MR. Acute renal failure associated with albendazole therapy in a patient with trichinosis. BMJ Case Rep. 2014;2014. http://dx.doi.org/10.1136/bcr-2013-200668. pii: bcr2013200668. [A].

[18] Awadzi K, Opoku NO, Attah SK, et al. A randomized, single-ascending-dose, ivermectin-controlled, double-blind study of moxidectin in Onchocerca volvulus infection. PLoS Negl Trop Dis. 2014;8(6):e2953 [c].

[19] van Westerloo DJ, Landman GW, Prichard R, et al. Persistent coma in Strongyloides hyperinfection syndrome associated with persistently increased ivermectin levels. Clin Infect Dis. 2014;58(1):143–4 [A].

[20] Long L, Song Y, Xu L, et al. Levamisole-induced leukoencephalopathy mimicking Baló disease. Neurology. 2015;84(3):328 [A].

[21] Valentino AMM, Fuentecilla K. Levamisole: an analytical profile. Microgram J. 2005;3(3–4):134–7 [r].

[22] Calpoison.org. Levamisole-contaminated cocaine. California Poison Control System 2014; 12(3). http://www.calpoison.org/hcp/2014/callusvol12no3.htm [Accessed 28th February, 2015] [r].

[23] Larocque A, Hoffman RS. Levamisole in cocaine: unexpected news from an old acquaintance. Clin Toxicol (Phila). 2012;50(4):231–41 [R].

[24] Eiden C, Diot C, Mathieu O, et al. Levamisole-adulterated cocaine: what about in European countries? J Psychoactive Drugs. 2014;46(5):389–92 [R].

[25] Lee KC, Ladizinski B, Federman DG. Complications associated with use of levamisole-contaminated cocaine: an emerging public health challenge. Mayo Clin Proc. 2012;87(6):581–6 [R].

[26] Michaud K, Grabherr S, Shiferaw K, et al. Acute coronary syndrome after levamisole-adultered cocaine abuse. J Forensic Leg Med. 2014;21:48–52 [A].

[27] Keith PJ, Joyce JC, Wilson BD. Pyoderma gangrenosum: a possible cutaneous complication of levamisole-tainted cocaine abuse. Int J Dermatol. 2014. http://dx.doi.org/10.1111/ijd.12212 [Epub ahead of print] [A].

[28] Gaertner EM, Switlyk SA. Dermatologic complications from levamisole-contaminated cocaine: a case report and review of the literature. Cutis. 2014;93(2):102–6 [A].

[29] Shawwa K, Alraiyes AH, Eisa N, et al. Cocaine-induced leg ulceration. BMJ Case Rep. 2013;2013. http://dx.doi.org/10.1136/bcr-2013-200507. pii: bcr2013200507 [A].

[30] Gillis JA, Green P, Williams J. Levamisole-induced vasculopathy: staging and management. J Plast Reconstr Aesthet Surg. 2014;67(1): e29–31 [A].

[31] Formeister EJ, Falcone MT, Mair EA. Facial cutaneous necrosis associated with suspected levamisole toxicity from tainted cocaine abuse. Ann Otol Rhinol Laryngol. 2015;124(1):30–4 [A].

[32] Polivka L, Peytavin G, Franck N, et al. Testing for levamisole and cocaine in hair samples for the diagnosis of levamisole-related panniculitis. J Eur Acad Dermatol Venereol. 2014. http://dx.doi.org/10.1111/jdv.12582 [Epub ahead of print] [A].

[33] Strazzula L, Brown KK, Brieva JC, et al. Levamisole toxicity mimicking autoimmune disease. J Am Acad Dermatol. 2013;69(6):954–9 [A].

[34] Auffenberg C, Rosenthal LJ, Dresner N. Levamisole: a common cocaine adulterant with life-threatening side effects. Psychosomatics. 2013;54(6):590–3 [A].

[35] James KT, Detz A, Coralic Z, et al. Levamisole contaminated cocaine induced cutaneous vasculitis syndrome. West J Emerg Med. 2013;14(5):448–9 [A].

[36] Crowe DR, Kim PS, Mutasim DF. Clinical, histopathologic, and immunofluorescence findings in levamisole/cocaine-induced thrombotic vasculitis. Int J Dermatol. 2014;53(5):635–7 [A].

[37] Lawrence LA, Jiron JL, Lin HS, et al. Levamisole-adulterated cocaine induced skin necrosis of nose, ears, and extremities: case report. Allergy Rhinol (Providence). 2014;5(3):132–6 [A].

[38] Ammar AT, Livak M, Witsil JC. Old drug new trick: levamisole-adulterated cocaine causing acute kidney injury. Am J Emerg Med. 2014. pii: S0735-6757(14)00549-X. [Epub ahead of print] [A].

[39] Álvarez Díaz H, Mariño Callejo AI, García Rodríguez JF, et al. ANCA-positive vasculitis induced by levamisole-adulterated cocaine and nephrotic syndrome: the kidney as an unusual target. Am J Case Rep. 2013;14:557–61 [A].

[40] Vos NS, Haak EA, Leeksma OC. Recurrent neutropenia due to adulterated cocaine [Article in Dutch]. Ned Tijdschr Geneeskd. 2014;158:A7430 [A].

[41] Pellegrini D, Young P, Grosso V, et al. Agranulocytosis induced by levamisole in association to cocaine [Article in Spanish]. Medicina (B Aires). 2013;73(5):464–6 [A].

[42] Lemaignen A, Goulenok T, Kalamarides S, et al. Agranulocytosis and vasculitis in a cocaine addict: levamisole, the hidden culprit [Article in French]. Rev Med Interne. 2014;35(10):676–9 [A].

[43] Hantson P1, Di Fazio V, Del Mar Ramirez Fernandez M, et al. Susac-like syndrome in a chronic cocaine abuser: could levamisole play a role? J Med Toxicol. 2015;11(1):124–8.

[44] Reta B, Erko B. Efficacy and side effects of praziquantel in the treatment for Schistosoma mansoni infection in school children in Senbete Town, northeastern Ethiopia. Trop Med Int Health. 2013;18(11):1338–43.

[45] Mekonnen A, Legesse M, Belay M, et al. Efficacy of Praziquantel against Schistosoma haematobium in Dulshatalo village, western Ethiopia. BMC Res Notes. 2013;6:392 [C].

[46] Keiser J, Silué KD, Adiossan LK, et al. Praziquantel, mefloquine-praziquantel, and mefloquine-artesunate-praziquantel against schistosoma haematobium: a randomized, exploratory, open-label trial. PLoS Negl Trop Dis. 2014;8(7):e2975 [C].

[47] Njenga SM, Ng'ang'a PM, Mwanje MT, et al. A school-based cross-sectional survey of adverse events following co-administration of albendazole and praziquantel for preventive chemotherapy against urogenital schistosomiasis and soil-transmitted helminthiasis in Kwale County, Kenya. PLoS One. 2014;9(2):e88315 [C].

[48] Kamsa-ard S, Laopaiboon M, Luvira V, et al. Association between praziquantel and cholangiocarcinoma in patients infected with Opisthorchis viverrini: a systematic review and meta-analysis. Asian Pac J Cancer Prev. 2013;14(11):7011–6 [M].

[49] Zwang J, Olliaro PL. Clinical efficacy and tolerability of praziquantel for intestinal and urinary schistosomiasis-a meta-analysis of comparative and non-comparative clinical trials. PLoS Negl Trop Dis. 2014;8(11):e3286 [M].

[50] Cai D, Zhang S, Wu J, et al. Efficacy and safety of different dosages of praziquantel for the treatment of Schistosoma japonicum: a systematic review and meta-analysis. Iran Red Crescent Med J. 2014;16(10):e9600 [M].

[51] Xu LL, Jiang B, Duan JH, et al. Efficacy and safety of praziquantel, tribendimidine and mebendazole in patients with co-infection of Clonorchis sinensis and other helminths. PLoS Negl Trop Dis. 2014;8(8):e3046 [c].

32

Vaccines

K.M. Damer*,[1], C.M. Jung*,[†], C.M. Maffeo*

*Butler University College of Pharmacy and Health Sciences, Indianapolis, IN, USA
[†]Eskenazi Health, Indianapolis, IN, USA
[1]Corresponding author: kmdamer@butler.edu

Abbreviations

9vHPV	9-valent human papillomavirus vaccine
aP	acellular pertussis
DTaP	diphtheria + tetanus toxoids + acellular pertussis vaccine
DTaP–Hib–IPV	diphtheria + tetanus toxoids + acellular pertussis + inactivated poliovirus + *Haemophilus influenzae* type B vaccine
DTaP–IPV	diphtheria + tetanus toxoids + inactivated poliovirus vaccine
HAV	hepatitis A virus
HBV	hepatitis B virus
Hib	*Haemophilus influenzae* type b
HPV	human papillomavirus
HZV	herpes zoster virus
IIV	inactivated influenza vaccine
IPV	inactivated poliovirus vaccine
JE vaccine	Japanese encephalitis vaccine
LAIV	live attenuated influenza vaccine
MCV4	quadrivalent (serogroups A, C, W, Y) meningococcal conjugate vaccine
MenB vaccine	monovalent serogroup B meningococcal vaccine
MenC	monovalent serogroup C meningococcal conjugate vaccine
MMR	measles + mumps + rubella virus
MMRV	measles + mumps + rubella + varicella virus
MPSV4	quadrivalent (serogroups A, C, W, Y) meningococcal polysaccharide vaccine
PCV13	13-valent pneumococcal conjugate vaccine
PPSV23	23-valent pneumococcal polysaccharide vaccine
qHPV	quadrivalent HPV vaccine
QIV	quadrivalent influenza vaccine
RV	rotavirus
Td	diphtheria + tetanus toxoids vaccine
Tdap	tetanus toxoid + diphtheria toxoid + acellular pertussis vaccine
VZV	varicella zoster virus
YF vaccine	yellow fever vaccine
YFV	yellow fever virus

GENERAL [SEDA-36, 465]

A consistent approach to the classification of adverse events following immunization (AEFI) is important for the determination of actual causality related to the adverse event. The Clinical Immunization Safety Assessment (CISA) Network defined terminology to be used in describing the causality of an AEFI which the World Health Organization (WHO) has similarly adopted [1H,2H]. In summary, it is the recommendation of the CISA Network to categorize AEFI as "consistent with", "inconsistent with", or "indeterminate". Additional details on the approach to determining how AEFI should be categorized with these terms have previously been described and readers should refer to the SEDA volume 36 for the detailed descriptions of definitions and criteria. A universal method to classifying AEFI is important to conveying correct education regarding immunization to patients and vital to ensuring immunization is maintained as a major public health initiative. Although not uniformly reported in the current literature, authors are encouraged to adopt the recommended classification system in order to more appropriately categorize AEFI in the future.

VIRAL VACCINES

Hepatitis B Vaccine [SED-15, 3565, 3566, 3568; SEDA-36, 466]

Organ and Systems

NEUROMUSCULAR FUNCTION

Isolated abducens nerve palsy was described in an 8-day-old infant. The infant exhibited normal abduction in both eyes on day 1 of life. He was administered the first-dose of HBV vaccine 10 mcg/mL on day 2 of life.

© 2015 Elsevier B.V. All rights reserved.

On day 4 of life, the patient was noted to have limited abduction in his right eye, which was confirmed on ophthalmological examination. A neurologic exam and workup were remarkable only for unilateral abducens nerve palsy [3A].

Susceptibility Factors

IMMUNOCOMPROMISED: HIV

Efficacy of HBV vaccination in HIV-positive individuals is comparatively less than healthy, HIV-negative individuals. A study comparing a standard three-dose vaccination series versus four doses and four double doses was completed to assess vaccine efficacy and safety in an HIV-infected population. Participants were randomized to receive either 20 mcg/mL of recombinant HBV vaccine at 0, 1, and 6 months, 20 mcg/mL of the HBV vaccine at 0, 1, 2, and 6 months, or 40 mcg/mL of the HBV vaccine at 0, 1, 2, and 6 months. All vaccine regimens were determined to be safe and effective, although patients in the double-dose group had higher rates of pain at the injection site. Of note, this study was completed in individuals with CD4 counts higher than 200 cells/mm^3 [4C].

Human Papillomavirus Vaccine [SEDA-34, 501; SEDA-35, 574; SEDA-36, 466]

General

The Global Advisory Committee on Vaccine Safety (GACVS) reviewed HPV vaccine safety during their December 2013 meeting with a focus on autoimmune disease and multiple sclerosis. GACVS found no increased risk of either type of disease among vaccination in girls. The committee recommended ongoing surveillance and epidemiological investigation of adverse events following HPV vaccination [5S].

The WHO also released an updated position paper on HPV vaccines in October 2014. They continue to recognize the efficacy of the bivalent and quadrivalent vaccines and report that both vaccines appear safe amongst immunocompromised and immunocompetent individuals [6S].

While the WHO and GACVS continue to support the safety of HPV vaccines, generalized concerns remain regarding increased risk of various types of adverse effects. A register-based cohort study in Denmark and Sweden reviewed safety of the quadrivalent HPV (qHPV) vaccine, specifically targeting the incidence of autoimmune, neurologic, and venous thromboembolic events. A cohort of nearly one million females aged 10–17 years was included in the study, of whom nearly 300 000 received a dose of qHPV vaccine. There was no difference in the rate of autoimmune, neurologic, or venous thromboembolic events between groups. This large cohort study supports the current WHO and GACVS statements on the safety of HPV vaccination [7C].

Organs and Systems

CARDIOVASCULAR: VENOUS THROMBOEMBOLISM

Previous literature suggested concern for venous thromboembolism (VTE) following HPV vaccination. A Danish study evaluated the risk of VTE following HPV vaccination in a self-controlled case-series. The study did not find an association between HPV vaccination and VTE [8r].

NERVOUS SYSTEM: ACUTE DISSEMINATED ENCEPHALOMYELITIS

Two females aged 12 and 13 were diagnosed with acute disseminated encephalomyelitis (ADEM) after a three-dose HPV series. Both girls were treated with high-dose steroids, which led to improvement of their symptoms [9r].

NERVOUS SYSTEM: AUTONOMIC DYSFUNCTION

Six cases of postural tachycardia syndrome (POTS) were reported. POTS is a disorder of the autonomic nervous system. The cases were reported in females between 12 and 22 years of age and varied from 6 days to 2 months following vaccination. All of the cases were treated with varying types of pharmacotherapy and improved over 15 months to 3 years [10A].

NERVOUS SYSTEM: CHOREA

An 11-year-old female presented with facial grimaces, ataxic gait, and dysarthria. She was diagnosed acute chorea. The patient had received her second HPV vaccine dose 1 month prior. All other causes were ruled out. The patient was treated with methylprednisolone and had resolution of her symptoms within 1 week [11r].

NERVOUS SYSTEM: GUILLAIN–BARRÉ SYNDROME

The International Federation of Gynecology and Obstetrics previously stated that despite Vaccine Adverse Event Reporting System (VAERS) reports suggesting an increased risk of Guillain–Barré syndrome (GBS) after HPV vaccination, there was insufficient evidence to conclude a causal relationship [12S]. An analysis of VAERS reports of GBS was completed to determine if there were any differences in reporting after administration HPV vaccine and other vaccines common to males and females 9–26 years of age. The analysis found no significant difference in the frequency of reporting GBS following HPV vaccination [13c].

SKIN

A 27-year-old female was diagnosed with lipoatrophy 9 months following the third dose in the HPV vaccine series. The authors presumed that the last injection was administered subcutaneously than intramuscularly [14r].

IMMUNOLOGIC

Concerns exist that HPV vaccination may be associated with various autoimmune diseases. A review of case reports and randomized controlled trials of HPV vaccine was completed to assess this relationship. The review included autoimmune diseases such as rheumatoid arthritis, juvenile idiopathic arthritis, primary ovarian failure, multiple sclerosis, GBS, and systemic lupus erythematosus. It was concluded that there is no decisive evidence to support a definitive causal relationship between HPV vaccination and the diseases studied [15R].

LONG-TERM EFFECTS

Boys and girls aged 9–15 years were randomized to receive three doses of either qHPV vaccine or placebo. Subjects were followed for 8 years post-vaccination to determine efficacy and safety long-term. For both genders, no new serious adverse events occurred throughout the study duration [16c].

Susceptibility Factors

IMMUNOCOMPROMISED: HIV

Patients with HIV are known to have a higher susceptibility to HPV infection. A limited number of efficacy and safety trials have been completed in this population. The safety and immunogenicity of the qHPV vaccine were compared between HIV-positive and HIV-negative individuals between the ages of 13–27 years. HPV type-specific antibody titers were assessed throughout the study at varying intervals, though the primary outcome were titers 1 month after completion of the vaccination series. Side effects were assessed within the 7-day follow-up period of each dose and CD4 and HIV viral loads were measured throughout the study period in HIV-positive individuals. There was no difference in the immunogenicity of the qHPV vaccine between HIV-positive and HIV-negative groups. The study did not have enough power to assess a difference in side effects between groups. The most common local side effect was pain at the injection site (32.6% in HIV-positive vs 18.8% in HIV-negative individuals) and the most common systemic side effect was headache (13.5% in HIV-positive vs 2.2% in HIV-negative individuals). This study adds to current literature suggesting the benefit and low risk of HPV vaccination in HIV-positive patients [17c].

Drug Administration

DRUG FORMULATIONS

A new 9-valent HPV (9vHPV) vaccine containing the four types in the quadrivalent (qHPV) vaccine (6, 11, 16, 18) and five additional oncogenic types (31, 33, 45, 52, 58) was recently released onto the market. The vaccine is given in a three-dose series. In the major approval trial, the 9vHPV vaccine was more likely to cause injection site reactions compared to the qHPV vaccine. There was no difference between systemic adverse effects between groups [18C].

DRUG DOSAGE REGIMENS

Safety and efficacy of the HPV vaccine when co-administered with other vaccines were reviewed in a recent analysis. Other vaccines included hepatitis A, hepatitis B, meningococcal conjugate, influenza, tetanus, diphtheria, pertussis, pneumococcal, Bacille Calmette–Guérin (BCG), typhoid, MMR, varicella, or poliovirus. No differences in safety were identified between the co-administration and control groups. The authors supported co-administration of the HPV vaccine with other vaccines as it may increase vaccine coverage rates [19M].

Influenza Vaccines [SED-15, 3565, 3569; SEDA-34, 501; SEDA-35, 574; SEDA-36, 467]

Organs and Systems

HEMATOLOGIC

A 29-year-old female was admitted to the hospital with complaints of headaches and fatigue. Her complaints began 2 days following vaccination with IIV. The patient was diagnosed with paroxysmal nocturnal hemoglobinuria (PNH) given the findings on physical and laboratory exam. Namely, a jaundiced appearance, hemoglobin level 6.9 g/dL, indirect hyperbilirubinemia (2.5 mg/dL), and lactate dehydrogenase level of ~6000 U/L. Flow cytometry revealed granulocytes and monocytes deficient in CD59. Findings were consistent with non-immune hemolytic anemia. The patient received one unit of packed red blood cells and a treatment course of oral prednisone. One week later, her hemoglobin level had stabilized. The authors did not perform a causality assessment to determine the association between IIV vaccination and the PNH in this patient. However, the temporal relationship between the events raised the question whether the PNH may have been associated with the influenza antigen(s) and/or the presence of adjuvant within the vaccine formulation. Further investigation was recommended [20A].

MUSCULOSKELETAL

Complications or adverse events following influenza vaccine may be associated with antigenic or adjuvant components of the vaccine and/or the administration technique. A series of four patients reported magnetic resonance imaging (MRI) following complaints of abnormal shoulder pain following influenza vaccine administration. The patients ranged from 36 to 66 years of age and half

(2/4) were female. The patients had non-contributory past medical histories and did not display any systemic symptoms related to the complaints. Laboratory testing was negative for infectious etiology in all patients. Two patients demonstrated MRI evidence of focal bone marrow edema-like signal changes within the humoral head. Three of the four patients required short-term treatment with systemic non-steroidal anti-inflammatory agents. All patients recovered. According to the authors, the most likely causes for the complaints and imaging findings include improper injection technique related to the needle length or the angle at which the vaccination was administered which may result in bursal or cortical penetration. These events may potentially occur more often in patients with lower body mass index (BMI). These results highlight the importance of utilizing appropriate injection technique [21A]. Another case of potential shoulder injury following influenza vaccination was presented in a 76-year-old male with severe pain and decreased range of motion 3 days following vaccine administration. An ultrasound of the patient's affected shoulder revealed subacromial bursa thickening and debris which was interpreted as "suggesting bursitis". The patient recovered following a steroid injection [22A]. This collection of cases will hopefully heighten awareness of the potential adverse events associated with not only the antigen and adjuvants but also the administration of IM vaccines.

NERVOUS SYSTEM

Acute disseminated encephalomyelitis (ADEM) is an immune-mediated inflammatory condition that has been reported as an adverse event associated with vaccination. A retrospective, observational study was performed utilizing the VAERS and EudraVigilance Post Authorization Module (EVPM) databases to characterize the features of ADEM. Cases defined by the WHO as "probable", "possible", and "unlikely" were evaluated from the VAERS database. The database searches identified 199 cases from VAERS and 205 "related" cases from EVPM. The demographics indicated that 48% of the patients were aged 0–17 years and there was a slightly increased percentage of females noted (51% and 60%) for VAERS and EVPM patients. The majority of cases reported occurred between 2 and 30 days following vaccination. Seasonal influenza and HPV vaccines were most frequently associated with ADEM in both VAERS and EVPM databases. Seasonal influenza was most frequently associated with ADEM in patients greater than 18 years of age (32% of total cases). The frequency did not equate to a higher risk, but rather a greater incidence of reporting. This may be connected to the significant numbers of seasonal influenza vaccines administered annually [23c].

One day following vaccination with quadrivalent influenza vaccine (QIV), a 50-year-old Caucasian male presented to the hospital with complaints of left-sided weakness and blurred vision. The patient reported left arm numbness and weakness which progressed to increasing left leg weakness with full left arm paresthesia. Other complaints included pruritus over the left face and blurred vision in the left eye. Upon presentation, the patient as afebrile with stable vital signs. Acute stroke and infection were ruled out with imaging studies and laboratory testing. A brain MRI revealed T2 flair signal changes in the peri- and non-periventricular region, deep hemispheric centrum, peritrigonal, and cortical/subcortical regions, indicative of demyelinating disease. The differential diagnosis included clinically isolated syndrome (CIS) or ADEM. Characteristics of both disorders were present and the authors did not state a definitive diagnosis. The patient was discharged and was able to perform all activities of daily living at either an independent or standby-assist level following treatment with corticosteroids and rehabilitation [24A].

Guillain–Barré Syndrome (GBS) is a peripheral neuropathy that is characterized by acute or sub-acute onset of weakness in the limbs and diminished or absent deep tendon reflexes. The cause of GBS is thought to be an autoimmune process resulting in nerve demyelination, axonal damage, or a combination of both. The annual incidence ranges between 0.4 and 4 per 100 000 persons [25c]. The majority of cases of GBS were preceded by a bacterial or viral infection. Cases of GBS have been associated with the administration of various vaccines, although no causal relationship has been distinctly determined. The highest risk of vaccine-associated GBS was noted in 1976 following vaccination with influenza vaccine when the estimated risk of GBS was one per 100 000 vaccines [25c,26c]. Beyond 1976, evidence is "inadequate to accept or reject a causal relationship between GBS and influenza vaccine" until data began to surface following vaccination with the monovalent influenza A H1N1 vaccine. A large retrospective, observational study was conducted utilizing the US Medicare population to evaluate the risk of GBS among patients who received the monovalent H1N1 vaccine during the 2009–2010 influenza season. Among a population of over three million elderly people vaccinated, 34 chart-confirmed cases of GBS met inclusion criteria. Results indicated a slightly statistically significant increased risk of GBS (Brighton level 1, 2, 3) within 6 weeks of receiving the monovalent H1N1 vaccine compared to the control period. The risk of GBS was highest in the 8–21 days following vaccination (75% of cases occurred within 7 days). The relative risk was lower than documented for the 1976 season [25c].

A large, international study was performed to demonstrate the feasibility of a global collaboration effort to assess vaccine safety and to assess the relative risk of GBS following vaccination with monovalent H1N1 vaccines. Data from 15 countries were included in the analysis. The pooled analysis produced a relative incidence of 2.42 (95% CI, 1.58–3.72) which indicated an increased risk of GBS following vaccination with monovalent H1N1 vaccines. The incidence of GBS was higher in males (RI, 2.75; CI, 1.65–4.57) and adults aged 65 years and older (RI, 4.3, 95% CI, 2.18–8.5), though these differences were not statically significant. Cases of GBS were more frequent in days 8–21 following vaccination; this time period has been identified in previous publications. The risk of GBS was higher following the administration of non-adjuvanted monovalent H1N1 vaccines. The relative incidence (RI) difference was not statistically significant between the adjuvanted and non-adjuvanted patients ($p=0.43$). A comparison between the two adjuvants was not possible due to limited use of the MF-59 adjuvant among patients in the available databases. While the study results indicated an association of GBS with monovalent H1N1 vaccination, the results imply a minimal increase in the overall incidence of GBS given the rarity of the condition [27C].

While the previous studies noted a slightly increased risk of GBS in a specific patient population, numerous other studies have reported a lack of increased risk of GBS associated with seasonal and monovalent H1N1 influenza vaccines. An observational study performed in the UK employed British Pediatric Surveillance Unit (BPSU) data to study the incidence of GBS in children 16 years of less who received monovalent H1N1 vaccine (Pandemrix®). The authors concluded that vaccination with Pandemrix® was not associated with an increased risk of GBS [28c].

The incidence of GBS potentially associated with the monovalent H1N1 vaccines as well as seasonal influenza vaccines continues to undergo examination. A retrospective, observational study examining GBS was performed using data obtained from electronic health records (EHR) of Vaccine Safety Datalink (VSD) children from eight managed care organizations in the United States. The study sought to report the incidence of outcomes in children receiving the 2012–2013 seasonal inactivated influenza vaccine (IIV). The outcomes of interest included seizures, GBS, encephalitis, and anaphylaxis. The authors did not identify a statically significant elevation in risk for any of the outcomes studied. Interestingly, the authors reported a statistically significant decreased risk of GBS in this patient population (RR, 0.5; 95% CI, 0.3–0.9). No safety concerns were identified and the study findings further support the administration of influenza vaccine among children aged 6 months and older [29c].

An 81-year-old male who recently received intradermal IIV during the 2012–2013 influenza season reported feelings of numbness and tingling in the soles of his feet 2 weeks after vaccination. Upon progression of paresthesia to his waistline, the patient presented to the hospital.

The patient complained of significant neuropathic pain but not weakness in his extremities. He did display a lack of deep tendon reflexes in his ankles on examination. The patient received a Brighton level 3 diagnostic certainties as he only met clinical criteria for GBS. The patient was treated with intravenous immunoglobulin (IVIG) for 5 days. He progressively improved and was discharged home after 10 days. Based on the WHO causality criteria, the influenza vaccine and GBS were "possibly" related in this patient [30A].

A healthy 15-year-old male presented to a neurologist following vaccination with IIV via the subcutaneous route. The patient experienced a choking on his saliva and difficulty swallowing solid food 7 days after vaccination. Symptoms progressed to include speech impairment. He was admitted to the hospital 29 days after vaccination. He was diagnosed with right glossopharyngeal and vagus nerve palsies. The patient's condition was categorized as a potential variant of GBS. The patient received IVIG for 5 days which resulted in a full recovery. Based on the WHO causality criteria, vaccination with IIV was "possibly" related to the patient's symptoms [31A].

The investigation surrounding the association of the monovalent H1N1 vaccine adjuvanted with ASO3 and narcolepsy continues. Additional study regarding this potential association is necessary to fully comprehend the disease state and observed increase in incidence following vaccination with the European ASO3 adjuvanted monovalent H1N1 vaccine. Narcolepsy remains a very rare adverse event but the association between the vaccine and disease state remains unclear [32R].

SKIN

A 46-year-old HIV-positive African American female presented to an outpatient clinic with complaints of a diffuse, highly pruritic rash that began to develop 1 day after receiving IIV. Physical exam was significant for a diffuse eruption of hyperpigmented, slightly violaceous polygonal papules and plaques with white, lacy reticulations involving the patient's face, palms, and soles of her feet. Histopathology revealed a lichenoid interface dermatitis with eosinophils; consistent with lichenoid drug eruption. The patient was treated with topical and oral corticosteroids, narrow band UVB therapy, topical tacrolimus, and even oral metronidazole therapy. Recovery occurred 6 months after therapy was completed; however, physical exam continued to reveal significant hyperpigmentation. Exact causality was not determined, but the temporal relationship with recent influenza vaccine implied an association [33A].

VASCULAR DISEASES

Two patients were diagnosed with antineutrophil cytoplasmic antibody associated vasculitis (AAV) 2 and 4 weeks following influenza vaccine. A 75-year-old female demonstrated an increase in serum creatinine from 0.7 to 1.8 mg/dL and up to 7.2 mg/dL along with proteinuria, hematuria, and positive perinuclear antineutrophil cytoplasmic antibody (ANCA). Renal biopsy noted necrotizing and crescentic pauci-immune glomerulonephritis. She was treated with hemodialysis, corticosteroids, cyclophosphamide, and plasmapheresis. A 50-year-old male presented with fatigue, fevers, joint pain, and muscle aches 2 days after IIV. Laboratory markers indicated an elevated erythrocyte sedimentation rate (ESR) of 56 mm/h, splinter hemorrhages, positive ANCA and an increase in serum creatinine (0.9–1.3 mg/dL). Renal biopsy revealed necrotizing vasculitis and focal necrotizing pauci-immune glomerulonephritis. He was treated with corticosteroids and cyclophosphamide and then azathioprine for maintenance of remission. A number of potential mechanisms for the association between IIV and AAV were discussed. No distinct causal relationship was determined, but the temporal association between AAV and IIV suggests that IIV vaccination may have potentially been associated with the development of these vasculitis cases [34A].

Second-Generation Effects

PREGNANCY

Given the potentially significant impact of prenatal influenza vaccination on maternal and fetal outcomes, a number of studies have been published providing supportive evidence for the safe use of influenza vaccines in pregnancy women. A retrospective, observational cohort study conducted with VSD studied pregnant women aged 14–49 years between 2002 and 2009 who received IIV. Results did not identify any concerning risks for adverse effects after IIV vaccination. The rate of gestational diabetes was statistically significantly reduced among pregnant women who received IIV (aRR, 0.89; 95% CI, 0.82–0.96; $p = 0.004$). There was a non-statistically significant increased risk of chorioamnionitis after IIV vaccination (aHR 1.08; 95% CI, 1.01–1.14; $p = 0.01$). The authors speculated if this increase could potentially be associated with the inflammatory responses associated with vaccination itself. Overall, the results provide additional support for the safety of IIV in pregnant women related to obstetrical outcomes [35c].

Another retrospective, observational cohort study utilized VSD data in pregnant women to assess pregnancy outcomes between 2004 and 2009. The primary outcomes of interest were preterm birth (before 37 weeks' gestation) and small for gestational age (SGA) birth (below the 10th and 5th percentiles). Vaccination with IIV was not associated with increased risk of SGA birth or preterm delivery. The study results add to the data supportive the safe use of IIV in pregnant women with regard to pregnancy outcomes of preterm and SGA birth [36c].

A recent review described the obstetric outcomes from eight observational studies involving pregnant women who received a variety of influenza vaccines (trivalent IIV, adjuvanted/non-adjuvanted, and monovalent H1N1 IIV vaccines). In addition, the authors reported results for two recent observational studies associated with VSD and the Pregnancy and Influenza Project (PIP). No significant associations between influenza vaccine and gestational diabetes, hypertension, preeclampsia/eclampsia, or chorioamnionitis were identified in the VSD and PIP studies. This body of evidence further supports the continued administration of influenza vaccine during pregnancy [37R].

Susceptibility Factors

AGE

The rates of adverse events associated with influenza vaccine continue to undergo study in the pediatric population. A review was recently published describing the risk of fever and febrile seizures following trivalent IIV vaccination reported from five published and 14 unpublished studies in children aged 6 months to less than 36 months. The unpublished trials reported an average weekly risk of fever of 26% (5.3–28.3%). The published trials represented a pooled average weekly risk of fever of 8% (95% CI, 5.9–10.6%) and 2.8% (95% CI, 1.3–5.1%) for severe fever (greater than or equal to 39 °C). Febrile seizures were reported in two unpublished studies and resulted in an average weekly risk of febrile seizures following IIV of 0.22% (95% CI, 0–1.24%) in infants less than 36 months of age. A key limitation of this review is associated with the heterogeneity in the design of studies assessed for risk of fever and febrile seizures following IIV vaccination. The authors recommend standardization of reporting with regard to the outcomes studies to enhance findings of future studies [38R].

The use of the live attenuated influenza vaccine (LAIV) is currently recommended in healthy children 2 years and older. A recent systematic review was performed to assess the safety and efficacy of LAIV in children less than 2 years of age. Nine studies were included in the review. The small number and heterogeneity of the study designs limited the assessment of results. LAIV demonstrated significant protection effects with regard to laboratory-confirmed cases of influenza infection when compared to placebo (RR, 0.36; 95% CI, 0.23–0.58; $p < 0.05$). In regards to safety, children who received LAIV had an increased risk of fever compared to placebo (RR, 1.16; 95% CI, 1.04–1.3; $p < 0.05$). When compared to IIV, subjects 6–11 months of age appeared to have an increased risk for hospitalization (any cause) following LAIV (RR, 0.92; 95% CI, 0.61–1.39; $p < 0.05$). Older infants (12–23 months) did not demonstrate this increased risk, and when all ages were combined, there was no statistically significant increase in hospitalization rate (RR, 0.92; 95% CI, 0.69–1.24; $p > 0.05$). Medically attended wheezing (MAW) was noted to have a statically significant increase in the children in the LAIV group (6–23 months) compared to IIV (5.9% versus 3.8%; $p = 0.002$). The results of the review indicated efficacy with regard to reducing the rates of laboratory-confirmed influenza; however, safety concerns were reported in the LAIV group of subjects. Further study with consistent methodology may provide a more clear description of the rates of these potential safety concerns in this patient population [39M].

IMMUNOCOMPROMISED: HUMAN IMMUNODEFICIENCY VIRUS (HIV)

A systematic review was performed to assess the efficacy and safety of trivalent IIV in HIV-positive patients. A total of six studies were included in the review. Outcomes of interest included all-cause mortality, all-cause hospitalization, all-cause pneumonia, laboratory-confirmed influenza infections, influenza-like illness (ILI), any respiratory illness, and any adverse event. In adult HIV-positive patients, the results related to efficacy of IIV included 85% (95% CI, 22–97%) for laboratory-confirmed influenza infection and 51% (95% CI, −439 to 96%) for all-cause mortality from the included randomized controlled trials. The efficacy of IIV reported for laboratory-confirmed influenza in a cohort study was 71% (95% CI, 44–85%). Adverse events in adults did not differ between IIV vaccine and placebo subjects (RR, 1.46; 95% CI, 0.66–3.21). In children, the efficacy of IIV was 11% (95% CI, −70 to 54%) to prevent laboratory-confirmed influenza infection. A small number of adverse events were reported, but this data did not include a comparison to controls. No serious adverse events were reported in HIV-positive children who received IIV. The results reported were obtained from a small number of studies with various study designs and methodology. Further study is necessary in the patient population to ascertain the efficacy and safety of IIV in HIV-positive patients [40M].

IMMUNOCOMPROMISED: CANCER PATIENTS RECEIVING CHEMOTHERAPY

It remains unclear if cancer patients undergoing systemic chemotherapy produce adequate antibody responses following vaccination with IIV. Furthermore, a lack of consensus exists with regard to IIV vaccination in patients receiving systemic chemotherapy. An observational review examined the safety and immunogenicity of IIV in solid and hematologic malignancies (subject ages were not reported). Antibody responses in subjects undergoing systemic chemotherapy were lower than those who had completed chemotherapy. A fourfold increase in antibody titer was observed in 17–52% of the chemotherapy subjects compared to 50–83% of the

subjects who completed chemotherapy, and 67–100% of healthy subjects. Limited specific safety data were reported. Adverse reactions were described as mild local reactions and mild fever [41R].

Two Cochrane reviews were recently published describing the results of IIV safety and immunogenicity in adults and children with cancer. Main results resulting from the review of studies pertaining to children with cancer receiving chemotherapy indicate that immune responses in this population were consistently weaker (fourfold titer rise of 38–65%) compared to children who completed chemotherapy (50–86%) and healthy children (53–89%). Adverse effects were generally mild local reactions and mild fever. The authors' conclusion stated the need for well-designed, randomized controlled trials to study the benefit with regard to clinical outcomes in this patient population [42M]. The main results from the Cochrane review of immunosuppressed adults with cancer included the effects of IIV on mortality from two studies. Overall, the included observational studies reported data suggestive of lower mortality with IIV as an adjusted HR, 0.88 (95% CI, 0.77–0.99) and OR of 0.43 (95% CI, 0.26–0.71), respectively. A randomized controlled trial also indicated a statically significant reduction in ILI. Various outcomes related to infection were lower or similar following IIV vaccination. The strength of the evidence was limited by the small number of studies and primary observational methodology. The results of the review favor continued IIV vaccination in immunosuppressed adults with cancer [43M].

RESPIRATORY DISEASES

In 2011, the Canadian National Advisory Committee on Immunization recommended the use of LAIV preferentially for healthy children and adolescents; however, use could be considered in children with chronic diseases. A prospective, observational study was conducted in children in Quebec, Canada aged 2–18 years with cystic fibrosis (CF) to determine the safety of LAIV. The primary outcome was a measurement of respiratory deteriorations resulting in a medical visit or hospitalization. There was no significant difference in the rate of respiratory deteriorations or all-cause hospitalizations during the at-risk period (0–28 days post LAIV) versus non-at-risk period (29–56 days post LAIV). A significant number of subjects reported at least one adverse event (64%) in the first week following LAIV vaccination. The most frequently reported adverse events included joint pain (RR, 10.5; 95% CI, 2.5–44.08), muscle aches (RR, 9.67; CI, 3–21.12), and vomiting (RR, 7.67; CI, 2.35–25.05). Fever was reported in 35% of patients during the first week following vaccination. An increased risk of wheezing was identified in the at-risk period (RR, 4.33; 95% CI, 1.26–14.93). There was no statistically significant difference for wheezing in the at-risk period. Wheezing did not occur beyond the day of vaccination. The authors recommended further study of LAIV in children with chronic conditions [44c].

Drug Administration

DRUG FORMULATIONS: QUADRIVALENT INFLUENZA VACCINE

The number of available quadrivalent influenza vaccines (QIV) continues to increase. Previous studies have reported safety data related to QIV in infants, children, and adults. The safety and immunogenicity of QIV were studied in a phase III, randomized, observer-blinded, active-controlled study in children aged 6 months to less than 9 years. Immune response rates met non-inferiority criteria for all strains compared to trivalent IIV and were superior related to the influenza B strain not contained in the IIV comparator. Reported local reactions were similar among all groups of subjects. The most common reactions were irritability and injection-site tenderness in subjects 6 months to less than 24 months of age. Among subjects 2 to less than 9 years of age, the most common reactions were myalgia, malaise, and pain. Most reactions were mild in intensity and resolved within 3 days. Three serious adverse events (SAE) were reported during the study period that were potentially related to the vaccines. Two patients who received trivalent IIV developed a febrile seizure 8 hours and 1 day following vaccination. Overall, QIV was well tolerated and produced significant immune response in this age group [45C].

The safety and immunogenicity of QIV were also reported in adult subjects aged greater than or equal to 18 years in a phase III, randomized, partially-blinded, international study. The QIV vaccine was highly immunogenic, producing seroconversion rates of 77.5%, 71.5%, 58.1%, and 61.7% against Influenza A/H1N1, H3N2, and Influenza B/Victoria, B/Yamagata, respectively. When the subjects were divided according to age, the resulting seroconversion rates for all strains were 66.9–82.7% in adults aged 18–64 years compared to 48–71.9% in those aged 65 years or older. Results met all criteria for non-inferiority and superiority in regards to immunogenicity. Reactogenicity of the QIV vaccine was comparable to the trivalent IIV vaccine. The most commonly reported local reaction was pain and the most commonly reported systemic reactions were fatigue, headache, and muscle ache. No reported SAEs were related to the vaccines. Vaccination with QIV appears to invoke a significant immune response with a comparable safety profile to that of trivalent IIV [46C].

DRUG ADMINISTRATION: DOSAGE REGIMEN

Data have been previously presented indicating lower antibody responses to the standard dose (SD) IIV in children with acute lymphoblastic leukemia (ALL). A phase I, prospective, randomized, double-blind safety study was conducted in children aged 3–17 years to determine the safety and immunogenicity of high dose (HD) IIV in this population. Of note, the study was not powered to determine immunogenicity. The most common local reaction reported were pain (43% and 40%) and tenderness (56% and 47%) in the SD and HD groups, respectively. The most common systemic reactions included fatigue (56% and 30%) and decrease in general activity level (44% and 33%), respectively. The majority of local and systemic reactions were mild in severity and quickly resolved. No SAEs were associated with vaccination. Safety data indicate that HD IIV is well tolerated in this population. A phase II study is necessary to determine immunogenicity of this formulation in children with ALL [47C].

DRUG ADMINISTRATION ROUTE: INTRADERMAL

A recent study supports previous study regarding the safety and immunogenicity of intradermal (ID) IIV administration in adult patients aged 18–64 years. A phase II, active-controlled, open-label study was conducted to evaluate the revaccination effects of ID IIV vaccine in regards to safety and immune response. The ID vaccine was associated with non-inferior immune responses compared to the IM vaccine regardless if the subject received IM or ID in the previous year. The local adverse events including erythema, swelling, induration, pruritus, and ecchymosis were more commonly reported among subjects revaccination with the ID vaccine (>50% of ID subjects). The most common systemic reactions were headache, myalgia, and malaise. One subject in the ID group did require a brief hospitalization for a grade three headache. No SAEs were related to the vaccines. The study results support the continued use of ID vaccine in adult patients and provide data to support consecutive year administration without negative implications with regard to safety or immune response [48C].

Another phase II study examining the safety and immunogenicity of two doses of ID IIV vaccine (15 or 21 mcg) was conducted in patients 65 years and older. Results indicated that the ID vaccines were more immunogenic than the standard dose IM IIV vaccine. However, the HD IIV vaccine demonstrated immune responses greater than either of the ID vaccines. The rates of local infection site reactions were similar in ID IIV vaccine subjects (76.5% for 15 mcg and 77.3% for 21 mcg dose), but higher than subjects receiving HD IIV (49.5%) or standard dose IIV (34.5%). The most common local reactions included erythema, induration, swelling, and pruritus. No SAEs related to the vaccines were reported. Study results support further study and consideration of the ID route of administration for elderly patients [49C].

The safety of ID IIV vaccine has also recently been studied in patients with cardiovascular disease (CVD) in an observational study. The mean patient age was 63 ± 12 years. Most of the patients were also receiving antithrombotic agents including aspirin (46.7%), clopido-grel (3.6%), dual antiplatelet therapy (13.6%), warfarin (25.4%), and warfarin plus antiplatelet therapy (1.1%). The most common reactions were local and included pruritus (11.9%) and swelling (5.7%). The most common systemic reaction was fatigue (5.7%). No local or systemic bleeding events occurred following vaccination with ID IIV. The data suggest ID IIV is safe and well tolerated among this patient population [50c].

MMR Vaccine [SED-15, 3555, 3566, 3567, 3569; SEDA-34, 503; SEDA-35, 575; SEDA-36, 473]

Susceptibility Factors

FEMALE SEX

Gender has been proposed as a prognostic indicator of vaccine reactions. A retrospective study compared emergency room visits or hospital admissions between males and females vaccinated between two through 12 months of age. Females had statistically significantly more emergency room visits or hospitalizations after vaccination at 12 months with MMR compared to males. The authors suggest this result correlates to an increase in adverse events in females following MMR vaccination [51c].

Measles–Mumps–Rubella–Varicella Vaccine [SEDA-35, 575; SEDA-36, 474]

General

Previous studies have demonstrated an increased risk of febrile seizures with administration of MMRV compared to receiving MMR + varicella vaccines separately. A retrospective cohort study found that children 12–15 months had a significantly lower incidence of fevers and seizures after MMRV vaccination compared to children 16–23 months at vaccination. The same study demonstrated that children vaccinated with MMRV are 1.4 times more likely to have fevers and twice as likely to develop seizures post-vaccination compared to MMR alone or with varicella administered separately; however, these results were not statistically significant [52A]. Additional studies confirm the increased incidence of febrile seizures after MMRV administration compared to MMR or MMR + varicella [53c,54c].

Rotavirus Vaccine [SED-15, 3554, 3555; SEDA-34, 504; SEDA-35, 576; SEDA-36, 473]

Organs and Systems

GASTROINTESTINAL

The risk of intussusception (IS) following rotavirus (RV) vaccination was identified after the first RV vaccine,

Rotashield®, was licensed. The occurrence of IS remains a central component of post-licensure safety surveillance worldwide for available RV vaccines, Rotateq® (RV5), Rotarix® (RV1), and Rotavac®.

In 2014, a novel monovalent human-bovine rotavirus vaccine, Rotavac®, was licensed in India. The efficacy and safety of this new RV vaccine were evaluated at 1 and 2 years. Among the RV vaccinated infants, 8 cases (0.2%, $n = 4532$) met Brighton Level 1 criteria for IS versus 3 cases (0.1%, $n = 2267$) in the placebo group ($p = 0.7613$). All cases were reported after the third dose and none of the cases occurred within 30 days of a vaccine dose. The incidence of any reported serious adverse events did not differ between the RV (20.9%, $n = 947$) or placebo (22.7%, $n = 515$) groups. Post-licensure studies are planned to assess the risk of IS and the new Rotavac® vaccine [55C].

An integrated analysis of 28 randomized, double-blinded, placebo-controlled phase II and III clinical trials of the RV vaccine (Rotarix®) was conducted and included 56 562 RV vaccine and 45 512 placebo recipients. A small number of IS cases was observed (11 and 7 in the RV and placebo groups, respectively; RR = 1.39 (95% CI: 0.49–4.27; $p = 0.66$). The study concluded that the overall risk of IS following RV vaccination was similar to placebo [56C].

Varicella Vaccine and Herpes Zoster Vaccine [SEDA-34, 506; SEDA-36, 474]

General

At the WHO GACVS June 2013 meeting, safety of herpes zoster virus (HZV) and varicella zoster virus (VZV) vaccination in immunocompromised populations was reviewed. It was determined that no new safety concerns with HZV vaccination exist in this population. The WHO confirmed that VZV vaccination should not occur in people with leukemia, or only under strict observation. VZV vaccination in other immunocompromised conditions may pose a higher risk of adverse reactions; however, benefits of standard VZV vaccination programs should be assessed [57S].

A review on the safety of vaccines used in the routine childhood immunization schedule for U.S. children was completed following the Institute of Medicine (IOM) consensus report on vaccine safety. HZV vaccination was determined to place individuals between 11 and 17 years at moderate risk for purpura [58M].

Organs and Systems

OPHTHALMIC

Ophthalmic complications following vaccination against HZV have previously been described. Two cases of optic neuritis following administration of HZV vaccine (Zostavax®) occurred 1 and 2 weeks after vaccination. Both women received high-dose IV steroids followed by a 6-week oral taper. Symptoms resolved partially in one woman and completely in the second within 1 week [59A].

SKIN

A case of granulomatous dermatitis at the site of a previous HZV vaccine was described. The dermatologic changes began soon after vaccination and persisted until presentation 9 months later. Infectious work-up was unremarkable. Granulomatous dermatitis has been described with administration of other vaccines as well as following HZV infections. This case report is the first to describe such a reaction following vaccination against zoster [60r].

INFECTION RISK

A 2-year-old boy developed herpes zoster following vaccination against VZV at his 12-month well-visit. He was treated with acyclovir and had a complete recovery. Development of herpes zoster in pediatric patients remains rare [61r].

DEATH

One death has previously been described following administration of VZV vaccine (Varivax®). A 15-month-old girl developed a vesicular rash 3 weeks after vaccination with Varivax®. The rash was confirmed positive for vaccine-strain VZV through polymerase chain reaction. The patient had a history of multiple prolonged hospitalizations due to infection, but no known immunodeficiency. After treatment with acyclovir for 2 months, the patient died after a course complicated by sepsis, acute respiratory distress syndrome, and multi-organ failure [62A].

Susceptibility Factors

IMMUNOCOMPROMISED: TRANSPLANT PATIENTS

Patients with hematopoietic stem-cell transplant (HSCT) are known to have an increased risk of VZV reactivation despite prophylaxis. Issa and colleagues describe their experience vaccinating HSCT patients against herpes zoster using a single dose of HZV vaccine (Zostavax®). Patients were at least 24 months from HSCT, without graft-versus-host disease, and on no immunosuppressive or prophylactic antiviral medications. Patients were followed for a median of 9.5 months (range 2–28 months). Two patients of one-hundred ten developed skin rashes consistent with HZV and VZV 10 and 24 days post-vaccination, respectively. The latter patient was vaccinated with both HZV vaccine and MMR on the same day. Neither patient had samples obtained to confirm VZV serology, determine wild-type or vaccine virus as the cause, or rule-out other causes. No other adverse events occurred during the observational period [63c].

ELDERLY

The safety of the HZV vaccine in elderly patients with a history of HZV was evaluated in a sub-study of the SPS trial. Patients who had received placebo during the SPS trial were offered vaccination with the zoster vaccine. Of these individuals, 420 had experienced an episode of HZV during the SPS trial. Safety of the vaccine in this group was compared to those who had not had an episode of HZV. The median age of vaccination was 74.2 years in both groups. There was no statistical difference in severe adverse events between groups. Of the severe adverse events that occurred, the majorities were general body or cardiovascular, using the COSTART body system. Non-serious adverse events and injection-site complications were not collected in the study. The study supports the current ACIP recommendation to vaccinate against HZV in all individuals 60 and older, despite previous history of HZV [64c].

The Long-Term Persistence Study (LTPS) was a continuation of the SPS and STPS trials. Vaccine efficacy for incidence of HZV decreased from 51.3% to 21.1% between SPS and LTPS. Efficacy of the vaccine for HZV burden of illness and incidence of post-herpetic neuralgia also decreased (61.1–37.3% and 66.5–35.4%, respectively). There were no serious adverse events which occurred during the LTPS. The results of the LTPS demonstrate long-term safety post-vaccination against HZV, but decreased efficacy [65C].

Yellow Fever Vaccine [SEDA-34, 506; SEDA-35, 577; SEDA-36, 475]

General

Serious adverse events associated with the yellow fever vaccination include viscerotropic disease (YEL-AVD), neurologic disease (YEL-AND), and anaphylaxis. During the yellow fever outbreaks in South America between December 2007 and April 2009 1 943 000 doses were administered in Argentina. A study utilizing Argentina's surveillance system identified that 165 AEs were reported, 49 of these were related to the YF vaccine. There were 24 SAEs and one death. Of these, 12 were classified as YEL-AVD and 12 classified as YEL-AND. The reported death 10 days post yellow fever vaccination was YEL-AVD confirmed from RNA sequencing from liver biopsy [66R].

In 2012, the Brighton Collaboration Viscerotropic Disease Work Group published guidelines for case definitions for YEL-AVD [67S]. A recent review was conducted to assess the number of previously published cases associated with SAEs following YF vaccination that met these criteria. One hundred and thirty-one cases met Brighton Collaboration criteria: 32 anaphylaxis, 41 YEL-AND (one death), 56 YEL-AVD (24 deaths),

2 YEL-AND and YEL-AVD, and 2 wild virus infections following travel to an endemic area. The number of yellow fever vaccinations associated with the reported SAE cases was not provided in this review; therefore, the rate of occurrence could not be calculated [68R].

Susceptibility Factors

ELDERLY

Retrospective reviews of previously published data continue to examine age as a risk factor for YEL-AVD following YF vaccination. A recent review supported previous data that the elderly population ($\geq$60 to 65 years old) is at higher risk for developing YEL-AVD than younger patients [69R]. The decision to provide YF vaccination in patients 60 years of age and older should include an assessment of the risks versus benefits.

Japanese Encephalitis Vaccine [SEDA-34, 503; SEDA-35, 575; SEDA-36, 475]

General

During the WHO GACVS December 2013 meeting, pre- and post-licensure safety data of the novel recombinant chimeric Japanese Encephalitis (JE) vaccine Imojev® was reviewed. This vaccine is licensed in four countries and pre-licensure data were limited with 2486 adults and 2248 children (age 9–18 months for first dose) receiving the vaccine. In adults, adverse reactions were significantly lower when compared to available mouse brain-derived inactivated JE vaccines [57S]. Further post-licensure safety data are necessary to evaluate and confirm the rate of adverse events for the new recombinant chimeric JE vaccine.

Postmarketing surveillance data of the live attenuated JE vaccine reviewed during the WHO GACVS June 2013 meeting was published. This report identified the most common AEFIs as fever and injection site reactions and observed a low rate of SAE's (1.12 per million doses). GACVS noted that the overall number of AEFI's reported was low and encouraged ongoing post licensure surveillance for all available JE vaccines [70R].

BACTERIAL VACCINES

Meningococcal Vaccines [372; SEDA-36, 476]

General

Invasive meningococcal disease (IMD) is most common amongst infants. Serogroups A, B, C, Y, and W-135 are responsible for the majority of IMD cases. A number of meningococcal vaccines are currently available that include various combinations of serogroups A, C, Y, and W-135. *Neisseria meningitidis* serogroup

B (MenB) accounts for a significant number of infections in the United States and Europe. Two monovalent MenB vaccines have been approved in the United States (Trumenba® and Bexsero®). The vaccines were approved for use in persons aged 10–25 years of age in October of 2014 and January 2015, respectively. Currently, there are no recommendations for routine vaccination against MenB. A randomized, phase 1/2 multicenter study was conducted in Spain to determine the safety and immunogenicity of a bivalent, recombinant lipoprotein (LP2086) meningococcal serogroup A and MenB vaccine (MnB rLP2086) administered with or without routine vaccines for infants. The results were limited due to early termination of the study. One subject developed aseptic meningitis following the 60 mcg dose of the vaccine. The adverse event was not considered vaccine related, but upon further examination, it was discovered that 80% of the subjects in the 60 mcg dose group experienced mild to moderate fever. Therefore, the study was terminated as the vaccine was deemed unfit for the infant group of subjects. Fever was less common and mild in toddlers (0–31.6%) and adolescents (0–12.5%). Further study of the rLP2086 vaccine is planned to determine the appropriate age for vaccination with this product [71c].

A bivalent meningococcal serogroup A and C polysaccharide conjugate vaccine has been utilized in China. A post-marketing assessment of safety of the vaccine described the adverse events among 10 609 healthy infants and children. Lower rates of adverse reactions were noted compared to previously published studies. None of the 253 subjects under active surveillance demonstrated local or systemic reactions. Of the 10 356 subjects under passive surveillance, only 0.183% of subjects reported mild local reactions and only 9 subjects reported systemic reactions which were mild to moderate in severity. The significantly lower numbers of adverse events may point to differences in definitions of events. While the data support the continued use of the vaccine in this population; the quantity of events may have been underestimated according to the authors [72r].

The current immunization recommendations primarily include quadrivalent meningococcal conjugate vaccines (MCV4) for routine vaccination in infants, adolescents, and adults at increased risk for IMD. Studies describing safety and immunogenicity of the MCV4 vaccines continue to provide supportive data for the recommended use of the vaccines. The quadrivalent meningococcal vaccine MenACYW-DT was recently studied in a multicenter, open-label, non-randomized, phase 3 clinical trial in children, adolescents, and adults in India. The vaccine produced high levels of immunogenicity with 92–100% of subjects achieving vaccine-type serogroup titers greater than or equal to 8 (serum bactericidal assay with baby rabbit complement [SBA-BR]) at

30 days following single-dose vaccination. Adverse events were reported in 38% of child subjects, 29% of adolescents, and 52% of adult subjects. Injection-site reactions were the most common and were typically mild. Systemic reactions were mostly mild in nature as well. No SAEs occurred during the study period. These results further support the use of quadrivalent conjugated meningococcal vaccine and the MenACYW-DT vaccine in this population [73C].

Organs and Systems

NERVOUS SYSTEM

A case of acute cerebellar ataxia was reported in a 12-year-old female following receipt of meningococcal group C conjugate vaccine (Menjugate®). Within 24 hours of receiving the vaccine, the patient was admitted to the hospital with progressive nausea, dizziness, and somnolence which progressed to difficulty walking until she could no longer stand or walk due to cerebellar ataxia. Infectious etiology was ruled out by laboratory analyses. The patient swiftly responded to intravenous corticosteroid therapy. The patient demonstrated improvement in symptoms, but at 1 year follow-ups remains with a mild neurological feature of ataxia. The authors utilized the WHO causality assessment criteria and classified the event as "very likely" to be vaccine related [74A].

Second-Generation Effects

PREGNANCY

Meningococcal serogroup A conjugate vaccine (MenAfriVac) utilization continues for the Meningitis Vaccine Project in the African meningitis belt. The WHO GACVS was recently presented with study results pertaining to the use of MenAfriVac in pregnant and lactating women in Ghana. A total of 1730 pregnant women received the vaccine and were matched to 3551 pregnant women in a historical unvaccinated control group to study outcomes including mortality, rates of spontaneous abortion, still births, perinatal deaths, prematurity, low birth weight, and rates of caesarean section. There was no significant difference reported in any of the outcomes studied. The GACVS commented that no concerns have been identified regarding the use of MenAfriVac in pregnancy over the course of its use these past 4 years [75S].

Interactions

DRUG–DRUG INTERACTIONS

The addition of vaccines to infant and child immunization schedules necessitates simultaneous administration; therefore, both safety and immunogenicity data must be demonstrated in order to support concomitant administration. A phase 3b, multicenter, open-label, randomized trial studied the safety of quadrivalent (serogroups A, C, W-135, and Y) meningococcal vaccine conjugated to CRM197 (MenACWY-CRM)) in healthy infants from six countries. Routine vaccines permitted during the study period included DTaP, inactivated polio (IPV), *H. influenzae* type b (Hib), PCV7, MMR, varicella, hepatitis A, and HBV vaccine based on national routine immunization schedules. The majority of subjects experienced at least one local or systemic reaction. Rates were similar among MenACWY-CRM plus routine vaccine group compared to the routine vaccines only group (75–89%). The most common local reactions were tenderness, erythema, and induration at the injection site. Results indicated a similar percentage of patients with reported severe systemic reaction by day 7 following vaccination with MenACWY-CRM plus routine vaccine compared to subjects who received routine vaccines only (16% versus 13%, respectively). The most common systemic reactions were irritability, sleepiness, and persistent crying. No new safety concerns were identified during the course of the study. The study results support the conclusion that MenACWY-CRM is safe and well tolerated when simultaneously administered with routine vaccinations in infants [76C].

The safety and immunogenicity of MenACWY-CRM have been demonstrated in infants, children, adolescents, and adults. A phase 3, randomized, open-label, controlled, multicenter study was performed in infants to determine the immunogenicity and safety of MenACWY-CRM vaccine when administered concomitantly with the pentavalent diphtheria–tetanus–acellular pertussis–inactivated poliovirus–*H. influenzae*-type b (DTaP–IPV–Hib), PCV (PCV7 or PCV13), HBV, and MMR vaccines. A significant immunogenic response was reported for all four vaccine serogroups (89%, 95%, 97%, and 96% of participants with serum bactericidal assay using human complement [hSBA] greater than or equal to 8%) for serogroups A, C, W-135, and Y, respectively. Immunogenic responses to routine vaccines were generally unaffected by MenACWY-CRM vaccine co-administration. Non-inferiority of immune response was obtained following the three-dose infant series and after the toddler dose at 12 months for all antigens except for pertussis antigens pertactin (PRN) and FIM, and pneumococcal serotypes 6B and 23F, although the clinical significance of these results is unclear given the achievement of non-inferiority based on GMT ratio. Adverse events were similar between the MenACWY-CRM plus routine vaccines group compared to the routine vaccines only group (39% in both groups). No SAEs were considered vaccine-related. Concomitant administration of MenACWY-CRM with routine vaccines was well tolerated and induced highly immunogenic effects without compromising the immunogenic responses to routine vaccines [77C].

Pneumococcal Vaccines [SEDA-36, 477]

General

The 13-valent pneumococcal conjugate vaccine (PCV13) was approved in 2010 and has replaced the 7-valent pneumococcal conjugate vaccine (PCV7) for the routine and catch-up immunization of infants and young children in the United States, Europe, and numerous other countries. Additional pneumococcal vaccines still employed for use in persons of varying ages include PCV7 and the 23-valent pneumococcal polysaccharide vaccine (PPSV23). A meta-analysis of nine studies including infant subjects from eight countries reported a safety profile of PCV13 that was comparable to PCV7. Most local and systemic reactions were mild to moderate in severity. Differences between the groups with regard to local reactions were not statistically significant. The most frequent local reactions included tenderness, redness, and swelling. Local reactions occurred in 26.71–53.25% of subjects in the PCV13 group compared with 27.89–58.20% in the PCV7 group. The most common systemic reactions reported were irritability and increased sleep. Systemic reactions occurred in 29.31–89.24% of subjects in the PCV13 group compared to 26.40–88.12% in the PCV7 group. Irritability occurred in 70.59% of PCV13 subjects versus 68.37% of PCV7 patients ($p = 0.04$). This was the only statistically significant difference between the two groups. No serious adverse events related to the study vaccines were reported [78M].

Susceptibility Factors

AGE: ADULTS & ELDERLY ADULTS

The safety and immunogenicity of PCV13 vaccine have been reported in adults ranging in age of 50–59 years, 60–64 years, and 65 years and older. Vaccination with PCV13 results in significant levels of opsonophagocytic activity (OPA) titers for all 12 common serotypes between PCV13 and PPSV23 vaccines [79R,80R]. Safety data indicate a higher proportion of local reactions following PPSV23 compared to PCV13 vaccine ($p = 0.003$ and 0.033). Systemic adverse effects were either similar between the groups or higher among the PPSV23 vaccine group [79R,80R]. One SAE considered to be related to the vaccine was reported in an 81-year-old male patient 132 days after receiving PCV13 vaccine. The PCV13 vaccine was administered 1 year after PPSV23 vaccine. The patient experienced idiopathic thrombocytopenia purpura (ITP). The ITP resolved following treatment [80R].

A recent study reported the effects of PCV13 vaccine on the outcomes of pneumonia in 42 240 persons 65 years and older in the Netherlands. Compared to placebo, the PCV13 vaccine demonstrated significant efficacy for the prevention of vaccine-type community-acquired pneumonia (CAP) and vaccine-type invasive pneumococcal disease ($p < 0.001$, CI = 21.8–62.5 and $p < 0.001$, CI = 41.4–90.8) [81C]. The results further support the utilization of PCV13 in adults.

AUTOIMMUNE DISEASE: SYSTEMIC LUPUS ERYTHEMATOSUS (SLE)

It has been suggested that both the humoral and cell-mediated immune response to pneumococcal vaccines is affected by SLE disease state and/or immunosuppressive drugs used to treat the condition. Antibody responses have been reported as similar or slightly decreased compared to control groups. A decrease in antibody response over time has also been described in this group of patients. Systemic adverse reactions are rare. The potential for triggering autoimmune reactions as a result of vaccination has been suggested but has not been confirmed. Furthermore, the risk of SLE exacerbation as a result of infection must be considered [82A].

HEMATOLOGIC DISEASE: SICKLE CELL DISEASE

A 5-year-old African American female with a history of sickle cell disease presented to the hematology clinic with arm pain, edema, erythema, nausea and fever the morning after she received PPSV23 vaccine. The patient's maximum temperature was 102.9 °F and the edema extended to the child's elbow, making it difficult to put a shirt sleeve over the arm. The event occurred after the second dose of PPSV23 (the last dose given 2.5 years prior to the event). Potential contributing factors include the shorter time between the previous dose and repeated exposure to PPSV23. In addition, the patient received the conjugated meningococcal vaccine concurrently, although in the other arm. Significant limb edema may occur in special populations, such as sickle cell disease [83A].

IMMUNOCOMPROMISED: RHEUMATOID ARTHRITIS (RA)

Antibody response to PPSV23 vaccine among 190 patients with RA receiving tocilizumab and/or methotrexate therapy was conducted as an open-label study in Japan. The results indicated a significant increase in antibodies to serotypes 6B and 23F in all groups. However, patients receiving combination tocilizumab and methotrexate or methotrexate monotherapy demonstrated a smaller increase in antibody production. The authors concluded that ongoing methotrexate therapy may affect the antibody response to PPSV23. Two patients developed fever and 12 developed local reactions. All adverse effects were mild [84c].

Antibody response to PCV7 was studied in 88 RA patients receiving immunosuppressive biologic therapies (other than anti-tumor necrosis factor alpha agents) in Sweden. The results demonstrated a decrease in immunologic response to the vaccine in patients receiving rituximab or abatacept therapy (with/without methotrexate). Methotrexate was identified as a predictor of impaired immune response. The vaccine was well tolerated. One patient reported significantly more joint pain, but no increased RA disease was noted [85c].

IMMUNOCOMPROMISED: CHRONIC LYMPHOCYTIC LEUKEMIA (CLL)

An adequate immune response rate to PPSV23 vaccine in CLL patients has been reported in only 20–25% of patients. A recent study reported the antibody response results of 24 patients with untreated CLL compared to a control group of 15 patients to determine the response to PCV13 vaccine. An adequate antibody response (at least twofold increase in antibody titer) was observed in 100% of controls and 58.3% of CLL patients ($p=0.037$). While a lower response rate was observed, the PCV13 vaccine demonstrated higher antibody titers compared to previously reported data with PPSV23 vaccine [86c].

Drug Administration

DRUG ADMINISTRATION: ROUTE

A phase 3, single-arm, open-label study was conducted to describe the safety and immunogenicity of PCV13 administered via the subcutaneous route in healthy infants from Japan. Local reactions did occur in a higher percentage of subjects in this study compared to previous studies utilizing the intramuscular route of administration. Local reactions were mild to moderate in severity. The most common local reactions were swelling and redness in 47.2–57.1% (infant series) and 68.1–74.4% (toddle dose) of subjects, respectively. The most common systemic reactions were irritability and increased sleep. One subject reported a fever >40 °C after dose two. No SAEs were considered to be related to the study vaccine [87c].

Interactions

DRUG–DRUG

Immunization schedules often include recommendations for multiple vaccines during a given age and/or visit for infants, children, and adults. Several studies have examined the safety and immunogenicity associated with the concomitant administration of pneumococcal vaccines with other vaccines, including influenza, meningococcal, and zoster vaccines. Fever following vaccination is commonly reported in studies with pneumococcal vaccines. Previous reports of fever and an increased risk for febrile seizures was associated with the simultaneous administration of trivalent IIV and PCV13. A prospective, observational study conducted in New York City sought to determine the frequency of fever following simultaneous administration of PCV13 and IIV in children 6–23 months of age. Results indicated that subjects who received both vaccines simultaneously were 2.7 times more likely to have a temperature of 38 °C or higher on the day 0 or day 1 following vaccination compared to those who did not receive the vaccines simultaneously. The adjusted risk relative risk was 0.2 (95% CI, 0.06–0.35) for simultaneous administration of PCV13 and IIV versus IIV alone and 0.23 (95% CI, 0.11–0.34) versus PCV13 alone. No hospitalizations or febrile seizures were noted for any study subject. These results indicate an increased risk of transient increases in temperature following concomitant administration of PCV13 and IIV [88c].

The product labeling regarding herpes zoster vaccine (Zostavax®) has undergone two updates since its approval in 2006; specifically regarding concomitant administration with pneumococcal vaccine. A blinded, controlled trial examining the safety and immunogenicity of concomitant administration of herpes zoster vaccine and PPSV23 described a potentially inadequate antibody response to VZV when the vaccines were co-administered. The question was raised as to whether the attained level of VZV antibodies would provide adequate protection against HZV infections. A large retrospective cohort study was performed to determine if concomitant administration of the vaccines was associated with an increased incidence of HZV infection. The hazard ratio in the concomitant versus non-concomitant cohort was 1.19 (95% CI, 0.81–1.74). The authors concluded that concomitant administration was not associated with an increased risk of HZV infection. Unfortunately, the VZV antibody titers were not assessed in this retrospective cohort study. Concomitant administration of PPSV23 and HZV vaccine continues to be recommended [89R].

Pertussis Vaccine (Including Diphtheria–Tetanus–Acellular Pertussis Vaccines) [SED-15, 3555, 3558, 3562, 3565, 3567, 3570; SEDA-35, 573; SEDA-36, 478]

General

The ACIP recommends routine vaccination with diphtheria–tetanus–acellular pertussis (DTaP) along with inactivated poliovirus (IPV) vaccine in children aged 4–6 years. In 2008, the combination vaccine product DTaP–IPV (Kinrix®) was licensed in the United States for use in children 4–6 years of age. A prospective observational study of the safety of DTaP–IPV was conducted utilizing four of the eight managed care organizations participating in the Vaccine Safety Datalink (VSD) surveillance system. Eight adverse events were evaluated including meningitis/encephalitis, seizures, stroke, GBS, Stevens–Johnson syndrome, anaphylaxis, serious allergic reactions other than anaphylaxis, and serious local reactions. There was no statistically significant increased risk of any adverse events studied when compared to historical incidence rates. One potential case each of GBS and anaphylaxis were reported; however, when the medical record was manually reviewed both GBS and anaphylaxis were ruled out. The risk of seizures was not elevated when compared to historical incidence rates (RR, 0.81). The rates of serious location reactions were not elevated in the DTaP–IPV group compared to the historical control group (RR, 0.76). The results support the continued study and utilization of DTaP–IPV vaccine in the ACIP recommended vaccination group [90c].

Organs and Systems

MUSCULOSKELETAL

A 49-year-old female presented to the hospital 11 days following vaccination with diphtheria–tetanus–acellular pertussis (Tdap) vaccine. The patient complained of severe myalgia, weakness, and dark urine. Over the course of following 3 days, the patient's symptoms progressed with increased pain, swelling, and weakness with dark urine. The patient had no significant medical history and was not taking any medications at the time of the event. The patient was diagnosed with rhabdomyolysis, evidenced by a significantly elevated creatinine kinase (CK) level of 91 000 U/L (maximum level 225 000 U/L) and alanine aminotransferase of 306 U/L on admission. Additional laboratory data included an elevated white blood cell count, low calcium, and elevated C-reactive protein (78 mg/L). The serum creatinine remained normal. Testing for autoimmune disorders and bacterial and viral infections were negative. The patient's symptoms and laboratory markers normalized 8 weeks later. The authors applied the Naranjo probability scale to the events which resulted in a score of five. The score indicated probable causality between the vaccination and the event of rhabdomyolysis [91A].

SKIN

Three previously healthy children aged 4–5 months developed cases of bullous pemphigoid (BP) 1–10 days following vaccination with diphtheria–tetanus–pertussis–poliovirus (Tetracoq®) with or without concomitant HBV, Hib, and/or meningococcal C vaccines. All three children developed itchy lesions on the palms and soles that spread to the trunk, face, and extremities. The lesions were described as tense blisters with surrounding erythema on the palms and soles and erythematous and edematous wheals on the trunk, face, and extremities. No lesions were observed on the oral mucosa, genitals, and perioral regions. Histological examination revealed sub-epidermal bullae and dermal inflammation with eosinophilic predominance. Patients were treated with oral corticosteroids which resulted in resolution of the lesions. None of the patients suffered recurrence following

subsequent vaccinations. The etiology of BP in these patients was not entirely clear and a causal relationship with vaccination is difficult to determine. Post vaccination BP in children is idiopathic and may occur following vaccination with diphtheria–tetanus–pertussis and other vaccines [92A].

Second-Generation Effects

PREGNANCY

In 2012, the Advisory Committee on Immunization Practices (ACIP) of the Centers for Disease Control and Prevention (CDC) recommended all pregnant women receive one dose of Tdap vaccine preferably between 27 and 36 weeks gestation during every pregnancy. The safety and immunogenicity of Tdap vaccine in pregnancy were studied in a phase 1/2, randomized, double-blind, placebo-controlled trial in the United States. Pain was the most common reaction following Tdap vaccination. Pain was reported in 75.8% of pregnant women, 73.3% of postpartum women, and 78.1% of non-pregnant women. Injection site reactions were common and not different among the groups including 78.8% for pregnant women, 80% for postpartum women, and 78.1% for non-pregnant women. Of the reported systemic reactions, fever was the only reaction that demonstrated statistical significant among the group with 26.7% of postpartum women reporting fever ($p = 0.04$). Most local and systemic reactions were mild following vaccination. No SAEs were determined to be attributed to vaccination with Tdap. There were no significance differences in the infants' outcomes including gestational age, birth weight, Apgar score, neonatal examinations, or complications. No cases of pertussis infections occurred in the mothers or infants included in the study. Women who received the Tdap vaccine during pregnancy demonstrated a significantly higher antibody response compared to those vaccinated postpartum. Infants born to women who received Tdap during pregnancy also demonstrated significantly higher pertussis antibodies at birth and at 2 months of age. The results of the study support the 2012 ACIP recommendations for Tdap vaccination in pregnancy [93C].

In response to a 2010 pertussis outbreak, California, USA began recommending Tdap during pregnancy and later conducted a retrospective, observational study utilizing the VSD and electronic health records (EHR) to report any increased risk of adverse events related to pregnancy or birth outcomes in pregnant women in California. The patients included were 14–49 years of age, were continuously insured through 6 weeks postpartum, had singleton pregnancies resulting in live births, and had at least one outpatient visit at a VSD affiliated site. The inclusion criteria for the study may limit the study's generalizability. The outcomes of interest in this study were chorioamnionitis, hypertensive disorders of pregnancy, pre-term birth (delivery before 37 weeks' gestation), and SGA births (less than 10th percentile). A diagnosis of chorioamnionitis occurred in 6.1% of vaccinated women compared to 5.5% of unexposed women (aRR, 1.19; 95% CI, 1.13–1.26). When analyzing the preterm births, there was no elevated risk of chorioamnionitis (aRR, 0.87; 95% CI, 0.64–1.16). Vaccination with Tdap was not associated with increased risk of pre-term or SGA births (SGA birth aRR, 1.00; 95% CI, 0.96–1.06). These results may indicate the presence of potential-confounders with regard to the occurrence of chorioamnionitis. Overall, the study results indicated the lack of increased risk of vaccination with Tdap on pregnancy and birth outcomes [94C].

In 2011, the UK implemented a temporary vaccination program with diphtheria–acellular pertussis–inactivated poliovirus (dTaP/IPV) targeting pregnant women between 28 and 38 weeks' gestation. A retrospective, observational study utilizing the Clinical Practice Research Datalink (CPRD) was conducted to report adverse events potentially related to the pertussis-containing vaccine in pregnant women. Outcomes of interest included stillbirth (intrauterine death after 24 weeks' gestation), maternal and neonatal death, pre-eclampsia, eclampsia, antepartum and postpartum hemorrhage, fetal distress, uterine rupture, placenta previa, vasa previa, cesarean delivery, low birth weight, and neonatal renal failure. The results indicated a lack of significant differences in the rates of any of the outcomes of interest. The 12 cases of stillbirth that occurred following vaccination resulted in a ratio of 0.85 when compared to national statistical data (95% CI, 0.44–1.61). The median birth weight in the vaccinated cohort was 3500 g (IQR, 3100–3800 g) compared with 3500 g (IQR, 3200–3800 g) in the matched unvaccinated cohort ($p = 0.81$). The study results provide further safety data to potentially expand the study and utilization of pertussis-containing vaccines in pregnant women in the UK [95C].

Susceptibility Factors

AGE & SEX: ADOLESCENT MALES

Pertussis-containing vaccine, dTaP/IPV (Repevax®) was offered to all students following a pertussis outbreak at a United Kingdom (UK) boarding school for boys aged 13–18 years. A prospective, observational study was conducted to identify self-reported adverse events 0–3 days following vaccination. Results were provided for only 22.8% of the students. The most commonly reported reactions included pain at the injection site (84.6%), headache (55.6%), muscle pain (55.4%), and feeling poorly (53.6%). Fever was reported in 19% of students; however, it is unclear if all students who reported fever had a temperature recording. All reported reactions were mild and self-limiting. Overall, the majority of student respondents reported at least one reaction following vaccination with dTaP/IPV. The low response rate of this study likely introduces bias; therefore, the results may not be applicable to all adolescent males. Additional limitations include the inclusion of only male subjects and the self-reporting of adverse events. The data presented from this study may provide guidance on future study design and the need for continued examination of the pertussis-containing vaccines in the adolescent population [96c].

References

[1] Halsey NA, Edwards KM, Dekker CL, et al. Algorithm to assess causality after individual adverse events following immunizations. Vaccine. 2012;30(39):5791–8 [H].

[2] Tozzi AE, Asturias EJ, Balakrishnan MR, et al. Assessment of causality of individual adverse events following immunization (AEFI): a WHO tool for global use. Vaccine. 2013;31(44):5041–6 [H].

[3] Grewal DS, Zeid JL. Isolated abducens nerve palsy following neonatal hepatitis B vaccination. J AAPOS. 2014;18:75–6 [A].

[4] Chaiklang K, Wipasa J, Chaiwarith R, et al. Comparison of immunogenicity and safety of four doses and four double doses vs. standard doses of hepatitis B vaccination in HIV-infected adults: a randomized, controlled trial. PLoS One. 2013;8(11):e80409 [C].

[5] Global advisory committee on vaccine safety, 11–12 December 2013. Wkly Epidemiol Rec. 2014;89(7):53–60 [S].

[6] Human papillomavirus vaccines: WHO position paper, October 2014. Wkly Epidemiol Rec. 2014;89(43):465–92 [S].

[7] Arnheim-Dahlstrom L, Pasternak B, Svanstrom H, et al. Autoimmune, neurological, and venous thromboembolic adverse vents after immunization of adolescent girls with quadrivalent human papillomavirus vaccine in Denmark and Sweden: cohort study. BMJ. 2013;347:f5906 [C].

[8] Scheller NK, Pasternak B, Svanstrom H, et al. Quadrivalent human papillomavirus vaccine and the risk of venous thromboembolism. JAMA. 2014;312(2):187–8 [r].

[9] Pellegrino P, Carnovale C, Perrone V, et al. Can HPV immunization cause ADEM? Two case reports and literature review. Mult Scler. 2014;20(6):762–3 [r].

[10] Blitshteyn S. Postural tachycardia syndrome following human papillomavirus vaccination. Eur J Neurol. 2014;21:135–9 [A].

[11] Decio A, Balottin U, De Giorgis V, et al. Acute chorea in a child receiving second dose of human papillomavirus vaccine. Pediatr Allergy Immunol. 2014;25:290–4 [r].

[12] Denny L. Safety of HPV vaccination: a FIGO statement. Int J Gynaecol Obstet. 2013;123(3):187–8 [S].

[13] Ojha RP, Jackson BE, Tota JE, et al. Guillain-Barre syndrome following quadrivalent human papillomavirus vaccination among vaccine-eligible individuals in the United States. Hum Vaccin Immunother. 2014;10(1):232–7 [c].

[14] Stephan F, Korkomaz J, Abadjian G, et al. A case of lipoatrophy following quadrivalent human papillomavirus vaccine administration. J Am Acad Dermatol. 2014;70(6):e132–3 [r].

[15] Pellegrino P, Carnovale C, Pozzi M, et al. On the relationship between human papilloma virus vaccine and autoimmune diseases. Autoimmun Rev. 2014;13:736–41 [R].

[16] Ferris D, Samakoses R, Block SL, et al. Long-term study of a quadrivalent human papillomavirus vaccine. Pediatrics. 2014;134(3):e657–65 [c].

[17] Giacomet V, Penagini F, Trabattoni D, et al. Safety and immunogenicity of a quadrivalent human papillomavirus vaccine

in HIV-infected and HIV-negative adolescents and young adults. Vaccine. 2014;32:5657–61 [c].

[18] Joura EA, Giuliano AR, Iversen OE, et al. A 9-valent HPV vaccine against infection and intraepithelial neoplasia in women. N Engl J Med. 2015;372:711–23 [C].

[19] Noronha AS, Markowitz LE, Dunne EF. Systematic review of human papillomavirus vaccine coadministration. Vaccine. 2014;32:2670–4 [M].

[20] Green H, Eliakim-Raz N, Zimra Y, et al. Paroxysmal nocturnal hemoglobinuria diagnosed after influenza vaccine: coincidence or consequence? Isr Med Assoc J. 2014;16(2):122–4 [A].

[21] Okur G, Chaney KA, Lomasney LM. Magnetic resonance imaging of abnormal shoulder pain following influenza vaccination. Skeletal Radiol. 2014;43:1325–31 [A].

[22] Cook IF. Subdeltroid/subacromial bursitis associated with influenza vaccination. Hum Vaccin Immunother. 2014;10(3):605–6 [A].

[23] Pellegrino P, Carnovale C, Perrone V, et al. Acute disseminated encephalomyelitis onset: evaluation based on vaccine adverse events reporting systems. PLoS One. 2013;8(10):e77766 [c].

[24] Sacheli A, Bauer R. Influenza vaccine-induced CNS demyelination in a 50-year-old male. Am J Case Rep. 2014;15:368–5923 [A].

[25] Polakowski LL, Sandhu SK, Martin DB, et al. Chart-confirmed Guillain-Barré syndrome after 2009 H1N1 influenza vaccination among the Medicare population, 2009–2010. Am J Epidemiol. 2013;178(6):962–73 [c].

[26] Baxter R, Bakshi N, Fireman B, et al. Lack of association of Guillain-Barré syndrome with vaccinations. Clin Infect Dis. 2013;57(2):197–204 [c].

[27] Dodd EN, Romio SA, Black S, et al. International collaboration to assess the risk of Guillain-Barré syndrome following influenza A (H1N1) 2009 monovalent vaccines. Vaccine. 2013;31:4448–58 [C].

[28] Verity C, Stellitano L, Winstone AM, et al. Pandemic A/H1N1 2009 influenza vaccination, preceding infections and clinical findings in UK children with Guillain-Barré syndrome. Arch Dis Child. 2014;99:532–8 [c].

[29] Kawai AT, Li L, Kulldorff M, et al. Absence of associations between influenza vaccines and increased risks of seizures, Guillain-Barré Syndrome, encephalitis, or anaphylaxis in the 2012–2013 season. Pharmacoepidemiol Drug Saf. 2014;23(5):548–53 [c].

[30] Finch NA, Guarascio AJ, Suda KJ. Guillain-Barré syndrome in an older man following influenza vaccination. J Am Pharm Assoc. 2014;54:188–92 [A].

[31] Ishii K, Kanazawa T, Tomidokoro Y, et al. Glossopharyngeal nerve and vagus nerve palsies associated with influenza vaccination. Intern Med. 2014;53:259–61 [A].

[32] Ahmed SS, Schur PH, MacDonald NE, et al. Narcolepsy, 2009 A (H1N1) pandemic influenza, and pandemic influenza vaccinations: what is known and unknown about the neurological disorder, the role for autoimmunity, and vaccine adjuvants. J Autoimmun. 2014;50:1–11 [R].

[33] de Golian EW, Brennan CB, Davis LS. Lichenoid drug reaction following influenza vaccination in an HIV-positive patient: a case report and literature review. J Drugs Dermatol. 2014;13(7):873–5 [A].

[34] Duggal T, Segal P, Shah M, et al. Antineutrophil cytoplasmic antibody vasculitis associated with influenza vaccination. Am J Nephrol. 2013;38:174–8 [A].

[35] Kharbanda EO, Vazquez-Benitez G, Lipkind H, et al. Inactivated influenza vaccine during pregnancy and risks for adverse obstetric events. Obstet Gynecol. 2013;122:659–67 [c].

[36] Nordin JD, Kharbanda EO, Vasquez-Benitez G, et al. Maternal influenza vaccine and risks for preterm or small for gestational age birth. J Pediatr. 2014;164:1051–7 [c].

[37] Naleway AL, Irving SA, Henninger ML, et al. Safety of influenza vaccination during pregnancy: a review of subsequent maternal obstetric events and findings from two recent cohort studies. Vaccine. 2014;32:3122–7 [R].

[38] Kaczmarek MC, Duong UT, Ware RS, et al. The risk of fever following one dose of trivalent inactivated influenza vaccine in children aged ≥6 months to <36 months: a comparison of published and unpublished studies. Vaccine. 2014;31:5359–65 [R].

[39] Prutsky GJ, Domecq JP, Elraiyah T, et al. Assessing the evidence: live attenuated influenza vaccine in children younger than 2 years. A systematic review. Pediatr Infect Dis J. 2014;33:e106–15 [M].

[40] Remschmidt C, Wichmann O, Harder T. Influenza vaccination in HIV-infected individuals: systematic review and assessment of quality of evidence related to vaccine efficacy, effectiveness and safety. Vaccine. 2014;32:5585–92 [M].

[41] Shehata MA, Karim NA. Influenza vaccination in cancer patients undergoing systemic therapy. Clin Med Insights Oncol. 2014;8:57–64 [R].

[42] Goossen GM, Kremer CM, van de Wetering MD. Influenza vaccination in children being treated with chemotherapy for cancer. Cochrane Database Syst Rev. 2013;(8). http://dx.doi.org/10.1002/14651858.CD006484.pub3. Art. No.:CD006484 [M].

[43] Eliakim-Raz N, Vinograd I, Zalmanovici Trestioreanu A, et al. Influenza vaccines in immunosuppressed adults with cancer. Cochrane Database Syst Rev. 2013;(10). http://dx.doi.org/10.1002/14651858.CD008983.pub2. Art.No.:CD008983 [M].

[44] Boikos C, De Serres G, Lands LC, et al. Safety of live-attenuated influenza vaccination in cystic fibrosis. Pediatrics. 2014;134:e983–91 [c].

[45] Greenberg DP, Robertson CA, Landolfi VA, et al. Safety and immunogenicity of an inactivated quadrivalent influence vaccine in children 6 months through 8 years of age. Pediatr Infect Dis J. 2014;33:630–6 [C].

[46] Kieninger D, Sheldon E, Lin WY, et al. Immunogenicity, reactogenicity and safety of an inactivated quadrivalent influenza vaccine candidate versus inactivated trivalent influenza vaccine: a phase III, randomized trial in adults aged ≥18 years. BMC Infect Dis. 2013;13:343 [C].

[47] McManus M, Frangoul H, McCullers JA, et al. Safety of high dose trivalent inactivated influenza vaccine in pediatric patients with acute lymphoblastic leukemia. Pediatr Blood Cancer. 2014;61:815–20 [C].

[48] Gorse GJ, Falsey AR, Johnson CM, et al. Safety and immunogenicity of revaccination with reduced dose intradermal and standard dose intramuscular influenza vaccines in adults 18–64 years of age. Vaccine. 2013;31:6034–40 [C].

[49] Tsang P, Gorse GJ, Strout CB, et al. Immunogenicity and safety of Fluzone® intradermal and high-dose influenza vaccines in older adults ≥65 years of age: a randomized, controlled phase II trial. Vaccine. 2014;32:2507–17 [C].

[50] Phrommintikul A, Wongcharoen W, Kuanprasert S, et al. Safety and tolerability of intradermal influenza vaccination in patients with cardiovascular disease. J Geriatr Cardiol. 2014;11:131–5 [c].

[51] Wilson K, Ducharme R, Ward B, et al. Increased emergency room visits or hospital admissions in females after 12-month MMR vaccination, but no difference after vaccinations given at a younger age. Vaccine. 2014;32:1153–9 [c].

[52] Rahbar AR, Fireman B, Lewis E, et al. Effect of age on the risk of fever and seizures following immunization with measles-containing vaccines in children. JAMA Pediatr. 2013;167(12):1111–7 [A].

[53] MacDonald SE, Dover DC, Simmonds KA, et al. Risk of febrile seizures after first dose of measles-mumps-rubella-varicella vaccine: a population-based cohort study. CMAJ. 2014;186(11):824–9 [c].

[54] Schink T, Holstiege J, Kowalzik F, et al. Risk of febrile convulsions after MMRV vaccination in comparison to MMR or MMR + V vaccination. Vaccine. 2014;32:645–50 [c].

[55] Bhandari N, Rongsen-Chandola T, Bavdekar A, et al. Efficacy of a monovalent human-bovine (116E) rotavirus vaccine in Indian children in the second year of life. Vaccine. 2014;32(Suppl 1): A110–6 [C].

[56] Buyse H, Vinals C, Karkada N, et al. The human rotavirus vaccine Rotarix™ in infants: an integrated analysis of safety and reactogenicity. Hum Vaccin Immunother. 2014;10:19–24 [C].

[57] Global advisory committee on vaccine safety, 12–13 June 2013. Wkly Epidemiol Rec. 2013;88(29):301–12 [S].

[58] Maglione MA, Das L, Raaen L, et al. Safety of vaccines used for routine immunization of US children: a systematic review. Pediatrics. 2014;134(2):325–37 [M].

[59] Han SB, Hwang JM, Kim JS, et al. Optic neuritis following Varicella zoster vaccination: report of two cases. Vaccine. 2014;32:4881–4 [A].

[60] Ferenczi K, Berke A, Cichon D, et al. Varicella-zoster virus vaccination-induced granulomatous dermatitis. J Am Acad Dermatol. 2014;71(4):e131–2 [r].

[61] Ulman CA, Trevino JJ, Gandhi RK. Herpes zoster in a 2-year-old vaccinated against varicella. Dermatol Online J. 2014;20(1):21259 [r].

[62] Leung J, Siegel S, Jones JF, et al. Fatal varicella due to the vaccine-strain varicella-zoster virus. Hum Vaccin Immunother. 2014;10(1):146–9 [A].

[63] Issa NC, Marty FM, Leblebjian H, et al. Live attenuated varicella-zoster vaccine in hematopoietic stem cell transplantation recipients. Biol Blood Marrow Transplant. 2014;20:279–87 [c].

[64] Morrison VA, Oxman MN, Levin MJ, et al. Safety of zoster vaccine in elderly adults following documented herpes zoster. J Infect Dis. 2013;208:559–63 [c].

[65] Morrison VA, Johnson GR, Schmader KE, et al. Long term persistence of zoster vaccine efficacy. Clin Infect Dis. 2015;60(6):900–9 [C].

[66] Biscayart C, Carrega ME, Sagradini S, et al. Yellow fever vaccine-associated adverse events following extensive immunization in Argentina. Vaccine. 2014;32:1266–72 [R].

[67] Gershman MD, Staples JE, Bentsi-Enchill AD, et al. Viscerotropic disease: case definition and guidelines for collection, analysis, and presentation of immunization safety data. Vaccine. 2012;30:5038–58 [S].

[68] Thomas RE, Spragins W, Lorenzetti DL. How many published cases of serious adverse events after yellow fever vaccination meet Brighton Collaboration diagnostic criteria? Vaccine. 2013;31:6201–9 [R].

[69] Rafferty E, Duclos P, Yactayo S, et al. Risk of yellow fever vaccine-associated viscerotropic disease among the elderly: a systematic review. Vaccine. 2013;31:5798–805 [R].

[70] Wang Y, Dong D, Cheng G, et al. Post-marketing surveillance of live-attenuated Japanese encephalitis vaccine safety in China. Vaccine. 2014;32:5875–9 [R].

[71] Martinon-Torres F, Gimenez-Sanchez F, Bernaola-Iturbe E, et al. A randomized, phase 1/2 trial of the safety, tolerability, and immunogenicity of bivalent rLP2086 meningococcal B vaccine in healthy infants. Vaccine. 2014;32:5206–11 [c].

[72] Fu C, Huang G, Cui M, et al. Post-marketing study on the safety of a meningococcal group A, C bivalent polysaccharide conjugate vaccine. Hum Vaccin Immunother. 2014;10(1):138–9 [r].

[73] Yadav S, Manglani MV, Narayan DHA, et al. Safety and immunogenicity of a quadrivalent meningococcal conjugate vaccine (MedACYW-DT): a multicenter, open-label, non-randomized, phase III clinical trial. Indian Pediatr. 2014;51(6):451–6 [C].

[74] Cutroneo PM, Italiano D, Trifirò G, et al. Acute cerebellar ataxia following meningococcal group C conjugate vaccination. J Child Neurol. 2014;29(1):128–30 [A].

[75] Global advisory committee on vaccine safety, 11–12 June 2014. Wkly Epidemiol Rec. 2014;89(29):325–35 [S].

[76] Abdelnour A, Silas PE, Valdés Lamas MR, et al. Safety of a quadrivalent meningococcal serogroups A, C, W, and Y conjugate vaccine (MenACWY-CRM) administered with routine infant vaccinations: results of an open-label, randomized, phase 3b controlled study in health infants. Vaccine. 2014;32:965–72 [C].

[77] Nolan TM, Nissen MD, Naz A, et al. Immunogenicity and safety of a CRM-conjugated meningococcal ACWY vaccine administered concomitantly with routine vaccines starting at 2 months of age. Hum Vaccin Immunother. 2014;10(2):280–9 [C].

[78] Ruiz-Aragón J, Peláez SM, Molina-Linde JM, et al. Safety and immunogenicity of 13-valent pneumococcal conjugate vaccine in infants: a meta-analysis. Vaccine. 2013;31:5349–58 [M].

[79] Jackson LA, Gurtman A, van Cleeff M, et al. Immunogenicity and safety of a 13-valent pneumococcal conjugate vaccine compared to a 23-valent pneumococcal polysaccharide vaccine in pneumococcal vaccine-naïve adults. Vaccine. 2013;31:3577–84 [R].

[80] Jackson LA, Gurtman A, Rice R, et al. Immunogenicity and safety of a 13-valent pneumococcal conjugate vaccine in adults 70 years of age and older previously vaccinated with 23-valent pneumococcal polysaccharide vaccine. Vaccine. 2013;31:3585–93 [R].

[81] Bonten MJM, Huijts SM, Bolkenbaas M, et al. Polysaccharide conjugate vaccine against pneumococcal pneumonia in adults. N Engl J Med. 2015;372:1114–25 [C].

[82] Murdaca G, Orsi A, Spano F, et al. Influenza and pneumococcal vaccinations of patients with systemic lupus erythematosus: current views upon safety and immunogenicity. Autoimmun Rev. 2014;13(2):75–84 [A].

[83] Daniels CC, Shelton CM, Bass PJ, et al. Limb swelling in a pediatric sickle cell patient after revaccination with pneumococcal vaccine. Int J Clin Pharm. 2014;36:261–3 [A].

[84] Mori S, Ueki Y, Akeda Y, et al. Pneumococcal polysaccharide vaccination in rheumatoid arthritis patients receiving tocilizumab therapy. Ann Rheum Dis. 2013;72:1362–6 [c].

[85] Kapetanovic MC, Saxne T, Jonsson G, et al. Rituximab and abatacept but not tocilizumab impair antibody response to pneumococcal conjugate vaccine in patients with rheumatoid arthritis. Arthritis Res Ther. 2013;15(5):R171 [c].

[86] Pasiarski M, Rolinski J, Grywalsa E, et al. Antibody and plasmablast response to 13-valent pneumococcal conjugate vaccine in chronic lymphocytic leukemia patients—preliminary report. PLoS One. 2014;9(12):e114966 [c].

[87] Togashi T, Yamaji M, Thompson A, et al. Immunogenicity and safety of a 13-valent pneumococcal conjugate vaccine in health infants in Japan. Pediatr Infect Dis J. 2013;32:984–9 [c].

[88] Stockwell MS, Broder K, LaRussa P, et al. Risk of fever after pediatric trivalent inactivated influenza vaccine and 13-valent pneumococcal conjugate vaccine. JAMA Pediatr. 2014;168(3): 211–9 [c].

[89] Wyman MJ, Sabi KL. Concomitant administration of pneumococcal-23 and zoster vaccines provides adequate herpes zoster coverage. Ann Pharmacother. 2013;47:1064–8 [R].

[90] Daley MF, Yih WK, Glanz JM, et al. Safety of diphtheria, tetanus, acellular pertussis and inactivated poliovirus (DTaP-IPV). Vaccine. 2014;32:3019–24 [c].

[91] Kulkarni H, Lenzo N, McLean-Tooke A. Causality of rhabdomyolysis and combined tetanus, diphtheria and acellular pertussis (Tdap) vaccine administration. J Clin Pharmacol. 2013;53(10):1099–102 [A].

[92] de la Fuente S, Hernández-Martín Á, de Lucas R, et al. Postvaccination bullous pemphigoid in infancy: report of three new cases and literature review. Pediatr Dermatol. 2013;30(6):741–4 [A].

[93] Munoz FM, Bond NH, Maccato M, et al. Safety and immunogenicity of tetanus diphtheria and acellular pertussis (Tdap) immunization during pregnancy in mother and infants. JAMA. 2014;311(17):1760–9 [C].

[94] Kharbanda EO, Vazquez-Benitez G, Lipkind HS, et al. Evaluation of the association of maternal pertussis vaccination with obstetric events and birth outcomes. JAMA. 2014;312(18):1897–904 [C].

[95] Donegan K, King B, Bryan P. Safety of pertussis vaccination in pregnant women in UK: observation study. BMJ. 2014;349: g4219 [C].

[96] McCann LJ, Ford KJ, Pollard AJ, et al. Self-reported adverse events in adolescents aged 13–18 years after mass vaccination with pertussis-containing vaccine, following a school outbreak. Public Health. 2013;127(12):1133–6 [c].

33

Blood, Blood Components, Plasma, and Plasma Products

Yekaterina Opsha*,†,1, Alison Brophy*,†

*Rutgers, the State University of New Jersey, Piscataway, NJ, USA
†Saint Barnabas Medical Center, Livingston, NJ, USA
1Corresponding author: kate.opsha@pharmacy.rutgers.edu

ALBUMIN AND DERIVATIVES [SEDA-15, 54; SEDA-33, 670; SEDA-34, 509; SEDA-35, 583;SEDA-36, 483]

Albumin [SEDA-15, 54; SEDA-33, 670; SEDA-34, 509; SEDA-35, 583; SEDA-36, 483]

Exogenous administration of human albumin has been used primarily for volume expansion. Albumin accounts for 70–80% of the oncotic pressure in plasma. Other proprieties of albumin include carrying hydrophobic substances, antioxidant activity, antithrombotic effects, anti-inflammatory effects, and endothelial stabilization. A recently published review article highlights these properties and indications for exogenous albumin administration [1r].

Comparative Studies

Albumin was compared to normal saline in 841 patients with acute ischemic stroke in the following international study. Albumin 25% at a dose 2 g/kg with a maximum volume of 750 mL or the equivalent volume of normal saline was administered within 5 hours of symptom onset. The study was terminated early for futility after finding no difference in the primary endpoint of neurological outcome at 90 days. Patients treated with albumin experienced more pulmonary edema (RR 10.8, 95% CI 4.37–26.72), shortness of breath (RR 2.58, 95% CI 1.09–6.12), and symptomatic intracranial hemorrhage within 24 hours (RR 2.42, 95% CI 2.42–5.78) [2C].

The randomized, multi-center, open-label ALBIOS trial compared 20% albumin, administered to maintain a serum albumin level of 3.0 g/dL, to crystalloid solution. The study of patients with severe sepsis found no difference in mortality at 28 or 90 days. Despite no difference in volume of fluid administered to the two groups, in the first 7 days of the study the net fluid balance was lower and the arterial blood pressure was higher in the albumin group compared to crystalloid group [3C].

A cohort study of 62 patients with bleeding peptic ulcers compared the following three groups: patients with normal serum albumin, patients with serum albumin less than 3 g/dL, and patients with serum albumin less than 3 g/dL treated with 1 or 2 days of 10 g of 20% albumin every 8 hours. Rebleeding was significantly lower in the patients with normal serum albumin compared to both groups with hypoalbuminemia. Duration of hospitalization was 7 versus 15 days ($p=0.01$) for patients treated with albumin compared to the untreated patients with low albumin [4c].

Systematic Reviews

Crystalloid versus colloid resuscitation including albumin was the subject of systematic reviews. A meta-analysis of 14 studies demonstrated possible benefit of albumin over crystalloids for mortality in sepsis with over 18 000 patients. The odds ratio for mortality was 0.83, 95% CI 0.65–1.04, not statistically significant [5M]. In patients with severe sepsis, a British meta-analysis of 16 trials with over 4000 patients demonstrated no mortality benefit for albumin over crystalloids and no signal for harm [6M].

Albumin for plasma expansion following paracentesis in patients with cirrhotic liver disease was associated with less circulatory dysfunction (OR 0.26, 95% CI 0.08–0.93) and no statistically significant effect on mortality, hyponatremia, encephalopathy, readmission, or renal

© 2015 Elsevier B.V. All rights reserved.

dysfunction. A statistically significant difference in death (OR 0.46, 95% CI 0.25–0.86) and renal dysfunction (OR 0.34, 95% CI 0.15–0.75) was found in cirrhotic patients with infection. This meta-analysis included 16 studies with 1518 patients [7M].

Respiratory

There is debate over resuscitation with crystalloids versus colloids, such as albumin, and the effect on the lungs. Pathophysiology, historic perspectives, and evidence are reviewed in a recent article. The authors concluded, despite theoretical benefit, resuscitation with albumin does not prevent respiratory dysfunction [8r].

Immunologic

Anaphylactic shock due to the human albumin found in fibrinogen and erythrocytes concentrates which was reported in a 40-year-old male patient under general anesthesia for prolapsed mitral valve replacement. Skin prick and intradermal testing was used to confirm reaction to albumin [9A].

Drug–Drug Interaction

Administration of human albumin with furosemide compared to furosemide alone was reviewed in a meta-analysis of 10 studies. At 8 hours, the combination of albumin and furosemide resulted in an increase of 231 mL (95% CI 135.5–326.5) urine output and 15.8 mEq (95% CI 4.9–26.8) of sodium excretion. There was no difference at 24 hours of treatment [10M].

BLOOD TRANSFUSION [SEDA-15, 529; SEDA-34, 509; SEDA-35, 583, SEDA-36, 483]

Erythrocytes

The clinical decision to transfuse patients should not be based solely on a single hemoglobin number. According to the American Cancer Society, blood transfusion can be life-saving; however, they are not without risks [11S]. There is substantial overutilization of transfusions based on the available hemovigilance programs. Blood transfusions have been cited as one of the top five most overutilized therapeutic procedures in the United States [12c]. The establishment of hemovigilance programs started over 20 years ago in France with the initiation of various monitoring systems by Blood Transfusion Committees which laid the foundation for a national hemovigilance system [13r]. Some of the most important factors to consider when evaluating a patient for transfusion suggested by hemovigilance systems include: goals of therapy, prior experiences with transfusions, and individualized risk–benefit analysis [14C]. Institutional experience and national databases suggest that a more

restrictive blood transfusion approach is being increasingly implemented as best practice [15R].

According to the Red Cross Blood Service organization, each blood product that is transfused carries a potential risk of causing a side effect [16r]. Typically, this risk or incidence is fairly small. The organization further classifies these reactions as acute, occurring within 24 hours of transfusion, or delayed, occurring 24 hours post-transfusion. The common acute immunological reactions are: hemolytic ABO/Rh mismatch which can occur in up to 1:40 000 patients and febrile nonhemolytic transfusion reactions which may affect 0.1–1% of patients. The latter can be treated with antipyretics. Other considerations include mild allergic reactions (urticaria) with up to 3% of patients being affected to more serious severe reactions of anaphylaxis with a much lower incidence of 1:50 000. Urticaria can be treated with antihistamines (diphenhydramine) or steroids. Reported delayed immunologic reactions include post-transfusion-related purpura and transfusion-associated graft versus host disease (TA-GVHD), both of which are reported to be rare [16r] but patients with weaker immune systems are more susceptible to TA-GVHD reactions [11S]. The more notable and commonly cited transfusion reactions that can occur are transfusion-related acute lung injury (TRALI) with a 1:1200–1:190 000 incidence and transfusion-associated circulatory overload (TACO) with a less than 1% reported incidence. Both of these reactions have been reported in adults and pediatric patient populations.

Respiratory

A recent retrospective Canadian study sought to evaluate the similarities and differences between adult and pediatric patients presenting with symptoms of TRALI after recent transfusions. A total of 284 cases of TRALI were reported and out of those 6% ($n = 17$) occurred in children. This retrospective trial demonstrated that the symptomatic presentation of TRALI in both of these patient populations is very similar and should not be overlooked. Although the numbers were small, there did not appear to be a difference in presentations or outcomes between adults and children with TRALI [17c]. By further stratifying the pediatric patients into age groups, the authors noted that most of the children who presented with TRALI were either teenagers or less than 1-year olds, potentially concluding that these two pediatric patient populations are at a higher risk. The American society of Hematology highlights that there is no single test to diagnose TRALI. It should be suspected if the patient has clinical findings (ex: hypoxemia, hypotension, fever, transient leucopenia and bilateral pulmonary edema) typically within 6 hours of transfusion [18S]. The treatment should include discontinuation of transfusion (if applicable) and supportive care where applicable including: ventilator support, maintenance of hemodynamic status and fever reducing agents. Most patients demonstrate clinical improvements within 96 hours from symptom onset. The reported overall fatality rate post-TRALI is 5% [18S].

Immunologic

Human Leucocyte Antigen (HLA) is one clinically implicated pathway in which TRALI is suspected to occur. Both the United Kingdom and the United States have demonstrated the benefit of excluding plasma collected from female donors as a means to reduce incidence of TRALI in the recipient [19r]. This resulted in a reduction of approximately half to two-thirds in TRALI incidences with fatalities almost disappearing [20S]. Previous studies have concluded that with each pregnancy comes an increased probability for HLA alloimmunization and this formed response appears to be long-lasting. These allo-antibodies tend to be present more frequently in females who have given birth to at least two children. Further reports indicate that the prevalence of HLA antibodies in the donor population is 2.3% in men and 17% in women [21c].

Hemotologic

Hemosiderosis (iron overload) is another potential complication of transfusions. The incidence of iron overload typically increases with number of transfusions. A retrospective chart analysis to determine the prevalence and risk factors for liver toxicity associated with Transfusion Related Iron Overload (TRIO) in pediatric oncology patients was recently published. The authors of this study also report their experience with Iron Chelating Therapy (ICT). The single major risk factor for TRIO was number of transfusions with a prevalence of greater than 35% in patients receiving over 10 transfusions. Four patients with TRIO and elevated liver function tests received chelation therapy. The study authors concluded that there was a significant decrease in serum ferritin levels and an improvement in liver function tests was observed with no serious adverse effect from iron chelation therapy [22c].

Death

Aggressive blood transfusion may affect long-term mortality. One hypothesis is that changing the immune function can potentially increase the risk of infections and risk of certain cancers. The authors sought to find a difference between a liberal transfusion strategy in which they received blood transfusion to maintain hemoglobin level at 100 g/L (10 g/dL) or higher vs. restrictive transfusion strategy in which they received blood transfusion when hemoglobin level was lower than 80 g/L (8 g/dL) or if they had symptoms of anemia [14C]. Over 2000 patients were enrolled in the study and randomly assigned in a 1:1 ratio to the liberal transfusion strategy

or restrictive transfusion strategy. The follow-up duration was 3 years, during which over 40% of patients died. However, the long-term mortality did not differ significantly between the liberal transfusion strategy (432 deaths) and the restrictive transfusion strategy (409 deaths) (hazard ratio 1.09 [95% CI 0.95–1.25]; $p=0.21$). These findings did not support idea that blood transfusions lead to long-term immunosuppression severe enough to affect long-term mortality rates [14C].

Another study provides interesting insight into a unique patient populations who otherwise are not candidates for blood transfusions but who are at the same time severely anemic. This was a retrospective study which analyzed the clinical outcomes of 293 patients 18 years and older who could not be transfused and had at least one hemoglobin measurement of ≤ 8 g/dL after surgery. The majority of the patients were self-identified as Jehovah's witnesses (98%) and female (74.1%). The odds ratio of death after adjustment for other significant factors was 1.82 with an overall mortality rate of 8.2%. This study confirms a very important clinical point that there is a low risk of mortality in patients with hemoglobin ranges from 7 to 8 g/dL. The risk substantially increases with lower hemoglobin ranges. The unadjusted odds ratio (OR) of death per each 1 g/dL decrease in the nadir postoperative Hgb was 2.04 (95% CI 1.52–2.74) although the number of patients who fell into this hemoglobin group was extremely small [23c].

Technology and Transfusions

The recent use of technology in medicine worldwide has substantially decreased the risks of side effects with many medications including therapeutic procedures such as blood transfusions. An observational study evaluated the impact of a computerized clinical decision support system to see if it would promote proper decision making strategies for transfusions of red blood cells (RBCs) by physicians. Patient outcomes (overall mortality, 30-day readmissions and length of stay) as well as the number of RBC transfusions were assessed before and after implementations of the computerized alert trigger for transfusions when hemoglobin levels were higher than 7 g/dL. The results were overwhelmingly positive [12c]. There was a significant improvement in RBC utilization and the clinical patient outcomes showed improvement as well (mortality, $p=0.034$; length of stay, $p=0.003$) or remained stable (30-day readmission rates, $p=0.909$). The mean number of units transfused per patient also declined (3.6 to 2.7, $p<0.001$). This also led to a reduction in acquisition costs of RBC units. The authors concluded that there was a statistically significant improvement in clinical patient outcomes when combined with an improved blood utilization protocol based on a computerized clinical decision support system [12c].

Granulocytes

Neutrophil granulocytes are the most abundant (50–75%) type of white blood cells in humans and form an essential part of the innate immune system. They are formed from stem cells in the bone marrow. Neutrophils play a critical role in preventing infections as part of the innate immune system. Reduction in neutrophils below an absolute count of 500 cells/pL is termed severe neutropenia or agranulocytosis [24H]. Neutrophils are able to phagocytize foreign substances such as bacteria. This blood product is used for patients with functionally defective granulocytes as well as neutropenic patients with life-threatening microbial infections. Occasionally, when transfused, this product is associated with hypoxia secondary to the high concentration of degrading cells.

Observational Study

In a study involving 128 patients with prolonged neutropenia and suspected invasive pulmonary aspergillosis (IA) patients were subdivided into two treatment groups. Group one received both granulocyte transfusion with antifungal therapy and group two only received antifungal therapy. Patients who received granulocyte transfusion were less likely to respond to antifungal therapy ($p=0.03$) and had a higher mortality rate ($p=0.009$). Among patients who received the granulocyte transfusion, 53% developed a pulmonary reaction characterized by worsening shortness of breath and pulmonary infiltrates within 48 hours of receiving the transfusion. This study suggests that granulocyte transfusion did not improve response to antifungal therapy and was associated with worse outcomes of invasive aspergillosis [25c].

Platelets

Observational Studies

Platelet transfusions prevent major haemorrhage and improve survival in thrombocytopenic patients [26c]. For many decades, advances in the preparation of platelets, including the introduction of pathogen reduction techniques, have been improved. Additionally, indications have been extended, for example to patients with drug-induced platelet dysfunction. However, platelet shortage is a serious medical concern. In November of 2014, the American Association of Blood Banks published guidelines for the administration of platelet transfusions in adult patients. These guidelines included only one strong recommendation on moderate quality evidence: platelets could be transfused prophylactically to reduce the risk of spontaneous bleeding in adult patients admitted to hospital with platelet counts of 10×10^9 cells/L or less, and low doses are equally effective as high doses [27r]. In 2012, the Society of Thoracic Surgeons recommended that patients should have transfusions after a coronary artery bypass only if their hemoglobin concentrations fell to less than 70 g/L (7 g/dL); before this time, some patients would automatically be transfused after surgery or when hemoglobin was at 100 g/L (10 g/dL). Due to these and other similar guidelines, the total number of transfusions each year has been falling according to the American Red Cross, which covers about 40% of the US blood bank market. This both decreases the medical costs as well as decreases the risk of unnecessary side effects [27r].

Allergic Reactions and Fever

Plasma constituents have been implicated in several types of platelet (PLT) transfusion reactions. Leukoreduced apheresis platelets stored in InterSol have 65% less plasma than apheresis platelets stored in 100% plasma (PPs). This open-label, nonrandomized retrospective study compared transfusion reaction rates in InterSol PLTs versus PPs. Over 14 000 transfusions from several sites were included with majority (9845 transfusions given to 2202 patients) were the apheresis platelets stored in 100% plasma (PP). A total of 165 adverse reactions were reported with majority appearing in the PP arm. The highest incidence transfusion reactions were allergic in nature as well as febrile nonhemolytic transfusion reactions (FNHTR's) at 0.66% and 0.40% of total transfusions reported, in the PP and InterSol groups, respectively [28c].

BLOOD SUBSTITUTES [SEDA-33, 672; SEDA-34, 511; SEDA-35, 586; SEDA-36, 485]

Hemoglobin-Based Oxygen Carriers [SEDA-33, 672; SEDA-34, 511; SEDA-35, 586; SEDA SEDA-36, 485]

Review of the properties of hemoglobin and the potential blood substitutes are discussed. While the authors offer no direct link to side effects, the potential for adverse outcomes could be linked to viscosity, vessel wall stress, and nitric oxide delivery [29r].

Comparative Studies

HBOC-201, a cell-free purified glutaraldehyde, cross-linked, and polymerized bovine hemoglobin, was compared to red cell transfusion in non-cardiac surgery patients during a study conducted from 1998 to 1999. Patients received up to seven units of HBOC-201 or red cells. The proportion of HBOC-201 group who avoided RBC transfusion was 0.427. There was no difference in 30-day mortality, serious adverse events, or time to hospital discharge between groups [30c].

PLASMA AND PLASMA PRODUCTS
[SEDA-15, 84; SEDA-34, 512; SEDA-35, 586, SEDA-36, 486]

α1-Antitrypsin

Alpha-1 antitrypsin (AAT) has broad anti-inflammatory and immunomodulating properties. Administration of human plasma-derived AAT is protective in models of acute myocardial infarction in mice. The objective of this prospective open-label, single-arm treatment study was to determine the safety and tolerability of human plasma-derived AAT and its effects on the acute inflammatory response in non-AAT deficient patients with ST-segment elevation myocardial infarction (STEMI). Ten patients with acute STEMI were enrolled and received AAT at 60 mg/kg IV within 12 hours of admission. C-reactive protein (CRP) and plasma AAT levels were determined at admission, 72 hours, and 14 days, and patients were followed clinically for 12 weeks for the occurrence of new onset heart failure, recurrent myocardial infarction, or death. Compared with historical controls, the area under the curve of CRP levels was significantly lower 14 days after admission in the study group (75.9 vs. 205.6 mg/L, $p = 0.048$). In conclusion, a single administration of study agent in patients with STEMI was well tolerated and was associated with a blunted acute inflammatory response [31c].

C1 Esterase Inhibitor Concentrate

Observational Studies

Hereditary angioedema (HAE) due to C1 esterase inhibitor (HAE-C1-INH) deficiency is a rare genetic disorder presenting with recurrent episodes of skin swellings, abdominal pain, and potentially fatal laryngeal edema. An observational study was designed to review the safety and efficacy of human, plasma-derived C1-INH concentrate for the treatment of patients with HAE-C1-INH. A systematic review of nearly 90 studies (2000 patients) was performed which investigated C1-INH for HAE. Replacement therapy with C1-INH significantly shortened time to onset of symptom relief in HAE attacks compared with placebo in many of the reviewed studies. C1-INH has been shown to be effective for patients receiving home therapy and short- and long-term prophylaxis. Treatment with C1-INH was generally well tolerated and administration of C1-INH was not associated with transmission of viruses or development of autoantibodies irrespective of treatment duration [32R]. Another observational study wanted to get a physician perspective on what they thought was a "true" incidence of side effects when administering C1-INH for HAE in their patients. This study was done via a survey to physicians who manage patients with HAE. The study was designed to determine the risk of thrombosis associated with C1-inhibitor (C1-INH) via a survey. The survey queried physicians about their observations while treating HAE. Of the 66 physicians who participated in the survey, 37 had patients (856 patients) who were on C1-INH but only 4 (total of 5 patients) had patients on C1-INH who experienced a thromboembolic episode [33c].

Dose Escalation Studies

Another study sought to evaluate the safety of escalating doses of Cintyze®, a nonfiltered C1 inhibitor, in patients who were not previously controlled on the standard doses (1000 units every 3–4 days). Eligible patients had to have >1 HAE attack/month. Dose escalation went up to 2500 units (max dose) in 12 of the 20 patients based on continued number of attacks per month. Eighteen of the patients experienced common and previously reported side effects. Four patients reported serious reactions including cerebral cystic hygroma, laryngeal angioedema attack, anemia, and bile duct stone) but these effects were considered by investigators to be unrelated to treatment. Notably, there were no systemic thrombotic events or discontinuations due to adverse events. Dose escalation of nanofiltered C1 inhibitor (human) up to 2500 units was well tolerated and reduced attack frequency in the majority of patients [34c].

Cryoprecipitate

Cryoprecipitate was originally developed as a therapy for patients with antihaemophilic factor deficiency or haemophilia A and has been used for nearly 50 years. With the production of recombinant and purified factor concentrates, the classical indications of hemophilia A and von Willebrand disease are no longer appropriate. Cryoprecipitate is now most commonly used to replenish fibrinogen levels in patients with acquired coagulopathy (ex: hemorrhage including cardiac surgery, trauma, organ transplantation, or obstetric hemorrhage).

This agent is a blood product that is manufactured from fresh frozen plasma. It contains a subset of coagulation factors namely: fibrinogen (minimum of 150 mg/unit), factor VIII (minimum 80 IU/unit), von Willebrand factor, and factor XIII. Currently, cryoprecipitate is used to treat hypofibrinogemia [35r].

Observational Study

The objective of this retrospective, non-controlled observational study was to determine the safety and efficacy of cryoprecipitate in improving plasma fibrinogen levels, coagulation parameters and clinical status in both acute and chronic acquired hypofibrinogenaemia. The average fibrinogen level before administration of cryoprecipitate was similar in the two disease groups (acute vs. chronic), and the amount of cryoprecipitate administered was comparable in the two cohorts. At 24 hours post-cryoprecipitate, the mean fibrinogen level was higher in the acute group when compared to the chronic group (2.02 vs. 1.45 g/L; $p = 0.0009$). Despite cohort differences, the increase in fibrinogen level was statistically significant for both cohorts between baseline and 24 hours (acute, $p \leq 0.0001$; chronic, $p = 0.0001$). On another very important note, there were no acute adverse transfusion reactions reported as a direct result of the cryoprecipitate administration; no cases of transfusion-associated circulatory overload (TACO) or transfusion-transmitted infection (TTI) were noted indicating that cryoprecipitate is an effective and safe method of increasing the plasma fibrinogen level in hypofibrinogenaemic patients [36c].

Fresh Frozen Plasma [SEDA-34, 513; SEDA-35, 587; SEDA-36, 487]

Systemic Review

A retrospective analysis was performed to identify the frequency of adverse reactions after transfusion on both per transfused patient and per transfused unit basis. The study evaluated red blood cells (RBCs), fresh frozen plasma (FFP), and platelet concentrates (PCs). The incidence of adverse reactions to RBCs, FFP, and PCs per transfused unit was 0.6%, 1.3%, and 3.8%, respectively. The incidence of adverse reactions to RBCs, FFP, and PCs per patient was 2.6%, 4.3%, and 13.2%, respectively—almost threefold higher. Most RBC associated adverse reactions were febrile nonhemolytic transfusion reactions and allergic reactions; whereas most FFP and PC associated adverse reactions were allergic reactions. This is consistent with what was found in prior literature [37R].

PLASMA SUBSTITUTES [SEDA-33, 675; SEDA-34, 513; SEDA-35, 587; SEDA-36, 487]

Dextrans [SEDA-15, 1082; SEDA-33, 675; SEDA-34, 513; SEDA-35,587; SEDA-36, 487]

Hematologic

Thrombolastometry analysis and extrinsic coagulation assay (EXTEM) was performed on blood samples from 10 healthy volunteers diluted first with 3% dextran 60, 6% dextran 60, buffered and unbuffered hydroxyethyl starch (HES) 130/0.4, 5% albumin and Ringers acetate. Correction of dilutional coagulopathy was then performed using fibrinogen concentrate on each sample. Samples diluted with HES or dextran demonstrated decreased correction of coagulopathy compared to those diluted with albumin ($p \leq 0.001$). The platelet component of clot strength was decreased more by the dextran solutions than albumin ($p \leq 0.001$) [38E].

Etherified Starches [SEDA-15, 1237; SEDA-33, 675; SEDA-34, 513; SEDA-35, 587; SEDA-36, 487]

Comparative Studies

Mortality in patients with hypovolemic shock treated with crystalloids or colloids was compared in the CRISTAL trial. In the colloid group, 68.8% of patients received HES. At 28 days, there was no difference in mortality but at 90 days, mortality was 30.7% in colloids group vs. 34.2% in crystalloids group (RR 0.92, 95% CI 0.86–0.99; $p = 0.03$) [39C].

Systematic Reviews

Crystalloid versus colloid resuscitation including use of HES was the subject of several systematic reviews [5M,6M]. One analysis included two studies which compared starch to albumin for sepsis and found albumin was associated with decreased risk of mortality OR 0.71 (95% CI 0.54–0.94) with moderate quality evidence. Comparisons between starches with gelatin and crystalloids were not statistically significant [5M].

Cardiovascular

Administration of 500 mL of 6% HES 130/0.4 and 500 mL of Ringer's Lactate (RL), was compared to 1000 mL of RL in 168 healthy mothers for elective caesarian section with spinal anesthesia. Use of HES + RL was associated with lower incidence of hypotension 36.6% compared to 55.3% ($p = 0.025$) in pure RL group. There was no difference in phenylephrine requirements, postoperative maternal hemoglobin, or neonatal outcomes. HES concentrations were undetectable in umbilical cord samples obtained from six of the neonates assigned to the HES group [40c].

Fluid Balance

Administration of 6% HES for volume replacement in a study of 61 pediatric open heart surgery patients resulted in less positive fluid balance than patients treated with albumin ($p = 0.050$) [41c].

Hematologic

Coagulation competence measured with thrombolastography and perioperative blood loss were compared in patients undergoing cystectomy administered 35 mL/kg of HES 130/0.4 or RL. There was reduced development and strength of clot in patients treated with HES. Perioperative blood loss was 2191 mL in the HES group compared to 1370 mL in the group treated with RL ($p = 0.038$) [42c]. In a similar comparison, cardiac surgery patients received HES, albumin, and RL as the major perioperative fluid with a maximal dose of 50 mL/kg/day. There was no difference in volume of chest tube drainage however 64% of patients treated with HES required transfusion compared to 62% and 35% of patients treated with albumin and RL, respectively (p-value HES vs. RL = 0.0003) [43c]. In a *post hoc* analysis of a Scandinavian starch for sepsis database, HES administration was associated with increased risk of bleeding when compared to Ringer's acetate (RR 1.55, 95% CI 1.16–2.08). This was also associated with an increased risk of death (RR 1.36, 95% CI 1.04–1.79; $p = 0.03$) [44c].

Urinary Tract

The role of HES in development of renal dysfunction was explored in a recent review in the surgical population [45r]. One study of on-pump cardiac bypass surgery patients compared normal saline to 7.2% NaCl/6% HES 200/0.5 resuscitation at a dose of 4 mL/kg in 30 minutes after the start of anesthesia. There was no difference in the rate of acute kidney injury between groups [46c]. However, in another a meta-analysis of 10 studies with more than 4600 patients with sepsis, the rate of acute kidney injury, requirement for renal replacement therapy was higher in treatment with HES. There was no difference in ICU or 28-day mortality but an increased rate of mortality in patients treated with HES compared to crystalloids [47R].

Skin

A retrospective study of 70 patients with electron microscopy-proven HES induced pruritus between 1993 and 2008 sought to characterize latency, duration, and severity. The majority of patients received HES 200/0.5 6% solutions. Patients experienced an average of 3.5 attacks per day with an onset of 3 weeks after HES administration. No clinical differences were seen between 200/0.5 and 130/0.4 HES associated pruritus nor in cumulative HES dose [48A].

Gelatin [SEDA-34, 514; SEDA-35, 584; SEDA 36–487]

Systematic Reviews

Crystalloid versus colloid resuscitation including use of gelatin was the subject of systematic reviews. Gelatin was compared with starch in one study included in the meta-analysis and no difference in mortality for sepsis resuscitation was noted [5M].

GLOBULINS

Immunoglobulins [SEDA-15, 1719; SEDA-33, 677; SEDA-34, 514; SEDA-35, 588; SEDA-36, 488]

Intravenous Immunoglobulin

The mechanism of immunoglobulin in primary and secondary immunodeficiency disorders is delivery of mature antibiotics in adequate concentrations against a variety of pathogens. The mechanism of action in other conditions is less understood but anti-inflammatory and immunomodulation effects are present. A variety of intravenous immunoglobulin (IVIG) products are available, each with different studied indications, formulations, and potential toxicities. The volume load, sugar content, osmolarity, sodium content, IgA content, and pH of preparations all influence these potential reactions [49R]. There are a variety of adverse reactions and management strategies for them related to intravenous immunoglobulin (IVIG). Infusion reactions such as headache, nausea, vomiting, musculoskeletal pain, flushing, and tachycardia many be prevented with premedication using NSAIDs, corticosteroids, antihistamines, and acetaminophen. These anaphylactoid reactions can appear like anaphylaxis but are differentiated due to a lack of hypotension and release of IgE. Anaphylaxis due to the IgA in IVIG products has also occurred. Thromboembolic events following treatment with IVIG have been associated with patient specific risk factors and formulations contaminated with coagulation factors XI, Xia, XIIa, and kallikrein. Acute renal dysfunction has been further linked with age, diabetes, sepsis, concomitant nephrotoxic agents, and products containing sucrose. Prehydration has been employed to decrease the chances of this toxicity. Hematologic adverse events including neutropenia and hemolysis have been described as well [50R,51R]. A series of proposed European consensus statements were published following the Kreuth III meeting [52R].

OBSERVATIONAL STUDIES

A single center retrospective review of 77 patients treated with IVIG over a 10-year period demonstrated an adverse event rate in 32% in this patient population. The most common reported adverse event was fever (30.5%) followed by rash (22.2%). Onset of fever was most frequently observed between 61 minutes and 6 hours from the initiation of the infusion [53c].

COMPARATIVE STUDIES

A prospective cohort of 1765 infusions of IVIG for 117 patients with primary immunodeficiency in Brazil was analyzed for adverse events. The incidence of reactions was 2.15% of infusions and 23.8% of patients. Pretreatment, infusion rate, and number of batches were not found to be significantly associated with increased or decreased infusion reactions. Only 7.9% of reactions were severe and there were no significant findings with respect to latency of reaction. There was a higher incidence of reactions with Tegeline® compared to Octagam® [54c].

MAJOR REVIEWS

In neonates, synthesis of immunoglobulin occurs several months after birth. Transfer of material immunoglobulin occurs after 32 weeks of gestation. Administration of exogenous IVIG in neonates with suspected sepsis was hypothesized to reduce morbidity and mortality. In a Cochrane review of 8 studies with 3871 infants, mortality was not improved in patients treated with IVIG (RR 0.94, 95% CI 0.80–1.12). No difference in morbidity at 2 years or length of stay was reported [55R]. A similar review of adult patients with sepsis and severe sepsis reviewed polyclonal IVIG and IgM-enriched polyclonal IVIG separately. In 10 trials of polyclonal IVIG trials with 1430 patients, reduction in mortality was confirmed when compared to placebo (RR 0.81, 95% CI 0.70–0.93). In the seven trials of 528 patients treated with IgM-enriched polyclonal IVIG reduction in mortality was also reported (RR 0.66, 95% CI 0.51–0.85). However, in those studies of low bias no mortality reduction was demonstrated [56R]. In a Cochrane review of seven trials with 623 patients with Guillain-Barre syndrome improvement, there was no difference, when compared to control treatments, in mean change in a validated disability scale. There was no difference in adverse effects between patients treated with IVIG or plasma exchange but more patients completed IVIG treatment [57R].

HEMATOLOGIC

The incidence of thromboembolic events in a retrospective cohort of 303 patients was 16.9% (95% CI 13–21.6). The study reviewed patients at a tertiary care center in Madrid over a 2-year period. The outcome of fatal thromboembolic events was observed in 16 patients, 32% of total thromboembolic cases. Patients who experienced thromboembolic events tended to be older, male gender, and treated with higher doses of IVIG ($p < 0.001$) [58C]. Hemolytic anemia was characterized in a study of 34 de novo and 50 maintenance patients treated for neurologic conditions. The fall in hemoglobin was 0.9 and 0.4 mM for the de novo and maintenance groups, respectively. There were no significant changes in reticulocytes, haptoglobin, and bilirubin. Lactate dehydrogenase was significantly increased [59c].

URINARY

A case report of severe antibody mediated rejection following IVIG for BK virus nephropathy in a Caucasian female recipient of a deceased donor transplant is discussed below. There were no donor specific antibodies present prior to IVIG infusion. Nephrectomy was performed and antibodies were present. Following IVIG infusion donor specific antibodies to HLA DR11 and HLA DQ7 were present in the recipient's serum. Twenty-five days after nephrectomy serum was negative for donor specific antibodies [60A].

SKIN

Erythematous rashes on the palms and chest are described in recipients of IVIG [61A,62A].

IMMUNOLOGIC

A prospective study of 21 patients receiving IVIG for primary antibody deficiency's tested plasma samples and drug lots of different IVIG products for antibodies to tetanus, diphtheria, measles and varicella. There was no significant difference between products or drug lots of IVIG with respect to antibodies for these diseases. There was fluctuation in the patients' plasma antibodies titers in the four blood samples drawn every 3 months [63c].

DRUG FORMULATIONS

BIVIGAM, a new IVIG formulation from Behring is reviewed [64r]. IVIG formulation is often implicated with renal toxicity. Osmotic nephrosis has been associated with glucose solutions. Maltose solutions are degraded in the brush boarder of the proximal tubule and therefore also implicated with nephrotoxicity. Mannitol, as an IVIG excipient, is suspected to cause renal vasoconstriction and osmotic nephrosis. Finally, D-sorbitol, glycine and L-proline IVIG products have little association with nephrotoxicity [65r].

Subcutaneous Immunoglobulin

OBSERVATIONAL STUDY

A prospective, open-label, multi-center, study of 24 adult and pediatric Japanese patients with primary immunodeficiency assessed serum IgG trough levels with IVIG treatment or IgPro20 (Hizentra®, L-proline stabilized 20% human subcutaneous IG). Patients were treated for three mandatory IVIG infusions, followed by a 12-week wash-out period with conversion to the IgPro20, followed by the 12-week study period of IgPro20. Dose equivalence was established as the primary efficacy endpoint. During the subcutaneous IG (SCIG) period, 52% of patients experienced a serious bacterial infection, with one patient requiring hospitalization. Overall, adverse event rates were 0.461 and 0.653 per treatment for the SCIG and IVIG, respectively. Local infusion site reactions occurred in 80% of patients during the SCIG treatment with decreasing incidence over time [66c].

SKIN

Two patients are described to have necrotic skin ulcers at the site of SCIG infusion. A 13-year-old boy treated with 20% SCIG for common variable immunodeficiency. After 3 years, with only local erythema at the site of injection the patient experienced a blister with necrotic center on the thigh which grew oxacillin-sensitive *Staphylococcus aureus*. He was treated with trimethoprim-sulfamethoxazole and erythromycin. The second patient, an 11-year-old girl treated for trichothiodystrophy and associated hypogammaglobulinemia. After 4 years of treatment, a blister at the site of infusion developed into a 4.5 × 5 cm area of induration with 1 cm necrotic center. She was hospitalized and treated initially with clindamycin, fluconazole, and piperacillin-tazobactam. She had resolution of infection after 9 days of antibiotic treatment. One month after her SCIG treatment she developed a blister at the injection site again, treated with clindamycin, but no development of necrosis of the skin [67A].

Anti-D immunoglobulin

The British Committee for Standards in Hematology (BCSH) published a guideline for use of Anti-D immunoglobulin to prevent hemolysis in newborns and fetuses. This statement reviews indications, dosage, administration, and monitoring. The low incidence of adverse events is emphasized with recommendations for surveillance for severe hypersensitivity reactions [68R].

COMPARATIVE STUDIES

A single center study comparing pediatric patients treated for immune thrombocytopenia before and after the March 2010 FDA warning regarding treatment with Anti-D immunoglobulin, demonstrated no statistical difference in adverse effects. Headache, nausea, vomiting, hematuria, anemia, fever, and chills were most frequently reported adverse events in 2186 patients before and 1782 patients after the warning [69c].

IMMUNOLOGIC

In a retrospective analysis of the Leukocyte Antibody Prevalence Study Database previously pregnant RhD negative and positive women were compared. HLA sensitization rate was lower in RhD negative women less than or equal to 40 years old (RR 0.58, 95% CI 0.40–0.84). Authors concluded this effect was associated with the routine use of RhIG prophylaxis [70c].

Suspected hypersensitivity reactions to Anti-D immunoglobulin in three pregnant women are described. A 18-year-old primigravida Rh(−) woman developed wheezing, severe dyspnea, and periorbital edema within 3 minutes of administration of Anti-D 500 IU (Rhophylac; CSL Behring, Haywards Health, UK). Upon subsequent pregnancy, skin prick and intradermal testing was negative. Empiric protocol was used with 10%, 30%, 60% of total 1500 IU if Rhophylac was administer on a subsequent Rh(−) pregnancy. A 25-year-old women, Rh(−) primigravida was administered 1500 IU Rhophylac at 28 weeks and 500 mcg of D-GAM (Anti-D; Bio Products Laboratory, Elstree, UK) upon delivery. Upon development of maternal hemorrhage, 7500 IU of Rhophylac was administered over 20 minutes. After 1 hour, the patient developed tremor, tachycardia, dyspnea, and desaturation to 80% on room air. After 6 months skin prick testing, intradermal testing, and challenge with 1500 IU of Rhophylac elicited no reaction. A 19-year-old Rh(−) r female who received three separate doses of Anti-D immunoglobulin. After the first dose of 250 IC D-Game she felt "unwell". Next she received 1500 IU of Rhophylac with reports of light-headedness, blurred vision, facial edema and pruritus. Skin prick testing and intradermal testing were negative 5 months later. After 300 IU of Rhophylac, she became dizzy with a headache and ocular pruritus. The additional 1200 IU of the full dose were well tolerated with no further reported reactions [71A].

DRUG INTERACTIONS

There is a risk of inadequate response to live vaccines, such as the influenza and MMR vaccines, when administered with Anti-D immunoglobulin. Because the obstetric population is a risk of co-administration of these products reminding patients to follow-up vaccine titers was the subject of a nursing quality initiative [72r].

COAGULATION PROTEINS [SEDA-15, 845; SEDA-33, 679; SEDA-34, 518; SEDA-36, 493]

Factor I

Fibrinogen (factor I) concentrate may be either plasma-derived or a recombinant product. It is the final protein in the common coagulation cascade.

Systemic Review

A systematic review identified 12 articles reporting fibrinogen concentrate (FC) usage in trauma patients: 4 case reports, 7 retrospective studies, and 1 prospective observational study were evaluated. Some of the available studies suggested that FC administration was associated with a reduced blood product requirement with minimally reported adverse events [73R].

Impact of Meals and Lab Levels

The authors of this research study hypothesized that fasting time for coagulation tests is not standardized and that this can decrease patient safety. The study evaluated the impact of whether a light meal (i.e. breakfast) can jeopardize laboratory coagulation tests. A blood sample was first collected from 17 fasting volunteers (12-hour fast). Immediately after blood collection, the volunteers consumed a light meal. Then samples were collected at 1, 2 and 4 hours after the light meal. Several coagulation tests were evaluated including, fibrinogen (Fbg) levels. The results of Fbg and PS test were not influenced by a light meal. The authors concluded that a light meal does not influence the laboratory coagulation tests, but they suggested that the laboratory quality managers standardize the fasting time for all blood tests at 12 hours, to completely metabolize the lipids intake [74c].

Factor II

A wide variety of topical agents are approved as potential therapies in the maintenance of hemostasis during surgical procedures. A multidisciplinary approach to the selection and application of these agents requires input from all members of the surgical team [75R].

Topical thrombin may be either from a bovine or recombinant source. Thrombin plays a central role in coagulation, both activating platelets and cleaving fibrinogen. It is often used intraoperative for hemorrhage control, but may also be used on superficial wounds.

Factor VIIa [SEDA-15, 1318; SEDA-34, 518; SEDA-35, 592; SEDA-36, 493]

Observational Studies

Severe bleeding, defined as the loss of 20% or more of the total blood volume, is associated with a markedly increased risk of morbidity and mortality [76c].

In severe post-partum hemorrhage refractory to standard treatment, the use of rFVIIa has been considered. Even though case reports suggest a potential benefit of this agent in this clinical setting, the lack of randomized controlled trials greatly limits the value of available favorable data [76c]. In a recent report published by the World Health Organization "Recommendations for Prevention and Treatment of Postpartum Hemorrhage", the group concluded that there is insufficient evidence to recommend rFVIIa for the treatment of post-partum hemorrhage, and that its use should be limited to women with licensed hematological indications. The group regarded rFVIIa as a potentially life-saving drug but noted that it is also associated with life-threatening adverse effects [77S].

Thromboembolic Events (TEs)

A *post hoc* analysis assessed the safety of rFVIIa dosing in congenital haemophilia and the impact of >240 µg/kg dosing. A total of 61 734 rFVIIa doses were reported in 481 patients treated for 3947 bleeding events. Over half (52%) exceeded 120 µg/kg, 37% exceeded 160 µg/kg

and 15% exceeded 240 µg/kg. No TEs were reported. The findings of this analysis show that high doses of rFVIIa are utilized clinically for treatment of patients [78R].

Factor VIII [SEDA-15, 1319; SEDA-34, 518; SEDA-35, 592; SEDA-36, 494]

Neurologic

Among 148 cases in a stroke registry, patients with acute ischemic stroke (AIS) were included if both FVIII and vWF were measured during admission. Out of the total 148 cases, 51 patients (34.5%) had FVIII+/vWF+. Patients with FVIII+/vWF+ had increased odds of inpatient complications (odds ratio, 8.6; 95% confidence interval, 1.58–46.85; $p=0.013$) and neurological worsening (odds ratio, 3.2; 95% confidence interval, 1.18–8.73; $p=0.022$) versus patients with FVIII−/vWF−. These findings suggest that FVIII and vWF levels may serve as clinically useful stroke biomarkers by providing risk profiles for patients with AIS [79E].

Factor IX [SEDA-15, 1324; SEDA-34, 518; SEDA-35, 592; SEDA-36, 494]

Drug Formulations

Multinational, randomized, single-blind trial investigated the safety and efficacy of a recombinant glycoPE-Gylated factor IX (FIX) with extended half-life, in 74 previously treated patients with Hemophilia B. Patients received prophylaxis for 52 weeks, randomized to either 10 or 40 IU/kg once weekly or to on-demand treatment of 28 weeks. Once-weekly prophylaxis with 40 IU/kg resolved target joint bleeds in 66.7% of the affected patients and improved health-related quality of life. No safety concerns were identified [80C].

Factor IX Gene Therapy

Another study evaluated long-term safety and efficacy of Factor IX gene therapy in Hemophilia B patients where gene therapy that is mediated by a novel adeno-associated virus serotype 8 vector has been shown to raise factor IX levels. The authors sought to evaluate if patients with severe Hemophilia B can benefit from gene therapy to raise factor IX levels and decrease rates of bleeding. The effects were found to be clinically positive with a significant decrease in rates of acute bleeding episodes with no reported acute or late toxic effects [81c].

Prothrombin Complex Concentrate [SEDA-34, 518; SEDA-35, 518; SEDA-36, 494]

There are three main types of Prothrombin Complex Concentrates (PCC) that are available on the market worldwide. The first one is an activated-PCC which contains activated forms of factors II, VII, IX, and X. Activated PCCs are used for bypass therapy in hemophilia patients who have developed inhibitor antibodies. The second type is a four-factor PCC which contains nonactivated forms of factors II, VII, IX, and X. And finally, three-factor PCC contains non-activated forms of factors II, IX, and X (while lacking factor VII). These three- and four-factor non-activated PCCs are most often used for anticoagulation reversal and severe hemorrhage in clinical practice.

Cardiac Surgery

Twenty-five patients who underwent cardiac surgery with coagulopathy and life-threatening bleeding refractory to conventional treatment received activated prothrombin complex concentrate FEIBA (factor VIII inhibitor bypassing activity). The mean FEIBA dose was 2154 units. The need for fresh frozen plasma and platelet transfusion decreased significantly after FEIBA administration ($p = 0.0001$ and $p < 0.0001$, respectively). The mean internationalized normalized ratio decreased from 1.58 to 1.13 ($p < 0.0001$). The study investigators report that the clinical outcomes were excellent with no patient returning to the operating room for re-exploration. There was no hospital mortality and all patients were discharged home [82C].

Haematologic

PCC is used as a reversal option for warfarin anticoagulation. This study compared warfarin reversal in patients who received either three-factor PCC (PCC3) or low-dose rFVIIa (LDrFVIIa) for reversal of warfarin anticoagulation. Seventy-four PCC3 and 32 LDrFVIIa patients were analyzed. Baseline demographics, reason for warfarin reversal, and initial INR were equivalent. There was no difference in the number of thromboembolic events (2 LDrFVIIa vs. 5 PCC3, $p = 1.00$), mortality, length of hospital stay, or cost [83c]. Similar results were found in a study from Spain which evaluated the use of PCC for reversal of vitamin K antagonists. The study reported that no infusion reactions were detected, and only 1 thrombotic episode was observed out of 31 patients who were included in the study [84c]. Another study sought to evaluate the safety and efficacy of nonactivated four-factor PCC versus plasma in patients experiencing major bleeding while taking vitamin K antagonists. The outcomes were both clinically and statistically positive in favor of using four-factor PCC. The safety profile was similar between groups; 66 of 103 (4F-PCC group) and 71 of 109 (plasma group) patients experienced ≥1 adverse event [85C].

von Willebrand Factor (VWF)/Factor VIII Concentrates [SEDA-34, 519; SEDA-35, 594; SEDA-36, 494]

Comparative Studies

Most studies on immune tolerance induction (ITI) therapy in haemophilia A patients are focused on primary ITI in children. The authors of this study report on the ITI outcome in a large retrospective cohort, including adult patients with rescue ITI, treated with a pdFVIII/VWF concentrate. Success rate of 87% was achieved in primary ITI and 74% in the higher risk profile of rescue ITI. Several safety concerns were observed including venous access complications consisting of seven infections, one case of haemarthrosis (bleeding into the joint spaces), one case of allergy to the pdFVIII/VWF concentrate that was considered a failure of therapy, and one case of pleural haemorrhage that resolved after treatment [86c].

Observational Study

The safety of recombinant von Willebrand factor (rVWF) combined at a fixed ratio with recombinant factor VIII (rFVIII) was investigated in 32 subjects with von Willebrand disease (VWD) in a prospective phase 1, multi-center, randomized clinical trial. The authors concluded that rVWF was well tolerated and no thrombotic events or serious adverse events were noted [87C].

ERYTHROPOIETIN AND DERIVATIVES [SEDA-34, 520; SEDA-35, 594; SEDA-36, 494]

Systematic Reviews

Erythropoiesis-stimulating agents are often used to attenuate blood transfusions among anemic patients receiving chemotherapy or those with chronic kidney disease (CKD). However, these agents are not without potentially serious side effects. They have been shown to be associated with venous thromboembolism and increased mortality. For these reasons, a recent Cochrane review discussed the potential adverse effects of these agents when used in the setting of CKD. Clinical guidelines recommend ESA treatment to avoid blood transfusions and anemia-related symptoms for patients with CKD. However, whether all the available ESAs are equally effective and safe has not been adequately evaluated by individual RCTs [88R].

Data for the effects of ESA treatment compared to placebo or no treatment on all-cause mortality was provided in 10 studies involving over 5000 participants. Three agents (epoetin alfa, epoetin beta and darbepoetin alfa) were assessed against placebo or no treatment with patients with underlying CKD. The odds of all-cause mortality, cardiovascular mortality and MI were not statistically significant with all three agents. However, when considering the odds of stroke, the results were not statistically significant in the epoetin alfa and beta groups, but were increased in darbepoetin alfa group when compared to placebo. Similar results were found with hypertension, where all three agents had a higher propensity to increase blood pressure in comparison to placebo [88R].

THROMBOPOIETIN AND RECEPTOR AGONISTS [SEDA-15, 3409; SEDA-36-495]

The ideal selection of thrombopoietin receptor agonists is an area of ongoing research. Eltrombopag and romiplostim are both efficacious in increasing platelet counts but differ in route of administration, dose titration, and potentially adverse effects [89r].

Observational Studies

An open-label extension trial of eltrombopag in Japanese patients with chronic immune thrombocytopenia (ITP) followed patients until the drug was commercially available or serious adverse events occurred. Median duration of therapy was 27.5 months with 15 patients treated for more than 2 years. Concomitant treatment was required in 79% ($n = 15$) of patients with 14 of those patients who were treated with corticosteroids. Adverse events included nasopharyngitis and headache. Two events of chest pain with normal ECG were determined to be associated with eltrombopag. Four events of cataract progression were reported in three patients during treatment and two were considered serious adverse events related to treatment. Five patient experienced elevation in liver enzymes. A total of 10 bone marrow biopsies were obtained from 7 patients which were normal or showed grade 1 bone marrow fibrosis [90c].

Systematic Review

A review of the French Pharmacovigilance Database from January 2009 to December 2013 identified 53 adverse drug reactions with romiplostim and 37 adverse drug reactions with eltrombopag. Twelve cases of venous thromboembolism occurred with romiplostim and 7 with eltrombopag, however 83% of the patients had at least one risk factor for thrombosis. Romiplastim was implicated with hematologic adverse reactions more frequently than eltrombopag, while eltrombopag was associated with gastrointestinal events [91R]. A systematic review of thrombopoietin receptor agonists (TPOs) for treatment of myelodysplasic disorder included 4 studies of romiplostim and 1 of eltrombopag.

Romiplastim was associated with decreased bleeding events and platelet transfusions when adjusted for time exposure. There was no increase in AML progression. The authors emphasized possible bias in reported data [92C].

Hematologic

Sixty six patients treated with TPOs were followed for a median of 29 months of treatment. At the beginning of treatment 67% of bone marrow biopsies showed no fibrosis which decreased to 22% at the end of treatment. High grade myelofibrosis, either 2 or 3, was associated with older age. Grade of myelofibrosis was not associated with initial marrow grade, TPO dose, TPO agent, or immature platelet fraction [93M].

Skin

Eltrombopag-induced hyperpigmentation of the skin is described in two patients. Tissue biopsies were Fontana-Masson stain and Prussian blue stain positive demonstrating increased melatonin deposition and hemosiderin deposition from red blood cell leakage, respectively [94A].

Pregnancy

Romiplostim was used in two pregnant patients with steroid resistant immune thrombocytopenia for 10 and 22 weeks during gestation. No neonatal complications were reported [95A].

Interference with Diagnostic Tests

Serum of patients treated with eltrombopag appears dark reddish brown and alters based on drug concentration and pH. Erroneous results for serum total bilirubin were described in patients treated with eltrombopag [96A].

TRANSMISSION OF INFECTIOUS AGENTS THROUGH BLOOD DONATION [SEDA-34, 521; SEDA-35, 596; SEDA-36, 495]

In 2009, the American Association of Blood Banks released a statement identifying emerging infectious disease agents with transfusion safety risks. The author of a recent review summarizes emerging infectious disease since the 2009 statement including MERS-CoV, Dengue viruses, Chikungunya virus, and Hepatitis E virus [97r].

Bacteria

Borrelia burgdorferi transmission by transfusion has not been widely described. Authors postulate, that is, it due to low bacterial low in infected humans and inability of host-adapted spirochetes to survive under blood storage conditions [98H].

Virus

Risk of arbovirus in South-East Asia is emerging due to limited resources and high incidence of the infection [99r]. In French Polynesia, during the 2013 outbreak of Zika virus, testing of 1505 asymptomatic blood donors was carried out. Three percent of donors were Zika virus positive using PCR testing [100c].

Transmission of hepatitis C virus from an Anti-HCV negative donor to two recipients in Turkey was described. The donor, a 33-year-old woman, was found to be HCV-RNA virus and Anti-HCV positive 3 weeks after donation. Initial donated blood was then tested for HCV-RNA with a viral load of 22 039 549 IU/mL. Two recipients were diagnosed with hepatitis C virus. One of the recipients, a 44-year-old female who received red blood cells for hemoglobin of 6.7 g/dL was successfully treated with interferon alpha. The other recipient, a 19-year-old male with myeloid leukemia, received platelets and was not treated for Hepatitis C virus due to comorbid disease. Authors highlight the need for nucleic acid amplification testing of donors to decrease risk of transmission [101A]. Hepatitis E virus was identified in 79 of 225 000 blood donations in England between October 2012 and September 2013. Follow up of 43 recipients identified 18 recipients or 43% with Hepatitis E viral infection [102R]. In the United States, testing of 1939 donated blood samples from 2006 to 2012, identified positive Ig Anti-HEV in 18.8% samples but no donations with HEV RNA. Two patients of the 362 recipients (0.6%) had positive post-transfusion blood samples for Hepatitis E virus however direct link to transfusion is not clear [103R].

Prion

Using predictive modeling based on United Kingdom prevalence of variant Creutzfeldt-Jakob disease (vCJD) estimates of transfusion-transmitted vVJD in the United States range from 1 in 134 million transfusions to 1 in 480 000 transfusions [104r].

STEM CELLS [*SEDA-34, 522; SEDA-35, 597; SEDA-36, 496*]

Endocrinology

At one center, 32 patients with history of type-2 diabetes and varying diabetic complications were administered autologous stem cells and observed for changes before and after therapy (improvement of symptoms, HgbA1c levels and 24 hours urine protein quantity). The researchers reported clinical improvement in hemoglobin levels and 24 hours urine protein quantity with no toxic side effects [105c].

Respiratory System

Literature suggests that hematopoietic stem cell transplantation (HSCT) is associated with more respiratory infections due to immunosuppression. In a retrospective trial, the researches aimed to investigate the frequency of rhinosinusitis after HSCT, and the association between rhinosinusitis and chronic graft vs. host disease (GVHD). Patients with GVHD had a higher frequency and recurrence of rhinosinusitis, in addition to more frequent need for endoscopic sinusectomy and decreased overall survival [106c].

Cardiovascular System

Hematopoietic cell transplantation (HCT) is an accepted treatment for many malignant disorders but may have side effects for several major organs, including the cardiovascular system. In this study, cardiac function was evaluated using echocardiography and levels of NT-proBNP in 18 patients, and in 18 matched controls. Patients in the HCT group had cardiac dimensions, and left ventricular ejection fractions within normal range. However, they also had lower measurements of left ventricular diastolic function and a significantly higher NT-proBNP levels. The investigators also reported that heart rate was significantly higher in the HCT group [107c].

References

[1] Caraceni P, Domenicali M, Tovoli A, et al. Clinical indications for the albumin use: still a controversial issue. Eur J Intern Med. 2013;24(8):721–8 [r].

[2] Ginsbery MD, Palesch YY, Hill MD, et al. High-dose albumin treatment for acute ischemic stroke (ALIAS) part 2: a randomized, double-blind, phase 3, placebo-controlled trial. Lancet Neurol. 2013;12:1049–58 [C].

[3] Caironi P, Tognoni G, Masson S, et al. Albumin replacement in patients with severe sepsis or septic shock. N Engl J Med. 2014;370:1412–21 [C].

[4] Cheng HC, Chang WL, Chen WY, et al. Intravenous albumin shortens the duration of hospitalization for patients with hypoalbuminemia and bleeding peptic ulcers: a pilot study. Dig Dis Sci. 2013;58:3232–41 [c].

[5] Rochwerg B, Alhazzani W, Sindi A, et al. Fluid resuscitation in sepsis. Ann Intern Med. 2014;161:347–55 [M].

[6] Patel A, Laffan MA, Waheed U, et al. Randomized trials of human albumin for adults with sepsis: systematic review and meta-analysis with trial sequential analysis of all-cause mortality. BMJ. 2014;349:g4561 [M].

[7] Kwok CS, Krupa L, Mahtani A, et al. Albumin reduces paracentesis-induced circulatory dysfunction and reduces death and renal impairment among patients with cirrhosis and infection; a systematic review and meta-analysis. Biomed Res Int. 2013;2013: 295153:1–8 [M].

[8] Polito C, Martin GS. Albumin physiologic and clinical effects on lung function. Minerva Anestesiol. 2013;79(10):1180–6 [r].

[9] Komericki P, Grims RH, Aberer W, et al. Near-fatal anaphylaxis caused by human serum albumin in fibrinogen and erythrocyte concentrations. Anaesthesia. 2014;69:176–8 [A].

[10] Kitsios GD, Mascari P, Ettunsi R, et al. Co-administration of furosemide with albumin for overcoming diuretic resistance in patients with hypoalbuminemia: a meta-analysis. J Crit Care. 2014;29(2):253–9 [M].

[11] Possible risks of blood transfusions. American Cancer Society. Last updated 7 October 2013 http://www.cancer.org/treatment/treatmentsandsideeffects/treatmenttypes/bloodproductdonationandtransfusion/blood-product-donation-and-transfusion-possible-transfusion-risks [S].

[12] Goodnough LT, Maggio P, Hadhazy E, et al. Restrictive blood transfusion practices are associated with improved patient outcomes. Transfusion. 2014;54(10):2753–9 [c].

[13] Jain A, Kaur R. Hemovigilance and blood safety. Asian J Transfus Sci. 2012;6(2):137–8 [r].

[14] Carson JL, Sieber F, Cook DR, et al. Liberal versus restrictive blood transfusion strategy: 3-year survival and cause of death results from the FOCUS randomised controlled trial. Lancet. 2015;385:1183–9 [C].

[15] Goodnough LT, Levy JH, Murphy MF. Concepts of blood transfusion in adults. Lancet. 2013;381(9880):1845–54 [R].

[16] Classification and incidence of adverse transfusion reactions. Australian Red Cross Blood Service. Last updated: 19 January, 2015. http://www.transfusion.com.au/adverse_transfusion_reactions/classification_and_incidence [r].

[17] Lieberman L, Petraszko T, Hannach B, et al. Transfusion-related lung injury in children: a case series and review of literature. Transfusion. 2014;54(1):57–64 [c].

[18] Weinstein R. Clinical practice guide on red blood cell transfusion. Ann Intern Med. 2012;157:49–58 [S].

[19] AuBuchon JP. TRALI: reducing its risk while trying to understand its causes. Transfusion. 2014;54:3021–5 [r].

[20] US Food and Drug Administration (FDA). Fatalities reported to FDA following blood collection and transfusion: annual summary for fiscal year 2012. FDA, Updated March 2014 [S].

[21] Frenette PS, Mohandas N. Bad blood: a trigger for TRALI. Nat Med. 2010;16(4):382–3 [c].

[22] Sait S, Zaghloul N, Patel A, et al. Transfusion related iron overload in pediatric oncology patients treated at a tertiary care center and treatment with chelation therapy. Pediatr Blood Cancer. 2014;61(12):2319–20 [c].

[23] Shander A, Javidroozi M, Naqvi S, et al. An update on mortality and morbidity in patients with very low postoperative hemoglobin levels who decline blood transfusion. Transfusion. 2014;54(10 Pt 2):2688–95 [c].

[24] Curtis BR. Drug-induced immune neutropenia/agranulocytosis. Immunohematology. 2014;30(2):95–101 [H].

[25] Raad II, Chaftari AM, Shuaibi Al, et al. Granulocyte transfusions in hematologic malignancy patients with invasive pulmonary aspergillosis: outcomes and complications. Ann Oncol. 2013;24(7):1873–9 [c].

[26] Holbro A, Infanti L, Sigle J, et al. Platelet transfusion: basic aspects. Swiss Med Wkly. 2013;143:1–10 [c].

[27] Editorial. Blood transfusions: optimizing resources. Lancet Haematol. 2014;1:85e [r].

[28] Cohn CS, Stubbs J, Schwartz J, et al. A comparison of adverse reaction rates for PAS C versus plasma platelet units. Transfusion. 2014;54(8):1927–34 [c].

[29] Cabrales P, Intaglietta M. Blood substitutes: evolution from non-carrying to oxygen and gas carrying fluids. ASAIO J. 2013;59(4):337–54 [r].

[30] Hemelrijck JV, Levien L, Veeckman L, et al. A safety and efficacy evaluation of hemoglobin-based oxygen carrier HBOC-201 in a randomized, multicenter, red blood cell controlled trial in noncardiac surgery patients. Anesth Analg. 2014;119:766–76 [c].

[31] Abbate A, Van Tassell BW, Christopher S, et al. Effects of prolastin C (plasma-derived alpha-1 antitrypsin) on the acute inflammatory response in patients with ST-segment elevation myocardial infarction (from the VCU-alpha 1-RT pilot study). Am J Cardiol. 2015;115:8–12 [c].

[32] Bork K, Steffensen I, Machnig T. Treatment with C1-esterase inhibitor concentrate in type I or II hereditary angioedema: a systematic literature review. Allergy Asthma Proc. 2013;34(4):312–27 [R].

[33] Kalaria S, Craig T. Assessment of hereditary angioedema treatment risks. Allergy Asthma Proc. 2013;34(6):519–22 [c].

[34] Bernstein JA, Manning ME, Li H, et al. Escalating doses of C1 esterase inhibitor (CINRYZE) for prophylaxis in patients with hereditary angioedema. J Allergy Clin Immunol Pract. 2014;2(1):77–84 [c].

[35] Nascimento B, Goodnough LT, Levy JH. Cryoprecipitate therapy. Br J Anaesth. 2014;113(6):922–34 [r].

[36] Besser M. The efficacy and safety or cryoprecipitate in the treatment of acquired hypofibrinogenaemia. Br J Haematol. 2014;166:449–67 [c].

[37] Kato H, Uruma M, Okuyama Y, et al. Incidence of transfusion-related adverse reactions per patient reflects the potential risk of transfusion therapy in Japan. Am J Clin Pathol. 2013; 140:219–24 [R].

[38] Winstedt D, Hanna J, Schott U. Albumin-induced coagulopathy is less severe and more effectively reversed with fibrinogen concentrate than is synthetic colloid induced coagulopathy. Scand J Clin Lab Invest. 2013;73:161–9 [E].

[39] Annane D, Siami S, Jaber S, et al. Effects of fluid resuscitation with colloids vs crystalloids on mortality in critically ill patients presenting with hypovolemic shock. JAMA. 2013;310(17): 1809–17 [C].

[40] Mercier FJ, Diemunsch P, Ducloy-Bouthors AS, et al. 6% Hydroxyethyl starch (130/0.4) vs Ringer's lactate preloading before spinal anaesthesia for caesarena delivery: the randomized, double-blind, multicenter CAESAR trial. Br J Anaesth. 2014;113(3): 459–67 [c].

[41] Van der Linden P, De Ville A, Hofer A, et al. Six percent hydroxyethyl starch 130/0.4 versus 5% human serum albumin for volume replacement therapy during elective open-heart surgery in pediatric patients. Anesthesiology. 2013;119:1296–309 [c].

[42] Rasmussen KC, Johansson PI, Hojskov M, et al. Hydroxyethyl starch reduces coagulation competence and increases blood loss during major surgery. Ann Surg. 2014;259:249–54 [c].

[43] Skhirtladze K, Base EM, Kassnigg A, et al. Comparison of the effects of albumin 5%, hydroxyethyl starch 130/0.4 6%, and Ringer's lactate on blood loss and coagulation after cardiac surgery. Br J Anaesth. 2014;112(2):255–64 [c].

[44] Haase N, Wettersev W, Winkel P, et al. Bleeding and risk of death with hydroxyethyl starch in severe sepsis: post hoc analysis of a randomized clinical trial. Intensive Care Med. 2013;39:2126–34 [c].

[45] Ishihara H. Kidney function after the intraoperative use of 6% tetrastarches (HES 130/0.4 and 0.42). J Anesth. 2014;28:249–56 [r].

[46] Lomivorotov VV, Fominskiy EV, Efremov SM, et al. Infusion of 7.2% NACL/6% hydroxyethyl starch 200/0.5 in on-pump coronary artery bypass surgery patients: a randomized, single-blind pilot study. Shock. 2014;41(3):193–9 [c].

[47] Neto AS, Veelo DP, Peireira VGM, et al. Fluid resuscitation with hydroxyethyl starches in patients with sepsis is associated with an

increased incidence of acute kidney injury and use of renal replacement therapy: a systematic review and meta-analysis of the literature. J Crit Care. 2014;29:185e1–7 [R].

[48] Stander S, Richter L, Osada N, et al. Hydroxyethyl starch-induced pruritus: clinical characteristics and influence of dose, molecular weight, and substitution. Acta Derm Venereol. 2014;94:282–7 [A].

[49] Saeedian M, Randhawa I. Immunoglobulin replacement therapy: a twenty year review and current update. Int Arch Allergy Immunol. 2014;164:151–66 [R].

[50] Berger M. Adverse effects of IgG therapy. J Allergy Clin Immunol Pract. 2013;1(6):558–66 [R].

[51] Stiehm ER. Adverse effects of human immunoglobulin therapy. Transfus Med Rev. 2013;27:171–8 [R].

[52] Carrock Sewell WA, Kerr J, Bejr-Gross ME, et al. European consensus proposal for immunoglobulin therapies. Eur J Immunol. 2014;44:2207–14 [R].

[53] Palabrica FRF, Kwong SL, Padua FR. Adverse events of intravenous immunoglobulin infusions: a ten year retrospective study. Asia Pac Allergy. 2013;3:249–56 [c].

[54] Bichuetti-Silva DC, Furlan FP, Nobre FA, et al. Immediate infusion-related adverse reaction to intravenous immunoglobulin in a prospective cohort of 1765 infusion. Int Immunopharmacol. 2014;23:442–6 [c].

[55] Ohlsson A, Lacy JB. Intravenous immunoglobulin for suspected or proven infection in neonates, Cochrane Database Syst Rev. 2013;(7), http://onlinelibrary.wiley.com/doi/10.1002/14651858.CD001239.pub4/abstract;jsessionid=3DBE6ED71D2AABCECB07BBB2CFCA744F.f03t03. Art. No.: CD001239. [R].

[56] Alejandria M, Lansang MAD, Dans LF, et al. Intravenous immunoglobulin for treating sepsis, severe sepsis and septic shock, Cochrane Database Syst Rev. 2013;(9), http://www.update-software.com/pdf/CD001090.pdf. Art. No.: CD001090. [R].

[57] Hughes RAC, Swan AV, van Doorn PA. Intravenous immunoglobulin for Guillain-Barré syndrome, Cochrane Database Syst Rev. 2014;(9), http://onlinelibrary.wiley.com/doi/10.1002/14651858.CD002063.pub6/otherversions. Art. No.: CD002063. [R].

[58] Ramirez E, Romero-Garrido JA, Lopez-Grandos E, et al. Symptomatic thromboembolic events in patients treated with intravenous-immunoglobulins: results from a retrospective cohort study. Thromb Res. 2014;133:1045–51 [C].

[59] Markvardsen LH, Christiansen I, Harbo T, et al. Hemolytic anemia following high dose intravenous immunoglobulin in patients with chronic neurologic disorders. Eur J Neurol. 2014;21:147–52 [c].

[60] Mainra R, Xu. Q, Chibbar R, et al. Severe antibody-mediated rejection following IVIG infusion in a kidney transplant recipient with BK-virus nephropathy. Transpl Immunol. 2013;28:145–7 [A].

[61] Hurelbrink CB, Spies JM, Yiannikas C. Significant dermatological side effects of intravenous immunoglobulin. J Clin Neurosci. 2013;20:1114–6 [A].

[62] Miyamoto J, Bockle BC, Zillikens D, et al. Eczematous reaction to intravenous immunoglobulin: an alternative cause of eczema. JAMA Dermatol. 2014;150(10):1120–1 [A].

[63] Nobre FA, da Silva Gonzalez IG, Simao RM, et al. Antibody levels to tetanus, diphtheria, measles, and varicella in patients with primary immunodeficiency undergoing intravenous immunoglobulin therapy: a prospective study. BMC Immunol. 2014;14:26 [c].

[64] Wasserman RL. A new intravenous immunoglobulin (BIVIGAM®) for primary humoral immunodeficiency. Expert Rev Clin Immunol. 2014;10(3):325–37 [r].

[65] Dantal J. Intravenous immunoglobulins: in-depth review of excipients and acute kidney injury. Am J Nephrol. 2013;38:275–84 [r].

[66] Kanegene H, Imai K, Yamada M, et al. Efficacy and safety of the IgPro20, a subcutaneous immunoglobulin in Japanese patients with primary immunodeficiency diseases. J Clin Immunol. 2014;34:204–11 [c].

[67] Datta R, Kuruvilla M, Gill M, et al. Association of skin necrosis with subcutaneous immunoglobulin therapy. Ann Allergy Asthma Immunol. 2014;113:227–38 [A].

[68] Qureshi H, Massey E, Kirwam D, et al. BCSH guideline for the use of Anti-D immunoglobulin for the prevention of haemolytic disease of the fetus and newborn. Transfus Med. 2014;24(1):8–20 [R].

[69] Thompson JC, Klima J, Despotovic JM, et al. Anti-D immunoglobulin therapy for pediatric ITP: before and after the FDA's black Box warning. Pediatr Blood Cancer. 2014;60:E149–E151 [c].

[70] Kaufman RM, Schlumpf KS, Wright DJ, et al. Does Rh immune globulin suppress HLA sensitization in pregnancy? Transfusion. 2013;53(9):2069–77 [c].

[71] Rutkowski K, Nasser SM. Management of hypersensitivity reactions to Anti-D immunoglobulin preparations. Allergy. 2014;69:1560–3 [A].

[72] Holmes A, Wright D. Potential drug interaction between Rho(D) immune globulin and live virus vaccine. Nurs Womens Health. 2014 Dec;18(6):519–22 [r].

[73] Aubron C, Reade MC, Fraser JF, et al. Efficacy and safety of fibrinogen concentrate in trauma patients—a systemic review. J Crit Care. 2014;29(3):471.e11–7 [R].

[74] Lima-Oliveira G, Salvagno LG, Lippi G, et al. Could light meal jeopardize laboratory coagulation tests? Biochem Med. 2014;24(3):343–9 [c].

[75] Gabay M, Boucher BA. An essential primer for understanding the role of topical hemostats, surgical sealants, and adhesives for maintaining hemostasis. Pharmacotherapy. 2013;33(9):935–55 [R].

[76] Franchini M, Crestani S, Frattini F, et al. Hemostatic agents for bleeding: recombinant-activated Factor VII and beyond. Semin Thromb Hemost. doi: http://dx.doi.org/10.1055/s-0034-1381234. ISSN 0094-6176 [c].

[77] WHO. WHO recommendations for the prevention and treatment of postpartum hemorrhage; http://apps.who.int/iris/bitstream/10665/75411/1/9789241548502_eng.pdf [S].

[78] Shapiro AD, Neufeld EJ, Blanchette V, et al. Safety of recombinant activated factor VII (rFVIIa) in patients with congenital haemophilia with inhibitors: overall rFVIIa exposure and intervals following high (>240 μg kg^{-1}) rFVIIa doses across clinical trials and registries. Haemophilia. 2014;20(1):e23–31 [R].

[79] Samai A, Monlezun D, Shaban A, et al. Von Willebrand factor drives the association between elevated factor VIII and poor outcomes in patients with ischemic stroke. Stroke. 2014;45(9):2789–91 [E].

[80] Collins PW, Young G, Knobe K, et al. Recombinant long-acting glycoPEGylated factor IX in Hemophilia B: a multinational randomized phase 3 trial. Blood. 2014;124(26):3880–6 [C].

[81] Nathwani AC, Reiss UM, Tuddenham EGD, et al. Long-term safety and efficacy of factor IX gene therapy in Hemophilia B. N Engl J Med. 2014;371:1994–2004 [c].

[82] Song HK, Tibayan FA, Kahl EA, et al. Safety and efficacy of prothrombin complex concentrates for the treatment of coagulopathy after cardiac surgery. J Thorac Cardiovasc Surg. 2014;147(3):1036–40 [C].

[83] Chapman SA, Irwin ED, Abou-Karam N, et al. Comparison of 3-factor prothrombin complex concentrate and low-dose recombinant factor VIIA for warfarin reversal. World J Emerg Surg. 2014;9:27 [c].

[84] Martínez-Calle N, Marcos-Jubilar M, Alfonso A, et al. Safety and efficacy of a prothrombin complex concentrate in patients with

coagulopathy and hemorrhage. An Sist Sanit Navar. 2014;37(3):363–9 [c].

[85] Sarode R, Milling TJ, Refaai M, et al. Efficacy and safety of a 4-factor prothrombin complex concentrate in patients on vitamin K antagonists presenting with major bleeding a randomized, plasma-controlled, phase IIIb study. Circulation. 2013;128:1234–43 [C].

[86] Oldenburg J, Jimenez-Yuste V, Peiro-Jordan R, et al. Primary and rescue immune tolerance induction in children and adults: a multicentre international study with a VWF-containing plasma-derived FVIII concentrate. Haemophilia. 2014;20:83–91 [c].

[87] Mannucci P, Kempton C, Millar C, et al. Pharmacokinetics and safety of a novel recombinant human von Willebrand factor manufactured with a plasma-free method: a prospective clinical trial. Blood. 2013;122(5):648–57 [C].

[88] Palmer SC, Saglimbene V, Mavridis D, et al. Erythropoiesis-stimulating agents for anaemia in adults with chronic kidney disease: a network meta-analysis (review). Cochrane Database Syst Rev. 2014;12:1–179 [R].

[89] Mitchell WB, Bussel JB. Thrombopoietin receptor agonists: a critical review. Semin Hematol. 2015;52(1):46–52 [r].

[90] Katsutani S, Tomiyama Y, Kimura A, et al. Oral eltrombopag for up to three years is safe and well-tolerated in Japanese patients with previously treated chronic immune thrombocytopenia: an open-label, extension study. Int J Hematol. 2013;98:323–30 [c].

[91] Moulis G, Bagheri H, Sailler L, et al. Are adverse drug reaction patients different between romiplostim and eltrombopag? 2009–2013 French PharmacoVigilance assessment. Eur J Intern Med. 2014;24:777–80 [R].

[92] Prica A, Sholzberg M, Buckstein R. Safety and efficacy of thrombopoietin-receptor agonists in myelodysplastic syndromes: a systematic review and meta-analysis of randomized controlled trials. Br J Haematol. 2014;167:626–38 [C].

[93] Ghanima W, Geyer JT, Lee CS, et al. Bone marrow fibrosis in 66 patients with immune thrombocytopenia treated with thrombopoietin-receptor agonists: a single-center long-term follow-up. Haematologica. 2014;99(5):937–44 [M].

[94] Braunstein I, Wanat KA, Elenitsas R, et al. Eltrombopag-associated hyperpigmentation. JAMA Dermatol. 2013;149(9):1112–5 [A].

[95] Decroocq J, Marcellin L, Le Ray C, et al. Rescue therapy with romiplostim for refractory primary immune thrombocytopenia during pregnancy. Obstet Gynecol. 2014;124:481–3 [A].

[96] Cardamone D, Milone MC, Glaser L, et al. Eltrombopag and serum of a different hue. Arch Pathol Lab Med. 2013;137:1175 [A].

[97] Stramer SL. Current perspectives in transfusion-transmitted infectious disease: emerging and re-emerging infectious. ISBT Sci Ser. 2014;9:30–6 [r].

[98] Ginzburg Y, Kessler D, Kang S, et al. Why has *Borrelia burgdorferi* not been transmitted by blood transfusion? Transfusion. 2014;53:2822–6 [H].

[99] Gan VCH, Leo YS. Current epidemiology and clinical practice in arboviral infections-implications on blood supply in south-east Asia. ISBT Sci Ser. 2014;9:262–7 [r].

[100] Musso D, Nhan T, Robin E, et al. Potential for zika virus transmission through blood transfusion demonstrated during an outbreak in French Polynesia, November 2013 to February 2014. Euro Surveill. 2014;19(14):1–3 [c].

[101] Biceroglu SU, Turhan A, Doskaya AD, et al. Probable hepatitis C virus transmission from a seronegative blood donor via cellular blood products. Blood Transfus. 2014;12(supple 1):s69–70 [A].

[102] Hewitt PE, Ijaz S, Brailsford SR, et al. Hepatitis E virus in blood components: a prevalence and transmission study in southeast England. Lancet. 2014;384:1766–73 [R].

[103] Xu C, Wang RY, Schechterly CA, et al. An assessment of hepatitis E virus in the US blood donors and recipients: no detectable HEV RNA in the 1939 donors tested and no evidence for HEV transmission to the 36 prospectively followed recipients. Transfusion. 2013;53(10 Pt 2):2505–11 [R].

[104] Yang H, Gregori L, Asher DM, et al. Risk assessment for transmission of variant Creutzfeldt-Jakob disease by transfusion of red blood cells in the United States. Transfusion. 2014;54:2194–201 [r].

[105] Xiaoxia S, Wei G, Dexue L, et al. Clinical observation of 32 cases with transplantation of autologous bone marrow stem cells on diabetes and its complications. Pak J Pharm Sci. 2014;27(6 Suppl):2083–5 [c].

[106] Bento LR, Ortiz E, Nicola EM, et al. Sinonasal disorders in hematopoietic stem cell transplantation. Braz J Otorhinolaryngol. 2014;80(4):285–9 [c].

[107] Genberg M, Öberg A, Andrén B, et al. Cardiac function after hematopoietic cell transplantation: an echocardiographic cross-sectional study in young adults treated in childhood. Pediatr Blood Cancer. 2015;62(1):143–7 [c].

34

Drugs That Affect Blood Coagulation, Fibrinolysis and Hemostasis

Michelle J. Taylor, Tahir Mehmood, Justin D. Kreuter[1]

Department of Laboratory Medicine and Pathology, Mayo Clinic, Rochester, MN, USA

[1]Corresponding author: kreuter.justin@mayo.edu

COUMARIN ANTICOAGULANTS [SED-15, 983; SEDA-34, 541; SEDA-35, 617; SEDA-36, 529]

Cardiovascular

Researchers analyzed a UK clinical practice research database, Datalink, and identified a total of 5519 patients who had stroke following a diagnosis of atrial fibrillation (70766 patients) between January 1, 1993 and December 31, 2008. The observational nested case–control analysis followed the patients for up to 16 years until ischemic stroke, death, or end of registration. The group used logistic regression to estimate the rate of stroke associated with and without current warfarin use. Compared to matched controls not taking warfarin, it was found that warfarin use was associated with a 71% increased risk of stroke in the first 30 days following treatment initiation (rate ratio 1.71 (95% confidence interval 1.39–2.12)), changing to a 50% reduction between days 31 and 90 (RR: 0.50, 95% CI: 0.34–0.75), then reduced by 45% beyond 90 days (RR: 0.55, 95% CI: 0.50–0.61). The authors noted that the increased stroke risk may stem from inadequate warfarin control, but because INR data were not consistently recorded in the database, this was only hypothesis-generating [1c].

An 85-year-old woman in atrial fibrillation presented with acute right middle cerebral artery infarct and underwent thrombolysis with tissue plasminogen activator. She was started on warfarin with enoxaparin bridging and was sent home. Three weeks after discharge, she developed fever, myalgia in the lower limbs, and a red macular rash on the shins and calves with painful purple discoloration of the toes and soles of the feet. Distal pulses were intact and capillary refill was normal. She had prolonged INR with new onset renal impairment. There was no evidence of thrombosis and normal arterial flow on Doppler. She was diagnosed with purple toe syndrome and cholesterol embolization syndrome secondary to oral anticoagulation. Warfarin was discontinued and enoxaparin (40 mg subcutaneous injection) was started. The INR lowered after 36 hours and she developed pregangrenous changes over the left great toe. She ultimately died from renal failure and sepsis. It is felt that her INR and thrombolysis that preceded the warfarin treatment were likely the precipitating factors for plaque destabilization and cholesterol embolization as well as purple toe syndrome [2A].

An 84-year-old female with a history of antiphospholipid antibody syndrome and bilateral lower extremity amputations receiving warfarin presented to the emergency department with bilateral necrotic changes over her arms and legs. Six days prior to admission, her INR was 6.04 and on admission her INR was 3.63. Warfarin was discontinued due to suspected involvement. She was diagnosed with warfarin-induced venous limb gangrene, which can present in the distal extremities with a paradoxical supratherapeutic INR (attributable to the concurrent depletion of protein C) in patients with hypercoagulable states such as antiphospholipid antibody syndrome and heparin-induced thrombocytopenia [3A].

HEPARINS [SED-15, 1590; SEDA-34, 543; SEDA-35, 618; SEDA-36, 530]

Hematologic

The global orthopedic registry was reviewed to identify patients who received either warfarin or

© 2015 Elsevier B.V. All rights reserved.

low-molecular-weight heparin for venous thromboembolism prophylaxis after hip or knee replacement surgery. Out of 15020 patients in the GLORY registry, 3775 patients were reviewed for rates of thromboembolism, infection, and other complications. 2194 patients received warfarin and 1561 received low-molecular-weight heparin. Warfarin was taken either preoperatively (40.0%) or within 24 hours postoperatively (60.0%) whereas low-molecular-weight heparin was administered in 81.0% of cases from 7 to 36 hours following surgery. A large portion of each group also received elastic stockings and/or intermittent pneumatic compression devices (85.0% of warfarin patients and 93.0% of low-molecular-weight heparin patients). The patients included in the study underwent elective primary total hip or knee arthroplasty, and had up to 90-day follow-up after discharge. Warfarin was used more frequently for hip arthroplasty with longer duration in patients with more preexisting comorbidities. Patients who received low-molecular-weight heparin had significantly higher rates of bleeding (6.2% vs. 2.1%), blood transfusion (29.4% vs. 22.0%), reoperation (2.4% vs. 1.3%), and infections (1.6% vs. 0.6%). However, propensity score-weighted analyses showed no differences in venous thromboembolism complications [4R].

In a retrospective single-center case series, five patients developed unexpectedly high partial thromboplastin times after receiving unfractionated heparin thromboprophylaxis following head and neck cancer surgery. All five patients received subcutaneous low-dose unfractionated heparin (SC-LDUH), 5000 units, three times daily, had a body mass index $\leq 20 \, kg/m^2$ and four had reduced kidney function (GFR 25–54 mL/min). The fifth patient had a GFR of 63 mL/min. Normal PTTs were observed at baseline, and were prolonged after surgery with a median of 90.0 seconds (ranging 52.8–127.0 seconds), which normalized with discontinuation of heparin. Bleeding complications associated with prolongation of the PTT was seen in 4 of the 5 patients, 3 developing a surgical site hematoma, 2 requiring operative drainage, and 1 requiring emergent reintubation. It was felt that the combination of TID dosing, low BMI, and impaired renal function led to increased risk of bleeding complications from SC-LDUH thromboprophylaxis [5c].

A 61-year-old male presented to the emergency department in acute respiratory distress requiring respiratory support and ventilation. He was diagnosed with a non-ST-segment elevation myocardial infarction and a left internal jugular central line was placed, through which heparin and vasopressors were initiated. After primary PCI, during which the placement of an intra-aortic balloon pump was required, the patient was noted to have a left parietal infarct on head CT. The patient's condition continued to deteriorate and a repeat CT scan revealed hemorrhagic conversion within the parietal infarct. The central line waveform was noted to be abnormal and a blood sample obtained through the central line found the oxygen saturation to be 95%. Repeat imaging confirmed that the central line catheter tip was located in the carotid artery. The misplaced central line was removed; however, the patient ultimately expired [6A].

Skin

An 83-year-old female with known chronic kidney disease was receiving thromboprophylaxis with subcutaneous nadroparin calcium, when she developed subcutaneous nodules at the injection sites. The diagnosis of subcutis calcinosis was confirmed by histological evaluation, which revealed calcium deposition in the dermis and hypodermis. The injections were discontinued and the lesions resolved. Several case reports exist in the literature, and should be kept in mind in patients with advanced kidney disease on calcium containing low-molecular-weight heparins [7A].

Immunologic

A 50-year-old male with work-related trauma was treated with open reduction and internal fixation and later developed chronic osteomyelitis and hardware infection. He was scheduled for thigh flap of chronic wound. Intraoperative, despite Doppler confirmation of flow, the flap appeared congested. Heparin drip and heparin soaks were initiated. The flap was re-explored and multiple venous and arterial thrombi were identified. Tissue plasminogen activator (tPA) was initiated and 3 days later, the flap was noted to be compromised and multiple thrombosis were identified. Multiple attempts were made to reestablish vascular flow to the flap. Ultimately, hematology was consulted to assess for subclinical coagulopathy and a positive result for heparin-PF4 antibodies was discovered. A diagnosis of heparin induced thrombocytopenia was made and the patient was transitioned off heparin. Literature review revealed 113 possible articles to be included, a total of 6 met inclusion criteria representing 477 patients. Of those cases, they identified 5 individual cases of heparin induced thrombocytopenia in a total of 8 flaps. The characteristics of the affected flaps included malperfusion, decreased Doppler signal, venous congestion, arterial thrombosis, and frank necrosis. The timing to flap failure ranged from post-operative day 1 to post-operative day 5 [8R].

A 62-year-old male with open comminuted distal tibial/fibula fracture underwent surgery with free gracilis muscle flap reconstruction; he had been receiving prophylactic subcutaneous unfractionated heparin 5000 IU twice daily. Post operatively, the flap showed signs of ischemia and the decision was made to re-explore.

Although the vein was patent the artery was thrombosed with no flow and the artery was washed and flushed with 5000 IU of intravenous heparin. Post-operatively the flap showed signs of failure and on re-operation the flap was removed. Repeat CT showed occlusion of the posterior tibial artery and the platelet count was decreasing. Heparin was discontinued, danaparoid was initiated, and the platelet count returned to within normal limits 3 days after the heparin was stopped [9A].

A 60-year-old male had a bilateral total knee replacement complicated by pulmonary embolism, and was treated with unfractionated heparin followed by dalteparin and warfarin at the time of discharge. Subsequently, he presented with fever, malaise, hypotension, diffuse abdominal pain, and he was noted to have bullous skin necrosis at the site of dalteparin injections. Post operatively, his symptoms progressed and he was found to have bilateral adrenal hemorrhage. Throughout his hospitalization his platelet count trended downward and heparin induced thrombocytopenia antibody and serotonin release assay were positive, confirming the diagnosis of adrenal hemorrhage secondary to heparin. He was transitioned to fondaparinux and recovered [10A].

A 33-year-old female with a mechanical prosthetic valve in the mitral position had been well controlled on warfarin and was admitted to the hospital due to pregnancy. After admission, IV heparin was started and warfarin was discontinued. She developed dyspnea with pulmonary congestion on X-ray 7 days after admission. Additionally, she had a diastolic rumble suggesting prosthetic valve stenosis. Transesophageal echocardiography revealed thrombus formation on the mitral prosthetic valve. After thrombolytic therapy with increased heparin dose, the thrombus increased in size. Heparin was replaced with argatroban and a mitral valve replacement was successfully performed. The patient was found to be positive for heparin antibodies and a diagnosis of HIT type II was made [11A].

A 72-year-old man being followed for a 6 cm asymptomatic abdominal aortic aneurysm had received low-molecular-weight heparin, followed by vitamin K antagonist, initiated 6 months earlier for a pulmonary embolism. Upon admission for elective endovascular aortic repair, he was placed on low-molecular-weight heparin. After successful graft placement, his postoperative course was uneventful, his platelet count was $160 \times 10^9/L$, and he was discharged. Low-molecular-weight heparin was maintained post-operatively and vitamin K antagonist was to be started on post-operative day 15. On post-operative day 10 he presented to the emergency department with bilateral lower limb ischemia, no femoral pulses, complete paralysis, and loss of sensation. His platelet count was noted to be $37 \times 10^9/L$ and he was positive for heparin antibodies, heparin

was discontinued and he was switched to danaparoid and emergent surgical conversion was performed. He received danaparoid throughout the procedure and at discharge and ultimately was discharged with a platelet count of $141 \times 10^9/L$. He re-presented on post-operative day 20 with subacute left limb ischemia and a platelet count of $59 \times 10^9/L$. Clots in the left popliteal artery were removed, followed by *in situ* alteplase fibrinolysis, and the post-operative course was uneventful. It was felt that cross reactivity of danaparoid with heparin immune complexes was the causes of the ischemia. Fondaparinux was used as a replacement when danaparoid was discontinued. Although rare cases of cross-reactivity to danaparoid have been reported, he was not tested for heparin-induced PF4 antibodies. His platelet count increased to $115 \times 10^9/L$ within 2 days and he was ultimately prescribed vitamin K antagonists and aspirin after discharge [12A].

A 51-year-old man presented with severe aortic stenosis and coronary artery disease for which the patient was scheduled for aortic valve replacement and coronary artery bypass graft. Prior to surgery, he was started on aspirin and low-molecular-weight heparin. Heparin coated, minimal extracorporeal circulation (CPB) was used, which was instituted after administration of unfractionated heparin, which resulted in an ACT of 309 seconds. Per institutional protocol, if the ACT was higher than the target range of 250–300 seconds, a tranexamic acid 10 mg/kg bolus, followed by 1 mg/kg/h was continued during CPB. After completion of CABG, subsequent aortic valve replacement was initiated, and another 10 000 IU of unfractionated heparin was added to keep the ACT in target range. The surgeon noted clotting at the valve prosthesis and an additional 10 000 IU of UFH and 1000 IU of antithrombin were given, which increased the ACT to 391 seconds. Upon repeat TEE, a new, large left ventricular thrombus was noted when weaning from cardiopulmonary bypass and the patient was screened for risk factors and found to be positive for PF4/heparin antibodies. Argatroban was initiated and maintained at a dose that increased the activated partial thromboplastin time to 45–50 seconds. Ultimately, the patient was switched to fondaparinux and recovered fully [13A].

A 64-year-old man was scheduled for elective catheter-directed ablation for his atrial fibrillation. He had been placed on warfarin anticoagulation after a cardioembolic cerebellar stroke, and received 6 days of dalteparin as bridging anticoagulation for a colonoscopy 5 months prior to his elective ablation procedure. The day prior to the procedure, he received one dose of dalteparin. During the procedure, unfractionated heparin was administered. Midway through ablation, he was noted to have fibrin strands attached to the ablation catheter, despite activated clotting time levels of mid to high 300 seconds and INR of 2.6; the procedure was aborted and the ablation catheter safely removed. The following day, the platelet count had decreased to a nadir of 118. Antibodies to heparin were strongly positive with an inhibitor and the diagnosis of heparin-induced thrombocytopenia was made. Compared to unfractionated heparin, the risk of developing heparin-induced thrombocytopenia with low-molecular-weight heparin is lower; however, the risk still exists and this case illustrates the development within 24 hours after heparin re-exposure. The patient completely recovered [14A].

A 62-year-old female with a history of complicated femur fracture and previous plate osteosynthesis underwent surgery to replace fractured femur nail. Postoperatively, she suffered a severe myocardial infarction involving lesions in three vessels. The patient developed cardiogenic shock and required cardiopulmonary resuscitation, and was stabilized with the placement of an intra-aortic balloon pump. She then developed acute renal failure and sepsis and although intra-aortic balloon had to be removed due to poor limb perfusion, the cardiogenic shock persisted and the patient was placed on extracorporeal membrane oxygenation (ECMO) with argatroban anticoagulation. On the first day on ECMO, she decompensated due to colonic necrosis requiring emergency bedside hemicolectomy and was noted to have spontaneous bleeding with a platelet count of 6×10^9/L. Heparin induced thrombocytopenia was suspected and confirmed by antibody testing. ECMO weaning began as the inner surfaces of modern ECMO systems are coated with heparin. HIT antibodies decreased and thrombocytopenia resolved with ECMO discontinuation. Unfortunately, the patient died 5 weeks later [15A].

A 56-year-old woman with 4 days of progressive dyspnea presented 14 days after total abdominal hysterectomy and bilateral salpingo-oophorectomy. During her initial stay at the institution, she received 2 days of subcutaneous unfractionated heparin post-operatively. At time of presentation for dyspnea, she underwent spiral computed tomography and was diagnosed with segmental pulmonary embolism and given a heparin bolus and started on a heparin drip. Five minutes after the infusion the patient became flushed with worsening dyspnea. She experienced a drop in blood pressure; she developed agonal respirations and went into cardiac arrest. Heparin was immediately discontinued and the advanced cardiac life support was started. Laboratory results showed a significant drop in platelets (nadir of 57×10^9/mL) and ELISA and serotonin release assays confirmed the presence of a PF4/heparin antibody and the patient was diagnosed with HIT-associated anaphylactoid reaction. With supportive management, including anticoagulation with argatroban, she successfully recovered [16A].

DIRECT THROMBIN INHIBITORS
[SED-15, 1142; SEDA-34, 544; SEDA-35, 619; SEDA-36, 531]

Dabigatran [SEDA-34, 544; SEDA-35, 620; SEDA-36, 531]

Cardiovascular

Two cases of mechanical valve thrombosis due to dabigatran were described. The first was a 72-year-old woman with a history of atrial fibrillation and remote history of mitral valve replacement that had recently been switched from acenocoumarol to dabigatran because of a single INR result of >5 (one of several national subsidized health care criteria for coverage of a non-warfarin anticoagulant prescription). She then presented with dysarthria and mild hemiparesis, was diagnosed with stroke, no cardiology consultation was sought, and she continued to receive dabigatran. She later presented with pulmonary edema and shock and was found to have a thrombus obstructing the mitral valve. The second case is that of a 73-year-old woman who was switched to dabigatran from warfarin with a history of mitral valve replacement, paroxysmal atrial fibrillation, and gastrointestinal bleeding. After switching therapy, she presented with pulmonary edema and cardiogenic shock and was found to have a thrombus obstructing the mitral valve leaflets. Both women died of complications. In both situations, it was felt that the likely cause was dabigatran therapy. Other reports of mechanical heart valve thrombosis occurring while on non-warfarin anticoagulation and the then-ongoing Phase II RE-ALIGN dabigatran 'heart valve' trial are also discussed [17A].

Hematologic

In a meta-analysis, five randomized controlled trials were reviewed to evaluate the bleeding risk with dabigatran compared to warfarin. Included in the meta-analysis were randomized controlled trials where treatment duration was ≥90 days. 18 615 patients had atrial fibrillation and 7998 patients had venous thromboembolism. Pooling data across the 4 trials with non-overlapping patient populations revealed that dabigatran was not associated with major risk of bleeding. However, when compared with vitamin K antagonists, dabigatran was associated with an increased risk of GI bleeding. Findings from the meta-analysis suggested that, compared to warfarin, dabigatran was associated with a 50% increased risk of GI bleeding, which was consistent across the two trials that evaluated GI bleeding as an outcome. In contrast, compared to warfarin, dabigatran patients had a lower risk of both intracranial bleeding and intra-articular or intramuscular bleeding and, although trial-specific all-cause mortality data were inconclusive in all but one trial, there was also a trend toward lower mortality in patients favoring dabigatran [18M].

A second meta-analysis was performed to evaluate the efficacy and safety of dabigatran for anticoagulation in atrial fibrillation ablation. 5513 patients undergoing catheter ablation were included in 17 observational studies and one randomized controlled trial. 150 mg dabigatran, twice daily, was the most frequently used dosing in the trials. Fourteen stroke or transient ischemic attacks (TIAs) were reported in the dabigatran group (0.65%, among 2137 patients), compared to 4 of 3376 (0.12%) in the warfarin group. The risk of all thromboembolic complications was higher in the dabigatran group (0.74%; 16 events) compared to the warfarin group (0.21%; 7 events). In the dabigatran group, 33 (1.54%) patients had major bleeding, compared to 53 (1.57%) in the warfarin group and a lower risk of minor bleeding was seen in the dabigatran group. Evaluation ultimately revealed that, compared to warfarin, periprocedural dabigatran use for atrial fibrillation ablation showed no significantly higher risk of pericardial tamponade, but was related to higher risk of thromboembolic complications including stroke and TIA. Outcomes with an incidence of <1% were analyzed using Peto's odds ratio estimates using a fixed-effects model did not show any statistical heterogeneity and a consistently high risk of stroke or TIA was observed with dabigatran in most of the sensitivity analyses. However, study sequential analysis, employed to limit type I error to ≤5% revealed that the numbers of events were too few to conclude firmly for a 150% increase in POR, and a high risk of random error was considered likely. The authors also noted that 3 recent comparatively smaller meta-analyses reported no increased risk of thromboembolic complications with dabigatran versus warfarin after atrial fibrillation ablation [19M].

Patients undergoing primary cemented total hip replacement for osteoarthritis or avascular necrosis of the femoral head were prospectively collected. These 122 patients were then divided into groups to receive either low-molecular-weight heparin (enoxaparin) or dabigatran. Minor and major bleeding events as well as thrombotic events were recorded. There were no significant differences in major bleeding events between the two groups, and no patients developed deep venous thromboembolism during the treatment period and follow-up. There were no differences in blood loss between the two groups and postoperative drainage did not differ significantly. The main differences in the two groups were the duration and intensity of serous wound drainage. The duration of discharge was longer in the dabigatran group (2.2 days) compared to the enoxaparin group (1.2 days) after drain removal. Higher intensity of wound drainage was also found in the dabigatran group. This was thought to potentially lead to longer hospitalizations and result in prolonged antibiotic prophylaxis [20C].

A 75-year-old man with a history of AF-related ischemic stroke 2 months prior to admission and on dabigatran presented with hemiparesis and dysarthria. A CT scan showed right sided parietal hemorrhage, the aPTT was 59 seconds and INR was 1.3. He deteriorated within 6 hours of admission, with hematoma expansion and penetration of blood into the ventricles with midline shift. He ultimately died 6 hours after the deterioration. Due to the prolonged aPTT, lack of other explanation, and the fact that large expansion is more commonly seen in coagulopathy, it was felt that the hematoma expansion was due to dabigatran [21A].

A 69-year-old woman who was being taking dabigatran for atrial fibrillation presented for dermabrasian for a scar secondary to Mohs surgery and flap repair of the nose. During infiltration of anesthetic she developed anxiety, and then began to feel uneasy with chest and shoulder discomfort and exhibited diaphoresis and pallor. Emergency services were notified and she was admitted to the hospital after a subarachnoid hemorrhage was noted which was felt to be related to dabigatran therapy [22A].

DIRECT FACTOR XA INHIBITORS [SEDA-34, 546; SEDA-35, 620; SEDA-36, 532]

Rivaroxaban [SEDA-34, 546; SEDA-35, 620, SEDA-36, 532]

Cardiovascular

A 75-year-old male with history of a dual chamber pacemaker and on rivaroxaban for AFib was admitted for chest pain and diagnosed with ST-segment elevation myocardial infarction. The rivaroxaban was continued and loading doses of aspirin and ticagrelor were given. Serial cardiac enzymes came back negative, a new diagnosis of pericarditis was made, the ticagrelor was stopped, and colchicine, ibuprofen and acetaminophen were initiated for the pericarditis. On hospital day 2, the patient became shocked and labs and imaging revealed hemopericardium with cardiac tamponade and acute ischemic hepatitis. The patient developed coagulopathy with an elevated INR and aPTT. Anti-factor Xa activity was 25 ng/mL. Rivaroxaban was discontinued and with supportive care, the coagulopathy gradually improved. Based on the clinical picture it was felt that the hemopericardium and cardiac tamponade were due to the antiplatelet, NSAID, and rivaroxaban therapies [23A].

Hematologic

An analysis of the ROCKET AF trial was performed to determine the efficacy and safety of rivaroxaban compared to warfarin in patients with peripheral artery disease and non-valvular atrial fibrillation. The ROCKET AF trial was a double blind randomized controlled trial comparing rivaroxaban and warfarin for prevention of stroke and systemic embolism. This analysis aimed to determine the rates of stroke and bleeding, effectiveness, and safety in patients with and without peripheral artery disease either on rivaroxaban versus warfarin. 14 264 patients with atrial fibrillation were randomly assigned to treatment within the ROCKET AF trial. 839 patients had a diagnosis of peripheral artery disease at the start of the study. The rate of stroke or non-CNS systemic embolism was not statistically different among patients with or without peripheral artery disease (2.41 vs. 2.09 events/100 patient-years). The rate of major or non-major clinically relevant bleeding was also not statistically different (17.81 vs. 14.54). The effect of rivaroxaban on primary efficacy outcome was similar when compared with warfarin in patients with or without peripheral arterial disease. The relative risk of rivaroxaban for the primary safety endpoint (major or non-major clinically relevant bleeding) was significantly higher in patients with peripheral artery disease (HR: 1.40, 95% CI: 1.06–1.86) than those without (HR: 1.03, 95% CI: 0.95–1.11; interaction $P = 0.037$) when compared with warfarin. Furthermore, in the rivaroxaban group, there was a non-statistically significant trend towards a higher risk of major bleeding when compared with warfarin in patients with peripheral artery disease than those without. Of note, there was no difference in the treatment efficacy when comparing rivaroxaban or warfarin in patients with or without peripheral arterial disease [24R].

A 67-year-old female on twice daily rivaroxaban (15 mg) for bilateral deep vein thrombosis experienced increased foot swelling, pain, and cyanosis. Duplex ultrasound revealed venous thrombosis of the entire leg. Laboratory investigation was consistent with intravascular coagulation and fibrinolysis. Rivaroxaban was discontinued and heparin was initiated. Additional diagnostic investigation revealed probable metastatic disease consistent with cancer. Although phase 3 clinical trials have shown rivaroxaban to be non-inferior in the treatment of acute venous thromboembolism, this case suggested that rivaroxaban may not be appropriate as sole therapy for prevention or treatment of cancer associated intravascular coagulation and fibrinolysis [25A].

A 67-year-old man taking once daily rivaroxaban (15 mg) for atrial fibrillation presented to the emergency department with acute abdominal pain. The patient was diagnosed with hemorrhagic shock secondary to spontaneous splenic rupture. Although supportive efforts were made, the patient remained in shock until splenectomy and ultimately developed multi system organ dysfunction with colic ischemia requiring a colectomy. In this patient, it was felt that his treatment with amlodipine (a weak CYP 3A4 inhibitor) and telmisartan/ hydrochlorothiazide (possibly contributing to hepatic/ renal hypoperfusion) likely increased the exposure to rivaroxaban leading to uncontrolled bleeding after spontaneous splenic rupture [26A].

THROMBOLYTIC DRUGS [SEDA-15, 3402; SEDA-35, 621; SEDA-36, 532]

Alteplase [SEDA-34, 547; SEDA-35, 621; SEDA-36, 532]

Currently alteplase is the only approved drug for thrombolytic therapy in acute ischemic strokes. The currently underway Norwegian Tenecteplase Stroke Trial (NOR-TEST) aims to compare the efficacy and safety of tenecteplase 0.4 mg/kg (single bolus) vs. alteplase 0.9 mg/kg (10% bolus + 90% infusion/60 minutes). This study will compare hemorrhagic transformation, symptomatic cerebral hemorrhage, major neurological improvements, recanalization and death in a prospective, randomized, open label and blinded endpoint trial. To date tenecteplase has been studied in small highly selected groups. This randomized, prospective, open-label, blinded endpoint trial will compare the similar patient populations and aims at establishing superiority of tenecteplase over alteplase [27C].

Cardiovascular

A 37-year-old male with acute pericarditis chest pain that was misdiagnosed as an acute myocardial infarction was reported in this study. He received thrombolytic therapy resulting in hemopericardium and cardiac tamponade with lethal consequences. These errors are rare and stress the importance of excluding underlying vascular etiologies that may lead to fatal complications [28A].

Nervous System

A 75-year-old man with acute right hemiparesis and no contraindication for thrombolysis underwent thrombolytic therapy with 72 mg of tissue plasminogen activator (tPA) 120 minutes after symptom onset. He showed recovery of functional deficits before the end of the infusion and within 24 hours he was able to ambulate. On third day of treatment he developed neck pain and right hemiparesis. MRI showed an acute c3–c6 level right posterolateral epidural spinal hematoma. He underwent bilateral microsurgical evacuation of hematoma and was eventually discharged in stable condition on month after the surgery. Epidural hematomas are the most common type of spinal hematomas in post thrombolytic period. Treating physicians should have a low threshold for evaluating neck or back pain in patients who recently have received tPA. Cervical and thoracic regions are the most common location for spinal hematoma in younger patients (16–45 years) and lower thoracic and lumbar regions are effected in a relatively older patient group (46–75 years) [29A].

Hematologic

Intracerebral hemorrhage (ICH) is the most feared complication of thrombolytic use in ischemic stroke patients. The Safe Implementation of Treatments in Stroke-International Stroke Thrombolysis Register (SITS-ISTR) is an internet-based prospective, ongoing, multinational, observational monitoring register of patients with acute ischemic strokes that were managed with thrombolysis. A study based on SITS-ISTR data compared the development of remote parenchymal hemorrhage (PHr) and parenchymal hemorrhage (PH) among 43 494 patients between 2002 and 2011. It was observed that 970 patients (2.2%) had PHr and 2325 patients (5.3%) had PH. A combination of PHr and PH was observed in 438 patients (1.0%). Risk of PHr was higher in subjects with female sex, higher age (74 vs. 70 years), and previous non-recent (>3 months) strokes. On the other hand risk of PH was higher among subjects with a hyperdense cerebral artery sign (HCAS), high National Institutes of Health Stroke Scale (NIHSS) score, hyperglycemia, diabetes, and atrial fibrillation. After thrombolysis, PHr was closely associated pre-existing vascular pathology, for example, cerebral amyloid angiopathy and prior stroke. Localized PH was associated with large vessel occlusions. Largely due to the less severe nature of stroke in PHr, the functional outcomes and mortality are lower when compared with PH [30M].

A retrospective study compared the risk factors associated with hemorrhagic transformation (HT) of ischemic stroke managed with intra-arterial thrombolysis. Regardless of the hemorrhagic conversion status, the mortality rates were similar. Patients who had high NIHSS score, elevated globulin level and prothrombin time activity (PTA) percentage were at higher risk of HT. Elevated globulin level is an independent risk factor for hemorrhagic transformation. It is postulated that acute phase reactants produced by liver, inflammatory cytokines, and matrix metalloproteinase 9, may play an important role [31M].

An 89-year-old female developed splenic hemorrhage after receiving alteplase for acute ischemic stroke. She was transferred to tertiary care. During MRI her vitals deteriorated and bedside abdominal ultrasound examination was performed by the emergency physician. A large perisplenic fluid collection was seen and, on surgical evaluation, it was determined that she did not require surgery and was managed conservatively [32A].

Musculoskeletal

A reported case of thrombolysis-induced sternocleidomastoid hematoma after acute ischemic stroke managed with intravenous alteplase was seen in an 83-year-old female. Notably the patient had lateral cervical extrapulmonary tuberculosis and an ipsilateral TB lymphadenitis proximal to the bleeding sternocleidomastoid muscle at the time of diagnosis. A possible relationship between chronic immune dysregulation and vascular inflammation was suggested to have contributed to formation of this skeletal muscle hematoma [33A].

Drug–Drug Interaction

An 80-year-old female with acute left hemiparesis received alteplase with improvement in her neurological function while receiving alteplase. A few minutes after the completion of alteplase she developed mild swelling of her tongue, uvula and lips. The airway was patent and did not require intubation. She received steroids with minimal improvement in tongue and lip swelling. She was receiving olmesartan for hypertension prior to alteplase therapy and was continued. Persistent swelling over next few days was suggestive of medication effect other than alteplase. Olmesartan was stopped promptly and swelling improved. Angioedema was attributed to the synergist effects of ARBs, alteplase and hypertension in the setting of elevated serum bradykinin levels [34A].

Streptokinase [SEDA-15, 62; SEDA-34, 547; SEDA-36, 533]

Hematologic

A 50-year-old male presented with acute chest pain. He received 1.2 MIU of streptokinase for STEMI. Subsequent EKG revealed successful thrombolysis. His hospital stay was complicated by the development of new onset left hemiparesis and progressive worsening in level of consciousness. CT head revealed hemorrhagic stroke in the right frontoparietal region. This case highlights the rare but well established risk associated with streptokinase therapy [35A].

Eyes

A limited number of cases of intraocular hemorrhage after intravenous streptokinase has been reported in the past. Patients had either pre-existing eye disorders (e.g., macular degeneration) or other risk factors (e.g., hypertension) prior to streptokinase therapy. A 46-year-old man underwent intravenous streptokinase for treatment of acute inferior myocardial infarction. During the infusion he developed blurry vision in the right eye but did not inform his physicians. The next day he was evaluated by ophthalmology for complete loss of vision. Detailed examination revealed massive intraocular hemorrhage leading to blindness. At 3 months interval he had no visual improvement. This case underlines the importance of urgent evaluation of any eye symptoms associated with streptokinase administration [36A].

GLYCOPROTEIN IIb–IIIa INHIBITORS
[SED-15, 2849; SEDA-33, 720; SEDA-34, 548; SEDA-35, 622]

Abciximab [SED-15, 2849; SEDA-34, 548; SEDA-35, 622]

Hematologic

A case report describes a 63-year-old man who received abciximab in the setting of percutaneous coronary intervention and developed critical thrombocytopenia, from $228\,000/mm^3$ to $9000/mm^3$, within 7 hours. The authors recommend checking the platelet count at 2 and 4 hours after initiating abciximab due to the rapid-onset of critical thrombocytopenia [37A].

Eptifibatide [SED-15, 2849; SEDA-34, 548; SEDA-35, 622; SEDA-36, 533]

Hematologic

A single-center, which uses a trans-radial over the trans-femoral approach for angioplasty in the setting of acute myocardial infarction, examined bleeding outcomes when using a combination of eptifibatide and unfractionated heparin [38c]. Consecutive patients ($n = 432$) were included based on HORIZONS-AMI criteria ($n = 350$). The authors note that in contrast to the HORIZONS-AMI study, these patients were older and had a higher rate of cardiogenic shock. Nonetheless, the authors found a trend towards decreased major bleeding, as defined by the HORIZONS-AMI definition (3.7% [2.0–6.3%] versus 4.9% [4.0–6.1%], $P = 0.32$), despite the use of eptifibatide. Similar results were found using the TIMI major bleeding and GUSTO severe or life-threatening bleeding classifications. The authors conclude that a trans-radial approach mitigates the increased bleeding risk normally seen with a glycoprotein inhibitor.

Another single-center study focused specifically on patients with left ventricular assist devices that develop pump thrombosis and treated with eptifibatide on top of aspirin and/or warfarin [39c]. 17 patients were retrospectively identified who had received 22 doses of eptifibatide (dose range 0.1–2 microgram/kg/min, determined by the renal function and perceived bleeding risk; most received ≤1 microgram/kg/min). The authors found active bleeding during infusion in 11 patients. Of these, intraparenchymal hemorrhage was the cause of death in 2 patients.

Two nearly identical case reports describe critical thrombocytopenia within hours of receiving eptifibatide, which required discontinuation of the drug and platelet transfusion. In one case the patient was discharged on aspirin alone [40A], while in the other case the patient was discharged on aspirin and clopidogrel [41A].

Sex

The EARLY ACS trial examined early versus delayed eptifibatide in acute coronary syndrome and failed to show any significant outcome differences. Therefore, a follow-up analysis of the pooled data examined bleeding rate and 30-day mortality in 2975 women compared with 6431 men [42C]. It is notable that since these groups are not random, but assigned by gender, there are several statistical differences in the patient characteristics by group. The authors identified a higher rate of bleeding in women (8.2% versus 5.5%, $P < 0.01$). Interestingly, the association between bleeding and 30-day mortality was significant for men only (odds ratio 5.8, 95% CI 3.9–8.8).

Tirofiban [SED-15, 2849; SEDA-34, 547; SEDA-35, 621; SEDA-36, 533]

Hematologic

A meta-analysis that included 8 randomized trials ($n = 1577$) was focused on early (given in the ambulance or emergency room) versus late (given in the catheterization laboratory) tirofiban in patients with acute ST-segment elevation myocardial infarction who were treated by percutaneous coronary intervention [43M]. Dosing of tirofiban varied based on the study. There were in-hospital major bleeding events reported in 13 of 412 patients and 15 of 434 patients with early and late tirofiban, respectively. There were 30-day major bleeding events reported in 13 of 305 patients and 10 of 311 patients with early and late tirofiban, respectively. There were in-hospital minor bleeding events reported in 15 of 185 patients and 14 of 187 patients with early and late tirofiban, respectively. The authors did not identify any statistically significant differences between in-hospital major bleeding (RR = 0.98, 95% CI: 0.46–2.10, $P = 0.96$), 30-day major bleeding (RR = 1.32, 95% CI: 0.59–2.97, $P = 0.49$), and in-hospital minor bleeding (RR = 1.08, 95% CI: 0.54–2.14, $P = 0.83$). Therefore, early and late administration of tirofiban has an equivalent bleeding risk.

A meta-analysis that examined the safety of intracoronary administration of tirofiban for "no-reflow" during percutaneous coronary intervention included 6 studies ($n = 183$) with bleeding data [44M]. Dosing of tirofiban varied based on the study. There were bleeding events with 20 of 183 and 14 of 176 patients, with tirofiban and conventional drugs, respectively. The authors identified a trend towards increased bleeding that was not statistically significant with tirofiban (OR 1.44, 95% CI: 0.69–3.0, $P = 0.32$), which may play a role in clinical decision-making.

A single-center consecutively enrolled 21 patients with recent stent placement who required surgery and were bridged for surgery with tirofiban [45c]. With aspirin and clopidogrel discontinued 5 days before surgery, the short-acting tirofiban was continued until 4 hours before surgery, and restarted after surgery before returning to the original regimen. Major bleeding was monitored during hospitalization and within 3 months. The surgical indications were: rectal cancer ($n=5$), early gastric cancer ($n=3$), cholecystitis ($n=3$), kidney cancer ($n=3$), prostate cancer ($n=3$), cholangitis ($n=2$), endometrial cancer ($n=1$) and ovarian cancer ($n=1$). None of the study patients experienced a TIMI major or minor bleeding event during the entire study period. Although a small study, the results encourage replication on a larger scale.

P2Y$_{12}$ RECEPTOR ANTAGONISTS *[SED-15, 821; SEDA-34, 548; SEDA-35, 622; SEDA-36, 533]*

Cangrelor

Cardiovascular

A study examined the electrophysiologic safety of cangrelor with 67 healthy volunteers [46c]. Both therapeutic (30 μg/kg IV bolus followed by 4 μg/kg per minute IV infusion for 3 hours) and supratherapeutic (60 μg/kg IV bolus followed by 8 μg/kg per minute IV infusion for 3 hours) doses were examined. Neither therapeutic nor supratherapeutic doses of cangrelor demonstrated significant QT changes (less than 5 ms with a 90% CI less than 10 ms). No additional adverse effects on electrocardiography were noted; however, this study utilized healthy volunteers.

Hematologic

A recent meta-analysis evaluated 3 randomized controlled trials ($n=25106$) [47M]. When co-administered with clopidogrel and/or low-dose aspirin, cangrelor demonstrated a significantly increased risk of major bleeding at 48 hours when using the ACUITY scale (RR: 1.51, 95% CI: 1.32–1.72, $P<0.00001$), but failed to show significance when the GUSTO (RR: 1.21, 95% CI: 0.70–2.11, $P=0.49$) and TIMI (RR: 1.00, 95% CI: 0.59–1.68, $P=0.99$) bleeding scales were used. The authors also observed that these results highlight the need for uniformity both in defining bleeding and how it is measured.

Clopidogrel *[SED-15, 821; SEDA-34, 548; SEDA-35, 622; SEDA-36, 533]*

Systematic Reviews

A recent review focused primarily on genetic factors that impact the pharmacology of clopidogrel (such as CYP2C19 polymorphism data), but nongenetic factors are covered as well [48R].

A recent meta-analysis, which integrated data from 21 studies ($n=23035$), examined how the CYP2C19 polymorphism impacts the risk of adverse events [49M]. Patients with a CYP2C19 variant were compared to those with non-variant alleles. The authors found an increased risk of adverse clinical events (OR 1.50, 95% CI: 1.21–1.87, $P=0.0003$), myocardial infarction (OR 1.62, 95% CI: 1.35–1.95, $P<0.00001$), stent thrombosis (OR 2.08, 95% CI: 1.67–2.60, $P<0.00001$), ischemic stroke (OR 2.14, 95% CI: 1.36–3.38, $P=0.001$) and repeat revascularization (OR 1.35, 95% CI: 1.10–1.66, $P=0.004$). In contrast, mortality and bleeding events were not statistically different between these groups. For mortality, the numbers for variant and non-variant alleles were 4089 and 6934, respectively. For bleeding events, the numbers for variant and non-variant alleles were 3609 and 7669, respectively, but it is unclear what criteria were used for the bleeding assessment.

Hematologic

A retrospective study involving military veterans sought to identify risk factors for gastrointestinal bleeding in patients prescribed clopidogrel due to recent acute myocardial infarction [50c]. A total of 107 out of 3218 patients did develop acute gastrointestinal bleeding. Statistically significant characteristics associated with bleeding were age greater than 65 years (HR 1.74, 95% CI: 1.16–2.61, $P=0.007$), concurrent warfarin use (HR 3.49, 95% CI: 2.18–5.58, $P<0.0001$), chronic liver disease (HR 3.28, 95% CI: 1.42–7.55, $P=0.005$), and chronic kidney disease (HR 2.41, 95% CI: 1.58–3.67, $P<0.0001$). Using this patient cohort, the authors propose a risk score that integrates these statistically significant aspects.

In an interesting *post hoc* analysis of the Rotterdam Scan Study, clopidogrel use and association with cerebral microbleeds found on MRI, authors analyzed 4408 individuals who had never experienced a stroke [51c]. Of these, 121 had taken clopidogrel previously and 4287 had never taken clopidogrel. Those who had taken clopidogrel demonstrated statistically increased prevalence of cerebral microbleeds (OR 1.55, 95% CI: 1.01–2.37), a higher number of microbleeds (OR 3.19, 95% CI: 1.52–6.72), and a higher number of infratentorial microbleeds (OR 1.90, 95% CI: 1.05–3.45). The authors suggested that the reported associations requires confirmation in further prospective study, especially given the small number of participants taking clopidogrel and the possibility of residual confounding.

Recently, the first case report of clopidogrel-associated pure red cell aplasia was reported in a 62-year-old woman with coronary atherosclerotic heart disease [52A]. The patient was prescribed a dose of 75 mg/day and approximately 4 days later the hemoglobin began to decrease. A complete evaluation of the patient failed to identify an alternative cause and clopidogrel was discontinued on the 14th day. Subsequently, the pure red cell aplasia resolved over the next 14 days.

Another case report describes bone marrow toxicity that was associated with clopidogrel [53A]. A 67-year-old female developed thrombocytopenia and leukopenia 13 days after starting clopidogrel at the daily dose of 75 mg. The complete blood count at a follow-up appointment 3 days later showed decrease in all the cell lineages. She showed improvement 8 days after discontinuing clopidogrel.

Skin

A recent case report implicated clopidogrel in an exacerbation of psoriasis [54A]. A 64-year-old man with a several year history of palmoplantar pustulosis had his lesions progress to palmoplantar pustular psoriasis after starting clopidogrel. This regressed with discontinuation of clopidogrel, but returned when re-challenged with the drug.

A letter described a case of clopidogrel-induced erythroderma that seemed to cross-react with ticlopidine [55r]. A 76-year-old man, negative for a history of dermatosis, developed erythroderma 20 days after starting clopidogrel at the daily dose of 75 mg. Clopidogrel was stopped and an equivalent dose of ticlopidine was started (250 mg twice daily), along with methylprednisolone. Six weeks later the patient was re-admitted with severe erythroderma. Subsequently, ticlopidine was discontinued; methylprednisolone was started, along with aspirin and low-molecular-weight heparin.

Another case report describes a 70-year-old man who after 2 weeks of 75 mg daily clopidogrel developed lip, hand, and foot swelling, erythematous popular non-pruritic lesions and arthralgias [56A]. The patient was first treated with a 3-hour slow infusion of clopidogrel, which ended when the patient developed a recurrence of symptoms on the fourth day. Next, the patient was treated with a modified desensitization protocol in which the dose was slowly increased over 2 months to the goal dose of 75 mg daily.

Musculoskeletal

A case of clopidogrel-associated polyarthritis was reported approximately 2 weeks after starting clopidogrel [57A]. The 72-year-old male was switched to prasugrel and his symptoms resolved over six days. Two weeks later the patient accidently took two doses of clopidogrel and experienced another episode of polyarthritis.

Genetic Factors

Authors studied 150 consecutive Chinese-Han patients for CYP2C19 gene influences on the response to clopidogrel [58c]. Results showed that CYP2C19 loss of function alleles (*2/*2, *2/*3, and *3/*3) were statistically significant independent predictors for clopidogrel resistance (OR 4.43, 95% CI: 3.28–6.37, $P < 0.05$). Furthermore, body-mass-index (OR 2.01, 95% CI: 1.63–3.71, $P < 0.05$) and type-2 diabetes mellitus (OR 2.76, 95% CI: 2.13–4.14, $P < 0.05$) were additional independent risk factors for resistance. The authors report a synergistic interaction between the genetic and comorbid conditions.

Race Factors

A recent analysis of CYP2C19 and CYP1A2 variants in patients receiving clopidogrel found racial differences in mortality [59C]. Using 2732 subjects from the multicenter TRIUMPH study, the authors found that white patients had a significant increase in 1-year mortality associated with the loss-of-function CYP2C19*2 allele (HR 1.70, 95% CI: 1.01–2.86, $P = 0.046$), whereas black patients had a significant increase in 1-year mortality associated with the gain-of-function CYP2C19*17 allele (HR 8.97, 95% CI: 3.34–24.10, $P < 0.0001$) and CYP1A2*1C allele (HR 4.96, 95% CI: 1.69–14.56, $P = 0.014$). Furthermore, a statistically significant increase in bleeding was associated with the CYP2C19*17 (homozygous OR 3.82, 95% CI: 1.17–12.42, $P = 0.027$) and CYP1A2*1C alleles (heterozygous OR 2.90, 95% CI: 1.41–5.93, $P = 0.0039$) in blacks.

Drug–Drug Interactions

Clopidogrel and angiotensin-converting enzyme inhibitors (ACEi) are both, in part, metabolized by hepatic carboxylesterase 1. To determine if there is any interaction, authors performed a novel study linking *in vitro* drug interaction studies to targeted pharmacoepidemiological studies of real-world patients recorded in nationwide Danish registries. A population of 70 934 patients with a first-time myocardial infarction over a 10-year period of time was identified [60C]. From this group, 29 043 had received clopidogrel and, of these, 9069 had received both clopidogrel and an ACEi. Of the 41 891 who did not receive clopidogrel, 6593 received ACEi. Co-treatment with clopidogrel and ACEi (95% was represented by ramipril, trandolapril, enalapril and perindopril) demonstrated a small, but statistically significant increase in the risk of bleeding (HRR 1.27, 95% CI: 1.09–1.49, $P = 0.002$).

Smoking

It has been shown that smoking enhances the effect of clopidogrel; however, the mechanism underlying this effect remains speculative. A study recruited 20 clopidogrel-naïve patients with stable coronary artery disease (10 smokers and 10 non-smokers) to elucidate if changes in the $P2Y_{12}$ receptor binding activity may mediate the differential clinical effect [61c]. Smokers demonstrated a 6.4-fold reduction in the $P2Y_{12}$ receptor binding activity compared with baseline; whereas, there were minimal changes in P2Y$_{12}$ receptor binding activity among the non-smokers. These pilot data support a future of follow-up pharmacodynamics studies with larger sample sizes. An overview of the published data is included in a recently published perspective piece [62r].

Prasugrel [SEDA-34, 549; SEDA-35, 624; SEDA-36, 535]

Review

Five major clinical trials and several case reports are discussed in this review, which extensively covers adverse events associated with prasugrel [63R].

Hematologic

A prospective, randomly controlled study enrolled 4033 patients to examine how the timing of prasugrel administration (30 mg at diagnosis of non-ST segment elevation acute coronary syndrome and another 30 mg at coronary angiography versus 60 mg at coronary angiography) impacts patient outcome [64C]. Patients in both study arms also received standard antithrombotic treatment which included aspirin (98%), unfractionated heparin (65%), low-molecular-weight heparin (30%), fondaparinux (4%), or bivalirudin (1%). No difference in ischemic events was demonstrated between treatment groups but with respect to thrombolysis in myocardial infarction (TIMI) major bleeding, early administration significantly increased bleeding (HR 1.90, 95% CI: 1.19–3.02, $P = 0.006$). Major and life-threatening bleeding events were noted to be predominantly associated with either the percutaneous coronary intervention (PCI) or coronary artery bypass graft surgery, and occurred early in patients who underwent PCI.

A single-center retrospective cohort study compared clinical outcomes between aspirin/clopidogrel and aspirin/prasugrel treatments in patients undergoing neurointerventional surgery performed by one interventionalist [65c]. The aspirin/clopidogrel group included 51 patients and 55 procedures. The aspirin/prasugrel group included 25 patients and 31 procedures. Notably, the procedures were similar, but the group who received aspirin/prasugrel were all known to be clopidogrel non-responders. A total of 8 hemorrhagic events documented in this trial; 2 (3.6%) in the clopidogrel group and 6 (19.4%) in the prasugrel group ($P = 0.02$). However, two of the hemorrhagic events in the aspirin/prasugrel group involved perforation of the involved arteries during coiling and pipeline embolization procedures. If these cases are excluded from the analysis, then the increased rate of bleeding associated with prasugrel was no longer statistically significant.

A recent study focused on prasugrel dosing in patients who are 75 years of age or older [66c]. The doses studied were 10 mg versus 5 mg of prasugrel. This Phase 1b blinded-crossover study enrolled 73 elderly subjects and 82 subjects who were less than 65 years of age. The authors report a statistically significant increase in the bleeding rate with the 10 mg dose for both age groups.

Skin

A case of prasugrel-induced diffuse, pruritic, maculopapular rash was recently reported effectively treated using a 'treating through' strategy [67A]. A 58-year-old man developed this rash after 7 days of treatment with 10 mg of prasugrel daily. Prasugrel was continued, but a 6-day tapered dose of methylprednisolone and diphenhydramine for pruritis was added. The rash began to improve on day 2 of this 'treating through' strategy and completely resolved by day 5. The authors have 3 months of follow-up that is absent of recurrence.

Ticagrelor [SEDA-34, 541; SEDA-35, 617]

REVIEW

Two excellent reviews have been recently published, which cover the major clinical studies as well as more general information regarding the common adverse events associated with Ticagrelor [68R,69C].

Respiratory

An analysis of pulmonary adverse events and sepsis from patients in the PLATO demonstrate lower mortality associated with ticagrelor relative to clopidogrel [70C]. All 18421 subjects were acute coronary syndrome patients. There were 9235 and 9186 adverse events associated with ticagrelor and clopidogrel, respectively. Ticagrelor was associated with fewer pulmonary adverse events (275 vs. 331, $P = 0.019$), fewer deaths after an adverse event (33 vs. 71, $P < 0.001$), and fewer sepsis cases (7 vs. 23, $P = 0.003$). Multivariable analysis showed that treatment-emergent pulmonary events were attributable to higher age, female gender and co-morbid conditions, such as asthma and chronic obstructive pulmonary disease, while the reduction in mortality remained significant after multivariate analysis.

A recent review highlights the challenge of untangling the cause of dyspnea in patients experiencing acute coronary syndrome and receiving ticagrelor, given that both are potential causes [71R].

Hematologic

A 56-year-old man was started on combination ticagrelor 90 mg bid and aspirin 100 mg daily following stent placement in the left circumflex coronary artery [72A]. Approximately 10 days later he presented with hemoptysis. His concomitant medications included rosuvastatin, fluticasone, salmeterol, and diltiazem. Coagulation studies were unremarkable and imaging showed diffuse pulmonary hemorrhage. Ticagrelor was temporarily stopped and eventually the patient underwent open lung biopsy and elective coronary artery bypass graft surgery. At that point ticagrelor could be permanently stopped, which finally led to resolution of the pulmonary hemorrhage. No predisposing risk was identified.

A 68-year-old man diagnosed with an inferior ST-elevated myocardial infarction was stented and started on ticagrelor 90 mg bid and aspirin 100 mg daily [73A]. While straining with a bowel movement the patient developed hypovolemic shock, which was subsequently identified due to omental bleeding. Surgical intervention was needed and the patient was switched from ticagrelor to clopidogrel.

Skin

A 65-year-old man developed a diffuse, pruritic, exanthematous rash 5 days after beginning ticagrelor [74A]. He was treated with a 3-week prednisone taper and switched to clopidogrel. His symptoms resolved and have not recurred.

Sex

A follow-up analysis of the PLATO data sought to identify ticagrelor-associated outcome differences [75C]. This analysis included 5288 women and 13336 men. The incidence of major bleeding complications was not different between women and men ($P = 0.43$–0.88).

HEMOSTATIC AGENTS [SEDA-34, 549; SEDA-35, 624; SEDA-36, 536]

Tranexamic Acid [SEDA-34, 549; SEDA-35, 625; SEDA-36, 536]

Nervous System

A retrospective analysis of previously collected prospective data of 11529 patients undergoing cardiopulmonary bypass was performed to assess the risk factors for seizures. Tranexamic acid was the only modifiable risk factor among age, female sex, cardiac surgery redo, calcifications of ascending aorta, congestive heart failure, deep hypothermic circulatory arrest, and duration of aortic cross-clamp. It was suggested that doses exceeding 80 mg/kg should be weighed against the risk of postoperative convulsions [76A].

Hematologic

A case controlled study based on the British General Practice Research Database assessed the thrombosis risks associated with use of tranexamic acid in various clinical situations. It was suggested that females had threefold higher risk of deep vein thrombosis risk when taking tranexamic acid. A major increase in the risk of thrombosis could not be ruled out due to the wide 95% confidence interval that ranged from 0.7 to 15.8. Previous studies lacked the statistical power needed to establish clear risk vs. benefit ratios. Tranexamic acid has been used in the settings of severe life threatening bleeding. In stable patients, however, there is a lack of data to support the use in the face of high thrombosis risk [77M].

A 45-year-old female with stage 4 chronic kidney disease developed menorrhagia and worsening renal failure. She received multiple units of pRBC and tranexamic acid was administered per vagina. Tranexamic acid was administered 1 g every 8 hours without adjustment for renal failure. Shortly after sixth dose she developed new onset generalized tonic clonic seizure. Tranexamic acid was discontinued and patient did not experience any recurrent seizure episode. She remained seizure free at 2 months follow-up. In the absence of any other triggers her seizure episode was attributed to the tranexamic acid use [78A].

Eyes

A 70-year-old female with bleeding gastric ulcer was treated with oral tranexamic acid. She presented with pale yellow pseudomembranous of the bilateral palpebral conjunctivae. Based on the lab result of hypoplasminogenemia and clinical findings, she was diagnosed with ligneous conjunctivitis. Patient continued to receive the tranexamic acid for additional 14 weeks. His conjunctival pseudomembranes regressed 6 weeks after the cessation of tranexamic acid. Her serum plasminogen levels returned to normal levels. This case suggests the association of tranexamic acid with unresolving ligneous conjunctivitis [79A].

References

[1] Azoulay L, Dell'Aniello S, Simon TA, et al. Initiation of warfarin in patients with atrial fibrillation: early effects on ischaemic strokes. Eur Heart J. 2014;35(28):1881–7 [c].

[2] Mooney T, Joseph P. Purple toes syndrome following stroke thrombolysis and warfarin therapy. Intern Med J. 2014;44(1):107–8. http://dx.doi.org/10.1111/imj.12327 [A].

[3] Sheng GH, Aronowitz P. The lesser known side-effect of warfarin: warfarin-induced venous limb gangrene. Mayo Clin Proc. 2014;89(5):037 [A].

[4] Wang Z, Anderson Jr. FA, Ward M, et al. Surgical site infections and other postoperative complications following prophylactic anticoagulation in total joint arthroplasty. PLoS One. 2014;9(4): e91755 [R].

[5] Blank SJ, Grindler DJ, Zerega J, et al. Systemic effects of subcutaneous heparin use in otolaryngology patients. Otolaryngol Head Neck Surg. 2014;151(6):967–71 [c].

[6] Khouzam RN, Soufi MK, Weatherly M. Heparin infusion through a central line misplaced in the carotid artery leading to hemorrhagic stroke. J Emerg Med. 2013;45(3):e87–9. http://dx.doi.org/10.1016/j.jemermed.2012.12.026 [A].

[7] Fatma LB, El Ati Z, Azzouz H, et al. Subcutis calcinosis caused by injection of calcium-containing heparin in a chronic kidney injury patient. Saudi J Kidney Dis Transpl. 2014;25(5):1068–71 [A].

[8] Tessler O, Vorstenbosch J, Jones D, et al. Heparin-induced thrombocytopenia and thrombosis as an under-diagnosed cause of flap failure in heparin-naive patients: a case report and systematic review of the literature. Microsurgery. 2014;34(2):157–63 [R].

[9] Zaman SR, Rawlins JM. Heparin induced thrombocytopaenia (HIT) as a cause of free flap failure in lower limb trauma. J Plast Reconstr Aesthet Surg. 2014;67(6):884–6. http://dx.doi.org/10.1016/j.bjps.2013.12.027. Epub 2013 Dec 31 [A].

[10] Maag RL, Chuang CH. Uncommon complications of heparin-induced thrombocytopenia. Am J Med. 2013;126(11):e5–e6. http://dx.doi.org/10.1016/j.amjmed.2013.06.032 [A].

[11] Higa T, Okura H, Tanemoto K, et al. Prosthetic valve thrombosis caused by heparin-induced thrombocytopenia thrombosis during pregnancy. Circ J. 2014;78(4):1004–5 [A].

[12] Canaud L, Hireche K, Marty-Ane C, et al. Heparin-induced thrombocytopenia with abdominal aortic stent-graft acute thrombosis. Ann Vasc Surg. 2013;27(6):801 [A].

[13] Ploppa A, Haeberle L, Schmid E, et al. Left ventricular thrombus during cardiopulmonary bypass as the primary manifestation of heparin-induced thrombocytopenia. J Cardiothorac Vasc Anesth. 2013;27(4):744–8 [A].

[14] Vaidya R, Pruthi R, Thompson C. An unusual presentation of heparin-induced thrombocytopenia in the setting of catheter-directed ablation of atrial fibrillation. Blood Coagul Fibrinolysis. 2014;25(2):188–90 [A].

[15] Welp H, Ellger B, Scherer M, et al. Heparin-induced thrombocytopenia during extracorporeal membrane oxygenation. J Cardiothorac Vasc Anesth. 2014;28(2):342–4 [A].

[16] Foreman JS, Daniels LM, Stettner EA. Heparin-induced anaphylactoid reaction associated with heparin-induced thrombocytopenia in the ED. Am J Emerg Med. 2014;32(12):11 [A].

[17] Atar S, Wishniak A, Shturman A, et al. Fatal association of mechanical valve thrombosis with dabigatran: a report of two cases. Chest. 2013;144(1):327–8 [A].

[18] Bloom BJ, Filion KB, Atallah R, et al. Meta-analysis of randomized controlled trials on the risk of bleeding with dabigatran. Am J Cardiol. 2014;113(6):1066–74 [M].

[19] Sardar P, Nairooz R, Chatterjee S, et al. Meta-analysis of risk of stroke or transient ischemic attack with dabigatran for atrial fibrillation ablation. Am J Cardiol. 2014;113(7):1173–7 [M].

[20] Gombar C, Horvath G, Gality H, et al. Comparison of minor bleeding complications using dabigatran or enoxaparin after cemented total hip arthroplasty. Arch Orthop Trauma Surg. 2014;134(4):449–57 [C].

[21] Simonsen CZ, Steiner T, Tietze A, et al. Dabigatran-related intracerebral hemorrhage resulting in hematoma expansion. J Stroke Cerebrovasc Dis. 2014;23(2):e133–e134 [A].

[22] Fakhouri TM, Harmon CB. Hemorrhagic complications of direct thrombin inhibitors-subarachnoid hemorrhage during dermabrasion for scar revision. Dermatol Surg. 2013;39(9):1410–2. http://dx.doi.org/10.1111/dsu.12256. Epub 2013 Jun 24 [A].

[23] Xu B, MacIsaac A. Life-threatening haemorrhagic pericarditis associated with rivaroxaban. Int J Cardiol. 2014;174(2):e75–e76. http://dx.doi.org/10.1016/j.ijcard.2014.04.151. Epub 2014 Apr 21. [A].

[24] Jones WS, Hellkamp AS, Halperin J, et al. Efficacy and safety of rivaroxaban compared with warfarin in patients with peripheral artery disease and non-valvular atrial fibrillation: insights from ROCKET AF. Eur Heart J. 2014;35(4):242–9 [R].

[25] Rosenbaum AN, Yu RC, Rooke TW, et al. Venous gangrene and intravascular coagulation and fibrinolysis in a patient treated with rivaroxaban. Am J Med. 2014;127(6):22 [A].

[26] Gonzva J, Patricelli R, Lignac D. Spontaneous splenic rupture in a patient treated with rivaroxaban. Am J Emerg Med. 2014;32(8):e3 [A].

[27] Logallo N, Kvistad CE, Nacu A, et al. The Norwegian tenecteplase stroke trial (NOR-TEST): randomised controlled trial of tenecteplase vs. alteplase in acute ischaemic stroke. BMC Neurol. 2014;14(106):1471–2377 [C].

[28] Irivbogbe O, Mirrer B, Loarte P, et al. Thrombolytic-related complication in a case of misdiagnosed myocardial infarction. Acute Card Care. 2014;16(2):83–7 [A].

[29] Ghadirpour R, Nasi D, Benedetti B, et al. Delayed cervical epidural hematoma after intravenous thrombolysis for acute ischemic stroke: case report and review of literature. Clin Neurol Neurosurg. 2014;122:50–3 [A].

[30] Mazya MV, Ahmed N, Ford GA, et al. Remote or extraischemic intracerebral hemorrhage—an uncommon complication of stroke thrombolysis: results from the safe implementation of treatments in stroke-international stroke thrombolysis register. Stroke. 2014;45(6):1657–63 [M].

[31] Xing Y, Guo ZN, Yan S, et al. Increased globulin and its association with hemorrhagic transformation in patients receiving intra-arterial thrombolysis therapy. Neurosci Bull. 2014;30(3):469–76 [M].

[32] Genthon A, Frasure S, Kinnaman K, et al. Bedside ultrasound diagnosis of a spontaneous splenic hemorrhage after tissue plasminogen activator administration. Am J Emerg Med. 2014;32(12):1553 [A].

[33] Giannantoni NM, Della Marca G, Broccolini A, et al. Spontaneous sternocleidomastoid muscle hematoma following thrombolysis for acute ischemic stroke. J Neurol Sci. 2014;341(1–2):189–90. http://dx.doi.org/10.1016/j.jns.2014.03.059 [A].

[34] Wang S, Bi X, Shan L, et al. Orolingual angioedema associated with olmesartan use after recombinant tissue plasminogen activator treatment of acute stroke. Ann Allergy Asthma Immunol. 2014;112(2):177–8 [A].

[35] Arzu J, Muqueet MA, Sweety SA, et al. Haemorrhagic stroke after thrombolysis with streptokinase. Mymensingh Med J. 2014;23(4):818–20 [A].

[36] Peyman M, Subrayan V. Irreversible blindness following intravenous streptokinase. JAMA Ophthalmol. 2013;131(10):1368–9 [A].

[37] Daley B, Miranda D, Kalra A, et al. Profound thrombocytopenia caused by abciximab infusion following. Minn Med. 2014;97(10):48–9 [A].

[38] Moody WE, Chue CD, Ludman PF, et al. Bleeding outcomes after routine transradial primary angioplasty for acute myocardial infarction using eptifibatide and unfractionated heparin: a single-center experience following the HORIZONS-AMI trial. Catheter Cardiovasc Interv. 2013;82(3):8 [c].

[39] Tellor BR, Smith JR, Prasad SM, et al. The use of eptifibatide for suspected pump thrombus or thrombosis in patients with left ventricular assist devices. J Heart Lung Transplant. 2014;33(1):94–101 [c].

[40] Pothineni NV, Watts TE, Ding Z, et al. Eptifibatide-induced thrombocytopenia-when inhibitor turns killer. Am J Ther. 2013;23:23 [A].

[41] Graidis C, Golias C, Dimitriadis D, et al. Eptifibatide-induced acute profound thrombocytopenia: a case report. BMC Res Notes. 2014;7:107 [A].

[42] Kaul P, Tanguay JF, Newby LK, et al. Association between bleeding and mortality among women and men with high-risk acute coronary syndromes: insights from the early versus delayed, provisional eptifibatide in acute coronary syndromes (EARLY ACS) trial. Am Heart J. 2013;166(4):723–8 [C].

[43] Liu Y, Su Q, Li L. Safety and efficacy of early administration of tirofiban in patients with acute ST-segment elevation myocardial

infarction undergoing primary percutaneous coronary intervention: a meta-analysis. Chin Med J (Engl). 2014;127(6):1126–32 [M].

[44] Qin T, Xie L, Chen MH. Meta-analysis of randomized controlled trials on the efficacy and safety of intracoronary administration of tirofiban for no-reflow phenomenon. BMC Cardiovasc Disord. 2013;13(68):1471–2261 [M].

[45] Xia JG, Qu Y, Shen H, et al. Short-term follow-up of tirofiban as alternative therapy for urgent surgery patients with an implanted coronary drug-eluting stent after ST-elevation myocardial infarction. Coron Artery Dis. 2013;24(6):522–6 [c].

[46] Green CL, Whellan DJ, Lambe L, et al. Electrocardiographic safety of cangrelor, a new intravenous antiplatelet agent: a randomized, double-blind, placebo- and moxifloxacin-controlled thorough QT study. J Cardiovasc Pharmacol. 2013;62(5):466–78 [c].

[47] Serebruany VL, Aradi D, Kim MH, et al. Cangrelor infusion is associated with an increased risk for bleeding: meta-analysis of randomized trials. Int J Cardiol. 2013;169(3):225–8 [M].

[48] Notarangelo MF, Bontardelli F, Merlini PA. Genetic and nongenetic factors influencing the response to clopidogrel. J Cardiovasc Med (Hagerstown). 2013;14(Suppl 1):s1–7 [R].

[49] Mao L, Jian C, Changzhi L, et al. Cytochrome CYP2C19 polymorphism and risk of adverse clinical events in clopidogrel-treated patients: a meta-analysis based on 23,035 subjects. Arch Cardiovasc Dis. 2013;106(10):517–27 [M].

[50] Cuschieri JR, Drawz P, Falck-Ytter Y, et al. Risk factors for acute gastrointestinal bleeding following myocardial infarction in veteran patients who are prescribed clopidogrel. J Dig Dis. 2014;15(4):195–201 [c].

[51] Darweesh SK, Leening MJ, Akoudad S, et al. Clopidogrel use is associated with an increased prevalence of cerebral microbleeds in a stroke-free population: the Rotterdam study. J Am Heart Assoc. 2013;2(5):000359 [c].

[52] Li G, Li ZQ, Yang QY, et al. Acquired pure red cell aplasia due to treatment with clopidogrel: first case report. J Thromb Thrombolysis. 2014;38(2):215–7 [A].

[53] Mauricio Adel C, Rosa MG, Cantadori L, et al. Bone marrow toxicity induced by clopidogrel. Int J Cardiol. 2014;174(3):e112–3. http://dx.doi.org/10.1016/j.ijcard.2014.04.194 [A].

[54] Mahajan VK, Khatri G, Prabha N, et al. Clopidogrel: a possible exacerbating factor for psoriasis. Indian J Pharmacol. 2014;46(1):123–4 [A].

[55] Ziakas A, Theofilogiannakos EK, Daniilidis M, et al. Clopidogrel and ticlopidine cross-reactivity-induced erythroderma following drug-eluting stenting. Cutis. 2013;92(6):E16–7 [r].

[56] Barreira P, Cadinha S, Malheiro D, et al. Desensitization to clopidogrel: a tailor-made protocol. Eur Ann Allergy Clin Immunol. 2014;46(1):53–5 [A].

[57] Williams MF, Maloof 3rd. JA. Resolution of clopidogrel-associated polyarthritis after conversion to prasugrel. Am J Health Syst Pharm. 2014;71(13):1097–100 [A].

[58] Liu T, Yin T, Li Y, et al. CYP2C19 polymorphisms and coronary heart disease risk factors synergistically impact clopidogrel response variety after percutaneous coronary intervention. Coron Artery Dis. 2014;25(5):412–20 [c].

[59] Cresci S, Depta JP, Lenzini PA, et al. Cytochrome p450 gene variants, race, and mortality among clopidogrel-treated patients after acute myocardial infarction. Circ Cardiovasc Genet. 2014;7(3):277–86 [C].

[60] Kristensen KE, Zhu HJ, Wang X, et al. Clopidogrel bioactivation and risk of bleeding in patients cotreated with angiotensin-converting enzyme inhibitors after myocardial infarction: a proof-of-concept study. Clin Pharmacol Ther. 2014;96(6):713–22 [C].

[61] Cho JR, Desai B, Haas MJ, et al. Impact of cigarette smoking on P2Y12 receptor binding activity before and after clopidogrel

therapy in patients with coronary artery disease. J Cardiovasc Transl Res. 2014;7(1):47–52 [c].

[62] Williams CD. Clopidogrel for smokers and aspirin for nonsmokers?: not so fast. Clin Pharmacol Ther. 2014;95(6):585–7 [r].

[63] Nanau RM, Delzor F, Neuman MG. Efficacy and safety of prasugrel in acute coronary syndrome patients. Clin Biochem. 2014;47(7–8):516–28 [R].

[64] Montalescot G, Bolognese L, Dudek D, et al. Pretreatment with prasugrel in non-ST-segment elevation acute coronary syndromes. N Engl J Med. 2013;369(11):999–1010 [C].

[65] Akbari SH, Reynolds MR, Kadkhodayan Y, et al. Hemorrhagic complications after prasugrel (Effient) therapy for vascular neurointerventional procedures. J Neurointerv Surg. 2013;5(4):337–43 [c].

[66] Erlinge D, Gurbel PA, James S, et al. Prasugrel 5 mg in the very elderly attenuates platelet inhibition but maintains noninferiority to prasugrel 10 mg in nonelderly patients: the GENERATIONS trial, a pharmacodynamic and pharmacokinetic study in stable coronary artery disease patients. J Am Coll Cardiol. 2013;62(7):577–83 [c].

[67] Yang DC, Feldman DN, Kim LK, et al. A strategy of "treating through" a prasugrel-induced rash. Int J Cardiol. 2013;168(4):4381–2 [A].

[68] Dobesh PP, Oestreich JH. Ticagrelor: pharmacokinetics, pharmacodynamics, clinical efficacy, and safety. Pharmacotherapy. 2014;34(10):1077–90 [R].

[69] Steiner JB, Wu Z, Ren J. Ticagrelor: positive, negative and misunderstood properties as a new antiplatelet agent. Clin Exp Pharmacol Physiol. 2013;40(7):398–403 [R].

[70] Storey RF, James SK, Siegbahn A, et al. Lower mortality following pulmonary adverse events and sepsis with ticagrelor compared to clopidogrel in the PLATO study. Platelets. 2014;25(7):517–25 [C].

[71] Parodi G, Storey RF. Dyspnoea management in acute coronary syndrome patients treated with ticagrelor. Eur Heart J Acute Cardiovasc Care. 2014; in press, pii: 2048872614554108 [R].

[72] Whitmore TJ, O'Shea JP, Starac D, et al. A case of pulmonary hemorrhage due to drug-induced pneumonitis secondary to ticagrelor therapy. Chest. 2014;145(3):639–41 [A].

[73] Cheng VE, Oppermen A, Natarajan D, et al. Spontaneous omental bleeding in the setting of dual anti-platelet therapy with ticagrelor. Heart Lung Circ. 2014;23(4):26 [A].

[74] Quinn KL, Connelly KA. First report of hypersensitivity to ticagrelor. Can J Cardiol. 2014;30(8):13 [A].

[75] Husted S, James SK, Bach RG, et al. The efficacy of ticagrelor is maintained in women with acute coronary syndromes participating in the prospective, randomized, PLATelet inhibition and patient Outcomes (PLATO) trial. Eur Heart J. 2014;35(23):1541–50 [C].

[76] Sharma V, Katznelson R, Jerath A, et al. The association between tranexamic acid and convulsive seizures after cardiac surgery: a multivariate analysis in 11 529 patients. Anaesthesia. 2014;69(2):124–30 [A].

[77] Tranexamic acid and thrombosis. Prescrire Int. 2013;22(140):182–3 [M].

[78] Bhat A, Bhowmik DM, Vibha D, et al. Tranexamic acid overdosage-induced generalized seizure in renal failure. Saudi J Kidney Dis Transpl. 2014;25(1):130–2 [A].

[79] Song Y, Izumi N, Potts LB, et al. Tranexamic acid-induced ligneous conjunctivitis with renal failure showed reversible hypoplasminogenaemia. BMJ Case Rep. 2014;19(10):2014–204138 [A].

35

Gastrointestinal Drugs

Karin Sandoval[1], Ken Witt

Department of Pharmaceutical Sciences, School of Pharmacy, Southern Illinois University Edwardsville,
Edwardsville, IL, USA

[1]Corresponding author: ksandov@siue.edu

ACID-IMPACTING AGENTS

Antacids [SED-15, 243; SEDA-34, 555; SEDA-35, 633; SEDA-36, 539]

Drug–Drug Interaction, Nemonoxicin

Nemonoxacin is a non-fluorinated quinolone antibiotic that is currently approved in Taiwan for treating community acquired pneumonia when given orally [1R]. Since drugs containing metal ions such as antacids can decrease the absorption of many quinolones, how antacids and other drugs containing metal ions (ferrous sulfate) could impact the absorption of nemonoxacin was investigated [2c]. Two randomized controlled trials in 24 healthy male Chinese volunteers (mean age 22.3 years old) were conducted. The first study was an open, randomized, four-way crossover study that investigated the impact of an antacid containing aluminum and magnesium (318 mg of aluminum and 496 mg of magnesium) when administered 2 hours before, concomitantly, or 4 hours after nemonoxacin (500 mg). The second study was an open, randomized, three-way crossover study which assessed the impact of ferrous sulfate (containing 60 mg of ferrous iron) or an antacid containing calcium carbonate (containing 600 mg of calcium) when given concurrently with nemonoxacin (500 mg). Administration of the magnesium and aluminum antacid concurrently as well as 4 hours after nemonoxacin administration decreased the area under the concentration-time curve (AUC 0–∞: 80.5% decrease concurrently and 58% decrease 4 hours later) and the maximum concentration of nemonoxacin (C_{max}:77.8% decrease concurrently, and 52.7% decrease 4 hours later). Data indicates antacids containing magnesium/aluminum should be administered at a minimum 2 hours prior to nemonoxacin administration.

Neoplasms

A prospective study assessed four different types of upper gastrointestinal cancer over 11 years in the NIH-AARP Diet and Health Study cohort with multivitamins or individual vitamin/mineral supplements [3C]. The use of calcium, a portion of which was noted to be in the form of antacids, was associated with an increased hazard of esophageal adenocarcinoma (HR=1.27, 95% CI=1.06–1.52) and gastric cardia adenocarcinoma (HR=1.27, 95% CI=1.03–1.56). However, calcium use as an antacid as compared to being a vitamin supplement was not delineated within the examination. Furthermore, gastroesophageal reflux disease itself is noted for being a primary risk factor for adenocarcinomas and was thought to account for this finding.

Histamine-2 Receptor Antagonists [SED-15, 1629; SEDA-34, 562; SEDA-35, 637; SEDA-36, 545]

Systematic Review

A systematic review was performed investigating the safety and efficacy of histamine-2 (H2) receptor antagonists in children (<15 years of age) with gastroesophageal reflux disease (GERD) [4M]. The systematic review included eight randomized controlled trials involving 276 children. For studies comparing H2 receptor antagonists to placebo, they were inadequately reported to where quantitative analyses for safety analyses could not be conducted. Three of the studies within the review reported no serious adverse outcomes. Adverse outcomes such as vomiting, nausea, abdominal pain, dizziness, and intermittent headache were reported only in children treated with H2 receptor antagonists. Four of the adverse events (non-specified) were identified as potentially treatment

© 2015 Elsevier B.V. All rights reserved.

related. The quality of the available evidence was low due to the high risk of bias, small sample sizes, and the clinical heterogeneity of the studies. Given the previously reported safety issues in newborns, H2 receptor antagonists were recommended to be prescribed with significant caution and only in confirmed acid-induced GERD.

Cognition

A retrospective cohort study was conducted to ascertain whether there was a relationship between starting a new standard dose of H2 receptor antagonist (40 mg/day famotidine or 300 mg/day ranitidine) and altered mental status in older adults (>65 years old) as compared to a low dose of a H2 receptor antagonist (20 mg/day famotidine or 150 mg/day ranitidine) within 30 days of starting the prescription [5C]. Exclusion criteria included those that were aged 65 since they were in their first year of eligibility for prescription drug coverage, those discharged from hospital in the 2 days prior to the index date to ensure prescriptions were initiated in an outpatient setting, those with end-stage renal disease, those living in long-term care facilities, and those with H2 receptor antagonist prescriptions 180 days prior to index date. The primary outcome was hospitalization with evidence of an urgent head computed tomography (CT) scan, which was felt by the authors to be a proxy measure for delirium. Only head CT scans performed in the emergency department preceding the hospital admission or within the first 5 days of a hospital admission were included in the analysis. Baseline characteristics, H2 receptor antagonist use and dose, and outcome data were ascertained using eight linked healthcare databases. There was not a significant difference in 27 baseline patient characteristics in those receiving the standard dose of H2 receptor antagonist compared to the low dose. In those taking the standard dose of an H2 receptor antagonist, this was associated with a higher risk of hospitalization with an urgent head CT scan (adjusted relative risk = 1.39, 95% CI: 1.17–1.65) compared to the low dose. This risk was not modified by the presence of chronic kidney disease (interaction p value = 0.71). In those taking the standard dose of a H2 receptor antagonist, this was also associated with a higher risk of all-cause mortality (adjusted relative risk = 1.38, 95% CI: 1.16–1.64) compared to the lower dose. Compared to a lower dose, initiation of the standard dose of H2 receptor antagonist in older adults was associated with a small absolute increase in the 30-day risk of altered mental status. This data suggested the risk of these outcomes may be reduced by initiating older adults on low doses of H2 receptor antagonist, with dosing titrated to maximize symptom control.

Peritonitis

A retrospective single-center study evaluated the association between gastric acid suppressants and prokinetic agents on peritonitis in adult peritoneal dialysis (PD) patients with end-stage renal disease [6c]. Exclusion criteria included those less than 20 years of age, individuals with incomplete data, peritonitis related to perforation of the gastrointestinal tract or gallbladder, liver cirrhosis, and those previously administered antibiotics within the last year. Individual episodes of recurrent or relapsing peritonitis were excluded to minimize bias. Medication use (H2 receptor antagonist, proton pump inhibitor (PPI) antacid, immunosuppressant) was determined from the records of the most recent clinical visits 1 year prior to the first episode of peritonitis. Use of gastric acid suppressants was defined by the authors as the use of any PPIs or H2 receptor antagonists for at least 2 days. Use of gastric acid suppressants was further classified into four groups: use within the previous 7 days, use within the previous 30 days but not within the past 7 days, use within the previous 1 year but not within the last 30 days, and no use of acid suppressants. Sixty-one patients had at least one occurrence of peritonitis (defined as group-A), and 59 patients did not experienced peritonitis (defined as group-B). Twenty-four of 61 patients (39.3%) in group A and 15 of 59 patients (25.4%) in group B used gastric acid suppressants. Fifteen out of 61 patients with peritonitis used H2 receptor antagonists within the last year, while only four that never experienced peritonitis used H2 receptor antagonists within the last year. In the multivariate analysis, H2 receptor antagonist use within 1 year prior to the development of peritonitis was a significant independent predictor for peritonitis (OR = 6.55; 95% CI: 1.64–26.26; p = 0.008). Of the agents assessed, only the use of H2 receptor antagonists was associated with significantly increased odds of PD-related peritonitis compared to the odds of non-users. However, the study did not include individual drug doses, reasons for gastric acid suppressant prescription, or potential confounding factors such as type of PD and exit-site infection. Additionally, the point estimates that were generated for H2 receptor antagonists were based on small counts (particularly amongst those that did not experience peritonitis) leading to very wide confidence intervals. Larger and further studies are required to delineate a clearer picture of this association, and the role of the dose and time-frame with this association.

Vitamin B12 Deficiency

A nested case–control study evaluated the association between vitamin B12 deficiency and use of H2 receptor antagonists or PPIs in adults within the Kaiser Permanente Northern California (KPNC) healthcare system [7C]. Patients were >18 years old, had to have been a member for at least 1 year, and had an initial diagnosis of vitamin B12 deficiency. Ten controls were randomly selected and matched per case by race/ethnicity, year of birth (within 1 year), sex, region, and membership duration (rounded to year) within 1 year. Medication exposure status was determined using the KPNC pharmacy database based on definitions established prior to assessment of exposure. PPI or H2 receptor antagonist exposure was defined as those who received at least a 2-year supply of PPIs or H2 receptor antagonists prior to their index date. Adherence and dose was investigated by using the number of dispensed pills divided by duration of use per day (mean daily dose). The unexposed reference group was defined as patients without current or prior prescriptions for either PPIs or H2 receptor antagonists. Conditional logistic regression was used to estimate the risk of vitamin B12 deficiency from the odds ratios. While many confounders were investigated, none were found to alter the odds ratio by more than 10%. Those with vitamin B12 deficiency were more likely to be supplied with greater than or equal to a 2-year supply of PPIs (OR = 1.65, 95% CI: 1.58–1.73) or H2 receptor antagonists (OR = 1.25, 95% CI: 1.17–1.34). Diagnosis of vitamin B12 deficiency in persons taking PPIs for 2 years or more was more likely in those taking PPIs for all mean daily doses (≥ 1.5 PPI pills/day OR = 1.95, 95% CI, 1.77–2.15; 0.75–1.49 PPI pills/day OR = 1.55, 95% CI: 1.46–1.64; <0.75 pills/day OR = 1.63, 95% CI: 1.48–1.78) when compared to non-users. The degree of the association between 2 and more years of PPI use and vitamin B12 deficiency was greater in women (OR = 1.84, 95% CI: 1.74–1.95) than in men (OR = 1.43, 95% CI: 1.33–1.53); and younger age groups (<30 years of age OR = 8.12, 95% CI: 3.36–19.59). Diagnosis of vitamin B12 deficiency in persons taking H2 receptor antagonists for 2 years or more was significantly more likely in those taking 0.75–1.49 pills/day (OR = 1.16, 95% CI: 1.04–1.28) and >1.5 pills/day (OR = 1.37, 95% CI: 1.23–1.52) compared to non-users. However, there was not a significant difference in vitamin B12 deficiency diagnosis in those receiving <0.75 pills/day of H2 receptor antagonists compared to non-users (OR = 1.19, 95% CI: 0.99–1.42). A subsequent point/counter-point series of "letters" identified concerns over several variables [8r,9r,10r], including lack of information as to over-the-counter PPI and H2 receptor antagonist use, lack of dietary data, defined daily dosing information, and definition of vitamin B12 deficiency. Nevertheless, the data are supportive of previous work identifying vitamin B12 deficiency with prolonged gastric acid suppression [11c], and the well-established dependency of vitamin B12 absorption with gastrointestinal pH.

Proton-Pump Inhibitors [SED-15, 2973; SEDA-34, 563; SEDA-35, 638; SEDA-36, 535]

Bone/Mineral Metabolism

PPIs given over a prolonged period of time may decrease bone mineral density, predisposing patients towards osteoporosis and fractures [12c]. Both the United States Food and Drug Administration (FDA) and the European Medicines Agency (EMA) have acknowledged that use of PPIs, especially at high doses and over prolonged time periods, may increase the risks of hip, wrist and spine fracture in the elderly, or in those with other risk factors that may predispose towards fracture.

A parallel randomized controlled trial investigated the effect of 8 weeks of treatment with either the PPI pantoprazole (40 mg/daily), or the potassium competitive acid blocker (PCAB) revaprazan (200 mg/daily), on parameters of bone turnover such as serum calcium, urine deoxypyridinoline (DPD), intact parathyroid hormone, fractional excretion of calcium and osteocalcin [12c]. This study was performed in Koreans with a mean age of ~63 years old with gastric ulcer. Thirteen patients were in each treatment group after withdrawal or exclusion from the study (pantoprazole group: five withdrew, two excluded due to low bone mineral density; revaprazan: five withdrew, one excluded due to low bone mineral density). In the pantoprazole group, there was a significant increase in serum corrected calcium (pre-pantoprazole: 8.8 ± 0.5, post-pantoprazole: 9.2 ± 0.6, $p = 0.046$) and urine DPD (pre-pantoprazole: 5.7 ± 2.2, post-pantoprazole: 6.5 ± 2.1, $p = 0.047$). No other significant changes for bone turnover markers including intact parathyroid hormone, fractional excretion of calcium, and osteocalcin were found in the pantoprazole group. No significant changes were found in any bone turnover parameters in the revaprazan group. This study suggested that even after only 8 weeks of treatment with pantoprazole (40 mg/daily) there were some significant changes in two bone turnover parameters, urine DPD and serum corrected calcium. However, the study did not account for dietary calcium intake. Thus, it is unclear whether differences in calcium intake could potentially explain these findings.

A prospective study was performed in gastroesophageal reflux disease (GERD) patients (18–56 years old) to investigate the association between treatment with PPIs and bone density [13c]. Patients with GERD were randomized into three treatment groups: lansoprazole 30 mg/day, pantoprazole 40 mg/day, or esomeprazole 40 mg/day. Exclusion criteria included chronic conditions that may affect bone density, medications known to modify fracture, and receiving PPI treatment for at least 1 month within a year before the study. The mean treatment duration for the study was 8.5 ± 2.3 months. In patients receiving PPIs, there was a significant reduction in all of the mean bone density measures post-treatment when compared to pre-treatment (L1 T score, L2 T score, L3 T score, L4 T score, L total T score, and femur neck T score, $p < 0.05$). When looking at each PPI, lansoprazole, pantoprazole and esomeprazole were found to significantly reduce L total T scores post-treatment when compared to pre-treatment ($p < 0.01$, for each PPI). When looking at femur neck T scores, only esomeprazole significantly reduced femur neck T scores post-treatment compared to pre-treatment ($p = 0.01$). While treatment with PPIs was shown as a whole to result in a significant reduction in bone density post-treatment compared to pre-treatment, some reductions in certain bone density measures were PPI specific. The authors note that monitoring of bone density for patients receiving long-term treatment with PPIs may be warranted.

A matched case–control study was conducted in pairs of men to determine the association between hip fracture and PPI use [14C]. Cases were men ($\geq$45 years old), who sustained a hip fracture from 1997–2006 identified from electronic medical records within the Southern California region of Kaiser Permanente (KPSC) healthcare system. Exclusion criteria included evidence of prior fracture preceding the study period. Controls were matched to cases 1:1 on age, race/ethnicity, medical center, and membership in the health plan on the fracture/index date. Exposure to PPIs was determined from pharmacy dispensing records from 1991 to 2006. Based on information obtained from the pharmacy dispensing records, PPI use was measured in terms of ever used versus never used, duration of use, recentness of use, as well as adherence. Adherence was based upon the medication possession ratio which calculates the total number of days the medication is supplied divided by the total number of days between the first and last prescription. In addition, information on other comorbid conditions for each subject was obtained from information in the medical record 2 years prior to the index date since this was thought to be a potential confounder. The overall comorbidity burden was calculated using the Deyo adaptation of the Charlson Index. Since matching was not performed using the comorbidity score, cases had significantly higher comorbidity than controls ($p < 0.001$). Before the index date, 13.2% of cases and 10.5% of controls had used omeprazole before index date. The odds of hip fracture were 13% higher in those ever exposed to omeprazole when adjusting for comorbidities (adjusted OR = 1.13, 95% CI: 1.01–1.27). The odds of hip fracture were significantly higher with greater omeprazole adherence (medication possession ratio >80% (adjusted OR = 1.33, 95% CI: 1.09–1.62)), longest of duration of use (adjusted OR, 1.23, 95% CI: 1.02–1.48), and most recent use (adjusted OR = 1.22; 95% CI, 1.02–1.47) compared to no omeprazole use and adjusting for comorbidities. For pantoprazole, 10.2% of cases and 8.5% of controls had used pantoprazole prior to the index date. The odds of hip fracture were the same in those that ever used pantoprazole when adjusting for comorbidities compared to never use (adjusted OR = 1.10; 95% CI: 0.97–1.24). The odds of hip fracture were significantly higher in those with the longest

duration of use of pantoprazole (adjusted OR = 1.25; 95% CI: 1.02–1.53) and most recent use (adjusted OR = 1.38, 95% CI: 1.12–1.71) when compared to the odds of no pantoprazole use and adjusted for comorbidities. However, the odds of hip fracture were the same with higher adherence (medication possession ratio >80% (adjusted OR = 1.07, 95% CI: 0.89–1.29)) compared to no pantoprazole use. The results suggested that omeprazole use and hip fractures were associated. Furthermore, it suggested that odds of hip fracture increased with longer duration of use and more recent use of PPIs. However, other injuries, over-the-counter use, dose, and dietary factors were not accounted for when looking at this association.

Cardiovascular

The association between PPIs and myocardial infarction was investigated in Taiwan retrospectively from 2000 to 2009 using both a propensity score matching analysis and a case–cross-over study [15C]. The primary outcome was hospitalization for myocardial infarction, which was obtained using ICD-9 codes from the Longitudinal Health Insurance Database (LHID). Information on prescriptions was also obtained from the LHID. Since the authors noted that the most common prescription for PPIs was 4 months in duration, they used a follow-up period of 120 days after prescription for PPIs, with the index date being the date of PPI prescription. Eligibility criteria included being 18–80 years old, no prior history of MI, acquired immunodeficiency syndrome, HIV infection, or cancer before prescription for PPIs, and no prior prescription for PPIs within 120 days. Exclusion criteria included the prescription of PPIs within 60 days after an episode of severe upper gastrointestinal bleeding requiring hospitalization, blood transfusion, or use of inotropic agents. For the propensity score analysis, a Cox proportional hazards model was used to calculate the hazard ratio (HR) for MI and 95% confidence intervals (CIs) in PPI users as compared to the PPI non-users. Hazard ratios were adjusted for the propensity score. For the case–cross-over analysis, a conditional logistic regression model was used to obtain point estimates for odds ratios (OR) and 95% CIs. The odds ratios were adjusted to control for confounding medication exposures. After 120 days of follow-up, the hazard of MI with PPI use was 1.58 times the hazard of MI for the control group (adjusted HR = 1.58, 95% CI = 1.11–2.25). In the case–cross-over study, MI risk was significantly increased with PPI use for the 7-day window period (adjusted OR = 4.61, 95% CI: 1.76–12.07) and the 14-day window period (adjusted OR = 3.47, 95% CI = 1.76–6.83). Although the results of this study suggested that use of PPIs may be independently associated with an increased risk of MI, it remains unclear whether this is a dose-dependent phenomenon. Furthermore, understanding the long-term effects of PPIs with MI should be ascertained since this study looked at a short time frame of duration.

A meta-analysis was performed using randomized and non-randomized studies that reported adverse cardiovascular events in patients taking PPIs (222 311 participants, average age 66.7 years old) and receiving clopidogrel. This analysis was done to determine whether the risk for cardiovascular events differed for individual PPIs when taken with clopidogrel [16M]. Pooled estimates of cardiovascular risk were significantly increased for individual PPIs such as omeprazole (OR = 1.24, 95% CI: 1.07–1.43, $I^2 = 74$%), esomeprazole (OR = 1.32, 95% CI: 1.09–1.60, $I^2 = 76$%), lansoprazole (OR = 1.39, 95% CI: 1.23–1.57, $I^2 = 26$%) and pantoprazole (OR = 1.41, 95% CI: 1.21–1.64, $I^2 = 75$%), but not rabeprazole (OR = 1.38, 95% CI: 0.78–2.45, $I^2 = 76$%) when used with clopidogrel. However, one of the issues with the pooled average estimates of risk for each PPI was that there was moderate to substantial heterogeneity between the studies. Meta-analysis of seven observational studies evaluating PPI therapy in the absence of clopidogrel found the odds of major adverse cardiac events were significantly higher in those receiving PPIs (OR = 1.28, 95% CI 1.14–1.44, $I^2 = 77$%) compared to the odds of those not receiving PPIs or clopidogrel. The authors noted that the marked heterogeneity from the meta-analysis assessing the cardiovascular risk without clopidogrel came from a single study. When this one study was removed, the heterogeneity dropped to 0% and the primary outcome remained similar (OR = 1.39; 95% CI: 1.32–1.46, $I^2 = 0$%). Meta-analysis of two randomized controlled trials showed no significant adverse cardiovascular effect from either esomeprazole or omeprazole. Within their analysis, they found a lack of consistent evidence on differential cardiovascular risk amongst PPIs. The authors felt that the results of their study raised serious questions about the clinical relevance of particular PPIs being labeled as safe or not safe when it comes to the PPI-clopidogrel interaction.

Another study assessed the association between hospitalizations for acute myocardial infarction or heart failure within 12 weeks of initiating PPI use in patients >66 years old [17C]. A self-matched case series method was used for both outcomes for both cohorts using population-based health care data from Ontario, Canada (1996–2008). The primary risk interval was defined as the initial 4 weeks of treatment, while the control interval was defined as the final 4 weeks of treatment. The index date was defined as the date of a first prescription for a PPI, which was obtained from the Ontario Drug Benefit Claims Database. Hospitalization for heart failure and acute myocardial infarction were obtained using ICD-9 codes from the Canadian Institute for Health Information's Discharge Abstract Database. Within 12 weeks of starting PPI therapy, there were 5550 hospital admissions for acute myocardial infarction and 6003 admissions for heart failure. Use of a PPI was associated with significantly higher odds of acute myocardial infarction (OR = 1.8; 95% CI: 1.7–1.9) and heart failure (OR = 1.8; 95% CI: 1.7–1.9) during the risk interval compared to odds of either event during the control interval. However, secondary analyses found similar measures of association for acute myocardial infarction for H2 receptor antagonists (OR = 1.8, 95% CI: 1.7–1.9; OR = 1.5, 95% CI: 1.4–1.6, respectively) and benzodiazepines (OR = 1.3, 95% CI: 1.3–1.4, OR = 1.6, 95% CI: 1.5–1.7, respectively), which are not affiliated with cardiotoxicity. While the authors found that use of PPIs was associated with a short-term increase in the odds of acute myocardial infarction and heart failure, given that similar odds were found with other drugs not suspected of cardiac toxicity, they felt the associations between PPIs and acute myocardial infarction and heart failure were spurious.

Clostridium difficile *Infection*

The association between PPIs and *Clostridium difficile* infection (CDI) has been noted by the Food and Drug Administration, which resulted in a safety announcement in November 2012, as well as a labeling change. The FDA safety announcement recommended for patients to use the lowest dose and shortest duration of PPI therapy appropriate to the condition being treated. However, determining which patient populations may be at greatest risk of CDI, risk factors that may predispose to CDI while on PPIs, and aspects relating to PPI dosing, continues to be investigated.

A retrospective case–control study evaluated the association between duration of PPI use in critically ill patients in the intensive care unit (ICU) and *Clostridium difficile* infection (CDI) [18c]. CDI cases were identified using ICD-9 secondary diagnosis codes for *Clostridium difficile* infection. Inclusion criteria included presence in an ICU for at least 48 hours prior to diagnosis of secondary CDI. Cases were matched 1:1 to patients without CDI using the ICD-9 primary diagnosis code, Sequential Organ Failure Assessment (SOFA) score (±1), and age (±5 years). Exclusion criteria for the study included CDI being listed as a primary diagnosis, a suitable match could not be found, or missing or incomplete data for the medication record. PPI exposure duration was classified as short (<2 days) or long (≥2 days). Of the 408 patients in the study, 81% received a PPI. The percentage of patients who had a long exposure (≥2 days) to PPIs was 83% in the CDI group compared to 73% with controls (p = 0.012). Considering confounding variables could distort the measure of association between CDI and PPIs, several conditional logistic regression models were built taking into account H2 receptor antagonist use, antimicrobial therapy, and immunosuppression as confounding variables. Only long-term PPI exposure (OR=2.03, 95% CI: 1.23–3.36) and antibiotic use (OR=2.52, 95% CI: 1.23–5.18) were identified as significant independent predictors of CDI, when adjusting for study duration. Considering there was a significant association between PPI use for greater than 2 days and CDI, but not a significant association with H2 receptor antagonist use and CDI, the authors suggested for clinicians to consider alternative forms of acid suppressive therapy for critically ill patients in the ICU.

A retrospective observational study looked at the association between PPIs being used to prevent gastrointestinal bleedings in critically ill patients in the intensive care unit (ICU) and *Clostridium difficile* associated diarrhea (CDAD) [19c]. Exclusion criteria included staying less than 48 hours in ICU or diagnosis of upper GI bleeding. Information about acid suppression medication use, type of antibiotics, and primary diagnosis was collected at admission. The outcome, development of CDAD, was collected from information obtained during the ICU stay. CDAD was defined as new onset of diarrhea using endoscopy and/or positive detection of *Clostridium difficile* antigen in feces, and/or positive *Clostridium difficile* toxin A/B DNA. The study included 3286 critically ill patients. Of those patients receiving stress ulcer prophylaxis, 55.6% received a PPI-only. One hundred and ten patients developed CDAD, which was associated with increased ICU mortality (OR=1.59, 95% CI: 1.06–2.41). Similar to fluoroquinolones (adjusted OR=1.87, 95% CI: 1.1–3.14) and cephalosporins, PPIs were identified as a significant independent predictor (adjusted OR=3.11, 95% CI: 1.11–8.74) for developing CDAD in the ICU when using multivariate logistic regression analysis. Considering PPI use was a significant positive predictor of CDAD and CDAD development in the ICU was associated with an increase in the odds of mortality, the authors suggested that further investigations are needed to identify which groups of patients may benefit most from PPI use for bleeding prophylaxis and to identify which patients are at highest risk for developing CDAD with PPIs.

A retrospective cohort study investigated the association between PPI or H2 receptor antagonist administration for ≥48 hours and *Clostridium difficile* infection (CDI), GI hemorrhage and pneumonia in intubated adult patients requiring mechanical ventilation for ≥24 hours [20C]. The outcomes were obtained using secondary ICD-9 diagnosis codes. Prior to data collection, exposure was defined as pharmacy dispensed H2 receptor antagonist or PPI within the first 48 hours of ventilation. Propensity score-adjusted and propensity-matched multivariate regression models were used control for confounders. Only the propensity score adjusted analyses will be presented here. Of 35 312 patients, 61.9% received PPIs and 38.1% received H2 receptor antagonists. The most common H2 receptor antagonist prescribed was famotidine, which accounted for 86.4% of those on H2 receptor antagonists. Of patients prescribed H2 receptor antagonists, 12.7% were classified as having received a high dose. The most common PPI prescribed was pantoprazole, which accounted for 74.7% of those on PPIs. Of patients prescribed PPIs, 47% of patients were classified as receiving high-dose PPIs. Mortality in the ICU was significantly higher in those receiving PPIs compared to H2 receptor antagonists (17.8% versus 10.8%, $p<0.001$). Development of CDI (3.8% versus 2.2%, respectively, $p<0.001$), gastrointestinal hemorrhage (5.9% versus 2.1%, respectively, $p<0.001$), or pneumonia (38.6% versus 27%, respectively, $p<0.001$) was significantly higher in the PPI group compared to the H2 receptor antagonist group. The odds of GI hemorrhage (OR=2.24, 95% CI: 1.81–2.76), CDI (OR=1.29, 95% CI: 1.04–1.64) and pneumonia (OR=1.2, 95% CI: 1.03–1.41) were significantly higher in those that received PPIs compared to the odds of these outcomes in the H2 receptor antagonist group after adjusting for the propensity score and covariates. This study demonstrated that use of PPIs for ≥48 hours compared to use of H2 receptor antagonists was associated with greater odds of GI hemorrhage, pneumonia, and CDI therapy in intubated adult patients requiring mechanical ventilation for ≥24 hours.

A retrospective cross-sectional analysis of 100 patients with CDI was performed, with assessment of risk factors, treatment, and clinical outcomes by reviewing electronic medical records [21c]. CDI diagnosis was based on a positive EIA for toxin A/B in the stool. The majority (87%) of the patients were >60 years of age, with 43% of patients presented from nursing facilities, and >50% with PPI use at the time of admission. Most of the patients had multiple co-morbidities, with 74% having taken antibiotics in the previous 6 months. Fifty-two patients were noted to be on a PPI at the time of CDI diagnosis. In those with CDI, a beta-lactam alone or in combination with other antibiotics was prescribed in 48%, quinolones in 13% and clindamycin in 4% of patients had been used in the last 6 months. Intensive care unit hospitalization was required in 33% of patients with CDI. Seventeen percent of patients with CDI died during hospitalization. Considering many of the patients were elderly, on PPIs and had been prescribed antibiotics in the last 6 months, the authors suggested that judicious use of PPIs and antibiotics in the elderly may help reduce the mortality and morbidity from CDI.

Drug–Drug Interaction, Cancer Chemotherapeutics

A recent review addressed the interaction between oral tyrosine kinase inhibitors and acid suppressive drugs [22R]. When tyrosine kinase inhibitors (generally weakly basic) are co-administered with acid suppressive drugs the pH in the stomach increases, resulting in a reduced bioavailability. The oral absorption of crizotinib, dasatinib, erlotinib, gefitinib, lapatinib, nilotinib, erlotinib, and pazopanib were noted to be substantially reduced by concomitant use of acid suppressive treatment. The degree of interaction was variable, and dependent on the form of gastric acid suppressor (i.e. antacid, H2 receptor antagonist, or PPI) and/or window of coadministration. Given the significance of these drugs respective to cancer treatment, concurrent use of acid suppressors with tyrosine kinase inhibitors warrants additional patient monitoring with potential need for dose adjustments.

Erlotinib is an epidermal growth factor receptor (EGFR) tyrosine kinase inhibitor used in the treatment of advanced non-small-cell lung cancer (NSCLC). Erlotinib has been shown to have pH dependent solubility. Drugs that suppress gastric acid secretion including the PPI omeprazole and the H2 receptor antagonist ranitidine have been shown to significantly decrease the C_{max} (omeprazole: 61%; ranitidine 300 mg: 54%; ranitidine 150 mg bid: 17%) and AUC (omeprazole: 46%; ranitidine 300 mg: 33%; ranitidine 150 mg bid: 15%) of erlotinib [23S]. Based on this interaction, the manufacturers of erlotinib recommended that PPIs should be avoided. Additionally, if treatment with an H2 receptor antagonist such as ranitidine was required, erlotinib was recommended to be taken 10 hours after the taking the H2 receptor antagonist and at least 2 hours prior to the next dose of the H2 receptor antagonist.

A retrospective analysis of the impact of gastric acid suppression on overall survival and progression free survival in patients that had taken erlotinib for ≥ 1 week was assessed ($n = 124$ acid suppressant, $n = 383$ no acid suppressant) [24c]. The majority of patients receiving acid suppressant therapy (93%) were on PPIs (pantoprazole 40 mg (43%), omeprazole 20 mg (29%), lansoprazole 30 mg (16%) and rabeprazole 20 mg, (5%)). Seven percent of patients were on 150 mg of a H2 receptor antagonist, ranitidine. Multivariate Cox proportional hazards regression was then used to ascertain the hazard of death when taking erlotinib with or without acid suppressants. When looking at progression free survival, the hazard of death in those taking erlotinib with acid suppressant therapy was ~70% higher (HR = 1.71, 95% CI: 1.48–2.25, $p < 0.0001$) than the hazard of those taking erlotinib without acid suppressant therapy when adjusting for female gender, squamous cell subtype, and Eastern Cooperative Oncology Group (ECOG) performance status (PS) 3-4. Median progression free survival time for those taking acid suppressant therapy with erlotinib was 1.4 months compared to 2.3 months for those that were not taking acid suppressant therapy with erlotinib. Respective to overall survival, the hazard of death in those taking acid suppressant therapy with erlotinib was 37% higher (HR = 1.37, 95% CI: 1.11–1.69, $p = 0.003$) than the hazard of those not taking acid suppressant therapy with erlotinib when adjusting for female gender, squamous cell subtype, and ECOG PS 3-4. The median overall survival time

in those receiving acid suppressant therapy and erlotinib was 12.9 months versus 16.8 months for those taking erlotinib without acid suppressant therapy. Out of 20 individuals tested for the EGFR mutation (specifically exon 19 deletion or exon 21 point mutation), four patients that had not received acid suppressant therapy had an EGFR mutation. Nonsmoking history, which was found to be a significant predictor of erlotinib efficacy in another study [25c] was not taken into account in this study. Thus, it is unclear whether differences in EGFR mutation status or non-smoking history could explain these findings. However, it is biologically plausible that changes in pharmacokinetics due to acid suppressant therapy impact survival probability in patients taking erlotinib for NSCLC.

An open-label, non-randomized, phase-I single site study examined the effect of lansoprazole on bosutinib pharmacokinetics in healthy subjects (18–50 years old) [26c]. Bosutinib is a Src and Abl tyrosine kinase inhibitor used for the treatment of Philadelphia chromosome-positive chronic myelogenous leukemia. On day 1, patients received bosutinib (400 mg). On day 14, patients received lansoprazole (60 mg). On day 15, patients received bosutinib (400 mg) co-administered with lansoprazole (60 mg). The mean maximum plasma concentration (C_{max}) of bosutinib decreased from 70.2 to 42.9 ng/mL when co-administered with lansoprazole. Additionally, the total area under the plasma concentration-time curve (AUC) for bosutinib decreased from 1940 to 1470 ng h/mL when co-administered with lansoprazole. Bosutinib pharmacokinetic parameters were significantly different when individuals received bosutinib alone compared to when they received bosutinib with lansoprazole, ($p < 0.05$ for C_{max}, AUC, and AUC_{last}). The least squares geometric mean ratio for C_{max} was 54% (90% CI: 42–70) and AUC was 74% (90% CI: 60–90). This demonstrated that compared with bosutinib alone, co-administration of bosutinib with lansoprazole decreased the C_{max} for bosutinib by 46% and AUC by 26%. The mean apparent total body clearance from plasma after oral administration was elevated from 237 to 330 L/h, and the median time to reach C_{max} (t_{max}) increased from 5 to 6 hours. However, the authors noted that there was moderate inter-subject variability of bosutinib pharmacokinetic parameters, with this variance increasing with the combination compared to botusinib alone. This study demonstrated that certain bosutinib pharmacokinetic parameters were significantly impacted by co-administration of lansoprazole with bosutinib compared to when bosutinib was administered alone. This suggested that absorption of bosutinib appeared to be reduced when co-administered with lansoprazole. The authors recommended that caution should be used when using PPIs with bosutinib, as it could impact the efficacy of bosutinib.

An interaction between PPIs and methotrexate has been documented in case reports and several retrospective studies [27A,28c,29c]. PPIs have been proposed to inhibit elimination of methotrexate through inhibition of human organic anion transporter-3 [30E], leading to increased drug levels of methotrexate through decreased elimination. Even though this interaction is listed as a drug–drug interaction on drug monographs for PPIs [31S], several recent studies have called this interaction into question [32c,33c].

A retrospective study assessed whether PPIs when administered with high-dose methotrexate (≥ 1000 mg m^{-2} intravenously (IV) over 3–4 hours or ≥ 200 mg m^{-2} IV bolus followed by ≥ 800 mg m^{-2} IV over 22–24 hours) resulted in delayed methotrexate elimination compared to patients not taking PPIs [33c]. Exclusion criteria for the study included being less than 18 years of age, not having methotrexate levels monitored or being pregnant. According to the author, the standard of care for checking methotrexate levels was assessing levels 24, 48 and 72 hours after the start of the methotrexate infusion and every morning thereafter, until the level of methotrexate was ≤ 0.1 µmol L^{-1}. In this study, it was possible for patients to have data collected on multiple cycles of methotrexate with multiple admissions. The analyses that were performed took this factor into account. Delayed methotrexate elimination was defined by the author as plasma methotrexate concentrations of >10 µmol L^{-1} with a bolus infusion (over 3–4 hours) or >20 µmol L^{-1} with infusional methotrexate (over 22–24 hours) at 24 hours after the start of methotrexate therapy, >1 µmol L^{-1} at 48 hours, and >0.1 µmol L^{-1} at 72 hours. A significant difference was found in the median methotrexate levels at 24 (8.0 vs. 3.9 µmol L^{-1}, respectively, $p = 0.013$) and 72 hours after methotrexate administration (0.08 vs. 0.05 µmol L^{-1}, respectively, $p = 0.037$) in those receiving a PPI compared to those not receiving a PPI. However, there were no differences in the proportion of patients experiencing delayed elimination in those receiving PPIs compared to those not taking PPIs at 24 (19.2% vs. 20.2%, respectively) and 72 hours (36.2% vs. 33.7%, respectively). PPI use was not found to be a significant predictor of time to methotrexate level of <0.1 µmol L^{-1} when controlling for multiple cycles of methotrexate for each patient. Co-administration of PPIs was not found to be a significant predictor of methotrexate level ($p = 0.969$) when the clustering effect of multiple cycles of methotrexate per patient was controlled for. The results of this study suggest that there may not be an interaction between PPIs and methotrexate. One of the limitations of this study is that it did not take into account the dose of the PPI or type of PPI.

A retrospective case–control study was performed to assess the relationship between high-dose methotrexate and delayed methotrexate clearance (serum MTX level ≥ 0.1 µmol/L at 72 hours) in adult oncology patients receiving their first cycle of high-dose methotrexate [32c]. Cases ($n = 23$) were patients who experienced delayed methotrexate clearance. Controls ($n = 50$) were patients who did not experience delayed methotrexate clearance. While baseline patient characteristics were generally similar, there was a significant difference between cases and controls in baseline renal impairment (5 cases or 23.1% of cases, compared to 0 controls, $p = 0.002$) and chemotherapy protocol ($p = 0.009$). The odds of exposure to PPIs in those with delayed methotrexate elimination were similar to the odds of exposure to PPIs in those without delayed methotrexate elimination when adjusting for baseline covariates (OR$= 1.50$, 95% CI: 0.55–4.06). Thus, this study did not find an association between PPIs and delayed methotrexate clearance.

While these studies did not find an association between delayed methotrexate elimination with PPIs, evidence for and against this interaction has only been ascertained using observational studies. Randomized controlled trials are likely needed to clarify this interaction.

Drug–Drug Interaction, Clopidogrel

Clopidogrel is an oral antiplatelet agent that requires hepatic activation by CYP2C19 to exert its antiplatelet effect. To date, omeprazole and esomeprazole have been identified to inhibit CYP2C19 at lower concentrations than that of other PPIs [34E]. FDA labeling currently recommends avoiding omeprazole and esomeprazole in patients taking clopidogrel. While many studies continue to support a drug–drug interaction between clopidogrel and esomeprazole or omeprazole [35R], the potential of other PPIs interacting with clopidogrel has not been fully elucidated. In addition, comorbidities, pharmacogenetics, duration of use, and dose of PPIs continue to be investigated in looking at the association between PPIs and clopidogrel with adverse cardiovascular events.

A randomized controlled trial looked at different treatment regimens (doubling clopidogrel dose or switching to prasugrel) to deal with the interaction between lansoprazole and clopidogrel on platelet aggregation [36c]. The primary endpoint for the study was the relative change in residual platelet reactivity (RPA: [(RPA$_{14\ day}$ − RPA$_{baseline}$)/RPA$_{baseline}$)], which was assessed by light transmission aggregometry using 20 µmol adenosine diphosphate (ADP) over the 14 day study period. Stable coronary artery disease patients ($n = 82$) that had been on 75 mg of aspirin and 75 mg of clopidogrel for a minimum of 3 months and without a PPI for 14 days had baseline platelet reactivity performed. They were then randomized to an open label 150 mg clopidogrel or 10 mg prasugrel with a double blind daily dose of lansoprazole 30 mg or placebo. Following 2 weeks of treatment, platelet reactivity testing was performed again. When looking at baseline residual platelet reactivity for all patients on 75 mg/day each of clopidogrel and aspirin, there was no significant difference between groups (ADP: clopidogrel placebo baseline: 24.6 ± 18.9 versus clopidogrel lansoprazole baseline: 21.1 ± 14.1, $p = 0.64$; prasugrel placebo baseline: 25.3 ± 18.4 versus prasugrel lansoprazole baseline: 20.9 ± 15.8). After 2 weeks of treatment, residual platelet reactivity decreased in patients receiving clopidogrel 150 mg/day with placebo (ADP: clopidogrel placebo day 14: 12.9 ± 15.3), but remained similar to baseline in patients assigned to clopidogrel 150 mg/day with lansoprazole (ADP: clopidogrel lansoprazole day 14: 22.4 ± 17.1). In contrast, residual platelet reactivity decreased in both groups of patients receiving prasugrel 10 mg/day with placebo or lansoprazole after 2 weeks of treatment (ADP: prasugrel placebo day 14: 6.5 ± 12.3, prasugrel lansoprazole day 14: 6.0 ± 7.9). There was a significant relative change in residual platelet reactivity between clopidogrel treatment groups (ADP: −53.6 ± 48.4% versus +0.8 ± 53.7% without and with lansoprazole, respectively, $p = 0.02$), suggesting lansoprazole interfered with clopidogrel. In contrast, there was no difference in the relative change in residual platelet reactivity in prasugrel treatment groups (ADP: −81.8 ± 24.8% vs. −72.9 ± 32.9% without and with lansoprazole, respectively, $p = 0.55$), suggesting lansoprazole did not interfere with prasugrel. While they did not perform any statistical analyses within groups looking at residual platelet activity compared to baseline since it was not the primary end point, it should be noted that the residual platelet reactivity was very similar to baseline when lansoprazole was administered with the double dose of clopidogrel. Considering baseline was obtained from the same patients taking clopidogrel with aspirin, this suggests that the double dose with lansoprazole was an effective regimen to keep platelet reactivity similar. In contrast, prasugrel treatment groups and the double dose of clopidogrel with placebo decreased platelet reactivity from baseline, suggesting a higher platelet inhibitory effect. Whether this further antiplatelet inhibitory activity would be desirable, was unclear.

A randomized three-period crossover study was performed to assess the interaction between rabeprazole and antiplatelet actions and pharmacokinetics of clopidogrel as compared to omeprazole or placebo in CYP2C19 genotyped adults [37c]. In the study, 36 healthy men (33.6 years ± 7.9) received clopidogrel (75 mg/day) with placebo, omeprazole (20 mg/day) or rabeprazole (20 mg/day) for 7 days separated by a wash-out period of 2–3 weeks. The antiplatelet effects of clopidogrel with combination placebo, omeprazole or rabeprazole, were assessed on the seventh day of therapy before and 4 hours after administration of the last dose of clopidogrel together with placebo, omeprazole, or rabeprazole. Of the subjects, 23 were extensive metabolizers (EMs) (CYP2C19*1/*1), 12 were heterozygous (CYP2C19*1/*2), and one was a poor metabolizer (CYP2C19*2/*2). While baseline platelet activity as measured through VASP index, which measures the activity of the P2Y12 receptor, was similar across treatment periods ($p = 0.60$), there was considerable interindividual variability in platelet function to where there were two distinct groups; good responders with a change of VASP index ≥30%, those with a VASP index <30%. Among the EMs (CYP2C19*1/*1), 15 were good clopidogrel responders. Among the heterozygotes (CYP2C19*1/*2), only three were good clopidogrel responders. Compared to heterozygotes (CYP2C19*1/*2), EMs had significantly greater baseline antiplatelet effects with clopidogrel when administered with placebo (VASP index: −39.3 ± 0.20% in CYP2C19*1/*1 versus −22 ± 0.15% in CYP2C19*1/*2, $p < 0.015$), demonstrating that the CYP2C19 genotype influenced the antiplatelet effects of clopidogrel. In good responders, there was a statistically significant increase in the VASP index compared to placebo with omeprazole (baseline: $p = 0.017$, 4 hours: $p = 0.009$), but not with rabeprazole when compared to placebo (baseline: $p = 0.26$, 4 hours: $p = 0.20$) at baseline. If subjects were grouped together, there was not a statistically significant effect with rabeprazole (baseline: $p = 0.85$, 4 hours $p = 0.82$, respectively) or omeprazole (baseline: $p = 0.34$, 4 hours: $p = 0.056$) on the VASP index compared to placebo at baseline or 4 hours. In those that were EMs (CYP2C19*1/*1), both rabeprazole and omeprazole significantly decreased the AUC_{0-24} (rabeprazole versus placebo: $p = 0.0009$, omeprazole versus placebo: $p < 0.0001$) and C_{max} (rabeprazole versus placebo: $p = 0.0008$, omeprazole versus placebo: $p = 0.0002$) of the clopidogrel active metabolite compared to placebo. The authors concluded that with the PPI doses that were used, that there was no significant pharmacodynamic interaction between rabeprazole or omeprazole and clopidogrel, even though there was significant decrease in the formation of clopidogrel active metabolite in all subjects. One of the major limitations was that this was a small study and there were not equal subjects of individuals by genotype. Another major limitation of the study was that they did not separate out the VASP analyses or the platelet aggregation assays for extensive metabolizers for omeprazole and rabeprazole as compared to placebo even though they did this for the pharmacokinetic analyses. For the VASP assay, they only separated it for those that were good responders, 15 of which were extensive metabolizers. Considering there was a significant effect on the VASP index with omeprazole, but not rabeprazole when compared to placebo in good responders, it is possible that the interaction between omeprazole and clopidogrel may be more relevant for those that are extensive metabolizers as compared to other genotypes. However, considering the significant interindividual variability, it also suggests there are factors beyond CYP2C19 metabolism and genotype contributing to the variability in clopidogrel response that have yet to be ascertained.

Drug–Drug Interaction, Mycophenolate

FDA required labelling revisions for all PPIs to include the interaction between PPIs and mycophenolate mofetil [38S]. A 78% reduction in the C_{max} and a 45% reduction in the AUC of mycophenolic acid were observed in transplant patients ($n = 21$) receiving both pantoprazole (40 mg/day) and MMF (~2000 mg/day) compared to transplant patients receiving approximately the same dose of MMF ($n = 12$) [31S], demonstrating that this interaction can occur and could potentially have very serious clinical consequences.

Considering PPIs have been documented to alter the pharmacokinetics of mycophenolate mofetil (MMF) in healthy volunteers [39c,40c], the clinical significance of this interaction on 1 year biopsy proven acute rejection (BPAR) rates in patients receiving kidney transplants was investigated using a retrospective cohort design [41r]. Kidney transplant patients received induction therapy with rabbit antithymocyte globulin, which was then followed with calcineurin inhibitors, mycophenolate mofetil and steroids. Patients prescribed PPIs ($n = 213$) were compared with patients on standard acid-suppressive therapy with ranitidine (150 mg/day, $n = 384$). BPAR occurred in similar rates in both groups (15% vs. 12%; $p = 0.31$) and PPI use was not found to be a significant predictor of BPAR using multivariable analysis (risk ratio (RR) = 1.41, 95% CI: 0.88–2.23). However, black race was associated with increased rejection (RR = 2.38; 95% CI: 1.41–4.03). While controlling for rejection risk factors, PPI exposure was associated with increased rejection in black patients (RR = 1.93, 95% CI: 1.18–3.16), but not in non-black patients (RR = 0.54, 95% CI: 0.19–1.49). This study demonstrated that PPI use in the first kidney transplant year in black patients, but not non-black patients, was associated with an increased BPAR compared to patients using ranitidine. Whether this increase in rejection in black patients was due to changes in mycophenolic acid concentrations was unclear since this was not assessed. Another recent similar study found no evidence of increased BPAR at three or 6 months of transplantation in kidney transplant recipients receiving pantoprazole (40 mg/day) compared to ranitidine (150 mg/day) [42c]. However, it should be noted that their population was over 98% Caucasian.

Drug–Drug Interaction, Tacrolimus

PPIs are often coadministered with calcineurin inhibitors to prevent upper GI complications. However, there is some concern for drug–drug interactions between PPIs and calcineurin inhibitors. The coadministration of PPIs with the calcineurin inhibitors tacrolimus or cyclosporin-A, in addition to the influence of the cytochrome P450 (CYP) 2C19 gene polymorphisms, on the blood concentrations of tacrolimus and cyclosporine-A in Japanese patients with connective tissue disease was investigated [43c]. Lansoprazole significantly increased the blood concentration of tacrolimus 12 hours after administration compared to rabeprazole ($p = 0.030$) or the control group ($p = 0.003$). In contrast, there were no significant differences in blood concentrations of tacrolimus between rabeprazole and control groups at 12 hours. Lansoprazole also significantly increased baseline blood concentration of cyclosporin-A compared to rabeprazole ($p = 0.047$) and the control group ($p = 0.014$). There were no significant differences in the mean cyclosporin-A blood concentration 2 hours after administration in patients with or without PPI treatment, in the incidence of adverse events, or in the CYP2C19 gene polymorphism status among the three groups. While the number of patients in the present was quite small, and the observation period was short, which are significant limitations, the study found that lansoprazole significantly elevated the blood concentrations of tacrolimus at 12 hours and tough levels of cyclosporine-A, suggesting a potential drug–drug interactions between lansoprazole and these calcineurin inhibitors. However, there was not a significant increase in adverse events to where the clinical relevance of this interaction remains unclear.

Hypomagnesemia

An adverse effect that continues to be investigated is the association between PPIs and hypomagnesemia. Hypomagnesemia is a rare but serious adverse effect in which low serum magnesium levels (<1.7 mg/dL) are accompanied by clinical symptoms ranging from the patient being asymptomatic to life threatening depending on the severity of the deficiency. In 2011, both the FDA and the Australian Medicines Safety Update of Therapeutic Goods Administration issued safety announcements regarding the association between proton pump inhibitors and hypomagnesemia [44c,45S,46S]. The FDA recommended obtaining serum magnesium levels in patients expected to be taking PPIs for long periods of time prior to initiating treatment and periodically monitoring their magnesium levels. The FDA also recommended monitoring serum magnesium levels in patients being prescribed PPIs when taking other drugs that predispose to hypomagnesemia (e.g. thiazide and loop diuretics). However, the role of PPIs in hypomagnesemia remains controversial as the studies reporting this finding have all been observational.

In a retrospective cross-sectional study done by Luk et al. [44c], hypomagnesemia was reported with all six PPIs available by prescription in the United States (lansoprazole, omeprazole, dexlansoprazole, rabeprazole, esomeprazole, and pantoprazole) using the FDA Adverse Event Reporting System database. Among those that reported one or more adverse effects while taking a PPI ($n = 66\,102$), 1.0% ($n = 69$) experienced hypomagnesemia.

The average age of those that experienced hypomagnesemia was 64.4 ± 12.9 years. When using multivariate logistic regression to determine which factors predicted hypomagnesemia in those that took PPIs, they found that the odds of hypomagenesemia were significantly higher in those that took pantoprazole (OR = 4.3; 95% CI 3.3–5.7; $p < 0.001$), lansoprazole (OR = 1.7; 95% CI 1.2–2.3, $p = 0.001$), or omeprazole (OR = 3.8; 95% CI 3.0–4.8, $p < 0.001$) when compared to the odds of hypomagnesemia taking esomeprazole, adjusting for gender and age. The odds of hypomagnesemia were significantly higher in those greater than 65 years of age (OR = 1.5; 95% CI 1.2–1.7; $p < 0.001$) compared to those 65 years of age and younger when also adjusting for gender and type of PPI. While this study suggested that the odds of hypomagnesemia were significantly higher in those that took pantoprazole, omeprazole and lansoprazole compared to those that took esomeprazole when also taking into account age and gender, it is important to note that other patient factors (co-morbidities and medications such as diuretics) that could predispose towards hypomagnesemia were not taken into account. Thus, it remains unclear whether these patient factors could explain the differences found between the PPIs in the odds of developing hypomagnesemia impacting the validity of the findings. Additionally, other relevant factors such as dose of PPI and length of treatment with the PPI were not assessed in this study.

A recent study looked at hypomagnesemia in hemodialysis patients being dialyzed with a dialysate magnesium concentration of 0.75–1 mEq/L taking PPIs [47c]. A 3-month chart review was performed on 62 hemodialysis male patients with a mean age of 64.3 ± 8.7 years at a single United States hospital. Most patients ($n = 22$) were treated with omeprazole (20–80 mg/day), while several patients ($n = 7$) were treated with pantoprazole (40–80 mg/day). A significant difference was found in patients who were hypomagnesemic (plasma Mg < 1.5 mEq/L) compared to non-hypomagnesemic in terms of plasma magnesium concentrations (1.37 ± 0.10 vs. 1.70 ± 0.20, respectively, $p < 0.001$), PPI use (16/24 or 67% vs. 13/38 or 34%, respectively, $p = 0.013$), and diuretic use (7/24 or 29% versus 3/38 or 8%, respectively, $p = 0.027$). While there was a significant difference in PPI use between those that were hypomagnesemic compared to non-hypomagnesemic, there was not a significant difference in the duration of PPI use (6.7 ± 2.3 years versus 5.8 ± 2.9 years, respectively, $p = 0.35$) or dose of the PPI (53 ± 24 mg/day versus 40 ± 24 mg/day, respectively, $p = 0.15$). Multivariable logistic regression was then used to determine which factors could predict hypomagnesemia when adjusting for PPI use, diuretic use, duration of dialysis, dialytic urea clearance, diabetes, plasma albumin, age, and dietary protein intake estimated by normalized protein catabolic rate. When adjusting for all these

factors, PPI use (OR = 4.20, 95% CI: 1.16–15.2, $p = 0.029$) and diuretic use (OR = 6.25, 95% CI: 1.05–37.1, $p = 0.044$) were significant predictors of hypomagnesemia. This study demonstrated that use of PPIs and diuretics in male hemodialysis patients (using a dialysate with a magnesium concentration off 0.75–1.0 mEq/L) were both associated with hypomagnesemia, suggesting that plasma magnesium concentrations should be monitored in male hemodialysis patients taking diuretics and/or PPIs.

A cross-sectional study was performed to determine whether PPI use was a predictor of hypomagnesemia (< 0.75 mM) in patients admitted to a large tertiary care emergency department in Bern, Switzerland and had serum magnesium levels available [48C]. Those with hypomagnesemia ($n = 1246$) were significantly older (56 ± 20 years compared to 54 ± 20), had significantly lower levels of sodium, calcium, chloride, phosphate and calcium even though these values were still within the normal range, tended to be sicker as measured by the Charlson comorbidity index (with higher scores reflecting more co-morbidities), had a greater percentage admitted to the hospital, and had significantly longer hospital stays (9.5 ± 11 versus 7.3 ± 9 days) than those with magnesium levels ≥ 75 mM ($n = 3872$). They then did multivariable regression to determine which factors predicted hypomagnesemia amongst patients in the emergency department using a model adjusting for PPI use, diuretic use, estimated glomerular filtration rate (eGFR), and Charlson co-morbidity index. PPI use (OR = 2.19, 95% CI: 1.54–2.86, $p < 0.0001$), diuretic use (OR = 1.35, 95% CI: 1.05–1.75, $p = 0.021$), and having a Charlson comorbidity of 2 (OR = 2.01, 95% CI 1.45–2.76, $p < 0.0001$) or 3 (OR = 1.70, 95% CI 1.13–2.55, $p = 0.010$) compared to a Charlson comorbidity score of 0 were significant predictors of hypomagnesemia when adjusting for other factors. This study suggested that PPI use was a significant predictor of hypomagnesemia in patients admitted to the emergency department even when adjusting for other factors.

A relatively recent case–control study did this retrospectively in a Korean population in patients with available serum magnesium levels [49c]. Ultimately, 105 PPI users were matched with 210 controls using propensity scores, although seven PPI users could not be matched with a control. Patients were matched with controls to adjust for various confounders using propensity scores for laboratory values (sodium, potassium, calcium, blood urea nitrogen, creatinine, albumin, but not magnesium) age, gender, comorbidities, and the use of other medications. When matched for potential confounders, there was not a significant difference in the mean serum magnesium levels between the matched PPI users and controls (0.85 ± 0.09 versus 0.86 ± 0.16 mM, respectively, $p = 0.297$). However, the majority of patients ($\sim 94\%$) in the PPI treatment group had received PPIs for less than a year. Thus, it is possible that this lack of relationship between PPI use and hypomagnesemia when using propensity scores could be related to the duration of use. This suggested that other factors were likely involved. When doing multivariable logistic regression to determine which factors predicted hypomagnesemia within PPI users, they found that using PPIs for over a year (OR = 5.388, 95% CI: 1.056–27.493, $p = 0.043$), age less than 45 years (OR = 4.710, 95% CI: 1.523–14.571, $p = 0.007$) and use of cisplatin or carboplatin (OR = 13.404, 95% CI: 2.066–86.952, $p = 0.007$) were significant predictors of hypomagnesemia when controlling for diuretic use and albumin. Interestingly, they did find a significant difference in serum magnesium levels between controls ($n = 1244$) and PPI users ($n = 112$) when controls were not matched using propensity scores (0.87 ± 0.19 versus 0.85 ± 0.11 mM, $p < 0.0001$), although whether this was clinically significant is debatable.

A matched case–control study in Ontario, Canada assessed the relationship between hospitalization with hypomagnesemia and current (most recent prescription within 90 days), recent (91–180 since most recent prescription) or remote (most recent prescription within 181–365 days) PPI use in those 66 or older when matching patients based on age, sex, kidney disease, and use of various diuretic classes using conditional logistic regression [50c]. PPIs that were included in the analysis included omeprazole, pantoprazole, lansoprazole, esomeprazole, and lansoprazole. The odds of being hospitalized for hypomagnesemia were 43% higher in those taking PPIs (OR = 1.43; 95% CI 1.06–1.93) compared to those that did not take PPIs when adjusting for diabetes, malignancy, congestive heart failure, steroid use, and a set of specific drugs used in the past year. Considering diuretic use could confound the relationship between PPI use and hypomagnesemia, they then assessed the relationship between current PPI use and being hospitalized for hypomagnesemia when stratified by diuretic use. In patients receiving diuretics, those currently taking PPIs were 73% more likely to be hospitalized for hypomagnesemia (adjusted OR = 1.73; 95% CI 1.11–2.70) compared to those not taking PPIs. In contrast for those not taking diuretics, current users of PPIs were not significantly more likely to be hospitalized with hypomagnesemia (adjusted OR = 1.25; 95% CI 0.81–1.91) compared to those not taking PPIs. This suggested that concurrent use of PPIs and diuretics were significantly more likely to be hospitalized with hypomagnesemia, but not when taking PPIs without diuretics.

Immunologic/Hypersensitivity

A retrospective study of PPI-induced subacute cutaneous lupus erythematosus (SCLE) was performed [51c]. Of the 24 PPI-induced SCLE cases evaluated, 19 were newly identified cases (mean age: 61 years old). The episodes of SCLE were associated with four groups of PPIs: lansoprazole (12), omeprazole (6), esomeprazole (4) and pantoprazole (2), with four patients having multiple episodes. The development period was on average 8 months, with average resolution period of 3 months. Positive anti-Ro/SSA antibodies were found in 73%, anti-La/SSB antibodies in 33%, and antihistone antibodies in 8% of cases at the time of the flare-up.

Case reports:

- A 74-year-old female was admitted with 8 hours history of shivering with fever (38.9 °C) after a single oral dose of 40 mg pantoprazole for heartburn 12 hours previously. The patient noted that four similar reactions had previously coincided with pantoprazole dosing that subsided within 24 hours. The incidence of this adverse reaction occurred in tandem with leukocytosis and increased serum C reactive protein (CRP) [52A].
- A 43-year-old female with respiratory arrest had dyspeptic complaints in the morning, and she took a capsule of 30 mg lansoprazole. She had allergic symptoms in minutes and lost consciousness. She had diabetes and a coronary angiography of mild stenosis in her medical history [53A].

Iron deficiency/case report:

- A 59-year-old male taking rabeprazole for GERD gradually developed iron-deficiency anemia [54A]. He had a history of angina, hypertension, type 2 diabetes, dyslipidemia, reflux esophagitis, atrophic gastritis and *Helicobacter pylori* infection. The anemia did not improve following ferrous fumarate administration, and endoscopic screening did not reveal the cause of the anemia. The patient was switched from rabeprazole to famotidine, with dissipation of the anemia.

Pneumonia

While several theories have emerged to explain the enhanced risk of pneumonia in patients using PPIs, the specific pathophysiological mechanism remains unclear [55R]. Observational studies have shown mixed results between PPIs and pneumonia over the past several years. Nevertheless, current evidence supports the association between PPIs and pneumonia, especially in older individuals. The FDA is continuing to evaluate this issue to determine the need for any regulatory action.

A replicated cohort study with meta-analysis was performed to look at the association between prophylactic PPI or H2 receptor antagonist use and cumulative 6-month incidence of hospitalization for community-acquired pneumonia (HCAP) in new users of non-steroidal anti-inflammatory drugs (NSAIDs) [56M]. Eight restricted cohorts consisted of new users of NSAIDs, aged ≥40 years old, using eight databases (1997–2010). High-dimensional propensity scores were constructed for each patient to minimize confounding by indication and other factors. Of the new users of NSAIDs ($n = 4238504$) 2.3% also started a PPI. The cumulative 6-month incidence of HCAP was 0.17% among patients prescribed PPIs, 0.16% in patients prescribed a H2 receptor antagonist, and 0.12% in unexposed patients. After adjusting multiple factors in addition to high-dimensional propensity score decile, when data were pooled across all databases, PPIs were not associated with increased odds of HCAP (adjusted OR = 1.05, 95% CI 0.89–1.25, $I^2 = 0$%). Pooled data with H2 receptor antagonists yielded similar results (adjusted OR = 0.95, 95% CI: 0.75–1.21, $I^2 = 0$%). Among new users of NSAIDs, there was no association between PPI use and HCAP. However, the reason for PPI use was not assessed nor was the dose taken into account.

A retrospective cohort population-based study examined the association between PPI use and pneumonia in patients (Taiwan) with non-traumatic intracranial hemorrhage (ICH) [57c]. Patients <18 years old and newly diagnosed with non-traumatic ICH complicated with pneumonia were excluded, leaving 2170 eligible participants. The adjusted HR for pneumonia in ICH patients who used PPIs was 1.61 (95% CI: 1.32–1.97, $p < 0.001$). The hazard of pneumonia in patients who used PPIs was 2.60 (95% CI: 2.01–3.38, $p < 0.001$) times the hazard of pneumonia in patients who did not use PPIs when the defined daily dose was <30. The hazard of pneumonia in patients who used PPIs was 2.04 (95% CI: 1.34–3.10, $p < 0.001$) times the hazard of pneumonia in patients who did not use PPIs when the defined daily dose was 30–60. Several potential confounders associated with pneumonia, such as smoking, alcohol use, weight, hygiene, were not included in the database to where there could still be residual confounding. Although there still could be residual confounding, the findings showed that use of PPIs in patients with non-traumatic ICH was associated with an increased hazard of pneumonia compared to those that did not take PPIs. However, whether this association would still hold or would be increased when these other confounding factors are taken into account remains to be elucidated.

Vitamin B12 Deficiency

In 2014, the FDA required for manufacturers of PPIs to include a risk of vitamin B12 deficiency when taken long term (>3 years) in the labelling information [31S,38S] (*See Section H2 receptor antagonist* above *for combined PPI/H2 antagonist study*).

ANTICONSTIPATION AND PROKINETIC AGENTS

Domperidone [SED-15, 1178; SEDA-34, 556; SEDA-35,633; SEDA-36, 541]

Cardiovascular

Data from preclinical studies identify domperidone as being able to produce significant hERG channel inhibition and action potential prolongation [58R]. Domperidone should not be given to patients with pre-existing QT prolongation/LQTS, receiving drugs that may inhibit CYP3A4, individuals with electrolyte abnormalities, or with other risk factors for QT-prolongation. The French medical journal *Prescrire* has called for the drug domperidone to be withdrawn after a study it conducted estimated that the drug may have caused 25–120 premature deaths in 2012 in France [59r]. Additionally, concerns over domperidone use in elderly, especially in those taking known CYP3A4 inhibitors have also been noted in Canada [60r,61C]. In August 2013, the FDA warned breastfeeding women and healthcare professionals not to use domperidone for the purposes of increasing lactation. FDA took these actions since some women are purchasing domperidone from compounding pharmacies and/or foreign sources. However, patients (≥12 years old) with certain gastrointestinal conditions may be able to receive domperidone through an expanded access investigational new drug application. Such conditions include gastroesophageal reflux disease with upper GI symptoms, chronic constipation, and gastroparesis. Patients who are eligible to receive domperidone in the US have generally failed standard therapies.

A recent review evaluated domperidone-associated sudden cardiac death in the general population and implications for use in patients specifically undergoing hemodialysis [62M]. Eligible studies included randomized controlled trials and cohort, cross-sectional, case–control, and other epidemiological studies comparing use of domperidone and sudden cardiac death in adults. No direct evidence applicable to patients with end-stage renal disease was found. However, given the gaps in the literature, use of domperidone for patients undergoing dialysis should be assessed on a case-by-case basis, with author noting for use of extreme caution for hemodialysis patients taking >30 mg/day of domperidone.

Linaclotide [SEDA-35, 646]

Meta-Analysis

A meta-analysis was conducted looking at the safety and efficacy of linaclotide compared to placebo in constipation-predominant irritable bowel syndrome (IBS-C) using randomized controlled trials [63M].

Inclusion criteria for the analysis were studies reporting clinical outcomes such as relief of abdominal pain/discomfort and bowel habits, treatment duration of at least 12 weeks, patients ($\geq$18 years) with IBS-C, and trials using 266, 290 or 300 µg doses of linaclotide. Exclusion criteria for the analysis included studies having patients with organic constipation, drug-induced constipation, or chronic idiopathic constipation. Three randomized controlled trials met the inclusion criteria. The incidence of diarrhea leading to treatment discontinuation was higher for linaclotide ($n = 1773$, risk ratio (RR) = 14.75; 95% CI: 4.04–53.81). Generalizability was limited by the study population (i.e. principally white female patients), limited data regarding prior therapy, and availability of few randomized control trials.

Lubiprostone [SEDA-35, 647; SEDA-36, 541]

Randomized Controlled Trial

A randomized, double-blind, placebo-controlled, phase-III trial was conducted to assess the efficacy and safety of oral lubiprostone for relieving symptoms of opioid-induced constipation in patients with chronic noncancer pain [64c]. Patients (mean age 50.4 years old) were randomized in two groups: oral lubiprostone 24 mcg BID (48 mcg daily, $n = 210$) or placebo capsules BID ($n = 208$), with the majority of patients completing the study (lubiprostone, 67.1%; placebo, 69.7%). The most common adverse effects with lubiprostone were nausea (16.8% compared to 5.8% for placebo), diarrhea (9.6% compared to 2.9% with placebo), and abdominal distention (8.2% compared to 2.4% for placebo). Lubiprostone did not interfere with opioid-induced analgesia.

Magnesium [SED-15, 2196; SEDA-34,569; SEDA-35, 645; SEDA-36, 553]

Drug–Drug Interaction, H2 Receptor Antagonists and PPIs

A retrospective observational study evaluated magnesium oxide (MgO) dosage levels and any concomitant use of H2 receptor antagonists or PPIs to determine whether the laxative effect of MgO was weakened with suppressed gastric acid secretion [65c]. Patients ($n = 112$) were prescribed MgO after colon surgery or total gastric resection as monotherapy ($n = 67$ colon surgery patients and $n = 4$ total gastric resection patients), or prescribed as a combination of MgO and a H2 receptor antagonist ($n = 14$), or PPI and MgO ($n = 27$). The daily dosage levels of MgO in the combination group with H2 receptor antagonist (1286 ± 257 mg/day) or with a PPI (1271 ± 421 mg/day) were significantly higher compared to MgO monotherapy (1019 ± 219 mg/day, $p < 0.01$). The combination use of H2 receptor antagonist or PPI with MgO significantly decreased the percentage of patients with good defecation control (36.4% controlled for both groups) compared to MgO monotherapy (72.2% controlled, $p < 0.05$). This study demonstrated that when patients received H2 receptor antagonists or PPIs with MgO, the laxative effect of MgO was decreased. The authors theorized this might be due to lower solubility of MgO at higher gastric pH.

Metoclopramide [SED-15, 2317; SEDA-34, 557; SEDA-35, 634; SEDA-36, 542]

Update

In December 2013, the EMA recommended for restrictions on metoclopramide use to minimize the risk of neurological and other adverse reactions. Restrictions included authorization for short-term use (5 days) only, reducing the maximum dose for adults to 30 mg/day or 0.5 mg/kg body weight/day and a ban on its use in individuals with chronic conditions such as gastroparesis [66R].

Case reports:

- A 50-year-old female with a history of transient ischemic attack, migraines, diabetes, hypertension, and hyperlipidemia developed a hypotensive episode after the administration intravenous metoclopramide (10 mg, i.v.) for the treatment of a migraine. Fifteen minutes after metoclopramide administration, her systolic blood pressure decreased from 138 to 84 mmHg. The patient was given 1 L of NaCl 0.9%. Patient did not reapproach baseline systolic blood pressure until 90 minutes after the metoclopramide. Subsequent contrast tomography of the head was negative [67A].
- Two cases of grand mal type seizures after heart transplant occurred, which were attributed to an interaction between metoclopramide and theophylline [68A]. The combination of dopamine-2 receptor inhibition in conjunction with possible impairment of theophylline metabolism through the CYP450 was noted as the cause of seizures.
  - A 26-year-old female with history of hypothyroidism was put on metoclopramide (20 mg daily, parenterally) for gastrointestinal disturbances and theophylline due to postoperative bradycardia following a heart transplant. The first seizure occurred on day 7 postoperatively, on the fourth day of anti-thymocyte globulin. The grand mal seizure was treated with benzodiazepines.
  - A 33-year-old male with two prior myocardial infarctions was placed on metoclopramide (20 mg daily, parenterally) for gastrointestinal disturbances and theophylline due to postoperative bradycardia following a heart transplantation. He experienced a self-limiting grand mal seizure day 15 postoperatively.

Pharmacogenetics

Several single nucleotide polymorphisms (SNPs) have been associated with the adverse effects of metoclopramide [69R]. A SNP in the CYP2D6 gene (rs3892097) was associated with increased incidence of adverse side effects in gastroparetic patients (OR = 2.134, lower confidence level (LCL)/upper confidence level (UCL): 1.001–4.55), while two SNPs were protective (rs1080985 OR = 0.508, LCL/UCL = 0.261–0.985; rs16947 OR = 0.467, 95% CI: 0.267–0.817) [70c]. A SNP (rs3815459) in the voltage gated voltage-gated potassium channel H (eag-related), member 2 gene (KCNH2) was also found to be protective against side effects (OR = 0.399, LCL/UCL = 0.191–0.835). A SNP (rs9325104), in the 5-HT$_4$ receptor gene was also found to be protective against side effects (OR = 0.499, LCL/UCL = 0.271–0.921) [70c].

Naloxegol

Update

Naloxegol is a new treatment for opioid-induced constipation (OIC) in adults with chronic non-cancer pain, FDA approved September 2014. Naloxegol is a peripherally acting mu-opioid receptor antagonist, designed to block the binding of opioids to the opioid receptors in the gastrointestinal tract without impacting the opioid receptors in the brain. Naloxegol is presently a schedule II controlled substance as it is structurally related to noroxymorphone. However, the FDA approved labeling that indicates that it has no risk of abuse or dependency.

Randomized Controlled Trial

A phase-II, randomized, double-blind, placebo-controlled, dose-escalation trial evaluated the safety, efficacy, and tolerability of naloxegol in patients with OIC [71c]. Patients ($n = 207$) on an opioid regimen (30–1000 mg/day morphine equivalents for ≥ 2 weeks) with <3 spontaneous bowel movements (SBMs) per week, were randomized to receive 4 weeks of naloxegol (5, 25, or 50 mg) or placebo once daily. The most common adverse events were diarrhea, abdominal pain, and nausea. The frequency and severity of these adverse events increased in the 50 mg cohort. There was not a significant increase in opioid use for the 25 and 50 mg cohorts compared to placebo. Additionally, there was not a significant increase from baseline in pain with naloxegol, or signs and/or symptoms of centrally mediated opioid withdrawal with naloxegol.

A 52-week phase-III, multicenter, randomized, parallel-group, safety and tolerability study on naloxegol was conducted in out-patients (≥ 18 to <85 years old) taking 30–1000 morphine-equivalent units per day for ≥ 4 weeks [72C]. Patients were randomized 2:1 to receive naloxegol (25 mg/day) or laxative regimen treatment for OIC. The safety set consisted of patients (naloxegol, $n = 534$; laxative regimen, $n = 270$). The occurrence of adverse events was 81.8% with naloxegol and 72.2% with laxative regimen. The adverse effects that occurred more frequently with naloxegol compared to the laxative regimen included abdominal pain (17.8% vs. 3.3% for laxative regimen), diarrhea (12.9% vs. 5.9%), nausea (9.4% vs. 4.1%), headache (9.0% vs. 4.8%), flatulence (6.9% vs. 1.1%), and upper abdominal pain (5.1% vs. 1.1%). According to the authors, primary naloxegol associated gastrointestinal adverse effects occurred early in the course of treatment, resolved during or after naloxegol discontinuation, and the severity of the adverse effects was mild or moderate.

Polyethylene Glycol [SEDA-34, 569; SEDA-35, 646; SEDA-36, 553]

Meta-Analysis

A meta-analysis was performed on the efficacy of polyethylene glycols for treatment of constipation in children compared to milk of magnesia (magnesium hydroxide), lactulose, oral liquid paraffin (mineral oil), or acacia fiber, psyllium fiber, and fructose and the safety of polyethylene glycol (PEG) [73M]. Adverse events reported in the seven studies for PEG including: diarrhea, nausea or vomiting, pain at defecation, abdominal pain, straining at defecation, hard stool consistency, bloating or flatulence, bad palatability, and rectal bleeding. Study limitations included children of different ages and criteria of constipation, different PEG forms, and different control arms comparators.

Prucalopride [SEDA-34, 557]

Meta-Analysis

A meta-analysis was conducted on the efficacy and safety of the 5-HT$_4$ receptor agonists, prucalopride, velusetrag and naronapride in adults with chronic constipation [74M]. Out of the 12 trials reporting adverse events, 11 involved prucalopride and only one involved velusetrag (experimental). The relative risk of adverse events in those that took prucalopride was 1.24 (95% CI: 1.12–1.38). The relative risk of adverse events with velusetrag was 1.35 (95% CI: 1.03–1.78). Although, the relative risks for adverse events were not significantly different between prucalopride and velusetrag ($p = 0.57$), it needs to be kept in mind that the estimate for velusetrag only came from one study. When looking at the relative risks for adverse events, the risk of headache (RR 1.77; 95% CI, 1.40–2.25), diarrhea (RR = 3.08, 95% CI, 2.31–4.09), nausea (RR = 2.19; 95% CI, 1.76–2.74), and abdominal pain (RR = 1.41, 95% CI, 1.10–1.81) were significantly higher in those receiving 5-HT$_4$ agonists compared to the control group. While this study showed that those receiving 5-HT$_4$ agonists were at significantly higher risk of developing several adverse effects, the adverse events had a favorable safety profile.

Systematic Review

A study investigated prucalopride (2 mg) adverse events in Asian and non-Asian patients with chronic constipation, pooling data from four 12-week randomized, double-blind, placebo-controlled, multicenter trials [75M]. Of the 1821 patients, Asians made up 26.1%, while Non-Asians made up 73.9%. In the Asian population, the most common adverse events with prucalopride treatment were diarrhea (22% versus 8.5% with placebo), headache (10% versus 2.1% with placebo), nausea (11.6% versus 2.5% with placebo), and abdominal pain (6.6% versus 2.1% with placebo). In non-Asians, the most common side effects with prucalopride treatment were headache (26.4% versus 14.2% with placebo), nausea (19.5% versus 10% with placebo), diarrhea (12.9% versus 4.6% with placebo), and abdominal pain (12.4% versus 10.6% with placebo). In both populations the odds of diarrhea (OR = 3.073, 95% CI: 2.194–4.305, $p < 0.05$), headache (OR = 2.420, 95% CI: 1.854–3.160, $p < 0.001$), and nausea (OR 2.480, 95% CI: 1.842–3.339, $p < 0.001$) were significantly higher in those treated with prucalopride compared to placebo when adjusting for race, gender, age, duration of chronic constipation, and prior laxative use. The odds of abdominal pain (OR = 0.301, 95% CI: 0.183, 0.497, $p < 0.001$), headache (OR = 0.205, 95% CI: 0.133–0.316, $p < 0.001$), and nausea (OR = 0.413, 95% CI: 0.274–0.622, $p < 0.001$) were significantly lower in Asians compared to Non-Asians when adjusted. The odds of diarrhea was significantly higher in Asians (OR = 1.911, 95% CI: 1.329–2.750, $p < 0.001$) compared to Non-Asians. Study identified the odds of diarrhea, headache, and nausea were significantly higher with prucalopride treatment. Secondly, the study demonstrated that Asian patients had significantly higher odds of diarrhea but significantly lower odds of headache, abdominal pain, and nausea when compared to non-Asians.

Case reports:

- A 75-year-old male developed chronic constipation following a Whipple's pancreaticoduodenectomy for pancreatic cancer was placed on prucalopride (2 mg/day). History included hypertension, dyslipidemia, and a cerebrovascular ischemic, stroke with minimal neurologic deficits. The patient was taking clopidogrel, pantoprazole, candesartan, indapamide, gabapentin, sennoside, and 30 g of fiber daily. Two months following initiation of prucalopride treatment, his creatinine was 165 µmol/L, and at 4-months increased to 270 µmol/L. He displayed no irritative or obstructive urinary symptoms. The patient was taken off of candesartan. At 4.5 months following the initiation of prucalopride creatinine was 285 µmol/L. The patient was then diagnosed with acute interstitial nephritis secondary to exposure to prucalopride. Prucalopride was discontinued, and prednisone initiated (40 mg/day for 1 week, followed by a taper of 5 mg weekly). At the 2-week follow-up, the patient's creatinine was at 310 µmol/L. The patient's renal function did not recover and his constipation returned [76A].

- A 61-year-old female experienced neuropsychiatric adverse effects when given prucalopride for chronic constipation. The patient experienced life-threatening neurological effects after oral administration of prucalopride (2 mg/day) with visual hallucination, disorientation, exhaustion, loss of balance and memory, and suicidal ideation. Symptoms disappeared after 24 hours after prucalopride was withdrawn. The patient had never before suffered from any other disorder or symptom affecting the nervous system [77A].

Sodium Picosulfate/Polyethylene Glycol [SEDA-34, 570]

Observational Study

A population-based retrospective cohort study assessed the association between sodium picosulfate and polyethylene glycol on the risk of hospitalization with hyponatremia within 30 days of the bowel preparation for colonoscopy (>65 years of age) [78C]. In addition, the association between these agents on the risk of urgent head CT scan, which was used to measure acute central nervous system disturbance, and mortality was assessed. Sodium picosulfate significantly increased the risk of hospitalization with hyponatremia (relative risk (RR): 2.4, 95% CI: 1.5–3.9), but did not significantly increase the risk of hospitalization with urgent computed tomography (CT) head (RR = 1.1, 95% CI: 0.7–1.4) or risk of mortality (RR: 0.9, 95% CI: 0.7–1.3) when compared to polyethylene glycol. While sodium picosulfate bowel preparations were associated with greater incidence of hyponatremia than polyethylene glycol, there was no evidence of increased acute neurologic symptoms or mortality with its use.

Case reports:

- A 75-year-old female ingested milk containing magnesium chloride (unknown concentration) to reduce weight. On the day before her death, she received two "treatments". Subsequently, she was unable to turn on her side and complained of severe diarrhea. She was carried to her bed and was found deceased the next day [79A].

- A 76-year-old female was given an oral prescription of MC-SP complex (10 mg sodium picosulfate, 3.5 g magnesium citrate) for the colonoscopy. She suffered diarrhea, nausea, and vomiting, followed by decreased energy and seizure. She had a history of seizure and dementia, and was taking thiazide and Synthroid for the treatment of hypertension and hypothyroidism, respectively. Following the diagnosis of hyponatremia, she was given 3% NaCl to normalize the sodium levels [80A].
- Three cases were noted for lactulose-associated lithium toxicity [81A]. In all cases patients were prescribed lithium for acute mania and lactulose for constipation:
  - A 47-year-old male on lithium (300 mg BID), divalproate (1500 mg/daily), and quetiapine (400 mg BID) was started on lactulose (30 mL BID, 10 g/15 mL solution) for constipation. After two doses of lactulose, it was discontinued. On day 3 lithium level was at 1.6 mEq/L and serum creatinine level of 0.57 mg/dL, with no physical signs of lithium toxicity.
  - A 45-year-old female on lithium carbonate (300 mg BID), risperidone (2 mg), lisinopril (25 mg), and hydrochlorothiazide (25 mg) had lithium levels at 0.5 mEq/L on day 5. Lithium dose was increased to 450 mg in the morning and 600 mg at night, due to mania, with lactulose (30 mL) for constipation 2 days later. After 3 days of lactulose, it was discontinued. Lithium level 9 days after the increase in lithium (1050 mg daily) was 2.4 mEq/L. While she reported mild fatigue, no changes in cognition, or other signs of overt lithium toxicity were observed. Lithium therapy and antihypertensives were discontinued.
  - A 48-year-old female was started on lithium (600 mg BID), quetiapine (400 mg BID), and benazepril (20 mg daily). On day 5, lithium dose was increased (900 mg BID). On day 11, she received five doses of lactulose (30 mL) for constipation for a 2-day period. On day 16, she developed a tremor and drowsiness (lithium levels at 1.6 mEq/L), and lithium dose was reduced to 300 mg in the morning and 600 mg in the evening, with lithium levels normalizing at 0.8 mEq/L.

Teduglutide

Randomized Controlled Trial

A tolerability and efficacy study of teduglutide in the reduction of parenteral nutrition dependency was conducted in patients with short bowel syndrome intestinal failure [82c]. Patients that received teduglutide (0.05 or 0.10 mg/kg/day) for 24 weeks in the first randomized

controlled trial were then eligible for a 28-week double-blind extension study. At week 52, safety, tolerability, and clinical efficacy were assessed. The most common adverse effects that were reported included abdominal pain (25%), nausea (31%), and headache (35%). Seven patients withdrew. Study suggested that the safety profile of teduglutide was sufficient for it to be considered for long-term use in patients with short bowel syndrome intestinal failure.

Systematic Review

A systematic review of the pharmacology, pharmacokinetics, clinical efficacy, and safety of teduglutide for short bowel syndrome (SBS) was performed [83M]. Teduglutide has been studied in short bowel syndrome (SBS) in three phase III trials [82C,84C,85C]. The most common adverse effects included upper-respiratory-tract infection (11.8%), abdominal distension (13.8%), headaches (15.9%), nausea (18.2%), injection site reactions (22.4%), and abdominal pain (30.0%). There were two cases of congestive heart failure. Since there has been concern of potential development of malignancy with teduglutide, a study investigated the large and small-intestine mucosa for dysplastic changes in patients that received either teduglutide (0.05 or 0.10 mg/kg/day) or placebo [86c]. After 6 months of treatment with either placebo or either dose of teduglutide, no dysplastic features were found in any biopsy from the large or small intestine of any treatment group. Because of the possibility of increased malignancy, it was not recommended in patients with active gastrointestinal malignancies by the authors of the systematic review.

ANTIDIARRHEAL AND ANTISPASMOTIC AGENTS

Bismuth Salts [SED-15, 518; SEDA-36, 551]

Case reports:

- A 21-year-old female had taken 20 tablets of colloidal bismuth subcitrate in a suicide attempt. The patient underwent gastric lavage and intravenous fluid therapy, followed by treatment with the chelating agent sodium-2,3-dimercapto-1-propanesulfonate (DMPS), 600 mg orally every 8 hours for 14 days. Hemodialysis was conducted daily for the first 4 days and then three times weekly. The patient's renal function (serum creatinine and BUN) test results remained high 8 weeks after discharge. The patient continued hemodialysis ~1 year later, indicative of irreversible renal damage [87A].
- A 56-year-old female presenting multiple fractures was initiated on warfarin due to inability to ambulate. Bismuth subsalicylate (30 mL) was taken every 4 hours

for diarrhea. Three days after starting bismuth subsalicylate therapy, the patient's international normalized ratio (INR) increased from 2.56 to 3.54. Discontinuation of bismuth subsalicylate stabilized the patient's INR into the target range on the same warfarin dose given at the time of the supratherapeutic INR. Bismuth subsalicylate may alter the anticoagulant effects of warfarin and other oral coumarin anticoagulants, and increase risk of bleeding [88A].

Loperamide [SED-15, 2159; SEDA-34, 573]

Case reports:

- A case report noted five patient cases with histories of loperamide abuse, with three of the patients exhibiting life-threatening cardiac arrhythmias, and one patient experiencing a second arrhythmia after subsequent use of loperamide [89A]. The loperamide levels obtained in four of the patients and were at least one order of magnitude greater than therapeutic concentrations. Loperamide discontinuation resulted in resolution of cardiac conduction disturbances.
- A 58-year-old female presented with abdominal pain, nausea, and vomiting over a 7-day period. She had a history of hypertension, hypothyroidism, and cholecystectomy. She did not smoke or drink alcohol. She had diarrhea 10 days before admission and took loperamide for 2 days, 10 mg on the first day and 6 mg on the second day. Her daily medications were atenolol, thyroxin, and hydrochlorothiazide. She had elevated lipase and amylase. WBC was 12.5 mmol/L and CRP was 63 mg/L. Calcium level was 2.22 mmol/L. CT scan showed the status after cholecystectomy and acute pancreatitis. Condition improved with discontinuation of loperamide [90A].

Otilonium Bromide

Randomized Controlled Trial

A dose-ranging randomized double-blind placebo-controlled trial evaluated the dose–response relationship of otilonium bromide and placebo on functional and/or clinical efficacy IBS variables [91c]. Patients ($n = 93$) with IBS symptoms complying with Rome II criteria (44.8 ± 12.6 years old) were administered otilonium bromide 20 mg ($n = 24$), 40 mg ($n = 23$) and 80 mg ($n = 23$) three times daily or placebo ($n = 23$) in four parallel groups for 4 weeks. After 4 weeks of treatment with otilonium bromide (80 mg), evacuation frequency was significantly reduced compared to placebo (-8.36% for placebo vs. -41.9% for 80 mg OB, $p < 0.01$). A dose-dependent reduction in frequency of diarrhea was found with otolonium bromide ($\chi^2 = 11.5$, $p < 0.001$) and an

increase in normal stool frequency was found. No significant difference was found between frequencies of adverse events for otilonium bromide vs. placebo. Nevertheless, owing to the small sample size, strong placebo effect, and variation in patient characteristics due to the natural history of IBS with cyclical variation of symptom intensity over time [92R], data for several individual endpoints had a degree of variability that resulted in lack of statistical significance.

Rifaximin

Systematic Review

The safety and tolerability of rifaximin in the treatment of IBS without constipation was conducted via a pooled analysis of randomized, double-blind, placebo-controlled trials [93M]. Analysis of the phase-IIb (rifaximin 275, 550, and 1100 mg BID for 2 weeks; 550 mg BID for 4 weeks) and phase-III (rifaximin 550 mg TID for 2 weeks) studies was performed. Patient follow-up was at 12 weeks and 10 weeks post-treatment in the phase-IIb and phase-III trials, respectively. In all trials, patients (≥ 18 years old) were diagnosed with IBS and met the criteria for non-C IBS. Exclusion criteria for the phase IIb and phase III trials included patients with symptoms of constipation during the ≥ 7-day eligibility period. Patients receiving rifaximin ($n = 1103$) and placebo ($n = 829$) had a similar incidence of drug-associated adverse effects (12.1% vs. 10.7%), serious adverse effects (1.5% vs. 2.2%), drug-related adverse effects resulting in study discontinuation (0.8% vs. 0.8%), gastrointestinal-associated adverse effects (12.2% vs. 12.2%) and infection-associated adverse effects (8.5% vs. 9.5%). The safety and tolerability profile of rifaximin was comparable to placebo. It was noted that rifaximin had only a 9% improvement in IBS symptoms compared to the placebo group [94r,95r]. This suggests that further data is needed to address the long-term management of IBS with rifaximin and/or viability of use therein.

ANTIEMETIC AGENTS

Aprepitant [SEDA-34, 561; SEDA-35,636; SEDA-36, 544]

Update

A safety label change including the addition of nervous system disorders as an adverse reaction of aprepitant when co-administered with ifosfamide was approved by the FDA (August 2014).

Case reports:

- Two case reports of fatal encephalopathy interaction were described in patients that received both aprepitant and ifosfamide [96A]:

o A 39-year-old female was given ifosfamide ($5\ g/m^2/day$), aprepitant (125 mg on day 1, 80 mg on days 2 and 3), and steroids after a relapse in her uterine leiomyosarcoma. Prior, she received doxorubicin ($75\ mg/m^2$). She then received doxorubicin ($60\ mg/m^2$) and ifosfamide ($9\ g/m^2$) for four cycles, and then ifosfamide alone for the fifth and sixth cycles without any incident of encephalopathy. Within several hours after the second cycle of ifosfamide, aprepitant, and steroids, the patient had obnubilation and troubles in awareness, and methylene blue treatment was begun. While there was transient improvement in the patient, the patient died 8 days later.

o A 75-year-old female that had underwent tumor resection and irradiation for pleomorphic rhabdomyosarcoma (FNCLCC grade III) of the left thigh was subsequently diagnosed bilateral pulmonary metastases. Prior to resection of the left and right metastasis, she received six cycles of doxorubicin ($60\ mg/m^2$ every 3 weeks). She then received three cycles of ifosfamide ($2\ g/m^2/day$ for 5 days, every 3 weeks) with aprepitant ($80\ mg/day \times 5$ days), and steroids, since the tumor was invading the left pleura. Eight days after the third cycle of ifosfamide, she was admitted for sepsis, renal insufficiency, pancytopenia, and lung infection. She then received methylene blue, but it was ineffective. While her blood counts and renal function were restored to normal levels, the coma worsened, and she subsequently died.

Observational Study

A retrospective study evaluated the safety and efficacy of aprepitant in cyclical vomiting syndrome (CVS) in children refractory to standard therapies [97c]. Patients ($n = 41$, median age 8 years old) were treated with either a prophylactic or acute regimen. In the prophylactic regimen ($n = 16$), aprepitant was administered when the patient was not having an episode of CVS (40 mg orally twice/week in <40 kg children, 80 mg in >40 to <60 kg children, and 125 mg in >60 kg children). Adverse effects were noted only in patients receiving the prophylactic regimen (5/16, 31%). Adverse effects included hiccough (3/16, 19%), asthenia/fatigue (2/16, 12.5%), mild headache (1/16, 6%), migraine (1/16, 6%) and increased appetite (2/16, 12.5%).

Droperidol [SED-15, 1192]

Cardiovascular

A prospective randomized-control study investigated the dose dependency of low-dose droperidol on the QTc interval and the interaction between low-dose droperidol

and propofol during anesthetic induction [98c]. Patients ($n = 72$) undergoing upper limb surgery were randomly allocated to one of three groups: group S ($n = 24$), which received 1 mL saline; group D1 ($n = 24$), which received 1.25 mg droperidol; or group D2 ($n = 24$), which received 2.5 mg droperidol. Fentanyl ($3\ \mu g/kg$) was administered 1 minute later, followed by propofol ($1.5\ mg/kg$) and vecronium. Saline or 1.25 mg droperidol did not prolong QTc interval, whereas 2.5 mg droperidol prolonged the QTc interval significantly compared to the saline group ($p < 0.05$), and propofol counteracted the prolongation of the QTc interval induced by 2.5 mg droperidol.

A retrospective observational study was to investigate the association between low-dose droperidol (0.625 mg) and torsade de pointes in the general surgical population (Mar 2007–Feb 2011) [99c]. Patients ($n = 20\,122$) were cross-matched with an electrocardiogram database and adverse outcome database. The cross-matched patients ($n = 858$) were then reviewed for reports of prolonged QTc (>440 ms), polymorphic ventricular tachycardia (VT) within 48 hours of receiving droperidol, or death within 7 days of receiving droperidol. Twelve patients had VT ($n = 4$; event rate $= 2.0$ per 10 000, 95% CI 0.5–5.1 per 10 000) or died ($n = 8$; event rate $= 4.0$ per 10 000, 95% CI 1.7–7.8 per 10 000). The authors noted that none of the patients who developed polymorphic VT or died due to droperidol administration ($n = 0$; event rate $= 0.0$ per 10 000, 95% CI 0.0–1.8 per 10 000). Additionally, it was noted that all of the patients that died were on palliative care and died of their disease.

Fosaprepitant [SEDA-34, 561; SEDA-35, 636]

Observational Studies

A retrospective study of patients ($n = 100$, ages 18–89 years old) was performed to investigate the incidence of infusion-site reactions with single-dose i.v. fosaprepitant when given through a peripheral line prior to administration of chemotherapy [100c]. Fosaprepitant was administered at a concentration of 1 mg/mL (150 mg/150 mL), in 0.9% sodium chloride over 20 minutes. A 15% incidence of infusion-site reactions occurred amongst all patients. An incidence rate of 28.7% (95% CI 21.6–36.6) was found per patient (95% CI: 21.6–36.6). They then determined which factors were associated with infusion-site reactions using univariate and multivariate regression. When using multivariate logistic regression, age (adjusted OR $= 0.97$, 95% CI 0.94–0.99), location of IV line compared to hand (adjusted OR forearm $= 0.41$, 95% CI 0.20–0.85; adjusted OR antecubital fossa $= 0.31$, 95% CI: 0.11–0.87), and simultaneous maintenance IV fluid rate $\geq 100\ mL/h$ during fosaprepitant infusion (adjusted OR $= 0.19$, 95% CI 0.08–0.44) were all significant predictors for infusion site reactions. The authors noted that the incidence of infusion-site reactions with peripherally administered fosaprepitant observed in their study was higher than that what was reported in the package insert. However, since they did not have a comparator arm, it remains unclear whether this increased incidence was a reflection of the combination of fosaprepitant and chemotherapy, or the chemotherapy alone.

Another retrospective investigation investigated the incidence of fosaprepitant (1 mg/mL, administered over 20–30 minutes) associated infusion site adverse events among a cohort of breast cancer patients ($n = 148$) receiving doxorubicin/cyclophosphamide (AC) chemotherapy [101c]. The incidence of fosaprepitant adverse effects was 34.7% ($n = 34$). The adverse effects included infusion site pain ($n = 26$), erythema ($n = 22$), swelling ($n = 12$), superficial thrombosis ($n = 8$), infusion site hives ($n = 5$), and phlebitis/thrombophlebitis ($n = 5$). Twenty-six patients experienced more than one type of adverse effect.

A retrospective study at two independent treatment centers of fosaprepitant site reactions was conducted in anthracycline-treated patients [102c]. Incidence of site reaction was compared between fosaprepitant group (1.5 mg/mL over 30 minutes, $n = 24$) and control group ($n = 32$). Frequency and symptoms *per injection* were also compared between fosaprepitant ($n = 61$) and control ($n = 98$). Both the site reaction incidence rate per patient and per injection were significantly higher in the fosaprepitant group than in the control group (67% vs. 16%; $p = 0.0002$, 34% vs. 8.2%; $p < 0.0001$, respectively). Multivariate analysis showed fosaprepitant injection was a significant predictor of infusion site reactions per injection (adjusted OR $= 4.565$, 95% CI: 1.750–11.908) and per patient (adjusted OR $= 10.476$, 95% CI: 2.282–48.091). Symptoms in 61 injections of fosaprepitant were pain ($n = 14$, 23%), erythema ($n = 10$, 16%), swelling ($n = 6$, 10%), and delayed drip infusion ($n = 6$, 10%). This study demonstrated that in patients treated with anthracyclines, infusion site reactions occurred more frequently with fosaprepitant compared to those without fosaprepitant. However, one of the limitations of this study was the small size, leading to very wide confidence intervals.

Netupitant/Palonosetron

Update

A combination fixed-dose capsule comprising two drugs netupitant and palonosetron (Akynzeo) to treat chemotherapy induced nausea and vomiting (CINV) was approved by the FDA in Oct 2014. Palonosetron is a second generation 5-HT$_3$ receptor antagonist used to prevent vomiting and nausea during the acute phase, after the start of cancer chemotherapy. Netupitant is used to prevent nausea and vomiting during both the acute phase and delayed phase (from 25 to 120 hours) after

the start of cancer chemotherapy. Common side effects of the combined drug in the clinical trials included headache, fatigue, weakness, indigestion, and constipation.

Randomized Controlled Trials

A phase-II randomized, double-blind, parallel group study was performed in chemotherapy naïve patients ($n = 694$, ≥ 18 years old) undergoing cisplatin-based chemotherapy for solid tumors. In this study, they compared different oral doses of netupitant (100, 200, and 300 mg) with palonosetron 0.50 mg (NEPA) compared to oral palonosetron (0.50 mg) [103c]. As an exploratory arm, a 3-day aprepitant (125 mg) with IV ondansetron (32 mg) regimen (APR) was included. All patients received dexamethasone on days 1–4. The efficacy endpoint was complete response (CR: no emesis, no rescue medication) during the overall (0–120 hours) phase. The overall incidence, type, frequency, and intensity of adverse events were comparable across treatment groups. There was no evidence of a dose-related increase in these adverse events for NEPA groups. At least one treatment-related adverse event was experienced by patients (15.6%). Five patients had a serious adverse event. One patient was NEPA200 patient who lost consciousness, but this was unrelated to the study treatment. A NEPA100 patient died during the study due to multiple organ failure. However, the death was not considered to be related to the study medication. The percentage of patients who developed treatment-emergent ECG abnormalities was comparable across groups.

A multinational randomized phase-III, double-blind, parallel group study evaluated the safety and efficacy of a single oral dose of netupitant (NEPA, 300 mg) versus a single oral dose (0.50 mg) of palonosetron. This study was performed in chemotherapy-naïve patients ($n = 1455$, ≥ 18 years old) receiving moderately emetogenic (anthracycline-cyclophosphamide) chemotherapy [104C]. Patients also received dexamethasone on day 1 only (12 mg in the NEPA arm and 20 mg in the palonosetron arm). There were no treatment-related adverse events leading to discontinuation. However, there were a few severe treatment-related adverse effects (0.7%) and no serious treatment-related adverse events for NEPA-treated patients.

Another multinational, double-blind, randomized phase-III study evaluated a fixed-dose combination of netupitant (NEPA), for prevention of chemotherapy-induced nausea and vomiting ($n = 413$, ≥ 18 years of age) [105C]. Patients were randomized using a 3:1 ratio to receive oral NEPA (netupitant (300 mg), palonosetron (0.50 mg), and dexamethasone) or oral APR (aprepitant (125 mg day 1, 80 mg days 2–3), oral palonosetron (0.50 mg), and dexamethasone). In highly emetogenic chemotherapy (HEC), dexamethasone was administered on days 1–4 and in moderately emetogenic chemotherapy (MEC) on day 1. Patients completed 1961 total chemotherapy cycles, with 76% receiving MEC and 24% HEC. 75% of patients completed ≥4 cycles. The incidence/type of adverse effects was comparable for both groups. Most frequent NEPA-related adverse effects included constipation (3.6%) and headache (1.0%). The number of patients who developed ECG abnormalities was comparable for the treatment groups. The most commonly reported abnormalities were flat T waves (16.9% for NEPA and 13.5% for APR) and ST depression (11.7% and 16.3%, respectively). Two (0.6%) NEPA-treated patients and one (1.0%) APR-treated patient experienced abnormal U waves.

Ondansetron [SED-1365; SEDA-34, 560; SEDA-35, 635; SEDA-36, 544]

Cardiovascular

Ondansetron is a 5-HT$_3$ receptor antagonist used to prevent nausea and vomiting with cancer chemotherapy. Over the past couple of years, there has been some concern with the cardiac safety profile of ondansetron [106R], specifically with ondansetron prolonging the QT interval of the electrocardiogram, which could predispose individuals towards the potentially fatal arrhythmia, torsades de pointes. Because of these safety concerns, the FDA issued several safety communications in regards to ondansetron prolonging the QT interval [107S,108S]. The 32 mg, single intravenous dose of ondansetron was subsequently withdrawn from the market due to cardiac safety concerns. Furthermore, the FDA advised that that the weight based dose for intravenous ondansetron should not exceed 16 mg due to cardiac safety concerns [109S]. Because of this, the cardiac safety concerns of ondansetron continue to be investigated. There has been some concern that the cardiac safety issue could extend to oral administration of ondansetron, especially in those with predisposing factors or in special populations.

A study investigated whether a single oral dose of ondansetron was associated with an arrhythmia or perceived/suspected arrhythmia since oral administration of ondansetron is commonly used in emergency departments. This study conducted a post-marketing analysis and systematic review of documented (or perceived) arrhythmia within 24 hours of receiving ondansetron administration in both the pediatric and adult populations [110M]. No reports describing an arrhythmia (or suspected arrhythmia) within 24 hours were identified using a single oral dose of ondansetron. For reports with documented or suspected arrhythmia, 80% of them were associated with intravenous route of administration. In most known or suspected cases, a significant medical history or concomitant use of a QT-prolonging medication was identified. This suggested that use of a single oral

dose of ondansetron was not associated with arrhythmia in those without predisposing risk factors.

A prospective study evaluated the prolongation of the QT interval by the combination of sevoflurane and ondansetron in pediatric patients ($n=41$) undergoing surgery [111c]. Patients (7.9 ± 2.8 year old) and were given 0.1 mg/kg intravenous ondansetron 30 minutes prior to the end of the surgery. The sevoflurane concentration was controlled based on vital signs. When patients were given sevoflurane, there was a significant increase in the QTc interval compared to the pre-induction period (sevoflurane: 432.5 (28.1) ms, pre-induction: 413.8 (20.8) ms, $p < 0.01$). When patients were given ondansetron with sevoflurane, there was a significant increase in the QTc and the peak and end of the T wave (TpE) interval compared to receiving sevoflurane alone (QTc: sevoflurane + ondansetron: 439.2(27.6) ms, sevoflurane: 432.5 (28.1) ms, $p < 0.01$, TpE: sevoflurane + ondansetron 55.6 (16.4), sevoflurane: 52.6 (17.0), $p < 0.05$). Of note, the TpE/QT ratio was not significantly different and there were no ECG abnormalities in any patient. Authors concluded that administration of sevoflurane and ondansetron (0.1 mg/kg, intravenous) appeared to be clinically safe, but recommended careful ECG monitoring. One of the limitations of this study was that this was not a randomized controlled trial and there was no comparator group.

Pharmacogenetic

The possibility that the adverse cardiac effects of ondansetron may be due to the $S(+)$ isomer of ondansetron, since ondansetron is a racemic mixture, has also been implicated [106R]. A study done by Stamer et al. in 2011 demonstrated that the genotype of an individual can affect the metabolism of specific isomers of racemic ondansetron [112c]. In this study, patients were given 4 or 8 mg of intravenous ondansetron. Blood was collected at 30, 90, and 180 minutes after the administration of ondansetron to obtain plasma concentrations of R- and S-ondansetron isomers using liquid chromatography–tandem mass spectrometry. Patients were then genotyped to determine how CYP2D6 and CYP3A genotypes influenced the AUC for plasma concentrations of ondansetron isomers. CYP2D6 activity scores were calculated for each subject, with the activity score being the sum of the values assigned to each single allele. CYP2D6 alleles *3, *4, *5, *6, *7, and *8 were given a value of 0, alleles *10 and *41 were given a value of 0.5, the wild-type allele was given a value of 1, and $*1 \times N$ was given a value of 2. CYP2D6-dependent activity score were classified as no activity (0), decreased activity (0.5–1), normal activity (1.5–2), or increased activity (3). For CYP2D6 activity scores, genotyping showed that 7.8% (11/141) had no activity, 35.5% (50/141) had decreased activity, 53.2% (75/141) had normal activity, and 5/141 (3.5%) had high activity. As CYP2D6 activity scores increased, the area under the plasma concentration-time curve for the *S*-isomer of ondansetron significantly decreased ($p = 0.01$ for 4 mg, $p = 0.03$ for 8 mg). In contrast, the AUCs for plasma concentrations for the *R*-isomer of ondansetron were unaffected by CYP2D6 activity scores.

Palonosetron [SED-15, 1365; SEDA-34, 561; SEDA-35, 636; SEDA-36, 544]

Cardiovascular

A randomized controlled trial of sevoflurane and palonosetron (0.075 mg, intravenous) on QTc intervals (QTcB, QTcF, and QTcH) in patients (age 20–75, $n = 100$) undergoing elective abdominal or gynecological surgery for a duration of greater than 1.5 hours was performed [113c]. Patients were randomly assigned to two groups: palonosetron administered prior to the induction of anesthesia ($n = 50$) or those who received palonosetron after surgery ($n = 50$). Placebos were administered to the group not receiving the palonosetron. Compared to baseline, the perioperative QTcF or QTcH intervals were found to significantly increased at all measured time points for both groups ($p < 0.05$). The perioperative QTcB interval was also found to be significantly higher starting around 10 minutes compared to baseline for both groups ($p < 0.05$). However, there were no significant differences in perioperative QTc changes over time between those receiving palonosetron prior to induction or following surgery. This study demonstrated that palonosetron appeared to have no significant impact on the QTc interval in patients undergoing elective abdominal or gynecological surgery with sevoflurane anesthesia.

ANTI-INFLAMMATORY AGENTS

Aminosalicylates [SED-15, 138; SEDA-34, 571; SEDA-35, 647; SEDA-36, 555]

Case reports:

- A 36-year-old male with ulcerative colitis presented with fever, dyspnea, pleuritic chest pain and fatigue. He had been diagnosed with ulcerative colitis 8 months prior, and had been placed on balsalazide 1.5 g (2 capsules) TID. After a flare-up in his ulcerative colitis 8–10 weeks prior to his admission, his dose of basalazide had been increased to 2.25 g (3 capsules) TID and was given mesalazine enemas (4 g) as needed. Pleuropericarditis was identified and the patient was started on a 5-day course of indomethacin, which had no effect on his symptoms. It was then suspected that his symptoms were due to a hypersensitivity reaction to balsalazide. Both oral balsalazide and mesalazine enema were discontinued. Following discontinuation of these agents, his symptoms significantly improved.

CT scan of his chest 1 month later showed complete resolution of pleural and pericardial effusions. One month later, his ulcerative colitis symptoms recurred, and he was restarted on balsalazide, 750 mg TID. His previously experienced fever, chest pain and shortness of breath reoccurred within 12 hours. The medication was stopped immediately with rapid resolution of his symptoms [114A].

- A 63-year-old female with abdominal distension and bloody stool was taking olsalazine (0.75 g/daily) for ulcerative colitis [115A]. She developed malaise, nausea, diarrhea and noted petechiae on her legs and topical chest. Hematologic evaluation had identified thrombocytopenia with blood platelet levels of 17×10^9/L. Her medications were stopped and within 2 weeks her platelet levels were 101×10^9/L. Within a month of restarting olsalazine 0.75 g daily, her platelet levels dropped again to 41×10^9/L. The olsalazine therapy was discontinued with subsequent near normalization of platelet levels.

- Three cases of mesalazine-induced pneumonitis were reported [116A]. In all three cases, CT images revealed upper lobe dominant bilateral peripherally localized consolidations.

  ○ A 15-year-old female was diagnosed with ulcerative colitis and prescribed 2.25 g/day. After 4 weeks of the oral mesalazine treatment, the patient noticed a dry cough, and self-diagnosed this as a common cold. The absolute eosinophil count was elevated to 1100 cells/μL. Mesalazine treatment was immediately ceased. A drug-induced lymphocyte stimulation test was positive for mesalazine.

  ○ A 48-year-old female with well-controlled asthma was on oral mesalazine (dose not provided) ulcerative colitis, exhibited fever and cough. Abnormal laboratories included an absolute eosinophil count of 9600 cells/μL, a C-reactive protein level of 4.64 mg/dL, and lactate dehydrogenase of 294 U/L. The mesalazine treatment was ceased. A drug-induced lymphocyte-stimulating test was negative for mesalazine.

  ○ A 50-year-old female was diagnosed with ulcerative colitis began treatment with oral mesalazine at 3.6 g/day. Two weeks later, owing to frequent diarrhea, the mesalazine was reduced to 2.4 g/day. Five weeks after the initiation of mesalazine treatment, the patient exhibited a cough, fever, and morning sputum. She was diagnosed with bacterial pneumonia on the basis of her clinical history, bilateral infiltration on radiography, and elevated inflammation markers. The patient's absolute eosinophil count was elevated to 4300 cells/μL. Mesalazine treatment was ceased. A drug-induced lymphocyte-stimulating test was negative for mesalazine.

Thiopurines (Azathioprine, 6-Thioguanine, 6-Mercaptopurine)

Update

The Clinical Pharmacogenetics Implementation Consortium (CPIC) guideline for thiopurine methyltransferase genotype and thiopurine dosing was recently reviewed. However, they found no new evidence to change the primary dosing recommendations that were provided in the original guideline [117S,118S]. The original dosing recommendations were to start with reduced doses of mercaptopurine in patients with one nonfunctional thiopurine-S-methyltransferase (TPMT) allele, or drastically reduce the doses for patients with malignancy and two nonfunctional alleles. Following this, the dose should be adjusted based on the degree of myelosuppression and disease-specific guidelines. They also recommended considering nonthiopurine immunosuppressant therapy for patients with nonmalignant conditions with two nonfunctional TPMT alleles as an alternative.

Cancer

A US retrospective cohort study evaluated the risk of lymphoma (ongoing, residual, and per year of therapy) in VA patients with ulcerative colitis treated with thiopurines [119c]. In total, 13% of patients were treated with thiopurines for a median of 1 year. Lymphoma occurred in 119 patients who had not been treated with thiopurines, in 18 who were treated with thiopurines, and in five patients who had discontinued treatment with thiopurines. The lymphoma incidence rates were higher among those treated with thiopurines (2.31 per 1000 person-years) compared to patients who had not been treated with thiopurines (0.60 per 1000 person-years), and patients who had discontinued treatment with thiopurines (0.28 per 1000 person-years). The incidence rates of lymphoma increased with years of thiopurine therapy (0.9, 1.6, 1.6, 5, and 8.9 per 1000 person-years for during the first, second, third, and fourth year, and >4 years of thiopurine therapy, respectively). The hazard of developing lymphoma while being treated with thiopurines was 4.2 (95% CI: 2.5–6.8) times the hazard of developing lymphoma when unexposed to thiopurines adjusting for age, sex and race. The hazard of developing lymphoma after discontinuing treatment with thiopurines was 0.5 (95% CI: 0.2–1.3) times the hazard of developing lymphoma when unexposed to thiopurines adjusting for age, sex and race. Additionally, in those that were over age 65, the hazard of lymphoma was significantly higher than the hazard of lymphoma in those younger than age 40 (HR: 2.6, 95% CI: 1.2–5.7). While the study showed that there was over a fourfold increase in hazard of lymphoma in patients being treated with thiopurines compared to those that were unexposed, the authors did not believe that their hazard ratios for lymphoma were overestimated since they were comparing patients within the same population and it adjusted for multiple factors such as age, race, and sex. However, since they were looking at a high-risk population, there was some concern by the authors that the standardized incidence rates and ratios for lymphoma were overestimated.

A prospective cohort study of IBD patients assessed the incidence of myeloid disorders in France [120c]. During follow-up, five patients were diagnosed with incident myeloid disorders. Four out of these five patients had been exposed to thiopurines. One of the patients had ongoing treatment, while three had past exposure to thiopurines. The risk of myeloid disorders among the IBD population was not significantly different compared to the general population (standardized incidence ratio (SIR) = 1.80, 95% CI: 0.58–4.20). The risk of myeloid disorders was not increased among IBD patients with ongoing thiopurine treatment (SIR = 1.54; 95% CI: 0.05–8.54). However, patients with past exposures to thiopurines were found to have a significantly increased risk of myeloid disorders (SIR = 6.98; 95% CI: 1.44–20.36). While the authors did find an association, given the small number of cases and the heterogeneous nature of the cases, this led to extremely wide confidence intervals to where the results of this study should be interpreted with caution. Further studies with larger numbers of patients are needed to ascertain the association between thiopurines and myeloid disorders.

A meta-analysis was conducted to examine the association between thiopurine use and nonmelanoma skin cancers (NMSC) in patients with IBD [121M]. Eight studies ($n = 60351$ patients) were used to assess the risk of developing NMSC in patients with IBD on thiopurines from three databases. The pooled adjusted hazards ratio of developing NMSC after exposure to thiopurines in IBD patients was 2.28 (95% CI: 1.50–3.45, $I^2 = 76\%$). However, there was significant heterogeneity ($I^2 = 76\%$) between the studies. The authors concluded that there was an increased risk of developing NMSC in patients with IBD on thiopurines.

Case reports:

- A 75-year-old male with a Crohn's disease with suspected sepsis, presented with fever and a maculopapular rash involving upper and lower extremities. Azathioprine (dose not given) had been initiated 2 weeks prior to hospitalization. A skin biopsy was performed, and the results were consistent with acute febrile neutrophilic dermatosis (Sweet's syndrome). Azathioprine was discontinued with subsequent resolution [122A].
- Three IBD cases (1-ulcerative colitis, 2-Crohn's disease) were noted for the development of thrombocytopenia and splenomegaly with use of azathioprine [123A]. In all cases, male patients >34-years-old received azathioprine for extended periods (range: 9 months to

7 years) over a range of doses. All patients were diagnosed with nodular regenerative hyperplasia (NRH), a form of noncirrhotic portal hypertension that can be caused by chronic use of medications (e.g. azathioprine, thioguanine, mercaptopurine, didanosine, stavudine, isoplatin, vitamin A). Two of the cases showed normal in liver function tests, a not uncommon feature of NRH. The same two cases were heterozygous for mutations in TPMT.

Pharmacogenetics

A retrospective cohort study examined whether gene polymorphisms in glutathione-S-transferases (GST) GSTM1, GSTT1 and TPMT combined with various clinical parameters, predicted thiopurine induced adverse effects [124c]. Patients ($n = 176$) with Crohn's Disease of predominantly Jewish descent (94.8%) were treated with thiopurines ($n = 131$ with 6-mercaptopurine, $n = 45$ with azathioprine) and were genotyped for common polymorphisms in GSTM1, GSTT1 and TPMT. Four patients (2.2%) were heterozygous for TPMT polymorphisms, 99 patients (56%) were GSTM1-null homozygotes and 48 patients (27%) were GSTT1-null homozygotes. The most common adverse effects were myelosuppression ($n = 11$), pancreatitis ($n = 7$) and hepatotoxicity ($n = 6$). There was no association was found between TPMT or GSTT1 polymorphisms and the development of adverse effects. While the authors reported a statistically significant association between the GSTM1-null genotype and serious adverse events, the p-values and confidence intervals indicate that while the association was bordering significance, there was not a significant association (OR = 2.63, 95% CI: 0.99–6.99, $p = 0.05$).

BIOLOGICS

See chapter-37 for further information

Update

The FDA approved (May 2014) the vedolizumab (Entyvio) injection to treat adult patients with moderate to severe ulcerative colitis or Crohn's disease [125S].

STEROIDS

See chapter-39 for further information.

References

[1] Poole RM. Nemonoxacin: first global approval. Drugs. 2014;74(12):1445–53 [R].
[2] Zhang YF, Dai XJ, Wang T, et al. Effects of an Al(3+)- and Mg(2+)-containing antacid, ferrous sulfate, and calcium carbonate on the absorption of nemonoxacin (TG-873870) in healthy Chinese volunteers. Acta Pharmacol Sin. 2014;35(12):1586–92 [c].
[3] Dawsey SP, Hollenbeck A, Schatzkin A, et al. A prospective study of vitamin and mineral supplement use and the risk of upper gastrointestinal cancers. PLoS One. 2014;9(2):1–7. e88774. [C].
[4] van der Pol R, Langendam M, Benninga M, et al. Efficacy and safety of histamine-2 receptor antagonists. JAMA Pediatr. 2014;168(10):947–54 [M].
[5] Tawadrous D, Dixon S, Shariff SZ, et al. Altered mental status in older adults with histamine2-receptor antagonists: a population-based study. Eur J Intern Med. 2014;25(8):701–9 [C].
[6] Kwon JE, Koh SJ, Chun J, et al. Effect of gastric acid suppressants and prokinetics on peritoneal dialysis-related peritonitis. World J Gastroenterol. 2014;20(25):8187–94 [c].
[7] Lam JR, Schneider JL, Zhao W, et al. Proton pump inhibitor and histamine 2 receptor antagonist use and vitamin B12 deficiency. JAMA. 2013;310(22):2435–42 [C].
[8] Corley D, Lam J, Schneider J. Gastric acid-inhibiting medications and vitamin B12 deficiency—reply. JAMA. 2014;311(14):1445–1446 [r].
[9] Dharmarajan TS, Norkus EP. Gastric acid-inhibiting medications and vitamin B12 deficiency. JAMA. 2014;311(14):1444–5 [r].
[10] Gonzalez-Gonzalez C, Figueiras A. Gastric acid-inhibiting medications and vitamin B12 deficiency. JAMA. 2014;311(14):1445 [r].
[11] Dharmarajan TS, Kanagala MR, Murakonda P, et al. Do acid-lowering agents affect vitamin B12 status in older adults? J Am Med Dir Assoc. 2008;9(3):162–7 [c].
[12] Jo Y, Park E, Ahn SB, et al. A proton pump inhibitor's effect on bone metabolism mediated by Osteoclast action in old age: a prospective randomized study. Gut Liver. 2014;1–8 [c].
[13] Ozdil K, Kahraman R, Sahin A, et al. Bone density in proton pump inhibitors users: a prospective study. Rheumatol Int. 2013;33(9):2255–60 [c].
[14] Adams AL, Black MH, Zhang JL, et al. Proton-pump inhibitor use and hip fractures in men: a population-based case-control study. Ann Epidemiol. 2014;24(4):286–90 [C].
[15] Shih CJ, Chen YT, Ou SM, et al. Proton pump inhibitor use represents an independent risk factor for myocardial infarction. Int J Cardiol. 2014;177(1):292–7 [C].
[16] Kwok CS, Jeevanantham V, Dawn B, et al. No consistent evidence of differential cardiovascular risk amongst proton-pump inhibitors when used with clopidogrel: meta-analysis. Int J Cardiol. 2013;167(3):965–74 [M].
[17] Juurlink DN, Dormuth CR, Huang A, et al. Proton pump inhibitors and the risk of adverse cardiac events. PLoS One. 2013;8(12):1–5. e84890. [C].
[18] Barletta JF, Sclar DA. Proton pump inhibitors increase the risk for hospital-acquired Clostridium difficile infection in critically ill patients. Crit Care. 2014;18(6):714 [c].
[19] Buendgens L, Bruensing J, Matthes M, et al. Administration of proton pump inhibitors in critically ill medical patients is associated with increased risk of developing Clostridium difficile-associated diarrhea. J Crit Care. 2014;29(4):696.e11–15 [c].
[20] MacLaren R, Reynolds PM, Allen RR. Histamine-2 receptor antagonists vs proton pump inhibitors on gastrointestinal tract hemorrhage and infectious complications in the intensive care unit. JAMA Intern Med. 2014;174(4):564–74 [C].
[21] Daniel A, Rapose A. The evaluation of Clostridium difficile infection (CDI) in a community hospital. J Infect Public Health. 2014;8(2):155–60 [c].
[22] van Leeuwen RW, van Gelder T, Mathijssen RH, et al. Drug-drug interactions with tyrosine-kinase inhibitors: a clinical perspective. Lancet Oncol. 2014;15(8):e315–26 [R].
[23] OSI Pharmaceuticals I. Tarceva (erlotinib) package insert. 2013; 1/19/2015. Available from: http://www.accessdata.fda.gov/drugsatfda_docslabel/2013/021743s018lbl.pdf. [S].

[24] Chu MP, Ghosh S, Chambers CR, et al. Gastric acid suppression is associated with decreased erlotinib efficacy in non-small-cell lung cancer. Clin Lung Cancer. 2015;16(1):33–9 [c].

[25] Tsao MS, Sakurada A, Cutz JC, et al. Erlotinib in lung cancer—molecular and clinical predictors of outcome. N Engl J Med. 2005;353(2):133–44 [c].

[26] Abbas R, Leister C, Sonnichsen D. A clinical study to examine the potential effect of lansoprazole on the pharmacokinetics of bosutinib when administered concomitantly to healthy subjects. Clin Drug Investig. 2013;33(8):589–95 [c].

[27] Beorlegui B, Aldaz A, Ortega A, et al. Potential interaction between methotrexate and omeprazole. Ann Pharmacother. 2000;34(9):1024–7 [A].

[28] Suzuki K, Doki K, Homma M, et al. Co-administration of proton pump inhibitors delays elimination of plasma methotrexate in high-dose methotrexate therapy. Br J Clin Pharmacol. 2009;67(1):44–9 [c].

[29] Santucci R, Leveque D, Lescoute A, et al. Delayed elimination of methotrexate associated with co-administration of proton pump inhibitors. Anticancer Res. 2010;30(9):3807–10 [c].

[30] Chioukh R, Noel-Hudson MS, Ribes S, et al. Proton pump inhibitors inhibit methotrexate transport by renal basolateral organic anion transporter hOAT3. Drug Metab Dispos. 2014;42(12):2041–8 [E].

[31] Pantoprazole revised label 2014; 3/1/2015. Available from: http://www.accessdata.fda.gov/drugsatfda_docs/label/2014/022020s011-020987s049lbl.pdf. [S].

[32] Chan AJ, Rajakumar I. High-dose methotrexate in adult oncology patients: a case-control study assessing the risk association between drug interactions and methotrexate toxicity. J Oncol Pharm Pract. 2014;20(2):93–9 [c].

[33] Reeves DJ, Moore ES, Bascom D, et al. Retrospective evaluation of methotrexate elimination when co-administered with proton pump inhibitors. Br J Clin Pharmacol. 2014;78(3):565–71 [c].

[34] Zvyaga T, Chang SY, Chen C, et al. Evaluation of six proton pump inhibitors as inhibitors of various human cytochromes P450: focus on cytochrome P450 2C19. Drug Metab Dispos. 2012;40(9):1698–711 [E].

[35] Johnson DA, Chilton R, Liker HR. Proton-pump inhibitors in patients requiring antiplatelet therapy: new FDA labeling. Postgrad Med. 2014;126(3):239–45 [R].

[36] Collet JP, Hulot JS, Abtan J, et al. Prasugrel but not high dose clopidogrel overcomes the lansoprazole neutralizing effect of P2Y12 inhibition: results of the randomized DOSAPI study. Eur J Clin Pharmacol. 2014;70(9):1049–57 [c].

[37] Funck-Brentano C, Szymezak J, Steichen O, et al. Effects of rabeprazole on the antiplatelet effects and pharmacokinetics of clopidogrel in healthy volunteers. Arch Cardiovasc Dis. 2013;106(12):661–71 [c].

[38] Administration FaD. Labelling revision letter for mycophenolic acid and vitamin B12 with pantoprazole; 2014. 3/1/2015. Available from: http://www.accessdata.fda.gov/drugsatfda_docs/appletter/2014/022020Orig1s011,020987Orig1s049ltr.pdf [S].

[39] Rupprecht K, Schmidt C, Raspe A, et al. Bioavailability of mycophenolate mofetil and enteric-coated mycophenolate sodium is differentially affected by pantoprazole in healthy volunteers. J Clin Pharmacol. 2009;49(10):1196–201 [c].

[40] Kees MG, Steinke T, Moritz S, et al. Omeprazole impairs the absorption of mycophenolate mofetil but not of enteric-coated mycophenolate sodium in healthy volunteers. J Clin Pharmacol. 2012;52(8):1265–72 [c].

[41] Knorr JP, Sjeime M, Braitman LE, et al. Concomitant proton pump inhibitors with mycophenolate mofetil and the risk of rejection in kidney transplant recipients. Transplantation. 2014;97(5):518–24 [r].

[42] van Boekel GA, Kerkhofs CH, van de Logt F, et al. Proton pump inhibitors do not increase the risk of acute rejection. Neth J Med. 2014;72(2):86–90 [c].

[43] Isoda K, Takeuchi T, Kotani T, et al. The proton pump inhibitor lansoprazole, but not rabeprazole, the increased blood concentrations of calcineurin inhibitors in Japanese patients with connective tissue diseases. Intern Med. 2014;53(13):1413–8 [c].

[44] Luk CP, Parsons R, Lee YP, et al. Proton pump inhibitor-associated hypomagnesemia: what do FDA data tell us? Ann Pharmacother. 2013;47(6):773–80 [c].

[45] Administration USFaD. FDA Drug Safety Communication: low magnesium levels can be associated with long-term use of Proton Pump Inhibitor drugs (PPIs); 2011. [updated 03/14/2011 cited 2015 1/12/15] Available from: http://www.fda.gov/Drugs/DrugSafety/ucm245011.htm#Data_Summary [S].

[46] Administration AGDoHTG. Risk of hypomagnesaemia with proton pump inhibitors. Medicines Safety Update [Internet]. 2011;2(3):81. 1/12/15. Available from: http://www.tga.gov.au/publication-issue/medicines-safety-update-vol-2-no-3-june-2011#risk [S].

[47] Alhosaini M, Walter JS, Singh S, et al. Hypomagnesemia in hemodialysis patients: role of proton pump inhibitors. Am J Nephrol. 2014;39(3):204–9 [c].

[48] Lindner G, Funk GC, Leichtle AB, et al. Impact of proton pump inhibitor use on magnesium homoeostasis: a cross-sectional study in a tertiary emergency department. Int J Clin Pract. 2014;68(11):1352–7 [C].

[49] Kim S, Lee H, Park CH, et al. Clinical predictors associated with proton pump inhibitor-induced hypomagnesemia. Am J Ther. 2013;22(1):14–21 [c].

[50] Zipursky J, Macdonald EM, Hollands S, et al. Proton pump inhibitors and hospitalization with hypomagnesemia: a population-based case-control study. PLoS Med. 2014;11(9):1–7. e1001736. [c].

[51] Sandholdt LH, Laurinaviciene R, Bygum A. Proton pump inhibitor-induced subacute cutaneous lupus erythematosus. Br J Dermatol. 2014;170(2):342–51 [c].

[52] Schiller D, Maieron A, Schofl R, et al. Drug fever due to a single dose of pantoprazole. Pharmacology. 2014;94(1–2):78–9 [A].

[53] Candar M, Gunes H, Boz BV, et al. Asystole after the first dose of lansoprazole. Am J Emerg Med. 2014;32(10). 1302.e3–4. [A].

[54] Hashimoto R, Matsuda T, Chonan A. Iron-deficiency anemia caused by a proton pump inhibitor. Intern Med. 2014;53(20):2297–9 [A].

[55] Fohl AL, Regal RE. Proton pump inhibitor-associated pneumonia: not a breath of fresh air after all? World J Gastrointest Pharmacol Ther. 2011;2(3):17–26 [R].

[56] Filion KB, Chateau D, Targownik LE, et al. Proton pump inhibitors and the risk of hospitalisation for community-acquired pneumonia: replicated cohort studies with meta-analysis. Gut. 2014;63(4):552–8 [M].

[57] Ho SW, Tsai MC, Teng YH, et al. Population-based cohort study on the risk of pneumonia in patients with non-traumatic intracranial haemorrhage who use proton pump inhibitors. BMJ Open. 2014;4(11):e006710 [c].

[58] Doggrell SA, Hancox JC. Cardiac safety concerns for domperidone, an antiemetic and prokinetic, and galactogogue medicine. Expert Opin Drug Saf. 2014;13(1):131–8 [R].

[59] Benkimoun P. French journal calls for domperidone to be withdrawn. BMJ. 2014;348:g1722 [r].

[60] Kanji S, Stevenson A, Hutton B. Sudden cardiac death and ventricular arrhythmias associated with domperidone: evidence supporting health Canada's warning. Can J Hosp Pharm. 2014;67(4):311–2 [r].

[61] Rojas-Fernandez C, Stephenson AL, Fischer HD, et al. Current use of domperidone and co-prescribing of medications that increase

its arrhythmogenic potential among older adults: a population-based cohort study in Ontario, Canada. Drugs Aging. 2014;31(11):805–13 [C].

[62] Makari J, Cameron K, Battistella M. Domperidone-associated sudden cardiac death in the general population and implications for use in patients undergoing hemodialysis: a literature review. Can J Hosp Pharm. 2014;67(6):441–6 [M].

[63] Atluri DK, Chandar AK, Bharucha AE, et al. Effect of linaclotide in irritable bowel syndrome with constipation (IBS-C): a systematic review and meta-analysis. Neurogastroenterol Motil. 2014;26(4):499–509 [M].

[64] Cryer B, Katz S, Vallejo R, et al. A randomized study of lubiprostone for opioid-induced constipation in patients with chronic noncancer pain. Pain Med. 2014;15(11):1825–34 [c].

[65] Yamasaki M, Funakoshi S, Matsuda S, et al. Interaction of magnesium oxide with gastric acid secretion inhibitors in clinical pharmacotherapy. Eur J Clin Pharmacol. 2014;70(8):921–4 [c].

[66] van der Meer YG, Venhuizen WA, Heyland DK, et al. Should we stop prescribing metoclopramide as a prokinetic drug in critically ill patients? Crit Care. 2014;18(5):502 [R].

[67] Nguyen TT, Petzel Gimbar RM. Sustained hypotension following intravenous metoclopramide. Ann Pharmacother. 2013;47(11):1577–80 [A].

[68] Urbanowicz T, Pawlowska M, Buczkowski P, et al. Seizures after heart transplantation–two cases of non-immunosuppressant drug interactions in young patients. Ann Transplant. 2014;19:417–20 [A].

[69] Porayette P, Flockhart D, Gupta SK. One size fits one: pharmacogenetics in gastroenterology. Clin Gastroenterol Hepatol. 2014;12(4):565–70 [R].

[70] Parkman HP, Mishra A, Jacobs M, et al. Clinical response and side effects of metoclopramide: associations with clinical, demographic, and pharmacogenetic parameters. J Clin Gastroenterol. 2012;46(6):494–503 [c].

[71] Webster L, Dhar S, Eldon M, et al. A phase 2, double-blind, randomized, placebo-controlled, dose-escalation study to evaluate the efficacy, safety, and tolerability of naloxegol in patients with opioid-induced constipation. Pain. 2013;154(9):1542–50 [c].

[72] Webster L, Chey WD, Tack J, et al. Randomised clinical trial: the long-term safety and tolerability of naloxegol in patients with pain and opioid-induced constipation. Aliment Pharmacol Ther. 2014;40(7):771–9 [C].

[73] Chen SL, Cai SR, Deng L, et al. Efficacy and complications of polyethylene glycols for treatment of constipation in children: a meta-analysis. Medicine (Baltimore). 2014;93(16):1–10. e65. [M].

[74] Shin A, Camilleri M, Kolar G, et al. Systematic review with meta-analysis: highly selective 5-HT4 agonists (prucalopride, velusetrag or naronapride) in chronic constipation. Aliment Pharmacol Ther. 2014;39(3):239–53 [M].

[75] Leelakusolvong S, Ke M, Zou D, et al. Factors predictive of treatment-emergent adverse events of prucalopride: an integrated analysis of four randomized, double-blind, placebo-controlled trials. Gut Liver. 2014;9(2):208–13 [M].

[76] Sivabalasundaram V, Habal F, Cherney D. Prucalopride-associated acute tubular necrosis. World J Clin Cases. 2014;2(8):380–4 [A].

[77] Carnovale C, Pellegrino P, Perrone V, et al. Neurological and psychiatric adverse events with prucalopride: case report and possible mechanisms. J Clin Pharm Ther. 2013;38(6):524–5 [A].

[78] Weir MA, Fleet JL, Vinden C, et al. Hyponatremia and sodium picosulfate bowel preparations in older adults. Am J Gastroenterol. 2014;109(5):686–94 [C].

[79] Torikoshi-Hatano A, Namera A, Shiraishi H, et al. A fatal case of hypermagnesemia caused by ingesting magnesium chloride as a folk remedy. J Forensic Sci. 2013;58(6):1673–5 [A].

[80] Cho YS, Nam KM, Park JH, et al. Acute hyponatremia with seizure and mental change after oral sodium picosulfate/magnesium citrate bowel preparation. Ann Coloproctol. 2014;30(6):290–3 [A].

[81] Bregman A, Fritz K, Xiong GL. Lactulose-associated lithium toxicity: a case series. J Clin Psychopharmacol. 2014;34(6):742–3 [A].

[82] O'Keefe SJ, Jeppesen PB, Gilroy R, et al. Safety and efficacy of teduglutide after 52 weeks of treatment in patients with short bowel intestinal failure. Clin Gastroenterol Hepatol. 2013;11(7):815–23. e1–3. [c].

[83] Wilhelm SM, Lipari M, Kulik JK, et al. Teduglutide for the treatment of short bowel syndrome. Ann Pharmacother. 2014;48(9):1209–13 [M].

[84] Jeppesen PB, Gilroy R, Pertkiewicz M, et al. Randomised placebo-controlled trial of teduglutide in reducing parenteral nutrition and/or intravenous fluid requirements in patients with short bowel syndrome. Gut. 2011;60(7):902–14 [C].

[85] Jeppesen PB, Pertkiewicz M, Messing B, et al. Teduglutide reduces need for parenteral support among patients with short bowel syndrome with intestinal failure. Gastroenterology. 2012;143(6):1473–81 e3. [C].

[86] Tappenden KA, Edelman J, Joelsson B. Teduglutide enhances structural adaptation of the small intestinal mucosa in patients with short bowel syndrome. J Clin Gastroenterol. 2013;47(7): 602–7 [c].

[87] Erden A, Karahan S, Bulut K, et al. A case of bismuth intoxication with irreversible renal damage. Int J Nephrol Renovasc Dis. 2013;6:241–3 [A].

[88] Bingham AL, Brown RO, Dickerson RN. Inadvertent exaggerated anticoagulation following use of bismuth subsalicylate in an enterally fed patient receiving warfarin therapy. Nutr Clin Pract. 2013;28(6):766–9 [A].

[89] Marraffa JM, Holland MG, Sullivan RW, et al. Cardiac conduction disturbance after loperamide abuse. Clin Toxicol (Phila). 2014;52(9):952–7 [A].

[90] Vidarsdottir H, Moller PH, Bjornsson ES. Loperamide-induced acute pancreatitis. Case Rep Gastrointest Med. 2013;2013:517414 [A].

[91] Chmielewska-Wilkon D, Reggiardo G, Egan CG. Otilonium bromide in irritable bowel syndrome: a dose-ranging randomized double-blind placebo-controlled trial. World J Gastroenterol. 2014;20(34):12283–91 [c].

[92] Evangelista S. Benefits from long-term treatment in irritable bowel syndrome. Gastroenterol Res Pract. 2012;2012:936960 [R].

[93] Schoenfeld P, Pimentel M, Chang L, et al. Safety and tolerability of rifaximin for the treatment of irritable bowel syndrome without constipation: a pooled analysis of randomised, double-blind, placebo-controlled trials. Aliment Pharmacol Ther. 2014;39(10):1161–8 [M].

[94] Cai ST, Yang YS. Editorial: safety and tolerability of rifaximin for IBS—more information is required. Aliment Pharmacol Ther. 2014;40(2):208 [r].

[95] Schoenfeld P, Pimentel M. Editorial: safety and tolerability of rifaximin for IBS—more information is required; authors' reply. Aliment Pharmacol Ther. 2014;40(2):209 [r].

[96] Sejourne A, Noal S, Boone M, et al. Two cases of fatal encephalopathy related to Ifosfamide: an adverse role of aprepitant? Case Rep Oncol. 2014;7(3):669–72 [A].

[97] Cristofori F, Thapar N, Saliakellis E, et al. Efficacy of the neurokinin-1 receptor antagonist aprepitant in children with cyclical vomiting syndrome. Aliment Pharmacol Ther. 2014;40(3):309–17 [c].

[98] Toyoda T, Terao Y, Oji M, et al. The interaction of antiemetic dose of droperidol with propofol on QT interval during anesthetic induction. J Anesth. 2013;27(6):885–9 [c].

[99] Nuttall GA, Malone AM, Michels CA, et al. Does low-dose droperidol increase the risk of polymorphic ventricular tachycardia or death in the surgical patient? Anesthesiology. 2013;118(2):382–6 [c].

[100] Lundberg JD, Crawford BS, Phillips G, et al. Incidence of infusion-site reactions associated with peripheral intravenous administration of fosaprepitant. Support Care Cancer. 2014;22(6):1461–6 [c].

[101] Leal AD, Kadakia KC, Looker S, et al. Fosaprepitant-induced phlebitis: a focus on patients receiving doxorubicin/cyclophosphamide therapy. Support Care Cancer. 2014;22(5):1313–7 [c].

[102] Sato Y, Kondo M, Inagaki A, et al. Highly frequent and enhanced injection site reaction induced by peripheral venous injection of fosaprepitant in anthracycline-treated patients. J Cancer Educ. 2014;5(5):390–7 [c].

[103] Hesketh PJ, Rossi G, Rizzi G, et al. Efficacy and safety of NEPA, an oral combination of netupitant and palonosetron, for prevention of chemotherapy-induced nausea and vomiting following highly emetogenic chemotherapy: a randomized dose-ranging pivotal study. Ann Oncol. 2014;25(7):1340–6 [c].

[104] Aapro M, Rugo H, Rossi G, et al. A randomized phase III study evaluating the efficacy and safety of NEPA, a fixed-dose combination of netupitant and palonosetron, for prevention of chemotherapy-induced nausea and vomiting following moderately emetogenic chemotherapy. Ann Oncol. 2014;25(7):1328–33 [C].

[105] Gralla RJ, Bosnjak SM, Hontsa A, et al. A phase III study evaluating the safety and efficacy of NEPA, a fixed-dose combination of netupitant and palonosetron, for prevention of chemotherapy-induced nausea and vomiting over repeated cycles of chemotherapy. Ann Oncol. 2014;25(7):1333–9 [C].

[106] Doggrell SA, Hancox JC. Cardiac safety concerns for ondansetron, an antiemetic commonly used for nausea linked to cancer treatment and following anaesthesia. Expert Opin Drug Saf. 2013;12(3):421–31 [R].

[107] Administration USFaD. FDA Drug Safety Communication: abnormal heart rhythms may be associated with use of Zofran (ondansetron); 2011. 1/28/15. Available from: http://www.fda.gov/Drugs/DrugSafety/ucm271913.htm [S].

[108] Administration USFaD. FDA Drug Safety Communication: new information regarding QT prolongation with ondansetron (Zofran); 2012. 1/28/2015. Available from: http://www.fda.gov/Drugs/DrugSafety/ucm310190.htm [S].

[109] Administration USFaD. FDA Drug Safety Communication: updated information on 32 mg intravenous ondansetron (Zofran) dose and pre-mixed ondansetron products; 2012. [S].

[110] Freedman SB, Uleryk E, Rumantir M, et al. Ondansetron and the risk of cardiac arrhythmias: a systematic review and postmarketing analysis. Ann Emerg Med. 2014;64(1):19–25. e6. [M].

[111] Lee JH, Park YH, Kim JT, et al. The effect of sevoflurane and ondansetron on QT interval and transmural dispersion of repolarization in children. Paediatr Anaesth. 2014;24(4):421–5 [c].

[112] Stamer UM, Lee EH, Rauers NI, et al. CYP2D6- and CYP3A-dependent enantioselective plasma concentrations of ondansetron in postanesthesia care. Anesth Analg. 2011;113(1):48–54 [c].

[113] Kim HJ, Lee HC, Jung YS, et al. Effect of palonosetron on the QTc interval in patients undergoing sevoflurane anaesthesia. Br J Anaesth. 2014;112(3):460–8 [c].

[114] Coman RM, Glover SC, Gjymishka A. Febrile pleuropericarditis, a potentially life-threatening adverse event of balsalazide–case report and literature review of the side effects of 5-aminosalicylates. Expert Rev Clin Immunol. 2014;10(5):667–75 [A].

[115] Rao Y, Zheng F. Thrombocytopenia associated with 5-aminosalicylate prodrug, olsalazine: is the devil still there? Int J Clin Pharm. 2013;35(4):529–31 [A].

[116] Inoue M, Horita N, Kimura N, et al. Three cases of mesalazine-induced pneumonitis with eosinophilia. Respir Investig. 2014;52(3):209–12 [A].

[117] Relling MV, Gardner EE, Sandborn WJ, et al. Clinical pharmacogenetics implementation consortium guidelines for thiopurine methyltransferase genotype and thiopurine dosing: 2013 update. Clin Pharmacol Ther. 2013;93(4):324–325 [S].

[118] Relling MV, Gardner EE, Sandborn WJ, et al. Clinical Pharmacogenetics Implementation Consortium guidelines for thiopurine methyltransferase genotype and thiopurine dosing. Clin Pharmacol Ther. 2011;89(3):387–91 [S].

[119] Khan N, Abbas AM, Lichtenstein GR, et al. Risk of lymphoma in patients with ulcerative colitis treated with thiopurines: a nationwide retrospective cohort study. Gastroenterology. 2013;145(5):1007–15. e3. [c].

[120] Lopez A, Beaugerie L, Peyrin-Biroulet L. Thiopurines and myeloid disorders: is more caution needed when treating inflammatory bowel disease patients? Expert Rev Clin Immunol. 2014;10(12):1563–5 [c].

[121] Ariyaratnam J, Subramanian V. Association between thiopurine use and nonmelanoma skin cancers in patients with inflammatory bowel disease: a meta-analysis. Am J Gastroenterol. 2014;109(2):163–9 [M].

[122] Grelle JL, Halloush RA, Khasawneh FA. Azathioprine-induced acute febrile neutrophilic dermatosis (Sweet's syndrome). BMJ Case Rep. 2013; http://dx.doi.org/10.1136/bcr-2013-200405 pii: bcr2013200405. [A].

[123] Dooremont D, Decaestecker J, De Wulf D, et al. Azathioprine induced serious portal hypertension: a case series of three IBD patients and review of the literature. Acta Gastroenterol Belg. 2013;76(3):342–6 [A].

[124] Mazor Y, Koifman E, Elkin H, et al. Risk factors for serious adverse effects of thiopurines in patients with Crohn's disease. Curr Drug Saf. 2013;8(3):181–5 [c].

[125] Administration USFaD. FDA approves Entyvio to treat ulcerative colitis and Crohn's disease; 2014 [S].

36

Drugs That Act on the Immune System: Cytokines and Monoclonal Antibodies

Lokesh K. Jha*, Sandeep Mukherjee[†,1]

*Sanford Center for Digestive Disease, Sanford Health, Sioux Falls, SD, USA
[†]Creighton University Medical Center, Omaha, NE, USA
[1]Corresponding author: smukherjee1168@gmail.com

CYTOKINES

Bone Morphogenic Proteins [SEDA-34, 579; SEDA-35, 659; SEDA-36, 561]

Musculoskeletal

In a randomized control trial comparing the efficacy of rh-BMP2 and synthetic silicate calcium phosphate (SiCaP) as bone graft substitutes on fusion rates and clinical outcomes in patients undergoing single-level lumbar stand-alone extreme lateral interbody fusion, higher rates of excessive bone formation and adjacent segment disease were found on the rh-BMP2 group [1C]. In a randomized controlled trial, one patient treated with BMP-2 for minimally invasive transforaminal lumbar interbody fusion developed symptomatic neuroforaminal bone growth [2C].

Colony-Stimulating Factors [SEDA-32, 675; SEDA-33, 769; SEDA-34, 581; SEDA-36, 563]

Granulocyte Colony-Stimulating Factor [SEDA-33, 769; SEDA-35, 659; SEDA-36, 563]

SKIN

A case report described occurrence of bullous Sweet's syndrome in a 20-month-old boy with congenital neutropenia for which he was being treated with granulocyte colony-stimulating factor [3A].

Filgrastim [SEDA-36, 563]

Hematologic

A case report described occurrence of extramedullary hematopoiesis as a complication of filgrastim usage in a 3-year-old boy with acute colchicine intoxication [4A].

Pegfilgrastim [SEDA-36, 563]

Musculoskeletal

In a randomized trial comparing efficacy and safety of lipegfilgrastim versus pegfilgrastim use in patients with breast cancer receiving doxorubicin/docetaxel chemotherapy, bone-pain-related symptoms were the most commonly reported adverse events in 16.8% pegfilgrastim patients and in 23.8% lipegfilgrastim patients, but the difference was not statistically significant [5C].

Hematologic

A case report described occurrence of fatal blast proliferation in a patient with acute myeloid leukemia following pegfilgrastim use [6A].

INTERFERONS [SEDA-32, 676; SEDA-33, 773; SEDA-34, 581; SEDA-35, 660; SEDA-36, 564]

Interferon Alfa [SEDA-32, 676; SEDA-33, 773; SEDA-34, 581; SEDA-36, 564]

Endocrine

Among 106 patients with chronic hepatitis B treated with PegIFNα-2a at a dose of 180 μg/week subcutaneously for 48 weeks, thyroid disorder occurred in seven patients (6.6%), six of them developed hypothyroidism and one developed hyperthyroidism [7c].

Eye

Among 22 patients with conjunctival intraepithelial neoplasia (CIN) treated with interferon alpha 2b

© 2015 Elsevier B.V. All rights reserved.

(1 million IU/mL) 4 times daily, 1 patient developed irritative conjunctivitis and 3 patients developed punctate keratitis [8c].

- In a prospective study of chronic hepatitis B patients treated with pegylated interferon-α (PEGIFN-α) monotherapy, a statistically significant increase in the retinal nerve fiber layer (RNFL) thickness was noted [9c].

Skin

In a phase II multicenter study, 55 patients with metastatic melanoma were treated with a combination of sorafenib (2 × 400 mg/day orally) and pegylated interferon alpha-2b (3 μg/kg body weight 1×/week subcutaneously). 41 patients (74.5%) developed cutaneous side effects, mainly exanthems (51.2%), hand-foot syndrome (36.5%), alopecia (36.5%) and pruritus (24.4%). 10 cases required dose reductions, 10 cases required interruption of therapy and 1 patient required permanent discontinuation of therapy due to extensive follicular-cystic lesions [10c].

Interferon Beta [SEDA-33, 776; SEDA-36, 566]

Skin

- Severe septal panniculitis occurred in a multiple sclerosis patient treated with subcutaneous interferon beta-1b [11A].
- In a case report, eosinophilic cellulitis was linked to subcutaneous administration of interferon beta in a patient with malignant melanoma [12A].

Hematologic

- The occurrence of thrombotic microangiopathy has been linked to the use of interferon beta in multiple case reports. In December 2013, the Medicines and Healthcare Products Regulatory Agency (MHRA) issued a drug-safety update regarding a possible link between interferon beta and thrombotic microangiopathy [13c].
- In a case report, hemolytic uremic syndrome (HUS) was linked to interferon beta use in a multiple sclerosis patient [14A].

Immunologic

In a case report, anaphylactic IgE mediated reaction to interferon beta 1a was described in a multiple sclerosis patient [15A].

Urinary Tract

In a case report, malignant hypertension was linked to interferon beta use in a multiple sclerosis patient [16A].

INTERLEUKINS [SEDA-33, 777; SEDA-34, 771; SEDA-36, 567]

Anakinra (Interleukin-1 Receptor Antagonist) [SEDA-32, 677; SEDA-33, 779; SEDA-34, 582]

Skin

In a case report, a 56-year-old man with diffuse large B-cell lymphoma who was treated with anakinra had exacerbation of interstitial granulomatous dermatitis with arthritis (IGDA) [17A].

Liver

In a case report, a 20-year-old man with Adult-onset Still disease treated with anakinra developed subacute liver failure. Liver function test normalized 5 months after stopping the drug and treated with prednisolone taper [18A].

Hematologic

In a retrospective study, out of 29 patients with Schnitzler syndrome (SchS) treated with IL1Ra, 3 patients developed grade 3–4 neutropenia [19c].

Tumor Necrosis Factor Alfa (TNF-α) and Its Antagonists [SEDA-33, 779; SEDA-34, 583; SEDA-36, 568]

Skin

- In a retrospective study, 4.9% of alopecia was found to occur during exposure to TNF-α antagonist (18 involved infliximab, 17 adalimumab, 15 etanercept and 2 certolizumab) [20c].
- A retrospective study analyzing the association between administration of TNFα and development of malignant melanoma showed significant relative risk for adalimumab use (RR 1.8, $P = 0.02$) and etanercept use (RR 2.35, $P = 0.0004 < 0.001$) [21c].

Adalimumab [SED-15, 2015; SEDA-32, 709; SEDA-33, 818; SEDA-34, 618; SEDA-35, 703; SEDA-36, 568]

Psychiatric

In a case report, a 53-year-old man treated with adalimumab for severe psoriasis, committed suicide [22A].

Respiratory

- In a case report, a 62-year-old female with rheumatoid arthritis developed acute interstitial lung disease which was thought to be due to adalimumab use [23A].

- In a case report, a 57-year-old male with rheumatoid arthritis developed hemidiaphragm paresis and granulomatous pneumonitis which was thought to be due to adalimumab use [24A].

Nervous System

- In a case report, adalimumab use was linked with the development of progressive multifocal leukoencephalopathy (PML) [25A].
- In a case report, a 67-year-old male with rheumatoid arthritis treated with adalimumab for 3 months developed cerebral toxoplasmosis without any other risk factors [26A].

Urinary Tract

A case report described the development of renal cell carcinoma in a 57-year-old female with rheumatoid arthritis who was taking adalimumab for 4 years [27A].

Skin

- In a case report, a 37-year-old female with psoriasis developed dermatomyositis after being treated with adalimumab [28A].
- A case report described exacerbation of cutaneous lesion of sarcoidosis in a patient treated with adalimumab [29A].
- A case report described deterioration of vitiligo and development of halo naevi with recalcitrant ankylosing spondylitis in two patients receiving adalimumab [30A].

Infection Risk

In a randomized, investigator-blinded study comparing safety, efficacy and radiographic outcomes of subcutaneous abatacept versus adalimumab, in combination with methotrexate (MTX), in patients with rheumatoid arthritis for 2 years, two cases of tuberculosis occurred in the adalimumab group [31C].

Liver

In an observational study, cholestatic liver disease occurring after rituximab and adalimumab use showed possible involvement of cross-reacting antibodies to Fab2 fragments [32c].

Certolizumab [SED-15, 2402; SEDA-32, 710; SEDA-33, 819; SEDA-34, 622; SEDA-35, 704]

Eye

In a case report, a 64-year-old female with rheumatoid arthritis developed bilateral uveitis, suggestive of sarcoidosis after being treated with certolizumab [33A].

Respiratory

- A case report described the development of severe acute pneumonitis in a patient with rheumatoid arthritis after treatment with certolizumab [34A].
- A case report described the development of interstitial lung disease in a patient with rheumatoid arthritis after treatment with certolizumab [35A].

Etanercept [SED-15, 3148; SEDA-32, 712; SEDA-33, 820; SEDA-34, 626; SEDA-35, 705]

Observational Study

In a 5-year Food and Drug Administration-mandated surveillance registry of 2510 patients with psoriasis treated with etanercept, the 5-year cumulative incidence for serious adverse events was 22.2% (95% confidence interval [CI] 20.3–24.2%); 6.5% (95% CI 5.4–7.7%) for serious infectious events; 3.2% (95% CI 2.3–4.1%) for malignancies excluding non-melanoma skin cancer; 3.6% (95% CI 2.7–4.5%) for non-melanoma skin cancer; 2.8% (95% CI 2.0–3.6%) for coronary artery disease; 0.7% (95% CI 0.3–1.2%) for psoriasis worsening; 0.2% (95% CI 0.0–0.4%) for central nervous system demyelinating disorder; 0.1% (95% CI 0.0–0.3%) for lymphoma and for tuberculosis; and 0.1% (95% CI 0.0–0.2%) for opportunistic infection and for lupus [36c].

Endocrine

In a letter to an editor, it was mentioned that primary thyroid marginal zone B-cell lymphoma occurred in a patient with psoriasis and psoriatic arthritis using etanercept for 4 years [37r].

Renal

A case report described the occurrence of lupus nephritis in a 57-year-old female patient taking etanercept for psoriasis which resolved with discontinuation of etanercept [38A].

Skin

- A case report described the occurrence of a rare form of skin tumor, epithelioma cuniculatum, while undergoing etanercept treatment for psoriatic arthritis [39A].
- In a letter to the editor, a case of lichen striatus associated with etanercept treatment in a 70-year-old female with rheumatoid arthritis was mentioned [40r].
- A case report described the occurrence of systemic sarcoidosis in a 50-year-old patient with rheumatoid arthritis treated with etanercept who initially presented with erythematous lesions surrounding a scar on the posterior region of thigh and gluteal area, followed by the emergence of painful erythematous

nodules on lower limbs and an increase of volume on the neck [41A].

- A case report described occurrence of nodular fasciitis in an otherwise healthy man with plaque psoriasis who was undergoing treatment with etanercept [42A].

Respiratory

A case report described the occurrence of sarcoidosis and hypercalcemia precipitated by treatment with etanercept for 5 years in a 39-years-old female with severe rheumatoid arthritis [43A].

Nervous System

A case report described the occurrence of neurosarcoidosis in a 40-year-old female treated with etanercept for 7 years for rheumatoid arthritis [44A].

Urinary Tract

A case report described the occurrence of retroperitoneal fibrosis in two patients with rheumatoid arthritis while being treated with etanercept [45A].

Eye

A case report described the occurrence of sarcoidosis uveitis in a 54-year-old woman being treated with etanercept for rheumatoid arthritis. Her condition improved, but did not recover completely after etanercept was stopped. After starting her on adalimumab, the uveitis recovered completely [46A].

Infection Risk

- A case report described occurrence of esophageal and intestinal tuberculosis during treatment with etanercept in an 88-year-old female with rheumatoid arthritis [47A].
- A case report described occurrence of Salmonella septic arthritis of the pubic symphysis while taking etanercept that resolved with cessation of etanercept [48A].
- A case report described occurrence of herpes simplex virus type 1 (HSV-1) encephalitis in a patient receiving etanercept [49A].

Golimumab [SED-15, 3279; SEDA-32, 714; SEDA-33, 821; SEDA-34, 629; SEDA-35, 705]

Skin

A case report described the development of leukocytoclastic vasculitis in the lower extremities in a 37-year-old female with ankylosing spondylitis after treatment with golimumab [50A].

Infliximab [SEDA-32, 716; SEDA-33, 824; SEDA-34, 632; SEDA-35, 707]

Retrospective Study

In a retrospective study of 32 inflammatory bowel disease patients treated with infliximab, the most common adverse effects were anaphylaxis (6%), mild acute infusion reaction (6%), hypotension (6%), respiratory distress (6%), skin rash and eruptions (6%), hypertension (3%) and tightness in the chest (3%) [51c].

Gastrointestinal

A case report described the occurrence of free bowel perforation in a Crohn's disease patient after an initial dose of infliximab [52A].

Liver

- In a letter to an editor, a case of 39-year-old female with ankylosing spondylitis treated with infliximab was reported to develop autoimmune hepatitis after 4 months of treatment [53r].
- In a letter to an editor, 2 cases of fulminant hepatic failure needing a liver transplant were described after the initiation with infliximab treatment [54r].
- A case report described a case of hepatitis due to infliximab use in a patient with ulcerative colitis [55A].
- A case report described the development of autoimmune hepatitis and lupus-like syndrome when infliximab was used to treat chronic plaque psoriasis [56A]. Due to multiple occurrences of autoimmune hepatitis, clinicians should be cautious about this side effect.

Hematologic

- A case report described the occurrence of malignant lymphoma in a 62-year-old male treated with infliximab for Behcet's disease after 4 years of treatment [57A].
- A case report described the development of acute promyelocytic leukemia in a patient on infliximab treatment for refractory Crohn's disease [58A].

Nervous System

- A case report described the occurrence of aseptic meningitis after a few days of treatment with infliximab [59A].
- A case report described the development of subacute sensory polyradiculopathy 1 month after infliximab treatment for psoriasis vulgaris [60A].

Infection Risk

- A case report described the occurrence of peritoneal tuberculosis causing renal failure in a patient with rheumatoid arthritis and initial negative PPD after treatment with infliximab [61A].

- A case report described the development of visceral leishmaniasis with cutaneous symptoms in a 44-year-old male treated with infliximab for Crohn's disease [62A].
- In a letter to the editor, a case of *Rothia dentocariosa* bacteremia was described in an ulcerative colitis patient receiving infliximab [63r].
- A case report described two cases of herpes zoster in a Crohn's disease patient while using infliximab alone [64A].

Teratogenicity

A case report described the occurrence of collodion membrane in a 2-day-old newborn of a mother who was treated for severe psoriasis and psoriatic arthritis with a 7.5-mg/kg infusion of infliximab every 6 weeks throughout pregnancy, and for 6 months before conception [65A].

Respiratory

A case report described the development of interstitial lung disease in a 64-year-old male with psoriasis 3 weeks after the initiation of infliximab treatment [66A].

Skin

- A case report described the development of segmental vitiligo after 2 months of treatment with infliximab in a 46-year-old patient with rheumatoid arthritis [67A].
- A case report described the development of intensely pruritic rash in a patient who had anti-infliximab antibodies from previous two infusions with Crohn's disease after the subsequent infusion of infliximab [68A].
  - In a letter to the editor, a case of alopecia areata was reported in a patient receiving infliximab for Crohn's disease [69r].

MONOCLONAL ANTIBODIES

Abciximab [SEDA-35, 672]

Respiratory

A case report described a 75-year-old female who had acute ST elevation myocardial infarction and was treated with percutaneous coronary intervention with adjunctive abciximab and heparin. The patient developed alveolar hemorrhage which was attributed to abciximab use. The patient was treated with extracorporeal membranous oxygenation (ECMO) [70A].

Hematologic

Acute profound thrombocytopenia has been attributed to abciximab use in multiple case reports [71A,72A].

Adalimumab—See above

Alemtuzumab [SEDA-34, 586; SEDA-35, 672; SEDA-36, 569]

Endocrine

A drug safety evaluation of alemtuzumab from open label, Phase II and Phase III trials in multiple sclerosis showed that thyroid disorders are the most common form of autoimmune adverse events and overt Graves' disease accounts for about half of these cases [73R].

Infection Risk

- A case report described the development of norovirus-related chronic diarrhea in a 62-year-old patient treated with alemtuzumab for chronic lymphocytic leukemia [74A].
- A retrospective study of 208 patients treated with alemtuzumab for advanced B-cell chronic lymphocytic leukemia (CLL) and prolymphocytic leukemia (B-PLL) showed that the main adverse effects were CMV reactivation (20%) and a broad spectrum of infections [75c].
- A case report described the development of prostatic and renal aspergillosis in a patient treated with alemtuzumab for chronic lymphocytic leukaemia [76A].

Bevacizumab [SEDA-34, 587; SEDA-36, 570]

Prospective Study

In a prospective study of 26 patients with recurrent malignant gliomas (rMGs) treated with a combination of bevacizumab and fotemustine, bevacizumab-related adverse events included grade 3 venous thromboembolic event (8%), grade 2 epistaxis (4%), hypertension (8%), and gastrointestinal perforation (4%) [77c].

Phase 3 Trial

In an open-label randomized phase, 3 trial evaluating maintenance capecitabine and bevacizumab after initial treatment with bevacizumab and docetaxel in HER2-negative metastatic breast cancer patients, the most common grade 3 or worse events were hand-foot syndrome (28 [31%] in the bevacizumab and capecitabine group vs. none in the bevacizumab alone group) and hypertension (eight [9%] vs. three [3%]), and proteinuria (three [3%] vs. four [4%]) [78C].

Meta-Analysis

In a meta-analysis of five studies comparing bevacizumab combined with the chemotherapy (1798 patients) and chemotherapy alone (1810 patients) in the treatment of ovarian cancer, toxicity analysis showed that the enterobrosis, hypertension, albuminuria, neutrophils, thrombosis, and bleeding were significantly increased in the bevacizumab combined with chemotherapy group [79M].

Gastrointestinal

A meta-analysis of 26 833 patients from 33 randomized control trials showed that bevacizumab-containing therapy significantly increased the risk of developing all-grade (RR 3.35, 95% CI 2.35–4.79, $P < 0.001$) and fatal GI perforation (RR 3.08, 95% CI 1.04–9.08, $P = 0.042$). The subgroup analysis showed significantly increased risk of GI perforation with bevacizumab in colorectal cancer (RR 2.84, 95% CI 1.43–5.61, $P = 0.003$), gynecologic cancer (RR 3.37, 95% CI 1.71–6.62, $P < 0.001$) and prostate cancer (RR 6.01, 95% CI 1.78–20.28, $P = 0.004$) [80M]. Due to increased risk of developing GI perforation, clinicians should be cautious about this fatal side effect.

Cardiovascular

In a retrospective study of 34 patients with non-small lung cancer (NSCLC) treated with bevacizumab-containing chemotherapy, cardiovascular adverse events, including hypertension and bleeding events were observed in 18 patients (53%). The median overall survival was significantly better in patients who experienced adverse cardiovascular events than those who did not (442 versus 304 days; $P = 0.012$) [81c].

Urinary Tract

A case report described that a 57-year-old female with advanced breast cancer who was treated with bevacizumab developed thrombotic microangiopathy (TMA) accompanied with glomerular subendothelial deposition of IgA [82A].

Skin

In a case report, a 74-year-old male with glioblastoma multiforme treated with partial resection, radiation, temozolomide, and bevacizumab developed crusted hemorrhagic ulcers and purpuric patches on the lower legs soon after starting bevacizumab. Skin biopsy showed an occlusive pauci-inflammatory thrombogenic vasculopathy associated with ischemic epidermal and dermal changes and accompanied by extensive vascular C5b-9 (complement C5b-9 membrane attack complex) deposition [83A].

Nervous System

A case report described the occurrence of reversible posterior leukoencephalopathy syndrome in a 67-year-old woman who was treated with bevacizumab and m-FOLFOX6 for metastatic colorectal cancer [84A].

Respiratory

- A case report described the occurrence of pneumothorax in a 62-year-old female treated with bevacizumab and paclitaxel for breast cancer and lung metastasis. The pneumothorax was attributed to bevacizumab use [85A].
- In a retrospective study of 72 patients with advanced colorectal cancer treated with bevacizumab-based chemotherapy, it was noted that five patients (6.9%) developed interstitial pneumonia [86c].

Liver

A case report described the occurrence of portal vein thrombosis and nodular regenerative hyperplasia in a 69-year-old male with colon cancer treated with bevacizumab and oxaliplatin [87A].

Infection Risk

In a retrospective study, there was an association between streptococcus mitis/oralis endophthalmitis after intravitreal injection with bevacizumab prepared by a single compounding pharmacy [88c].

Skin

A case report described the occurrence of subacute cutaneous lupus erythematosus 6 weeks after two intravitreal injections of bevacizumab in a 63-year-old female with central serous choroidopathy [89A].

Eye

A case report indicated the occurrence of vascular congestion and subepithelial infiltrates in the peripheral cornea on day 2 following the first intravitrous bevacizumab injection in a 66-year-old man who presented with visual acuity loss due to cystic macular edema secondary to branch retinal vein occlusion [90A].

Cetuximab [SEDA-34, 590; SEDA-35, 673]

Meta-Analysis

A meta-analysis of the randomized controlled trials evaluating efficacy and toxicity of adding cetuximab to oxaliplatin-based or irinotecan-based chemotherapeutic regimens for the treatment of patients with mCRC with wild-type/mutated KRAS tumors showed that the occurrence of grade 3/4 adverse events, including skin toxicity, diarrhea, hypertension, anorexia, and mucositis/stomatitis, was slightly higher in the combined therapy group than in the chemotherapy-only group [91M].

Skin

- In an observational study of cetuximab use in metastatic colorectal cancer, clinically non-relevant skin toxicity was observed in 50% and clinically relevant in 50% of the patients. Grade 4 skin toxicity was documented in 1 patient [92c].

- In an observational study of 50 gastrointestinal cancer patients treated with cetuximab in combination with either FOLFIRI or FOLFOX, acneiform follicular skin exanthema occurred in more than 80% of patients. Severe exanthema (grade III/IV) developed in about 9–19% of patients with the necessity of cetuximab dose reduction or cessation [93c].

Gastrointestinal

A case report described the occurrence of esophageal ulcers in a 59-year-old man with metastatic rectal cancer after five cycles of treatment with cetuximab [94A].

Respiratory

A case report described the occurrence of interstitial lung disease in a patient with metastatic colorectal cancer within first 4 weeks of treatment with cetuximab that led to patient's death [95A].

Daclizumab [SEDA-34, 591; SEDA-35, 675; SEDA-36, 574]

Observational Study

In a retrospective study of 20 multiple sclerosis patients treated with daclizumab, 3 patients developed adverse events which were diffuse rash and alopecia, diffuse lymphadenopathy, and breast nodules [96c].

Natalizumab [SEDA-34, 593; SEDA-35, 676; SEDA-36, 578]

Pregnancy

In a case series, 12 women with 13 pregnancies and highly active multiple sclerosis who were treated with natalizumab during their third trimester of pregnancy, mild to moderate hematologic changes were noted in 10 of 13 infants including thrombocytopenia and anaemia [97c].

Hematologic

A case report described the occurrence of drug-induced thrombocytopenia in a 52-year-old woman treated with natalizumab for relapsing-remitting multiple sclerosis [98A].

Skin

A case report described the occurrence of eosinophilic fasciitis in a 40-year-old man treated with natalizumab for multiple sclerosis [99A].

Nervous System

- A case report described the occurrence of primary central nervous system lymphoma (PCNSL) after treatment with natalizumab [100A].
- In a letter to an editor, a case of a 45-year-old patient with relapsing-remitting multiple sclerosis who was treated with natalizumab developed progressive multifocal leukoencephalopathy starting in the brainstem which was attributed to natalizumab use [101r].
- Another case report also described the development of progressive multifocal leukoencephalopathy in a 55-year-old woman with relapsing-remitting multiple sclerosis while on natalizumab [102A].

Ranibizumab [SEDA-34, 762; SEDA-35, 877; SEDA-36, 580]

Eye

- A case report described the occurrence of marginal keratitis in a 56-year-old man who received intravitreal injection of ranibizumab for diffuse diabetic macular edema. It resolved with topical corticosteroids and antibiotics [103A].
- A case report described the occurrence of *Burkholderia cepacia* endophthalmitis 15 days after injection of ranibizumab for neovascular age-related macular degeneration [104A].

Rituximab [SEDA-34, 594; SEDA-35, 678; SEDA-36, 581]

Liver

In a prospective study of 260 Chinese patients diagnosed with hematologic malignancies and receiving rituximab-containing chemotherapy who had HBsAg-negative, anti-HBc-positive and undetectable serum HBV DNA (<10 IU/mL), the 2-year cumulative rate of HBV reactivation was 41.5%, at a median of 23 weeks (range, 4–100 weeks) after rituximab treatment [105c].

Skin

A case report described the occurrence of psoriatic lesions in a 69-year-old patient with rheumatoid arthritis on her trunk and arms, 3 months after the second course of rituximab [106A].

Cardiovascular

- A case report described 2 cases of patients with stage IV non-Hodgkin lymphoma who experienced cardiovascular accidents temporally related to rituximab infusion (one with atrial fibrillation and the other one had chest pain with fever and chills) [107A].

- A case report described the occurrence of myocardial infarction in a 52-year-old man, without cardiovascular risk factors, who was treated for seronegative myasthenia with rituximab infusions [108A].
- A case report described occurrence of fulminant myocarditis due to enterovirus in a 7-year-old boy with high-degree steroid-dependent idiopathic nephrotic syndrome who was treated with rituximab [109A].

Tocilizumab [SEDA-35, 668; SEDA-36, 582]

Hematologic

In a case series of 8 patients with severe and refractory non-infectious uveitis treated with tocilizumab, side effects noted were grade 1 leukopenia ($n=1$), thrombocytopenia ($n=1$) and bronchitis ($n=1$) [110c].

Trastuzumab [SEDA-34, 595; SEDA-35, 680; SEDA-36, 582]

Cardiovascular

In a cohort study of 2046 early breast cancer patients treated with trastuzumab, 53 (2.6%) experienced at least one hospitalization for a cardiac event, and there were two cardiac deaths [111c].

References

[1] Rostaing L, Sanchez-Fructuoso A, Franco A, et al. Conversion to tacrolimus once-daily from cyclosporin in stable kidney transplant recipients: a multicenter study. Transpl Int. 2012;25(4):391–400 [C].

[2] Nandyala SV, Marquez-Lara A, Fineberg SJ, et al. Prospective, randomized, controlled trial of silicate-substituted calcium phosphate versus rhBMP-2 in a minimally invasive transforaminal lumbar interbody fusion. Spine. 2014;39(3):185–91 [C].

[3] Akilov OE, Desai N, Jaffe R, et al. Bullous Sweet's syndrome after granulocyte colony-stimulating factor therapy in a child with congenital neutropenia. Pediatr Dermatol. 2014;31(2):e61–2 [A].

[4] Kilic SC, Alaygut D, Unal E, et al. Acute colchicine intoxication complicated with extramedullary hematopoiesis due to filgrastim in a child. J Pediatr Hematol Oncol. 2014;36(7):e460–2 [A].

[5] Bondarenko I, Gladkov OA, Elsaesser R, et al. Efficacy and safety of lipegfilgrastim versus pegfilgrastim: a randomized, multicenter, active-control phase 3 trial in patients with breast cancer receiving doxorubicin/docetaxel chemotherapy. BMC Cancer. 2013;13:386 [C].

[6] Duval C, Boucher S, Moulin JC, et al. Fatal stimulation of acute myeloid leukemia blasts by pegfilgrastim. Anticancer Res. 2014;34(11):6747–8 [A].

[7] Kozielewicz D, Zalesna A, Dybowska D. Can pegylated interferon alpha 2a cause development of thyroid disorders in patients with chronic hepatitis B? Expert Opin Drug Saf. 2014;13(8):1009–14 [c].

[8] de Escalona Munoz E, Rojas JE, Garcia Serrano JL, et al. Application of interferon alpha 2b in conjunctival intraepithelial neoplasia: predictors and prognostic factors. J Ocul Pharmacol Ther. 2014;30(6):489–94 [c].

[9] Koktekir BE, Sumer S, Bakbak B, et al. Ocular effects of pegylated interferon-alpha in patients with chronic hepatitis B. Cutan Ocul Toxicol. 2013;32(4):275–8 [c].

[10] Degen A, Weichenthal M, Ugurel S, et al. Cutaneous side effects of combined therapy with sorafenib and pegylated interferon alpha-2b in metastatic melanoma (phase II DeCOG trial). J Dtsch Dermatol Ges. 2013;11(9):846–53 [c].

[11] Mazzon E, Guarneri C, Giacoppo S, et al. Severe septal panniculitis in a multiple sclerosis patient treated with interferon-beta. Int J Immunopathol Pharmacol. 2014;27(4):669–74 [A].

[12] Kambayashi Y, Fujimura T, Ishibashi M, et al. Eosinophilic cellulitis induced by subcutaneous administration of interferon-beta. Acta Derm Venereol. 2013;93(6):755–6 [A].

[13] Hunt D, Kavanagh D, Drummond I, et al. Thrombotic microangiopathy associated with interferon beta. N Engl J Med. 2014;370(13):1270–1 [S].

[14] Nerrant E, Charif M, Ramay AS, et al. Hemolytic uremic syndrome: an unusual complication of interferon-beta treatment in a MS patient. J Neurol. 2013;260(7):1915–6 [A].

[15] Cortellini G, Amadori A, Comandini T, et al. Interferon beta 1a anaphylaxis, a case report. Standardization of non-irritating concentration for allergy skin tests. Eur Ann Allergy Clin Immunol. 2013;45(5):181–2 [A].

[16] Rubin S, Lacraz A, Galantine V, et al. Malignant hypertension and interferon-beta: a case report. J Hum Hypertens. 2014;28(5):340–1 [A].

[17] Michailidou D, Voulgarelis M, Pikazis D. Exacerbation of interstitial granulomatous dermatitis with arthritis by anakinra in a patient with diffuse large B-cell lymphoma. Clin Exp Rheumatol. 2014;32(2):259–61 [A].

[18] Aly L, Iking-Konert C, Quaas A, et al. Subacute liver failure following anakinra treatment for adult-onset Still disease. J Rheumatol. 2013;40(10):1775–7 [A].

[19] Neel A, Henry B, Barbarot S, et al. Long-term effectiveness and safety of interleukin-1 receptor antagonist (anakinra) in Schnitzler's syndrome: a French multicenter study. Autoimmun Rev. 2014;13(10):1035–41 [c].

[20] Bene J, Moulis G, Auffret M, et al. Alopecia induced by tumour necrosis factor-alpha antagonists: description of 52 cases and disproportionality analysis in a nationwide pharmacovigilance database. Rheumatology (Oxford). 2014;53(8):1465–9 [c].

[21] Nardone B, Hammel JA, Raisch DW, et al. Melanoma associated with tumour necrosis factor-alpha inhibitors: a Research on Adverse Drug events And Reports (RADAR) project. Br J Dermatol. 2014;170(5):1170–2 [c].

[22] Ellard R, Ahmed A, Shah R, et al. Suicide and depression in a patient with psoriasis receiving adalimumab: the role of the dermatologist. Clin Exp Dermatol. 2014;39(5):624–7 [A].

[23] Dias OM, Pereira DA, Baldi BG, et al. Adalimumab-induced acute interstitial lung disease in a patient with rheumatoid arthritis. J Bras Pneumol. 2014;40(1):77–81 [A] por.

[24] Abdallah T, Abdallah M, Saifan C, et al. Hemidiaphragm paresis and granulomatous pneumonitis associated with adalimumab: a case report. Heart Lung. 2014;43(1):84–6 [A].

[25] Ray M, Curtis JR, Baddley JW. A case report of progressive multifocal leucoencephalopathy (PML) associated with adalimumab. Ann Rheum Dis. 2014;73(7):1429–30 [A].

[26] Nardone R, Zuccoli G, Brigo F, et al. Cerebral toxoplasmosis following adalimumab treatment in rheumatoid arthritis. Rheumatology (Oxford). 2014;53(2):284 [A].

[27] Kobak S, Karaarslan A, Aktakka Y. Renal cell carcinoma in a patient with rheumatoid arthritis treated with adalimumab. Curr Drug Saf. 2014;9(1):69–72 [A].

[28] Dicaro D, Bowen C, Dalton SR. Dermatomyositis associated with anti-tumor necrosis factor therapy in a patient with psoriasis. J Am Acad Dermatol. 2014;70(3):e64–5 [A].

[29] Santos G, Sousa LE, Joao AM. Exacerbation of recalcitrant cutaneous sarcoidosis with adalimumab—a paradoxical effect? A case report. An Bras Dermatol. 2013;88(6 Suppl 1):26–8 [A].

[30] Maruthappu T, Leandro M, Morris SD. Deterioration of vitiligo and new onset of halo naevi observed in two patients receiving adalimumab. Dermatol Ther. 2013;26(4):370–2. PubMed PMID: 23914896. Epub 2013/08/07.eng [A].

[31] Schiff M, Weinblatt ME, Valente R, et al. Head-to-head comparison of subcutaneous abatacept versus adalimumab for rheumatoid arthritis: two-year efficacy and safety findings from AMPLE trial. Ann Rheum Dis. 2014;73(1):86–94 [C].

[32] Latus J, Klein R, Koetter I, et al. Cholestatic liver disease after rituximab and adalimumab and the possible role of cross-reacting antibodies to Fab 2 fragments. PLoS One. 2013;8(11): e78856 [c].

[33] Moisseiev ESS. Certolizumab-induced uveitis: a case report and review of the literature. Case Rep Ophthalmol. 2014;5(1):54–9 [A].

[34] Lager J, Hilberg O, Lokke A, et al. Severe interstitial lung disease following treatment with certolizumab pegol: a case report. Eur Respir Rev. 2013;22(129):414–6 [A].

[35] Glaspole IN, Hoy RF, Ryan PF. A case of certolizumab-induced interstitial lung disease in a patient with rheumatoid arthritis. Rheumatology (Oxford). 2013;52(12):2302–4 [A].

[36] Kimball AB, Rothman KJ, Kricorian G, et al. OBSERVE-5: observational postmarketing safety surveillance registry of etanercept for the treatment of psoriasis final 5-year results. J Am Acad Dermatol. 2015;72(1):115–22 [c].

[37] Jin H, Cho HH, Kim WJ, et al. Primary thyroid marginal zone B-cell lymphoma in a patient with psoriatic arthritis treated with etanercept. J Am Acad Dermatol. 2014;71(4):e152–3 [r].

[38] Yahya TM, Dhanyamraju S, Harrington TM, et al. Spontaneous resolution of lupus nephritis following withdrawal of etanercept. Ann Clin Lab Sci. 2013;43(4):447–9 [A].

[39] Tchernev G, Guarneri C, Bevelacqua V, et al. Carcinoma cuniculatum in course of etanercept: blocking autoimmunity but propagation of carcinogenesis? Int J Immunopathol Pharmacol. 2014;27(2):261–6 [A].

[40] Lora V, Kanitakis J, Latini A, et al. Lichen striatus associated with etanercept treatment of rheumatoid arthritis. J Am Acad Dermatol. 2014;70(4):e90–2 [r].

[41] Unterstell N, Bressan AL, Serpa LA, et al. Systemic sarcoidosis induced by etanercept: first Brazilian case report. An Bras Dermatol. 2013;88(6 Suppl 1):197–9 [A].

[42] Vine K, Dacko A, Weinberg JM. Nodular fasciitis: a possible side effect of etanercept? Cutis. 2013;92(4):199–202 [A].

[43] Watrin A, Royer M, Legrand E, et al. Severe hypercalcemia revealing sarcoidosis precipitated by etanercept. Rev Mal Respir. 2014;31(3):255–8. Hypercalcemie majeure revelatrice d'une sarcoidose induite par etanercept. fre [A].

[44] Durel CA, Feurer E, Pialat JB, et al. Etanercept may induce neurosarcoidosis in a patient treated for rheumatoid arthritis. BMC Neurol. 2013;13:212 [A].

[45] Couderc M, Mathieu S, Dubost JJ, et al. Retroperitoneal fibrosis during etanercept therapy for rheumatoid arthritis. J Rheumatol. 2013;40(11):1931–3 [A].

[46] Dragnev D, Barr D, Kulshrestha M, et al. Sarcoid panuveitis associated with etanercept treatment, resolving with adalimumab. BMJ Case Rep. 2013;2013: [A].

[47] Anazawa R, Suzuki M, Miwa H, et al. A case of esophageal and intestinal tuberculosis that occurred during treatment of rheumatoid arthritis with etanercept. Kekkaku. 2014;89(8):711–6 [A].

[48] Sky K, Arroyo RA, Collamer AN. Salmonella septic arthritis in a patient receiving etanercept: case report and review of the literature. Mil Med. 2013;178(12):e1384–7 [A].

[49] Crusio RH, Singson SV, Haroun F, et al. Herpes simplex virus encephalitis during treatment with etanercept. Scand J Infect Dis. 2014;46(2):152–4 [A].

[50] Pamies A, Castro S, Poveda MJ, et al. Leucocytoclastic vasculitis associated with golimumab. Rheumatology (Oxford). 2013;52(10):1921–3 [c].

[51] Uyanikoglu A, Ermis F, Akyuz F, et al. Infliximab in inflammatory bowel disease: attention to adverse events. Eur Rev Med Pharmacol Sci. 2014;18(16):2337–42 [c].

[52] Lim CS, Moon W, Park SJ, et al. A rare case of free bowel perforation associated with infliximab treatment for structuring Crohn's disease. Korean J Gastroenterol. 2013;62(3):169–73 [A].

[53] Yilmaz B, Roach EC, Koklu S. Infliximab leading to autoimmune hepatitis: an increasingly recognized side effect. Dig Dis Sci. 2014;59(10):2602–3 [r].

[54] Rowe BW, Gala-Lopez B, Tomlinson C, et al. Fulminant hepatic failure necessitating transplantation following the initiation of infliximab therapy: a cautionary tale times two. Transpl Int. 2013;26(12):e110–2 [r].

[55] Colina F, Molero A, Casis B, et al. Infliximab-related hepatitis: a case study and literature review. Dig Dis Sci. 2013;58(11):3362–7 [A].

[56] Dang LJ, Lubel JS, Gunatheesan S, et al. Drug-induced lupus and autoimmune hepatitis secondary to infliximab for psoriasis. Australas J Dermatol. 2014;55(1):75–9 [A].

[57] Sonoda KH, Fukuhara T, Yoshikawa H, et al. A case report of malignant lymphoma receiving infliximab therapy with Behcet's disease. Nippon Ganka Gakkai Zasshi. 2014;118(5):440–5 [A].

[58] Mohammad F, Vivekanandarajah A, Haddad H, et al. Acute promyelocytic leukaemia (APL) in a patient with Crohn's disease and exposure to infliximab: a rare clinical presentation and review of the literature. BMJ Case Rep. 2014;2014 [A].

[59] Shah R, Shah M, Bansal N, et al. Infliximab-induced aseptic meningitis. Am J Emerg Med. 2014;32(12):1560.e3–1560.e4 [A].

[60] Naruse H, Nagashima Y, Maekawa R, et al. Successful treatment of infliximab-associated immune-mediated sensory polyradiculopathy with intravenous immunoglobulin. J Clin Neurosci. 2013;20(11):1618–9 [A].

[61] Sharma A, Dubey D, Janga K, et al. A case of peritoneal TB causing renal failure in a patient with rheumatoid arthritis and initial negative PPD after treatment with infliximab. Ren Fail. 2014;36(6):948–50 [A].

[62] Juzlova K, Votrubova J, Kacerovska D, et al. Visceral leishmaniasis with cutaneous symptoms in a patient treated with infliximab followed by fatal consequences. Dermatol Ther. 2014;27(3):131–4 [A].

[63] Yeung DF, Parsa A, Wong JC, et al. A case of Rothia dentocariosa bacteremia in a patient receiving infliximab for ulcerative colitis. Am J Gastroenterol. 2014;109(2):297–8 [r].

[64] Wang X, Zhao J, Zhu S, et al. Herpes zoster in Crohn's disease during treatment with infliximab. Eur J Gastroenterol Hepatol. 2014;26(2):237–9 [A].

[65] Offiah M, Brodell RT, Campbell LR, et al. Collodion-like membrane in a newborn exposed to infliximab. J Am Acad Dermatol. 2014;71(1):e22–3 [A].

[66] Kakavas S, Balis E, Lazarou V, et al. Respiratory failure due to infliximab induced interstitial lung disease. Heart Lung. 2013;42(6):480–2 [A].

[67] Carvalho CL, Ortigosa LC. Segmental vitiligo after infliximab use for rheumatoid arthritis—a case report. An Bras Dermatol. 2014;89(1):154–6 [A].

[68] Ladizinski B, Lee KC. Infliximab-induced urticaria. J Emerg Med. 2014;46(5):691–2 [A].

[69] Ormaechea-Perez N, Lopez-Pestana A, Munagorri-Santos AI, et al. Alopecia areata in a patient receiving infliximab. Indian J Dermatol Venereol Leprol. 2013;79(4):529–31 [r].

[70] Choi AW, Blair JE, Flaherty JD. Abciximab-induced alveolar hemorrhage treated with rescue extracorporeal membranous oxygenation. Catheter Cardiovasc Interv. 2015;85(5):828–31 [A].

[71] Park S, Lee J, Lee SY, et al. Acute profound thrombocytopenia after using abciximab for no-reflow during primary percutaneous coronary intervention for ST-segment elevation myocardial infarction. Korean Circ J. 2013;43(8):557–60 [A].

[72] Daley B, Miranda D, Kalra A, et al. Profound thrombocytopenia caused by abciximab infusion following. Minn Med. 2014;97(10):48–9 [A].

[73] Willis M, Robertson NP. Drug safety evaluation of alemtuzumab for multiple sclerosis. Expert Opin Drug Saf. 2014;13(8):1115–24 [R].

[74] Ronchetti AMHB, Ambert-Balay K, Pothier P, et al. Norovirus-related chronic diarrhea in a patient treated with alemtuzumab for chronic lymphocytic leukemia. BMC Infect Dis. 2014;14:239 [A].

[75] Fiegl M, Stauder R, Steurer M, et al. Alemtuzumab in chronic lymphocytic leukemia: final results of a large observational multicenter study in mostly pretreated patients. Ann Hematol. 2014;93(2):267–77 [c].

[76] Roux C, Thyss A, Gari-Toussaint M. Prostatic and renal aspergillosis due to Aspergillus fumigatus in a patient receiving alemtuzumab for chronic lymphocytic leukaemia. J Mycol Med. 2013;23(4):270–3 [A].

[77] Vaccaro V, Fabi A, Vidiri A, et al. Activity and safety of bevacizumab plus fotemustine for recurrent malignant gliomas. BioMed Res Int. 2014;2014:351252 [c].

[78] Gligorov J, Doval D, Bines J, et al. Maintenance capecitabine and bevacizumab versus bevacizumab alone after initial first-line bevacizumab and docetaxel for patients with HER2-negative metastatic breast cancer (IMELDA): a randomised, open-label, phase 3 trial. Lancet Oncol. 2014;15(12):1351–60 [C].

[79] Wang TS, Lei W, Cui W, et al. A meta-analysis of bevacizumab combined with chemotherapy in the treatment of ovarian cancer. Indian J Cancer. 2014;51(Suppl 3):e95–8 [M].

[80] Qi WX, Shen Z, Tang LN, et al. Bevacizumab increases the risk of gastrointestinal perforation in cancer patients: a meta-analysis with a focus on different subgroups. Eur J Clin Pharmacol. 2014;70(8):893–906 [M].

[81] Koyama N. Adverse cardiovascular events predict survival benefit in non-small lung cancer patients treated with bevacizumab. Cancer Biomark. 2014;14(4):259–65 [c].

[82] Tomita M, Ochiai M, Shu S, et al. A case of thrombotic microangiopathy with glomerular subendothelial IgA deposition due to bevacizumab. Nihon Jinzo Gakkai Shi. 2014;56(5):612–7 [A].

[83] Kiuru M, Schwartz M, Magro C. Cutaneous thrombogenic vasculopathy associated with bevacizumab therapy. Dermatol Online J. 2014;20(6) [A].

[84] Miyamoto S. Bevacizumab-induced reversible posterior leukoencephalopathy syndrome in a patient with metastatic colorectal cancer. Nihon Shokakibyo Gakkai Zasshi. 2014;111(4):743–7 [A].

[85] Makino T, Kudo S, Ogata T. Pneumothorax after treatment with bevacizumab-containing chemotherapy for breast cancer—a case report. Gan To Kagaku Ryoho. 2014;4(2):233–5 [A].

[86] Tamura S, Kusaba H, Kubo N, et al. Interstitial pneumonia during bevacizumab-based chemotherapy for colorectal cancer. Med Oncol. 2014;31(3):856 [c].

[87] Fluxa CD, Salas MS, Regonesi MC, et al. Portal vein thrombosis and nodular regenerative hyperplasia associated with the use of bevacizumab and oxaliplatin. Report of one case. Rev Med Chil. 2013;141(10):1344–8 [A].

[88] Matthews JL, Dubovy SR, Goldberg RA, et al. Histopathology of streptococcus mitis/oralis endophthalmitis after intravitreal injection with bevacizumab: a report of 7 patients. Ophthalmology. 2014;121(3):702–8 [c].

[89] Cleaver N, Ramirez J, Gildenberg S. Cutaneous lupus erythematosus in a patient undergoing intravitreal bevacizumab injections: case report and review of the literature. J Drugs Dermatol. 2013;12(9):1052–5 [A].

[90] Yamato F, Imai D, Mori K, et al. Corneal subepithelial infiltrates that developed following intravitreous injection of bevacizumab. Nippon Ganka Gakkai Zasshi. 2013;117(7):558–60 [A].

[91] Lv ZC, Ning JY, Chen HB. Efficacy and toxicity of adding cetuximab to chemotherapy in the treatment of metastatic colorectal cancer: a meta-analysis from 12 randomized controlled trials. Tumour Biol. 2014;35(12):11741–50 [M].

[92] Cvetanovic A, Vrbic S, Filipovic S, et al. Clinical benefit of cetuximab and prognostic value of cetuximab-related skin toxicity in metastatic colorectal cancer: a single institution analysis. J BUON. 2014;19(1):83–90 [c].

[93] Wehler TC, Graf C, Mohler M, et al. Cetuximab-induced skin exanthema: prophylactic and reactive skin therapy are equally effective. J Cancer Res Clin Oncol. 2013;139(10):1667–72 PubMed PMID: 23918349 [c].

[94] Babacan T, Turkbeyler IH, Dag MS, et al. Cetuximab-induced esophageal ulcer: the first report in literature. Libyan J Med. 2014;9:23723 [A].

[95] Shablak A, Conn A. A case of fatal cetuximab-induced interstitial lung disease during the first weeks of treatment. Target Oncol. 2014;9(2):177–80 [A].

[96] Oh J, Saidha S, Cortese I, et al. Daclizumab-induced adverse events in multiple organ systems in multiple sclerosis. Neurology. 2014;82(11):984–8 [c].

[97] Haghikia A, Langer-Gould A, Rellensmann G, et al. Natalizumab use during the third trimester of pregnancy. JAMA Neurol. 2014;71(7):891–5 [c].

[98] Cachia D, Izzy S, Berriosmorales I, et al. Drug-induced thrombocytopenia secondary to natalizumab treatment. BMJ Case Rep. 2014;2014 [A].

[99] Bujold J, Boivin C, Amin M, et al. Eosinophilic fasciitis occurring under treatment with natalizumab for multiple sclerosis. J Cutan Med Surg. 2014;18(1):69–71 [A].

[100] Na A, Hall N, Kavar B, et al. Central nervous system lymphoma associated with natalizumab. J Clin Neurosci. 2014;21(6):1068–70 [A].

[101] Havla J, Hohlfeld R, Kumpfel T. Unusual natalizumab-associated progressive multifocal leukoencephalopathy starting in the brainstem. J Neurol. 2014;261(1):232–4 [r].

[102] Thaker AA, Schmitt SE, Pollard JR, et al. Natalizumab-induced progressive multifocal leukoencephalopathy. Clin Nucl Med. 2014;39(7):e365–6 [A].

[103] Aslan Bayhan S, Bayhan HA, Adam M, et al. Marginal keratitis after intravitreal injection of ranibizumab. Cornea. 2014;33(11):1238–9 [A].

[104] Saffra N, Moriarty E. Burkholderia cepacia endophthalmitis, in a penicillin allergic patient, following a ranibizumab injection. BMJ Case Rep. 2014;2014 [A].

[105] Seto WK, Chan TS, Hwang YY, et al. Hepatitis B reactivation in patients with previous hepatitis B virus exposure undergoing rituximab-containing chemotherapy for lymphoma: a prospective study. J Clin Oncol. 2014;32(33):3736–43 [c].

[106] Guidelli GM, Fioravanti A, Rubegni P, et al. Induced psoriasis after rituximab therapy for rheumatoid arthritis: a case report and review of the literature. Rheumatol Int. 2013;33(11):2927–30 [A].

[107] Passalia C, Minetto P, Arboscello E, et al. Cardiovascular adverse events complicating the administration of rituximab: report of two cases. Tumori. 2013;99(6):288e–92e [A].

[108] Renard D, Cornillet L, Castelnovo G. Myocardial infarction after rituximab infusion. Neuromuscul Disord. 2013;23(7):599–601 [A].

[109] Sellier-Leclerc AL, Belli E, Guerin V, et al. Fulminant viral myocarditis after rituximab therapy in pediatric nephrotic syndrome. Pediatr Nephrol. 2013;28(9):1875–9 [A].

[110] Papo M, Bielefeld P, Vallet H, et al. Tocilizumab in severe and refractory non-infectious uveitis. Clin Exp Rheumatol. 2014;32 (4 Suppl 84):S75–9 [c].

[111] Bonifazi M, Franchi M, Rossi M, et al. Trastuzumab-related cardiotoxicity in early breast cancer: a cohort study. Oncologist. 2013;18(7):795–801 [c].

37

Drugs that Act on the Immune System: Immunosuppressive and Immunostimulatory Drugs

Calvin J. Meaney[1]

Department of Pharmacy Practice, School of Pharmacy and Pharmaceutical Sciences, State University of
New York at Buffalo, Buffalo, NY, USA
[1]Corresponding author: cjmeaney@buffalo.edu

BELATACEPT [SEDA 34–609]

Belatacept is a first in class biologic immunosuppressive drug that inhibits co-stimulation of T cells and is used in the prevention of renal transplant rejection. A systematic review of available randomized controlled trial evidence revealed similar efficacy of belatacept compared to calcineurin inhibitor therapy [1M]. There was less allograft nephropathy, hypertension, hyperlipidemia, and new onset diabetes mellitus with belatacept compared to calcineurin inhibitor controls. However, incidence of post-transplant lymphoproliferative disorder (PTLD) was 0–4% in randomized controlled trials and has prompted additional investigation [2R]. The risk appeared highest in Epstein Barr Virus negative patients and with more intensive belatacept dosing [3C]. Recent data indicate that incidence of PTLD is similar between belatacept and calcineurin inhibitor regimens [1M]. As clinical experience with belatacept increases, additional information regarding rare but serious adverse effects and drug interactions will be revealed.

Successful use of belatacept in pediatric transplantation was reported in a patient with microangiopathic hemolytic anemia secondary to calcineurin inhibitors [4A]. Belatacept was investigated for use following liver transplantation but was associated with poor efficacy compared to calcineurin inhibitors [5C]. Two cases of PTLD and one case of progressive multifocal leukoencephalopathy occurred in belatacept treated patients. However, belatacept used as bridging therapy in seven liver transplant recipients with perioperative renal dysfunction demonstrated acceptable efficacy without significant toxicity [6c].

Comparative Studies

A patient-reported outcomes sub-study of two large, randomized, controlled, clinical trials followed 1209 patients for the first 3-years post-renal transplant [7C]. Compared to cyclosporine, belatacept treatment was associated with improved health-related quality of life (HRQoL) and a lower total number of side effects at each time point assessed. The improvement in HRQoL observed for belatacept treatment was likely the result of better renal function in this group.

The BENEFIT-EXT was a randomized controlled phase III trial comparing belatacept to cyclosporine for immunosuppression following renal transplant [8C]. In a 3-year follow-up of 323 patients, belatacept treated patients had improved renal function (11 ml/min increase in glomerular filtration rate) but more PTLD and tuberculosis than cyclosporine treated patients.

Infection Risk

In a single-center, prospective study, monitoring of viral replication in 42 renal transplant recipients receiving belatacept revealed that Epstein Barr virus replication occurred more frequently than in 20 cyclosporine treated patients [9c]. Replication of other viruses (JC, BK, and cytomegalovirus) was similar between the two treatments.

ISSN: 0378-6080
http://dx.doi.org/10.1016/bs.seda.2015.06.015
© 2015 Elsevier B.V. All rights reserved.

CYCLOPHOSPHAMIDE [SED-15, 1025; SEDA-34, 612; SEDA-35, 700; SEDA-36, 592]

Observational Studies

In a single center, retrospective study, 419 Chinese patients with systemic auto-immune diseases were assessed for adverse effects of cyclophosphamide treatment [10c]. Occurrence of adverse effects was: gastrointestinal (GI) discomfort 21.5%, alopecia 12.4%, myelosuppression 7.4%, abnormal liver function 3.1%, and menstrual disturbance 30.3%. Alopecia, GI discomfort, and myelosuppression were more likely in females and with intravenous (IV) administration. Hemorrhagic cystitis did not occur in this trial which could be a result of adequate hydration pre-treatment or possibly a racial difference in this adverse effect manifestation.

A pharmacogenetic analysis of a phase 3 trial investigated the impact of *CYP2B6* polymorphisms on treatment response and adverse effects of fludarabine-cyclophosphamide (FC) in 428 patients with chronic lymphocytic leukemia [11c]. The *CYP2B6*6* variant allele is associated with reduced mRNA and protein expression, which may impact the enzymatic activation of the prodrug cyclophosphamide to active metabolite, 4-hydroxycyclophosphamide. The *CYP2B6*6* allele was associated with less cumulative adverse effects (a collection of 10 categories; $P = 0.002$) compared to *1/*1 carriers after treatment with FC.

A prospective observational study compared short-interval lower-dose cyclophosphamide to conventional dosing in lupus nephritis patients [12c]. Menstrual disturbances, GI adverse effects, and leukopenia occurred significantly less in the short-interval lower-dose group, suggesting a dose dependency to these side effects in this population.

Comparative Studies

In a randomized clinical trial, autologous hematopoietic stem cell transplantation was compared to cyclophosphamide for the treatment of diffuse cutaneous systemic sclerosis [13c]. Grade 3 or 4 adverse events which were severe or life-threatening occurred in 30/77 (37%) patients on cyclophosphamide compared to 51/79 (63%) patients that underwent transplantation ($P = 0.002$).

Cardiovascular

Cyclophosphamide was suspected to be the cause of cardiotoxicity in a 66-year-old female receiving treatment for lymphoma [14A].

Central Nervous System

A 33-year-old female with lupus nephritis being treated with cyclophosphamide developed posterior reversible encephalopathy syndrome (PRES) [15A]. Following the second cyclophosphamide dose of 500 mg, the patient experienced repeated generalized tonic clonic seizures and MRI confirmed PRES.

Electrolyte Balance

Elazzazy and colleagues reported a 43-year-old female with breast cancer that developed symptomatic hyponatremia with serum sodium 112 mEq/l following treatment with cyclophosphamide 600 mg/m^2 [16A]. Serum sodium persistently declined following cyclophosphamide administration during each cycle of chemotherapy. The patient was also receiving chlorthalidone which may have contributed to the severity of hyponatremia.

Hematologic

A prospective pharmacogenomic study evaluated the effect of multiple cytochrome P450 enzyme polymorphisms on the myelotoxicity of cyclophosphamide treatment in 234 breast cancer patients [17c]. Myelosuppression, categorized as any hematologic grade 2–4 toxicity, exhibited no association to 8 individual polymorphisms. The CYP2C8*3 (rs1057910)-CYP2C9*2 (rs1799853)-CYP2C9*3 (rs1057910)-CYP2C19*2 (rs4244285) haplotype on chromosome 10 had an association between the G-*1-*3-G haplotype and overall myelosuppresion ($P = 0.024$) and grade 2–4 leukopenia ($P = 0.03$).

Liver

A case report described a 48-year-old male that developed acute hepatic failure within 24 hours of receiving 200 mg IV cyclophosphamide [18A]. Alanine transaminase (ALT) peaked at 568 U/L from a baseline of 27 U/L following the first dose, and resolved to 104 U/L after 2 weeks. A second dose of 200 mg cyclophosphamide was administered at this time and a similar hepatotoxic reaction occurred with ALT peaking at 1253 U/L within 48 hours.

Immunologic

Late-onset anaphylactic reaction occurred following IV cyclophosphamide treatment in a 46-year-old female with scleroderma lupus overlap syndrome [19A]. The onset of reaction became quicker and severity of symptoms worsened with each subsequent dose. This reaction is believed to be a response to cyclophosphamide metabolites.

SPECIAL REVIEWS - CYCLOSPORINE (CICLOSPORIN) *[SED-15, 743; SEDA-34, 609; SEDA-35, 699; SEDA-36, 591]*

Cardiovascular

The mechanisms underpinning the hypertensive effect of cyclosporine were reviewed with comparison to other immunosuppressive drugs [20R].

In a cardiovascular risk sub-study to a prospective, open-label, single center, controlled trial, 119 stable renal transplant recipients were randomized to late withdrawal of the calcineurin inhibitor ($n = 81$ on cyclosporine) or mycophenolate mofetil [21c]. Late withdrawal from a calcineurin inhibitor significantly reduced ambulatory blood pressure but did not change carotid intima thickness. Cardiovascular outcomes were not measured. Acute rejection rates were low in both groups. Cyclosporine-induced hypercholesterolemia was noted in 47.2% of ulcerative colitis patients [22c]. Successful treatment of cyclosporine-induced thrombotic microangiopathy and thrombocytopenia-associated multiple organ failure with therapeutic plasma exchange was described in a 13-year-old [23A].

Nervous System

A case report describes an 18-year-old female treated with cyclosporine and voriconazole following stem cell transplantation that developed leukoencephalopathy likely due to voriconazole-mediated inhibition of cyclosporine metabolism [24A].

Endocrine

The diabetogenic effects of cyclosporine and tacrolimus were investigated in an *in vitro* study of human adipocytes [25E]. Glucose transporter 4 (GLUT4) endocytosis was increased thereby impairing glucose uptake which offers a novel mechanism for cyclosporine- and tacrolimus-induced diabetes. New onset diabetes after transplantation was more frequent among tacrolimus treated kidney transplant recipients (26%) compared to cyclosporine counterparts (14%, $P = 0.0002$) [26c]. A 48-year-old male patient developed painful gynecomastia following cyclosporine administration for focal segmental glomerulosclerosis [27A]. Gynecomastia recurred with subsequent tacrolimus use.

Mouth and Teeth

The impact of cytosine–adenine–guanine (CAG) repeat length of androgen receptor (*AR*) gene on cyclosporine-induced gingival overgrowth was evaluated in a case–control study [28c]. There was a smaller allele size in the gingival overgrowth group ($n = 50$) compared to controls ($P < 0.001$). This smaller CAG repeat length may be associated with increased transcriptional activity of *AR* with a subsequent increase in cell growth and extracellular matrix formation, worsening gingival overgrowth.

While gingival overgrowth is commonly associated with calcineurin inhibitors, particularly cyclosporine, a recent study showed that the occurrence of gingival overgrowth declined from 56.5% to 34.8% ($P = 0.063$) and was less severe after 44 months of continuous cyclosporine therapy [29c]. Gingival overgrowth occurs more commonly in patients treated with cyclosporine, which was demonstrated in 84 liver transplant recipients [30c]. Those also receiving calcium channel blockers exhibited greater risk of developing gingival overgrowth. In a cross-sectional study of 73 renal transplant recipients, the ratio of cyclosporine to cyclophilin A concentrations were a significant risk factor for development of gingival overgrowth and may provide predictive ability [31c].

Gastrointestinal

Occurrence of *Clostridium difficile* infections was no different between lung transplant recipients treated with cyclosporine ($n = 106$) and tacrolimus ($n = 111$) in a retrospective chart review (18.9% vs. 27.9%, $P = 0.16$, respectively) [32c].

Liver

A pharmacogenetic study of 339 Chinese renal transplant recipients investigated the association between *CYP3A4*18B* and *CYP3A5*3* polymorphisms with cyclosporine-induced liver injury [33c] Liver injury, according to Hy's law, occurred in 37% of patients (125/339). *CYP3A4*18 GG* genotype was associated with a 5-fold and 2.5-fold increased risk of liver injury compared to *AA* and *GA* genotypes, respectively. There were no associations with *CYP3A5*3* genotypes and liver injury.

Urinary Tract   ℞

Nephrotoxicity is a significant treatment complication that has limited the clinical utility of cyclosporine. A number of recent studies have examined novel pathways and potential therapeutic targets in the prevention of cyclosporine nephrotoxicity.

Inhibition of protein kinase A pathway reduced the degree of cyclosporine-induced nephrotoxicity in renal cell lines, likely through inhibition of interleukin-6 and/or stimulation of nitric oxide activity [34E]. The use of PPARγ agonists (rosiglitazone and PGDJ2) ameliorated some of the nephrotoxic effects of cyclosporine in a rat study [35E]. N-acetylcysteine administered with cyclosporine preserved Klotho gene expression and mitigated cyclosporine nephrotoxicity in mice [36E]. A novel tissue protective peptide, helix B surface peptide, ameliorated renal damage in a rat model of cyclosporine nephrotoxicity [37E]. Celecoxib, a cyclooxygenase-2 inhibitor, was associated with less cyclosporine nephrotoxicity in a rat model, suggesting that the cyclooxygenase pathway plays an important role in cyclosporine mediated renal damage [38E]. Co-administration of mizoribine and valsartan decreased markers of chronic cyclosporine nephrotoxicity in a rat study [39E].

Empiric conversion of cyclosporine to sirolimus in 16 pediatric heart transplant recipients improved glomerular filtration rate from 86±37 to 130±49 ml/min (P = 0.02) [40c]. While improvement in renal function following cyclosporine conversion has been noted in a number of prior studies, this was the first among pediatric heart transplant recipients.

Hair

A retrospective care series ($n=25$) described the use of cyclosporine in the treatment of alopecia areata [41c]. While 3 patient (16%) discontinued cyclosporine due to adverse effects, 10 of the remaining 22 (45.4%) experienced significant hair growth.

Drug Administration Route

Continuous infusion of IV cyclosporine had a higher incidence of hypertension than IV twice daily administration among 70 pediatric hematopoietic stem cell transplant recipients [42c]. Incidence of hyperglycemia, nephrotoxicity, or hyperbilirubinemia was no different between administrations.

Drug–Drug Interactions

In a case series of four liver transplant recipients with recurrent hepatitis C, telaprevir was successfully administered during concurrent cyclosporine immunosuppressive therapy [43c]. Telaprevir is a potent inhibitor of CYP3A4 and 3A5, for which cyclosporine is a substrate. Through frequent therapeutic drug monitoring of cyclosporine trough (target 150–200 ng/ml) and 2 hour concentrations combined with cyclosporine dose adjustments, telaprevir was successfully administered for a full treatment course in all patients. Cyclosporine dose was decreased by approximately 60% after initiation of telaprevir and ranged 25–50 mg/day. Chinese herbal tea inhibited cyclosporine metabolism leading to toxic concentrations in a renal transplant recipient [44A].

Dose-normalized cyclosporine trough concentrations were increased following administration of nicardipine and amlodipine, but not lacidipine among 51 pediatric bone marrow transplant patients [46c]. An increase in cyclosporine dose-normalized trough concentration was also

observed following imatinib administration in 6 pediatric patients [47c]. Cyclosporine inhibition of organic anion transporting polypeptides (OATP) was evaluated in 17 healthy subjects administered danoprevir, a hepatitis C anti-viral drug that is a substrate for OATP 1B1 and 1B3 [48c]. Substantial increases in danoprevir exposure were observed when co-administered with cyclosporine, indicating that a clinically relevant drug–drug interaction exists. In an open-label, cross-over, pharmacokinetic study of 26 healthy volunteers, cyclosporine administration was shown to more than double the exposure of ticagrelor and its active metabolite [50c]. A case series of 9 liver transplant recipients evaluated rivaroxaban pharmacokinetics and bleeding events between cyclosporine ($n=5$) and tacrolimus ($n=4$) co-administration [53c]. Rivaroxaban trough level was elevated above the therapeutic range in cyclosporine treated patients ($131.7±119.5$ ng/ml) compared to tacrolimus group ($20.3±14.4$, $P=0.014$). Bleeding complications occurred in 3/5 cyclosporine treated patients compared to 1/4 in the tacrolimus group. This interaction may be the result of cyclosporine inhibition of P-glycoprotein, for which rivaroxaban is a known substrate.

Acute kidney injury occurred after a 29-year-old male treated with cyclosporine for atopic dermatitis after he started taking methyl-1-testosterone, an over-the-counter supplement [45A]. This was associated with elevated cyclosporine blood concentration of 322 μmol/l. Kidney injury resolved after discontinuation of both medications.

A case report of a 60-year-old heart transplant patient revealed a potential interaction between argatroban and IV cyclosporine [49A]. An abrupt decline in cyclosporine blood concentrations was observed following argatroban administration and recovery of cyclosporine level was achieved after argatroban discontinuation. The author's suggested a pharmacokinetic mechanism, such as CYP450 enzyme induction, but this remains to be fully elucidated. An interaction between ciprofibrate, interferon-α, and cyclosporine (50 mg twice daily) was believed to contribute to rhabdomyolysis in a 47-year-old male liver transplant recipient [51A]. Rhabdomyolysis and acute kidney injury occurred in an 81-year-old female likely the result of an interaction between cyclosporine and simvastatin [52A]. A 14-year-old male treated with cyclosporine developed neurotoxicity after addition of itraconazole [54A]. Cyclosporine may have caused an elevation in cibenzoline in a 64-year-old female that resulted in ventricular tachycardia [55A].

EVEROLIMUS [SED-15, 1306; SEDA-34, 614; SEDA-35, 701; SEDA 36, 592]

Systematic Reviews

The concentration-effect relationship for everolimus was investigated in a meta-analysis of 5 phase II/III clinical trials [56M]. A doubling of trough everolimus concentrations (Cmin) increased the relative risk of stomatitis, pulmonary and metabolic events by 30–93%. This was also associated with a 40% relative reduction in tumor size. A meta-analysis of 9 randomized controlled trials demonstrated an increased incidence of fatal adverse events with everolimus compared to non-everolimus treatment in cancer patients (OR 3.8, 95% CI: 1.6–9.1) [57M]. Stomatitis, skin rash, pruritus, and mouth ulceration were the most prevalent adverse effects associated with everolimus treatment of solid tumors in a systematic review and meta-analysis of 10 clinical trials [58M]. Everolimus adverse effect profile was also reviewed for renal transplant breast and renal cancer populations [59R,60R,61R,62R].

Observational Studies

Eight children under the age of 3 years with tuberous sclerosis complex treated with everolimus were followed for a mean of 35 months [63c]. Adverse effects such as stomatitis, skin rash, GI disturbances, and hyperlipidemia were common but no different than those for older children or adult and did not lead to permanent drug discontinuation. Decreased growth rate was observed in one patient. A similar adverse effect profile was observed in a phase I/II trial of 20 tuberous sclerosis complex patients (median age: 8 years), although effect of growth rate was not discussed [64c]. Lastly, a series of 7 children (median age: 5 years) with tuberous sclerosis complex were treated with everolimus and followed for 36 weeks [65c]. One patient discontinued therapy due to flushing, although they later re-started everolimus without recurrence of symptoms. Adverse effect profile was mild-moderate in severity and similar to that observed in the previous two studies.

℞

Use of everolimus in the treatment of breast cancer has dramatically increased in recent years. The adverse effect profile in this patient population has not been well documented until now. A timely review article described everolimus adverse effects in cancer treatment, including incidence from large randomized controlled trials and management strategies [66R].

A phase III, double-blind, randomized, placebo-controlled trial investigated the effects of everolimus in treatment of breast cancer with and without visceral metastases [67C]. While adverse effects were more prevalent with everolimus compared to placebo, overall adverse effect profile was similar between patients with and without visceral metastases. Health-related quality of life was similar between everolimus and placebo in a follow-up study [68c]. This may indicate that the clinical benefit of everolimus outweighs the increased adverse effects experienced.

Hematologic toxicities of everolimus were evaluated in a phase II clinical trial of 31 metastatic breast cancer patients [69c]. While adverse effects were common (71% anemia, 55% thrombocytopenia, and 45% leukopenia), they were generally mild and did not require dose reduction. Microcytosis was observed with reductions in mean corpuscular volume and mean corpuscular hemoglobin after treatment initiation which resolved within 1 month of discontinuation.

In an 18-month follow-up of the BOLERO-2 clinical trial, the adverse effects of everolimus for treatment of breast cancer were evaluated 720 patients [70C]. Most adverse effects occurred quickly after initiation of everolimus and were mild-to-moderate in severity. Treatment interruption or dose reduction due to adverse effects was required in 62% of the everolimus group compared to 12% in the placebo group. When everolimus was held or dose reduced, the adverse effect resolved within 2 weeks 76% of the time and 44% of the episodes were followed by full dose re-initiation. This study provides clinically useful data on the management of everolimus related adverse effects. In particular, temporary dose reduction or interruption is an option for successful treatment of the adverse effect.

Cardiovascular

Compared to cyclosporine, everolimus was not associated with improvement in echocardiographic measures of left ventricular systolic function or mass after 1 year of treatment in 44 renal transplant recipients [71c]. Everolimus treatment was associated with increased von Willebrand factor, prothrombin fragment $1+2$, thrombin-activatable fibrinolysis inhibitor and plasminogen activator inhibitor-1 compared to control immunosuppression in renal transplant recipients [73c]. This general procoagulant state may impose an increased risk of venous thromboembolic events in patients treated with everolimus.

A report described chylothorax associated with everolimus in a 36-year-old male heart transplant recipient [72A].

Respiratory

In a case–control study, 12.7% of 103 renal transplant recipients treated with everolimus developed interstitial pneumonitis [74c]. This side effect was also noted in 23% of renal cell carcinoma patients [75c] and was observed in breast cancer patients [76c].

Diffuse alveolar hemorrhage was reported in a 65-year-old female treated with everolimus for stage 4 breast cancer [77A].

Neuromuscular Function

Treatment related fatigue for everolimus and temsirolimus was compared to placebo in a meta-analysis of 56 clinical trials of 9650 cancer patients [78M]. A higher incidence of all-grade fatigue (RR 1.22, 95% CI 1.03–1.38, $P=0.002$) and high-grade fatigue (RR 1.92, 95% CI 1.24–2.69, $P=0.002$) occurred with treatment compared to placebo. Everolimus was associated with a higher incidence of all-grade fatigue compared to temsirolimus (RR 1.85, 95% CI 1.71-2.01, $P<0.001$).

Urinary Tract

Acute kidney injury (AKI) occurred in 23% (21/93) of renal cell carcinoma patients treated with everolimus in a retrospective study [79c]. However, only 14/21 cases were believed to be associated with everolimus and only 1 patient discontinued therapy because of AKI. Baseline glomerular filtration rate was the single independent risk factor for everolimus-associated AKI.

Conversion from calcineurin inhibitor based regimen to everolimus resulted in significant proteinuria in a renal transplant recipient which resolved following everolimus discontinuation and steroid administration [80A].

Immunologic

In a 52-year-old female renal transplant recipient, everolimus was associated with severe angioedema necessitating discontinuation of therapy [81A]. The patient recovered well after switching to tacrolimus. A fatal case of hepatitis B reactivation occurred in a patient receiving everolimus for breast cancer [82A].

Liver

A 76-year-old male treated with everolimus for neuroendocrine carcinoma of the ileum developed severe steatohepatitis [83A].

Drug–Drug Interactions

Everolimus is subject to a number of clinically relevant drug–drug and drug–food interactions because it is a substrate for CYP3A4 and P-glycoprotein (Pgp). Grabowsky provided a thorough review of everolimus drug interactions in cancer patients [84R]. A randomized, open-label, cross-over study in 20 renal transplant recipients evaluated the drug interaction between everolimus and atorvastatin [88c]. There were no predictable changes in everolimus area under the concentration-time curve (AUC), maximum concentration or time or maximum concentration after administration of atorvastatin suggesting a negligible drug interaction. A case series of liver transplant recipients with hepatocellular carcinoma demonstrated a poor tolerability of the combination of everolimus and sorafenib, including grade 3 adverse events in 7 out of the 15 patients and possible drug toxicity related mortality in 2 patients [89c].

A case report described a drug interaction between everolimus and voriconazole in a 66-year-old male renal transplant recipient [85A]. Voriconazole, a potent CYP3A4 inhibitor, was initiated for treatment of *Aspergillus fumigatus* pneumonia. Everolimus trough concentration increased approximately fivefold despite an empiric 33% dose reduction following voriconazole initiation. The patient had worsening pulmonary function, with chest X-ray and lung computer tomography showing everolimus-associated pneumonia, although worsening of the underlying *Aspergillus* infection secondary to excess immunosuppression could not be ruled out. The authors suggest an empiric 80% dose reduction of everolimus when co-administered with voriconazole to maintain therapeutic drug concentrations.

A 57-year-old female with breast cancer was treated with everolimus at 10 mg daily with a trough concentration of 10.1 ng/ml [86A]. Fenofibrate was started due to hyperlipidemia. Two weeks later, everolimus trough concentration was 4.2 ng/ml, suggesting fenofibrate induction of CYP3A4 metabolism. After discontinuation of fenofibrate, the everolimus trough concentration increased to 11.5 ng/ml without dose adjustment.

The addition of maribavir to everolimus immunosuppression in a 59-year-old renal transplant patient increased the everolimus trough concentration from 6 to 17.2 ng/ml within 5 days [87A]. Following a 30% everolimus dose reduction, the trough concentration was within target range and maribavir continued. No toxicities occurred.

FINGOLIMOD [SEDA-34, 616; SEDA-35, 703; SEDA-36, 593]

Placebo-Controlled Studies

The safety of fingolimod was assessed in a randomized, double-blind, phase III clinical trial comparing 0.5 and 1.25 mg daily doses to placebo in 1083 patients with relapsing-remitting multiple sclerosis [90C]. Adverse effects were frequent with discontinuation due to adverse effects 20% in the 1.25 mg arm, 18% in the 0.5 mg arm, and 10% in the placebo arm. Hypertension, lymphopenia, macular edema, herpes zoster infection, lower respiratory tract infection, bradycardia, first degree AV block, and elevated lifer function tests were more common in the fingolimod groups compared to placebo. The 1.25 mg arm had increased incidence of cardiac adverse effects following the first dose including bradycardia and first-degree AV block compared to 0.5 mg arm.

Cardiac safety following fingolimod initiation was assessed in 2282 patients with multiple sclerosis [91c]. Bradycardia adverse events occurred in 0.6% of patients and were more frequent with beta-blocker or calcium channel block co-treatment. Second degree AV block was more frequent in patients with pre-existing cardiac conditions in the 6-hour post dose period (4.1% vs. 2.0%). Other real-world studies showed a similar cardiac safety profile [92c].

Cardiovascular

A 42-year-old male developed paroxysmal atrial fibrillation within 3 hours of fingolimod administration on two separate occasions [93A]. First degree AV block progressed into second degree AV block (Mobitz type I) 4 hours after the first dose of fingolimod 0.5 mg in a 24-year-old female [94A]. A case report described type I and II AV block in a 4-year-old male between 2 and 10 hours post accidental ingestion of a 0.5 mg fingolimod tablet. No prolonged effects after 24 hours of observation were noted [95A].

Ear, Nose, Throat

Macular edema is a rare but serious adverse effect of fingolimod use identified in large phase III clinical trials [90C]. Discontinuation of fingolimod leads to resolution of this untoward effect, but many choose to remain on therapy because of its beneficial impact on relapse rates. Management of macular edema on fingolimod therapy has not been well described, but Thoo and colleagues report two cases successfully managed with intravitreal triamcinolone [96A]. Both patients received fingolimod 0.5 mg daily and failed topical corticosteroid treatment for macular edema prior to intravitreal triamcinolone.

Hematologic

Lower pre-treatment lymphocyte count and body mass index less than 18.5 kg/m^2 in females were predictive of lymphopenia related to fingolimod [97c]. Autoimmune hemolytic anemia developed in a 19-year-old female treated with fingolimod [98A]. Improvement in symptoms and laboratory parameters occurred only after fingolimod discontinuation.

Skin

Within 3 days of starting fingolimod, a 26-year-old female developed a large ecchymotic angioedema-like lesion on her knee [99A]. Additional lesions developed on her back and arms. All lesions completely resolved 10 days after discontinuation of fingolimod and no other plausible cause was identified.

Infection Risk

A 37-year-old female being treated with fingolimod for multiple sclerosis developed visceral leishmaniasis from *Leishmani infantum* infection 29 months into treatment [100A]. She made a full recovery after amphotericin treatment.

Teratogenicity

Karlsson and colleagues reviewed 89 pregnancies that occurred during clinical trials of fingolimod [101c]. Of the 66 pregnancies with *in utero* exposure to fingolimod, 2 infants were born with malformations and 5 cases of abnormal fetal development were reported. A total of 24 elective abortions (3 of which with serious fetal abnormalities) and 9 spontaneous abortions occurred.

GLATIRAMER *[SEDA-34, 617; SEDA-35, 703; SEDA-36]*

Hematologic

A 59-year-old female developed leukocytosis and eosinophilia while on glatiramer [102A]. This progressed to respiratory depression, shock, and myocarditis. White blood cell count peaked at 77 000 cells/mm^3 and eosinophils peaked at 69%. Discontinuation of glatiramer 6 days after initial presentation resulted in a resolution of leukocytosis and eosinophilia within 9 days. Glatiramer was re-started and after 1 month, eosinophilia recurred, prompting permanent discontinuation.

Liver

A 17-year-old female developed hepatotoxicity following glatiramer initiation for multiple sclerosis which was confirmation as drug-induced disease on biopsy [103A]. A similar hepatotoxicity reaction was observed in a 28-year-old female receiving glatiramer [104A].

LEFLUNOMIDE *[SED-15, 2015; SEDA-34, 618; SEDA-35, 703; SEDA-36, 594]*

Respiratory

A case series described 5 patients receiving leflunomide in combination with methotrexate that developed interstitial lung disease [105A]. All patients had been on methotrexate therapy (range: 20–146 months) without pulmonary complications or pre-existing lung disease. Leflunomide 20 mg daily was added to therapy and between 3.3 and 5.3 months later, pulmonary complications were diagnosed. All patients discontinued lefluonomide therapy; 3 out of the 5 recovered. Leflunomide was included in a recent review of drug-induced interstitial lung disease in rheumatoid arthritis patients [106R].

Skin

A 78-year-old female developed multiple keratoacanthomas following leflunomide treatment [107A].

Genetic Factors

The C1858T polymorphism in the protein tyrosine phosphatase non-receptor type 22 (*PTPN22*) gene is involved in T-cell responses and rheumatoid arthritis susceptibility [108c]. Association between the C1858T polymorphism and leflunomide in 94 rheumatoid arthritis patients revealed no relationship between C and T alleles and discontinuation of treatment or reduction of dose due to adverse effects.

MYCOPHENOLIC ACID [SED-15, 2402; SEDA-34, 622; SEDA-35, 704; SEDA-36, 594]

Mycophenolic acid is an immunosuppressive drug that acts by inhibiting guanosine nucleotide biosynthesis in lymphocytes. It is available in two distinct formulations: (1) mycophenolate mofetil, a prodrug which is rapidly hydrolyzed in the GI tract to mycophenolic acid and (2) enteric-coated mycophenolate sodium, which has delayed absorption due to enteric coating. While these formulations are not bioequivalent, the safety and efficacy profiles of the drugs are similar. Initials reports of less GI toxicity with the enteric-coated mycophenolate sodium have not been substantiated by large randomized controlled trials.

Systematic Reviews

A systematic review compared mycophenolate mofetil to methotrexate in 177 patients undergoing allogeneic hematopoietic stem cell transplantation [109M]. Mycophenolate mofetil had a lower incidence of severe mucositis compared to methotrexate (RR 0.48, 95% confidence interval 0.32–0.73). Dose reductions in mycophenolate mofetil occurred in 365 out of 749 renal transplant recipients and were due to hematologic toxicity (46.5%), GI toxicity (12.3%), infection (16.1%) and malignancy (2.1%) [110c].

Hematologic

Mycophenolic acid is well known to cause leukopenia and anemia. Shin and colleagues report two cases of severe leukopenia from mycophenolate mofetil that resolved after conversion to sirolimus [111A]. Both patients were renal transplant recipients treated with mycophenolate mofetil 1.5 g/day. White blood cell count returned to within normal range and 7–14 days of sirolimus conversion, suggesting this as a management option for severe mycophenolate mofetil associated leukopenia.

Mycophenolic acid glucuronide (MPAG), the primary inactive metabolite of mycophenolic acid, had a negative correlation with hemoglobin and hematocrit values (range of correlation coefficient: -0.27 to -0.36) in 51 renal transplant recipients [112c]. However, this may have reflected anemia secondary to reduced renal function wherein mycophenolic acid glucuronide would also be elevated as renal clearance is its primary route of elimination.

Genetic associations with hematologic toxicities were observed in 189 renal transplant recipients [113c]. The CYP2C8 rs11572076 wild-type genotype was associated with lower risk of leukopenia (HR 0.14, 95% CI 0.03–0.59), a higher dose and UGT2B7 c.-840G > A polymorphism was associated with higher risk of anemia (GG vs. AA HR 1.88, 95% CI 1.23–2.88).

Gastrointestinal

Gastrointestinal disturbances, primarily nausea, vomiting, and diarrhea, are the most common adverse effects of mycophenolic acid drugs. These often lead to dose reduction or disruption, which increases the risk of allograft rejection in solid organ transplant recipients [114R]. Despite the high frequency of GI adverse effects and their negative impact on outcomes, the mechanism is poorly understood. An *in vitro* study demonstrated the mycophenolic acid increased myosin light chain 2 (MLC2) expressions which is associated with disruption in epithelial tight junctions and may partly explain the mechanism of gastrotoxicity [115E].

In a pharmacogenomic study, polymorphisms in UGT1A8 (rs1042597, 518 C > G), UGT1A9 (rs6744284), and HNF1α (rs1169288; I27L A > G) were assessed in relation to GI adverse effects in 109 renal transplant recipients [116c]. UGT1A8 alleles were associated with overall gastrointestinal symptoms at weeks 1 and 2 but not months 3 and 6 (worse symptoms with GG compared to CC genotypes). HNF1α was associated with overall GI symptoms at 1 week but also abdominal pain sub-scores at months 3 and 6 (worse symptoms with AA compared to CC genotypes). Fifteen patients completed a pharmacokinetic sub-study, which revealed that decreased clearance of MPAG was associated with increased acid reflux and constipation.

Lung

A heart transplant recipient developed pulmonary hemorrhage with capillaritis which resolved after discontinuation of mycophenolate mofetil, the proposed cause of this adverse event [117A].

Drug Formulations

After conversion from brand name *CellCept* to a generic equivalent of mycophenolate mofetil, 8/154 liver transplant recipients reported drug-related complications [118c]. A large majority of patients (>90%) reported feeling "about the same" after conversion on quality of life and overall treatment effect scales. This study indicates that generic substitution of mycophenolate mofetil can occur with little complication.

In a prospective case series, 34 liver transplant recipients with GI complications from mycophenolate mofetil treatment were converted to equivalent doses of enteric-coated mycophenolate sodium [119c]. After conversion, improvement in GI symptoms and HRQOL was observed. In another study of liver transplant recipients, conversion from mycophenolate mofetil to enteric-coated mycophenolate sodium was associated with improvement in GI symptoms [120c]. However, in a randomized, prospective, double-blind sub-study, no differences were noted between formulations. While these studies suggests that conversion from mycophenolate mofetil to enteric-coated mycophenolate sodium improves GI adverse effects, the selection bias of patients already experiencing adverse effects and lack of placebo-control or randomization are important limitations to consider.

Drug–Drug Interactions

Proton pump inhibitors have been shown to decrease exposure to mycophenolic acid. A retrospective cohort study examined the effect of proton pump inhibitors on outcomes following renal transplantation with mycophenolate mofetil immunosuppression [121c]. Biopsy proven acute rejection (BPAR) occurred in 32/213 patients on proton pump inhibitor compared to 46/384 on the control treatment of ranitidine ($P = 0.31$). On multivariable analysis, use of proton pump inhibitor was associated with increased risk of BPAR in African-American patients (RR 1.93, 95% CI 1.18–3.16) suggesting a possible ethnic predisposition to the clinical relevance of the drug interaction.

In 88 Chinese renal transplant recipients, the interaction with proton pump inhibitors was evaluated between the mycophenolate mofetil and enteric-coated mycophenolate sodium formulations [122c]. Exposure to mycophenolic acid was increased in the enteric-coated mycophenolate sodium group ($P < 0.01$) despite equimolar dosing. This indicates that the proton pump inhibitor drug interaction is more clinically relevant for mycophenolate mofetil administration than the enteric-coated formulation which bypasses the stomach and avoids any effect of acid suppression. The primary metabolite, mycophenolic acid glucuronide (MPAG), undergoes enterohepatic circulation via the biliary system with de-glucuronidation in the GI tract to active mycophenolic acid that is systemically absorbed and contributes to 10–60% of overall drug exposure. This process was interrupted by ciprofloxacin, which was shown to inhibit β-glucuronidase and subsequent mycophenolic acid production in an *in vitro* study [123E].

SIROLIMUS (RAPAMYCIN) [SED-15, 3148; SEDA-34, 626; SEDA-35, 705; SEDA-36, 594]

Systematic Reviews

Sirolimus has been investigated as a potential disease modifying drug for autosomal-dominant polycystic kidney disease (ADPKD). Adverse effects in this population are not well defined. A meta-analysis of four randomized controlled trials evaluated sirolimus for ADPKD and included safety endpoints [124M]. Increased prevalence of stomatitis, pharyngitis, overall infections, and hyperlipidemia was observed for sirolimus treatment, consistent with the known adverse effects in other disease states. No differences in leukocytes, hemoglobin, platelets, or blood pressure were found compared to control treatments. Verhave and colleagues reviewed the side effect profile of sirolimus in 219 renal transplant recipients [125c].

Skin

Chronic lymphedema was reported in 2 renal transplant recipients treated with sirolimus [126A]. Sirolimus associated mucocutaneous disorders was evaluated in a case–control study of 100 renal transplant recipients [127c]. Herpes simplex infections and seborrheic dermatitis were more common in sirolimus treated patients ($P < 0.05$ for both).

Genetic Factors

Polymorphisms *CYP3A4*22* (rs3559367), *POR*28* (rs1057868) and *PPARα* (rs4253728) were analyzed in 113 renal transplant recipients with assessment of sirolimus trough concentrations and adverse effects [128c]. There were no significant associations between the three polymorphisms and adverse effects measured. Median sirolimus dose was 3 mg/day.

Drug–Drug Interactions

A 64-year-old female developed rhabdomyolysis and acute kidney injury while receiving sirolimus 2 mg/day, simvastatin 20 mg/day, and chemotherapy containing cisplatin and gemcitabine [129A]. The most plausible mechanism was sirolimus competitive inhibition of CYP3A4 leading to decreased simvastatin metabolism. However, given the patient's stage 4 lung cancer and active chemotherapy, other causes could not be ruled out.

Following addition and dose titration of ranolazine, a 57-year-old male renal transplant recipient experienced a sixfold increase in sirolimus trough concentrations, from 10 to greater than 60 ng/ml [130A]. After holding repeated doses of sirolimus and a 50% dose reduction (6–3 mg/day) trough concentrations returned to target range of 8–12 ng/ml. No acute adverse events occurred. Ranolazine mediated inhibition of P-glycoprotein and CYP3A4 is the probable mechanism for this clinically significant drug–drug interaction. Empiric sirolimus dose reductions may be necessary when initiating and titrating ranolazine.

TACROLIMUS [SED-15, 3279; SEDA-34, 629; SEDA-35, 705; SEDA-36, 596]

Placebo-Controlled Studies

Tacrolimus was evaluated in a randomized, placebo-controlled, double-blind fashion in 40 patients with IgA nephropathy [131c]. Adverse effects were similar to other indications, generally mild, and primarily related to the GI and neurologic systems. One subject discontinued treatment due to weakness and myalgia.

Observational Studies

In a prospective, open-label, controlled trial, 60 renal transplant recipients were evaluated for change in renal function and regulatory T cell (T_{reg}) populations following 1:1 randomized conversion from a calcineurin inhibitor (CNI) to sirolimus [132c]. Tacrolimus was the CNI in 90% (54/60) of the patients whereas cyclosporine was used in the remaining 10%. At 6 months, estimated glomerular filtration (eGFR) was 88.9 ± 11.8 ml/min in the sirolimus group compared to 80.6 ± 16.5 ml/min the CNI group ($P = 0.038$); T_{reg} populations were increased in the sirolimus group ($6.3 \pm 2.6\%$) compared to the CNI group ($3.9 \pm 1.8\%$; $P = 0.004$). A randomized trial evaluated dyslipidemia in cyclosporine compared to tacrolimus in renal transplant recipients [133c]. Dyslipidemia was observed in 115 out of 182 patients and was no different between CNI regimens. A retrospective analysis of 32 liver transplant recipients investigated the relationship between tacrolimus trough concentrations and neurotoxicity, nephrotoxicity, and diabetes [134c]. Results suggested that a trough concentration range of 5–8 ng/ml was associated with least adverse effects, although diabetes did not appear concentration dependent. A retrospective study compared low-dose tacrolimus (0.05 mg/kg/day for 1 year, then 0.03 mg/kg/day thereafter) to normal-dose tacrolimus (0.1 mg/kg/day for 1 year, then 0.05 mg/kg/day thereafter) in 66 living-donor liver transplant recipients [135c]. Infection, hypertension, hyperglycemia, and renal insufficiency were less frequent in the low-dose compared to normal-dose group at 1-and 3-year follow-ups ($P < 0.05$ for all). However, 3-year survival rate was improved in the normal-dose group (88%) compared to low-dose (82%, $P < 0.05$). Tacrolimus was evaluated in 44 steroid resistant nephrotic syndrome patients in a single-center, open-label, prospective study [136c]. Adverse effects included diarrhea (22.7%), hyperglycemia (22.7%), and nephrotoxicity (reversible: 15.9%, irreversible: 9.0%).

Pulmonary

A 51-year-old female developed pleural effusion, peripheral edema, and ascites following renal transplantation with tacrolimus based immunosuppression [137A]. Tacrolimus dose was 3.5–4.5 mg/day with trough 11.9 ng/ml. Conversion from tacrolimus to sirolimus was done as tacrolimus related fluid retention was the likely diagnosis. Pleural effusion, edema, and ascites subsequently resolved and had not recurred within 7 months of follow-up.

Nervous System

A prospective cohort study investigated peripheral nerve dysfunction associated with calcineurin inhibitor (CNI) treatment in 38 renal transplant recipients [138c]. Clinical neuropathy was present in 68% (13/19) of the CNI group compared to 37% (7/19) of the CNI-free group. Neuropathy scores revealed more severe disease in the CNI group (7.9 ± 6.5) compared to the CNI-free group (3.6 ± 5.0; $P < 0.018$). Mechanistic investigation using nerve excitability measures revealed a pattern consistent with depolarization of the nerve membrane potential in the CNI group. Of note, in the CNI group 7 patients were on cyclosporine and 12 on tacrolimus; no differences in nerve dysfunction between these medications were noted. Three cases of posterior reversible encephalopathy syndrome (PRES) were associated with tacrolimus used in bone marrow transplant patients [139A]. All patients were maintained within the therapeutic range of tacrolimus trough concentrations (10–17 ng/ml) prior to PRES diagnosis. Resolution of neurologic symptoms occurred in all patients following discontinuation of tacrolimus and alternative immunosuppression. A renal transplant recipient developed altered mental status, new-onset bilateral foot drop, and had common peroneal nerve demyelination following and inadvertent overdose of tacrolimus [140A]. All symptoms resolved within 5 months after conversion to cyclosporine. Sudden hearing loss developed in 2 pediatric renal transplant recipients treated with tacrolimus [141A]. High concentrations of tacrolimus were observed at the time of development of hearing loss, which did not progress following dose reduction. Trough concentration of tacrolimus was an independent predictor of seizure development in pediatric liver transplant recipients [142c].

Endocrine

Recent advances in pancreatic transplant have improved outcomes in diabetics. Tacrolimus based immunosuppression presents a challenge in this setting due to diabetogenic effects. A timely review by Rangel discusses mechanisms of tacrolimus-induced diabetes, drug interactions, and management strategies [143R].

A 12-year-old female receiving tacrolimus for nephrotic syndrome developed diabetic ketoacidosis [144A].

Hematologic

Severe tacrolimus-induced neutropenia was suspected in a 3-year-old male cardiac transplant recipient after numerous other causes were ruled out [145A].

Urinary Tract

Acute and chronic nephrotoxicity are a major concern with tacrolimus therapy. Renal function was monitored over 5-years in 48 pancreatic islet-cell transplant recipients treated with tacrolimus [146c]. An initial mean decline in eGFR by 19 ml/min/1.72 m^2 occurred during the first 1–2 weeks of tacrolimus but remained stable throughout follow-up. Decline in eGFR was associated with higher tacrolimus dose and trough concentrations, consistent with acute concentration dependent vasoconstriction of renal arterioles. Tacrolimus was discontinued in 21/48 patients and eGFR returned to pre-transplant baseline.

Genetic Factors

Tacrolimus is a substrate of CYP3A5 and P-glycoprotein, which contribute to interpatient variability in pharmacokinetics and drug response. The polymorphisms CYP3A5*3 (A6986G) and ABCB1 C3435T were associated with tacrolimus adverse effects in 38 pediatric renal transplant recipients [147c]. CYP3A5 non-expressors (A6986G, rs776746) had double the time-dependent risk of adverse effects compared to expressors (CYP3A5*1) over 12 months. Mean tacrolimus dose was 7.2 mg/day. Dose-normalized trough concentrations were higher in CYP3A5 non-expressors during the first 3 months, which may have attributed to higher adverse effects observed in this group. ABCB1 3435TT genotype was associated with a lower probability of adverse effects in the first 3 months but this did not persist over the 12-month study period. Therefore, CYP3A5 genotype and phenotype characteristics are important in determining optimal initial tacrolimus dosing and impact adverse effects experienced in the first year post-transplant.

In 101 renal transplant recipients, single nucleotide polymorphisms in peroxisome proliferator-activated receptor alpha (PPARα; rs4253728 and rs4823613) and P450 oxidoreductase (POR; rs1057868; POR*28) were evaluated as risk factors for development of new-onset diabetes after transplantation (NODAT) [148c]. The variant alleles in both PPARα rs4253728 and POR rs1057868 were independently associated with increased risk of NODAT (OR 8.6, 95% CI: 1.4–54.2; OR 8.1, 95% CI: 1.1–58.3, respectively).

A case–control study of 312 renal transplant recipients evaluated mitochondrial DNA haplogroups and associations to new-onset diabetes after transplantation [149c]. Haplogroup H was associated with a higher incidence of new-onset diabetes (50% vs. 35%, $P=0.01$, OR 1.82) which may provide a pre-transplant screening tool to predict diabetes risk and determine optimal immunosuppression selection.

Drug Formulations

Recently, a once-daily formulation of tacrolimus has become widely available. A prospective cohort study evaluated treatment satisfaction and adherence following conversion from twice-daily to once-daily formulations [150c]. Based on a validated survey, treatment satisfaction significantly increased ($P<0.001$) and self-reported adherence improved from 80% to 95% ($P<0.001$).

Topical tacrolimus administration was associated with increased systemic concentrations in two patients being treated for graft-versus-host disease [151A]. While both patients were also receiving oral tacrolimus, topical absorption was believed to be increased by use of occlusive dressings.

Drug–Drug Interactions

The use of ketoconazole in combination with tacrolimus was studied in 30 renal transplant recipients

[152c]. Median tacrolimus dose reduction of 63% was necessary to maintain therapeutic trough concentration of 5–7 ng/ml after initiation of ketoconazole (100 mg/day) due to CYP3A4 inhibition. This strategy reduced monthly tacrolimus costs by $150USD and was not associated with new onset adverse effects.

The combination of colchicine and tacrolimus in a 62-year-old renal transplant recipient caused myopathy with elevations in aspartate aminotransferase and creatine phosphokinase [153A]. Symptoms and laboratory elevations resolved following discontinuation of colchicine. Tacrolimus-mediated competitive inhibition of P-glycoprotein may have led to elevated colchicine concentrations and this adverse effect.

A 9-year-old female renal transplant recipient experienced tacrolimus toxicity with a trough of 32 ng/ml that was treated with corticosteroids and phenytoin [154A]. Within 24 hours, the trough declined the 5 ng/ml and symptoms such as acute kidney injury and neurotoxicity resolved. Induction of CYP3A4 metabolism with phenytoin and induction of P-glycoprotein with corticosteroids was the postulated mechanism for rapid correction of toxicity.

Carbajal and colleagues described a potential herbal interaction between boldo (*Peumus boldus* Mol.) a tree leaf extract, and tacrolimus [155A]. A 78-year-old male renal transplant recipient on tacrolimus 4 mg/day had an undetectable tacrolimus trough (<3 ng/ml) after initiation of boldo 600 mg/day. Following boldo discontinuation, tacrolimus trough concentration rose to 6.1 ng/ml on the same 4 mg/day dose.

The interaction between interleukin-2 receptor antagonists (basiliximab and daclizumab) and tacrolimus was evaluated in a sub-analysis of a randomized, controlled trial in 386 patients [156C]. During the first-week post-transplant, tacrolimus trough concentrations were higher and weight-based doses were lower to achieve target trough concentration among patients treated with interleukin-2 receptor antagonists (IL2RA) compared to anti-thymocyte globulin. After 1 week, tacrolimus troughs were similar between groups but doses remained lower in the IL2RA group. IL2RA may down-regulate CYP enzymes causing increased tacrolimus exposure early post-transplant.

An interaction between dronedarone and tacrolimus was described in a 63-year-old male renal transplant recipient [157A]. The initial tacrolimus dose was 0.15 mg/kg (12 mg/day) which required a 90% dose reduction to 0.75 mg/day over the first 2 months post-transplant. At one point, dronedarone was held (or was a help; or helped?) and tacrolimus trough concentrations decreased, but quickly rose upon re-initiation. Dronedarone mediated inhibition of P-glycoprotein and CYP3A4 is the likely mechanism for this drug interaction. Concomitant use of dronedarone and tacrolimus should be done cautiously with close monitoring of tacrolimus trough concentrations.

Telaprevir is a potent CYP3A4 inhibitor and has been shown to markedly increase tacrolimus exposure. A case series of 17 liver transplant recipients described a successful protocol to manage this drug–drug interaction to prevent tacrolimus toxicity and maintain telaprevir efficacy [158c]. Following initiation of telaprevir, tacrolimus was held until trough concentrations began to decline. Then, tacrolimus was re-initiated at 0.1 mg once or twice daily with frequent monitoring of trough concentrations. This protocol maintained tacrolimus trough concentrations within the target range of 5–7 ng/ml for a majority of patients over the 48-week study period. Mean tacrolimus dose was 3 mg/day (range 0.5–7 mg/day) prior to telaprevir, which reflects an average 30-fold dose reduction to maintain target tacrolimus exposure. Nephrotoxicity did not occur and no patient experienced acute rejection.

The nephrotoxic potential of tacrolimus and teicoplanin combination was evaluated in a retrospective analysis of 67 patients [159c]. A doubling of serum creatinine occurred in 3% of patients which was reversible, indicating that with appropriate tacrolimus concentration management, nephrotoxicity with the combination is low.

Increased tacrolimus concentrations (from 8 to 22 ng/ml) were observed in a 16-year-old male after initiation of berberine, an isoquinoline alkaloid found in herbal remedies, for treatment of diarrhea [160A]. This interaction was proposed to be the result of berberine inhibition of CYP3A4. However, the causality of the interaction is confounded by the presenting symptom of diarrhea, which has also been associated with increased tacrolimus concentrations.

TEMSIROLIMUS [SEDA-34, 632; SEDA-35, 707; SEDA-36, 597]

Systematic Reviews

Recent reviews have included adverse effects of temsirolimus in the treatment of renal cell carcinoma [61R,161R] and focused on hematologic toxicities [62R].

Neuromuscular Function

A case series of 16 cancer patients treated with temsirolimus evaluated body composition [162c]. Sarcopenia (skeletal muscle index lower than 38.5 cm^2/m^2 for females and 52.4 cm^2/m^2 for males) occurred in 44% (7/16) of patients. While weight loss is a potential side effect of temsirolimus, but many factors contributing to sarcopenia were not addressed in this study and cannot be directly correlated with temsirolimus treatment.

Gastrointestinal

A retrospective review of 87 temsirolimus treated patients showed a 64.4% occurrence of mucositis and 9.2% occurrence of grade 3 mucositis [164c]. A dose–response to this side effect was not observed and with no difference in mucositis between three dosing levels.

A case report of bowel perforation was graded to be a probable relationship to temsirolimus therapy in a 45-year-old female with uterine leiomyosarcoma [163A]. Diffuse mucosal GI bleeding was observed in a 47-year-old female treated with temsirolimus for renal cell carcinoma and associated with a hemoglobin decline from 10.1 to 2.9 g/dl [165A].

THIOPURINES [SED-15, 377; SEDA-34, 633; SEDA-35, 709; SEDA-36, 598]

Observational Studies

A prospective cohort study examined adverse effects of azathioprine in 82 pediatric atopic dermatitis patients [166c]. Myelosuppression, elevated liver enzymes, and cutaneous viral infections were the most common adverse effects. Five (6%) patients discontinued therapy due to adverse effects. A prospective monitoring algorithm was proposed by authors based on their experience and results of the study.

Nervous System

Bilateral tremor occurred in a 48-year-old female with Crohn's disease following dose increase of azathioprine from 100 to 150 mg/day [167A]. Tremors were most severe 2 hours after administration and stopped within 24 hours of discontinuation, suggesting a dose dependent adverse effect.

Ear, Nose, and Throat

A 47-year-old female renal transplant recipient developed sensorineural hearing loss 10 days after starting azathioprine 75 mg/day [168A]. She experienced a full recovery following discontinuation of azathioprine.

Hematologic

Myelosuppression is a well-known adverse effect of 6-mercaptopurine. A 15-year-old female with acute lymphoblastic leukemia patient developed severe pancytopenia despite a 6-mercaptopurine reduction to 5% of the standard dose [169A]. She was found to have the *3A/*3C polymorphism in thiopurine S-methyltransferase (TPMT) gene which could have contributed to severe myelosuppression due to accumulation of active thioguanine nucleotide metabolites.

A retrospective cohort study from the Veterans Affairs health care system evaluated the risk of lymphoma in patients with ulcerative colitis treated with thiopurines [170c]. There was an increased risk of lymphoma among 4734 patients treated with thiopurines (HR 4.2, 95% CI: 2.5–6.8, $P < 0.001$) compared to those not treated with thiopurines. Interestingly, in a small subset of patients who had discontinued thiopurine treatment, lymphoma risk was similar to those never exposed, suggesting the risk declines after discontinuation.

Skin

The risk of thiopurine associated melanoma and non-melanoma skin cancer was evaluated in a retrospective cohort study of 14 527 ulcerative colitis patients [171c]. Treatment with thiopurines was associated with an increased risk of skin cancer compared to no thiopurine treatment (HR 2.1, 95% CI: 1.6–2.6, $P < 0.001$). Similar risk for non-melanoma skin cancer was observed in a meta-analysis of inflammatory bowel disease patients (HR 2.28, 95% CI: 1.50–3.45) [172M]. Overall malignancy risk was also increased for thiopurine treatment compared to anti-tumor necrosis factor antibody treatment in 666 inflammatory bowel disease patients (HR 4.15, 95% CI: 1.82–9.44, $P = 0.0007$) [173c].

Body Temperature

Azathioprine-induced fever was diagnosed in a 53-year-old female with autoimmune hepatitis [174A]. The patient's fever resolved following discontinuation of all medications. Azathioprine 50 mg/day was re-started and fever recurred within a few hours. Extensive diagnostic testing revealed no other likely source.

Genetic Factors

The associations of inosine triphosphate pyrophosphohydrolase (ITPA) polymorphisms with 6-mercaptopurine toxicities were investigated in 95 pediatric leukemia patients [175c]. Those with 94A allele in exon 2 had lower odds of overall toxicity compared to CC genotype (OR 0.34, 95% CI 0.12–0.98).

A case–control study in 401 inflammatory bowel disease patients investigated the association between PACSIN2 rs2413739, SLCO1B1 rs11045879, and TPMT*2 polymorphisms and thiopurine toxicity (GI, liver, hematologic, and skin) [176c]. No associations were observed for PACSIN2 polymorphism and thiopurine toxicity, regardless of TPMT*2 or SLCO1B1 genotype.

A genome-wide association study of 172 cases of pancreatitis secondary to thiopurine use and 2035 controls without pancreatitis sought to identify genetic factors that predispose patients to this rare complication [177c]. The class II Human Leukocyte Antigen (HLA) polymorphism rs2647087 demonstrated the strongest association with pancreatitis (OR 2.59, 95% CI: 2.07–3.26, $P = 2 \times 10^{-16}$) which conferred a 9% risk of pancreatitis with heterozygosity and 17% risk with homozygosity. The HLA-DQA1*02:01-HLA-DRB1*07:01 haplotype was also significantly associated with pancreatitis risk.

Polymorphisms in glutathione *S*-transferase mu 1 (*GSTM1*), active smoking, and older age were risk factors for development of serious adverse effects of thiopurines in a retrospective cohort study of 176 Crohn's disease patients [178c].

Drug–Drug Interactions

Allopurinol inhibits xanthine oxidase, which is one metabolic pathway of azathioprine inactivation. A study in 11 inflammatory bowel disease patients investigated this drug interaction to minimize doses of azathioprine [179c]. Combination of allopurinol 50 mg/day and azathioprine 50 mg/day was safe and effective with only one patient discontinuing therapy due to nausea.

VOCLOSPORIN

Voclosporin is a novel calcineurin inhibitor in development for immunosuppression in auto-immune diseases and following solid organ transplantation. It is a more potent inhibitor of calcineurin than (perhaps 'than?') cyclosporine but possesses many of the adverse effects and drug-interaction potential of traditional calcineurin inhibitor agents.

Drug–Drug Interactions

The interactions between voclosporin and inhibitors/inducers of CYP3A4 and P-glycoprotein (Pgp) were evaluated in 24 healthy subjects [180c]. Voclosporin 0.4 mg/kg dose was studied in combination with ketoconazole (CYP3A4 and Pgp inhibitor), rifampin (CYP3A4 inducer), midazolam (CYP3A4 substrate), verapamil (Pgp inhibitor), and digoxin (Pgp substrate). Ketoconazole increased voclosporin exposure by 18-fold. Rifampin decreased voclosporin exposure by 90%. Therefore, strong CYP3A4 inhibitors and inducers should not be co-administered with voclosporin. No changes in midazolam exposure were observed suggesting the voclosporin does not inhibit CYP3A4. Verapamil increased voclosporin exposure by 2.7-fold. Digoxin exposure

was increased 25% by voclosporin. These data suggest that voclosporin is a substrate and competitive inhibitor of Pgp and therapeutic drug monitoring should be performed if these agents are co-administered.

IMMUNOENHANCING DRUGS

LEVAMISOLE [SED-15, 2028; SEDA-34, 638; SEDA-35, 710; SEDA-36, 460]

Levamisole is an immunostimulant associated with vascular toxicity and agranulocytosis. It is a common adulterant in cocaine and therefore distinguishing causality between levamisole and adverse effects is difficult in many cases. In some cases, levamisole and cocaine may act synergistically to contribute to a negative manifestation.

Cardiovascular

In a postmortem case report, eosinophilic inflammatory coronary arteries causing acute coronary syndrome and death occurred with confirmed levamisole-adulterated cocaine [181A]. Inflammatory changes in the coronary arteries were consistent with levamisole-induced vasculitis.

A case series of 6 patients provides insights into diagnosis with a focus on differentiating levamisole vasculopathy from auto-immune disorders [182A]. All patients presented with purpuric lesions and vasculitis changes on biopsy with positive antineutrophil cytoplasmic antibody. Assessment of cocaine use in the history and physical may have aided in the diagnosis and prevented 5 of the 6 patients from being treated for auto-immune disease prior to final diagnosis of levamisole-induced vasculopathy. Levamisole-associated vasculopathy has been reported by others and often included neutropenia and vasculitis with necrosis [183A,184A,185A,186A,187A].

Nervous System

A 40-year-old female developed recurrent episodes of leukoencephalopathy from cocaine presumably containing levamisole [188A]. Complete recovery after each episode occurred while in the hospital, but upon discharge the patient continued cocaine use and developed subsequent episodes. Levamisole was likely the culprit in this case as cocaine alone is not associated with leukoencephalopathy and prior reports also implicate levamisole.

Urinary Tract

Pauci immune glomerulonephritis was described in four patients with recent history of cocaine use and signs of levamisole contamination (neutropenia or cutaneous manifestations) [189A]. Two patients recovered following prednisone and cyclophosphamide treatment, but the two others developed end-stage renal disease and dialysis dependence.

Skin

Facial cutaneous necrosis developed in a 29-year-old female cocaine abuser with suspected levamisole toxicity [190A]. A case series described four patients with known cocaine abuse that developed retiform purpura [191c]. Levamisole was proposed to be associated with worsening of this syndrome due to vasculitis effects. This has also been observed in other case reports [192A,193A].

References

[1] Masson P, Henderson L, Chapman JR, et al. Belatacept for kidney transplant recipients. Cochrane Database Syst Rev. 2014;11: Cd010699 [M].

[2] Martin ST, Tichy EM, Gabardi S. Belatacept: a novel biologic for maintenance immunosuppression after renal transplantation. Pharmacotherapy. 2011;31(4):394–407 [R].

[3] Grinyo J, Charpentier B, Pestana JM, et al. An integrated safety profile analysis of belatacept in kidney transplant recipients. Transplantation. 2010;90(12):1521–7 [C].

[4] Reynolds BC, Talbot D, Baines L, et al. Use of belatacept to maintain adequate early immunosuppression in calcineurin-mediated microangiopathic hemolysis post-renal transplant. Pediatr Transplant. 2014;18(5):E140–5 [A].

[5] Klintmalm GB, Feng S, Lake JR, et al. Belatacept-based immunosuppression in de novo liver transplant recipients: 1-year experience from a phase II randomized study. Am J Transplant. 2014;14(8):1817–27 [C].

[6] LaMattina JC, Jason MP, Hanish SI, et al. Safety of belatacept bridging immunosuppression in hepatitis C-positive liver transplant recipients with renal dysfunction. Transplantation. 2014;97(2):133–7 [c].

[7] Dobbels F, Wong S, Min Y, et al. Beneficial effect of belatacept on health-related quality of life and perceived side effects: results from the BENEFIT and BENEFIT-EXT trials. Transplantation. 2014;98(9):960–8 [C].

[8] Pestana JO, Grinyo JM, Vanrenterghem Y, et al. Three-year outcomes from BENEFIT-EXT: a phase III study of belatacept versus cyclosporine in recipients of extended criteria donor kidneys. Am J Transplant. 2012;12(3):630–9 [C].

[9] Bassil N, Rostaing L, Mengelle C, et al. Prospective monitoring of cytomegalovirus, Epstein-Barr virus, BK virus, and JC virus infections on belatacept therapy after a kidney transplant. Exp Clin Transplant. 2014;12(3):212–9 [c].

[10] Li J, Dai G, Zhang Z. General adverse response to cyclophosphamide in Chinese patients with systemic autoimmune diseases in recent decade—a single-center retrospective study. Clin Rheumatol. 2015;34(2):273–8 [c].

[11] Johnson GG, Lin K, Cox TF, et al. CYP2B6*6 is an independent determinant of inferior response to fludarabine plus cyclophosphamide in chronic lymphocytic leukemia. Blood. 2013;122(26):4253–8 [c].

[12] Zhang XW, Li C, Ma XX, et al. Short-interval lower-dose intravenous cyclophosphamide as induction and maintenance therapy for lupus nephritis: a prospective observational study. Clin Rheumatol. 2014;33(7):939–45 [c].

[13] van Laar JM, Farge D, Sont JK, et al. Autologous hematopoietic stem cell transplantation vs intravenous pulse cyclophosphamide in diffuse cutaneous systemic sclerosis: a randomized clinical trial. JAMA. 2014;311(24):2490–8 [c].

[14] Atalay F, Gulmez O, Ozsancak Ugurlu A. Cardiotoxicity following cyclophosphamide therapy: a case report. J Med Case Rep. 2014;8:252 [A].

[15] Jayaweera JL, Withana MR, Dalpatadu CK, et al. Cyclophosphamide-induced posterior reversible encephalopathy syndrome (PRES): a case report. J Med Case Rep. 2014;8:442 [A].

[16] Elazzazy S, Mohamed AE, Gulied A. Cyclophosphamide-induced symptomatic hyponatremia, a rare but severe side effect: a case report. Onco Targets Ther. 2014;7:1641–5 [A].

[17] Tulsyan S, Agarwal G, Lal P, et al. Significant role of CYP450 genetic variants in cyclophosphamide based breast cancer treatment outcomes: a multi-analytical strategy. Clin Chim Acta. 2014;434:21–8 [c].

[18] Subramaniam SR, Cader RA, Mohd R, et al. Low-dose cyclophosphamide-induced acute hepatotoxicity. Am J Case Rep. 2013;14:345–9 [A].

[19] Taniguchi T, Asano Y, Tamaki Z, et al. Late-onset anaphylactic reactions following i.v. cyclophosphamide pulse in a patient with systemic sclerosis and systemic lupus erythematosus overlap syndrome. J Dermatol. 2014;41(10):912–4 [A].

[20] El-Gowelli HM, El-Mas MM. Central modulation of cyclosporine-induced hypertension. Naunyn Schmiedebergs Arch Pharmacol. 2015;388(3):351–61 [R].

[21] Mourer JS, de Koning EJ, van Zwet EW, et al. Impact of late calcineurin inhibitor withdrawal on ambulatory blood pressure and carotid intima media thickness in renal transplant recipients. Transplantation. 2013;96(1):49–57 [c].

[22] Balint A, Farkas K, Szucs M, et al. Long-term increase in serum cholesterol levels in ulcerative colitis patients treated with cyclosporine: an underdiagnosed side effect frequently associated with other drug-related complications. Scand J Gastroenterol. 2014;49(1):59–65 [c].

[23] Odek C, Kendirli T, Yaman A, et al. Cyclosporine-associated thrombotic microangiopathy and thrombocytopenia-associated multiple organ failure: a case successfully treated with therapeutic plasma exchange. J Pediatr Hematol Oncol. 2014;36(2):e88–90 [A].

[24] Caihong Q, Weimin L, Jieming Z. Elevation of blood ciclosporin levels by voriconazole leading to leukoencephalopathy. J Pharmacol Pharmacother. 2013;4(4):294–7 [A].

[25] Pereira MJ, Palming J, Rizell M, et al. Cyclosporine A and tacrolimus reduce the amount of GLUT4 at the cell surface in human adipocytes: increased endocytosis as a potential mechanism for the diabetogenic effects of immunosuppressive agents. J Clin Endocrinol Metab. 2014;99(10):E1885–94 [E].

[26] Borda B, Lengyel C, Varkonyi T, et al. Side effects of the calcineurin inhibitor, such as new-onset diabetes after kidney transplantation. Acta Physiol Hung. 2014;101(3): 388–94 [c].

[27] Borrego-Utiel FJ, Perez-del Barrio Mdel P, Polaina-Rusillo M, et al. Painful gynaecomastia secondary to cyclosporine A and tacrolimus in a patient with focal segmental glomerulosclerosis. Nefrologia. 2013;33(6):866–7 [A].

[28] Al Sayed AA, Al Sulaiman MH, Mishriky A, et al. The role of androgen receptor gene in cyclosporine induced gingival overgrowth. J Periodontal Res. 2014;49(5):609–14 [c].

[29] Costa LC, Costa FO, Cortelli SC, et al. Gingival overgrowth in renal transplant subjects: a 44-month follow-up study. Transplantation. 2013;96(10):890–6 [c].

[30] Helenius-Hietala J, Ruokonen H, Gronroos L, et al. Oral mucosal health in liver transplant recipients and controls. Liver Transpl. 2014;20(1):72–80 [c].

[31] Jiang L, Gao MJ, Zhou J, et al. Serum cyclophilin A concentrations in renal transplant recipients receiving cyclosporine A: clinical implications for gingival overgrowth. Oral Surg Oral Med Oral Pathol Oral Radiol. 2013;116(4):447–54 [c].

[32] Lee JT, Whitson BA, Kelly RF, et al. Calcineurin inhibitors and Clostridium difficile infection in adult lung transplant recipients: the effect of cyclosporine versus tacrolimus. J Surg Res. 2013;184(1):599–604 [c].

[33] Xin HW, Liu HM, Li YQ, et al. Association of CYP3A4*18B and CYP3A5*3 polymorphism with cyclosporine-related liver injury in Chinese renal transplant recipients. Int J Clin Pharmacol Ther. 2014;52(6):497–503 [c].

[34] Franca FD, Ferreira AF, Lara RC, et al. Role of protein kinase A signaling pathway in cyclosporine nephrotoxicity. Toxicol Mech Methods. 2014;24(6):369–76 [E].

[35] Korolczuk A, Maciejewski M, Smolen A, et al. The role of peroxisome-proliferator-activating receptor gamma agonists: rosiglitazone and 15-deoxy-delta(12,14)-prostaglandin J2 in chronic experimental cyclosporine A-induced nephrotoxicity. J Physiol Pharmacol. 2014;65(6):867–76 [E].

[36] Piao SG, Kang SH, Lim SW, et al. Influence of N-acetylcysteine on Klotho expression and its signaling pathway in experimental model of chronic cyclosporine nephropathy in mice. Transplantation. 2013;96(2):146–53 [E].

[37] Wu Y, Zhang J, Liu F, et al. Protective effects of HBSP on ischemia reperfusion and cyclosporine a induced renal injury. Clin Dev Immunol. 2013;2013:758159 [E].

[38] El-Gowelli HM, Helmy MW, Ali RM, et al. Celecoxib offsets the negative renal influences of cyclosporine via modulation of the TGF-beta1/IL-2/COX-2/endothelin ET(B) receptor cascade. Toxicol Appl Pharmacol. 2014;275(2):88–95 [E].

[39] Endo A, Someya T, Nakagawa M, et al. Synergistic protective effects of mizoribine and angiotensin II receptor blockade on cyclosporine A nephropathy in rats. Pediatr Res. 2014;75(1–1):38–44 [E].

[40] Loar RW, Driscoll DJ, Kushwaha SS, et al. Empiric switch from calcineurin inhibitor to sirolimus-based immunosuppression in pediatric heart transplantation recipients. Pediatr Transplant. 2013;17(8):794–9 [c].

[41] Acikgoz G, Caliskan E, Tunca M, et al. The effect of oral cyclosporine in the treatment of severe alopecia areata. Cutan Ocul Toxicol. 2014;33(3):247–52 [c].

[42] Umeda K, Adachi S, Tanaka S, et al. Comparison of continuous and twice-daily infusions of cyclosporine A for graft-versus-host-disease prophylaxis in pediatric hematopoietic stem cell transplantation. Pediatr Blood Cancer. 2014; http://dx.doi.org/10.1002/pbc.25243 [Epub ahead of print] [c].

[43] Kikuchi M, Okuda Y, Ueda Y, et al. Successful telaprevir treatment in combination of cyclosporine against recurrence of hepatitis C in the Japanese liver transplant patients. Biol Pharm Bull. 2014;37(3):417–23 [c].

[44] Kwan LP, Mok MM, Ma MK, et al. Acute drug toxicity related to drinking herbal tea in a kidney transplant recipient. Ren Fail. 2014;36(2):309–12 [A].

[45] Al-Niaimi F, Lyon CC. Acute kidney injury due to interaction of methyl-1-testosterone with ciclosporin metabolism in a patient with severe atopic dermatitis. Dermatol Ther (Heidelb). 2013;3(2):211–4 [A].

[46] Bernard E, Goutelle S, Bertrand Y, et al. Pharmacokinetic drug-drug interaction of calcium channel blockers with cyclosporine in hematopoietic stem cell transplant children. Ann Pharmacother. 2014;48(12):1580–4 [c].

[47] Bleyzac N, Kebaili K, Mialou V, et al. Pharmacokinetic drug interaction between cyclosporine and imatinib in bone marrow transplant children and model-based reappraisal of imatinib drug interaction profile. Ther Drug Monit. 2014;36(6):724–9 [c].

[48] Brennan BJ, Moreira SA, Morcos PN, et al. Pharmacokinetics of a three-way drug interaction between danoprevir, ritonavir and the organic anion transporting polypeptide (OATP) inhibitor ciclosporin. Clin Pharmacokinet. 2013;52(9):805–13 [c].

[49] Sanchez R, Picard N, Mouly-Bandini A, et al. Severe decrease of cyclosporine levels in a heart transplant recipient receiving the direct thrombin inhibitor argatroban. Ther Drug Monit. 2014;36(3):273–7 [A].

[50] Teng R, Kujacic M, Hsia J. Pharmacokinetic interaction study of ticagrelor and cyclosporine in healthy volunteers. Clin Drug Investig. 2014;34(8):529–36 [c].

[51] dos Santos AG, Guardia AC, Pereira TS, et al. Rhabdomyolysis as a clinical manifestation of association with ciprofibrate, sirolimus, cyclosporine, and pegylated interferon-alpha in liver-transplanted patients: a case report and literature review. Transplant Proc. 2014;46(6):1887–8 [A].

[52] Scarfia RV, Clementi A, Granata A. Rhabdomyolysis and acute kidney injury secondary to interaction between simvastatin and cyclosporine. Ren Fail. 2013;35(7):1056–7 [A].

[53] Wannhoff A, Weiss KH, Schemmer P, et al. Increased levels of rivaroxaban in patients after liver transplantation treated with cyclosporine A. Transplantation. 2014;98(2):e12–3 [c].

[54] Bayers SL, Arkin L, Bohaty B, et al. Neurotoxicity in the setting of pediatric atopic dermatitis treated with modified cyclosporine and itraconazole. J Am Acad Dermatol. 2013;69(4):e177–8 [A].

[55] Kojima T, Imai Y, Fujiu K, et al. An elevated cibenzoline level interacted with cyclosporine caused ventricular tachyarrhythmia and high defibrillation threshold in hypertrophic cardiomyopathy. Int J Cardiol. 2013;168(1):e24–6 [A].

[56] Ravaud A, Urva SR, Grosch K, et al. Relationship between everolimus exposure and safety and efficacy: meta-analysis of clinical trials in oncology. Eur J Cancer. 2014;50(3):486–95 [M].

[57] Wesolowski R, Abdel-Rasoul M, Lustberg M, et al. Treatment-related mortality with everolimus in cancer patients. Oncologist. 2014;19(6):661–8 [M].

[58] Abdel-Rahman O, Fouad M. Risk of mucocutaneous toxicities in patients with solid tumors treated with everolimus; a systematic review and meta-analysis. Expert Rev Anticancer Ther. 2014;14(12):1529–36 [M].

[59] Zaza G, Tomei P, Ria P, et al. Systemic and nonrenal adverse effects occurring in renal transplant patients treated with mTOR inhibitors. Clin Dev Immunol. 2013;2013:403280 [R].

[60] Barroso-Sousa R, Santana IA, Testa L, et al. Biological therapies in breast cancer: common toxicities and management strategies. Breast. 2013;22(6):1009–18 [R].

[61] Soulieres D. Side-effects associated with targeted therapies in renal cell carcinoma. Curr Opin Support Palliat Care. 2013;7(3):254–7 [R].

[62] Xu J, Tian D. Hematologic toxicities associated with mTOR inhibitors temsirolimus and everolimus in cancer patients: a systematic review and meta-analysis. Curr Med Res Opin. 2014;30(1):67–74 [R].

[63] Kotulska K, Chmielewski D, Borkowska J, et al. Long-term effect of everolimus on epilepsy and growth in children under 3 years of age treated for subependymal giant cell astrocytoma associated with tuberous sclerosis complex. Eur J Paediatr Neurol. 2013;17(5):479–85 [c].

[64] Krueger DA, Wilfong AA, Holland-Bouley K, et al. Everolimus treatment of refractory epilepsy in tuberous sclerosis complex. Ann Neurol. 2013;74(5):679–87 [c].

[65] Wiegand G, May TW, Ostertag P, et al. Everolimus in tuberous sclerosis patients with intractable epilepsy: a treatment option? Eur J Paediatr Neurol. 2013;17(6):631–8 [c].

[66] Aapro M, Andre F, Blackwell K, et al. Adverse event management in patients with advanced cancer receiving oral everolimus: focus on breast cancer. Ann Oncol. 2014;25(4):763–73 [R].

[67] Campone M, Bachelot T, Gnant M, et al. Effect of visceral metastases on the efficacy and safety of everolimus in postmenopausal women with advanced breast cancer: subgroup analysis from the BOLERO-2 study. Eur J Cancer. 2013;49(12):2621–32 [C].

[68] Campone M, Beck JT, Gnant M, et al. Health-related quality of life and disease symptoms in postmenopausal women with HR(+), HER2(−) advanced breast cancer treated with everolimus plus exemestane versus exemestane monotherapy. Curr Med Res Opin. 2013;29(11):1463–73 [c].

[69] Chen A, Chen L, Al-Qaisi A, et al. Everolimus-induced hematologic changes in patients with metastatic breast cancer. Clin Breast Cancer. 2015;15(1):48–53 [c].

[70] Rugo HS, Pritchard KI, Gnant M, et al. Incidence and time course of everolimus-related adverse events in postmenopausal women with hormone receptor-positive advanced breast cancer: insights from BOLERO-2. Ann Oncol. 2014;25(4):808–15 [C].

[71] Murbraech K, Holdaas H, Massey R, et al. Cardiac response to early conversion from calcineurin inhibitor to everolimus in renal transplant recipients: an echocardiographic substudy of the randomized controlled CENTRAL trial. Transplantation. 2014;97(2):184–8 [c].

[72] Fukushima N, Saito S, Sakata Y, et al. A case of everolimus-associated chylothorax in a cardiac transplant recipient. Transplant Proc. 2013;45(8):3144–6 [A].

[73] Baas MC, Gerdes VE, Ten Berge IJ, et al. Treatment with everolimus is associated with a procoagulant state. Thromb Res. 2013;132(2):307–11 [c].

[74] Baas MC, Struijk GH, Moes DJ, et al. Interstitial pneumonitis caused by everolimus: a case-cohort study in renal transplant recipients. Transpl Int. 2014;27(5):428–36 [c].

[75] Atkinson BJ, Cauley DH, Ng C, et al. Mammalian target of rapamycin (mTOR) inhibitor-associated non-infectious pneumonitis in patients with renal cell cancer: predictors, management, and outcomes. BJU Int. 2014;113(3):376–82 [c].

[76] Willemsen AE, Grutters JC, Gerritsen WR, et al. Caution for interstitial lung disease as a cause of CA 15–3 rise in advanced breast cancer patients treated with everolimus. Int J Cancer. 2014;135(4):1007 [c].

[77] Junpaparp P, Sharma B, Samiappan A, et al. Everolimus-induced severe pulmonary toxicity with diffuse alveolar hemorrhage. Ann Am Thorac Soc. 2013;10(6):727–9 [A].

[78] Peng L, Zhou Y, Ye X, et al. Treatment-related fatigue with everolimus and temsirolimus in patients with cancer-a meta-analysis of clinical trials. Tumour Biol. 2015;36(2):643–54 [M].

[79] Ha SH, Park JH, Jang HR, et al. Increased risk of everolimus-associated acute kidney injury in cancer patients with impaired kidney function. BMC Cancer. 2014;14:906 [c].

[80] Miura M, Yanai M, Fukasawa Y, et al. De novo proteinuria with pathological evidence of glomerulonephritis after everolimus induction. Nephrology (Carlton). 2014;19(Suppl 3):57–9 [A].

[81] Belliere J, Guilbeau-Frugier C, Del Bello A, et al. Beneficial effect of conversion to belatacept in kidney-transplant patients with a low glomerular-filtration rate. Case Rep Transplant. 2014;2014:190516 [A].

[82] Teplinsky E, Cheung D, Weisberg I, et al. Fatal hepatitis B reactivation due to everolimus in metastatic breast cancer: case report and review of literature. Breast Cancer Res Treat. 2013;141(2):167–72 [A].

[83] Schieren G, Bolke E, Scherer A, et al. Severe everolimus-induced steatohepatis: a case report. Eur J Med Res. 2013;18:22 [A].

[84] Grabowsky JA. Drug interactions and the pharmacist: focus on everolimus. Ann Pharmacother. 2013;47(7–8):1055–63 [R].

[85] Lecefel C, Eloy P, Chauvin B, et al. Worsening pneumonitis due to a pharmacokinetic drug-drug interaction between everolimus and voriconazole in a renal transplant patient. J Clin Pharm Ther. 2015;40(1):119–20 [A].

[86] Mir O, Poinsignon V, Arnedos M, et al. Pharmacokinetic interaction involving fenofibrate and everolimus. Ann Oncol. 2015;26(1):248–9 [A].

[87] Verdier MC, Patrat-Delon S, Lemaitre F, et al. Suspicion of interaction between maribavir and everolimus in a renal transplant recipient. Transplantation. 2014;98(3):e20–1 [A].

[88] Wanitchanont A, Somparn P, Vadcharavivad S, et al. Effects of atorvastatin on the pharmacokinetics of everolimus among kidney transplant recipients. Transplant Proc. 2014;46(2):418–21 [c].

[89] Perricone G, Mancuso A, Belli LS, et al. Sorafenib for the treatment of recurrent hepatocellular carcinoma after liver transplantation: does mTOR inhibitors association augment toxicity? Eur J Gastroenterol Hepatol. 2014;26(5):577–8 [c].

[90] Calabresi PA, Radue EW, Goodin D, et al. Safety and efficacy of fingolimod in patients with relapsing-remitting multiple sclerosis (FREEDOMS II): a double-blind, randomised, placebo-controlled, phase 3 trial. Lancet Neurol. 2014;13(6):545–56 [C].

[91] Gold R, Comi G, Palace J, et al. Assessment of cardiac safety during fingolimod treatment initiation in a real-world relapsing multiple sclerosis population: a phase 3b, open-label study. J Neurol. 2014;261(2):267–76 [c].

[92] Fragoso YD, Arruda CC, Arruda WO, et al. The real-life experience with cardiovascular complications in the first dose of fingolimod for multiple sclerosis. Arq Neuropsiquiatr. 2014;72(9):712–4 [c].

[93] Rolf L, Muris AH, Damoiseaux J, et al. Paroxysmal atrial fibrillation after initiation of fingolimod for multiple sclerosis treatment. Neurology. 2014;82(11):1008–9 [A].

[94] Voon V, Saiva L, O'Kelly S, et al. Fingolimod-induced atrioventricular conduction defects in a young lady with multiple sclerosis—insights into possible drug mechanism. Eur J Clin Pharmacol. 2014;70(3):373–5 [A].

[95] Hojer J, Olsson E. AV block II in a toddler after ingestion of a single tablet fingolimod. Clin Toxicol (Phila). 2014;52(6):644 [A].

[96] Thoo S, Cugati S, Lee A, et al. Successful treatment of fingolimod-associated macular edema with intravitreal triamcinolone with continued fingolimod use. Mult Scler. 2015;21(2):249–51 [A].

[97] Warnke C, Dehmel T, Ramanujam R, et al. Initial lymphocyte count and low BMI may affect fingolimod-induced lymphopenia. Neurology. 2014;83(23):2153–7 [c].

[98] Lysandropoulos AP, Benghiat F. Severe auto-immune hemolytic anemia in a fingolimod-treated multiple sclerosis patient. Mult Scler. 2013;19(11):1551–2 [A].

[99] Masera S, Chiavazza C, Mattioda A, et al. Occurrence of ecchymotic angioedema-like cutaneous lesions as a possible side effect of fingolimod. Mult Scler. 2014;20(12):1666–7 [A].

[100] Artemiadis A, Nikolaou G, Kolokythopoulos D, et al. Visceral leishmaniasis infection in a fingolimod-treated multiple sclerosis patient. Mult Scler. 2015;21(6):795–6 [A].

[101] Karlsson G, Francis G, Koren G, et al. Pregnancy outcomes in the clinical development program of fingolimod in multiple sclerosis. Neurology. 2014;82(8):674–80 [c].

[102] Michaud CJ, Bockheim HM, Nabeel M. Diagnosis of exclusion: a case report of probable glatiramer acetate-induced eosinophilic myocarditis. Case Rep Neurol Med. 2014;2014:786342 [A].

[103] Makhani N, Ngan BY, Kamath BM, et al. Glatiramer acetate-induced acute hepatotoxicity in an adolescent with MS. Neurology. 2013;81(9):850–2 [A].

[104] Antezana A, Herbert J, Park J, et al. Glatiramer acetate-induced acute hepatotoxicity in an adolescent with MS. Neurology. 2014;82(20):1846–7 [A].

[105] Rutanen J, Kononoff A, Arstila L, et al. Five cases of interstitial lung disease after leflunomide was combined with methotrexate therapy. Scand J Rheumatol. 2014;43(3):254–6 [A].

[106] Roubille C, Haraoui B. Interstitial lung diseases induced or exacerbated by DMARDS and biologic agents in rheumatoid arthritis: a systematic literature review. Semin Arthritis Rheum. 2014;43(5):613–26 [R].

[107] Frances L, Guijarro J, Marin I, et al. Multiple eruptive keratoacanthomas associated with leflunomide. Dermatol Online J. 2013;19(7):18968 [A].

[108] Hopkins AM, O'Doherty CE, Foster DJ, et al. The rheumatoid arthritis susceptibility polymorphism PTPN22 C1858T is not associated with leflunomide response or toxicity. J Clin Pharm Ther. 2014;39(5):555–60 [c].

[109] Kharfan-Dabaja M, Mhaskar R, Reljic T, et al. Mycophenolate mofetil versus methotrexate for prevention of graft-versus-host disease in people receiving allogeneic hematopoietic stem cell transplantation. Cochrane Database Syst Rev. 2014;7: CD010280 [M].

[110] Vanhove T, Kuypers D, Claes KJ, et al. Reasons for dose reduction of mycophenolate mofetil during the first year after renal transplantation and its impact on graft outcome. Transpl Int. 2013;26(8):813–21 [c].

[111] Shin BC, Chung JH, Kim HL. Sirolimus: a switch option for mycophenolate mofetil-induced leukopenia in renal transplant recipients. Transplant Proc. 2013;45(8):2968–9 [A].

[112] Sobiak J, Kaminska J, Glyda M, et al. Effect of mycophenolate mofetil on hematological side effects incidence in renal transplant recipients. Clin Transplant. 2013;27(4):E407–14 [c].

[113] Woillard JB, Picard N, Thierry A, et al. Associations between polymorphisms in target, metabolism, or transport proteins of mycophenolate sodium and therapeutic or adverse effects in kidney transplant patients. Pharmacogenet Genomics. 2014;24(5):256–62 [c].

[114] Staatz CE, Tett SE. Pharmacology and toxicology of mycophenolate in organ transplant recipients: an update. Arch Toxicol. 2014;88(7):1351–89 [R].

[115] Qasim M, Rahman H, Ahmed R, et al. Mycophenolic acid mediated disruption of the intestinal epithelial tight junctions. Exp Cell Res. 2014;322(2):277–89 [E].

[116] Vu D, Tellez-Corrales E, Yang J, et al. Genetic polymorphisms of UGT1A8, UGT1A9 and HNF-1alpha and gastrointestinal symptoms in renal transplant recipients taking mycophenolic acid. Transpl Immunol. 2013;29(1–4):155–61 [c].

[117] Gorgan M, Bockorny B, Lawlor M, et al. Pulmonary hemorrhage with capillaritis secondary to mycophenolate mofetil in a heart-transplant patient. Arch Pathol Lab Med. 2013;137(11):1684–7 [A].

[118] Kim JM, Kwon CH, Yun IJ, et al. A multicenter experience with generic mycophenolate mofetil conversion in stable liver transplant recipients. Ann Surg Treat Res. 2014;86(4):192–8 [c].

[119] Sterneck M, Settmacher U, Ganten T, et al. Improvement in gastrointestinal and health-related quality of life outcomes after conversion from mycophenolate mofetil to enteric-coated mycophenolate sodium in liver transplant recipients. Transplant Proc. 2014;46(1):234–40 [c].

[120] Lopez-Solis R, DeVera M, Steel J, et al. Gastrointestinal side effects in liver transplant recipients taking enteric-coated mycophenolate sodium vs. mycophenolate mofetil. Clin Transplant. 2014;28(7):783–8 [c].

[121] Knorr JP, Sjeime M, Braitman LE, et al. Concomitant proton pump inhibitors with mycophenolate mofetil and the risk of rejection in kidney transplant recipients. Transplantation. 2014;97(5):518–24 [c].

[122] Xu L, Cai M, Shi BY, et al. A prospective analysis of the effects of enteric-coated mycophenolate sodium and mycophenolate mofetil co-medicated with a proton pump inhibitor in kidney transplant recipients at a single institute in China. Transplant Proc. 2014;46(5):1362–5 [c].

[123] Kodawara T, Masuda S, Yano Y, et al. Inhibitory effect of ciprofloxacin on beta-glucuronidase-mediated deconjugation of mycophenolic acid glucuronide. Biopharm Drug Dispos. 2014;35(5):275–83 [E].

[124] Liu YM, Shao YQ, He Q. Sirolimus for treatment of autosomal-dominant polycystic kidney disease: a meta-analysis of randomized controlled trials. Transplant Proc. 2014;46(1):66–74 [M].

[125] Verhave J, Boucher A, Dandavino R, et al. The incidence, management, and evolution of rapamycin-related side effects in kidney transplant recipients. Clin Transplant. 2014;28(5):616–22 [c].

[126] Baliu C, Esforzado N, Campistol JM, et al. Chronic lymphedema in renal transplant recipients under immunosuppression with sirolimus: presentation of 2 cases. JAMA Dermatol. 2014;150(9):1023–4 [A].

[127] Ozcan D, Seckin D, Ada S, et al. Mucocutaneous disorders in renal transplant recipients receiving sirolimus-based immunosuppressive therapy: a prospective, case–control study. Clin Transplant. 2013;27(5):742–8 [c].

[128] Woillard JB, Kamar N, Coste S, et al. Effect of CYP3A4*22, POR*28, and PPARα rs4253728 on sirolimus in vitro metabolism and trough concentrations in kidney transplant recipients. Clin Chem. 2013;59(12):1761–9 [c].

[129] Hong YA, Kim HD, Jo K, et al. Severe rhabdomyolysis associated with concurrent use of simvastatin and sirolimus after cisplatin-based chemotherapy in a kidney transplant recipient. Exp Clin Transplant. 2014;12(2):152–5 [A].

[130] Masters JC, Shah MM, Feist AA. Drug interaction between sirolimus and ranolazine in a kidney transplant patient. Case Rep Transplant. 2014;2014:548243 [A].

[131] Kim YC, Chin HJ, Koo HS, et al. Tacrolimus decreases albuminuria in patients with IgA nephropathy and normal blood pressure: a double-blind randomized controlled trial of efficacy of tacrolimus on IgA nephropathy. PLoS One. 2013;8(8):e71545 [c].

[132] Bansal D, Yadav AK, Kumar V, et al. Deferred pre-emptive switch from calcineurin inhibitor to sirolimus leads to improvement in GFR and expansion of T regulatory cell population: a randomized, controlled trial. PLoS One. 2013;8(10):e75591 [c].

[133] Fazal MA, Idrees MK, Akhtar SF. Dyslipidaemia among renal transplant recipients: cyclosporine versus tacrolimus. J Pak Med Assoc. 2014;64(5):496–9 [c].

[134] Varghese J, Reddy MS, Venugopal K, et al. Tacrolimus-related adverse effects in liver transplant recipients: its association with trough concentrations. Indian J Gastroenterol. 2014;33(3):219–25 [c].

[135] Wu Z, Meng Q, Xia Y, et al. A retrospective analysis of the safety and efficacy of low dose tacrolimus (FK506) for living donor liver transplant recipients. J Biomed Res. 2013;27(4): 305–9 [c].

[136] Ramachandran R, Kumar V, Rathi M, et al. Tacrolimus therapy in adult-onset steroid-resistant nephrotic syndrome due to a focal segmental glomerulosclerosis single-center experience. Nephrol Dial Transplant. 2014;29(10):1918–24 [c].

[137] Nayagam LS, Vijayanand B, Balasubramanian S. Massive pleural effusion in a renal transplant recipient on tacrolimus. Indian J Nephrol. 2014;24(5):318–20 [A].

[138] Arnold R, Pussell BA, Pianta TJ, et al. Association between calcineurin inhibitor treatment and peripheral nerve dysfunction in renal transplant recipients. Am J Transplant. 2013;13(9):2426–32 [c].

[139] Apuri S, Carlin K, Bass E, et al. Tacrolimus associated posterior reversible encephalopathy syndrome—a case series and review. Mediterr J Hematol Infect Dis. 2014;6(1):e2014014 [A].

[140] Wu G, Weng FL, Balaraman V. Tacrolimus-induced encephalopathy and polyneuropathy in a renal transplant recipient. BMJ Case Rep. 2013, http://dx.doi.org/10.1136/bcr-2013-201099. pii: bcr2013201099 [A].

[141] Gulleroglu K, Baskin E, Bayrakci U, et al. Sudden hearing loss associated with tacrolimus after pediatric renal transplant. Exp Clin Transplant. 2013;11(6):562–4 [A].

[142] Xie M, Rao W, Sun LY, et al. Tacrolimus-related seizure after pediatric liver transplantation—a single-center experience. Pediatr Transplant. 2014;18(1):58–63 [A].

[143] Rangel EB. Tacrolimus in pancreas transplant: a focus on toxicity, diabetogenic effect and drug-drug interactions. Expert Opin Drug Metab Toxicol. 2014;10(11):1585–605 [R].

[144] Sarkar S, Mondal R, Nandi M, et al. Tacrolimus induced diabetic ketoacidosis in nephrotic syndrome. Indian J Pediatr. 2013;80(7):596–7 [A].

[145] Amorim J, Costa E, Teixeira A, et al. Tacrolimus-induced neutropenia in a cardiac transplant patient. Pediatr Transplant. 2014;18(1):120–1 [A].

[146] Gillard P, Rustandi M, Efendi A, et al. Early alteration of kidney function in nonuremic type 1 diabetic islet transplant recipients under tacrolimus-mycophenolate therapy. Transplantation. 2014;98(4):451–7 [c].

[147] Sy SK, Heuberger J, Shilbayeh S, et al. A Markov chain model to evaluate the effect of CYP3A5 and ABCB1 polymorphisms on adverse events associated with tacrolimus in pediatric renal transplantation. AAPS J. 2013;15(4):1189–99 [c].

[148] Elens L, Sombogaard F, Hesselink DA, et al. Single-nucleotide polymorphisms in P450 oxidoreductase and peroxisome proliferator-activated receptor-alpha are associated with the development of new-onset diabetes after transplantation in kidney transplant recipients treated with tacrolimus. Pharmacogenet Genomics. 2013;23(12):649–57.

[149] Tavira B, Gomez J, Diaz-Corte C, et al. Mitochondrial DNA haplogroups and risk of new-onset diabetes among tacrolimus-treated renal transplanted patients. Gene. 2014;538(1):195–8 [c].

[150] van Boekel GA, Kerkhofs CH, Hilbrands LB. Treatment satisfaction in renal transplant patients taking tacrolimus once daily. Clin Ther. 2013;35(11) 1821–9.e1 [c].

[151] Olson KA, West K, McCarthy PL. Toxic tacrolimus levels after application of topical tacrolimus and use of occlusive dressings in two bone marrow transplant recipients with cutaneous graft-versus-host disease. Pharmacotherapy. 2014;34(6):e60–4 [c].

[152] Nadeem A, Sayed-Ahmed MM, Alabidy AD, et al. Co-administration of ketoconazole and tacrolimus to kidney transplant recipients: cost minimization and potential metabolic benefits. Biomed Res Int. 2014;25(4):814–8 [A].

[153] Yousuf Bhat Z, Reddy S, Pillai U, et al. Colchicine-induced myopathy in a tacrolimus-treated renal transplant recipient: case report and literature review. Am J Ther. 2014; http://dx.doi.org/10.1097/mjt.0000000000000044 [Epub ahead of print] [A].

[154] Bax K, Tijssen J, Rieder MJ, et al. Rapid resolution of tacrolimus intoxication-induced AKI with a corticosteroid and phenytoin. Ann Pharmacother. 2014;48(11):1525–8 [A].

[155] Carbajal R, Yisfalem A, Pradhan N, et al. Case report: boldo (Peumus boldus) and tacrolimus interaction in a renal transplant patient. Transplant Proc. 2014;46(7):2400–2 [A].

[156] Lin S, Henning AK, Akhlaghi F, et al. Interleukin-2 receptor antagonist therapy leads to increased tacrolimus levels after kidney transplantation. Ther Drug Monit. 2015;37(2):206–13 [C].

[157] Marin-Casino M, Perez-Saez MJ, Crespo M, et al. Significant tacrolimus and dronedarone interaction in a kidney transplant recipient. Transplantation. 2014;98(4):e33–4 [A].

[158] Papadopoulos-Kohn A, Achterfeld A, Paul A, et al. Daily low-dose tacrolimus is a safe and effective immunosuppressive regimen during telaprevir-based triple therapy for hepatitis C virus recurrence after liver transplant. Transplantation. 2015;99(4):841–7 [c].

[159] Mori T, Shimizu T, Kato J, et al. Nephrotoxicity of concomitant use of tacrolimus and teicoplanin in allogeneic hematopoietic stem cell transplant recipients. Transpl Infect Dis. 2014;16(2):329–32 [c].

[160] Hou Q, Han W, Fu X. Pharmacokinetic interaction between tacrolimus and berberine in a child with idiopathic nephrotic syndrome. Eur J Clin Pharmacol. 2013;69(10):1861–2 [A].

[161] Hirsch BR, Harrison MR, George DJ, et al. Use of "Real-World" data to describe adverse events during the treatment of metastatic renal cell carcinoma in routine clinical practice. Med Oncol. 2014;31(9):156 [R].

[162] Veasey-Rodrigues H, Parsons HA, Janku F, et al. A pilot study of temsirolimus and body composition. J Cachexia Sarcopenia Muscle. 2013;4(4):259–65 [c].

[163] Mach CM, Urh A, Anderson ML. Bowel perforation associated with temsirolimus use in a recently irradiated patient. Am J Health Syst Pharm. 2014;71(11):919–23 [A].

[164] Liu X, Lorusso P, Mita M, et al. Incidence of mucositis in patients treated with temsirolimus-based regimens and correlation to treatment response. Oncologist. 2014;19(4):426–8 [c].

[165] Fujihara S, Mori H, Kobara H, et al. Life-threatening gastrointestinal bleeding during targeted therapy for advanced renal cell carcinoma: a case report. BMC Nephrol. 2013;14:141 [A].

[166] Fuggle NR, Bragoli W, Mahto A, et al. The adverse effect profile of oral azathioprine in pediatric atopic dermatitis, and recommendations for monitoring. J Am Acad Dermatol. 2015;72(1):108–14 [c].

[167] Karaahmet F, Akinci H, Ayte R, et al. Tremor as dose dependent side-effect of azathioprine in remission patient with ileal Crohn's disease. J Crohns Colitis. 2013;7(9):e404 [A].

[168] Jenkinson PW, Syed MI, McClymont L. Progressive, reversible sensorineural hearing loss caused by azathioprine. J Laryngol Otol. 2014;128(9):838–40 [A].

[169] Belen BF, Gursel T, Akyurek N, et al. Severe myelotoxicity associated with thiopurine S-methyltransferase*3A/*3C polymorphisms in a patient with pediatric leukemia and the effect of steroid therapy. Turk J Haematol. 2014;31(4):276–85 [A].

[170] Khan N, Abbas AM, Lichtenstein GR, et al. Risk of lymphoma in patients with ulcerative colitis treated with thiopurines: a nationwide retrospective cohort study. Gastroenterology. 2013;145(5) 1007–15.e3 [c].

[171] Abbas AM, Almukhtar RM, Loftus Jr. EV, et al. Risk of melanoma and non-melanoma skin cancer in ulcerative colitis patients treated with thiopurines: a nationwide retrospective cohort. Am J Gastroenterol. 2014;109(11):1781–93 [c].

[172] Ariyaratnam J, Subramanian V. Association between thiopurine use and nonmelanoma skin cancers in patients with inflammatory bowel disease: a meta-analysis. Am J Gastroenterol. 2014;109(2):163–9 [M].

[173] Beigel F, Steinborn A, Schnitzler F, et al. Risk of malignancies in patients with inflammatory bowel disease treated with thiopurines or anti-TNF alpha antibodies. Pharmacoepidemiol Drug Saf. 2014;23(7):735–44 [c].

[174] Khoury T, Ollech JE, Chen S, et al. Azathioprine-induced fever in autoimmune hepatitis. World J Gastroenterol. 2013;19(25):4083–6 [A].

[175] Ma X, Zheng J, Jin M, et al. Inosine triphosphate pyrophosphohydrolase (ITPA) polymorphic sequence variants in Chinese ALL children and possible association with mercaptopurine related toxicity. Int J Clin Exp Pathol. 2014;7(7):4552–6 [c].

[176] Roberts RL, Wallace MC, Seinen ML, et al. PACSIN2 does not influence thiopurine-related toxicity in patients with inflammatory bowel disease. Am J Gastroenterol. 2014;109(6):925–7 [c].

[177] Heap GA, Weedon MN, Bewshea CM, et al. HLA-DQA1-HLA-DRB1 variants confer susceptibility to pancreatitis induced by thiopurine immunosuppressants. Nat Genet. 2014;46(10):1131–4 [c].

[178] Mazor Y, Koifman E, Elkin H, et al. Risk factors for serious adverse effects of thiopurines in patients with Crohn's disease. Curr Drug Saf. 2013;8(3):181–5 [c].

[179] Curkovic I, Rentsch KM, Frei P, et al. Low allopurinol doses are sufficient to optimize azathioprine therapy in inflammatory bowel disease patients with inadequate thiopurine metabolite concentrations. Eur J Clin Pharmacol. 2013;69(8):1521–31 [c].

[180] Ling SY, Huizinga RB, Mayo PR, et al. Cytochrome P450 3A and P-glycoprotein drug-drug interactions with voclosporin. Br J Clin Pharmacol. 2014;77(6):1039–50 [c].

[181] Michaud K, Grabherr S, Shiferaw K, et al. Acute coronary syndrome after levamisole-adultered cocaine abuse. J Forensic Leg Med. 2014;21:48–52 [A].

[182] Strazzula L, Brown KK, Brieva JC, et al. Levamisole toxicity mimicking autoimmune disease. J Am Acad Dermatol. 2013;69(6):954–9 [A].

[183] Auffenberg C, Rosenthal LJ, Dresner N. Levamisole: a common cocaine adulterant with life-threatening side effects. Psychosomatics. 2013;54(6):590–3 [A].

[184] Belfonte CD, Shanmugam VK, Kieffer N, et al. Levamisole-induced occlusive necrotising vasculitis in cocaine abusers: an unusual cause of skin necrosis and neutropenia. Int Wound J. 2013;10(5):590–6 [A].

[185] Gillis JA, Green P, Williams J. Levamisole-induced vasculopathy: staging and management. J Plast Reconstr Aesthet Surg. 2014;67(1):e29–31 [A].

[186] Tsai MH, Yang JH, Kung SL, et al. Levamisole-induced myopathy and leukocytoclastic vasculitis: a case report and literature review. Dermatol Ther. 2013;26(6):476–80 [A].

[187] Crowe DR, Kim PS, Mutasim DF. Clinical, histopathologic, and immunofluorescence findings in levamisole/cocaine-induced thrombotic vasculitis. Int J Dermatol. 2014;53(5):635–7 [A].

[188] Gonzalez-Duarte A, Williams R. Cocaine-induced recurrent leukoencephalopathy. Neuroradiol J. 2013;26(5):511–3 [A].

[189] Carlson AQ, Tuot DS, Jen KY, et al. Pauci-immune glomerulonephritis in individuals with disease associated with levamisole-adulterated cocaine: a series of 4 cases. Medicine (Baltimore). 2014;93(17):290–7 [A].

[190] Formeister EJ, Falcone MT, Mair EA. Facial cutaneous necrosis associated with suspected levamisole toxicity from tainted cocaine abuse. Ann Otol Rhinol Laryngol. 2015;124(1):30–4 [A].

[191] Magro CM, Wang X. Cocaine-associated retiform purpura: a C5b-9-mediated microangiopathy syndrome associated with enhanced apoptosis and high levels of intercellular adhesion molecule-1 expression. Am J Dermatopathol. 2013;35(7):722–30 [c].

[192] Gaertner EM, Switlyk SA. Dermatologic complications from levamisole-contaminated cocaine: a case report and review of the literature. Cutis. 2014;93(2):102–6 [A].

[193] Souied O, Baydoun H. Levamisole-contaminated cocaine: an emergent cause of vasculitis and skin necrosis. Case Rep Med. 2014;2014:434717 [A].

38

Corticotrophins, Corticosteroids, and Prostaglandins

Alison Brophy[*,†,1], *Sidhartha D. Ray*[‡]

*Clinical Assistant Professor, Rutgers, the State University of New Jersey, NJ, USA
[†]Critical Care Clinical Pharmacist, Saint Barnabas Medical Center, Livingston, NJ, USA
[‡]Professor of Pharmaceutical Sciences, Manchester University College of Pharmacy, Fort Wayne, IN, USA
[1]Corresponding author: aabrophy@pharmacy.rutgers.edu

EDITOR'S NOTES

In this chapter adverse effects and reactions that arise from the oral or parenteral administration of corticosteroids (glucocorticoids and mineralocorticoids) are covered. Other routes of administration are discussed with in the sections after that; inhalation and nasal administration are dealt with in Chapter 16, topical administration to the skin in Chapter 14, and ocular administration in Chapter 47.

All the uses of prostaglandins are covered in this chapter, apart from topical administration to the eyes, which is covered in Chapter 47.

CORTICOTROPHINS [SED-15, 906; SEDA-33, 841; SEDA-34, 653; SEDA-35, 719; SEDA-36, 603]

Adrenalcorticotropic hormone (ACTH) is most commonly used for infantile spasm; corticosteroids are the alternative therapy for this condition. ACTH therapy is administered intramuscularly and is associated with significant cost. Therefore, ACTH is often used after failure to achieve electroencephalography (EEG) remission with steroids [1r]. ACTH has been evaluated for other indications including renal diseases [2c,3c].

Psychological

A pilot study of ACTH for nephrotic syndrome due to idiopathic membranous nephropathy included 20 patients who received 40 or 80 units subcutaneously twice weekly for 12 weeks. Six patients noted increased irritability, depression, and mood disturbance which improved when therapy was discontinued. Additionally, six patients reported transient insomnia. Other reported side effects included: Cushingoid appearance, hyperglycemia, acne, flushing, weight gain, and bruising at the injection site [2c].

Endocrine

An open-label study evaluating the effect of ACTH on proteinuria in diabetic adults compared treatment with daily subcutaneous injection of 16 or 32 units for 6 months. Partial or complete remission of proteinuria (<300 mg/24 hours) occurred in 57% of patients. In patients treated with the 32 unit dose, hemoglobin A1c rose from $8.0 \pm 0.5\%$ to $8.7 \pm 0.4\%$. A total of 14 patients completed 6 months of therapy, four patients developed refractory edema, and three patients developed hyperglycemia. Upon withdrawal of ACTH, one patient developed hypotension requiring treatment with corticosteroids and slow taper of ACTH [3c].

Infection Risk

A late, preterm, 1720 g female, twin, neonate exhibited poor response to stimuli and suck reflex despite normal EEG and negative sepsis evaluation. On day seven of life, a brain ultrasound demonstrated minimal brain edema. A follow up MRI exhibited diffuse bilateral ischemic brain damage of the basal ganglia and cystic encephalomalacia without hemorrhage. EEG on day 35 of life demonstrated no cortical activity. The patient developed seizures at 2 months treated with phenobarbital initially. After treatment escalation with phenobarbital, vigbatrin,

© 2015 Elsevier B.V. All rights reserved.

and prednisone the patient did not improve. The patient had severe microcephaly, hyperreflexia, and EEG demonstrated hypsarrhythmia. High dose ACTH (150 units/m^2) was initiated. After 7 daily doses EEG hypsarrhythmia resolved. The patient was maintained on phenobarbital, vigabatrin, and ACTH 2 doses per week for 2 weeks then 1 dose per week for 1 week. At 8 months, 1 week after completing ACTH treatment the patient was admitted to the pediatric intensive care unit requiring intubation for pneumonia. The endotracheal tube secretions were positive by PCR for *Legionella pneumophila* but also for *Pneumocystis jirovecii*. The patient was treated with meropenem, vancomycin, trimethoprim/sulfamethoxazole, immunoglobulin, and corticosteroids but ultimately expired on hospital day 10 from multiorgan failure and severe acute respiratory distress syndrome. While HIV testing was negative, flow cytometry demonstrated low T lymphocytes, including CD4+ count of 124 cells/mm^3. Authors attribute the development of infection with these pathogens to high dose ACTH therapy and the infant's complex medical history. ACTH increases release of endogenous corticosteroids which decrease innate and adaptive immunity [4A].

SYSTEMIC GLUCOCORTICOIDS [SED-15, 906; SEDA-33, 841; SEDA-34, 653; SEDA-35, 719; SEDA-36, 604]

Glucocorticoids are used extensively for a variety of both short-term and long-term indications as immunosuppressant or anti-inflammatory agents. Both prescribers and patients report a wide variety of side effects: weight gain, edema, diabetes, hypertension, psychiatric disturbances, infections, increased appetite, lipodystrophy, dyslipidaemia, development of cataracts, adrenal suppression, and infections [5c]. Recent reports of study results, reviews of existing data, and adverse reactions are presented below.

Observational Studies

An analysis of the World Health Organization multicountry survey on maternal and newborn health database included birth outcomes in 29 countries between 2010 and 2011. Antenatal steroids were given in 52%, 19%, and 24% of women who gave birth at 26–34 weeks, 22–25 weeks, and 35–36 weeks gestation, respectively. The database included over 300 000 deliveries. Authors determined this represented underutilization of the therapy in cases where potential fetal benefit was probable. Antenatal steroids have demonstrated improvement in fetal lung maturity without significant increase in maternal adverse events. [6C].

Comparative Studies

A cohort study of 230 patients with systemic lupus erythematosus compared rate of glucocorticoid damage by dosage. Patients were divided into groups receiving no prednisone, less than 7.5 mg per day (low dose), greater than 7.5 mg per day (medium-high dose), or pulse dose therapy with methylprednisolone. Avascular osteonecrosis, osteoporotic fractures, diabetes and cataracts were considered glucocorticoid related damage. Patients with medium-high dose therapy compared to no prednisone were at an increased risk of accrual of corticosteroid damage over the 5 year period (odds ratio 5.39, 95% CI 1.59–18.27). There was no difference between the subjects receiving no predinsone, the low dose group, or pulse dose therapy for damage accrual [7r].

Systematic Reviews

Use of systemic steroids for pulmonary conditions has been the subject of many reviews. Short low dose courses of steroids were determined to be efficacious for COPD exacerbations while mitigating the risk of adverse effects such as superinfection and hyperglycaemia by the authors of a recent review article. This was not a systematic review but incorporated guidelines and pertinent studies [8r]. For pediatric asthma exacerbation in the emergency department, systematic steroid therapy compared to inhaled steroid therapy resulted in no difference in rate of hospital admission or rate of unscheduled asthma visits. In the eight studies with 797 patients, there was no difference in reported vomiting between systemic and inhaled steroid groups [9r].

A Cochrane review evaluated the use of steroids for sinusitis and included 5 studies with over 1000 patients. Monotherapy with corticosteroids was associated with no benefit. However, when combined with antibiotics, steroids were associated with short-term improvement of symptoms compared to control treatments. The risk ratio for day 3 compared to day 7 resolution was 1.3 (95% CI 1.1–1.6) in favor of steroid treatment [10R].

Hypothalamic–pituitary injury which occurs after brain death, is often treated with corticosteroids to improve outcomes in organ donations. A systematic review of 25 randomized and observational studies indicated improved donor hemodynamics, oxygenation, and increased in organ procurement with corticosteroids. The most commonly used agent was methylprednisolone [11R].

A Cochrane review of corticosteroids for viral myocarditis found no mortality benefit in eight studies with 719 patients. In two studies, with 200 children, there was an increase in left ventricular ejection fraction at 3 months in the corticosteroid treated patients; however, the authors cautioned there was substantial heterogeneity in the sample population [12R].

Cardiovascular

A retrospective review of 85 percutaneous epicardial mapping and ablation procedures for ventricular tachycardia compared no corticosteroid therapy with systemic or intrapericardial steroids. Pericarditic chest pain occurred in 21.1%, 43.4%, and 58.8% of patients treated with intrapericardial, systemic or no steroids, respectively. There was a statistically significant difference between the intrapericardial steroid group and the group without steroids ($p = 0.006$). Triamcinolone 2 mg/kg was administered to the intrapericardial steroid group [13c].

Nervous System

Dexamethasone 0.1 mg/kg, 0.2 mg/kg, or placebo was administered to 1000 patients undergoing microvascular decompression surgery for facial spasm. The group which was administered 0.2 mg/kg of dexamethasone experienced a statistically significant higher incidence of postoperative cognitive dysfunction compared to the placebo and lower dose of dexamethasone. Cognitive decline included measures of attention, concentration, learning, and memory [14c]. Another study assessed cognitive functioning in young adults and adolescents who were exposed to 2–9 weeks of antenatal betamethasone compared to patients matched for age, sex, and gestational age at birth, without steroid exposure. Scores in tests of attention and speed were significantly lower in patients exposed to more than 2 courses of steroids *in utero* ($p < 0.05$). There were no differences in higher cognitive functions, self-reported attention, adaptability, or overall psychological function [15c].

Psychiatric

A literature review of 45 articles evaluated psychiatric symptoms in pediatric patients treated with steroids. The authors concluded that there was no clear correlation in timing or dose of steroids and the development of adverse psychiatric events. Corticosteroid use in acute lymphoblastic leukemia appears to be associated with negative psychiatric and behavioral effects [16r]. A prospective study evaluating 520 mechanically ventilated adults with acute lung injury identified 330 patients who developed acute delirium. Systemic corticosteroid therapy in the previous 24 hours was associated with transition to delirium, odds ratio 1.52 (95% CI 1.05–2.21) [17r]. The risk of severe neuropsychiatric disturbances during corticosteroid use is described, including a patient case vignette in a recent review. Suicide, mania, depression, panic disorder, delirium, and disorientation were described potential glucocorticoid induced adverse effects. Mechanisms include impairment from recovery of neuronal damage, decreased glucose availability in the hippocampus, and attenuation of synaptic strengthening for memory function. The authors recommend counseling

and monitoring patients for side effects. The primary treatment should be to decrease or withdrawal glucocorticoid therapy [18r].

Endocrine

A French study of 60 patients receiving long-term prednisone therapy for systemic inflammatory disorders were tested for adrenal insufficiency. After a bolus dose of 0.25 mg, 1–24 ACTH (Synacthen) was administered to patients in the morning after an overnight fast. Adrenal insufficiency was defined as plasma cortisol less than 100 nmol/L at baseline, or less than 550 nmol/L 1 hour after ACTH injection. Cumulative steroid dose and exposure were predictive for adrenal insufficiency. In those patients without adrenal insufficiency, prednisone therapy was stopped and no hydrocortisone replacement therapy was required during a mean follow up of 10 months [19c].

Hematologic

A retrospective cohort study reviewed 61 430 patients who underwent tonsillectomy between 2007 and 2013. Children who received steroids had a high rate of reoperation for bleeding compared to those who did not receive steroids 1.2% vs 0.5%, $p < 0.001$. The rates of reoperation for adults were not significantly different [20C].

Gastrointestinal

A prospective cohort study of 36 586 middle-aged women with diverticular disease evaluated medication associated risks for hospitalization. In a multivariate analysis oral corticosteroid intake was associated with increased risk of hospitalization, RR 1.37 (95% CI 1.06–1.78; $p = 0.012$) [21c]. Treatment with corticosteroids is associated with decreased wound healing in colorectal surgery. A review of 12 studies with 9564 patients identified patients who received corticosteroids and experienced anastomotic leakage. In the group receiving steroid the rate of anastomotic leak was 6.77% compared to 3.25% in the non-steroid group [22r].

Skin

A review of literature evaluating wound healing in surgical patients concluded that high dose steroids for less than 10 days had no effect. However, chronic steroid therapy for 30 days prior to surgery was associated with two to five times more wound complications. Authors speculated the mechanisms included decreased macrophage infiltration of the wound, impaired re-epithelialization, and impaired collagen turnover [23r].

Musculoskeletal

In patients treated with corticosteroids for ulcerative colitis, between 2001 and 2011 in the Veterans Affairs system, 1.4% of the 5736 patients developed fragility fractures. Dual-energy X-ray absorptiometry (DXA) screening guideline adherence rate was 23%. Patients who received DXA screening were more likely to receive calcium or bisphosphonate therapy [24c].

Sensory Systems

A total 59 eyes with cataracts in 30 children treated with chronic steroid therapy were followed for an average of 7.9 years. Progression of cataracts occurred in 34% of eyes. Three patients required bilateral cataract surgery for loss of visual acuity and progression [25c].

Infection Risk

In elderly patients with irritable bowel syndrome the rate of serious infections was higher when exposed to corticosteroids in the last 6 months, relative risk 2.3(95% CI 1.8–2.9). More than 3500 patients were included in the analysis of Canadian healthcare databases [26c]. A case report of herpes simplex associated esophagitis with total dysphagia was reported in a 72-year-old woman treated with 3 days of oral corticosteroids [27A].

Death

Three statistical models were used to evaluate the risk of death in patients from the National Emphysema Treatment trial, with stable COPD treated with long-term oral corticosteroids. All three models demonstrated statistically significant increased risk of death when steroids were administered; however, it appeared as though the patients treated with corticosteroids had more severe COPD [28r]. In a study of 779 patients treated for rheumatoid arthritis risk of cardiovascular death was greater in patients treated with 8–15 mg per day of prednisone compared to no steroids, HR 1.78 (95% CI 1.22–2.60). The minimal total exposure prednisone dose associated with all-cause mortality increase was 40 g, HR 1.74(95% CI 1.25–2.44) [29c].

Tumorgenicity

The authors of an editorial discussing castration resistant prostate cancer highlighted that androgen receptors could be activated by corticosteroids in the absence of testosterone. Corticosteroids should be avoided in advanced androgen receptor positive prostate cancers to avoid tumor growth [30r].

Drug Interactions

A 48-year-old female patient was treated for Crohn's disease with oral budesonide 9 mg per day and developed fluconazole resistant *Candida albicans* esophagitis. Treatment with voriconazole 200 mg every 12 hours for 3 weeks was prescribed. After recurrent symptoms of dysphagia a second course was started. The patient presented to her physician with hypertension, edema, and weight gain. Six weeks later she presented again with hypertension, moon face, posterior cervical fat pad prominence and pitting edema. Voriconazole is a cytochrome P450 3A4 substrate and inhibitor. Budesonide has low systemic activity due to first pass metabolism by the 3A4 enzyme. The combination resulted in iatrogenic Cushing's syndrome which regressed over the following 2 months [31A].

Pharmacogenomics

The response to corticosteroid treatment was evaluated in 35 Korean children and 70 Korean adults after screening for single nucleotide polymorphisms (SNP) in histone deacetylase (HDAC) 1 and HDAC2. RS1741981, was a SNP in HDAC1, associated with asthma severity ($p = 0.036$). Response to corticosteroid therapy, defined as percent increase in FEV1, was decreased in adult patients who were heterozygous or homozygous for the major allele 12.7% vs 37.4%, $p = 0.018$. Similar findings were reported in children, 14.1% vs 19.4%, $p = 0.035$ [32C].

PROSTAGLANDINS AND ANALOGUES
[SED-15, 2955; SEDA-33, 846; SEDA-34, 660; SEDA-35, 725]

See also Chapter 47.

Prostaglandin and prostaglandin therapy is associated with a variety of indications including pulmonary arterial hypertension, glaucoma, and obstetrical diseases. Pulmonary artery hypertension (PAH) is the increase in pulmonary vascular pressures which can be complicated by right heart failure and progress until death. A variety of pulmonary dilating therapies are available for PAH; however, prostanoids are a mainstay of treatment. Prostanoids have vasodilating, antithrombotic, antiproliferative, and anti-inflammatory properties. Prostanoid epoprostenol and the analogs iloprost, and treprostinil are available products for PAH therapy [33r].

Systematic Reviews

A meta-analysis of 14 trials with 2244 patients evaluated prostanoid therapy. All-cause mortality rate was reduced by 44%, RR 0.56 (95% CI 0.35–0.88; $p = 0.01$). In a subgroup analysis, only IV therapy showed survival benefit, RR 0.36 (95% CI 0.16–0.79; $p = 0.011$). Risk of clinical worsening, 6-minute walk distance, and hemodynamic parameters were all improved by prostanoid therapy. In 10 of the studies, 5.86% of patients withdrew from treatment with prostanoids due to adverse effects. In a subgroup analysis, subcutaneous and oral administration routes were associated with increased withdrawal from therapy due to adverse side effects. Intravenous therapy was not associated with this risk [34R].

Observational Studies

A study of 8 adult patients sought to evaluate long-term effects of prostanoid therapies in patient with PAH from congenital heart disease. The average duration of therapy was 1 year. Improvements in pulmonary artery pressures and oxygenation were significant. There was no significant decline in systemic blood pressure or systemic oxygen saturation [35c].

Epoprostenol (PGI$_2$)

Observational Studies

A review of the FDA database for adverse events in the treatment of PAH in children identified 554 records from 1997 to 2009. A total of 157 events were identified in treatment with epoprostenol. Pulmonary hemorrhage (13.1%) and cardiac failure (9.7%) were unique events noted by the authors [36c].

Cardiovascular

Hypotension is a common adverse event associated with initiation of epoprostenol therapy. A prospective study of initiation of epoprostenol therapy in 71 patients evaluated the use of dobutamine and dopamine to treat hypotension or hypoxia. A total of 46 patients required hemodynamic support which was not associated with short-term mortality risk [37c].

A 30-year-old women was treated for PAH with epoprostenol over 2 years. Her dose was increased to 75 ng/kg/min and she developed ascites which accumulated over several months and led to hospitalization. Large volume paracentesis was performed but fluid re-accumulated. The fluid was a transudate and alternative causes of ascites were ruled out: lymphoma, hypoproteinemia, portal hypertension, and lymph vessel obstruction. The dose of epoprostenol was reduced to 66 ng/kg/min leading to reduction patients waist circumference and weight with no worsening of PAH symptoms. The right heart catheterization procedure at the time identified high cardiac output failure which was attributed to the high dose of epoprostenol [38A].

Drug Formulations

Continuous infusion of epoprostenol was initially limited due to product stability at room temperature. The EPITOME-1 study compared treatment with epoprostenol formulated with arginine–mannitol (EPO-AM) to epoprostenol formulated with glycine–mannitol (EPO-GM). EPO-AM is stable at room temperature while EPO-GM is not and requires cooling with ice packs. This prospective, open-label, multicenter study randomized 30 patients with PAH. The adverse effects reported included flushing, headache, jaw pain, and nausea [39c]. The EPITOME-2 study transitioned patients treated with EPO-GM to epoprostenol with arginine and sucrose excipients. This was an open-label, prospective, single arm, phase IIIb study including 41 patients. No differences in efficacy or toxicity were observed with the arginine–sucrose product. Reported adverse effects included headache, nasopharyngitis, jaw pain, flushing, dyspnea, device connection issues, epistaxis, extremity pain, and palpitations [40c].

Iloprost (PGI$_2$ Analogue) [SED-15, 1716; SEDA-33, 847; SEDA-34, 660; SEDA-35, 726]

Comparative Studies

Patients with stage IIb peripheral arterial disease were randomized to receive standard care or standard care and iloprost continuous infusion for 6 hours per day over 10 days. Treatment was re-administered every third month for 1 year. Iloprost increased exercise capacity compared to standard care. Three patients (5.9%) patients withdrew due to adverse events which were drug related. Adverse effects included flushing, headache, and gastrointestinal bleeding [41c].

Cardiovascular

Iloprost was evaluated for preterm neonates and newborns with PAH. In 33 neonates oxygenation was improved with continuous infusion of iloprost. However, after the initiation of iloprost there was a statistically significant increase in the need for inotropic medications to treat hypotension ($p < 0.01$) [42c].

Pulmonary

Twenty patients with acute respiratory distress syndrome were administered nebulized iloprost. Improvement in PaO$_2$:FiO$_2$ ratio from a mean of 177–213 was statistically significant. No significant alternations in air pressures, systemic blood pressure, or heart rate were identified [43c].

Infection Risk

Catheter related bloodstream infections (CR-BSI) have been reported in patients receiving continuous prostanoid therapy. A study of one United Kingdom hospital records reviewed all patients with iloprost therapy between 2007 and 2012. A rate of 0.65 CR-BSI per 1000 treatment days was identified. More Gram-negative infections were identified [44c].

Treprostinil

Skin

Subcutaneous administration of treprostinil is associated with local skin pain and hypersensitivities. A single center, double-blind, randomized, placebo controlled crossover study assessed the use of single capsaicin 8% patch before treatment with treprostinil. Two weeks after the patch was administered there was a statistically significant difference in patient pain scores in the capsaicin group ($p = 0.01$) [45c].

Liver

A study of four cohorts explored pharmacokinetics of treprostinil in liver failure. The findings after a single 1 mg oral sustained release dose included decreased mean treprostinil clearance values with the severity of hepatic impairment. Compared to healthy volunteer subjects, mean area under the curve from time zero to 24 h after dosing interval (AUC0-24) values in subjects with mild, moderate and severe hepatic impairment increased by approximately 2.2, 4.9, and 7.6 times, respectively [46c].

Drug Formulations

A small study of 9 patients evaluated the safety of transitioning from subcutaneous treprostinil to intravenous epoprostenol or intravenous treprostinil. It was determined that upon transition from subcutaneous to intravenous therapy a decrease in dose was required for both intravenous products [47c].

Drug Administration Routes

A placebo controlled study of twice daily oral treprostinil in 310 patients demonstrated improvement in 6-minute walk test in patients with PAH. Most common adverse events in the group treated with oral treprostinil were headache (71%), diarrhea (55%), nausea (46%), flushing (35%), and jaw pain (25%) [48c].

Latanoprost (PGF$_{2\alpha}$ Analogue) [SED-15, 2002; SEDA-33, 847; SEDA-34, 660; SEDA-35, 726]

In a retrospective review of patients receiving at least 1 month prostaglandin therapy, 41.4% of patients treated with latanoprost developed periorbitopathy [49c]. Other findings associated with ophthalmic use of latanoprost will be reviewed in chapter 47.

Misoprostol (PGE$_1$ Analogue) [SED-15, 2357; SEDA-33, 847; SEDA-34, 660; SEDA-35, 726; SEDA-36, 612]

Systematic Reviews

Misoprostol was evaluated in several *Cochrane* reviews for indications of labor induction, post-partum hemorrhage, neonatal respiratory distress, and delivery of retained placenta [50R,51R,52R,53R,54R,55R].

Hematologic

A double-blind randomized controlled trial evaluated oxytocin 20 units in 1000 mL Ringer's solution or 400 mcg oral misoprostol in 400 pregnant women after vaginal delivery. The amount of hemorrhage was 182.4 g vs 157.0 g in the oxytocin and misoprostol groups, respectively, $p = 0.007$. There was no difference in hemoglobin change between the two groups. Misoprostol was associated with fever in 14.5% of patients compared to 2% of patients with oxytocin, $p < 0.001$ [56c].

Immunologic

Anaphylaxis and tachysystole developed in a 21-year-old woman administered buccal misoprostol for cervical ripening. Administration of epinephrine and emergent caesarean delivery lead to safe delivery of the neonate and minimal maternal morbidity [57A].

Fertility

A historical-prospective study reviewed all patients with missed abortion treated by misoprostol between 2005 and 2011. Pregnancy rates 2 years after treatment were 90.8% in patients who were interested in future pregnancy. Lower rates of pregnancy were observed in the first 3 months following treatment [58c].

References

[1] Mytinger JR, Heyer JL. Oral corticosteroids versus adrenocorticotrophic hormone for infantile spasms-an unfinished story. Pediatr Neurol. 2014;51:13–4 [r].

[2] Hladunewich M, Cattran D, Beck LH, et al. A pilot study to determine the dose and effectiveness of adrenocorticotropic hormone in nephrotic syndrome due to idiopathic membranous nephropathy. Nephrol Dial Transplant. 2014;29:1570–7 [c].

[3] Tumlin JA, Galphin CM, Rovin BH. Advanced diabetic nephropathy with nephrotic range proteinuria: a pilot study of the long-term efficacy of subcutaneous ACTH gel on proteinuria, progression of CKD, and urinary levels of VGF and MCP-1. J Diabetes Res. 2013;2013:489869 [c].

[4] Musallam N, Bamberger E, Srugo I, et al. Legionella pneumophila and pneumocystis jirovecii coinfection in an infant treated with adrenocorticotropic hormone form infantile spasm: case report and literature review. J Child Neurol. 2014;29(2):240–2 [A].

[5] Nassar K, Janani S, Roux C, et al. Long-term systemic glucocorticoid therapy: patients' representations, prescribers perceptions, and treatment adherence. Joint Bone Spine. 2014;81:68 [c].

[6] Vogel JP, Souza JPm Gulmezoglu AM, et al. Use of antenatal corticosteroids and tocolytic drugs in preterm births in 29 countries: an analysis of the WHO multicountry survey on maternal and newborn health. Lancet. 2014;384:1869–77 [C].

[7] Ruiz-Arruza I, Ugarte A, Cabezas-Rodriguez I, et al. Glucocorticoids and irreversible damage in patients with systemic lupus erythematosus. Rheumatology. 2014;53:1470–6 [r].

[8] Woods JA, Wheeler JS, Finch CK, et al. Corticosteroids in the treatment of acute exacerbations of chronic obstructive pulmonary disease. Int J Chron Obstruct Pulmon Dis. 2014;9:421–30 [r].

[9] Beckhaus AA, Riutort MC, Castro-Rodriguez JA. Inhaled versus systemic corticosteroids for acute asthma in children. A systematic review. Pediatr Pulmonol. 2014;49:326–34 [r].

[10] Venekamp RP, Thompson MJ, Hayward G, et al. Systemic corticosteroids for acute sinusitis. Cochrane Database Syst Rev. 2014;3:CD008115 [R].

[11] Dupuis S, Amiel JA, Desgroseilliers M, et al. Corticosteroids in the management of brain-dead potential organ donors: a systematic review. Br J Anaesth. 2014;113(3):346–59 [R].

[12] Chen HS, Wang W, Wu SN, et al. Corticosteroids for viral myocarditis. Cochrane Database Syst Rev. 2013;(Issue 10), Art. No.: CD004471. [R].

[13] Dyrada K, Piers SR, van Huls van Taxis CF, et al. Influence of steroid therapy on the incidence of pericarditis and atrial fibrillation after percutaneous epicardial mapping and ablation for ventricular tachycardia. Circ Arrhythm Electrophysiol. 2014;7:671–6 [c].

[14] Fang Q, Qian X, An J, et al. Higher dose dexamethasone increase early postoperative cognitive dysfunction. J Neurosurg Anesthesiol. 2014;26(3):220–3 [c].

[15] Stalnacke J, Diaz Heijtz R, Norberg H, et al. Cognitive outcome in adolescents and young adults after repeat course of antenatal corticosteroids. J Pediatr. 2013;163:441–6 [c].

[16] Drozdowicz LB, Bostwick JM. Psychiatric adverse effects of pediatric corticosteroid use. Mayo Clin Proc. 2014;89(6):817–34 [r].

[17] Schreiber MP, Colantuoni E, Bienvenu OJ, et al. Corticosteroids and transition to delirium in patients with acute lung injury. Crit Care Med. 2014;42:1480–6 [r].

[18] Judd LL, Schettler PJ, Brown ES, et al. Adverse consequences of glucocorticoid medication: psychological, cognitive, and behavioural effects. Am J Psychiatry. 2014;171:1045–51 [r].

[19] Sacre K, Dehoux M, Chauveheid MP, et al. Pituitary-adrenal function after prolonged use of glucocorticoid therapy for systematic inflammatory disorders: an observational study. Endocrinol Metab. 2013;98:3199–205 [c].

[20] Suzuki S, Yasunaga H, Matsui H, et al. Impact of systemic steroids on posttonsillectomy bleeding. JAMA Otolaryngol Head Neck Surg. 2014;140(10):906–10 [C].

[21] Hjern F, Mahmood MW, Abraham-Nordling M, et al. Cohort study of corticosteroid use of risk of admission for diverticular disease. Br J Surg. 2015;102:119–24 [c].

[22] Eriksen TF, Lassen CB, Gogenur I. Treatment of corticosteroids and risk of anastomotic leakage following lower gastrointestinal surgery: a literature survey. Colorectal Dis. 2014;16(5): O154–O160 [r].

[23] Wang AS, Armstrong EJ, Armstrong AW. Corticosteroids and wound healing: clinical considerations in the perioperative period. Am J Surg. 2013;206:410–7 [r].

[24] Khan N, Abbas AM, Almukhtar RM, et al. Adherence and efficacy of screening for low bone mineral density among ulcerative colitis patients treated with corticosteroid. Am J Gastroenterol. 2014;109:572–8 [c].

[25] Suh SY, Kim JH, Kim SJ, et al. Systemic steroid-induced cataracts in children: long-term changes in morphology and visual acuity. J AAPOSS. 2013;17:371–3 [c].

[26] Brassard P, Bitton A, Suissa A, et al. Oral corticosteroids and the risk of serious infections in patients with elderly-onset inflammatory bowel disease. Am J Gastroenterol. 2014;109:1795–802 [c].

[27] Jette-cote I, Oiellette D, Beliveau C, et al. Total dysphagia after short course of systemic corticotherapy: herpes simplex virus esophagitis. World J Gastroenterol. 2013;19(31):5178–81 [A].

[28] Horita N, Miyazawa N, Morita S, et al. Evidence suggesting that oral corticosteroids increase mortality in stable chronic obstructive pulmonary disease. Respir Res. 2014;15:37 [r].

[29] del Rincon I, Battafarano DF, Restrepo JF, et al. Glucocorticoid dose thresholds associated with all-cause and cardiovascular mortality in rheumatoid arthritis. Arthritis Rheum. 2014;66(2):264–72 [c].

[30] Rescigno P, di Lorenzo G. The potential detrimental effect of corticosteroids in prostate cancer. Future Oncol. 2014;10(3):325–7 [r].

[31] Jones W, Chastain CA, Wright PWl. Iatrogenic Cushing syndrome secondary to a probable interaction between voriconzole and budesonide. Pharmacotherapy. 2014;34(7):e116–e119 [A].

[32] Kim MH, Kim SH, Kim YK, et al. A polymorphism in the histone deacetylase 1 gene is associated with the response to corticosteroids in asthmatics. Korean J Intern Med. 2013;28:708–14 [C].

[33] Seferian A, Simonneau G. Therapies for pulmonary arterial hypertension: where are we today, where do we go tomorrow? Eur Respir Rev. 2013;22:217–26 [r].

[34] Zheng Y, Yang T, Chen G, et al. Prostanoid therapy for pulmonary arterial hypertension: a meta-analysis of survival outcomes. Eur J Clin Pharmacol. 2014;70:13–21 [R].

[35] Thomas IC, Glassner-Kolmin C, Gomber-Maitland M. Long-term effects of continuous prostacyclin therapy in adults with pulmonary hypertension associated with congenital heart disease. Int J Cardiol. 2013;168:4117–21 [c].

[36] Maxey DM. Food and drug administration postmarket reported side effects and adverse events associated with pulmonary hypertension therapy in pediatric patients. Pediatr Cardiol. 2013;34(7):1628–36 [c].

[37] Akagi S, Ogawa A, Miyaji K, et al. Catecholamine support at the initiation of epoprostenol therapy in pulmonary arterial hypertension. Ann Am Thorac Soc. 2014;11(5):719–27 [c].

[38] Kataoka M, Yanagisawa R, Yoshino H, et al. Massive ascites in pulmonary arterial hypertension caution with epoprostenol. Ann Am Thorac Soc. 2013;10(6):726–7 [A].

[39] Chin KM, Badesch DB, Robbins IM, et al. Two formulations of epoprostenol sodium in the treatment of pulmonary arterial hypertension: EPITOME-1. Am Heart J. 2014;167:218–25 [c].

[40] Sitbon O, Delcroix M, Bergot E, et al. EPITOME-2: an open-label study assessing the transition to a new formulation of intravenous epoprostenol in patients with pulmonary arterial hypertension. Am Heart J. 2014;167:210–7 [c].

[41] Mazzone A, Di Salvo M, Mazzuca S, et al. Effects of iloprost on pain-free walking distance and clinical outcome in patients with severe stage IIb peripheral arterial disease: the FADOI 2bPILOT Study. Eur J Clin Invest. 2013;43(11):1163–70 [c].

[42] Janjindamai W, Thatrimontrichai A, Maneenil G, et al. Effectiveness of safety of intravenous iloprost for severe persistent pulmonary hypertension of the newborn. Indian Pediatr. 2013;50:934–9 [c].

[43] Sawheny E, Ellis AL, Kinasewitz GT. Iloprost improves gas exchange in patients with pulmonary hypertension and ARDS. Chest. 2013;144(1):55–62 [c].

[44] Sammut D, Elliot CA, Kiely DG, et al. Central venous catheter-related blood stream infections in patients receiving intravenous iloprost for pulmonary hypertension. Eur J Clin Microbiol Infect Dis. 2013;32:883–9 [c].

[45] Libri V, Gibbs JS, Pinato DJ, et al. Capsaicin 8% patch for treprostinil subcutaneous infusion site pain in pulmonary hypertension patients. Br J Anaesth. 2014;112(2):337–47 [c].

[46] Peterson L, Marbury T, Marier J, et al. An evaluation of the pharmacokinetics of treprostinil diolamine in subjects with hepatic impairment. J Clin Pharm Ther. 2013;38:518–23 [c].

[47] Tapson VF, Jing ZC, Xu KF, et al. Oral treprostinil for the treatment of pulmonary hypertension in patients receiving background endothelin receptor antagonist and phosphodiesterase type 5 inhibitor threapy (the FREEDOM-C2 study). Chest. 2013;144(3):952–8 [c].

[48] Alkukhun L, Bair ND, Dweik RA, et al. Subcutaneous to intravenous prostacyclin analogue transition in pulmonary hypertension. J Cardiovasc Pharmacol. 2014;63:4–8 [c].

[49] Kucukevcilioglu M, Bayer A, Uysal Y, et al. Prostaglandin associated periorbitopathy in patients using bimatoprost, latanoprost, and travaprost. Clin Experiment Ophthalmol. 2014;42(2):126–31 [c].

[50] Alfirevic Z, Aflaifel N, Weeks A. Oral misoprostol for induction of labour. Cochrane Database Syst Rev. 2014;(Issue 6), Art. No.: CD001338. [R].

[51] Vogel JP, West HM, Dowswell T. Titrated oral misoprostol for augmenting labour to improve maternal and neonatal outcomes. Cochrane Database Syst Rev. 2013;(Issue 9), Art. No.: CD010648. [R].

[52] Motaze NV, Mbuagbaw L, Young T. Prostaglandins before caesarean section for preventing neonatal respiratory distress. Cochrane Database Syst Rev. 2013;(Issue 11), Art. No.: CD010087. [R].

[53] Mousa HA, Blum J, Abou El Senoun G, et al. Treatment for primary postpartum haemorrhage. Cochrane Database Syst Rev. 2014;(Issue 2), Art. No.: CD003249. [R].

[54] Grillo-Ardila CF, Ruiz-Parra AI, Gaitan HG, et al. Prostaglandins for management of retained placenta. Cochrane Database Syst Rev. 2014;(Issue 5), Art. No.: CD010312. [R].

[55] Thomas J, Fairclough A, Kavanagh J, et al. Vaginal prostaglandin (PGE2 and PGF2a) for induction of labour at term. Cochrane Database Syst Rev. 2014;(Issue 6), Art. No.: CD003101. [R].

[56] Rajaei M, Karimi S, Shahboodaghi Z, et al. Safety and efficacy of misoprostol versus oxytocin for the prevention of postpartum haemorrhage. J Pregnancy. 2014, Article ID 713879. [c].

[57] Schoen C, Campbell S, Maratas A, et al. Anaphylaxis to buccal misoprostol for labor induction. Obstet Gynecol. 2014;124(2 Pt 2 Suppl 1):466–8 [A].

[58] Bord I, Gdalevich M, Nahum R, et al. Misoprostol treatment for early pregnancy failure does not impair future fertility. Gynecol Endocrinol. 2014;30(4):316–9 [c].

39

Sex Hormones and Related Compounds, Including Hormonal Contraceptives

Marta Martín Millán*,1, Santos Castañeda†,1

*Department of Internal Medicine, IFIMAV, Hospital Universitario Marqués de Valdecilla, Santander, Cantabria, Spain
†Department of Rheumatology, IIS-IPrincesa, Hospital Universitario de La Princesa, Madrid, Spain
1Corresponding authors: martinmma@unican.es; mmmillan1974@hotmail.com; scastas@gmail.com

GENERAL

Sex hormones, particularly estrogens and progestogens, can be used separately or in combination, and for various purposes. It is often not possible to determine to which compound or combination a particular adverse reaction can be attributed. Thus, it is important to comment on particular types of adverse reactions; therefore, this topic has been explained under a series of differing headings.

ESTROGENS [SED-15, 1253; SEDA-34, 663; SEDA-35, 731; SEDA-36, 615]

Diethylstilbestrol [SED-15, 1119; SEDA-34, 665; SEDA-35, 731; SEDA-36, 615]

Diethylstilbestrol (DES) is a synthetic estrogen which was used to prevent miscarriages in the mid-twentieth century. Cohort studies have shown that women who were prenatally exposed to DES >40 years ago are at risk of developing a broad spectrum of gynecological and non-gynecological adverse conditions during adulthood, as well as an increased incidence of hypospadias in male children of women who had exposure during their pregnancy [1C].

Reproductive System

A couple of animal studies were designed to shed light on deleterious effects of both neonatal and prenatal DES exposure. Neonates of C57BL/6J mice were orally administered DES at different doses. Reproductive function was monitored as the animals aged. Female pups who received 5 µg/kg/day exhibited abnormal estrous cycles such as persistent estrus at 8 weeks of age. Treated females also developed spontaneous endocrine-related pituitary tumors, which were causal factors in their accelerated mortality. Thus, investigators found that exposure to low-dose DES early on in life induced early onset of spontaneous abnormalities in the estrous cycle in female mice [2E].

The effect of prenatal DES exposure has been observed postnatally in children of exposed mothers but also in grandchildren. A recent paper analyzed the transgenerational effects of prenatal DES exposure in two generations, and in two different strains (CD1 and C57BL/6) of mice. Animals were examined at birth, and 5–120 days postnatally to assess external genitalia malformations. Of 23 adult males (>60 days) prenatally exposed to DES, incidence of features indicative of urethral meatal hypospadias was very high. These features ranged from 18% to 100% in CD-1 males, and 31–100% in C57BL/6 males when prenatally exposed to DES. Thus, the strains differed only slightly in the incidence of male urethral hypospadias. Ninety-one percent of DES-exposed CD-1 and 100% of DES-exposed C57BL/6 females exhibited urethral–vaginal fistula. The clitoris was absent in all female animals who received DES, regardless of their strain [3E].

Second-Generation Effects

None of the F1 DES-treated females were fertile in the second generation. Nine out of 10 prenatally DES-exposed CD-1 males produced offspring with untreated females, giving rise to 55 male and 42 female pups. Of the F2 DES-lineage adult males, 20% had urethral meatal hypospadias. Five of 42 (11.9%) F2 DES lineage females

© 2015 Elsevier B.V. All rights reserved.

had urethral–vaginal fistula. Thus the study concluded that prenatal DES exposure induces malformations of external genitalia in both sexes and strains of mice, and certain malformations are transmitted to the second generation [3E].

HORMONE REPLACEMENT THERAPY
[SED-15, 1684, 1686, 1692; SEDA-34, 666; SEDA-35, 732; SEDA-36, 616]

General Information

A recent overview of the most recent findings from the Women's Health Initiative (WHI) hormone therapy (HT) trials has been published [4R]. Cardiovascular disease, cancer outcomes, all-cause mortality, and other major endpoints in the two WHI HT trials (conjugated equine estrogens [CEEs 0.625 mg/day] with or without medroxyprogesterone acetate [MPA 2.5 mg/day]) are reported and the role of age and other clinical risk factors is highlighted. The hazard ratio (HR) for coronary heart disease (CHD) was 1.18 (95% CI=0.95, 1.45) in the CEE +MPA trial and 0.94 (95% CI=0.78, 1.14) in the CEE-alone trial. In both HT trials, there was an increased risk of stroke and deep vein thrombosis and a lower risk of hip fractures and diabetes. The HT regimens had divergent effects on breast cancer. CEE+MPA increased breast cancer risk (cumulative HR=1.28; 95% CI=1.11, 1.48), while CEE alone had a protective effect (cumulative HR=0.79; 95% CI=0.65, 0.97). The absolute risks of HT were low in younger women (ages 50–59 years) and those who were within 10 years of menopause date. Furthermore, for CHD, the risks were elevated for women with metabolic syndrome or high low-density-lipoprotein cholesterol concentrations but not for women without these risk factors. Factor V Leiden genotype was associated with elevated risk of venous thromboembolism on HT women [4R,5c].

Women in early menopause have low absolute risks of chronic disease outcomes on HT. Therefore, it seems that use of HT for management of menopausal symptoms remains appropriate, and risk stratification will help to identify women in whom benefits would be expected to outweigh risks [4R].

Increased life expectancy makes many women spend a large part of their lives in a post-menopausal state. Apart from causing degeneration of the cardiovascular, skeletal and central nervous systems, estrogen deficiency also increases the risk for metabolic syndrome and type 2 diabetes. The role of estrogen deficiency as a mechanism which induces chronic diseases in women is emerging as a novel therapeutic challenge that parallels the increased risk associated with conventional estrogen replacement strategies. The new trend in menopausal therapy consists of using a tissue selective estrogen complex (TSEC) which combines estrogens with a selective estrogen receptor modulator. These compounds represent a novel strategy approach to treat menopausal symptoms in women with a uterus. The goal of a TSEC regimen containing bazedoxifene (BZA) with CEE is to provide the benefits of estrogen, such as reducing hot flashes and vulvar–vaginal atrophy, preventing menopausal osteoporosis, and promoting favorable effects on the cardiovascular system, while simultaneously protecting the endometrium and breast from estrogen stimulation without the need for a progestin. Clinical trials with CEE/BZA in postmenopausal women have shown improvement in vasomotor symptoms, vulvo–vaginal atrophy, and bone mineral density, without stimulation of the endometrium or breast tissue, with a generally favorable safety and tolerability profile [6R,7R,8R].

Hypertension

It is believed that sex steroids protect fertile women from hypertension, and that the loss of estrogens may play a role in blood pressure control. In fact, the role played by steroid withdrawal at menopause is still controversial. A review about this issue was published last year explaining that different studies consistently show a reduction of blood pressure with the use of transdermal estradiol. With regard to progestin association, they do not affect or favor the hypotensive effect of estrogens, and it seems that drospirenone (DRSP) provides the best anti-hypertensive effects [9R].

Metabolism

Recently, a study in rodents was designed to investigate the effect of TSEC on glucose and energy homeostasis in ovariectomized (OVX) mice fed with a high-fat diet [10E]. Female C57BL/6J mice were randomly divided into seven treatment groups as follows: (1) sham vehicle, (2) OVX+vehicle, (3) OVX+CEE, (4) OVX+estradiol (E2), (5) OVX+BZA, (6) OVX+CE+BZA, (7) OVX+E2 +BZA. All estrogen treatments and BZA prevented body weight increase, visceral adipose tissue accumulation, and adipocyte hypertrophy induced by OVX. Treating OVX mice with E2, CE, BZA and TSEC markedly decreased markers of insulin resistance and atherogenesis, such as the leptin/adiponectin ratio—with the strongest effect observed in mice treated with CE and CE +BZA. In conclusion, the study demonstrated that BZA exhibits estrogen-mimetic action with regard to glucose and energy homeostasis. It also shows that TSEC prevents estrogen deficiency-induced visceral adiposity, systemic inflammation, insulin resistance, and glucose intolerance as efficiently as CE or E2 alone, and importantly, without causing endometrial hyperplasia. All these observations provide novel insights into the mechanisms underlying the beneficial effects of TSEC in reversing postmenopausal metabolic abnormalities, and suggest that clinical studies in postmenopausal women are warranted [10E].

HORMONAL CONTRACEPTIVES [SED-15, 1642, 1645; SEDA-34, 667; SEDA-35, 733; SEDA-36, 618]

Oral contraceptives (OC) not only prevent undesired pregnancy, but also provide other benefits such as treatment of menstrual cycle irregularity, heavy menstrual bleeding, premenstrual syndrome, perimenopausal vasomotor symptoms and acne or hirsutism. It is calculated that 82% of sexually active women aged between 15 and 44 years are currently consuming OC in the United States. The vast majority use a combined formula composed of estrogen and progestin, and less than 1% use only progestin. OC have been in the market since 1960, however, today´s formulations contain much lower hormone doses compared with those used in the past. In spite of the formulation improvement, it is established that women who smoke, suffer from hypertension, diabetes or obesity and consume OC have higher cardiovascular risk, which is why potential candidates for OC use can be screened for cardiovascular risk before receiving the prescription by their physician.

Cardiovascular

The use of OC has been associated with an increased risk of adverse cardiovascular events, which is why several studies are trying to elucidate the real risk of new formulations. A recent study investigated whether contraceptives which contained 20 mcg of ethinyl estradiol and 3 mg of drospirenone alter the cardiac autonomic nervous system. Researchers analyzed heart rate variability, baroreflex sensitivity and blood pressure in 69 healthy women in a prospective controlled trial. Women were tested before initiating the contraceptive method and 6 months afterwards. Multiple ANOVA were used to analyze the data. No differences were detected in autonomic clinical parameters. The same group also performed another prospective controlled trial in hypertensive women. The purpose was to evaluate the effect of combined OC (COC) containing DRSP plus ethinyl estradiol on the systemic blood pressure, metabolic variables and neurohumoral axis. Women were allocated to two groups: 30 volunteers received COC and 26 volunteers were given non-hormonal contraceptive methods. Patients were followed up for 6 months and no significant changes in clinical and autonomic parameters, metabolic variables and the neurohumoral axis were detected [11c].

Thromboembolism

It is well established that women using COC are exposed to a higher risk of venous and arterial thromboembolism, although the latter is much less frequent than the former. Contrary to the risk of arterial thromboembolism, the risk of venous thromboembolism varies among combined oral contraceptives, and depending on which type of progestogen they contain, the risk can increase. A study was designed to estimate the number of venous thromboembolic events and related premature deaths due to pulmonary embolism (including immediate in-hospital lethality) attributable to the use of COC in exposed women of childbearing age. The follow-up covered 11 years, from 2000 to 2011. French data on sales of COC and on contraception behaviors from two national surveys were combined to estimate the number of exposed women according to contraceptive generation and age. Absolute risk of first-time venous thromboembolism in non-users of hormonal contraception and increased risk of thromboembolism in users vs. non-users of hormonal contraception were estimated on the basis of literature data [12R].

Finally, immediate in-hospital lethality due to pulmonary embolism and premature mortality due to recurrent venous thromboembolism were estimated from the French national database of hospitalization and literature data [13C]. Authors estimated that in France more than four million women are exposed daily to COC. The mean annual number of venous thromboembolic events attributable to their use was 2529 (778 of them were associated with the use of first- and second-generation contraceptives, while 1751 to the use of third- and fourth-generation contraceptives), corresponding to 20 premature deaths (six with first- and second-generation contraceptives and 14 with third- and fourth-generation contraceptives), of which there were eight to nine immediate in-hospital deaths. Therefore, it seems that exposure to third- and fourth-generation contraceptives led to a mean annual excess of 1167 venous thromboembolic events and nine premature deaths (including three immediate in-hospital deaths) as compared to the use of first- and second-generation contraceptives. This data should be considered in order to limit the use of third- and fourth-generation contraceptives and optimize the benefit-risk ratio of combined oral contraceptives [13C].

- A dangerous triplet condition has been reported.
  A 14-year-old female diagnosed with polycystic ovary syndrome was under oral contraceptive treatment. After 3 months of using OC she experienced chest pain and skin itching. Eosinophils and troponin levels were increased and T wave inversion in lead III was detected. The presence of normal coronary arteries suggested Kounis syndrome. Drug-related Kounis syndrome has been reported on several occasions. However, this patient was only receiving OC [14A].

Psychiatric

Prevalence of autism spectrum disorder has increased over the past 60 years, as has the use of hormonal contraceptives. Although there is not much research into potential neurodevelopmental effects of oral contraceptive use on progeny, some authors have hypothesized that there might be a relationship between autism spectrum disorders and hormonal contraceptive use. Compounds used in oral contraceptives may modify some conditions of the oocyte. It has been proposed that epigenetic changes could explain some side effects of some drugs [15H].

Metabolism

In line with the aforementioned studies, another group designed a study to determine whether consuming contraceptives containing non-androgenic progestins in association with estradiol or ethinyl estradiol (EE) influences glucose metabolism and body composition. A group of 16 women took estradiol valerate (E2V)/dienogest (DNG) in a quadriphasic regimen while another group of 16 women received 30 µg EE/2 mg chlormadinone acetate (CMA) in a monophasic regimen. Both groups were evaluated at the third cycle for modifications in lipoproteins, apolipoproteins and homeostatic model assessment for insulin resistance (HOMA-IR), and at the sixth cycle for body composition and bone turnover markers, such as osteocalcin and C-telopeptide X. HOMA-IR remained stable in those whose treatment was E2V/DNG [16c]. During EE/CMA treatment, total-cholesterol ($p=0.003$), high-density lipoprotein (HDL)-cholesterol ($p=0.001$), triglycerides ($p=0.003$), Apoprotein-A1 (Apo-A1) ($p=0.001$) and Apo B ($p=0.04$) increased. However, low-density lipoprotein/HDL ($p=0.039$) decreased and total-cholesterol/HDL and Apoprotein-B/Apo-A1 ratio did not change. HOMA-IR slightly increased from 1.33 ± 0.87 to 1.95 ± 0.88 ($p=0.005$). There was a reduction of markers of bone metabolism in both groups with no modification of body composition. The authors concluded that E2V/DNG administration does not influence lipid and glucose metabolism, while mixed effects are found with EE/CMA treatment. Both preparations reduce bone metabolism without influencing the short-term effect on body composition [16c].

It is believed that depot MPA increases low-density lipoprotein cholesterol. In Ghana, most of the women who attend family planning clinics use this kind of injectable contraceptive. The impact of injectable contraceptives (IC) on obesity and metabolic syndrome was studied in females (aged 20–49) who were receiving OC ($n=19$), injectable contraceptives (IC) ($n=19$) and subdermal implants ($n=6$) for a period of 60 months. A total of 24 non-users served as controls and lipid profiles, such as total cholesterol (TC), high-density lipoprotein cholesterol (HDLC), low-density lipoprotein cholesterol (LDLC), and very-low-density lipid lipoprotein cholesterol (VLDLC), were determined. Castelli index I and II were calculated. The body mass index (BMI) of the OC and IC groups was significantly different from the control group ($p=0.003$ and $p=0.008$, respectively). TC levels for the control and case groups were 3.35 ± 0.62 and 4.07 ± 0.91 mmol/L, respectively ($p=0.002$). LDLC levels for the control and case groups were 1.74 ± 0.57 and 2.38 ± 0.84 mmol/L, respectively ($p=0.003$). Castelli index I (TC/HDLC) and II (LDLC/HDLC) were significantly different between the control and OC groups ($p=0.026$ and $p=0.014$, respectively). Spearman's rho correlation showed significant influence of HC use on TG ($p=0.026$), TC ($p=0.000$), LDLC ($p=0.004$), and VLDLC ($p=0.026$) over time. The authors concluded that some of the potential CVD risk of hormonal contraceptive use is especially due to their effect on increasing BMI, which seems to be the most consistent marker [17c].

Hypertriglyceridemia

Estrogen combined with progestins is known to have a negative effect on triglycerides and high-density lipoprotein (HDL) cholesterol levels. Two cases of high levels of hypertriglyceridemia associated with OC have been reported in the past year [18A,19A].

- *A 17-year-old girl with a history of congenital human immunodeficiency virus (HIV) infection and lipodystrophy secondary to highly active antiretroviral therapy (HAART) developed severe worsening of preexisting hypertriglyceridemia after treatment with oral contraceptive pills (OCP) for polycystic ovary syndrome. Her hypertriglyceridemia improved upon OCP discontinuation. Little had been reported about the association of HAART-related lipodystrophy and severe hypertriglyceridemia with OCP, although triglycerides should be monitorized in this kind of patients [18A].*
- *Another case of severe, acute hypertriglyceridemia was reported in a 24-year-old woman who was using norethindrone acetate/ethinyl estradiol (Estrostep). This is an "estrophasic" oral contraceptive, which combines a continuous low progestin dose with a gradually increasing estrogen dose. The patient developed acute pancreatitis which required intensive medical care for aggressive volume resuscitation and management of severe electrolyte abnormalities. Laboratory studies obtained on admission indicated severe hypertriglyceridemia (2200 mg/dL), hyponatremia (120 mEq/L), and hypocalcemia (0.78 mmol/L). Amylase and lipase levels were also elevated (193 and 200 U/L, respectively). Ranson score calculated after 48 hours of admission was 4, and her Acute Physiology and Chronic Health Evaluation (APACHE) IV score was 35. Treatment included an insulin infusion, ω-3 fatty acid esters, and gemfibrozil [19A].*

Death

A very valuable prospective cohort (The Nurses' Health Study), which started in 1976 and ended in 2012, was followed to determine whether OC use was associated with high mortality. Follow-up questionnaires were sent biennially in order to update about risk factors and newly diagnosed diseases. Overall, 121 701 participants were included, and Cox proportional hazards models were used to calculate the relative risk of mortality. Ever use of OC was not associated with all causes of mortality. However, it was associated with specific causes of death including an increased rate of deaths due to violent or accidental death (HR=1.20; 95% CI=1.04, 1.37) and breast cancer (HR=1.08; 95% CI=0.98, 1.18). On the other hand, the authors observed a decreased rate due to ovarian cancer [20C].

Tumorigenicity

Evidence from previous studies suggests that recent OC use is associated with a small increase in breast cancer risk. However, continued surveillance and pooled analysis of OC are still necessary to improve breast cancer risk according to genetic background. A case–control study of 2492 matched pairs of women with a deleterious BRCA1 mutation was conducted to elucidate whether early oral contraceptive use increases the risk of breast cancer among young women with a breast cancer susceptibility gene 1 (BRCA1) mutation. Breast cancer cases and unaffected controls were matched on year of birth and country of residence. Detailed information about oral contraceptive use was collected from a routinely administered questionnaire [21C]. Conditional logistic regression was used to estimate the odds ratios (OR) and 95% confidence intervals (CI) for the association between oral contraceptives and breast cancer, by age at first use and by age at diagnosis. Among BRCA1 mutation carriers, OC use was significantly associated with an increased risk of breast cancer for women who started the pill prior to age 20 (OR=1.45; 95% CI=1.20, 1.75; $p=0.0001$) and possibly between ages 20 and 25 as well (OR=1.19; 95% CI=0.99, 1.42; $p=0.06$). The effect was limited to breast cancers diagnosed before age 40 (OR=1.40; 95% CI=1.14, 1.70; $p=0.001$); the risk of early-onset breast cancer increased by 11% with each additional year of pill use when initiated prior to age 20 (OR=1.11; 95% CI=1.03, 1.20; $p=0.008$). By contrast, increased risk for women diagnosed at or after the age of 40 (OR=0.97; 95% CI=0.79, 1.20; $p=0.81$) was not observed. The researchers concluded that OC use before age 25 increases the risk of early-onset breast cancer among women with a BRCA1 mutation and the risk increases with duration of use. Therefore, the data of this study claim that caution is warranted when advising women with a BRCA1 mutation to take oral contraceptives prior to age 25 [21C].

Other studies have tried to address whether current OC are associated with certain breast cancer molecular subtypes. A population-based case–control study of invasive breast cancer among women ages 20–44 from 2004 to 2010 (985 cases and 882 controls) was conducted in the Seattle-Puget Sound area. Information on contraceptive use and participant characteristics via an in-person interview was collected. Multivariable-adjusted logistic regression was used to calculate odds ratios and 95% CI. The authors found that lifetime duration of OC use for ≥15 years was associated with an increased breast cancer risk (OR=1.5; 95% CI=1.1, 2.2). Current OC use (within 1 year of reference date) for ≥5 years was associated with an increased risk (OR=1.6; 95% CI=1.1, 2.5). There were no statistically significant differences in risk by OC preparation [22C]. Risk magnitudes were generally greater among women ages 20–39, and for estrogen receptor-negative (ER(−)) and triple-negative breast cancer (current use for ≥5 years among ages 20–39: ER(−) OR=3.5; 95% CI=1.3, 9.0; triple-negative OR=3.7; 95% CI=1.2, 11.8), although differences between groups were not statistically significant. Therefore, long-term use of contemporary OC and current use for ≥5 years was associated with an increased breast cancer risk especially in women ages 20–44 [22C].

Contrary to what happens regarding breast cancer, OC seems to reduce the risk of ovarian cancer. A recent study analyzed if the benefit extends to higher risk women from families who have suffered ovarian cancer. Participants proceeded from the three clinic-based sites of the Breast Cancer Family Registry (BCFR). The eligibility criteria for each site included being a male with breast cancer, being a female diagnosed with breast cancer at a young age, being a female diagnosed with breast and ovarian cancer at any age, having multiple affected relatives with breast or ovarian cancer or being a BRCA1/2 mutation carrier. Overall, there were 2375 families from the three clinic-based sites, and 101 families who have at least two sisters discordant for ovarian cancer status. All sisters were included in the analyses. The authors used generalized estimating equations to obtain the population average effect across all families ($n=389$ cases, $n=5643$ controls) and conditional logistic regression to examine within-family differences in a subset with at least two sisters discordant on ovarian cancer status ($n=109$ cases, $n=149$ unaffected sister controls). In the multivariable generalized estimating equation model, a reduced risk of ovarian cancer forever use of oral contraceptives compared with never use (OR=0.58, 95% CI=0.37, 0.91) was found. In the conditional logistic model, a similar inverse association was detected; however, it was not statistically significant (OR=0.52, 95% CI=0.23, 1.17). They examined this association by BRCA1/2 status and observed a statistically significant reduced risk in the non-carriers only. Therefore, the researchers concluded that a decreased risk of ovarian cancer with OC use supports that the association observed in unrelated women extends to related women at higher risk [23C].

Emergency Contraception [SEDA-34, 668; SEDA-35, 734; SEDA-36, 618]

Emergency contraception (EC) offers women an important strategy to prevent unintended pregnancy following intercourse. Despite the constant improvement of availability of different molecules and techniques already existing (Yuzpe regimen, levonorgestrel, intrauterine device) and the emergence of ulipristal acetate, the numbers of unintended pregnancies and unplanned births could still be reduced.

This review will evaluate all the information about the potential adverse effects and tolerability of each method of EC by putting them in balance with their safety and effectiveness. A literature search until December 2013 was recently performed to identify all trials studying the safety data available concerning EC [24R].

ANTI-ESTROGENS AND SELECTIVE ESTROGEN RECEPTOR MODULATORS [SEDA-34, 669; SEDA-35, 735; SEDA-36, 619]

Aromatase Inhibitors [SEDA-35, 735; SEDA-36, 619]

Anastrazole [SEDA-35, 735; SEDA-36, 619]

LIVER

Although tamoxifen and anastrozole, agents widely used as adjuvant treatment for early stage breast cancer, may induce hepatotoxicity, this side effect has not been fully defined. A recent study compared hepatotoxicity of anastrozole with tamoxifen in the adjuvant setting in postmenopausal breast cancer patients [25c]. Three hundred and fifty-three Chinese postmenopausal women with hormone receptor-positive early breast cancer were randomized to receive either anastrozole or tamoxifen after optimal primary therapy. The primary end-point was fatty liver disease and the secondary end-points included abnormal liver function and treatment failure during the 3-year follow up. The cumulative incidence of fatty liver disease after 3 years was lower in the anastrozole arm than that of tamoxifen (14.6% vs. 41.1%, $p < 0.0001$; relative risk $= 0.30$; 95% CI $= 0.21$, 0.45). However, there was no difference in the cumulative incidence of abnormal liver function (24.6% vs. 24.7%, $p = 0.61$). Interestingly, a higher treatment failure rate was observed in the tamoxifen arm compared with anastrozole and median times to treatment failure were 15.1 months and 37.1 months, respectively ($p < 0.0001$; HR $= 0.27$; 95% CI $= 0.20$, 0.37). The most commonly

reported adverse events were "reproductive system disorders" in the tamoxifen group (17.1%), and "musculoskeletal disorders" in the anastrozole group (14.6%). Postmenopausal women with hormone receptor-positive breast cancer receiving adjuvant anastrozole displayed less fatty liver disease, suggesting that this drug had a more favorable hepatic safety profile than tamoxifen and may be preferable for patients at risk of hepatic dysfunction [25c].

Bazedoxifene Plus CEEs [SEDA-34, 665; SEDA-35, 735; SEDA-36, 619]

Estrogen is well known to favorably regulate body composition and glucose homeostasis; however, its use to prevent obesity and type 2 diabetes in postmenopausal women is limited due to sex steroid-responsive cancer development.

METABOLISM

Bazedoxifene acetate (BZA) uniquely antagonizes both breast cancer development as well as estrogen-related changes in the female reproductive tract. However, whether BZA combined with conjugated estrogen (CE) or alone impacts metabolism is still to be determined. The effects of BZA alone or CE plus BZA on body composition and glucose homeostasis were assessed in ovariectomized female mice which were fed a Western diet for 10–12 weeks. In contrast to the vehicle, E2, CE, BZA, and CE + BZA equally prevented body weight gain by 50%. All treatments caused equal attenuation of the increase in body fat mass invoked by the diet as well as the increases in subcutaneous and visceral white adipose tissue. Diet-induced hepatic steatosis was attenuated by E2 or CE, and BZA alone or with CE provided even greater steatosis prevention. All interventions improved pyruvate tolerance tests. Glucose tolerance tests and HOMA-IR were improved by E2, CE, and CE + BZA. Whereas E2 or CE alone invoked a uterotrophic response, BZA alone or CE + BZA had a negligible impact on the uterus. Thus, CE + BZA afford protection from diet-induced adiposity, hepatic steatosis, and insulin resistance with minimal impact on the female reproductive tract in mice [26E].

Exemestane [SEDA-36, 620]

MUSCULOSKELETAL

Adjuvant therapy with an aromatase inhibitor improves outcomes, as compared with tamoxifen, in postmenopausal women with hormone-receptor-positive breast cancer. In 2003, the International Breast Cancer Study Group (IBCSG) initiated two randomized phase 3 trials. The Tamoxifen and Exemestane Trial (TEXT) and the Suppression of Ovarian Function Trial (SOFT), involving premenopausal women with hormone-receptor-positive early breast cancer. The trials were designed to determine whether adjuvant therapy with the aromatase inhibitor exemestane improved disease-free survival, as compared with premenopausal women treated with tamoxifen plus ovarian suppression, and to determine the value of ovarian suppression in women who were suitable candidates for treatment with adjuvant tamoxifen. At 5 years, 92.8% (95% CI=91.6, 93.9) of the patients assigned to receive exemestane plus ovarian suppression were free from breast cancer, as compared with 88.8% (95% CI=87.3, 90.1) of those assigned to receive tamoxifen plus ovarian suppression (hazard ratio for recurrence, 0.66; 95% CI=0.55, 0.80; $p < 0.001$). The recurrence of breast cancer at a distant site was reported in 325 patients (6.9%), and at 5 years the rate of freedom from distant recurrence was 93.8% (95% CI=92.7, 94.8) among patients assigned to receive exemestane plus ovarian suppression, as compared with 92.0% (95% CI=90.7, 93.1) among those assigned to receive tamoxifen plus ovarian suppression (HR for recurrence, 0.78; 95% CI=0.62, 0.97; $p=0.02$). The events of grade 3 or 4 that were reported most frequently were hot flushes, musculoskeletal symptoms and hypertension. Specifically, osteoporosis (T-score less than −2.5) was reported in 13.2% of the patients assigned to exemestane plus ovarian suppression, but in only 6.4% of those assigned to tamoxifen plus ovarian suppression [27C].

Raloxifene [SEDA-36, 620]

CARDIOVASCULAR

Knowledge of the effects of raloxifene on myocardial hypertrophy in postmenopausal women has not been investigated; therefore, an open-label prospective-randomized-controlled study was designed to address this matter. A total of 22 postmenopausal osteoporotic women were included. Women were randomized into two groups: 11 of the patients were treated with raloxifene 60 mg/day, and another 11 patients were defined as the control group. Echocardiographic examination was performed in all patients at baseline, and at the end of the 6-month follow-up period. Left ventricle mass (LVM) and left ventricle mass index (LVMI) were calculated. The authors did not find differences in echocardiographic parameters of LVM and LVMI compared with the control group (201.2 ± 25.9 g vs. 169.7 ± 46.2 g, $p=0.14$ and 120.4 ± 25.9 g/m² vs. 105.5 ± 26.3 g/m², $p=0.195$, respectively). Therefore, it was concluded that raloxifene therapy does not affect myocardial hypertrophy in postmenopausal women, at least after 6 months of treatment [28c].

Tamoxifen [SED-15, 3296; SEDA-34, 669; SEDA-35, 736; SEDA-36, 621]

CARDIOVASCULAR

In order to explain the mechanism by which tamoxifen increases thrombotic risk, a study was performed to assess if tamoxifen induces acquired resistance to activated protein C (APC). Blood samples were collected prospectively from 25 women with breast cancer before and monthly after the start of adjuvant treatment. APC resistance was evaluated on basis of the effect of APC on the endogenous thrombin generation potential. APC plasma levels were measured using a highly sensitive oligonucleotide-based enzyme capture assay, and routine hemostasis parameters were measured additionally. APC sensitivity decreased by 41% ($p=0.001$) compared to baseline after 1 month of tamoxifen treatment and remained significantly decreased during the study period. Free protein S increased ($p=0.008$) while other analyzed procoagulant factors, inhibitors, and activation markers of coagulation decreased or did not change significantly. In five patients, the APC concentration increased to non-physiological levels but an overall significant increase of APC was not observed [29c].

TUMORIGENICITY

The risk of endometrial cancer has been reported for postmenopausal women who were receiving tamoxifen therapy for a long period of time.

A largest population-based study was designed to further assess the potential association between tamoxifen use for breast cancer treatment and the risk for developing endometrial cancer in Taiwan. A total of 74 280 women treated for breast cancer between January 1, 1997 and December 31, 2004 were included in the study. Of the 74 280 patients, 39 411 (53.1%) received tamoxifen treatment, and 34 869 (46.9%) did not. A total of 222 patients developed endometrial cancer, 153 out of them (69%) were seen in patients with tamoxifen treatment, and 69 (31%) in patients without tamoxifen. The incidence of endometrial cancer was 0.388% (153/39 411) in patients under tamoxifen treatment, while it was 0.198% (69/34 869) in patients without tamoxifen treatment ($p < 0.001$). Among patients under tamoxifen therapy, the mean duration of tamoxifen use was 2.91 years in patients who developed endometrial cancer, while the average was 1.67 years in patients who did not develop endometrial cancer. Logistic regression analysis demonstrated that tamoxifen use and age over 35 years were significantly correlated with development of endometrial cancer ($p < 0.001$ and $p=0.002$, respectively). The OR was 2.94 (95% CI=2.13, 4.06) for 3 years or longer tamoxifen use. The OR was 4.08 (95% CI=1.67, 9.93) for women older than 35 years compared to those 35 or younger. It was different from the Western countries. The incidence peak of Taiwanese female breast cancer is also different form the Western countries. Therefore, further studies are needed in order to evaluate real clinical implications [30C].

PROGESTOGENS [SED-15, 2930; SEDA-34, 671; SEDA-35, 736; SEDA-36, 622]

Drospirenone [SEDA-35, 736; SEDA-36, 622]

Endocrine

Women who suffer from polycystic ovary syndrome (PCOS) have increased adrenal androgen production, enhanced peripheral metabolism of cortisol and elevated urinary excretion of its metabolites. Increased cortisol clearance in PCOS is followed by a compensatory over-drive of the hypothalamic–pituitary–adrenocortical (HPA) axis. Macut et al. hypothesized that oral contraceptives containing ethinyl estradiol and drospirenone (EE-DRSP) could affect HPA axis activity in PCOS patients. A total of 12 women with PCOS (aged 24.17 ± 4.88 years; body mass index 22.05 ± 3.97 kg/m^2) treated for 12 months with EE-DRSP and 20 BMI matched controls were studied. Testosterone, dehydroepiandrosterone sulfate (DHEAS), sex hormone binding globulin (SHBG), cortisol (basal and after dexamethasone), concentrations of glucocorticoid receptor (GR) protein, phospo-GR211 protein, number of GR per cell and its equilibrium dissociation constant (KD) were measured before and after treatment. Increased concentrations of testosterone and DHEAS ($p < 0.001$, respectively), unaltered basal cortisol and an increased sensitivity ($p < 0.05$) of the HPA axis to dexamethasone were observed in PCOS women in comparison to controls at baseline. After treatment, testosterone ($p < 0.01$), DHEAS ($p < 0.05$) and cortisol suppression after dexamethasone ($p < 0.01$) were decreased in PCOS women. There were changes neither in GR protein concentration, GR phosphorylation nor in the receptor functional parameters Bmax and KD in women with PCOS before and after the therapy in comparison to controls. Therefore, the researcher concluded that prolonged treatment with EE-DRSP in PCOS women decreased serum androgens and increased cortisol in the presence of decreased sensitivity of the HPA axis and did not exert changes in GR expression and function [31c].

Etonogestrel [SEDA-36, 622]

Respiratory

It is established that women with cystic fibrosis (CF) have worse lung function with faster function decline, earlier onset of bacterial colonization, frequent pulmonary exacerbations (PE), greater bronchial hyper-responsiveness, and higher mortality rates after puberty than men. The reason for this gender disparity remains unknown, but it has been suggested that female hormones might be implicated.

- Lamas et al. report the case of a 20-year-old female with CF with severe recurrent pulmonary exacerbations with lung function decline and requiring multiple courses of intravenous antibiotics, related to the menstrual cycle since menarche. Treatment with a subcutaneous implant with 68 mg of etonogestrel was initiated and cessation of pulmonary exacerbations was observed, suggesting that the sex differential between men and women contributes to morbidity/mortality in patients with CF and that hormonal manipulation might be an effective therapy for women with CF [32A].

Medroxyprogesterone [SEDA-15, 2225; SEDA-35, 737; SEDA-36, 623]

Infection Risk

An important issue in women's health in developing countries is choosing a contraceptive with minimal effects on susceptibility to infectious diseases, in particular to human immunodeficiency virus (HIV)-1 acquisition via the female reproductive tract. Genital epithelial cells are the first line of defense against pathogens and serve not only as a physical barrier but also express a wide variety of immune mediators aiding in both innate and adaptive immunity. These cells may determine the outcome to virus exposure. A recent paper reported that HIV uptake by genital epithelial cells increased significantly in the presence of MPA and progesterone and that uptake occurred primarily via endocytosis. No productive infection was detected, but an endocytosed virus was released into apical and basolateral compartments. Significantly higher viral transcytosis was observed in the presence of MPA. When genital epithelial cells and T-cells were co-cultured, maximum viral replication in T cells was observed in the presence of MPA, which also broadly upregulated chemokine production by these cells, suggesting that MPA may play a significant role in regulating susceptibility to HIV [33E].

PROGESTERONE ANTAGONISTS [SEDA-34, 671; SEDA-35, 738; SEDA-36, 625]

Mifepristone [SED-15, 2344; SEDA-34, 671; SEDA-35, 738; SEDA-36, 625]

Second-Generation Effects

REPRODUCTIVE SYSTEM

Mifepristone is a synthetic steroid compound that induces abortion. It has recently been found that mifepristone can pass into human milk. A study was designed to determine the effects of mifepristone administration to lactating mice on the development and reproduction of their progeny. Therefore, lactating mice were gavage fed with mifepristone daily for 4 days either from days 1–4 or from days 7–10 of lactation. Controls received only peanut oil. Growth, mortality rate, organ weight to body weight ratio, sex hormones at 20, 40 and 60 days, fertility of these F1 progeny and litter size, sex ratio and mortality rate of the second generation were recorded. The authors did not observe significant differences in the average body weight, mortality rate of the female or male pups, and organ coefficient of uterus and ovaries of females in adulthood in comparison with controls. However, the organ coefficient of testis at days 20 and 40 and testosterone concentration at day 60 were increased in male pups. Reproductive capacity of the F1 pups was unaffected by 4 days exposure to mifepristone via their mother's milk: time to birth of F2 pups, litter size, sex ratio and mortality rate were similar to control F1 pups. The authors conclude that mifepristone influenced only on the organ coefficient of testis at day 40 and the testosterone concentration in male pups at day 60; however, the development and fertility of female and male pups were not affected [34E].

Ulipristal [SEDA-36, 626]

Reproductive System

Internal sales data estimate that over 1 400 000 individual women have been exposed to UPA for emergency contraception worldwide. Between October 1, 2009 and May 14, 2013, 553 women from 23 countries reported 1049 suspected adverse drug reactions, among which the most frequent events reported were pregnancies and gastrointestinal (nausea, abdominal pain, vomiting), nervous (headache, dizziness) and reproductive (metrorrhagia/genital hemorrhage, menses delay, breast symptoms) system disorders. All 20 delivered babies were declared to be healthy by the reporter. Data from more than 5000 exposed women during clinical development of emergency contraception (EC) and uterine fibroid treatment and more than 1.4 million women in EC post-marketing surveillance indicate that the use of UPA 30 mg for EC seems to be safe [35C].

ANABOLIC STEROIDS, ANDROGENS AND RELATED COMPOUNDS [SED-15, 216; SEDA-34, 672; SEDA-35, 738; SEDA-36, 627]

Anabolic Steroids [SEDA-35, 738; SEDA-36, 627]

Cardiovascular

Anabolic-androgenic steroid (AAS) consumption is a widespread practice among bodybuilders. Structural changes within the myocardium such as hypertrophy,

restricted diastolic function as well as systolic dysfunction and impaired ventricular inflow have been reported among users. A recent review has been published with all the known adverse cardiovascular effects induced by chronic AAS use; reduction in HDL cholesterol, increased inflammatory markers and oxidative stress, hypertension and cardiac dysfunction. Epidemiological and autopsy studies demonstrated the relation between AAS use and early mortality [36R].

- Recently, a case report illustrated the use of cardiovascular magnetic resonance (CMR) to detect heart damage in an AAS user. A 39-year-old bodybuilder with over 20 years of AAS abuse developed dyspnea and fatigue. A CMR was performed and it showed a patchy midwall enhancement in the septal and posterolateral region of the left ventricle. Normal coronary arteries were found, suggesting that this test might be useful in detecting damage in this group of patients [37A].

Atrial fibrillation (AF) is the most frequently observed arrhythmia in bodybuilders who are using AAS, which suggests a causal link between these conditions. A recent paper investigated the effect of long-term supraphysiologic doses of AAS on atrial electromechanical delay (AEMD) in male bodybuilders. AEMD was measured as the interval between the onset of the P wave on the electrocardiogram and the beginning of late diastolic Am wave at the lateral mitral annulus [PA (atrial electromechanical coupling) lateral], septal mitral annulus (PA septum), and right ventricular tricuspid annulus (PA tricuspid) [38c]. The authors found that inter-AEMD and intra-atrial electromechanical delay (AEMD) were significantly increased in AAS using bodybuilders compared with nonusers that are known to be related to various arrhythmias, especially AF. The PA lateral and PA septum were significantly higher in the AAS user than in nonusers (65.55 ± 7.50 ms versus 49.08 ± 6.66 ms, $p < 0.01$; 49.27 ± 7.88 ms versus 42.71 ± 4.39 ms, $p < 0.01$, respectively). Inter-atrial and intra-atrial EMD values were significantly higher in the AAS using bodybuilders compared with those in the nonusers (26.15 ± 6.54 ms versus 12.42 ± 6.58 ms, $p < 0.01$; 9.88 ± 5.23 ms versus 6.04 ± 3.21 ms, $p < 0.05$, respectively). The authors conclude that these findings may be markers of subclinical cardiac involvement in AAS using bodybuilders [38c].

Urinary Tract

Cholemic nephrosis represents a spectrum of renal injury from proximal tubulopathy to intrarenal bile cast formation found in patients with severe liver dysfunction. Most often, patients with severe obstructive jaundice develop this lesion, which is thought to occur due to direct bile acid injury to tubular cells, as well as obstructing bile acid casts. In these circumstances, acute tubular injury develops from a combination of hemodynamic changes with some contribution from direct bile acid-related tubular toxicity and obstructive bile casts. The authors presented the case of acute kidney injury due to bile acid nephropathy in a bodybuilder who developed severe cholestatic liver disease in the setting of anabolic androgenic steroid use [39A].

Nandrolone

Psychological

Nandrolone decanoate has been reported to induce psychiatric side effects, such as aggression and depression. Adolescence represents an extremely sensitive neurodevelopmental period to influence by detrimental effects of drug abuse. A group of investigators provide some evidence regarding the effects of nandrolone decanoate on the emotional profile of animals exposed during adolescence.

Adolescent rats received daily injections of nandrolone decanoate for 14 days. Behavioral tests such as forced swim, sucrose preference, open field and elevated plus maze tests were performed at early adulthood on separate groups of animals. *In vivo* electrophysiological recordings were carried out to monitor changes in electrical activity of serotonergic neurons of the dorsal raphe nucleus (DRN) and noradrenergic neurons of the locus coeruleus (LC). What the authors observed was that after early exposure to nandrolone, rats displayed depression-related behavior, characterized by increased immobility in the forced swim test and reduced sucrose intake in the sucrose preference test. In addition, adult rats presented anxiety-like behavior characterized by decreased time and number of entries in the central zone of the open field and decreased time spent in the open arms of the elevated plus maze, suggesting that nandrolone decreased the firing rate of spontaneously active serotonergic neurons in the DRN while increasing the firing rate of noradrenergic neurons in the LC. Nandrolone decanoate is not recommended in adolescents, and public health measures should be taken to prevent the abuse of this compound in the developing population [40E].

Testosterone [SEDA-35, 739; SEDA-36, 628]

Tumorigenicity

Patients with prostate cancer can have hypogonadism and experience health and quality-of-life declines related to low testosterone levels. Despite generations of urological dogma suggesting that testosterone supplementation therapy (TST) for hypogonadism causes prostate-cancer progression, a review of the contemporary literature provides evidence to the contrary. The prostate saturation model suggests that the androgen receptor (AR) is

saturated at serum testosterone levels of 150–200 ng/dL; therefore, additional serum testosterone above this level has limited effects within the prostate. Indeed, studies in the modern era of PSA assessments indicate that TST does not affect prostate size, intraprostatic testosterone levels or prostate-cancer progression, provided the baseline serum testosterone level is greater than this AR saturation point. However, one should consider that the vast majority of the data on this issue comes from a small number of cases; therefore, risks and benefits should be considered when TST is administered to patients with prostate cancer [41R].

ANTIANDROGENS [SEDA-34, 674; SEDA-35, 740; SEDA-36, 628]

Bicalutamide [SEDA-34, 674; SEDA-35, 740; SEDA-36, 629]

Liver

Bicalutamide is a nonsteroidal anti-androgen which is used during the initiation of androgen deprivation therapy with a luteinizing hormone-releasing hormone agonist to reduce the symptoms of tumor flare in patients with metastatic prostate neoplasm. Since this is a competitive androgen receptor ligand it can induce gynecomastia, hot flashes, fatigue and decreased libido. Liver injury is a rare secondary effect which it generally mild and transitory. However, a symptomatic acute liver injury secondary to its use is reported [42A].

- *An 81-year-old African American male with metastatic prostate neoplasm presented nonspecific symptoms along with jaundice. Three weeks earlier he had started to take bicalutamide. On physical examination, scleral icterus was noted. Workup revealed acutely elevated liver transaminases (>5 times the upper limit of normal), alkaline phosphatase, conjugated hyperbilirubinemia, and coagulopathy. Other etiologies, including viruses, common toxins, drugs, autoimmune, and copper-induced hepatitis, were considered. Bicalutamide was discontinued and the patient was treated with supportive care. He showed improvement of clinical and laboratory abnormalities within days [42A].*

Enzalutamide [SEDA-35, 740; SEDA-36, 629]

It is a potent androgen receptor antagonist used in the treatment of metastatic castration-resistant prostate cancer. Enzalutamide has been previously linked to the increased risk of seizures. Clinicians should be aware that, in rare cases, patients treated with enzalutamide could potentially be at risk for posterior reversible encephalopathy syndrome (PRES) characterized by a clinical/radiological syndrome which included seizure, headache, impaired vision and hypertension. Diagnosis is generally confirmed by magnetic resonance imaging. The list of medications linked to PRES includes traditional cytotoxic chemotherapeutics, newer agents that target the vascular endothelial growth factor pathway, and supportive care mediations. If symptoms suggestive of PRES arise in patients receiving enzalutamide, the drug should be discontinued immediately and the diagnostic process should be initiated [43A].

5α-Reductase Inhibitors

Dutasteride & Finasteride [SED-15, 3132; SEDA-34, 675; SEDA-35, 740; SEDA-36, 629]

PSYCHIATRIC

Finasteride has been approved since 1992 by the United States Food and Drug Administration (FDA) for the treatment of benign prostatic hyperplasia and since 1997 for the treatment of men with male pattern hair loss (MPHL) or androgenetic alopecia (AGA). Since that time, more than 2230 articles have been published regarding the use of this medication. Of these articles, 250 were considered as randomized controlled trials. A recent article performed a critical review of the literature taking into account a paper which addressed potential adverse effects [44R]. The authors conclude that the reports of potential irreversible sexual dysfunction and severe depression do raise concerns about the safety of finasteride; however, given the data from the hundreds of randomized, controlled trials, finasteride should still be considered a safe and well-tolerated medication. Further research should be performed to further evaluate if there are any unique characteristics in these individuals suffering from prolonged sexual dysfunction and severe depression after using finasteride [44R].

MUSCULOSKELETAL

Dihyrotestosterone (DHT) is the main prostatic androgen. It is generated by a reduction in testosterone by two isoenzymes of 5alpha-reductase. Finasteride and dutasteride are 5alpha-reductase inhibitors (5ARIs) commonly used in the treatment of benign prostatic hyperplasia. A recent case–control study was conducted to explore the possible association between the use of two typical 5ARIs (finasteride and dutasteride) and osteoporosis. A total of 1352 men with a diagnosis of osteoporosis were identified and 5387 control cases without osteoporosis were recruited from the claims data for patients with benign prostate hyperplasia (BPH). Four controls were frequency-matched to each case according to age (every 5 years) and diagnosis date. We measured the effect of

5ARIs and determined the adjusted ORs with 95% CI. 1.52-fold increase in osteoporosis diagnosis among patients with BPH using finasteride (95% CI = 1.01, 2.30) was detected. Moreover, a dosage analysis showed that higher doses of finasteride were associated with higher osteoporosis diagnosis risk (OR = 1.68; 95% CI = 1.01, 2.81), relative to the patients not using 5ARIs [45C].

By contrast, another small study analyzed the bone mineral density (BMD) in 50 men treated with finasteride and 50 men treated with dutasteride. Another 50 men served as controls. Bone mineral density of spine and hip was measured using dual energy X-ray absorptiometry and what the researcher found was that men in the dutasteride group had significantly higher BMD than controls, suggesting that long-term 5alpha-reductase suppression does not adversely affect BMD [46c].

BREASTS

Breast Cancer A case–control study was conducted with data from the United Kingdom Clinical Practice Research Datalink database among all men aged 45 years and older in the period January 1, 1992 to December 31, 2011 in order to quantify the association between use of 5-ARIs and the risk for male breast cancer. Cases of men diagnosed with breast cancer were matched to 10 controls on age and general practice. Crude and adjusted odds ratios were estimated for the risk of breast cancer associated with the use of 5-ARIs. Three hundred and ninety-eight cases were identified and matched to 3930 controls. Ever use of 5-ARIs was associated with an adjusted OR for breast cancer of 1.08 (95% CI = 0.62, 1.87) compared to non-users. Increasing cumulative duration of treatment showed no increasing risks: adjusted odds ratios for use for less than 280, for 280 to 1036 and for more than 1036 days were 1.21 (95% CI = 0.47, 3.10), 0.94 (95% CI = 0.36, 2.41) and 1.29 (95% CI = 0.54, 3.08), respectively. All these data suggest that no evidence of an association between short- or long-term treatment with 5-ARIs and the risk for breast cancer in older men is found [47C].

Leuprolide [SEDA-36, 631]

Long-acting gonadotropin-releasing hormone agonists (GnRHa) are considered a treatment of choice for pediatric central precocious puberty (CPP). Prolonged administration of GnRHa suppresses the pituitary–gonadal axis activity with a subsequent decrease of sex hormones. Lee et al. reported the prevalence rate of adverse reactions among patients with CPP who were using long-acting GnRHa in a pediatric tertiary medical center. Among the total 621 patients, 469 girls (8.78 ± 0.45 years) were treated with monthly depot leuprolide acetate. Six drug-related serious side effects were observed in 5 girls among the total patients (0.9%). Sterile abscess formation was seen in 3 patients. Anaphylaxis happened in one patient, and unilateral slipped capital femoral epiphysis in another patient. The authors recommend being aware of these potential adverse effects related to GnRHa therapy in CPP [48c].

Acknowledgements

The authors thank Justin Peterson for their contributions and help in translating this manuscript.

References

[1] Klip H, Verloop J, van Gool JD, et al. OMEGA Project Group. Lancet. 2002;359(9312):1102–7 [C].

[2] Ohta R, Ohmukai H, Toyoizumi T, et al. Ovarian dysfunction, obesity and pituitary tumors in female mice following neonatal exposure to low-dose diethylstilbestrol. Reprod Toxicol. 2014;50:145–51 [E].

[3] Mahawong P, Sinclair A, Li Y, et al. Prenatal diethylstilbestrol induces malformation of the external genitalia of male and female mice and persistent second-generation developmental abnormalities of the external genitalia in two mouse strains. Differentiation. 2014;88(2-3):51–69 [E].

[4] Bhupathiraju SN, Manson JE. Menopausal hormone therapy and chronic disease risk in the women's health initiative: is timing everything? Endocr Pract. 2014;20(11):1201–13 [R].

[5] Bergendal A, Persson I, Odeberg J, et al. Association of venous thromboembolism with hormonal contraception and thrombophilic genotypes. Obstet Gynecol. 2014;124(3):600–9 [c].

[6] Sharifi M, Lewiecki EM. Conjugated estrogens combined with bazedoxifene: the first approved tissue selective estrogen complex therapy. Expert Rev Clin Pharmacol. 2014;7(3):281–91 [R].

[7] Pinkerton JV, Thomas S. Use of SERMs for treatment in postmenopausal women. J Steroid Biochem Mol Biol. 2014;142:142–54 [R].

[8] Komm BS, Mirkin S, Jenkins SN. Development of conjugated estrogens/bazedoxifene, the first tissue selective estrogen complex (TSEC) for management of menopausal hot flashes and postmenopausal bone loss. Steroids. 2014;90:71–81 [R].

[9] Cannoletta M, Cagnacci A. Modification of blood pressure in postmenopausal women: role of hormone replacement therapy. Int J Womens Health. 2014;6:745–57 [R].

[10] Kim JH, Meyers MS, Khuder SS, et al. Tissue-selective estrogen complexes with bazedoxifene prevents metabolic dysfunction in female mice. Mol Metab. 2014;3(2):177–90 [E].

[11] Nisenbaum MG, de Melo NR, Giribela CR, et al. Effects of a contraceptive containing drospirenone and ethinyl estradiol on blood pressure and autonomic tone: a prospective controlled clinical trial. Eur J Obstet Gynecol Reprod Biol. 2014;175:62–6 [c].

[12] Lidegaard Ø. Hormonal contraception, thrombosis and age. Expert Opin Drug Saf. 2014;13(10):1353–60 [R].

[13] Tricotel A, Raguideau F, Collin C, et al. Estimate of venous thromboembolism and related-deaths attributable to the use of combined oral contraceptives in France. PLoS One. 2014;9(4): e93792 [C].

[14] Erol N, Karaagac AT, Kounis NG. Dangerous triplet: polycystic ovary syndrome, oral contraceptives and Kounis syndrome. World J Cardiol. 2014;6(12):1285–9 [A].

[15] Strifert K. The link between oral contraceptive use and prevalence in autism spectrum disorder. Med Hypotheses. 2014;83(6):718–25 [H].

[16] Grandi G, Piacenti I, Volpe A, et al. Modification of body composition and metabolism during oral contraceptives containing non-androgenic progestins in association with estradiol or ethinyl estradiol. Gynecol Endocrinol. 2014;30(9):676–80 [c].

[17] Asare GA, Santa S, Ngala RA, et al. Effect of hormonal contraceptives on lipid profile and the risk indices for cardiovascular disease in a Ghanaian community. Int J Womens Health. 2014;6:597–603 [c].

[18] Patni N, Diaz EG, Cabral MD, et al. Worsening hypertriglyceridemia with oral contraceptive pills in an adolescent with HIV-associated lipodystrophy: a case report and review of the literature. J Pediatr Endocrinol Metab. 2014;27(11-12): 1247–51 [A].

[19] Abraham M, Mitchell J, Simsovits D, et al. Hypertriglyceridemic pancreatitis caused by the oral contraceptive agent estrostep. J Intensive Care Med. 2015;30(5):303–7 [PMID: 24671004] [A].

[20] Charlton BM, Rich-Edwards JW, Colditz GA, et al. Oral contraceptive use and mortality after 36 years of follow-up in the Nurses' health study: prospective cohort study. BMJ. 2014;349: g6356 [C].

[21] Kotsopoulos J, Lubinski J, Moller P, et al. Hereditary breast cancer clinical study group. Timing of oral contraceptive use and the risk of breast cancer in BRCA1 mutation carriers. Breast Cancer Res Treat. 2014;143(3):579–86 [C].

[22] Beaber EF, Malone KE, Tang MT, et al. Oral contraceptives and breast cancer risk overall and by molecular subtype among young women. Cancer Epidemiol Biomarkers Prev. 2014;23(5):755–64 [C].

[23] Ferris JS, Daly MB, Buys SS, et al. Oral contraceptive and reproductive risk factors for ovarian cancer within sisters in the breast cancer family registry. Br J Cancer. 2014;110(4):1074–80 [C].

[24] Thomin A, Keller V, Daraï E, et al. Consequences of emergency contraceptives: the adverse effects. Expert Opin Drug Saf. 2014;13(7):893–902 [R].

[25] Lin Y, Liu J, Zhang X, et al. A prospective, randomized study on hepatotoxicity of anastrozole compared with tamoxifen in women with breast cancer. Cancer Sci. 2014;105(9):1182–8 [c].

[26] Barrera J, Chambliss KL, Ahmed M, et al. Bazedoxifene and conjugated estrogen prevent diet-induced obesity, hepatic steatosis, and type 2 diabetes in mice without impacting the reproductive tract. Am J Physiol Endocrinol Metab. 2014;307(3): E345–E354 [E].

[27] Pagani O, Regan MM, Walley BA, et al. TEXT and SOFT Investigators; International Breast Cancer Study Group. Adjuvant exemestane with ovarian suppression in premenopausal breast cancer. N Engl J Med. 2014;371(2):107–18 [C].

[28] Bal UA, Atar I, Oktem M, et al. The effect of raloxifene on left ventricular hypertrophy in postmenopausal women: a prospective, randomized, and controlled study. Anatol J Cardiol. 2015;15(6):480–4 [c].

[29] Rühl H, Schröder L, Müller J, et al. Tamoxifen induces resistance to activated protein C. Thromb Res. 2014;133(5):886–91 [c].

[30] Chen JY, Kuo SJ, Liaw YP, et al. Endometrial cancer incidence in breast cancer patients correlating with age and duration of tamoxifen use: a population based study. J Cancer. 2014;5(2):151–5 [C].

[31] Macut D, Božić Antić I, Nestorov J, et al. The influence of combined oral contraceptives containing drospirenone on hypothalamic-pituitary-adrenocortical axis activity and glucocorticoid receptor expression and function in women with polycystic ovary syndrome. Hormones (Athens). 2015;14(1):109–17 [c].

[32] Lamas A, Máiz L, Ruiz de Valbuena M, et al. Subcutaneous implant with etonogestrel (Implanon®) for catamenial exacerbations in a

patient with cystic fibrosis: a case report. BMC Pulm Med. 2014;14:165 [A].

[33] Ferreira VH, Dizzell S, Nazli A, et al. Medroxyprogesterone acetate regulates HIV-1 uptake and transcytosis but not replication in primary genital epithelial cells, resulting in enhanced T-cell infection. J Infect Dis. 2015;211(11):1745–56 [E].

[34] Su QQ, Huang XL, Qin J, et al. Assessment of effects of mifepristone administration to lactating mice on the development and fertility of their progeny. J Obstet Gynaecol Res. 2015;41(4):575–81 [PMID: 25331362] [E].

[35] Levy DP, Jager M, Kapp N, et al. Ulipristal acetate for emergency contraception: postmarketing experience after use by more than 1 million women. Contraception. 2014;89(5):431–3 [C].

[36] Santos MA, Oliveira CV, Silva AS. Adverse cardiovascular effects from the use of anabolic-androgenic steroids as ergogenic resources. Subst Use Misuse. 2014;49(9):1132–7 [R].

[37] Baumann S, Jabbour C, Huseynov A, et al. Myocardial scar detected by cardiovascular magnetic resonance in a competitive bodybuilder with longstanding abuse of anabolic steroids. Asian J Sports Med. 2014;5(4):e24058 [A].

[38] Akçakoyun M, Alizade E, Gündoğdu R, et al. Long-term anabolic androgenic steroid use is associated with increased atrial electromechanical delay in male bodybuilders. Biomed Res Int. 2014;2014:451520 [c].

[39] Luciano RL, Castano E, Moeckel G, et al. Bile acid nephropathy in a bodybuilder abusing an anabolic androgenic steroid. Am J Kidney Dis. 2014;64(3):473–6 [A].

[40] Rainer Q, Speziali S, Rubino T, et al. Chronic nandrolone decanoate exposure during adolescence affects emotional behavior and monoaminergic neurotransmission in adulthood. Neuropharmacology. 2014;83:79–88 [E].

[41] Dupree JM, Langille GM, Khera M, et al. The safety of testosterone supplementation therapy in prostate cancer. Nat Rev Urol. 2014;11(9):526–30 [R].

[42] Hussain S, Haidar A, Bloom RE, et al. Bicalutamide-induced hepatotoxicity: a rare adverse effect. Am J Case Rep. 2014;15:266–70 [A].

[43] Crona DJ, Whang YE. Posterior reversible encephalopathy syndrome induced by enzalutamide in a patient with castration-resistant prostate cancer. Invest New Drugs. 2015;33(3):751–4 [PMID: 25467090] [A].

[44] Singh MK, Avram M. Persistent sexual dysfunction and depression in finasteride users for male pattern hair loss: a serious concern or red herring? J Clin Aesthet Dermatol. 2014;7(12):51–5 [R].

[45] Lin WL, Hsieh YW, Lin CL, et al. A population-based nested case-control study: the use of 5-alpha-reductase inhibitors and the increased risk of osteoporosis diagnosis in patients with benign prostate hyperplasia. Clin Endocrinol (Oxf). 2015;82(4):503–8 [C].

[46] Mačukat IR, Spanjol J, Orlič ZC, et al. The effect of 5alpha-reductase inhibition with finasteride and dutasteride on bone mineral density in older men with benign prostatic hyperplasia. Coll Antropol. 2014;38(3):835–9 [c].

[47] Duijnhoven RG, Straus SM, Souverein PC, et al. Long-term use of 5α-reductase inhibitors and the risk of male breast cancer. Cancer Causes Control. 2014;25(11):1577–82 [C].

[48] Lee JW, Kim HJ, Choe YM, et al. Significant adverse reactions to long-acting gonadotropin-releasing hormone agonists for the treatment of central precocious puberty and early onset puberty. Ann Pediatr Endocrinol Metab. 2014;19(3):135–40 [c].

40

Thyroid Hormones, Iodine and Iodides, and Antithyroid Drugs

Vicky V. Mody*,[1], *Ajay N. Singh*[†], *Rahul Deshmukh*[‡], *Samit Shah*[§]

*Associate Professor of Pharmaceutical Sciences, PCOM School of Pharmacy, Suwanee, GA, USA

[†]Department of Pharmaceutical Sciences, South University School of Pharmacy, Appalachian College of Pharmacy, Oakwood, VA, USA

[‡]Department of Pharmaceutical Sciences, Rosalind Franklin University of Medicine and Science, College of Pharmacy, North Chicago, IL, USA

[§]Department of Biopharmaceutical Sciences, KGI School of Pharmacy, Claremont, CA, USA

[1]Corresponding author: vickymody@gmail.com

THYROID HORMONES [SED-15, 3409; SEDA-31, 687; SEDA-32, 763; SEDA-33, 881; SEDA-34, 679; SEDA-35, 747; SEDA-36, 635]

Subclinical hypothyroidism is defined as elevated levels of serum thyroid stimulating hormone (TSH), whereas, overt hypothyroidism presents with elevated TSH levels and low levels of free triiodothyronine (fT3) and free levothyroxine (fT4). Patients presenting with overt or subclinical hypothyroidism are at increased risk of developing cardiovascular disease. Consequently, thyroid hormones mimetics (eprotirome), levothyroxine (T4), and triiodothyronine (liothyronine, T3) hold promise in the treatment of both overt and subclinical hypothyroidism.

Eprotirome

Eprotirome, a liver-selective thyroid hormone mimetic specific for the hepatic β receptor, has been shown to lower serum low-density lipoprotein (LDL) cholesterol concentrations in patients with dyslipidemia [1R]. Abnormal lipid levels put patients at risk for cardiovascular disease, which sometimes becomes difficult to reverse with stand-alone statin therapy. The use of thyroid hormone mimetics in these patients can help lower levels of LDL cholesterol.

Hepatotoxicity

In a randomized, double-blind, placebo-controlled, multicenter phase 3 clinical trial, 236 patients were enrolled with an aim to analyze the LDL cholesterol lowering effect of eprotirome [2C]. The patients enrolled had not reached target LDL cholesterol concentrations after at least 8 weeks of statin therapy with or without ezetimibe. Patients were divided into three groups, 80 patients in group 1 received placebo, 79 patients in group 2 received 50 μg eprotirome, and 77 patients in group 3 received 100 μg eprotirome. Among 236 patients, only 69 patients reached the 6-week time point (23 taking placebo, 24 taking 50 μg eprotirome, and 22 taking 100 μg eprotirome). It was found that the mean LDL cholesterol concentration increased by 9% in the placebo group and decreased by 12% and 22% in the 50 and 100 μg eprotirome groups, respectively. All of these patients also showed an increase in serum aspartate aminotransferase (AST; $P < 0.0001$), alanine aminotransferase (ALT; $P < 0.0001$), conjugated bilirubin ($P = 0.0006$), and gamma-glutamyltranspeptidase ($P < 0.0001$) levels, which may suggest that eprotirome has the potential to induce liver injury. The trial was prematurely terminated as it was also found in another study that eprotirome also causes cartilage damage in dogs [3S].

Levothyroxine

Levothyroxine remains the mainstay of current treatment for hypothyroidism, and the mean dosage prescribed for levothyroxine therapy is 1.6 μg/kg/day. Intestinal absorption of levothyroxine varies from

© 2015 Elsevier B.V. All rights reserved.

patient to patient and is usually in the range of 60–80% of the dose administered.

Rheumatoid Arthritis (RA)

The use of levothyroxine to manage hypothyroidism has been shown to increase the risk of developing rheumatoid arthritis for patients with autoimmune disorders [4M]. In a population based case controlled study, 1998 patients along with 2252 controls with incident RA cases were analyzed. The individuals reporting use of thyroxine substitute (levothyroxine) were compared with those who were not taking thyroxine substitute. It was found that the patients taking thyroxine substitution were at two fold increased risk of both anti-citrullinated peptide antibodies (ACPA)-positive (OR=1.9, 95%, CI 1.4–2.6) and ACPA-negative (OR=2.1, 95%, CI 1.5–3.1) RA. The risk also increased if the patients were smokers or had HLA-DRB1 shared epitope alleles (SE) [4M].

Cardiovascular Disorders

Bakiner et al. conducted a controlled, single-blind study to evaluate plasma Fetuin A levels in hypothyroid patients ($n = 39$) before and after treatment with levothyroxine and to determine if there is an association between Fetuin A levels and cardiovascular risk in those patients [5c]. The results indicated that there was no correlation between Fetuin A levels and cardiovascular risk factors and that Fetuin A levels were restored to normal levels for patients taking levothyroxine. Additionally, the study found that the mean LDL cholesterol levels of patients taking levothyroxine substantially decreased from 113.0 (59.0–214.0) to 101 (66.8–207). However, the mean HDL cholesterol levels also decreased from 49.3 (23–83.9) to 44 (28.3–69.0) among these patients [5c].

Drug Overdose

It is known that low doses of levothyroxine can contribute to cardiovascular effects, arrhythmias, and fractures and high doses of levothyroxine can result in acute detrimental effects on the patient. For example, a 23-year-old woman who attempted suicide by ingesting 25 mg of levothyroxine experienced hypercoagulation and a hypofibrinolytic effect, reflecting an increased risk of venous thrombosis [6A]. In another case, a 61-year-old woman accidentally ingested 50 mg of levothyroxine rather than the 50 µg actual dose [7A]. The high dose of levothyroxine in the serum lead to a thyroid storm, and patient exhibited acute respiratory failure, atrial fibrillation, and altered mental consciousness [7A].

Drug–Drug Interaction

Levothyroxine absorption can be affected by the coadministration of other drugs. The effect on the absorption of levothyroxine, when coadministered along with ciprofloxacin or rifampin, was assessed via a double-blind, randomized, placebo-controlled study on 8 healthy volunteers who received 1000 µg of levothyroxine combined with placebo, ciprofloxacin 750 mg, or rifampin 600 mg as single doses [8c]. The total plasma T4 concentrations over a 6-hour period were measured using liquid chromatography-tandem mass spectrometry (LCMS). Results indicated that the coadministration of ciprofloxacin significantly decreased the area under the curve (AUC) AUC of T4 [AUC of T4 reduced by 39% ($P = 0.035$)], whereas, rifampin coadministration significantly increased the AUC of T4 [AUC by 25% ($P = 0.003$)].

IODINE AND IODIDES [SED-15, 1896; SEDA-32, 764; SEDA-33, 883; SEDA-34, 680; SEDA-35, 752; SEDA-36]

Dietary Iodine

Iodine is an essential component of thyroid hormones, which regulate many important biochemical processes in the body. Iodine deficiency can have multiple adverse effects on growth and development, and it also can critically jeopardize children's mental health and often their very survival. Iodine deficiency disorders (IDD) in pregnant women can result in stillbirth, spontaneous abortion, and congenital abnormalities such as cretinism, a grave, irreversible form of mental retardation that affects people mostly living in iodine-deficient areas of Africa and Asia. Iodine deficiency is routinely surveyed in developed nations and has recently been found in young and pregnant women in UK [9M,10M,11c]. The World Health Organization (WHO) recommends that iodine deficiency in patients should be corrected through salt iodization. Moreover, iodine deficiency and its side effects are commonly reported and can be easily accessed from the WHO website [12S].

Iodine-Containing Solutions

Excessive iodine intake due to a long-term topical exposure like iodine solution dressings or by intravenous administration of iodine-containing agents can lead to hyperthyroidism [13A,14A]. Excessive iodine intake can also lead to hypothyroidism.

Hypothyroidism

Three cases of iodine-induced hypothyroidism were reported in full-term neonates after cardiac angiography and topical application of iodine-containing antiseptics [15A]. Two of these infants had transient hypothyroidism, and 1 infant had severe hypothyroidism requiring ongoing thyroid replacement therapy. All infants were asymptomatic; hypothyroidism was detected incidentally in the inpatient setting due to repeat newborn screening mandated by the long duration of hospitalization in these infants.

Iodine-125 Brachytherapy

Iodine-125 has a relatively long half-life (59.4 days) and emits low-energy photons (35 keV), making it a preferred isotope for radiation therapy (brachytherapy, BT) to treat prostate cancer and brain tumors.

Inflammation

Iodine-125 brachytherapy was used to treat 114 tumors from 1994 to 2010. Brachytherapy alone was used for 72 tumors, 39 post-surgery and 33 *de novo* [16R]. A brachytherapy boost together with external beam radiotherapy was used for 42 tumors, eight post-surgery and 34 *de novo*. Tumors were in the tongue, floor of mouth, soft palate, and tonsils. Brachytherapy was administered via an applicator or in plastic tubes implanted into the soft tissues or submandibular region. Complications of soft tissue ulceration occurred in 21 patients (18.4%) and healed spontaneously in 20 patients. There was no mandibular necrosis.

Nausea and Vomiting

Efficacy of interstitial brachytherapy (IBT) was evaluated for intracranial ganglioglioma in 8 patients [17R]. Patients ($m/f = 5/3$, median age 30.4 years, age range 7–42.5 years) were treated with IBT using stereotactically implanted ^{125}I seeds. The median follow-up time was 41.5 months (range 16.7–140.1 months). The cumulative tumor surface dose ranged between 50 and 65 Gy (permanent implantation) and the median tumor volume was 5.6 ml (range 0.9–26 ml). After BT, follow-up magnetic resonance imaging (MRI) revealed complete remission in 1 patient, partial remission in 3 patients, and stable disease in the remaining 4 patients. Five of 8 patients who presented with seizures were either seizure-free (1/5) or improved (4/5) after treatment. Temporary treatment-related headache, nausea, and vomiting occurred in 1 patient only and resolved completely after 4 weeks of steroid medication. No treatment-related mortality was observed.

Iodine-131

Iodine-131 (^{131}I) is the most commonly used iodine radioisotope, and it decays mostly by beta-emission (606 keV; 90%). It is well-known for causing death of cells because it can penetrate other cells up to several millimeters away. For this reason, ^{131}I is used for the treatment of thyrotoxicosis (hyperthyroidism) and some types of thyroid cancer that absorb iodine. The ^{131}I isotope is also used as a radioactive label for certain radiopharmaceutical therapies, e.g. ^{131}I-metaiodobenzylguanidine (^{131}I-MIBG) for treating pheochromocytoma and neuroblastoma. Iodine-131 also emits high energy gamma radiation (364 keV; 10%) that can be used for imaging [18E]. Adverse reactions with the use of ^{131}I include myelotoxicity, swelling and tenderness of salivary glands, nausea, vomiting, dry mouth, and hypothyroidism [19c].

Hypothyroidism

The clinical outcome of 153 Graves' disease patients treated with varying doses of radioactive iodine-131 (RAI, as NaI) during 1999–2001 was analyzed, retrospectively [20R]. This study suggested that the treatment outcome was dependent on the initial thyroid volume (17, 26, 33 and 35 ml, $P < 0.001$) or activity per gram tissue retained at 24 hours (6.02, 4.95, 4.75, and 4.44 MBq/g, $P = 0.002$). Treatment with a higher radiation dose (>6 MBq/g) showed an 80% cure rate, and a lower dose t ($\leq$6 MBq/g, cure rate 46%) showed a 46% cure rate ($P < 0.001$). Six to 9 months after the first dose of RAI, 39% of patients ($n = 60$) showed hypothyroidism (or rather thyroxine-substituted), 17% of patients ($n = 26$) were euthyroid, and 44% of patients ($n = 67$) did not respond properly [20R].

Leukopenia

A randomized trial evaluated the role of a single dose of postoperative adjuvant intra-arterial ^{131}I-lipiodol (vs. unlabeled lipiodol) in reducing the rate of intrahepatic recurrence. Fifty-eight patients who underwent curative treatment for hepatocellular carcinoma (HCC) and recovered within 6 weeks were inducted in the study [median age of 63 years (range, 23–85 years)]. Half of the patients ($n = 29$) received a single 2200-MBq intra-arterial ^{131}I-lipiodol dose and the remaining half ($n = 29$) received a single unlabeled lipiodol dose on a 1:1 basis. Recurrence-free and overall survival rates were analyzed. Two years after treatment, the rate of patients with intrahepatic recurrence was 28% in the ^{131}I-lipiodol group and 56% in the lipiodol group ($P = 0.0449$). The Kaplan–Meier analysis confirmed that the 2-year recurrence-free survival in the ^{131}I-lipiodol and lipiodol groups was 73% and 45%, respectively ($P = .0259$). The 5-year recurrence-free survival rates in the ^{131}I-lipiodol and lipiodol groups were 40% and 0%, respectively ($P = 0.0184$). The overall and specific survivals were not significantly different between groups ($P = 0.9378$ and $P = 0.1339$, respectively). ^{131}I-lipiodol had no severe toxic effects due to radioactive iodine, with exception of lowering white blood cell count [21R].

Radioactive Iodine

Of 37 known iodine isotopes, four isotopes (^{123}I, ^{124}I, ^{125}I, and ^{131}I) are routinely used in medical settings for diagnosis or therapeutic applications [22R,23S]. Preferential uptake of iodine by the thyroid led to the application of radioiodine in imaging and treatment of dysfunctional thyroid tissues [24S].

ANTITHYROID DRUGS [SEDA-32, 765; SEDA-33, 884; SEDA-34, 681; SEDA-35, 754, SEDA-36, 638]

Thionamides, a class of antithyroid drugs (ATDs), are compounds that are known to inhibit thyroid hormone synthesis via the inhibition of organification of iodine to tyrosine residues in thyroglobulin and the coupling of iodotyrosines [25R]. The commonly available thionamides are Propylthiouracil (PTU) and methimazole (MMI). Carbimazole (CBZ), which is a prodrug of methimazole, is currently not available in the Unites States. MMI has some intrinsic pharmacokinetic advantages over propylthiouracil in terms of longer half-life, resulting in once daily dosing and higher patient compliance. MMI also tends to exhibit less hepatotoxicity compared to PTU.

Common Side-Effects

Some of the common side effects associated with PTU and MMI include pruritus, rash, urticaria, arthralgias, arthritis, fever, abnormal taste sensation, nausea, and vomiting. These adverse effects were observed in 13% of patients ($n = 389$) taking thionamide drugs in one study [26R].

Agranulocytosis

Agranulocytosis, although not common, is a serious complication of thionamide therapy. A prevalence of as high as 0.5% has been observed within the first 2 months of treatment with thionamide drugs [27R,28R]. The risk of agranulocytosis is higher for ATDs when compared to 20 other classes of drugs associated with this rare complication [29R]. A Japanese case study looking at 754 cases of ATD-induced agranulocytosis over a period of 30 years noted that agranulocytosis developed within 90 days of starting ATD therapy in most patients (84.5%). The mean age of patients was 43.4 ± 15.2 years (mean $\pm$ SD), and the

male to female ratio was 1:6.3. The MMI dose given at onset was 25.2 ± 12.8 mg/day and in some patients the development of agranulocytosis was gradual. The analysis of physician reports for 30 fatal cases revealed that some deaths might have been prevented through appropriate intervention [30R]. Another Japanese study evaluated the characteristics of agranulocytosis as an adverse event of ATDs in the second or later course of treatment. The study concluded that when ATD treatment is resumed, patient follow-up is essential in order to monitor for the development of agranulocytosis [31R]. For the first time, a Korean study reported that a patient with Graves' disease developed post-infectious Guillain-Barre syndrome (GBS) during a course of MMI-induced agranulocytosis [32A]. MMI induced neutropenia and ecthyma was also reported in a pregnant patient with hyperthyroidism. The patient subsequently had to undergo a thyroidectomy [33A]. A 37-year-old female who was started on MMI for hyperthyroidism was presented to medical facility for evaluation of suspected thyroid storm. The patient was diagnosed with sepsis mimicking thyroid storm as a result of MMI-induced agranulocytosis [34A]. Recently, a 27-year-old woman who was previously prescribed MMI for 9 months presented with a 4-day history of a sore throat. She was initially diagnosed with febrile agranulocytosis and later with *S. pneumoniae* infection. She was successfully treated with intubation, intravenous antibiotics, and granulocyte colony-stimulating factor. Antithyroid drug-induced agranulocytosis contributed to the complications associated with pneumococcal sepsis and upper airway obstruction [35A]. The EIDOS and DoTS descriptions of thionamide induced agranulocytosis are shown in Figure 1.

ANCA-Positive Vasculitis

Antineutrophil cytoplasmic antibody (c-ANCA) positive vasculitis, a potentially life-threatening disease, has been reported with use of PTU. A case of perinuclear c-ANCA developed during treatment with PTU for Grave's disease was reported recently [36R]. In another case, a 42-year-old woman presented with acute renal and hepatic failure. The failure was attributed to PTU-induced c-ANCA production [37A]. In another case study, a 27-year-old woman presenting with refractory hypoxaemic respiratory failure, haemoptysis, and thyrotoxicosis was attributed by the authors as a rare manifestation of propylthiouracil therapy resulting from the development of c-ANCA [38A]. A 35-year-old woman with Graves' disease who wished to get pregnant was switched for MMI to PTU. The patient developed symptoms of hemoptysis and dyspnea after 3 weeks and her c-ANCA level increased to 259 Elisa units after PTU

FIGURE 1 EIDOS and DoTS description of thionamide-induced agranulocytosis.

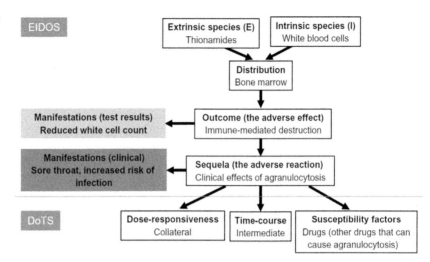

treatment. Her clinical condition improved with the discontinuation of PTU and with immunosuppressive therapy [39A]. A 34-year-old female was being treated for autoimmune hyperthyroidism, 6 weeks later she exhibited purpuric plaques with central necrosis on the gluteal areas [40A]. Laboratory results showed the presence of cryoglobulin, cryofibrinogen, and c-ANCA. PTU is considered to be the most common inducer of ANCA-associated microscopic polyangiitis [41R]. When PTU was stopped and the patient was prescribed MMI, the skin lesions improved within a week, but the cryoglobulins, cryofibrinogens, c-ANCA and anti-SSA remained positive even after 5 months. In another study, a 56-year-old female patient who was diagnosed with toxic nodular goiter was prescribed PTU 100 mg. After 6 months, she was seen for rash on both legs and bloody urine. The patient was diagnosed with PTU-induced p-ANCA positive vasculitis. PTU was discontinued and a regimen of methlyprednisolone 32 mg/day, azathioprine 150 mg/day, and ACE inhibitor (for proteinuria) was initiated in this patient [42A]. To investigate renal involvement in PTU-associated antineutrophil cytoplasmic autoantibody (ANCA) vasculitis (PTU-AAV), Chen et al. studied 12 patients who developed ANCA associated vasculitis after treatment with PTU [43R]. Seven of 12 (58.3%) patients had renal dysfunction, and 3 among them needed initial renal replacement therapy. The renal biopsy showed the presence of pauci-immune segmental necrotizing crescentic glomerulonephritis in 10 patients and 2 of the 12 patients also showed the presence of segmental necrotizing glomerulonephritis superimposed on membranous nephropathy.

Hepatotoxicity

Hepatotoxicity is a rare complication of thionamide therapy. Although MMI has been associated with liver disease, it is typically due to cholestatic dysfunction, not hepatocellular inflammation [44R]. Recently, a 33-year-old woman was treated at the University Hospital Fundación Santa Fe de Bogota, and the condition was induced by a MMI-based treatment for Graves' disease. According to the authors, the causal diagnosis of MMI-induced hepatotoxicity was supported by the results of a liver biopsy [45A]. A case report of a patient with Graves' disease exhibiting thyrotoxicosis and signs of severe hepatotoxicity induced by propylthiouracil suggested that plasmapheresis could be an important treatment option to rapidly reduce thyroid hormones, in preparation for total thyroidectomy [46A].

Pancreatitis

Pancreatitis has very rarely been reported in association with MMI treatment [47A].

Teratogenicity and Birth Defects

MMI has been associated with a rare fetal scalp defect, aplasia cutis [48R]. More serious congenital malformations such as choanal atresia and tracheoesophageal fistulas, also called MMI embryopathy, have also been associated with MMI use. A recent review article analyzed 92 papers discussing use of MMI and birth defects. The review concludes that MMI use in early pregnancy may lead to birth defects in 2–3% of the exposed children, and that the defects are often severe. Proposals are given on how to minimize the risk of birth defects in fertile women treated for hyperthyroidism with ATDs [49R]. Another study explored the association of genetics with MMI/CBZ therapy. The case reports 2 siblings with physical features consistent with carbimazole/MMI embryopathy. Also reported is a previously unreported minor dental anomaly in this sibling pair with antenatal exposure of CBZ [50A]. A Danish study looked at the use of MMI/CMZ and PTU in early pregnancy, and its association with an increased prevalence of birth defects. The prevalence of birth defects was higher in children exposed to ATDs in early pregnancy (PTU, 8.0%; MMI/CMZ, 9.1%; MMI/CMZ and PTU, 10.1%; no ATD, 5.4%; nonexposed, 5.7%; $P < 0.001$). Both maternal use of MMI/CMZ (adjusted odds ratio = 1.66 [95%, CI 1.35–2.04]) and PTU (1.41 [1.03–1.92]) and maternal shift between MMI/CMZ and PTU in early pregnancy (1.82 [1.08–3.07]) were associated with an increased odds ratio (OR) of birth defects. MMI/CMZ and PTU toxicities were also associated with the urinary system. Choanalatresia, esophageal atresia, omphalocele, omphalomesenteric duct anomalies, and aplasia cutis were common in MMI/CMZ-exposed children (combined, adjusted OR = 21.8 [13.4–35.4]) [27R]. Another study discussed case of a newborn exposed to MMI during the first 4 weeks of gestation, leading to MMI embryopathy consisting of esophageal atresia, small omphalocele, and ileal prolapse through a patent omphalomesenteric duct [51A]. A Chinese study examined the incidence of CMZ embryopathy in the Hong Kong Chinese population and the factors associated with its development. The study concluded that the incidence of CMZ embryopathy in the study group was 11.1%. Critical factors for its development are exposure to a CMZ dosage of ≥ 20 mg/day before 7 weeks of gestation. Genetic susceptibility may also play a role [52R].

References

[1] France M, Schofield J, Kwok S, et al. Treatment of homozygous familial hypercholesterolemia. Clin Lipidol. 2014;9(1):101–18 [R].

[2] Sjouke B, Langslet G, Ceska R, et al. Eprotirome in patients with familial hypercholesterolaemia (the AKKA trial): a randomised, double-blind, placebo-controlled phase 3 study. Lancet Diabetes Endocrinol. 2014;2(6):455–63 [C].

[3] Karo Bio terminates the eprotirome program. www.karobio.com/investormedia/pressreleaser/pressrelease?pid=639535 [S].

[4] Bengtsson C, Padyukov L, Källberg H, et al. Thyroxin substitution and the risk of developing rheumatoid arthritis; results from the Swedish population-based EIRA study. Ann Rheum Dis. 2014;73(6):1096–100 [M].

[5] Bakiner O, Bozkirli E, Ertugrul D, et al. Plasma fetuin—a levels are reduced in patients with hypothyroidism. Eur J Endocrinol. 2014;170(3):411–8 [c].

[6] Stuijver DJ, van Zaane B, Squizzato A, et al. The effects of an extremely high dose of levothyroxine on coagulation and fibrinolysis. J Thromb Haemost. 2010;8(6):1427–8 [A].

[7] Kreisner E, Lutzky M, Gross JL. Charcoal hemoperfusion in the treatment of levothyroxine intoxication. Thyroid. 2010;20(2):209–12 [A].

[8] Goldberg AS, Tirona RG, Asher LJ, et al. Ciprofloxacin and rifampin have opposite effects on levothyroxine absorption. Thyroid. 2013;23(11):1374–8 [c].

[9] Bath SC, Button S, Rayman MP. Availability of iodised table salt in the UK—is it likely to influence population iodine intake? Public Health Nutr. 2014;17(2):450–4 [M].

[10] Bath SC, Rayman MP. Iodine deficiency in the U.K.: an overlooked cause of impaired neurodevelopment? Proc Nutr Soc. 2013;72(2):226–35 [M].

[11] Bath SC, Sleeth ML, McKenna M, et al. Iodine intake and status of UK women of childbearing age recruited at the University of Surrey in the winter. Br J Nutr. 2014;112(10):1715–23 [c].

[12] World Health Organization, Vitamin and Mineral Nutrition Information System, The Association; c1946-2015 [updated 2015]. Geneva, Switzerland http://www.who.int/vmnis/database/iodine/countries/en/ [S].

[13] Dunne P, Kaimal N, MacDonald J, et al. Iodinated contrast-induced thyrotoxicosis. Can Med Assoc J. 2013;185(2):144–7 [A].

[14] Brotfain E, Koyfman L, Frenkel A, et al. Iodine-induced hyperthyroidism—an old clinical entity that is still relevant to daily ICU practice: a case report. Case Rep Endocrinol. 2013;2013:792745 [A].

[15] Thaker VV, Leung AM, Braverman LE, et al. Iodine-induced hypothyroidism in full-term infants with congenital heart disease: more common than currently appreciated? J Clin Endocrinol Metab. 2014;99(10):3521–6 [A].

[16] Stannard C, Maree G, Tovey S, et al. Iodine-125 brachytherapy in the management of squamous cell carcinoma of the oral cavity and oropharynx. Brachytherapy. 2014;13(4):405–12 [R].

[17] El Majdoub F, Rezk E, Hunsche S, et al. Intracranial ganglioglioma WHO I: results in a series of eight patients treated with stereotactic interstitial brachytherapy. J Neurooncol. 2014;118(2):345–50 [R].

[18] Rault E, Vandenberghe S, Van Holen R, et al. Comparison of image quality of different iodine isotopes (I-123, I-124, and I-131). Cancer Biother Radiopharm. 2007;22(3):423–30 [E].

[19] Alexander C, Bader JB, Schaefer A, et al. Intermediate and long-term side effects of high-dose radioiodine therapy for thyroid carcinoma. J Nucl Med. 1998;39(9):1551–4 [c].

[20] Cepkova J, Horacek J, Vizda J, et al. Radioiodine treatment of Graves' disease—dose/response analysis. Acta Medica (Hradec Kralove). 2014;57(2):49–55 [R].

[21] Dumortier J, Decullier E, Hilleret M-N, et al. Adjuvant intraarterial lipiodol or 131I-lipiodol after curative treatment of hepatocellular carcinoma: a prospective randomized trial. J Nucl Med. 2014;55(6):877–83 [R].

[22] Finn R. Chemistry applied to iodine radionuclides. Handbook of radiopharmaceuticals. Chichester, UK: John Wiley & Sons, Ltd.; 2005. p. 423–40 [R].

[23] Silberstein EB, Alavi A, Balon HR, et al. The SNMMI practice guideline for therapy of thyroid disease with 131I 3.0. J Nucl Med. 2012;53(10):1633–51 [S].

[24] Meier DA, Brill DR, Becker DV, et al. Procedure guideline for therapy of thyroid disease with 131Iodine. J Nucl Med. 2002;43(6):856–61 [S].

[25] Cooper DS. Antithyroid drugs. N Engl J Med. 2005;352(9): 905–17 [R].

[26] Werner MC, Romaldini JH, Bromberg N, et al. Adverse effects related to thionamide drugs and their dose regimen. Am J Med Sci. 1989;297(4):216–9 [R].

[27] Andersen SL, Olsen J, Wu CS, et al. Birth defects after early pregnancy use of antithyroid drugs: a Danish nationwide study. J Clin Endocrinol Metab. 2013;98(11):4373–81 [R].

[28] Watanabe N, Narimatsu H, Noh JY, et al. Antithyroid drug-induced hematopoietic damage: a retrospective cohort study of agranulocytosis and pancytopenia involving 50,385 patients with Graves' disease. J Clin Endocrinol Metab. 2012;97(1):E49–53 [R].

[29] Van Staa TP, Boulton F, Cooper C, et al. Neutropenia and agranulocytosis in England and Wales: incidence and risk factors. Am J Hematol. 2003;72(4):248–54 [R].

[30] Nakamura H, Miyauchi A, Miyawaki N, et al. Analysis of 754 cases of antithyroid drug-induced agranulocytosis over 30 years in Japan. J Clin Endocrinol Metab. 2013;98(12):4776–83 [R].

[31] Kobayashi S, Noh JY, Mukasa K, et al. Characteristics of agranulocytosis as an adverse effect of antithyroid drugs in the second or later course of treatment. Thyroid. 2014;24(5): 796–801 [R].

[32] Cho YY, Joung JY, Jeong H, et al. Postinfectious Guillain-Barre syndrome in a patient with methimazole-induced agranulocytosis. Korean J Intern Med. 2013;28(6):724–7 [A].

[33] Thomas SK, Sheffield JS, Roberts SW. Thionamide-induced neutropenia and ecthyma in a pregnant patient with hyperthyroidism. Obstet Gynecol. 2013;122(2 Pt 2):490–2 [A].

[34] Rayner SG, Hosseini F, Adedipe AA. Sepsis mimicking thyroid storm in a patient with methimazole-induced agranulocytosis. BMJ Case Rep. 2013;2013:1–3 [A].

[35] Ishimaru N, Ohnishi H, Nishiuma T, et al. Antithyroid drug-induced agranulocytosis complicated by pneumococcal sepsis and upper airway obstruction. Int Med (Tokyo, Japan). 2013;52(20):2355–9 [A].

[36] Criado PR, Grizzo Peres Martins AC, Gaviolli CF, et al. Propylthiouracil-induced vasculitis with antineutrophil cytoplasmic antibody. Int J Low Extrem Wounds. 2014;14(2):187–91 [R].

[37] Khan TA, Yin Luk FC, Uqdah HT, et al. A fatal case of propylthiouracil-induced ANCA-associated vasculitis resulting in rapidly progressive glomerulonephritis, acute hepatic failure, and cerebral angiitis. Clin Nephrol. 2014;83(5):309–14.

[38] Ortiz-Diaz EO. A 27-year-old woman presenting with refractory hypoxaemic respiratory failure, haemoptysis and thyrotoxicosis: a rare manifestation of propylthiouracil therapy. BMJ case rep. 2014;2014:167 [A].

[39] Kimura M, Seki T, Ozawa H, et al. The onset of antineutrophil cytoplasmic antibody-associated vasculitis immediately after methimazole was switched to propylthiouracil in a woman with Graves' disease who wished to become pregnant. Endocr J. 2013;60(3):383–8 [A].

[40] Akkurt ZM, Ucmak D, Acar G, et al. Cryoglobulin and antineutrophil cytoplasmic antibody positive cutaneous vasculitis due to propylthiouracil. Indian J Dermatol Venereol Leprol. 2014;80(3):262–4 [A].

[41] Bonaci-Nikolic B, Nikolic MM, Andrejevic S, et al. Antineutrophil cytoplasmic antibody (ANCA)-associated autoimmune diseases induced by antithyroid drugs: comparison with idiopathic ANCA vasculitides. Arthritis Res Ther. 2005;7(5):R1072–81 [R].

[42] Bes C, Dikbas O, Keskin E, et al. A case of propylthiouracil-induced antineutrophilic cytoplasmic antibody-positive vasculitis successfully treated with radioactive iodine. Reumatismo. 2013;65(3):131–3 [A].

[43] Chen Y, Bao H, Liu Z, et al. Clinico-pathological features and outcomes of patients with propylthiouracil-associated ANCA vasculitis with renal involvement. J Nephrol. 2014;27(2):159–64 [R].

[44] Arab DM, Malatjalian DA, Rittmaster RS. Severe cholestatic jaundice in uncomplicated hyperthyroidism treated with methimazole. J Clin Endocrinol Metab. 1995;80(4):1083–5 [R].

[45] Lopez PRP, Forero JD, Sierra F. Methimazole-induced cholestatic jaundice in a hyperthyroid patient. Acta Gastroenterol Latinoam. 2014;44(1):52–8 [A].

[46] Almeida RF, Comarella AP, Silveira MB, et al. Plasmapheresis before thyroidectomy in a patient with thyrotoxicosis and hepatotoxicity by propylthiouracil: case report. Arq Bras Endocrinol Metabol. 2013;57(4):322–6 [A].

[47] Yang M, Qu H, Deng HC. Acute pancreatitis induced by methimazole in a patient with Graves' disease. Thyroid. 2012;22(1):94–6 [A].

[48] Mandel SJ, Cooper DS. The use of antithyroid drugs in pregnancy and lactation. J Clin Endocrinol Metab. 2001;86(6):2354–9 [R].

[49] Laurberg P, Andersen SL. Therapy of endocrine disease: antithyroid drug use in early pregnancy and birth defects: time windows of relative safety and high risk? Eur J Endocrinol. 2014;171(1):R13–20 [R].

[50] Goel H, Dudding T. Carbimazole/methimazole embryopathy in siblings: a possible genetic susceptibility. Birth Defects Res A Clin Mol Teratol. 2013;97(11):755–8 [A].

[51] Panait N, Michel F, D'Ercole C, et al. Esophageal atresia, small omphalocele and ileal prolapse through a patent omphalomesenteric duct: a methamizole embryopathy? J Pediatr Surg. 2013;48(6):E9–E11 [A].

[52] Ting YH, Zhou Y, Lao TT. Carbimazole embryopathy in a Chinese population: case series and literature review. Birth Defects Res A Clin Mol Teratol. 2013;97(4):225–9 [R].

41

Insulin, Other Hypoglycemic Drugs, and Glucagon

Alisa K. Escaño[1]

Department of Pharmacotherapy & Outcomes Science, Virginia Commonwealth University
School of Pharmacy, Falls Church, VA, USA
[1]Corresponding author: Alisa.Escano@inova.org

Glucagon [SEDA-15, 1510; SEDA-31, 689; SEDA-32, 769; SEDA-33, 889; SEDA-36, 645]

Metabolism

APPETITE REDUCTION

A double-blind crossover study, evaluated the effects of glucagon 2.8 pmol/kg/min and GLP-1 0.4 pmol/kg/min infusions of each peptide alone, both peptides in combination, or placebo on reduction of appetite. Glucagon or GLP-1, given individually at these doses, did not significantly reduce food intake; however, coinfusion at the same doses led to a significant reduction in food intake of 13%. Furthermore, the addition of GLP-1 protected against glucagon-induced hyperglycemia, and an energy expenditure increase of 53 kcal/day was reported on coinfusion. These observations support the concept of GLP-1 and glucagon dual agonism as a possible treatment for obesity and diabetes [1C].

Insulin [SED-15, 1761; SEDA-31, 689; SEDA-32, 769; SEDA-33, 889; SEDA-34, 685; SEDA-36, 645]

Endocrine

HYPOGLYCEMIA

The debates over choosing the right basal insulin therapy in patients focus on efficacy by reducing basal blood glucose and safety by producing minimal nocturnal hypoglycemia. The efficacy and safety of two, once daily basal insulin formulations, a long acting lispro protamine suspension (ILPS) vs. insulin glargine (glargine), were studied when added to oral antihyperglycemic medications

(OAMs) or exenatide twice daily in patients with type 2 diabetes (T2DM). Patients were randomized to bedtime ILPS ($n = 171$) or glargine ($n = 168$) in addition to their OAMs or exenatide therapy. Overall, the rates of hypoglycemia (ILPS 120/171; glargine 125/168, $P = 0.394$) and rates of severe hypoglycemia (ILPS 3/171; glargine 0/168, $P = 0.249$) were similar and not statistically significant. Patients who were treated with ILPS had a more occurrences of nocturnal hypoglycemia versus glargine (4.88 ± 8.43 episodes/patient/year vs. 3.01 ± 7.21 4.88 ± 8.43 episodes/patient/year; $P = 0.004$) [2C].

The occurrence of hypoglycemia in patients with severe cardiac disease and the potential impact on mortality has been on an ongoing discussion in the literature. To determine whether insulin glargine therapy posed a significant hypoglycemic risk, a meta-analysis analyzed studies of patients who had baseline cardiovascular risk factors (CVRFs), who added insulin glargine to ongoing OAM treatment compared to other treatment interventions (e.g. lifestyle modifications, additional OAMs, adding insulin NPH, lispro, or premixed insulins in patients failing OAM therapy). Nine randomized controlled comparator trials of glargine use in insulin-naive patients with T2DM inadequately controlled on OAMs were analyzed. From the nine studies analyzed, patient data was pooled and broken down to compare results in patients treated with glargine ($n = 1462$) compared to overall pooled (glargine compared to all treatment arms in the RCTs analyzed) ($n = 1476$) and individual comparators (glargine compared to the individual treatment arms in the RCTs analyzed) for efficacy of treatment (goal HbA1c level $\leq 7.0\%$ or decrease $\geq 1.0\%$ change from baseline) and rates of hypoglycemia (symptomatic, confirmed,

© 2015 Elsevier B.V. All rights reserved.

nocturnal, or severe). Patients with hypertension (~69%), dyslipidemia (~58%), history of cardiovascular disease (~25%), or any CVRF (~83%) at baseline were identified and efficacy and safety were also compared. Patients treated with glargine had greater reductions in HbA1c and higher rates of hypoglycemia compared to patients treated with OAMs and in patients with any CVRF. However, reductions in HbA1c level were greater and hypoglycemia rates lower with use of glargine compared with premixed insulin and in patients with any CVRF. Overall, the authors concluded that the benefits of glargine use compared with alternative therapeutic options on lowering HbA1c and glucose are maintained without excess hypoglycemia in patients with CVRFs [3M].

NOCTURNAL HYPOGLYCEMIA

A study concerning the long-term safety and efficacy of the basal insulin analogue, insulin degludec, as compared to insulin glargine (both with insulin aspart) in patients with type 1 diabetes, was conducted. The rate of nocturnal hypoglycemia was 25% lower with insulin degludec than with insulin glargine (3.9 vs. 5.3 episodes/patient-year of exposure; estimated rate ratio (insulin degludec/insulin glargine): 0.75 [95% CI 0.59–0.95]; $P = 0.02$). Rates of hypoglycemia, severe hypoglycemia, and reductions in HbA1c and fasting plasma glucose were similar between both groups [4C].

Endocrine

LIPOTROPHY

A 62-year-old woman with T2DM presented with 4-month history of a depressed area of skin (15×10 cm) on her abdomen. She had been treating her T2DM with insulin detemir and insulin aspart injected at various sites on her abdomen for 6 years. A biopsy of the tissue was obtained from the lipotropic area. Prominent atrophy of the subcutaneous fatty tissue was seen, associated with disappearance of the subcutaneous fat and replaced by loose, partially myxoid connective tissue. Numerous foamy macrophages, including multinucleated giant cells of the Touton and foreign body type, were present surrounding atrophic fat lobules and within connective tissue septa along with focal areas of hemosiderin deposition and aggregates of lymphocytes. The patient's localized lipotrophy remained unchanged with continued insulin treatment, although the patient was instructed to use a different site on her abdomen for her insulin injections [5c].

Metabolism

WEIGHT GAIN

The efficacy and safety of two, once daily basal insulin formulations [insulin lispro protamine suspension (ILPS) vs. insulin glargine (glargine)] added to oral antihyperglycemic medications (OAMs) and exenatide twice daily in suboptimally controlled T2DM patients was studied. Patients were randomized to bedtime ILPS ($n = 171$) or glargine ($n = 168$). Weight gain was similar between groups (ILPS: 0.27 ± 3.38 kg; glargine: 0.66 ± 3.93 kg, $P = $NS) [2].

Metabolism

APPETITE REGULATION

A study aimed to examine the effects of insulin detemir compared to insulin NPH on appetite regulation and weight loss in type 1 diabetic (T1DM) patients. Due to the lipophilic nature of insulin detemir, the investigators proposed that insulin detemir enters the brain more readily than insulin NPH and may differentially modify brain activation in response to food stimuli. Patient responses to viewing food and non-food pictures were measured in the brain using functional Magnetic Resonance Imaging (MRI) in T1DM patients ($n - 32$) and cerebral spinal fluid (CSF) insulin levels were measured after two 12-week treatment periods with insulin detemir and insulin NPH. Patients treated with insulin detemir demonstrated a mean weight loss of 0.8 kg while patients treated with insulin NPH experienced a mean 0.5 kg weight gain ($P = 0.02$ for difference). MRI reports indicate that brain activation was significantly lower in bilateral insula, an appetite-regulating brain region, in response to visual food stimuli in the insulin detemir group compared to insulin NPH ($P = 0.02$ for right and $P = 0.05$ for left insula) with higher levels of insulin in the CSF in the insulin detemir treated group compared to those treated with insulin NPH ($P = 0.003$). The authors concluded that, in T1DM patients, the weight sparing effect of insulin detemir may be mediated by its enhanced action on the central nervous system, resulting in blunted activation in bilateral insula in response to food stimuli [6C].

Tumorigenicity

The risk of breast, prostate, colorectal, or all cancers combined and the association with insulin glargine use was examined in a population-based cohort study among patients with diabetes aged ≥18 years from 2001 to 2009. Cox regression modeling compared the risk of cancer in users of insulin glargine ($n = 27418$) to users of NPH ($n = 100757$). Patients taking NPH did not have an increased risk of breast, prostate, colorectal, or all cancers combined before switching to glargine. Insulin glargine was not associated with an increased risk of prostate, colorectal, or all cancers combined; however, the hazard ratio (HR) for breast cancer with the use of glargine was 1.3 (95% CI 1.0–1.8) in patients who were only treated with glargine. The HR for breast cancer associated with the use of glargine for ≥2 years was 1.6 if NPH had also been used at baseline or 1.7 if the glargine users had not used NPH. These results are not absolute and do not indicate a direct cause and effect relationship [7c].

A nested case–control study was conducted in 275 164 T2DM patients in Barcelona. The aim of the study was to evaluate the risk of cancer in patients on glucose-lowering agents. In patients ($n = 1040$) with a diagnosis of cancer between 2008 and 2010, the investigators matched three control subjects for each case ($n = 3120$) based on age, sex, diabetes duration, and geographical area. The treatments analyzed for the risk of causing cancer were: insulin glargine, insulin detemir, human insulin, fast-acting insulin and analogues, metformin, sulfonylureas, repaglinide, thiazolidinediones, dipeptidyl peptidase IV inhibitors, and alpha-glucosidase inhibitors. No significant increases in the risk of cancer were observed for any of the types of insulin and oral agents analyzed. Specifically when glargine was used alone or in combination with metformin. The investigators concluded that the type of treatment used did not influence the risk of cancer in T2DM patients [8c].

Alpha-Glucosidase Inhibitors [SEDA-15, 85; SEDA-30, 496; SEDA-31, 691; SEDA-32, 772; SEDA-33, 893; SEDA-36, 647]

Cardiovascular

Acarbose has demonstrated the ability to decrease progression of carotid intima-media thickness (CIMT) in pre-diabetes patients. In a randomized trial of acarbose versus placebo, patients ($n = 219$) were enrolled if: glucose values over 11.1 mmol/L 2 hours after a 75 g oral glucose load and a mean HbA1c of 6.3%. CIMT was measured at baseline and annually. Follow-up was discontinued if participants progressed to the study glucose endpoints defined as a fasting blood glucose >140 mg/dL observed at quarterly visits. CIMT readings were available for a median of 2 years, with 72 subjects followed for 5 years. While CIMT progression occurred in both groups, patients in the acarbose group had a reduction in progression of CIMT ($P = 0.047$); however, changes in glucose were not important determinants of CIMT progression [9C].

Endocrine

Administration of miglitol 30 minutes before a meal can be effective in preventing hyperinsulinemic hypoglycemia in patients who are post-gastrectomy. A case report was published of a 45-year-old woman who had undergone total gastrectomy for gastric cancer and presented with a history of post-prandial hypoglycemic episodes with loss of consciousness after meals. Laboratory findings revealed marked hyperinsulinemia and hypoglycemia after a meal. After treatment with octreotide and diazoxide, the patient continued to experience hypoglycemia induced by hyperinsulinemia. When miglitol was administered prior to a meal, insulin secretion was suppressed, although hypoglycemia was not prevented. The authors concluded that administration of miglitol 30 minutes before a meal prevented post-prandial hypoglycemia by slowing the increase of the blood glucose and serum insulin levels following the meal to a greater degree than administration just before a meal [10c].

Gastrointestinal

A case report published described the interference of acarbose with treatment with helical tomotherapy. The authors determined that the alpha-glucosidase inhibitor caused persistent gas production and internal organ motion in a 68-year-old Japanese man with prostate cancer. The acarbose was not held prior to the routine treatment planning computed tomography, which showed a large volume of rectal gas; an enema was given to void the rectum. Subsequent computed tomography showed a large volume of gas accumulation following previous removal. The patient was asked to discontinue his acarbose. Four days after discontinuation, the fourth attempted computed tomography was performed without noted gas accumulation. The authors concluded that the use of acarbose caused the accumulation of intestinal gas, which may have caused unexpected organ motion, untoward reactions, and insufficient doses to clinical targets [11c].

In another case series, two female patients, aged 53 and 26 years, experienced post-prandial reactive hypoglycemia due to primary accelerated gastric emptying. Both patients continued to experience post-prandial hypoglycemia despite dietary intervention of small, frequent meals. The authors concluded that the addition of acarbose to the dietary interventions resulted in a resolution of hypoglycemia [12c].

Biguanides [SEDA-15, 506; SEDA-31, 692; SEDA-32, 773; SEDA-33, 893; SEDA-34, 687; SEDA-36, 647]

Anti-Tumorigenicity

REDUCTION OF CANCER RISK

A number of studies published indicate metformin may affect cancer incidence in subjects with T2DM. Several meta-analyses have been published in an attempt to quantify this effect. One meta-analysis reviewed studies that assessed the effects of metformin and/or sulfonylureas on cancer risk in subjects with T2DM. Twenty-four studies showed that metformin use is associated with reduced risk for the development of cancer, in both cohort (RR = 0.70 [95% CI = 0.67–0.73]) and case–control studies (OR = 0.90 [95% CI = 0.84–0.98]), but this finding was not supported by randomized controlled trials

(RCTs) (RR=1.01 [95% CI=0.81–1.26]). Data from 18 studies in T2DM subjects showed that sulfonylurea use is associated with an increase in all-cancer risk in cohort studies (RR=1.55 [95% CI=1.48–1.63]); however, data from RCTs (RR=1.17 [95% CI=0.95–1.45]) and case–control studies (OR=1.02 [95% CI=0.93–1.13]) failed to demonstrate a statistically significant effect. This meta-analysis suggests that metformin use reduces, while sulfonylurea use may be associated with an increased cancer risk in subjects with T2DM [13M].

A second meta-analysis of 12 randomized controlled trials (21 595 patients) and 41 observational studies (1 029 389 patients) aimed to summarize the evidence on the association between metformin and cancer risk or mortality in patients with diabetes. Outcomes were cancer mortality, all malignancies and site-specific cancers. The results suggest that metformin might be associated with a significant reduction in the risk of cancer and cancer-related mortality. In observational studies, there was a significant association between metformin exposure and the risk of cancer death [6 studies, 24 410 patients, OR: 0.65, 95% CI, 0.53–0.80], all malignancies [18 studies, 561 836 patients, OR: 0.73, 95% CI, 0.61–0.88], liver [8 studies, 312 742 patients, OR: 0.34; 95% CI, 0.19–0.60] colorectal [12 studies, 871 365 patients, OR: 0.83, 95% CI, 0.74–0.92], pancreas [9 studies, 847 248 patients, OR: 0.56, 95% CI, 0.36–0.86], stomach [2 studies, 100 701 patients, OR: 0.83, 95% CI, 0.76–0.91], and esophagus cancer [2 studies, 100 694 patients, OR: 0.90, 95% CI, 0.83–0.98]. Metformin was not associated with the risk of: breast cancer, lung cancer, ovarian cancer, uterus cancer, prostate cancer, bladder cancer, kidney cancer, and melanoma [14M].

HEPATOCELLULAR CARCINOMA BENEFIT

A meta-analysis of eight studies was reviewed to evaluate the safety and efficacy of metformin in patients with T2DM and chronic hepatitis C virus (HCV) with or without cirrhosis and hepatocellular carcinoma (HCC). An increased benefit on virological response was seen in metformin-treated patients with insulin resistance receiving HCV treatment. A significant reduction in the occurrence of HCC, liver-related death, and liver transplant, and a decreased risk of HCC was seen in metformin-treated patients with T2DM and chronic liver disease. This observation indicates that metformin may provide benefit in the treatment of HCV and in reducing the risk of HCC in patients with T2DM and HCV. Although diarrhea was increased in patients receiving metformin, no serious adverse effects, including lactic acidosis, were reported [15M].

ENDOMETRIAL CANCER ANTI-PROLIFERATION BENEFIT

A study of 11 newly diagnosed, untreated, non-diabetic patients with endometrial cancer (EC) received metformin 500 mg orally three times daily from the point of a diagnostic biopsy to surgery with a mean of 36.6 days of treatment. Fasting plasma insulin, insulin-like growth factor 1 (IGF-1), insulin-like growth factor binding protein 1 (IGFBP-1) and insulin-like growth factor binding protein 7 (IGFBP-7) measurements were taken before and after metformin treatment. Ki-67, pAMPK, and pS6 immunohistochemistry staining was performed on the endometrial cancer before and after metformin treatment and was compared to a control group of 10 women with EC who did not receive metformin. Mean plasma insulin (P=0.0005), IGF-1 (P=0.001), and IGFBP-7 (P=0.0098) were significantly reduced after metformin treatment. A clear reduction in ki-67 and pS6 expression was observed with a significant mean reduction in percentage of cells staining for ki-67 (9.7%, P=0.02) and pS6 (31%, P=0.03). Study results indicate biological evidence consistent with the anti-proliferative effects of metformin in women with EC [16c].

COLORECTAL CANCER

A meta-analysis of 15 studies reported 13 871 cases of colorectal cancer in patients (n=840 787) with diabetes mellitus. The authors observed a protective association between metformin use and the risk of colorectal cancer. An 11% reduction in colorectal cancer risk associated with metformin use (n=9 studies; OR, 0.89; 95% CI, 0.81–0.99) was observed, whereas thiazolidinedione use was not associated with an increased colorectal cancer risk (n=5 studies; OR, 0.96; 95% CI, 0.87–1.05). Conversely, a trend toward higher colorectal cancer risk was observed with use of sulfonylurea (n=7 studies; OR, 1.11; 95% CI, 0.97–1.26) and insulin (n=9 studies; OR, 1.33; 95% CI, 0.91–1.94), although these associations were not statistically significant [17M].

LUNG CANCER REDUCTION

A meta-analysis found that metformin therapy was associated with significantly lower risk for cancers of the lung (4 studies; pooled relative risk=0.71, 95% confidence interval (CI): 0.55, 0.95; P=0.02) and respiratory system (6 studies; pooled relative risk=0.85, 95% CI, 0.75, 0.96; P=0.01) in diabetic patients [18M].

Cardiovascular

ENDOTHELIAL FUNCTION

A randomized, placebo-controlled trial investigated whether metformin can improve endothelial function and decrease inflammatory activity, thereby decreasing the risk of atherothrombotic disease. A total of 390 patients with T2DM treated with insulin were included and treated with add-on therapy of either metformin 850 mg or placebo. Metformin significantly reduced levels of von Willebrand factor, soluble vascular adhesion molecule-1, tissue-type plasminogen activator, plasminogen activator inhibitor-1, C-reactive protein (CRP) and soluble intercellular adhesion molecule-1, which, except for CRP, remained significant after adjustment for baseline differences in age, sex, smoking and severity of previous cardiovascular (CV) disease. A 34% reduction in the risk of CV morbidity and mortality associated with metformin treatment was associated with improvements in vWf and sVCAM-1, which may explain the decreased risk of CV disease in T2DM [19C].

Dermatology

ROSACEA-LIKE RASH

A case report of a 29-year-old woman that developed a non-vasculitis facial skin rash during the treatment with metformin found that discontinuation of metformin resulted in an improvement of symptoms, while the rechallenge resulted in a recurrence of the skin rash [20c].

Hematology

HEMOLYTIC ANEMIA

A case report of hemolytic anemia in a 17-year-old boy hospitalized receiving chemotherapy was given metformin for presumed steroid-induced hyperglycemia. On the second day of metformin treatment, the patient's hemoglobin level decreased, and a direct Coombs test was positive for immunoglobulin G but negative for complement and an indirect Coombs test was negative. The metformin was discontinued after it was suspected to have induced the hemolytic anemia. Upon metformin discontinuation, the jaundice resolved and the patient did not require red blood cell transfusions [21c].

Nephrology

LACTIC ACIDOSIS

The relationship between metformin accumulation and lactate increase is still debated in the literature. Several case reports and case series suggest that a true relationship exists between metformin and lactic acidosis occurrence. An observational case series was published of 66 patients with metformin accumulation and lactic acidosis from 2007 to 2011. The cases were reviewed to evaluate the correlation between metformin plasma levels and pH, lactate, creatinine, and the mortality rate. A correlation between metformin plasma concentrations, creatinine ($P = 0.002$, $R = 0.37$), pH ($P < 0.0001$, $R = -0.43$) and plasma lactate levels ($P = 0.001$, $R = 0.41$) was observed. Lactate and metformin concentrations had mean levels not statistically different in surviving and deceased patients. The authors concluded that patients on chronic metformin therapy may develop a mitochondrial-related toxicity that should be considered when patients present with lactic acidosis and renal failure at hospital admission [22c].

A case report of a 76-year-old male with a past medical history of chronic renal failure and intermittent dialysis, hypertension, and type 2 diabetes mellitus (T2DM) treated with metformin 2 g daily for 4 weeks presented with altered mental status. The patient had been hospitalized 10 days prior where a blood gas analysis revealed a pH 6.84, pCO_2 14.4 mmHg, HCO_3 2.5 mEq/L, and lactate level was measured but not reported. Upon admission, his respiratory rate was 22 breaths per minute while his other vital signs were within normal range. The patient was diagnosed with metformin-induced lactic acidosis and acute renal failure and was treated with intermittent hemodialysis with a bicarbonate buffer solution for 6 hours for 3 days. The metformin was discontinued and he was transitioned to insulin for treatment of his T2DM [23]. A second report highlights a case of a 66-year-old Caucasian woman that was initially thought to be ischemic gut but later determined to be metformin-induced lactic acidosis [24c].

Nutrition

VITAMIN B12 DEFICIENCY

Metformin is associated with reduced serum vitamin B12 concentrations in patients with long-term use in the treatment of T2DM. Several studies have attempted to quantify the degree of vitamin B12 deficiency over time. One study evaluated the effects of metformin and insulin treatment on vitamin B12 and homocysteine (Hcy) levels in women with gestational diabetes mellitus (GDM). Fasting serum total vitamin B12 (TB12), holotranscobalamin (HoloTC), a marker of functional B12 status and plasma Hcy levels were measured at 20–34 weeks (at randomization), 36 weeks gestation, and 6–8 weeks postpartum. Circulating TB12, HoloTC and Hcy were similar in both treatment groups at each time point. The investigators found that women who were taking dietary folate supplements had higher serum TB12 and HoloTC at randomization than those not taking folate. Overall, serum TB12 decreased more between randomization and 36 weeks gestation in the metformin group than in the insulin group (metformin: -19.7 ± 4.7 pmol/L, insulin: -6.4 ± 3.6 pmol/L, $P = 0.004$). The decrease in serum TB12 was greater with longer treatment duration in metformin-treated ($P < 0.001$), but not in insulin-treated women [25C].

In a second study, the cross-sectional observational design objective was to determine the prevalence of vitamin B12 deficiency in people with T2DM on metformin therapy. Positive correlations were observed between B 12 concentration, age and dosage and duration of metformin treatment. The investigators concluded since low serum B12 concentration is a common occurrence in people with T2DM treated with metformin, periodic screening should occur [26C].

A third study aimed to clarify the relationship between metformin-induced vitamin B12 deficiency, hyperhomocysteinemia and vascular complications in patients with T2DM. Serum B12 concentrations, homocysteine plasma levels, the presence of retinopathy and history of macroangiopathy (stroke or coronary heart disease) were analyzed in patients without renal dysfunction (serum creatinine <115 µmol/L). Among the 62 metformin-treated patients, the investigators found that the higher the metformin dose, the lower the B12 level ($P=0.02$, Spearman's $\rho=-0.30$). Metformin-induced B12 lowering in T2DM was associated with an elevation of homocysteine resulting in hyperhomocysteinemia ($P<0.01$, $r=-0.34$) and was independently related to retinopathy ($P=0.02$, OR 1.26, 95% CI 1.04–1.52). Patients concurrently treated with B12 supplementation had a recovery of their B12 levels [27C].

Metabolism

WEIGHT LOSS

A 16-week study examining the effects of metformin in clinically stable, overweight outpatients with chronic schizophrenia or schizoaffective disorder was modestly effective in reducing weight and other risk factors for cardiovascular disease with minimal gastrointestinal side effects. The primary outcome measure was change in body weight from baseline to the end of the study period. The mean change in body weight was −3.0 kg (95% CI = −4.0 to −2.0) for the metformin group and −1.0 kg (95% CI = −2.0 to 0.0) for the placebo group, with an absolute difference of −2.0 kg (95% CI = −3.4 to −0.6). Metformin also demonstrated a significant between-group treatment advantage for BMI (−0.7; 95% CI = −1.1 to −0.2), triglyceride level (−20.2 mg/dL; 95% CI = −39.2 to −1.3), and hemoglobin A1c level (−0.07%; 95% CI = −0.14 to −0.004) [28C].

CHILDHOOD OBESITY

Because childhood obesity has become an important public health problem with increasing prevalence, studies to evaluate pharmacologic treatment options are of interest to help combat this growing epidemic. A meta-analysis reviewed studies using metformin for the treatment of obesity in children aged 18 years and younger without a diagnosis of diabetes mellitus. The primary outcome measure was a change in body mass index (BMI). A statistically significant reduction in BMI was observed in metformin-treated patients when combined with lifestyle interventions. In the context of other options for treating childhood obesity, metformin has not been shown to be clinically superior. With regards to side effects, the meta-analysis indicated that 26% of the patient populations reported a gastrointestinal event with metformin compared to 13% of patients in the control groups

(relative risk, 2.05; 95% CI, 1.19–3.54), although there was no difference in discontinuations due to adverse events [29M].

Reproductive System

ENDOMETRIAL HYPERPLASIA

A 57-year-old woman with the diagnoses of hypertension and dyslipidemia was prescribed metformin 500 mg twice daily for pre-diabetes and metabolic syndrome. Within 1 week of therapy initiation, the patient experienced vaginal bleeding. Bleeding stopped following discontinuation of metformin, and recurred on rechallenge. The symptoms were dose dependent as bleeding did not occur at a dose of 500 mg orally once daily, but recurred at a total dose of 1000 mg orally daily. The patient was found to have complex endometrial hyperplasia. Female patients initiated on metformin therapy should be aware that any changes to their menstrual cycle following metformin initiation might indicate endometrial disease [30c].

Teratogenicity

In order to estimate the overall rate of major birth defects, a meta-analysis aimed to review nine prospective and retrospective studies of women with polycystic ovarian syndrome (PCOS) or pre-pregnancy T2DM and first trimester exposure to metformin. A random effects model was used for the meta-analysis of data, using odds ratios. Studies not fulfilling the inclusion criteria for the meta-analysis but reporting relevant data on major malformations in women diagnosed with PCOS were then used to estimate the overall birth defects rate. The authors concluded that there was insufficient evidence to associate a risk of major birth defects in the offspring of women treated with metformin for PCOS during the first trimester [31M].

Dipeptidyl Peptidase 4 (DDP-4) Inhibitors [SEDA-31, 693; SEDA-32, 774; SEDA-33, 894; SEDA-34, 688; SEDA-36, 648]

Linagliptin

HEPATOTOXICITY

Liver injury with linagliptin has not been reported in the literature despite the fact that its excretion is mainly biliary. One case report describes the first case of probable linagliptin-induced liver toxicity in a 58-year-old Japanese woman presenting with fatigue, nausea, jaundice and marked elevations of hepatic enzymes 4 weeks after starting linagliptin 5 mg orally daily as monotherapy. Imaging studies revealed no other obvious causes of hepatic injury and tests for viral serology and antinuclear antigen were negative. Upon discontinuation of linagliptin, symptoms disappeared and hepatic enzyme levels slowly recovered. Healthcare providers should consider monitoring for hepatotoxicity in patients at risk when managing linagliptin therapy [32c].

IMMUNOLOGIC

Angioedema A case report describes angioedema in a patient treated with an angiotensin converting enzyme inhibitor (ACEi), lisinopril 10 mg orally daily, and sitagliptin. Once the ACEi was withdrawn, the angioedema decreased but did not fully resolve until the sitagliptin was discontinued [33]. Another case in a 60-year-old man was reported with the initiation of anagliptin 200 mg orally daily. In this case, the patient was not on any other medication, such as an ACEi. While the patient's blood glucose and HgA1c moved closer to goal, severe edema of the hands and face developed. Upon discontinuation of anagliptin, the edema promptly and completely disappeared within 2 weeks. The authors hypothesized the mechanism of angioedema to be linked to the mechanism of action of the DPP-IV inhibitor. By inhibiting the DPP-IV enzyme which inactivates incretins and influences the degradation of bradykinin, the DPP-IV inhibitors may increase the half-life of bradykinin, a crucial mediator of ACE inhibitor-induced angioedema [34c].

MUSCULOSKELETAL

Arthralgia In a clinical trial assessing the effectiveness of linagliptin in elderly patients with T2DM, arthralgia occurred in 3.1% (5/162) of the linagliptin group and none in the placebo group. Back pain was reported more frequently in the linagliptin group at 4.1% (7/162) than the placebo group [35C].

VERTIGO

In the same study of elderly patients, vertigo occurred 3.1% (5/162) in the linagliptin group and none in the placebo group [35C].

Saxagliptin

CARDIOVASCULAR

Heart Failure A large clinical trial of patients ($n = 16492$) with T2DM who had a history of, or were at risk for, cardiovascular events were randomly assigned treatment with saxagliptin or placebo to assess for cardiovascular safety and efficacy. The patients were followed for a median of 2.1 years. Treatment with saxagliptin did not increase or decrease the rate of ischemic events, though the rate of hospitalization for heart failure was increased. The primary end point was a composite of cardiovascular death, myocardial infarction, or ischemic stroke which occurred in 613 patients in the saxagliptin group and in 609 patients in the placebo group (7.3% and 7.2%, respectively, according to 2-year Kaplan–Meier estimates; hazard ratio with saxagliptin, 1.00; 95%

confidence interval [CI], 0.89–1.12; $P = 0.99$ for superiority; $P < 0.001$ for non-inferiority) with similar results in the "on-treatment" analysis (hazard ratio, 1.03; 95% CI, 0.91–1.17). The secondary composite end point of cardiovascular death, myocardial infarction, stroke, and hospitalization for unstable angina, coronary revascularization, or heart failure occurred 12.4% (1059 patients) in the saxagliptin group versus 12.8% (1034 patients) in the placebo group (hazard ratio, 1.02; 95% CI, 0.94–1.11; $P = 0.66$). More hospitalizations for heart failure occurred in saxagliptin group than in the placebo group (3.5% vs. 2.8%; hazard ratio, 1.27; 95% CI, 1.07 to 1.51; $P = 0.007$) [36C].

In the same study, the authors attempted to further analyze the data on heart failure leading to hospitalizations. In 12301 patients, in whom a baseline N-terminal pro B-type natriuretic peptide was measured, patients treated with saxagliptin (289, 3.5%) had an increased incidence of hospitalization for heart failure compared with placebo (228, 2.8%; hazard ratio, 1.27; 95% confidence interval, 1.07–1.51; $P = 0.007$). Patients with a previous history of heart failure, an estimated glomerular filtration rate ≤ 60 mL/min, or elevated baseline levels of N-terminal pro B-type natriuretic peptide had the greatest risk for hospitalization [37C].

Sitagliptin

MUSCULOSKELETAL

Achilles Tendonitis A case report of a 56-year-old female who developed bilateral Achilles tendonitis 4 months after restarting sitagliptin was described. Sitagliptin was discontinued and the patient reported complete resolution of her tendonitis in the left foot and >50% improvement in the right after 4 weeks. The patient has not restarted sitagliptin and reports no further incidents of tendonitis [38c].

RHEUMATOLOGIC

Polyarthritis In a case series of DPP-IV inhibitor-induced polyarthritis, three patients presented with bilateral, symmetrical, seronegative polyarthritis after introduction of a DPP-IV inhibitor [sitagliptin ($n = 2$) and vildagliptin ($n = 1$)]. Two patients treated with sitagliptin developed xerostomia and laboratory test results showed normal values of CRP and erythrocyte sedimentation rate. One patient treated with sitagliptin was diagnosed with primary Sjögren's syndrome and treated with hydroxychloroquine, methotrexate and prednisone, with poor efficacy. Once the sitagliptin was stopped, all symptoms disappeared, leading to methotrexate and prednisone discontinuation within a month. There were no immunological abnormalities in the other two patients, but discontinuation of sitagliptin led to resolution of symptoms in 1 and 3 weeks for both patients. The patient treated with vildagliptin experienced knee and ankle arthralgias and synovitis of both wrists. X-rays of the joints were normal as were all laboratory tests with the exception of the patient's Hepatitis B panel, which was positive with a viral load of 30 copies/mL. Discontinuation of vildagliptin leads to complete resolution of arthralgias 1 month later. As suggested by clinical and in vitro studies, the DPP-IV enzyme is expressed on many cells including lymphocytes and fibroblasts, and its inhibition may lead to an immunomodulation effect [39c].

Vildagliptin

ENDOCRINE

Hypoglycemia A multinational, non-interventional study attempted to assess the effects of vildagliptin on hypoglycemia when compared with sulphonylurea (SU) treatment in patients who were Muslim with T2DM and fasting during Ramadan. The primary objective was to compare the proportion of patients with ≥1 hypoglycemic event (HE) during fasting. Significantly fewer patients experienced ≥1 HE with vildagliptin compared with those receiving SUs (5.4% vs. 19.8%, respectively; $P < 0.001$); no vildagliptin-treated patients reported a grade 2 HE, vs. 4 SU-treated patients ($P = 0.053$). Mean HbA1c changes from baseline were: vildagliptin −0.24%, SUs +0.02% ($P < 0.001$). Mean body weight reductions from baseline were: vildagliptin −0.76 kg, SUs −0.13 kg ($P < 0.001$). A higher proportion of SU-treated patients experienced adverse events (AEs) such as hypoglycemia compared with vildagliptin (22.8% vs. 10.2%). Overall, the investigators concluded that vildagliptin was associated with good glycemic and weight control when used in a fasting population [40C].

ENDOCRINE

Post-Prandial Lipemia and Insulinemia A randomized, double-blind study attempted to evaluate the effects of vildagliptin 50 mg orally twice daily compared to glimepiride 2 mg orally three times daily plus metformin therapy on glycemic control, insulin resistance and post-prandial lipemia. Overall, the investigators found that vildagliptin plus metformin reduced post-prandial lipemia and insulinemia compared to glimepiride plus metformin [41C].

ENDOCRINE

Pancreatitis To investigate the risk of pancreatitis associated with the use of incretin-based treatments in patients with T2DM, a meta-analysis was conducted to compare treatment with a glucagon-like peptide-1 (GLP-1) receptor agonists or dipeptidyl peptidase-4 (DPP-4) inhibitors with placebo, lifestyle modification, or active anti-diabetic drugs. Fifty-five RCTs ($n = 33\,350$) and five observational studies (three retrospective cohort

studies, two case–control studies; $n = 320\,289$) were included in the analysis. Pooled estimates of the RCTs did not suggest an increased risk of pancreatitis with incretins versus control (placebo or active drug) (odds ratio 1.11, 95% confidence interval 0.57–2.17). Additionally, the risk of pancreatitis was not increased in three retrospective cohort studies; two associated with exenatide (adjusted odds ratios: 0.93 (0.63–1.36) or 0.9 (0.6–1.5)) and one associated with sitagliptin (adjusted hazard ratio: 1.0 (0.7–1.3)). One case–control study suggested use of either exenatide or sitagliptin was associated with significantly increased odds of acute pancreatitis within two years of beginning therapy (adjusted odds ratio 2.07, 1.36–3.13). The evidence from this meta-analysis suggests the incidence of pancreatitis among patients using incretins is low and that incretins do not increase the risk of pancreatitis [42]. Similar results were observed comparing saxagliptin to placebo with the rates of acute and chronic pancreatitis being similar in the two groups (acute pancreatitis, 0.3% in the saxagliptin group and 0.2% in the placebo group; chronic pancreatitis, <0.1% and 0.1% in the two groups, respectively) [36M].

Incretin Mimetic [SEDA-31, 695; SEDA-32, 775; SEDA-33, 896; SEDA-34, 690; SEDA-36, 650]

GASTROINTESTINAL

Nausea, Vomiting, Diarrhea, Dyspepsia In a phase 3, randomized, open-label, parallel-group non-inferiority study, the safety and efficacy of once-weekly dulaglutide (1.5 mg) was compared to once daily liraglutide (1.8 mg) in metformin-treated patients with uncontrolled T2DM. The most common adverse events were nausea (20% in dulaglutide group vs. 18% in liraglutide group), diarrhea (12% vs. 12%), dyspepsia (8% vs. 6%), and vomiting (7% vs. 8%) [43C].

A case report was published on a 67-year-old patient who experienced repeated nausea, vomiting, and diarrhea while taking liraglutide 18 mg daily in addition to pioglitazone 45 mg. His intended prescribed liraglutide dose was 1.8 mg once daily. Due to a transcription error, he received a 10-fold overdose for about 6 months. The patient did not complain of signs of hypoglycemia or have low serum glucose levels when measured during his repeat visits to the hospital. A second case report was published on a woman who attempted suicide by injecting liraglutide 72 mg subcutaneously. While she experienced severe nausea and vomiting after injection, she did not have hypoglycemia and therefore did not experience death as a result of liraglutide overdose. This case report adds an additional report of liraglutide overdose with the only adverse effects being gastrointestinal effects [44,45c].

METABOLISM

Appetite Reduction A double-blind crossover study evaluated the effects of glucagon 2.8 pmol/kg/min and GLP-1 0.4 pmol/kg/min infusions alone, in combination, or placebo on reduction of appetite. Glucagon or GLP-1, given individually at these doses, did not significantly reduce food intake; however, coinfusion of glucagon and GLP-1 at the doses described above led to a significant reduction in food intake (13%). Furthermore, the addition of GLP-1 protected against glucagon-induced hyperglycemia and an increase in energy expenditure of 53 kcal/day was seen on coinfusion. These observations support the concept of GLP-1 and glucagon dual agonism as a possible treatment for obesity and diabetes [1C].

METABOLISM

Weight Loss Patients treated with GLP-1 receptor agonists for diabetes have been associated with significant weight loss. Trials examining the effects of GLP-1 receptor agonists for weight loss have compared exenatide, liraglutide, and orlistat in patients without diabetes. In a study of once-weekly exenatide, patients experienced significantly lower glycosylated hemoglobin (HbA1c) levels (decreased 1.5–1.9%) and more weight loss (decreased 2.3–3.7 kg) compared to those receiving sitagliptin or pioglitazone ($P < 0.05$). The most common adverse events reported were injection-site reactions and transient nausea [46].

A review article examined the studies completed to date and found that both exenatide 10 μg twice daily and liraglutide in dosages of up to 3 mg daily resulted in significant weight loss in patients without diabetes. Nausea and vomiting were the most frequently reported adverse events in patients from these studies [47].

Albiglutide
GASTROINTESTINAL

An open-label, non-inferiority study compared the effects of albiglutide to liraglutide on HgA1c reduction in adult patients ($n = 841$) with inadequately controlled T2DM and a BMI between 20 and 45 kg/m². The doses were albiglutide 30 mg once-weekly titrated to 50 mg at week 6, or liraglutide 0.6 mg once daily titrated to 1.2 mg at week 1 and 1.8 mg at week 2. Gastrointestinal events such as nausea and vomiting occurred more in liraglutide patients than in the albiglutide patients (49% versus 35.9%; treatment difference −13.1% [95% CI −19.9 to −6.4]; $P = 0.00013$). However, diarrhea occurred more often in albiglutide patients, although not statistically significant [48C].

DERMATOLOGY

Injection Site Reactions In the same study, more injection-site reactions occurred in patients given albiglutide than liraglutide (12.9% vs. 5.4%; absolute difference 7.5% [95% CI 3.6–11.4]; $P = 0.0002$) [48C].

Dulaglutide
CARDIOVASCULAR

Blood Pressure The effects of dulaglutide on the reduction in systolic blood pressure and heart rate were investigated using ambulatory monitoring in patients ($n = 755$; 56 ± 10 years; 81% white; 48% women) randomized to dulaglutide (1.5 or 0.75 mg) or placebo subcutaneously for 26 weeks. The primary end point was change from baseline to week 16 in mean 24-hour SBP. Overall, dulaglutide 1.5 mg was associated with a reduction in 24-hour SBP and an increase in 24-hour heart rate. Non-inferiority was seen in both doses of dulaglutide compared to placebo for changes in 24-hour SBP and diastolic blood pressure. Dulaglutide 1.5 mg significantly reduced SBP (least squares mean difference [95% confidence interval], −2.8 mm Hg [−4.6, −1.0]; $P \leq 0.001$). Non-inferiority was seen with dulaglutide 0.75 mg compared to placebo (1.6 bpm; [0.3, 2.9]; $P \leq 0.02$) for 24-hour heart rate, but not with the 1.5 mg dose (2.8 bpm [1.5, 4.2]) [49].

Exenatide
REDUCTION OF INFARCT

Investigators examined whether routine use of exenatide at the time of primary percutaneous coronary intervention would reduce infarct size in patients with ST-segment-elevation myocardial infarction. Patients were randomly assigned to receive either exenatide or placebo subcutaneously. Infarct size was assessed by measuring the release of creatine kinase-MB and troponin I during 72 hours and by performing cardiac magnetic resonance imaging 1 month after infarction. Overall, the patients with ST-segment-elevation myocardial infarction had a reduction of infarct size and improvement of subclinical left ventricular function when administered exenatide with primary percutaneous coronary intervention. Patients did not experience significant adverse effects with exenatide administration [50].

NEPHROLOGY

Acute Interstitial Nephritis Several case reports have been published concerning the cause of interstitial nephritis in exenatide and liraglutide treated patients. Severe vomiting and/or diarrhea or dehydration was common symptoms in patients that presented with acute renal failure. Hematuria and proteinuria, favoring an acute interstitial nephritis, has also been present in these cases. In the case where the patient had liraglutide associated acute renal failure, the patient was also receiving a diuretic and ACEi, which may have contributed to dehydration and renal hypoperfusion leading to acute renal failure. Administration of an ACEi, diuretics or NSAIDs should be considered a risk factor for development of acute renal failure in GLP-1 treated patients. Acute interstitial nephritis should be documented by renal biopsy, as steroid therapy may be indicated [51]. A case report was published of an 83-year-old male patient with a diagnosis of acute interstitial nephritis, likely induced by liraglutide with a possible cross-reaction to exenatide. The patient had received exenatide initially then switched to liraglutide for convenience. The patient received steroids and transient dialysis, and liraglutide therapy was discontinued which led to a progressive improvement in kidney function (serum creatinine, 3.58 mg/dL; eGFR, 18 mL/min/1.73 m^2) [52].

Liraglutide

AUTOIMMUNE HEPATITIS

Hepatotoxicity may be an incretin analogue class effect with a long latency period, however, not been frequently reported in the literature. A case report of a young woman with T2DM presented with a 10-day history of acute hepatitis after 4 months of liraglutide therapy. She reported no changes in medication therapy and no use of supplements. The patient's symptoms worsened after liraglutide therapy was discontinued. Laboratory tests and a liver biopsy demonstrated massive hepatic necrosis and interface hepatitis with prominent eosinophils and rare plasma cells. The patient was started on oral prednisone therapy for presumed liraglutide-induced marker-negative autoimmune hepatitis [53].

Lixisenatide

GASTROINTESTINAL

Nausea, Vomiting, Diarrhea In a study examining the effects of lixisenatide added to basal insulin therapy, the incidence of adverse events was lower in the lixisenatide cohort ($n=45$ patients, 58.4%) compared to the liraglutide cohort ($n=52$, 73.2%). The most common adverse events reported were nausea and vomiting. There were two cases of treatment discontinuation relating to adverse events (2.8%) in the liraglutide cohort resulting from adverse gastrointestinal events. No cases of symptomatic hypoglycemia were reported [54C].

Pancreatitis

Several meta-analyses have been published in an attempt to determine the effect of GLP-1 agonists on the incidence of pancreatitis. The first meta-analysis consisted of 41 trials ($n=14972$). The overall risk of pancreatitis was not significant between glucagon-like peptide-1 receptor agonists (GLP-1RA) and comparators (MH-OR: 1.01 [0.37; 2.76]; $P=0.99$). The results did not suggest any increase in the risk of pancreatitis with the use of GLP-1RA [55M].

A second meta-analysis consisted of sixty trials ($n=353\,639$), which examined treatment with a GLP-1RA or dipeptidyl peptidase-4 (DPP-4) inhibitors in adults with T2DM as compared to placebo, lifestyle modification, or active anti-diabetic drugs to determine the risk of pancreatitis. The pooled estimates of 55 RCTs did not suggest an increased risk of pancreatitis with incretins versus placebo (odds ratio 1.11, 95% confidence interval 0.57–2.17). The authors did not see a significant difference in pancreatitis incidence between the GLP-1RAs and the DPP-IV. Overall, the authors concluded the available evidence suggests that the GLP-1RA and the DPP-IV inhibitors do not increase the incidence of pancreatitis among patients using the medications for diabetes treatment [42M].

A case report of an obese lady with T2DM was prescribed liraglutide for glycemic control and reduction of weight. She developed severe abdominal pain, nausea and vomiting 8 weeks after initiation of liraglutide. Elevated pancreatic enzymes and a CT scan revealed she had acute pancreatitis. Liraglutide was discontinued with resolution of her symptoms and a return to normal levels of pancreatic enzymes [56c].

Sodium–Glucose Transporter Type 2 (SGLT2) Inhibitors [*SEDA-33, 898; SEDA-34, 695; SEDA-36, 652*]

Canagliflozin

CARDIOVASCULAR

Blood Pressure Reduction The reduction in blood pressure by canagliflozin could be a potential benefit to patients with T2DM and metabolic syndrome. Multiple studies evaluating the safety and efficacy of canagliflozin as monotherapy and in combination therapy have observed this effect without significant variation in results. Two studies reviewed here include a study where canagliflozin (100 and 300 mg) was compared to metformin and pioglitazone and a monotherapy study of canagliflozin (100 or 200 mg) to placebo. Both studies found that patients treated with canagliflozin had statistically significant reductions in systolic blood pressure with the effects maintained after discontinuation of the study [57,58C].

Electrolyte Imbalances

In a single center, open-label, fixed-sequence, two-period study the effects of HCTZ on the pharmacokinetic and pharmacodynamic properties and tolerability of canagliflozin were evaluated in healthy participants. The investigators found that the coadministration of canagliflozin and HCTZ resulted in a greater increase in sodium excretion. However, serum sodium and potassium levels were unchanged with canagliflozin treatment alone, and both levels were slightly decreased after treatment with HCTZ alone. Other laboratory imbalances included a marked decrease in uric acid levels with canagliflozin alone but increased with HCTZ alone. This result is consistent with the known effect of HCTZ to inhibit uric acid excretion [59C].

ENDOCRINE

Hypoglycemia In the same study, there were no reports of hypoglycemia from either the canagliflozin alone or the canagliflozin and HCTZ combination [59C].

In a double-blind, multi-center study comparing canagliflozin therapy (100 or 200 mg) once daily to placebo for effects on HbA1c in 24 weeks, the most common adverse effect was asymptomatic hypoglycemia (4.4%, 5.6% and 2.2%, respectively), but not symptomatic hypoglycemia (2.2%, 1.1% and 1.1%, respectively) [58C].

GENITOURINARY

Infections In a double-blind, multi-center study comparing canagliflozin therapy (100 or 200 mg) once daily to placebo for effects on HbA1c in 24 weeks the most common adverse effect was genital mycotic infections in females (6.5%, 6.3% and 0%, respectively) [58C].

A 12-week, randomized, double-blind study was conducted to evaluate the effects of canagliflozin on body weight in overweight and obese subjects (body mass index [BMI] $\geq$27 and <50 kg/m^2). Patients ($n = 376$) without diabetes mellitus received canagliflozin 50, 100, or 300 mg or placebo once daily. The most common adverse effect was a higher rate of genital mycotic infections in women treated with canagliflozin [60C].

METABOLISM

Weight Loss In the same study describe above, the primary endpoint was the percent change in body weight from baseline through week 12. Canagliflozin produced statistically significant reductions in body weight compared with placebo (least squares mean percent changes from baseline of −2.2%, −2.9%, −2.7%, and −1.3% with canagliflozin 50, 100, and 300 mg and placebo; $P < 0.05$ for all comparisons) [60C].

In a double-blind, multi-center study to compare canagliflozin therapy (100 or 200 mg) orally daily to placebo for 24 weeks, the change in body weight (percent change: −3.76% and −4.02% vs. −0.76%) was significantly greater with 100 and 200 mg canagliflozin than with placebo ($P < 0.05$) [58C].

A study examined the safety and efficacy of canagliflozin in Japanese patients with T2DM undergoing diet and exercise therapy. Body weight was significantly decreased by canagliflozin with a low incidence of hypoglycemia. There was no dose-dependent increase in the adverse effect incidence in the canagliflozin groups [61C].

Empagliflozin

GENITOURINARY

Infections In a 12-week, double-blind, placebo-controlled trial comparing empagliflozin to sitagliptin in 495 patients with T2DM inadequately controlled on metformin, the most common adverse effects reported for empagliflozin were urinary tract infections (4.0% vs. 2.8% with placebo) and pollakiuria (2.5% vs. 1.4% with placebo). Only patients treated with empagliflozin experienced genital infections (4.0%) [62C].

Tofogliflozin

NEPHROLOGY/UROLOGY

Tofogliflozin, a newer SGLT-2 inhibitor, is approved for use in Japanese patients with T2DM. A multi-center, placebo-controlled, randomized, double-blind parallel-group study involving patients with T2DM ($n = 230$) and inadequate glycemic control on diet/exercise therapy evaluated the safety and efficacy of tofogliflozin. Like the other SGLT-2 inhibitors, tofogliflozin decreases fasting blood glucose, 2-hour post-prandial glucose, and body weight in all tofogliflozin groups compared with the placebo group. The main adverse effects observed were hyperketonemia, ketonuria, and pollakiuria [63C].

Sulphonylureas [SED-15, 3230; SEDA-31, 695; SEDA-32, 777; SEDA-33, 898; SEDA-34, 695; SEDA-36, 652]

CARDIOVASCULAR DISEASE

A meta-analysis for clinical and observational studies was conducted to determine if there was a direct relationship between sulphonylureas and cardiovascular disease events. A total of 33 studies ($n = 1325446$ patients), followed for a range of 0.46–10.4 years were included in the analysis. In all studies, a significantly increased risk of cardiovascular death (relative risk 1.27 [95% CI 1.18–1.34]; $n = 27$ comparisons) and composite cardiovascular event (including myocardial infarction, stroke, cardiovascular-related hospitalization or cardiovascular death) (relative risk 1.10 [95% CI 1.04–1.16]; $n = 43$ comparisons) was associated with use of a sulphonylurea. In studies comparing a sulphonylureas to metformin, the relative risks were 1.26 ([95% CI 1.17–1.35]; $n = 17$ comparisons) and 1.18 ([95% CI 1.13–1.24]; $n = 16$ comparisons), respectively, suggesting that use of a sulphonylurea may increase the risk of cardiovascular disease among patients with T2DM [64M].

Ischemic Preconditioning In patients with a history of acute coronary syndrome or other severe cardiovascular disease, remote ischemic pre-conditioning attenuates myocardial injury. Investigators aimed to determine if sulphonylureas interfered with ischemic and anesthetic pre-conditioning effects. Troponin I concentration area under curve (measurements: baseline, 1, 6, 12, 24, 48, and 72 hours post-operatively) were assessed in T2DM patients treated with sulfonylureas ($n=27$) and in non-diabetics ($n=230$) with or without remote ischemic pre-conditioning (three 5-minute periods of left upper arm ischemia with 5-minute reperfusion each) during isoflurane anesthesia before two- to three-vessel coronary artery surgery. A decrease in the troponin I concentration area under curve (AUC) of 41% (514 ng/mL ×72 hours ± 600 vs. 302 ± 190, $P=0.001$) in non-diabetic patients was observed compared to no change (404 ng/mL × 72 hours ± 224 vs. 471 ± 383, $P=0.62$) in sulphonylurea-treated patients suggesting that remote ischemic pre-conditioning is lost in patients treated with sulphonylureas [65C].

NEUROLOGY

Investigators aimed to determine if intravenous (IV) glyburide (3 mg IV daily) was safe and effective in preventing edema and improving outcome after focal ischemia in patients with severe stroke based off of hypotheses generated from pre-clinical and retrospective clinical data. Ten patients (mean age 50.5 years) with acute ischemic stroke and baseline diffusion-weighted imaging lesion volumes of 82 to 210 cm^3, +/− treatment with recombinant tissue-type plasminogen activator, administration of intravenous glyburide ≤10 hours were enrolled. The baseline diffusion-weighted image lesion volume was 102 ± 23 cm^3. Intravenous glyburide did not cause any serious adverse events or symptomatic hypoglycemia. The increase in ipsilateral hemisphere volume was 50 ± 33 cm^3, lower than previously reported historical controls of 72 ± 27 cm^3. The proportion of 90-day modified Rankin Scale ≤4 was 90% (40% modified Rankin Scale, ≤3) [66C].

VASCULAR

Leukocytoclastic vasculitis is a medication-induced small-vessel vasculitis that most commonly manifests with palpable purpuric lesions on gravity dependent areas. The vasculitis develops within weeks after the initial administration of a medication, with clearance upon withdrawal of the medication. A case report of a rare occurrence of glyburide-associated leukocytoclastic vasculitis in a 71-year-old man with T2DM was published. The patient presented with palpable purpura on his lower extremities. Cutaneous biopsy revealed superficial small-vessel vasculitis with IgA perivascular deposits. The patient revealed he had three prior episodes of palpable purpura after restarting his glyburide, with clearance upon discontinuation [67c].

Thiazolidinediones [SED-15, 3380; SEDA-31, 697; SEDA-32, 779; SEDA-33, 899; SEDA-34, 696; SEDA-36, 653]

Pioglitazone

AUTOIMMUNE

Rheumatoid Arthritis Investigators aimed to determine if pioglitazone 45 mg orally daily could promote vasculoprotective and anti-inflammatory effects in patients with rheumatoid arthritis (RA). Patients ($n=143$) on a stable RA standard of care therapy were enrolled in a randomized, double-blind placebo-controlled crossover trial of pioglitazone versus placebo. When added to standard of care RA therapy, pioglitazone significantly improved aortic elasticity, decreased inflammation and disease activity as well as significantly reduced RA disease activity ($P=0.02$) and CRP levels ($P=0.001$), while improving lipid profiles [68].

ENDOCRINE

Bone Mineral Density Meta-analyses have demonstrated that the use of thiazolidinediones increases the risk of bone fractures in women. A randomized double-blind, placebo-controlled study designed to evaluate the effects of pioglitazone on bone mineral density (BMD) and turnover in postmenopausal women ($n=156$) with impaired fasting glucose or impaired glucose tolerance. Percentage changes were measured from baseline to month 12 as well as from month 12 to month 18 in BMD in total proximal femur (primary end point), total body, femoral neck, lumbar spine, and radius. No statistically significant between-group differences were observed for any BMD or bone remodeling marker end point. Pioglitazone appeared to increase body fat, which may affect bone density measurements, especially in the lumbar spine. Only one pioglitazone-treated and three placebo-treated women experienced confirmed fractures. The authors concluded that patients on maximum dose pioglitazone had no effects on BMD or bone turnover, while improving glycemic control in postmenopausal women with impaired fasting glucose or impaired glucose tolerance [69M].

A smaller double-blind, randomized controlled trial ($n=86$) of patients with T2DM or impaired glucose tolerance (IGT) attempted to evaluate the effects of pioglitazone 30 mg orally daily on BMD. The primary outcome was change in lumbar spine BMD; secondary outcomes included changes in BMD at other sites and in biochemical markers of bone turnover. The mean difference in lumbar spine BMD was −0.7% [95% CI, −2.1–0.7] and total hip BMD was −1.2% [95% CI, −2.1–0.2] at 1 year with an increased loss of bone at the proximal femur (=0.03) was observed. Pioglitazone did not alter the BMD at other skeletal sites, nor did it affect changes in the levels of either of the biochemical markers of bone turnover, procollagen type 1 N-terminal propeptide, or β-C-terminal telopeptide of type 1 collagen [70C].

ENDOCRINE

Inflammation A randomized, placebo-controlled, double-blind, crossover study of 18 obese and non-obese individuals with T2DM treated with pioglitazone found an improvement in insulin resistance and reduced adipose tissue inflammation. Patients underwent pair of crossover euglycemic-hyperinsulinemic clamp studies after receiving either 21 days of treatment with 45 mg orally daily of pioglitazone or placebo. Subcutaneous adipose tissue biopsies were taken during the last 30 minutes of the clamp study. A euglycemic-hyperglycemic clamp study is a study in which the subject receives a continuous infusion of insulin (usually 100 μU/mL) along with a variable glucose infusion to maintain constant serum glucose levels. The clamp study's goal is to measure the subject's insulin sensitivity. Significant decreases in insulin resistance and many adipose inflammatory parameters were seen in obese patients treated with pioglitazone. Additionally, the study found significant improvements in glucose infusion rates, suppression of hepatic glucose production, and whole fat expression of certain inflammatory markers (IL-6, IL-1B, and inducible nitric oxide synthase) were observed in the obese patients only. Adipose tissue from the obese subjects demonstrated reduced infiltration of macrophages, dendritic cells, and neutrophils as well as increased expression of factors associated with fat "browning" (peroxisome proliferator-activated receptor gamma coactivator-1α and uncoupling protein-1) [71C].

The effect of pioglitazone on glucose metabolism and the inflammatory state in obese individuals with T2DM was evaluated in a randomized, double-blind, placebo-controlled, trial ($n = 29$) in patients previously treated with metformin and/or sulfonylurea. Patients were randomized to pioglitazone 15 mg orally daily or placebo. Patients were tested for: (1) OGTT; (2) muscle biopsy to evaluate expression of tumor necrosis factor-α (TNF-α), tissue inhibitor of metalloproteases 3 (TIMP-3) levels, TNF-α converting enzyme (TACE) expression and enzymatic activity; (3) euglycemic-hyperinsulinemic clamp; (4) measurement of plasma high-sensitivity C-reactive protein (hsCRP), plasminogen activator inhibitor type-1 (PAI-1), TNF-α, IL-6, monocyte chemotactic protein-1 (MCP-1), adiponectin and fractalkine (FRK) at baseline and after 6 months of treatment. In patients treated with pioglitazone, a modest decrease in fasting plasma glucose and HbA1c was observed ($P < 0.05$). Decreases in the inflammatory markers, MCP-1, IL-6, FRK, hsCRP and PAI-1 in patients on pioglitazone were also observed. While TNF-α levels remained unchanged throughout

the study, pioglitazone therapy significantly reduced the TNF-α protein expression and TACE enzymatic activity in muscle. This effect was not seen in the placebo arm. Overall, the investigators concluded that pioglitazone 15 mg orally daily improves glucose metabolism and inflammatory state in obese patients with T2DM [72].

METABOLISM

Weight Gain A randomized, open-label study evaluated the efficacy and safety of add-on pioglitazone orally 30 mg daily ($n = 59$) versus sitagliptin 100 mg orally daily ($n = 60$) in patients with T2DM inadequately controlled on metformin and a sulfonylurea (SU). Patients in the pioglitazone group had more weight gain compared to sitagliptin (absolute difference of 1.6 kg, $P < 0.01$) [73].

PSYCHIATRY

Depression A study attempted to assess if pioglitazone (15–30 mg orally daily) could reduce bipolar depression symptom severity in patients ($n = 34$) with bipolar disorder (I, II, or not otherwise specified) and metabolic syndrome/insulin. The secondary objective was to determine if C-reactive protein and interleukin (IL)-6 levels predicted treatment outcome. Pioglitazone therapy was associated with an improvement in mood and depression shown by the decrease in the patient's self-reported depressive symptom severity ($P < 0.001$), clinician-rated anxiety symptom severity ($P < 0.001$), and total Inventory of Depressive Symptomatology (IDS-C30) score from 38.7 ± 8.2 at baseline to 21.2 ± 9.2 at week 8 ($P < 0.001$). A decrease in depression severity was seen in patients with a higher baseline level of IL-6 (parameter estimate $\beta = -3.89$, standard error [SE] $= 1.47$, $P = 0.015$). The investigators concluded that pioglitazone was associated with an improvement in depression and a reduced cardio-metabolic risk [74].

TUMORIGENICITY

A meta-analysis to evaluate the magnitude of an increased risk of bladder cancer in patients with diabetes was conducted in response to the suggestion in several observational studies. Six studies ($n = 215142$) were included with a median period of follow-up of 44 months. The authors found that the hazard of developing bladder cancer was significantly higher in patients using pioglitazone (hazard ratio 1.23; 95% CI 1.09–1.39; $I^2 = 0\%$) compared with control groups. The rate of bladder cancer incidence was 20.8 per 100 000 person years, with a number needed to harm of five additional cases of bladder cancer. Overall, the authors concluded that patients treated with pioglitazone have a slight increased risk of bladder cancer compared to the general population and those with a history of bladder cancer must discontinue pioglitazone treatment [75M].

In a randomized, open-label study evaluated the efficacy and safety of add-on pioglitazone 30 mg daily ($n=59$) versus sitagliptin 100 mg daily ($n=60$) in patients with T2DM inadequately controlled on metformin and a sulfonylurea (SU). Pioglitazone was associated with a significant decrease in high-sensitive C-reactive protein (hsCRP) while sitagliptin was not [73].

Rosiglitazone

METABOLISM

In a small, prospective study of patients with both T2DM and coronary heart disease, the effect of rosiglitazone on serum metabolic and lipoprotein subclass changes was evaluated. Patients were given either placebo ($n=26$) or treated with rosiglitazone 4–8 mg ($n=25$). Circulating low-molecular-weight metabolites, lipoprotein subclasses, and lipids associated with T2DM before and after 16 weeks of treatment were measured. Compared to placebo, patients treated with rosiglitazone had significantly increased circulating glutamine and decreased lactate concentrations, with circulating lactate concentrations inversely correlated to increases in myocardial glucose uptake reflecting improvements in insulin sensitivity [76C].

MUSCULOSKELETAL

An increase in fracture risk was observed in patients taking rosiglitazone versus patients not taking a thiazolidinedione in a randomized controlled trial designed to examine the cardiovascular effects of rosiglitazone on patients with coronary artery disease and being considered for revascularization therapy. While no significant effects on cardiac function were observed, the authors noted an increase rate of bone fractures. The rate of bone fractures was significantly higher among patients who received rosiglitazone than among patients who were not receiving a thiazolidinedione (adjusted HR $=1.62$; 95% CI, 1.05–2.51; $P=0.03$). When stratified by sex, the relative risk for fractures in women appeared greater than for men (RR 1.82 vs. 1.47; $P=0.55$). A Kaplan–Meier time-to-event analysis showed that with long durations of rosiglitazone therapy, the risk of bone fracture increases [77C].

Thiazolidinediones and HIV/HAART-Associated Lipodystrophy Syndrome

The use of HAART in HIV-1 infected patients has been associated with adverse effects, including metabolic dysregulation and changes in body fat deposition, known as HIV/HAART-associated lipodystrophy syndrome (HALS). Insulin resistance, dyslipidemia, lipodystrophy, and increased visceral adiposity characterize HALS, which contribute to an increased risk of cardiovascular

disease for these patients. The peroxisome proliferator-activated receptor (PPAR) is involved in the regulation of insulin sensitivity and lipid metabolism. Expression of these receptors are found to be reduced in HAART treated patients, likely due to an interaction with protease inhibitors. A number of clinical trials have analyzed whether thiazolidinediones could affect the HIV/HAART-associated lipodystrophy syndrome in HAART treated patients. Based on the results of these short-term trials, thiazolidinediones appear to up-regulate peroxisome proliferator-activated receptor-dependent genes such as adiponectin, which could have important physiological benefits in the long-term for HIV/HAART-associated lipodystrophy syndrome patients. In addition, the few studies on the thiazolidinedione pioglitazone showed a beneficial effect on limb fat mass not associated with a pro-atherogenic lipid profile. Based on these studies, a large-scale clinical trial of pioglitazone use in HIV/HAART-associated lipodystrophy syndrome patients is warranted [78R].

Peroxisome Proliferator Activated Dual Receptor Agonists [SEDA-32, 782; SEDA-33, 902; SEDA-34, 698; SEDA-36, 655]

Aleglitazar

Aleglitazar, a dual peroxisome proliferator-activated receptor agonist, has been shown to have insulin-sensitizing and glucose-lowering actions in addition to favorable effects on lipid profiles. A phase 3, multi-center, randomized, double-blind, placebo-controlled study was conducted to determine whether aleglitazar reduces cardiovascular morbidity and mortality among patients with T2DM and a recent acute coronary syndrome (ACS) when added to standard treatment. Patients ($n=7226$) hospitalized for ACS (myocardial infarction or unstable angina) with T2DM were randomized to receive aleglitazar 150 µg or placebo daily. The primary efficacy end point was time to cardiovascular death, nonfatal myocardial infarction, or nonfatal stroke. Principal safety end points were hospitalization due to heart failure and changes in renal function. A data and safety monitoring board terminated the trial on July 2, 2013, after a median follow-up of 104 weeks, due to futility for efficacy at an unplanned interim analysis and increased rates of safety end points. The primary end point occurred in 344 patients (9.5%) in the aleglitazar group and 360 patients (10.0%) in the placebo group (hazard ratio 0.96 [95% CI, 0.83–1.11]; $P=0.57$). Rates of serious adverse events were increased including heart failure (3.4% for aleglitazar vs. 2.8% for placebo, $P=0.14$), gastrointestinal hemorrhages (2.4% for aleglitazar vs. 1.7% for placebo, $P=0.03$), and renal dysfunction (7.4% for aleglitazar vs.

2.7% for placebo, $P < 0.001$). Overall, the use of aleglitazar did not reduce the risk of cardiovascular outcomes among patients with T2DM and recent ACS [79C].

References

[1] Cegla J, Troke RC, Jones B, et al. Coinfusion of low-dose GLP-1 and glucagon in man results in a reduction in food intake. Diabetes. 2014;63(11):3711–20 [C].

[2] Arakaki RF, Blevins TC, Wise JK, et al. Comparison of insulin lispro protamine suspension versus insulin glargine once daily added to oral antihyperglycaemic medications and exenatide in type 2 diabetes: a prospective randomized open-label trial. Diabetes Obes Metab. 2014;16(6):510–8 [C].

[3] Blonde L, Baron MA, Zhou R, et al. Efficacy and risk of hypoglycemia with use of insulin glargine or comparators in patients with cardiovascular risk factors. Postgrad Med. 2014;126(3):172–89 [M].

[4] Bode BW, Buse JB, Fisher M, et al. Insulin degludec improves glycaemic control with lower nocturnal hypoglycaemia risk than insulin glargine in basal-bolus treatment with mealtime insulin aspart in Type 1 diabetes (BEGIN((R)) Basal-Bolus Type 1): 2-year results of a randomized clinical trial. Diabet Med. 2013;30(11):1293–7 [C].

[5] Breznik V, Kokol R, Luzar B, et al. Insulin-induced localized lipoatrophy. Acta Dermatovenerol Alp Pannonica Adriat. 2013;22(4):83–5 [c].

[6] van Golen LW, Veltman DJ, IJzerman RG, et al. Effects of insulin detemir and NPH insulin on body weight and appetite-regulating brain regions in human type 1 diabetes: a randomized controlled trial. PLoS One. 2014;9(4):e94483 [C].

[7] Habel LA, Danforth KN, Quesenberry CP, et al. Cohort study of insulin glargine and risk of breast, prostate, and colorectal cancer among patients with diabetes. Diabetes Care. 2013;36(12):3953–60 [c].

[8] Simo R, Plana-Ripoll O, Puente D, et al. Impact of glucose-lowering agents on the risk of cancer in type 2 diabetic patients. The Barcelona case-control study. PLoS One. 2013;8(11):e79968 [c].

[9] Patel YR, Kirkman MS, Considine RV, et al. Effect of acarbose to delay progression of carotid intima-media thickness in early diabetes. Diabetes Metab Res Rev. 2013;29(7):582–91 [C].

[10] Shirakawa J, Murohashi Y, Okazaki N, et al. Using miglitol at 30 min before meal is effective in hyperinsulinemic hypoglycemia after a total gastrectomy. Endocr J. 2014;61(11):1115–23 [c].

[11] Nishimura T, Yamazaki H, Iwama K, et al. Potential risk of alpha-glucosidase inhibitor administration in prostate cancer external radiotherapy by exceptional rectal gas production: a case report. J Med Case Rep. 2014;8:136. http://dx.doi.org/10.1186/1752-1947-8-136 [c].

[12] Playford RJ, Pither C, Gao R, et al. Use of the alpha glucosidase inhibitor acarbose in patients with 'Middleton syndrome': normal gastric anatomy but with accelerated gastric emptying causing postprandial reactive hypoglycemia and diarrhea. Can J Gastroenterol. 2013;27(7):403–4 [c].

[13] Thakkar B, Aronis KN, Vamvini MT, et al. Metformin and sulfonylureas in relation to cancer risk in type II diabetes patients: a meta-analysis using primary data of published studies. Metabolism. 2013;62(7):922–34 [M].

[14] Franciosi M, Lucisano G, Lapice E, et al. Metformin therapy and risk of cancer in patients with type 2 diabetes: systematic review. PLoS One. 2013;8(8):e71583 [M].

[15] Harris K, Smith L. Safety and efficacy of metformin in patients with type 2 diabetes mellitus and chronic hepatitis C. Ann Pharmacother. 2013;47(10):1348–52 [M].

[16] Laskov I, Drudi L, Beauchamp MC, et al. Anti-diabetic doses of metformin decrease proliferation markers in tumors of patients with endometrial cancer. Gynecol Oncol. 2014;134(3):607–14 [c].

[17] Singh S, Singh H, Singh PP, et al. Antidiabetic medications and the risk of colorectal cancer in patients with diabetes mellitus: a systematic review and meta-analysis. Cancer Epidemiol Biomarkers Prev. 2013;22(12):2258–68 [M].

[18] Zhang ZJ, Bi Y, Li S, et al. Reduced risk of lung cancer with metformin therapy in diabetic patients: a systematic review and meta-analysis. Am J Epidemiol. 2014;180(1):11–4 [M].

[19] de Jager J, Kooy A, Schalkwijk C, et al. Long-term effects of metformin on endothelial function in type 2 diabetes: a randomized controlled trial. J Intern Med. 2014;275(1):59–70 [C].

[20] Mumoli L, Gambardella A, Labate A, et al. Rosacea-like facial rash related to metformin administration in a young woman. BMC Pharmacol Toxicol. 2014;15:3. http://dx.doi.org/10.1186/2050-6511-15-3 [c].

[21] Kirkiz S, Yarali N, Arman Bilir O, et al. Metformin-induced hemolytic anemia. Med Princ Pract. 2014;23(2):183–5 [c].

[22] Vecchio S, Giampreti A, Petrolini VM, et al. Metformin accumulation: lactic acidosis and high plasmatic metformin levels in a retrospective case series of 66 patients on chronic therapy. Clin Toxicol (Phila). 2014;52(2):129–35 [c].

[23] Altun E, Kaya B, Paydas S, et al. Lactic acidosis induced by metformin in a chronic hemodialysis patient with diabetes mellitus type 2. Hemodial Int. 2014;18(2):529–31.

[24] Ncomanzi D, Sicat RM, Sundararajan K. Metformin-associated lactic acidosis presenting as an ischemic gut in a patient who then survived a cardiac arrest: a case report. J Med Case Rep. 2014;8:159. http://dx.doi.org/10.1186/1752-1947-8-159 [c].

[25] Gatford KL, Houda CM, Lu ZX, et al. Vitamin B12 and homocysteine status during pregnancy in the metformin in gestational diabetes trial: responses to maternal metformin compared with insulin treatment. Diabetes Obes Metab. 2013;15(7):660–7 [C].

[26] Haeusler S, Parry-Strong A, Krebs JD. The prevalence of low vitamin B12 status in people with type 2 diabetes receiving metformin therapy in New Zealand—a clinical audit. N Z Med J. 2014;127(1404):8–16 [C].

[27] Sato Y, Ouchi K, Funase Y, et al. Relationship between metformin use, vitamin B12 deficiency, hyperhomocysteinemia and vascular complications in patients with type 2 diabetes. Endocr J. 2013;60(12):1275–80 [C].

[28] Jarskog LF, Hamer RM, Catellier DJ, et al. Metformin for weight loss and metabolic control in overweight outpatients with schizophrenia and schizoaffective disorder. Am J Psychiatry. 2013;170(9):1032–40 [C].

[29] McDonagh MS, Selph S, Ozpinar A, et al. Systematic review of the benefits and risks of metformin in treating obesity in children aged 18 years and younger. JAMA Pediatr. 2014;168(2):178–84 [M].

[30] Lyster RL, Houle SK. Abnormal vaginal bleeding following pharmacist prescribing of metformin leads to the detection of complex endometrial hyperplasia. Ann Pharmacother. 2013;47(11):1581–3 [c].

[31] Cassina M, Dona M, Di Gianantonio E, et al. First-trimester exposure to metformin and risk of birth defects: a systematic review and meta-analysis. Hum Reprod Update. 2014;20(5):656–669 [M].

[32] Kutoh E. Probable linagliptin-induced liver toxicity: a case report. Diabetes Metab. 2014;40(1):82–4 [c].

[33] Beaudouin E, Defendi F, Picaud J, et al. Iatrogenic angioedema associated with ACEi, sitagliptin, and deficiency of 3 enzymes

catabolizing bradykinin. Eur Ann Allergy Clin Immunol. 2014;46(3):119–22.

[34] Hamasaki H, Yanai H. The development of angioedema in a patient with type 2 diabetes due to a novel dipeptidyl peptidase-IV inhibitor, anagliptin. Int J Cardiol. 2013;168(3):e106 [c].

[35] Barnett AH, Huisman H, Jones R, et al. Linagliptin for patients aged 70 years or older with type 2 diabetes inadequately controlled with common antidiabetes treatments: a randomised, double-blind, placebo-controlled trial. Lancet. 2013;382(9902):1413–23 [C].

[36] Scirica BM, Bhatt DL, Braunwald E, et al. Saxagliptin and cardiovascular outcomes in patients with type 2 diabetes mellitus. N Engl J Med. 2013;369(14):1317–26 [C].

[37] Scirica BM, Braunwald E, Raz I, et al. Heart failure, saxagliptin, and diabetes mellitus: observations from the SAVOR-TIMI 53 randomized trial. Circulation. 2014;130(18):1579–88 [C].

[38] Bussey MR, Emanuele MA, Lomasney LM, et al. Sitagliptin-induced bilateral Achilles tendinitis. Rheumatology (Oxford). 2014;53(4):630 [c].

[39] Crickx E, Marroun I, Veyrie C, et al. DPP4 inhibitor-induced polyarthritis: a report of three cases. Rheumatol Int. 2014;34(2):291–2 [c].

[40] Al-Arouj M, Hassoun AA, Medlej R, et al. The effect of vildagliptin relative to sulphonylureas in Muslim patients with type 2 diabetes fasting during Ramadan: the VIRTUE study. Int J Clin Pract. 2013;67(10):957–63 [C].

[41] Derosa G, Bonaventura A, Bianchi L, et al. Vildagliptin compared to glimepiride on post-prandial lipemia and on insulin resistance in type 2 diabetic patients. Metabolism. 2014;63(7):957–67 [C].

[42] Li L, Shen J, Bala MM, et al. Incretin treatment and risk of pancreatitis in patients with type 2 diabetes mellitus: systematic review and meta-analysis of randomised and non-randomised studies. BMJ. 2014;348:g2366 [M].

[43] Dungan KM, Povedano ST, Forst T, et al. Once-weekly dulaglutide versus once-daily liraglutide in metformin-treated patients with type 2 diabetes (AWARD-6): a randomised, open-label, phase 3, non-inferiority trial. Lancet. 2014;384(9951):1349–57 [C].

[44] Bode SF, Egg M, Wallesch C, et al. 10-Fold liraglutide overdose over 7 months resulted only in minor side-effects. J Clin Pharmacol. 2013;53(7):785–6.

[45] Nakanishi R, Hirose T, Tamura Y, et al. Attempted suicide with liraglutide overdose did not induce hypoglycemia. Diabetes Res Clin Pract. 2013;99(1):e3–4 [c].

[46] Ryan GJ, Moniri NH, Smiley DD. Clinical effects of once-weekly exenatide for the treatment of type 2 diabetes mellitus. Am J Health Syst Pharm. 2013;70(13):1123–31.

[47] Ottney A. Glucagon-like peptide-1 receptor agonists for weight loss in adult patients without diabetes. Am J Health Syst Pharm. 2013;70(23):2097–103.

[48] Pratley RE, Nauck MA, Barnett AH, et al. Once-weekly albiglutide versus once-daily liraglutide in patients with type 2 diabetes inadequately controlled on oral drugs (HARMONY 7): a randomised, open-label, multicentre, non-inferiority phase 3 study. Lancet Diabetes Endocrinol. 2014;2(4):289–97 [C].

[49] Ferdinand KC, White WB, Calhoun DA, et al. Effects of the once-weekly glucagon-like peptide-1 receptor agonist dulaglutide on ambulatory blood pressure and heart rate in patients with type 2 diabetes mellitus. Hypertension. 2014;64(4):731–7.

[50] Woo JS, Kim W, Ha SJ, et al. Cardioprotective effects of exenatide in patients with ST-segment-elevation myocardial infarction undergoing primary percutaneous coronary intervention: results of exenatide myocardial protection in revascularization study. Arterioscler Thromb Vasc Biol. 2013;33(9):2252–60.

[51] Dubois-Laforgue D, Boutboul D, Levy DJ, et al. Severe acute renal failure in patients treated with glucagon-like peptide-1 receptor agonists. Diabetes Res Clin Pract. 2014;103(3):e53–5.

[52] Gariani K, de Seigneux S, Moll S. Acute interstitial nephritis after treatment with liraglutide. Am J Kidney Dis. 2014;63(2):347.

[53] Kern E, VanWagner LB, Yang GY, et al. Liraglutide-induced autoimmune hepatitis. JAMA Intern Med. 2014;174(6):984–7.

[54] Brown DX, Butler EL, Evans M. Lixisenatide as add-on therapy to basal insulin. Drug Des Devel Ther. 2013;8:25–38 [C].

[55] Monami M, Dicembrini I, Nardini C, et al. Glucagon-like peptide-1 receptor agonists and pancreatitis: a meta-analysis of randomized clinical trials. Diabetes Res Clin Pract. 2014;103(2):269–75 [M].

[56] Jeyaraj S, Shetty AS, Kumar CR, et al. Liraglutide-induced acute pancreatitis. J Assoc Physicians India. 2014;62(1):64–6 [c].

[57] Forst T, Guthrie R, Goldenberg R, et al. Efficacy and safety of canagliflozin over 52 weeks in patients with type 2 diabetes on background metformin and pioglitazone. Diabetes Obes Metab. 2014;16(5):467–77.

[58] Inagaki N, Kondo K, Yoshinari T, et al. Efficacy and safety of canagliflozin monotherapy in Japanese patients with type 2 diabetes inadequately controlled with diet and exercise: a 24-week, randomized, double-blind, placebo-controlled. Phase III study. Expert Opin Pharmacother. 2014;15(11):1501–15 [C].

[59] Devineni D, Vaccaro N, Polidori D, et al. Effects of hydrochlorothiazide on the pharmacokinetics, pharmacodynamics, and tolerability of canagliflozin, a sodium glucose co-transporter 2 inhibitor, in healthy participants. Clin Ther. 2014;36(5):698–710 [C].

[60] Bays HE, Weinstein R, Law G, et al. Canagliflozin: effects in overweight and obese subjects without diabetes mellitus. Obesity (Silver Spring). 2014;22(4):1042–9 [C].

[61] Inagaki N, Kondo K, Yoshinari T, et al. Efficacy and safety of canagliflozin in Japanese patients with type 2 diabetes: a randomized, double-blind, placebo-controlled, 12-week study. Diabetes Obes Metab. 2013;15(12):1136–45 [C].

[62] Rosenstock J, Seman LJ, Jelaska A, et al. Efficacy and safety of empagliflozin, a sodium glucose cotransporter 2 (SGLT2) inhibitor, as add-on to metformin in type 2 diabetes with mild hyperglycaemia. Diabetes Obes Metab. 2013;15(12):1154–60 [C].

[63] Kaku K, Mori M, Kanoo T, et al. Efficacy and safety of alogliptin added to insulin in Japanese patients with type 2 diabetes: a randomized, double-blind, 12-week, placebo-controlled trial followed by an open-label, long-term extension phase. Expert Opin Pharmacother. 2014;15(15):2121–30 [C].

[64] Phung OJ, Schwartzman E, Allen RW, et al. Sulphonylureas and risk of cardiovascular disease: systematic review and meta-analysis. Diabet Med. 2013;30(10):1160–71 [M].

[65] Kottenberg E, Thielmann M, Kleinbongard P, et al. Myocardial protection by remote ischaemic pre-conditioning is abolished in sulphonylurea-treated diabetics undergoing coronary revascularisation. Acta Anaesthesiol Scand. 2014;58(4):453–62 [C].

[66] Sheth KN, Kimberly WT, Elm JJ, et al. Pilot study of intravenous glyburide in patients with a large ischemic stroke. Stroke. 2014;45(1):281–3 [C].

[67] Henley JK, Blackmon JA, Fraga GR, et al. A case of glyburide-induced leukocytoclastic vasculitis. Dermatol Online J. 2013;19(9):19619 [c].

[68] Marder W, Khalatbari S, Myles JD, et al. The peroxisome proliferator activated receptor-gamma pioglitazone improves vascular function and decreases disease activity in patients with rheumatoid arthritis. J Am Heart Assoc. 2013;2(6):e000441.

[69] Bone HG, Lindsay R, McClung MR, et al. Effects of pioglitazone on bone in postmenopausal women with impaired fasting glucose or impaired glucose tolerance: a randomized, double-blind, placebo-controlled study. J Clin Endocrinol Metab. 2013;98(12):4691–701 [M].

[70] Grey A, Bolland M, Fenwick S, et al. The skeletal effects of pioglitazone in type 2 diabetes or impaired glucose tolerance: a randomized controlled trial. Eur J Endocrinol. 2013;170(2):255–62 [C].

[71] Esterson YB, Zhang K, Koppaka S, et al. Insulin sensitizing and anti-inflammatory effects of thiazolidinediones are heightened in obese patients. J Investig Med. 2013;61(8):1152–60 [C].

[72] Tripathy D, Daniele G, Fiorentino TV, et al. Pioglitazone improves glucose metabolism and modulates skeletal muscle TIMP-3-TACE dyad in type 2 diabetes mellitus: a randomised, double-blind, placebo-controlled, mechanistic study. Diabetologia. 2013;56(10):2153–63.

[73] Liu SC, Chien KL, Wang CH, et al. Efficacy and safety of adding pioglitazone or sitagliptin to patients with type 2 diabetes insufficiently controlled with metformin and a sulfonylurea. Endocr Pract. 2013;19(6):980–8.

[74] Kemp DE, Schinagle M, Gao K, et al. PPAR-gamma agonism as a modulator of mood: proof-of-concept for pioglitazone in bipolar depression. CNS Drugs. 2014;28(6):571–81.

[75] Ferwana M, Firwana B, Hasan R, et al. Pioglitazone and risk of bladder cancer: a meta-analysis of controlled studies. Diabet Med. 2013;30(9):1026–32 [M].

[76] Badeau RM, Honka MJ, Lautamaki R, et al. Systemic metabolic markers and myocardial glucose uptake in type 2 diabetic and coronary artery disease patients treated for 16 weeks with rosiglitazone, a PPARgamma agonist. Ann Med. 2014;46(1):18–23 [C].

[77] Bach RG, Brooks MM, Lombardero M, et al. Rosiglitazone and outcomes for patients with diabetes mellitus and coronary artery disease in the Bypass Angioplasty Revascularization Investigation 2 Diabetes (BARI 2D) trial. Circulation. 2013;128(8):785–94 [C].

[78] Edgeworth A, Treacy MP, Hurst TP. Thiazolidinediones in the treatment of HIV/HAART-associated lipodystrophy syndrome. AIDS Rev. 2013;15(3):171–80 [R].

[79] Lincoff AM, Tardif JC, Schwartz GG, et al. Effect of aleglitazar on cardiovascular outcomes after acute coronary syndrome in patients with type 2 diabetes mellitus: the AleCardio randomized clinical trial. JAMA. 2014;311(15):1515–25 [C].

42

Miscellaneous Hormones

Vasileios Chortis, Kristien Boelaert[1]

Centre for Endocrinology, Diabetes and Metabolism, University of Birmingham, Birmingham, United Kingdom

[1]Corresponding author: k.boelaert@bham.ac.uk

INTRODUCTION

This chapter aims to provide an overview of all recent information on adverse effects of various hormonal drugs that have not been covered in other chapters of this volume, including calcitonin, gonadotropins, gonadotrophin-releasing hormone antagonists, human recombinant growth hormone (somatropin), growth hormone receptor antagonists (pegvisomant), parathyroid hormone analogues (teriperatide), melatonin and analogues, oxytocin and analogues, somatostatin and analogues, vasopressin and analogues. For each section, all relevant original clinical studies are presented first, followed by reviews and meta-analyses. Case reports on new or rare side effects are presented at the end of each section.

CALCITONIN [SEDA-34, 703; SEDA-35, 789; SEDA-36, 659]

Clinical Studies

Liver Cancer

A recent population-based, nested case-control study suggested an association of salmon calcitonin nasal spray use with increased risk of hepatic cancer. 1925 osteoporotic patients with cancer were used as the study population. 3727 non-cancer patients, matched according to age, sex, comorbidity, index-year, and osteoporosis-year comprised the control group. Calcitonin use was associated with an increased risk of liver cancer (odds ratio 1.94, 95% confidence interval 1.23–3.05) and a lower breast cancer risk (OR 0.35, 95% CI 0.15–0.80). In male patients, the difference was not statistically significant. The risk was higher in patients receiving high daily doses. An increased risk of lung cancer was also reported in the high daily dose group (OR 2.04, 95% CI 1.21–3.44) [1C].

Systematic Reviews and Meta-Analyses

Carcinogenic Potential

In 2013, the United States Food and Drug Administration and the European Medicines Agency's Committee for Medicinal Projects for Human Use withdrew their approval for salmon calcitonin use for osteoporosis, in view of concerns regarding the drug's carcinogenic potential. A systematic review of 18 published randomized-controlled trials explored the existing literature regarding this association. Overall, the authors considered the evidence suggesting an increased risk of cancer with calcitonin use weak and underlined several methodological shortcomings of many of the pertinent studies (inclusion of patients with past medical history of malignancy, limited duration of follow-up, use of higher doses than the ones approved in most countries). They agree, however, that it is reasonable to avoid the use of calcitonin in osteoporosis, given its limited efficacy in comparison to other available treatment options [2M].

GONADOTROPINS (GONADORELIN, GnRH AND ANALOGUES) [SEDA-35, 789; SEDA-36, 660]

Prostate Cancer and Chemical Castration Studies

A randomized, crossover study assessed the tolerability and adverse events profiles of intramuscular triptorelin pamoate (GnRH analogue: 22.5 mg) and subcutaneous leuprolide acetate (GnRH analogue: 45 mg) in 107 male patients with advanced prostate cancer. No serious

© 2015 Elsevier B.V. All rights reserved.

adverse events were reported. Injection site pain was reported by one triptorelin-treated patient and two leuprolide-treated patients. A case of cystitis and a case of urinary retention in the triptorelin group, as well as an episode of diarrhea in the leuprolide groups completed the adverse events list, with unlikely causality [3c].

A non-comparative clinical trial assessed the efficacy and safety of high-dose leuprorelin acetate in prostate cancer patients. 42 patients were given two subcutaneous injections of leuprorelin acetate 22.5 mg subcutaneously every 12 weeks, for a total period of 24 weeks. Hot flushes ($n = 4$) and pain ($n = 2$) were the most common treatment-emergent adverse events. A case of hepatitis and a case of pruritis were also noted. Overall, the incidence of adverse events (20/42) was not higher than previous studies using lower leuprorelin doses [4c].

Acute Kidney Injury

A large retrospective study in a group of 69 292 patients diagnosed with non-metastatic prostate cancer revealed a 10-year risk of acute kidney injury of 31.1% for patients treated with goserolin (GnRH agonist) vs. 26% in patients treated with bilateral orchidectomy and 24.9% in patients not subjected to any form of androgen deprivation. On multivariate analysis, GnRH analogue treatment, but not orchidectomy, was a risk factor for acute kidney injury. Further research is required to elucidate the mechanisms underlying this association [5C].

The role of combination treatment with leuprolide and abiretarone was assessed in a randomized, phase II trial. 58 patients with localized prostate cancer were randomized to receive leuprolide or leuprolide plus abiretarone and prednisone for 12 weeks, followed by 12 additional weeks of combination treatment. Prostate biopsy at 12 weeks showed that combination therapy was more effective in reducing intratumoral levels of androgens. The adverse events profile was similar between the two groups. The most common side effects reported included hot flushes, elevated transaminases and fatigability [6c].

A population-based study used a large national cohort of prostate cancer patients to explore the cardiovascular and cerebrovascular risks of androgen deprivation therapy. 31 571 patients (median age: 71 years) were identified, 9204 of whom had received medical androgen deprivation therapy with GnRH analogues, while 2060 had been orchidectomized. Follow-up observation was for a median duration of 3.3 years. GnRH treatment conferred an increased risk of myocardial infarction (adjusted hazard ratio 1.31, 95% CI 1.16–1.49) and cerebrovascular accident (adjusted hazard ratio 1.19, 95% CI 1.06–1.35) in comparison to patients not subjected to androgen deprivation. Interestingly, this was not the case for patients treated with orchidectomy, who had the same risk of myocardial infarction or stroke as other prostate cancer patients. An important limitation of this study is its failure to control for lifestyle risk factors for coronary artery disease and cerebrovascular disease. These findings corroborate previous observational studies demonstrating an increased risk of thrombotic events in patients receiving androgen deprivation treatment, possibly in the context of higher metabolic syndrome rates. However, randomized-controlled trials comparing androgen deprivation treatment to no androgen deprivation exposure have not demonstrated such an effect [7C].

A prospective, cross-sectional study assessed the efficacy and safety of chemical castration in 38 Korean sex offenders who had undergone voluntary androgen deprivation therapy. Patients experienced a reduction in sexual drive and frequency of sexual fantasies. Leuprolide acetate depot 3.75 mg subcutaneous injections were administered for 3 months, followed by an observation period of 14 months. Most common side effects included flushes ($n = 17$, 45%), weight gain ($n = 11$, 29%) and decreased testicular volume ($n = 8$, 24%). Reduction in bone mineral density was noted in 4 patients (11%). 8 patients (24%) developed depressive symptoms. Other commonly reported adverse events included injection site pain ($n = 7$), myalgia ($n = 4$) and decreased body hair ($n = 2$) [8c].

Clinical Studies on Endometriosis

A randomized, controlled trial assessed the effectiveness and safety of combined laparoscopy plus gonadotropin-releasing hormone agonist in patients with endometriosis ($n = 198$). Patients were randomized to laparoscopy alone ($n = 52$) laparoscopy combined with domestic Leuprolide acetate at a dose of 3.75 mg every 28 days ($n = 76$) or laparoscopy combined with imported Goserelin acetate with dose of 3.6 mg every 28 days ($n = 70$). Combination treatment was superior to laparoscopy alone. The incidence of adverse events was 21% (15/70) with Leuprolide acetate and 20% (13/66) with Goserelin acetate, including irregular vaginal bleeding due to hypoestrogenism [9c].

Fertility Studies

A prospective study explored the gastrointestinal side effects of busorelin in 124 women in the context of in vitro fertilisation. 2 age- and sex-matched controls were used per patient. There was a statistically significant correlation of busorelin treatment with constipation, nausea, vomiting and impaired psychological well-being. At 5-year follow-up, psychological well-being in busorelin-treated patients was improved, but there was still an increased incidence of abdominal pain and 15% of women had gastrointestinal symptoms consistent with development or deterioration of irritable bowel syndrome [10c].

Pediatric Studies

A retrospective study examined the use of long-acting GnRH agonists in the treatment of central precocious puberty and early-onset puberty ($n = 621$). 6 severe adverse events were observed in 5 patients; of these, 4 pertained to the development of sterile abscesses (0.6%). One anaphylactic reaction was reported, while another patient developed slipped capital femoral epiphysis [11C].

A prospective extension study evaluated the safety of long-term leuprolide acetate depot in children with central precocious puberty. 72 children received 3 monthly leuprolide acetate depot injections at a dose of 11.25 mg ($n = 34$) or 30 mg ($n = 38$) for a period of 32 months. Adverse events were similar between the two groups. Injection site pain was the most common side effect ($n = 19$ overall). No participants had to stop treatment due to side effects [12C].

The safety of histrelin (GnRH analogue) capsule implantation in children with precocious puberty has been reviewed in a retrospective study of 114 patients. Two cases of systemic allergic reaction requiring explantation were reported. One child developed insertion site infection requiring antibiotics. Implant fracture was observed in 16/58 removals (28%) [13c].

A retrospective study evaluated the association of various maternal hormonal treatments with the subsequent risk of Autism Spectrum Disorders (ASD) for the offspring. 480 cases of 2–10-year-old children with ASD were reviewed. A healthy control group was included for comparison. 12.3% of mothers in the ASD group (59 cases) had undergone hormonal fertility interventions. The corresponding percentage in the control population was only 4.4%. Hormonal interventions included estrogens, progesterone, gonadotropins, HMG, clomiphene and GnRH. The odds ratio on logistic regression analysis for hormonal interventions was 2.24 (CI 95% 1.309–3.835, $p = 0.003$). No separate analyses were performed for individual agents [14C].

Literature Reviews and Meta-Analyses

A meta-analysis evaluated the use of GnRH analogues in the treatment of endometriosis. Hot flushes were the most commonly observed side effect and were only mild in 80% of cases [15M].

A meta-analysis of studies reporting on the incidence of alopecia with hormonal treatments estimated a 9.5% risk of all-grade alopecia with leuprorelin and 25% with goserelin plus anastrazole [16M].

A systematic review analysed the adverse effect profile of Luteinizing Hormone-Releasing Hormone (LHRH) Agonists. Genital shrinkage (93%), mild anaemia (77–90%), erectile dysfunction (77.3–95.0%), loss of libido (58.0–91.4%) and flushing (44–88%) were the most commonly reported side effects. Weight gain/increased fat mass was reported in 14–70% of patients. Depression was reported in some studies (14.4–26.5%), but not consistently [17M].

Case Reports

Hypertension During Triptorelin in Childhood

Hypertension in association with triptorelin treatment was reported in a 7-year-old girl with precocious puberty. Triptorelin was administered at 3.75 mg/month. At the age of 10 years and 8 months, she was diagnosed with severe hypertension (150/110 mmHg, >99th centile for age), which was confirmed on 24-hour monitoring. Echocardiogram revealed concentric left ventricular hypertrophy. She was started on nifedipine and ramipril, while gonadorelin was stopped. Other secondary causes of hypertension were excluded. Her blood pressure improved and antihypertensives were stopped over the next 8 months [18A].

Pituitary Apoplexy

A case of pituitary apoplexy post-GnRH agonist treatment was reported, the first described in the Asian population. A 77-year-old patient with a 6-month history of prostate cancer developed acute headache and visual blurring, a few hours after receiving 3.75 mg subcutaneous leuprorelin. Ophthalmological assessment was consistent with left III nerve palsy, with ptosis and ophthalmoplegia; MRI pituitary showed an enlarged pituitary, with evidence of infarction. Trans-sphenoidal surgery was performed 10 days later and resulted in complete recovery [19A].

Drug-Induced Rash

A rare case of leuprolide acetate-induced rash has been reported. A 65-year-old man with a 4-year history of prostate cancer on chronic treatment with 4–6 monthly leuprolide acetate injections developed a generalized papular rash 3 weeks after receiving his leuprolide injection. The eruption resolved with 5 days of prednisolone and antihistamines, but re-emerged 3 weeks after his next leuprolide injection. A punch biopsy revealed a histological picture of eosinophilic dermatitis, consistent with drug-induced rash [20A].

Traumatic Hematoma

Massive traumatic subcutaneous hematoma was caused by goserelin acetate injection in an 87-year-old man with prostate cancer. Blood transfusion was required. Arteriography identified injury to a branch of the lower epigastric artery, which was embolized [21A].

GONADOTROPHIN-RELEASING HORMONE ANTAGONISTS [SEDA-35, 790; SEDA-36, 661]

Case Reports

Ovarian Hyperstimulation Syndrome

Two cases of severe ovarian hyperstimulation syndrome (OHSS) after ovarian stimulation with combined GnRH agonist–GnRH antagonist course followed by GnRH agonist trigger have been described. A 29-year-old woman was subjected to the following ovulation induction protocol: recombinant FSH 150 IU in days 2–11 of the menstrual cycle, accompanied by ganirelix (GnRH antagonist) from day 5 of stimulation. Final follicular maturation induction was completed with a bolus of triptorelin (GnRH agonist, 0.3 mg). She developed abdominal pain and distension with severe ascites, ovarian enlargement and hemoconcentration 1 day after oocyte retrieval. 2.5 l of ascitic fluid was drained. She recovered within 3 days. The second patient was a 27-year-old woman who underwent ovarian stimulation on days 2–11 of her menstrual cycle with rFSH (187.5 IU starting dose) plus cetrorelix acetate from day 5 of stimulation. Finally, a bolus of Decapeptyl (GnRH agonist, 0.2 mg) was given to induce follicular maturation. 6 days after oocyte retrieval, she also developed abdominal pain and distension, associated with ovarian enlargement and ascites. 3.7 l of ascitic fluid was drained. She was discharged 4 days later. This is only the second report of severe OHSS associated with GnRH agonist 'trigger' protocols so far [22A].

SPECIAL REVIEW - SOMATROPIN (HUMAN GROWTH HORMONE, hGH) [SEDA-35, 791; SEDA-36, 661]

Cancer Risk in Growth Hormone-Treated Patients

The potential carcinogenic risk of growth hormone replacement was explored in two retrospective studies. The first was a retrospective cohort study with longitudinal follow-up. 338 pediatric cancer survivors who reported use of growth hormone, as well as 11760 who never underwent GH treatment, were compared. GH treatment was not associated with increased risk of CNS tumors (adjusted rate ratio 1, CI 95%

0.6–1.8, $p = 0.94$) [23C]. The second study included 164 patients with growth hormone deficiency post cure of acromegaly (acroGHD) and 2469 with non-functioning pituitary adenomas (NFPA), also treated with growth hormone. Patients were followed up for 5 years. Various cohorts from the general population were used as external control groups (including the World Health Organization Global Burden of Disease). The two GH treatment groups did not have a different overall cancer mortality risk than the general population. The risk of brain malignancies was higher in GH treated patients than the general population; however, previous radiotherapy is a likely confounding factor in this relationship. Indeed, on stratification analysis the increased incidence of malignant brain tumors only applied to patients with previous radiotherapy (SIR for malignant brain tumors in patients with a history of RT was 6.07 (CI 95% 1.96–14.17) in patients with a history of radiotherapy vs. 3.32 (CI 95% 0.89–8.49) in those without history of radiotherapy) [24C]. Overall, there does not seem to be convincing evidence of an association between growth hormone relationship and cancer risk.

Clinical Studies in Adults

Stroke Risk

A large retrospective observation study explored the risk of stroke in young adults who had received growth hormone replacement in childhood ($n = 6874$), using two other population-based studies on cerebrovascular events to derive control groups. 11 cases of stroke were identified in the GH-treated group: 5 pertained to subarachnoid hemorrhage, 3 to intracerebral hemorrhage and 3 to ischemic stroke. The mean patient age at the time of the stroke was 24.2 years. Four patients died, including three cases of subarachnoid hemorrhage. There was a significantly higher risk of stroke among patients treated with GH in childhood than in the control populations (standardized incidence ratio 2.2, 95% CI 1.3–3.6). Most of this increased risk was attributable to subarachnoid hemorrhage [25C].

Long-Acting Growth Hormone

A novel recombinant growth hormone preparation (NNC0195-0092), with the ability to reversibly bind to plasma albumin achieving longer bioavailability, was assessed in a randomized, placebo-controlled trial in healthy volunteers. Five cohorts of eight volunteers received a single dose of NNC0195-0092 (0.01–0.32 mg/kg) ($n = 6$) or placebo ($n = 2$). 16 volunteers were randomized to receive once-weekly doses of NNC0195-0092 (0.02–0.24 mg/kg; $n = 12$) or placebo ($n = 4$) for 4 weeks. No severe adverse events were noted. Headaches, myalgia, and peripheral edema were the most frequently reported side effects. The risk of adverse events was greatest with the highest NNC0195-0092 dose levels and similar to placebo for the lowest NNC0195-0092 dose levels. One patient withdrew due to electrocardiographic changes but no further details were provided. Glucose levels were not affected by the study drug, although a transient increase in insulin levels was noted in some subjects [26c].

Sustained-Release Growth Hormone

A 26-week extension study assessed the safety of long-term treatment with once weekly, sustained-release growth hormone in adults with GH deficiency. Patients who had already received 26 weeks of GH in the context of a previous RCT ($n=93$, 'throughout group'), as well as patients who had been on the placebo arm of the said trial ($n=42$, 'switch group'), received sustained-release GH (LB03002) for 26 weeks (starting doses 1–3 mg/week). The most common treatment-emergent adverse events included peripheral edema ($n=5$ in the 'throughout' group vs. 7 in the switch group) and headache ($n=3$ vs. 9) [27c].

Long-Term Safety

A retrospective study looked at the safety of long-term growth hormone replacement in adults using 164 patients with growth hormone deficiency post cure of acromegaly (acroGHD) and 2469 with non-functioning pituitary adenomas (NFPA). Various cohorts from the general population were used as external control groups (including the World Health Organization Global Burden of Disease). Cardiovascular mortality was higher in the acroGHD than the general population, but lower in the GH-treated NFPA patients than the general population. Cerebrovascular morbidity was not different from the general population. The two GH treatment groups did not have a different overall cancer mortality risk than the general population. The incidence of diabetes mellitus was higher in the two treatment groups than in the control population. Metabolically, GH replacement was associated with lower total and LDL cholesterol and higher HDL cholesterol; this effect was more pronounced in the previously acromegalic group [24C].

A randomized, placebo-controlled, crossover trial investigated the effects of growth hormone in patients with spinal muscular atrophy. 19 patients with type II/III spinal muscular atrophy were randomized to receive somatropin subcutaneously (0.03 mg/kg/day) or placebo for 3 months. Somatropin did not improve muscle power or respiratory function. 11 patients reported side effects with somatropin (headache, arthralgia, myalgia and peripheral edema). Two patients stopped treatment due to severe adverse events, namely myalgia and progressive headache [28c].

Pediatric Clinical Studies

A randomized, controlled trial assessed the long-term metabolic effects of growth hormone treatment in patients with short stature born small for gestational age. 65 children, 3–8 years of age, received 33 μg/kg/day ($n=31$) or 67 μg/kg/day ($n=34$) GH for 260 weeks. The treatment had a favorable metabolic impact with regard to lipid profile, with no adverse effects on insulin and glucose levels, body mass index or vital signs [29C].

Central Corneal Thickness

A prospective study aimed to evaluate the effects of growth hormone replacement on central corneal thickness and intraocular pressure in 74 pre-pubertal children with growth hormone deficiency (median age: 10.4 years). 50 healthy children (matched for age, sex and body mass index) were used as controls. After 12 months of growth hormone treatment, children with growth hormone deficiency showed greater central corneal thickness (564.7 ± 13.1 μm) than both baseline values (535.7 ± 17 μm; $p < 0.001$) and control subjects (536.2 ± 12.5 μm; $p < 0.001$). Intraocular pressure was also higher post growth hormone treatment (15.6 ± 0.7 mmHg) than both baseline (12.5 ± 0.8 mmHg; $p < 0.001$) and controls (12.3 ± 0.5 mmHg; $p < 0.001$). This was the first prospective study demonstrating these ocular effects of growth hormone, suggesting the need for ophthalmological assessment during follow-up of growth hormone treated children [30c].

A prospective, uncontrolled intervention trial assessed the efficacy and safety of short-term growth hormone treatment in children with idiopathic short stature. 36 patients received subcutaneous injections of GH (0.37 mg/kg/week) for 26 weeks. Nasopharyngitis was the most commonly reported adverse event during the study ($n=12$), followed by abdominal pain ($n=4$) and otitis media ($n=3$). Limb pain and urticaria were also reported in 2 patients. Biochemically, mild rises in alkaline phosphatase were noted (presumably due to bone growth). Mean HbA1c also increased (5.45 at 24 weeks vs. 5.28 at baseline, $p < 0.0001$) [31c].

The use of sustained-release growth hormone was assessed in a 2-year randomized trial in pre-pubertal children. This involved administration of once weekly, sustained-release GH ($n=87$) or daily GH ($n=87$) for 1 year, followed by sustained-release GH for all for an additional year. There was no statistically significant difference in the incidence of adverse events or severe adverse events between the two modes of GH administration. 90% of patients reported mild-moderate injection site reactions and 8% reported severe site reactions in the sustained-release GH treated group [32C].

A retrospective cohort study on childhood cancer survivors who developed subsequent growth hormone deficiency post radiotherapy ($n=119$) aimed to assess the known risk of slipped capital femoral epiphysis (SCPE) during recombinant growth hormone treatment in this population. 57 patients received total body irradiation, while 62 only received cranial irradiation. A national registry of children receiving growth hormone for idiopathic growth hormone replacement was used as control group. 16 events of SCPE were observed in patients who had received total body irradiation, but none in the cranial irradiation only group. SCPE was much more prevalent among patients having received total body irradiation than in the control group of idiopathic GHD patients (incidence rate 35.9 vs. 0.17 events per 1000 person-years, respectively). The data suggests that the reported excess risk of SCPE in childhood cancer survivors is not due to GH treatment alone [33c].

A randomized-controlled trial assessed the importance of timing of recombinant growth hormone treatment to improve height and muscle strength in children receiving glucocorticoids. 30 children with short stature and at least 1 year of glucocorticoid treatment were randomized to receive growth hormone immediately or 6 months later. rhGH was administered at a dose of 0.065 mg/kg/day for 6 months and then at a dose maintaining serum IGF-I levels below 2 standard deviation scores for their age for a further 12 months. Growth hormone was associated with increased height and lean mass and was well tolerated with no serious adverse events. Treatment was interrupted due to headaches in one patient but reintroduced successfully after 2 weeks with no headache recurrence. Fasting glucose and 2-hour post-load glucose did increase after 12 months of growth hormone replacement and five patients developed impaired glucose tolerance; however, no cases of diabetes mellitus were reported [34c].

Literature Reviews and Meta-Analyses

The use of growth hormone in children outside the context of idiopathic growth hormone deficiency has been reviewed, including conditions such as Turner syndrome, chronic renal insufficiency, Prader-Willi syndrome (PWS), Noonan syndrome, SHOX (short stature homeobox containing gene) deficiency, children born small for gestational age (SGA) and children with idiopathic short stature (ISS). No significant adverse events have been noted with growth hormone treatment in these patient groups. The only caveat underlined in the review pertains to the need for polysomnographic exclusion of severe sleep apnea before embarking on growth hormone replacement in severely obese Prader-Willi patients, in view of the sudden deaths that have been previously reported in this group of patients [35R].

The safety of growth hormone replacement in adults was the subject of two systematic literature reviews. Of the six studies that have commented on the incidence of malignancies, none identified a higher risk in GH treated patients; the follow-up periods may not have been long enough to conclusively exclude such a risk though. Two post-marketing databases and one national study explored the risk of diabetes mellitus as a result of GH replacement. The results were contradictory, with increased risk identified in one of the databases only. Differences in the reference populations may account for this discrepancy; further research is required. The effects of exogenous GH on glucose metabolism have been explored in 11 studies. Of these, seven found no effect on glucose levels, three an increase, while one study reported a transient increase only during the first year of treatment. Insulin levels were increased in one study. HbA1c was assessed in three studies, two of which showed a decrease with growth hormone replacement, while the other showed no change. Insulin sensitivity was assessed in three studies, none of which found a significant effect. 10 cases of new-onset diabetes mellitus during GH treatment have been reported overall [36R,37M].

A meta-analysis focused on randomized controlled trials assessing the role of growth hormone in the treatment of burns in children and adults. 13 RCTs were identified (6 in children and 7 in adults), including 701 patients in total. Hyperglycemia was more frequent in adults receiving rhGH treatment compared with placebo (risk ratio (RR) 2.43, 95% CI 1.54–3.85), but not in children [38M].

Case Reports

Chiari I Malformation

Two cases of Chiari I malformation progression on growth hormone were reported. The first patient was a 4-year-old girl who was diagnosed with growth hormone deficiency. MRI brain revealed Chiari I malformation without syringomyelia. She received growth hormone replacement (0.7 mg subcutaneously 6 days per week initially, titrated up to 1.3 mg subcutaneously 6 days per week). Follow-up imaging 6 months later revealed a new syrinx; this was not, however, associated with any symptoms. The second case involved a 5-year-old girl with growth hormone deficiency and Chiari I malformation without syringomyelia. She received treatment with somatropin 0.7 mg subcutaneously 6 days per week, titrated up to 1.0 mg subcutaneously 6 days per week. On 6-month follow-up imaging, an asymptomatic cervical syrinx was discovered. 3 months later, she developed bulbar palsy and bilateral abducens nerve palsy. She underwent neurosurgery with removal of the posterior arch of C1 and duraplasty. The neurological symptoms resolved and she continued growth hormone replacement. Follow-up MRI 2 years later revealed a decrease in the size of the syrinx. Previous reports on the effect of growth hormone replacement on Chiari I malformations have shown contradictory results, ranging from deterioration to improvement [39A].

Hemangioma Enlargement

Increased erythema and prominence of vasculature in a pre-existing hemangioma in response to growth hormone treatment was reported in a 20-month-old girl with PHACE syndrome, a few weeks after she was started on growth hormone replacement (0.15 mg/kg/week) for partially empty sella with GH deficiency. The hemangioma did stabilize by the end of the second month of GH however and treatment did not have to be withdrawn. She went on to have GH for 9 years, with no change in the size of her hemangioma. A similar event was reported in another young female patient with the same condition, who was started on growth hormone at the age of 5 years. GH was stopped after 3 months as there were concerns that her facial hemangioma appeared to be more prominent. However, on follow-up assessment 1 year later her hemangioma had continued to grow despite GH withdrawal [40A].

GROWTH HORMONE RECEPTOR ANTAGONISTS [SEDA-34, 708; SEDA-35, 792; SEDA-36, 664]

Clinical Studies

Combination Pegvisomant and Somatostatin Analogues

Combination treatment of acromegaly with somatostatin analogues and pegvisomant was the subject of a prospective, uncontrolled trial. 141 acromegalic patients who had failed to attain normal IGF-1 levels or quality of life with 6 months of monotherapy with somatostatin analogues (Sandostatin LAR 30 mg or Lanreotide Autogel 120 mg every 28 days), were started on additional treatment with pegvisomant for a median duration of 5 years. The starting dose was 25 mg weekly ($n = 27$), 40 mg weekly ($n = 18$), while 67 patients received an adjusted dose based on their IGF-1 levels. Treatment dose was adjusted every 6–8 weeks aiming to normalize IGF-1. Four patients developed hypertrophy at injection sites; in three of these cases, the problem resolved with regular rotation of injection sites, while the fourth patient had to resort to cosmetic surgery. Transient transaminasemia more than three times above the upper normal range was observed in 19 patients (13.5%). The vast majority of these events occurred within the first year of combination treatment. Liver function returned to normal within a few months of drug withdrawal (median 5.5 months). Two patients experienced a recurrence of hypertransaminasemia when pegvisomant was restarted [41C].

A single-dose, crossover study compared single 30 mg/ml pegvisomant subcutaneous injections to two 15 mg/ml subcutaneous injections in 14 healthy volunteers. No serious adverse events were observed. The number of adverse events was similar in the two groups. The only moderate-severity adverse event pertained to musculoskeletal chest pain after two doses of 15 mg/ml. Overall, the tolerability was similar between the two administration strategies [42c].

Case Reports

Type I Hypersensitivity Reaction

The first case of a severe type I hypersensitivity reaction to pregvisomant has been reported. A 26-year-old female patient with surgically treated acromegaly was commenced on pegvisomant for persistent disease. Within 3 min of receiving her first, 40 mg subcutaneous injection, she developed upper body and facial flushing and a blanching erythematous rash. Conjunctival congestion, eyelid and lip swelling ensued, followed by chest tightness. There was no stridor, but a few polyphonic rhonchi were noted on chest auscultation. She was managed with intravenous hydrocortisone, salbutamol inhalers and supplemental oxygen. She responded well, with the rash, angioedema and bronchospasm subsiding over the next hour. She recovered fully and did not receive pegvisomant again [43A].

MELATONIN AND ANALOGUES [SED-15, 2245; SEDA-35, 792; SEDA-36, 664]

Clinical Studies on Pharmacokinetics and Tolerability

Mild transient somnolence was the only side effect reported in a prospective, dose escalation study assessing the tolerability and pharmacokinetics of 20, 30, 50, and 100 mg oral doses of melatonin in healthy volunteers [44c].

Clinical Studies on Sleep Quality

Another randomized, controlled study examined the efficacy of melatonin in improving sleep quality and cognitive function in patients with mild-moderate Alzheimer's disease ($n = 80$). Patients were treated for 2 weeks with placebo and then randomized (1:1) to receive 2 mg of prolonged-release melatonin or placebo nightly for 24 weeks, followed by 2 weeks of placebo. Melatonin treatment resulted in improved sleep quality and cognitive function. The adverse events profile of melatonin was similar to placebo [45C].

Clinical Studies on Anxiety and Depression

A randomized, double-blind, placebo-controlled trial assessed the effects of melatonin on depressive symptoms in breast cancer patients undergoing surgery. 44 patients received 6 mg oral melatonin daily or placebo for 3 months, starting 1 week pre-operatively. Melatonin decreased the incidence of depressive symptoms with a similar adverse effects profile to placebo. Of note, perioral or limb paresthesiae were reported in 3 melatonin-treated patients (10%) but not in placebo-treated patients [46c].

A randomized, controlled trial explored the efficiency of alprazolam, melatonin and a combination thereof in allaying pre-operative anxiety. 80 patients were randomised to receive alprazolam 0.5 mg, melatonin 3 mg, combination of the two or placebo orally 90 min before anesthesia. Combination treatment was more effective at reducing anxiety scores than monotherapy. Mild adverse events such as nausea, headache and dizziness were reported in all groups at similar frequency, including the placebo arm [47C].

A randomized, controlled trial examined the effects of melatonin and gabapentin pre-medication on anxiety and pain in adult patients undergoing retrobulbar eye block for cataract surgery ($n = 120$). Melatonin was associated with improvements in anxiety levels. Mild headache in one patient was the only reported melatonin-associated side effect [48c].

Other Clinical Studies

The role of melatonin in pediatric migraine prophylaxis was assessed in an observation study of 60 children, reporting a decrease in the frequency and severity of headaches. Mild side effects were observed in 14 children (23%), including somnolence, vomiting, mild hypotension and constipation [49c].

A parallel-group, randomized, placebo-controlled trial examined the efficacy of melatonin (3 mg) at reducing the metabolic side effects of olanzapine in 48 patients (11–17 year old) with bipolar disorder. Patients were treated with a combination of olanzapine, lithium carbonate, and melatonin, or olanzapine, lithium carbonate and placebo for 12 weeks. Melatonin-treated patients demonstrated a smaller increase in systolic blood pressure and plasma cholesterol, as well as a non-statistically significant trend towards lower triglycerides and fasting blood glucose. No adverse events were reported [50c].

Literature Reviews and Meta-Analyses

A European consensus conference reviewed the role of melatonin in pediatric sleep disturbances. The expert committee reported morning somnolence, enuresis, headache, dizziness, diarrhea, rash, and hypothermia as the most commonly occurring side effects, endorsing the safety of melatonin for short-term and long-term treatment. Attention was drawn to the potential

interaction between melatonin and CYP1A2 inhibitors. It is known that melatonin is metabolized by CYP11A2 and CYP2C19; consequently, concurrent treatment with CYP11A2 inhibitors such as tricyclic antidepressants or cimetidine may increase circulating melatonin levels, potentially resulting in a decrease in blood pressure or serum glucose levels [51M].

A systematic review assessed the efficacy of various pharmacological interventions for delirium based on prospective studies. Overall, only 2 out of 72 patients treated with melatonin experienced side effects mandating treatment cessation. These included recurrent nightmares and perceptual disturbances [52M].

The role of melatonin in patients with autism spectrum disorders was assessed in a systematic review of alternative treatments. Studies on the use of melatonin, including five randomized, controlled trials, have demonstrated the safety of doses up to 10 mg daily [53M].

A meta-analysis assessing the efficacy of a number of drugs at improving sleep in Alzheimer's patients based on randomized, controlled trials found no evidence that melatonin is beneficial. Only one study compared the occurrence of adverse effects between melatonin and placebo; this revealed no differences in frequency or severity [54,55M].

Ramelteon

The role of the melatonin receptor agonist ramelteon as insomnia treatment in adults was reviewed in a meta-analysis, which identified 13 relevant randomized, controlled trials and ascertained a statistically significant improvement in several parameters associated with sleep duration and quality in melatonin-treated patients. Somnolence was more commonly reported in ramelteon-treated patients than in placebo-treated patients (10 studies; relative risk 1.97 [95% CI 1.21–3.20]). The incidence of other adverse events was not significantly different between melatonin and placebo-treated groups [56M].

OXYTOCIN AND ANALOGUES [SEDA-35, 793; SEDA-36, 665]

Clinical Studies on Active Labor and Post-Partum Hemorrhage Prevention

A randomized, controlled trial compared the efficacy and safety of misoprostol and oxytocin in the active management of third-stage labor. 200 women were randomized 1:1 to receive misoprostol 600 mcg orally or oxytocin 10 IU intramuscularly. Obstetric outcomes were similar between the two treatment arms. Adverse events were more common in the misoprostol group overall. The most commonly reported side effects in the oxytocin group included abdominal pain ($n=22$), shivering ($n=8$) and nausea ($n=8$) [57C].

A randomized, placebo-controlled trial compared per rectum misoprostol to intravenous oxytocin in the context of post-cesarean section hemorrhage prevention. 192 women were randomized to receive 800 mg of rectal misoprostol or intravenous oxytocin infusion at the end of the procedure. Treatments were equally effective in preventing post-partum hemorrhage. The frequency of commonly reported adverse effects (pyrexia, shivering, vomiting) was not different between the two groups. Oxytocin infusion was associated with lower mean arterial pressure (96 vs. 91 mmHg; $p=0.0002$) and higher heart rate post-operatively, as compared with the preoperative vital signs [58C].

A randomized trial compared the use of misoprostol and oxytocin in the prevention of post-partum hemorrhage. 100 women were randomized to receive 600 mg sublingual misoprostol ($n=50$) or 10 IU intravenous oxytocin ($n=50$). Mean blood loss was lower in the oxytocin group and the only observed adverse effects included nausea ($n=3$) and vomiting ($n=1$) [59c].

Carbetocin monotherapy was compared to combined sublingual misoprostol and oxytocin infusion in the context of post-partum hemorrhage prevention in high-risk patients. 380 patients undergoing Cesarean section were randomized to receive either combined sublingual misoprostol 400 µg before surgery plus 20 IU oxytocin after delivery ($n=190$) or intravenous carbetocin 100 µg ($n=190$). Efficacy in post-partum hemorrhage prevention was similar between the two treatment strategies. Combination treatment was associated with higher rates of shivering ($n=47$ vs. 6, $p<0.001$) and fever ($n=17$ vs. 2, $p<0.001$) than carbetocin alone. Other treatment-emergent adverse effects included flushing, vomiting, nausea, hypotension and headache and they were not different between the two groups [60C].

A prospective, observational study in 74 women showed that oxytocin treatment is associated with higher levels of lactate in the amniotic fluid during active labor [61c].

A large retrospective observation study in 260 174 Japanese women showed that the use of uterotonics, including oxytocin ($n=53 925$) is not associated with increased risk of abruption placentae or eclampsia [62c].

Clinical Studies on Cardiovascular Effects

A randomized, placebo-controlled trial assessed the cardiovascular effects of oxytocin and carbetocin, administered in the context of cesarean delivery with spinal anesthesia. 76 women were randomized to oxytocin 5 U ($n=26$), carbetocin 100 mcg ($n=25$) or placebo ($n=25$). There was a transient increase in blood pressure, heart rate and cardiac output in the two treatment arms compared to placebo. Blood pressure returned to baseline within 1 hour, while heart rate and cardiac output returned to baseline measurements within 5 min [63c].

QT Prolongation

A prospective observation study assessed the effects of carbetocin on the electrocardiographic QT interval. 20 women received carbetocin 100 mg intravenous bolus during Cesarean delivery. Serial electrocardiograms were recorded; including a baseline electrocardiogram obtained 3 min after stable anesthesia had been established. QTcf (corrected QT) was prolonged from 5 to 15 min post-carbetocin, with peak prolongation at 7 min ($+18\pm4$ ms, $p=0.01$). No arrhythmias occurred and the heart rate remained stable. Carbetocin was also associated with a 19% drop in arterial blood pressure, with a maximum decrease from baseline of 23 ± 4 and 22 ± 3 mmHg for systolic and diastolic blood pressure, respectively (both $p<0.0001$), observed after 15 min [64c].

Other Clinical Studies

Uterine Tachysystole

A retrospective cohort study explored the risk factors for tachysystole (frequent uterine contractions) in term labor using a large population of 48 529 women. Oxytocin use was associated with a doubling of tachysystole risk, and a dose–response relationship was demonstrated. Tachysystoles were accompanied by fetal heart rate changes in a quarter of cases, and associated with higher neonatal morbidity [65C].

A randomized, controlled trial assessed the use of intranasal oxytocin in fibromyalgic patients. 14 female patients were randomised to 3 weeks of daily intranasal oxytocin or 3 weeks of daily intranasal placebo. No therapeutic effect was demonstrated. There was no significant difference in side effects between the two groups. The most common adverse events included headache, nausea or abdominal pain, drowsiness, unsteadiness and local irritation [66c].

Dose-Escalation Study

A prospective study aimed to estimate the dose of carbetocin required to produce effective uterine contraction in 90% of women undergoing elective Cesarean delivery (ED^{90}), administering incremental doses of intravenous carbetocin (10, 15 and 20 mcg) to a group of 40 women. The estimated ED^{90} of carbetocin was 14.8 mcg, much less than the commonly used dose of 100 mcg. Overall, hypotension ($n=15$), tachycardia ($n=12$), nausea ($n=11$) and hypertension ($n=5$) were the most commonly encountered side effects. Less commonly reported adverse events included flushing ($n=4$), vomiting ($n=3$), chest pain ($n=2$), bradycardia ($n=1$) and headache ($n=1$) [67c]. Another study by the same group randomized 120 women undergoing Cesarean section to receive 20, 40, 60, 80 or 100 mcg carbetocin ($n=24$ per group). There was no difference in effectiveness between different doses. The side effects profile was similar to the one described in the previous study, with no difference across the various dosing regimens [68c].

Literature Reviews and Meta-Analyses

A systematic review evaluated a number of uterotonics, including carbetocin and oxytocin, in regard to their efficacy and safety for post-partum haemorrhage prevention. Carbetocin has demonstrated superior efficacy to other agents. Authors underline the potential haemodynamic effects of oxytocin and carbetocin and advice against their use in patients with hypertension, pre-eclampsia, and cardiac abnormalities. Abdominal pain (40%), nausea (21–27%), flushing (26%), itching (10%), vomiting (7–9%) headache (3–14%) and tremor (11%) were listed as the most commonly reported adverse effects of intravenous carbetocin [69M].

A meta-analysis evaluated the effects of early discontinuation of oxytocin post active-phase labor on maternal and neonatal outcomes. 8 studies were identified, involving 1232 deliveries. Early discontinuation of oxytocin was associated with lower rates of Cesarean section and uterine hyperstimulation. Moreover, cases of abnormal fetal heart rates were less frequent [70M].

Two meta-analyses compared high- and low-dose oxytocin infusion regimens for labor induction. In the first one, low dose was defined as less than 100 mU oxytocin in the first 40 min, and increments delivering less than 600 mU total doses in the first 2 hours. Nine randomized and quasi-randomized trials were identified, involving 2391 women. No difference was identified in serious maternal morbidity or death, serious neonatal morbidity or perinatal death between the two regimens. Various secondary obstetric outcomes, including uterine rupture or hemorrhage, were also similar between the two groups [71M]. The second meta-analysis evaluated the efficacy of high-dose versus low-dose regimens of oxytocin for labor augmentation. High-dose oxytocin was defined as starting dose and increment of equal to or more than 4 mU per minute. Four randomized-controlled and one quasi-randomized trial were identified, including 644 women overall. High-dose oxytocin was associated with lower Cesarean section rates, higher rates of spontaneous vaginal birth and faster progress of labor, with no difference in adverse events between the two regimens [72M].

Autism Spectrum Disorders

A systematic review of oxytocin use in the management of autism spectrum disorders (7 randomized-controlled trials, $n=101$ patients) identified no effect of treatment duration or mode of administration on the occurrence of adverse events. These were generally mild and included drowsiness, anxiety/irritability, depression, headache, tingling, backache, trembling, restlessness, stomach cramps and enuresis [73M].

Case Reports

Oxytocin-Induced Hypoxia

The first case of hypoxia following oxytocin administration has been reported. A 35-year-old primigravida with a background of primary ciliary dyskinesia was admitted for elective Cesarean section. Intravenous oxytocin was commenced after delivery of the fetus and the placenta at a rate of 0.3 U/min. A minute later, a precipitous drop in oxygen saturations from 95% to 84% was noted (PaO_2 51 mmHg on arterial blood gas). She remained hypoxic despite supplemental oxygen (PaO_2 79 mmHg on 10 l/min oxygen). Oxytocin infusion was slowed down and 60 Units were infused over the first 20 hours. Oxygen saturation returned to 94% 20 hours after oxytocin initiation. Computed tomography pulmonary arteriogram excluded pulmonary embolism. She was discharged after 3 days. Pulmonary vasodilatation resulting in increased shunting towards poorly ventilated alveoli is hypothesized as a potential mechanism for this effect [74A].

Myocardial Ischemia

A case of myocardial ischemia following oxytocin was reported. A 38-year-old pregnant woman underwent cesarean section, during which she received oxytocin infusion. She immediately developed chest and bilateral shoulder pain, accompanied by ST depression on electrocardiogram and blood pressure drop. Phenylephrine intravenous bolus and continuous infusion of nicorandil and noradrenaline was administered. The episode resolved by the end of surgery [75A].

PARATHYROID HORMONE AND ANALOGUES [SEDA-34, 711; SEDA-35, 794; SEDA-36, 661]

Clinical Studies

A randomized, dose-escalation trial assessed the safety and tolerability of teriperatide in 42 healthy volunteers, who were randomized to receive a single dose of teriperatide (10, 20, 30, 40, 50, or 60 µg) or a 7-day course (10 and

20 μg once daily for 7 consecutive days). No side effects were reported with 10 and 20 μg as a single dose and 10 μg in multiple doses. Injection site infection was the most common side effect, followed by nausea and vomiting [76c].

A randomized, placebo-controlled trial evaluated the efficacy and safety of low-dose teriperatide (28.2 μg/week) in fracture risk reduction in osteoporotic patients, over a median observation period of 48 weeks ($n=158$ each treatment arm). This regimen was effective, resulting in a relative risk reduction for vertebral fractures of 66.4%. Adverse events were more common in the teriperatide group ($n=38$ vs. 5 in the placebo group, $p=0.001$). Nausea ($n=9$) and vomiting ($n=6$) were the most common side effects [77C].

A randomized study compared teriperatide, denosumab and combination thereof in 100 women at high risk of fractures. Study participants received 20 μg teriparatide daily ($n=36$), 60 mg denosumab every 6 months ($n=34$), or both ($n=30$). Combination treatment was more effective at increasing bone mineral density. Mild asymptomatic hypercalcaemia was detected in one woman in the teriparatide group, one in the denosumab group, and three in the combination treatment group [78C].

Combination Treatment with Teriperatide and Risedronate

29 adult male patients with osteoporosis (idiopathic, steroid-induced or secondary to hypogonadism) were randomised to receive oral risedronate (25 mg weekly) plus placebo injection ($n=10$), subcutaneous teriparatide (20 μg daily) plus oral placebo ($n=9$), or oral risedronate plus subcutaneous teriparatide ($n=10$). All strategies were effective at increasing bone mineral density at several points (total hip, femoral neck, lumbar spine); combination treatment was actually more effective than either monotherapy at increasing total hip bone density. Adverse events were not significantly different across the three groups. In the teriperatide-only group, these included injection site irritation ($n=2$) and leg cramps ($n=1$) [79c].

Case Reports

Calciphylaxis

A fatal case of nonuremic calciphylaxis has been reported in a teriperatide-treated patient. A 66-year-old woman with rheumatoid arthritis presented with a 3-month history of indurated leg nodules and purpura, 5 months after commencing teriperatide. Her medications included leflunomide, warfarin and prednisolone (2 mg). Biopsy of a thigh lesion was consistent with thrombotic vasculopathy. Teriperatide was stopped

and warfarin was replaced by low-molecular-weight heparin. Repeat histology was obtained in view of progressive clinical signs and revealed intramural calcium deposition in subcutaneous arterioles, consistent with calciphylaxis. Intravenous sodium thiosulphate was administered to no avail and she eventually died. A limited number of calciphylaxis cases associated with teriperatide had been previously described, but warfarin and glucocorticoids are also potential offending drugs for such events [80A].

Subungual Exostosis

Subungual exostosis in association with teriperatide treatment was reported for the first time. A 54-year-old female patient with severe osteoporosis and multiple fractures was commenced on teriperatide (20 μg subcutaneously once daily). After 16 months of treatment, she presented with a 4-month history of pain and atraumatic swelling of her right thumb. X-ray imaging indicated trabecular bony overgrowth. Surgical excision revealed endochondral bone formation with reactive atypia, confirming the diagnosis of subungual exostosis [81A].

SOMATOSTATIN (GROWTH HORMONE RELEASE-INHIBITING HORMONE) AND ANALOGUES [SED-15, 3160; SEDA-35, 794; SEDA-36, 666]

LANREOTIDE

Clinical Studies

A randomized, placebo-controlled study of lanreotide in patients with advanced neuroendocrine tumors showed longer progression-free survival with the study drug versus placebo. Half the patients in the lanreotide group had drug-emergent adverse events (versus 28% in the placebo group), predominantly diarrhea ($n=26$ vs. 9). Less frequent adverse events included hyperglycemia (5 lanreotide-treated patients vs. 0 placebo-treated patients) and cholelithiasis (10 lanreotide-treated patients vs. 3 placebo-treated patients) [82C].

The efficacy of lanreotide autogel in the treatment of polycystic liver disease was assessed by pooled analysis of data from three trials ($n=132$). Lanreotide autogel was administered at 90 mg monthly and 120 mg monthly, and a placebo arm was included. Both doses were shown to be effective in reducing liver volume, but the lower dose treatment arm experienced less side effects. In the 90 mg group, four patients (7%) developed serious adverse events (severe abdominal cramps and steatorrhea). One patient experienced severe hair loss. In the

LAN 120 mg group, eight patients (16%) developed steatorrhea [83C].

A prospective, uncontrolled, phase II trial explored the role of lanreotide in the treatment of patients with well-differentiated but progressive neuroendocrine tumors, including 30 adult patients who received lanreotide autogel 120 mg every 28 days, for a mean duration of 291 days. Treatment led to disease stabilization in most patients. 63% patients reported treatment-related adverse effects. Diarrhea (40% of patients) was the most common side effect, followed by asthenia, flatulence and injection site pain. Two severe adverse events were reported: aerophagia and acute renal failure; both resolved without any long-term clinical consequences [84c].

Literature Reviews and Meta-Analyses

A systematic review and meta-analysis of treatments for polycystic kidney disease included three trials (141 patients) using somatostatin analogues (octreotide LAR or lanreotide). Somatostatin analogues were associated with an increased risk of diarrhea (relative risk (RR) 3.09, 95% confidence interval (CI) 1.2–8.00) and other gastrointestinal symptoms (RR 3.32, 95% CI 1.57–7.04). Injection site reactions were also common (RR 11.50, 95% CI 1.57–84.05) [85M].

The risk of cholecystitis with somatostatin analogues has been evaluated in a systematic review. Two studies exploring the risks of long-term treatment with somatostatin analogues ($n=44$ and $n=144$) were identified. These reported percentages of patients developing gallstones of 52% and 63%, symptomatic gallstones 6.8% and 15% and cholecystectomy rates 18% and 15%, respectively. Average time to development of gallstones was 44–55 months [86M].

OCTREOTIDE AND OCTREOTIDE LONG-ACTING RELEASE (LAR)

Clinical Studies

A randomized, prospective phase III trial compared octreotide implant ($n=122$) to octreotide long acting release (LAR) injections ($n=41$) in adult acromegalic patients, demonstrating similar efficacy in IGF-1 control and comparable safety profiles. Local reaction to the implant was reported in 13% of patients. Diarrhea and headache were more frequently reported in the implant arm than in the injectable treatment arm (9.8% vs. 7.9% and 9.8% vs. 4.9%, respectively), whereas cholecystitis and hypertension were more frequent with octreotide LAR. 32 of 122 implants were broken at explantation, but this did not have any adverse clinical sequelae [87C].

The effects of short-term preoperative octreotide treatment for TSH-secreting pituitary adenomas were examined retrospectively in a cohort of 44 patients, 19 of whom had received octreotide as a subcutaneous injection (2–3 times per day) and 24 as a long-acting release (LAR) injection. One patient was excluded due to drug intolerance (headaches, nausea, bradycardia). A significant effect on tumor size and thyroid function was observed after a median treatment duration of 33 months. Three patients became clinically hypothyroid requiring replacement pre-operatively, while two developed transient painless thyroiditis. Other side effects included transient mild diarrhea ($n=5$), and constipation, transient nausea and mild bilirubin elevation ($n=1$ each) [88c].

A retrospective study reviewed 98 patients who had received somatostatin analogue treatment to control angiodysplasia hemorrhage (octreotide 0.1 mg three times a day for 28 days followed by 6 months of long acting release-octreotide 20 mg monthly). Mild gastrointestinal side effects were again the most common and self-resolved within a few weeks. Only one patient developed gallbladder sludge during the treatment period. One case of impaired glucose tolerance was also reported [89c].

Polycystic Kidney Disease

The effect of somatostatin analogues on kidney and cyst growth in patients with polycystic kidney disease was explored in a large randomized, placebo-controlled trial. Patients were randomized to 3-year treatment with two 20 mg intramuscular injections of octreotide long-acting release (LAR) ($n=40$) or placebo ($n=39$) every 28 days. Severe adverse events were similarly distributed between the two groups. Four cases of cholelithiasis or cholecystitis were reported in the octreotide-LAR group (none in the placebo group). Hypoglycemic episodes were noted in two participants in the octreotide LAR group; this is a side effect not previously reported with this somatostatin analogue. Uterine leiomyomas were noted in five patients in the octreotide LAR group, but drug causality is unlikely [90c].

A randomised, phase III trial examined the role of octreotide long-acting release in the prevention of chemotherapy-induced diarrhoea in colorectal cancer patients. 139 patients were randomly assigned to octreotide LAR 30 mg intramuscularly every 4 weeks, or the physician's drug of choice in the event of diarrhea (control arm). No protective effect was observed. No serious adverse events were reported [91c].

Systematic Reviews and Meta-Analyses

Alopecia

Somatostatin analogues were included in a systematic review of the risk of alopecia with endocrine treatments. The review was limited to phase II and III clinical trials. One study reporting low-grade alopecia with octreotide

LAR treatment (30 mg IM every 4 weeks) was identified (1/15 patients) [16M].

Case Reports

Head and Neck Paragangliomas

A case series of four patients with progressive head and neck paragangliomas on octreotide long-acting release (30 mg monthly intramuscularly) for 12 months reported side effects in two of them. This included debilitating vertigo in a 53-year-old patient after 4 months of treatment resulting in drug withdrawal and *de novo* cholelethiasis in a 66-year-old female [92A].

PASIREOTIDE

Clinical Studies

A randomized, open-label study examined the pharmacokinetics and safety of subcutaneous pasireotide and intramuscular pasireotide long-acting release (LAR) in healthy male volunteers ($n = 45$). Each volunteer was randomized to receive 300, 600, or 900 μg of pasireotide subcutaneously on day 1, followed by the same dose twice daily from day 15–19, and then a single intramuscular dose of 20, 40, or 60 mg of pasireotide LAR on day 33. No severe adverse events were reported. One participant discontinued treatment due to recurrent supraventricular extrasystoles after receiving a single dose of 300 μg of pasireotide subcutaneously. Another volunteer stopped his treatment because of moderate diarrhea and abdominal pain during treatment with 600 μg subcutaneously twice daily. Overall, 44 of 45 participants reported at least one adverse event, including injection site reaction, nausea or dizziness. On follow-up, gallbladder polyp was detected on ultrasound in 3 volunteers; all were small (<0.5 cm) and did not require medical intervention [93c].

Another randomized, open-label study looked into the best combination treatment options to manage pasireotide-induced hyperglycemia. 90 healthy male volunteers were randomized to receive pasireotide 600 μg subcutaneously twice daily, alone or co-administered with metformin, nateglinide or liraglutide. An oral glucose tolerance test (OGTT) was performed on days 1 and 7. Plasma glucose 2 hours post glucose administration was 99.9% and 90.2% higher than baseline in the pasireotide-only group at day 1 and day 7, respectively. This increase was ameliorated in all combination treatment arms. Vildagliptin and liraglutide were associated with the lowest plasma glucose measurements. Hypoglycemia was reported in 12 volunteers (66.7%) receiving pasireotide with nateglinide. Drug-related adverse events were most common with liraglutide and nateglinide. Diarrhea, nausea and abdominal discomfort were

the most common side effects in the pasireotide-only group. The only severe adverse event pertained to the development of jaundice in a patient in the pasireotide-plus-liraglutide group, after 1 week of treatment. Liver biopsy indicated toxic cholestasis. Treatment was stopped and liver function spontaneously returned to normal within 3 months of the first pasireotide dose [94C].

An open-label, single-arm, open-ended extension study aimed to assess the efficacy and safety of pasireotide in acromegalic patients at 6 and 9 months from treatment induction ($n = 30$). Treatment doses varied from 400 to 1800 μg daily. Most reported side effects were mild, usually involving the gastrointestinal system (diarrhoea, nausea, abdominal pain, flatulence). 12 patients experienced hyperglycemic episodes, while 5 were diagnosed with diabetes mellitus; however, 4 of these were already known with 'glucose disorders' before treatment initiation. Mean HbA1c levels increased from a mean $\pm$ SD value of $6.16 \pm 0.56\%$ at extension baseline to $6.82 \pm 1.51\%$ at 6 months and $6.32 \pm 0.68\%$ at 9 months. Two patients suffered severe drug-related adverse events (deteriorating diabetes mellitus and cholecystitis). Two patients presented new gallstones during the extension study. One patient presented a new finding of prolonged QT interval, which returned to normal at follow-up. Sinus bradycardia was reported in 9 patients [95c].

Glucose Metabolism

72.8% of patients experienced drug-related hyperglycaemia in a randomized, phase III trial of pasireotide in Cushing's patients ($n = 162$). Patients were randomised to receive either 600 or 900 μg of the study drug twice daily; at 3 months, the dose was up-titrated by 300 μg twice daily in all patients who had unsatisfactory biochemical response and treatment continued up to 12 months. Hypocortisolism-related events were reported in 13 participants (8%). Otherwise, the side effects profile was similar to previous studies, with a predominance of mild gastrointestinal symptoms [96C].

A prospective, dose-escalation study evaluated the safety and tolerability of once-daily and twice-daily pasireotide, as well as its metabolic effects on glucose regulation. Pasireotide was administered subcutaneously at 150, 300, 600, 900, 1200, or 1500 μg once daily, or 150, 300, 450, 600, or 750 μg twice daily, for 8 days ($n = 6$ patients/ dose). Treatment at all doses was well tolerated, with predominantly gastrointestinal side effects of mild-moderate severity. Pasireotide was associated with higher fasting and post-prandial plasma glucose levels in a dose-dependent pattern. Insulin concentrations were markedly lower. Glucagon was also suppressed [97C].

Pasireotide-induced hyperglycemia was also investigated in a randomized trial in 45 healthy male volunteers, who were randomized to receive pasireotide 600, 900, or 1200 μg subcutaneously twice a day for 7 days. The

1200 μg treatment arm had to discontinue treatment due to unduly high gastrointestinal intolerance rates. Glucose metabolism was investigated by means of an oral glucose tolerance test (OGTT), a hyperglycemic clamp test and a hyperinsulinemic-euglycemic clamp test. Pasireotide treatment was associated with suppression of insulin and glucagon levels, without changes in peripheral tissue sensitivity to insulin [98c].

Dumping Syndrome

The effects of pasireotide on post-operative dumping symptom were investigated in the context of a placebo-controlled, cross-over study in 9 adult patients. Participants received 2 weeks of pasireotide 300 μg subcutaneously three times per day or placebo. 2 patients stopped pasireotide treatment due to gastrointestinal intolerance (abdominal cramps, nausea and diarrhea). 6 patients developed diarrhea during pasireotide treatment (2 during placebo treatment). No biliary symptoms were reported [99c].

Dose-Limiting Nausea

A randomized, placebo-controlled trial evaluated the use of perioperative pasireotide to prevent the formation of pancreatic fistula in patients undergoing pancreatoduodenectomy or distal pancreatectomy. Patients were randomized to receive 900 μg of subcutaneous pasireotide ($n = 152$) or placebo ($n = 148$) twice daily for 7 days, starting from the morning of the operation. Pasireotide reduced the risk of post-operative pancreatic fistula formation or abscess. Adverse events were similar between treatment and placebo, with the only exception of nausea ($n = 87$ with pasireotide vs. 61 with placebo) and vomiting ($n = 43$ vs. 32). Nausea was dose-limiting in 16 patients in the pasireotide arm. Such a high incidence of severe nausea has not been reported in previous pasireotide studies but the authors note patients had no oral intake for several days post-operatively, which may have contributed to this accentuated effect [100C].

VASOPRESSIN RECEPTOR ANTAGONISTS [SEDA-34, 713; SEDA-35, 797; SEDA-36, 668]

Clinical Studies

A prospective, observational study assessed the efficacy and safety of the vasopressin type 2 receptor antagonist tolvaptan in the treatment of heart failure patients with fluid overload ($n = 1057$). Tolvaptan was used in variable doses (3.5–15 mg) and duration (1–60 days). Side effects were reported in 18.7% of patients. Thirst was reported by 10% of patients, independent of tolvaptan dose. Other adverse events included hypernatremia (3.3%), renal impairment (1.4%), hyperkalemia (0.8%)

and hyperuricemia (0.6%). Only 6 cases of deranged liver function were observed. Most major adverse events occurred in the first 3 days of treatment. One case of death as an adverse event is reported, without any elaborating details on this incident. With regard to hypernatremia, serum sodium ≥ 142.0 mEq/l, starting dosage of tolvaptan of at least 15 mg/day and serum potassium < 3.8 mEq/l were identified as independent predictors on multivariate analysis [101C].

A prospective observational study assessed the effects of low-dose tolvaptan (15 mg) on acute decompensated heart failure with hyponatremia ($n = 40$). Tolvaptan was associated with an increase in sodium concentration and symptomatic improvement. Side effects included dry mouth ($n = 16$), thirst ($n = 12$), vomiting ($n = 14$), abdominal pain ($n = 8$) and muscle cramps ($n = 6$). 4 patients developed hypernatremia and 6 suffered deterioration in their renal function, although the magnitude and clinical significance of these effects is not clarified [102c].

Literature Reviews and Meta-Analyses

A meta-analysis evaluated the use of vasopressin receptor antagonists in the treatment of heart failure, identifying 13 relevant trials (5525 participants). There was no improvement in mortality. The risk of drug-related adverse events was increased by 14% in comparison to placebo. Thirst and oral dryness were the most commonly reported side effects [103M].

The efficacy and safety of tolvaptan was reviewed in a recent article on vasopressin receptor antagonists. The authors discuss the evidence underlying the recent US Food and Drug Administration guidance that tolvaptan should not be used for longer than 30 days or in patients with underlying liver disease, in view of rare reports of liver failure. Such reports derive from polycystic kidney disease patients exposed to prolonged courses of high-dose tolvaptan, which raises questions regarding their applicability in different populations (e.g. patients with liver congestion secondary to heart failure) [104R].

VASOPRESSIN AND ANALOGUES [SEDA-33, 915; SEDA-34, 714; SEDA-35, 798; SEDA-36, 669]

DESMOPRESSIN (N-DEAMINO-8-D-ARGININE VASOPRESSIN, DDAVP) [SEDA-34, 714; SEDA-35, 798; SEDA-36, 669]

Clinical Studies on Nocturia

A randomized, controlled trial explored the benefits of add-on desmopressin in patients treated with tamsulosin for benign prostatic hyperplasia with nocturia. 248

patients were randomized to receive tamsulosin 0.4 mg and desmopressin 60 mcg, or tamsulosin 0.4 mg alone. Combination treatment was associated with fewer episodes of nocturia and better sleep quality over 3 months. No serious adverse events were reported. Only one desmopressin-treated patient developed clinical hyponatremia [105C].

A prospective, uncontrolled study explored the role of desmopressin in the treatment of nocturia and enuresis in patients undergoing radical cystectomy with orthotopic urinary diversion. 52 Patients were treated with oral desmopressin 0.1 mg at bedtime for 30 days. A positive effect was observed in approximately 50% of participants. Three patients withdrew from the study due to headaches and anxiety. No cases of hyponatremia were identified [106c].

A randomized, controlled trial assessed the efficacy and safety of low-dose desmopressin orally disintegrating tablets in men with nocturia. 385 patients were randomized to receive 50 mg of desmopressin ($n = 119$), 70 mg of desmopressin ($n = 124$), or placebo ($n = 142$). Treatment was well tolerated. 50 mg desmopressin was associated with less frequent adverse events than 70 mg. Dry mouth, headaches, constipation and hyponatremia were the most common side effects. 2 cases of Na < 130 mmol/l were reported in the 50 mg treatment arm vs. 9 cases in the 70 mg arm [107C].

Pediatric Studies

A retrospective study assessed the risk of hyponatremia in pediatric patients with bleeding disorders undergoing surgery. 107 patients with platelet function defects or von Willebrand's disease, aged 2–19 years, were included in the study. 11 patients had post-operative sodium levels $\leq$ 130 mEq/l. Significant complications included post-operative bleeding in a 6-year-old and post-DDAVP tonic-clonic seizures in a 2-year-old [108C].

Literature Reviews and Meta-Analyses

A systematic review examined the role of desmopressin and other non-surgical interventions in the treatment of menorrhagia. Two studies comparing side effects in melatonin-treated patients to placebo-treated patients found no statistically significant difference. Headaches, flushing and nausea were the most frequently reported side effects [109M].

The efficacy of desmopressin as a treatment for nocturia in adults was the subject of a systematic review, pooling data from 10 randomized, controlled trials. Desmopressin in doses of at least 25 mg appeared to afford modest benefits, with some improvement in terms of numbers of nocturnal voids and time to first void. Headaches and hyponatremia were the two most commonly reported side effects (relative risk 3.3 and 3.6,

respectively). The risk did not appear to be dose or gender dependent. One study reported the development of respiratory failure in two patients treated with desmopressin; the first patient returned to normal upon drug withdrawal, while underlying pneumonia was identified as the trigger in the second case [110M].

A systematic review reported headaches, nausea, diarrhoea, abdominal pain, dry mouth and hyponatremia as the most commonly observed adverse effects in clinical trials using desmopressin for nocturia management [111M].

A review of published reports on severe hyponatremic symptoms (epileptic seizures, altered mental state) in the context of desmopressin use for enuresis has been published, identifying 54 relevant cases (age range 2–37 years). Headache, nausea and vomiting were the most common early warning symptoms, reported in the majority of patients. In 47 out of 54 cases, desmopressin had been administered intranasally. Excessive fluid intake was present as a contributing factor in 22 patients; three of them were on treatment with oxybutynin which can cause mucosal dryness. Intranasally treated patients had lower blood sodium than their orally treated counterparts, of similar demographics and morbidity, by 8 mmol/l ($p < 0.02$). One fatal case of head injury caused by hyponatremic seizures after desmopressin and alcohol consumption was reported; other than this, no long-term adverse effects were identified [112M].

A systematic review evaluated the use of desmopressin in the management of nocturia. Seven clinical trials and two review articles were identified. Desmopressin seemed to be associated with short-term improvement, but no studies explored long-term treatment effects. Mild hyponatremia and fluid retention were the main side effects (46)M [113M].

Case Reports

ST-Elevation Myocardial Infarction

The first case of ST-elevation myocardial infarction following desmopressin administration has been described. A 67-year-old male patient with a drug-eluting stent in his proximal left anterior descending artery was treated with intravenous desmopressin for traumatic subgaleal hematoma. 5 hours later he developed chest pain with 2 mm ST elevation in the anterior leads. Urgent cardiac catheterization revealed total occlusion of the proximal left anterior descending stent. A new stent was inserted successfully, but the patient had to be intubated in view of hypoxia during the procedure. He recovered after a prolonged intensive care stay [114A].

Diabetes Insipidus Post-Vasopressin

Transient diabetes insipidus post-vasopressin cessation was reported in a 3-year-old girl undergoing surgery for transposition of the great vessels. She was started on an intravenous vasopressin infusion at a rate 0.0003 units/kg/min due to hemodynamic instability. On post-operative day 4, vasopressin was tapered off. Over the next 7 hours, she became polyuric (1300 ml output over 7 hours) and her sodium increased suddenly from 130 to 142 mmol/l. Vasopressin infusion was restarted at a lower dose, resulting in a prompt reduction of her urine output. She was successfully weaned off vasopressin over 24 hours maintaining a normal urine output. A similar case of post-vasopressin diabetes insipidus had been previously described in a septic patient [115A].

TERLIPRESSIN [SEDA-34, 714; SEDA-35, 798; SEDA-36, 669]

Clinical Studies

A randomized trial compared terlipressin and adrenaline in the treatment of type 2 hepatorenal syndrome. 46 patients were randomized to receive terlipressin (0.5 mg intravenously three times a day) or adrenaline for up to 15 days. In the terlipressin-treated group, 2 patients suffered abdominal pain, one developed cyanosis of the toe and another patient developed transient ventricular extrasystoles. All adverse events were self-limiting. Both treatments were effective at improving renal function [116A].

A randomized trial compared high-dose to low-dose terlipressin in the treatment of type I hepatorenal syndrome. 56 cirrhotic patients with type I HRS were randomly assigned to terlipressin 1 mg every 6–8 hours ($n = 27$) or terlipressin 1 mg every 12 hours ($n = 29$). No difference in efficiency or adverse events was observed between the 2 groups [117c].

Case Reports

Prolonged QT

A 47-year-old alcoholic female patient was admitted with jaundice. Two days later, she developed upper gastrointestinal bleeding and was commenced on terlipressin. 24 hours after terlipressin initiation, she developed torsades-de-pointes, escalating to cardiac arrest. She reverted to sinus rhythm with DC shock. Post-cardioversion, she had a prolonged QT interval of 542 mm (normal baseline electrocardiograph on admission). Serum biochemistry revealed mild hypokalemia (3.3 mmol/l) and hypomagnesemia (0.58 mmol/l), which would not be expected to account for this rhythm disturbance. This was the third case report of ventricular arrhythmias associated with terlipressin use [118A].

Ischemic Bowel Necrosis

Ischemic bowel necrosis was reported in a 46-year-old cirrhotic male patient who was commenced on terlipressin 1 mg four times daily. After 2 doses, he developed abdominal pain. Terlipressin was stopped and urgent bowel resection was performed; however, the patient died after developing profound hypotension and metabolic acidosis. Three cases of terlipressin-induced bowel ischemia have been reported previously, but this was the first that occurred after only two doses and did not reverse upon drug discontinuation [119A].

Severe Hyponatremia

Two cases of severe terlipressin-induced hyponatremia have been described. A 39-year-old female patient with a background of pancreatic neuroendocrine tumor with liver metastases complicated by portal hypertension and esophageal varices presented with hematemesis. She was commenced on terlipressin 1 mg four times a day. After 6 mg total injected dose, she developed delirium. Serum biochemistry revealed acute severe hyponatremia (Na 116 mmol/l, baseline 136 mmol/l). Her serum osmolality was low, with an inappropriately high urine Na and osmolality. Terlipressin was stopped and urgent treatment with hypertonic saline was administered. Her Na increased to 130 mmol/l after 12 hours and she gradually returned to her baseline cognitive state. The second case pertained to a 7-year-old male patient presenting with hematemesis from esophageal varices. He was commenced on terlipressin 1 mg four times daily. Two days later, he developed tonic-clonic seizures; serum biochemistry revealed profound hyponatremia (110 mmol/l, baseline 142 mmol/l). Intravenous saline for 2 days failed to improve his sodium sufficiently. Terlipressin was withdrawn and his sodium returned to normal within the next 4 days. Hyponatremia is a known side effect of terlipressin, due to the drug's slow metabolism to vasopressin in the liver. Vasopressin activates the arginine-vasopressin type 2 receptor in the kidneys, promoting water retention [120A,121A].

Ischemic skin necrosis

Extensive skin necrosis was reported during intravenous infusion of terlipressin (1 mg every 4 hours) in a 65-year-old man with variceal esophageal hemorrhage, affecting his arm and hand. Erythema developed from day 2 of terlipressin use and deteriorated despite treatment cessation, requiring skin grafting. 20 other similar cases have been previously reported in the literature [122A].

VASOPRESSIN [SEDA-34, 715; SEDA-35, 798; SEDA-36, 669]

Clinical Studies on Cardiovascular Effects

A randomized, controlled trial showed that vasopressin can increase the blood pressure in patients being operated in the beach chair position, reducing the procedural risk of hypotension. 30 patients undergoing arthroscopic shoulder surgery were randomized to receive intravenous AVP 0.07 U/kg or placebo. Despite its positive effects on blood pressure, vasopressin was associated with regional cerebral desaturation [123c].

A randomized, controlled trial compared vasopressin to catecholamines for cerebral perfusion pressure maintenance in the context of severe brain injury ($n = 30$). The incidence of side effects was similar between the two groups [124c].

Other Clinical Studies

Hyponatremia in Infants

A retrospective study ($n = 13$) explored the ability of vasopressin to stabilize infants with systemic hypotension secondary to congenital diaphragmatic hernia (CDH). Vasopressin increased mean arterial pressure and decreased the pulmonary/systemic pressure ratio; however, prolonged treatment for over 24 hours was invariably associated with hyponatremia [125c].

References

[1] Sun LM, Lin MC, Muo CH, et al. Calcitonin nasal spray and increased cancer risk: a population-based nested case-control study. J Clin Endocrinol Metab. 2014;99(11):4259–64 [C].

[2] Overman RA, Borse M, Gourlay ML. Salmon calcitonin use and associated cancer risk. Ann Pharmacother. 2013;47(12):1675–84 [M].

[3] Shore ND, Sieber P, Schimke L, et al. Comparison of tolerability and adverse events following treatment with two GnRH agonists in patients with advanced prostate cancer. Urol Nurs. 2013;33(5):236–44. 48 [c].

[4] Lee SH, Lee HM, Kim SW, et al. Is high-dose leuprorelin acetate effective and safe in Asian men with prostate cancer? An open-label, non-comparative, multi-center clinical trial. Yonsei Med J. 2014;55(2):310–5 [c].

[5] Gandaglia G, Sun M, Hu JC, et al. Gonadotropin-releasing hormone agonists and acute kidney injury in patients with prostate cancer. Eur Urol. 2014;66(6):1125–32 [C].

[6] Taplin ME, Montgomery B, Logothetis CJ, et al. Intense androgen-deprivation therapy with abiraterone acetate plus leuprolide acetate in patients with localized high-risk prostate cancer: results of a randomized phase II neoadjuvant study. J Clin Oncol. 2014;32(33):3705–15 [c].

[7] Jespersen CG, Norgaard M, Borre M. Androgen-deprivation therapy in treatment of prostate cancer and risk of myocardial infarction and stroke: a nationwide Danish population-based cohort study. Eur Urol. 2014;65(4):704–9 [C].

[8] Koo KC, Shim GS, Park HH, et al. Treatment outcomes of chemical castration on Korean sex offenders. J Forensic Legal Med. 2013;20(6):563–6 [c].

[9] Song JH, Lu H, Zhang J, et al. Clinical study on the effectiveness and safety of combined laparoscopy and gonadotropin-releasing hormone agonist in the treatment of endometriosis. Zhonghua Fu Chan Ke Za Zhi. 2013;48(8):584–8 [c].

[10] Hammar O, Roth B, Bengtsson M, et al. Autoantibodies and gastrointestinal symptoms in infertile women in relation to in vitro fertilization. BMC Pregnancy Childbirth. 2013;13:201 [c].

[11] Lee JW, Kim HJ, Choe YM, et al. Significant adverse reactions to long-acting gonadotropin-releasing hormone agonists for the treatment of central precocious puberty and early onset puberty. Ann Pediatr Endocrinol Metab. 2014;19(3):135–40 [C].

[12] Lee PA, Klein K, Mauras N, et al. 36-Month treatment experience of two doses of leuprolide acetate 3-month depot for children with central precocious puberty. J Clin Endocrinol Metab. 2014;99(9):3153–9 [C].

[13] Davis JS, Alkhoury F, Burnweit C. Surgical and anesthetic considerations in histrelin capsule implantation for the treatment of precocious puberty. J Pediatr Surg. 2014;49(5):807–10 [c].

[14] Mamidala MP, Polinedi A, Kumar PT, et al. Maternal hormonal interventions as a risk factor for Autism Spectrum Disorder: an epidemiological assessment from India. J Biosci. 2013;38(5):887–92 [C].

[15] Kamath MS, Kalampokas EE, Kalampokas TE. Use of GnRH analogues pre-operatively for hysteroscopic resection of submucous fibroids: a systematic review and meta-analysis. Eur J Obstet Gynecol Reprod Biol. 2014;177:11–8 [M].

[16] Saggar V, Wu S, Dickler MN, et al. Alopecia with endocrine therapies in patients with cancer. Oncologist. 2013;18(10):1126–34 [M].

[17] Walker LM, Tran S, Robinson JW. Luteinizing hormone-releasing hormone agonists: a quick reference for prevalence rates of potential adverse effects. Clin Genitourin Cancer. 2013;11(4):375–84 [M].

[18] Calcaterra V, Mannarino S, Corana G, et al. Hypertension during therapy with triptorelin in a girl with precocious puberty. Indian J Pediatr. 2013;80(10):884–5 [A].

[19] Huang TY, Lin JP, Lieu AS, et al. Pituitary apoplexy induced by gonadotropin-releasing hormone agonists for treating prostate cancer-report of first Asian case. World J Surg Oncol. 2013;11:254 [A].

[20] Burris K, Ding CY, Lim GF. Leuprolide acetate-induced generalized papular eruption. J Drugs Dermatol. 2014;13(6):755–7 [A].

[21] Tashiro K, Kimura S, Naruoka T, et al. Giant subcutaneous hematoma with hemorrhagic shock induced by goserelin acetate injection for prostate cancer: report of a case. Hinyokika Kiyo. 2014;60(9):455–8 [A].

[22] Fatemi HM, Popovic-Todorovic B, Humaidan P, et al. Severe ovarian hyperstimulation syndrome after gonadotropin-releasing hormone (GnRH) agonist trigger and "freeze-all" approach in GnRH antagonist protocol. Fertil Steril. 2014;101(4):1008–11 [A].

[23] Patterson BC, Chen Y, Sklar CA, et al. Growth hormone exposure as a risk factor for the development of subsequent neoplasms of the central nervous system: a report from the childhood cancer survivor study. J Clin Endocrinol Metab. 2014;99(6):2030–7 [C].

[24] Tritos NA, Johannsson G, Korbonits M, et al. Effects of long-term growth hormone replacement in adults with growth hormone deficiency following cure of acromegaly: a KIMS analysis. J Clin Endocrinol Metab. 2014;99(6):2018–29 [C].

[25] Linglart A, Tauber M, Bougneres P, et al. Growth hormone treatment for childhood short stature and risk of stroke in early adulthood. Neurology. 2015;84(10):1062–3 [C].

[26] Rasmussen MH, Olsen MW, Alifrangis L, et al. A reversible albumin-binding growth hormone derivative is well tolerated and possesses a potential once-weekly treatment profile. J Clin Endocrinol Metab. 2014;99(10):E1819–29 [c].

[27] Biller BM, Ji HJ, Ahn H, et al. 12-month effects of once-weekly sustained-release growth hormone treatment in adults with GH deficiency. Pituitary. 2013;16(3):311–8 [c].

[28] Kirschner J, Schorling D, Hauschke D, et al. Somatropin treatment of spinal muscular atrophy: a placebo-controlled, double-blind crossover pilot study. Neuromuscul Disord. 2014;24(2):134–42.

[29] Kappelgaard AM, Kiyomi F, Horikawa R, et al. The impact of long-term growth hormone treatment on metabolic parameters in

Japanese patients with short stature born small for gestational age. Horm Res Paediatr. 2014;81(4):272–9 [C].

[30] Ciresi A, Morreale R, Radellini S, et al. Corneal thickness in children with growth hormone deficiency: the effect of GH treatment. Growth Horm IGF Res. 2014;24(4):150–4.

[31] Kim HS, Yang SW, Yoo HW, et al. Efficacy of short-term growth hormone treatment in prepubertal children with idiopathic short stature. Yonsei Med J. 2014;55(1):53–60 [c].

[32] Khadilkar V, Radjuk KA, Bolshova E, et al. 24-Month use of once-weekly GH, LB03002, in prepubertal children with GH deficiency. J Clin Endocrinol Metab. 2014;99(1):126–32 [C].

[33] Mostoufi-Moab S, Isaacoff EJ, Spiegel D, et al. Childhood cancer survivors exposed to total body irradiation are at significant risk for slipped capital femoral epiphysis during recombinant growth hormone therapy. Pediatr Blood Cancer. 2013;60(11): 1766–71 [c].

[34] Simon D, Alberti C, Alison M, et al. Effects of recombinant human growth hormone for 1 year on body composition and muscle strength in children on long-term steroid therapy: randomized controlled, delayed-start study. J Clin Endocrinol Metab. 2013;98(7):2746–54 [c].

[35] Loche S, Carta L, Ibba A, et al. Growth hormone treatment in non-growth hormone-deficient children. Ann Pediatr Endocrinol Metab. 2014;19(1):1–7 [R].

[36] van Bunderen CC, van Varsseveld NC, Erfurth EM, et al. Efficacy and safety of growth hormone treatment in adults with growth hormone deficiency: a systematic review of studies on morbidity. Clin Endocrinol. 2014;81(1):1–14 [R].

[37] Appelman-Dijkstra NM, Claessen KM, Roelfsema F, et al. Long-term effects of recombinant human GH replacement in adults with GH deficiency: a systematic review. Eur J Endocrinol. 2013;169(1):R1–R14 [M].

[38] Breederveld RS, Tuinebreijer WE. Recombinant human growth hormone for treating burns and donor sites. Cochrane Database Syst Rev. 2014;9:CD008990 [M].

[39] Naftel RP, Tubbs RS, Menendez JY, et al. Progression of Chiari I malformations while on growth hormone replacement: a report of two cases. Childs Nerv Syst. 2013;29(12):2291–4 [A].

[40] Uihlein LC, Garzon MC, Goodwin G, et al. Growth hormone replacement in patients with PHACE association and hypopituitarism. Pediatr Dermatol. 2014;31(3):337–40 [A].

[41] Neggers SJ, Franck SE, de Rooij FW, et al. Long-term efficacy and safety of pegvisomant in combination with long-acting somatostatin analogs in acromegaly. J Clin Endocrinol Metab. 2014;99(10):3644–52 [C].

[42] Jen J, LaBadie RR, Liang Y, et al. Pegvisomant bioavailability of single 30 mg/mL subcutaneous injection compared to two 15 mg/mL subcutaneous injections: a pharmacokinetic, safety and tolerability study. Growth Hormon IGF Res. 2013;23(4):114–9 [c].

[43] Jacob JJ, Bevan JS. Type 1 drug hypersensitivity following first dose of pegvisomant. Clin Endocrinol. 2014;80(2):315 [A].

[44] Galley HF, Lowes DA, Allen L, et al. Melatonin as a potential therapy for sepsis: a phase I dose escalation study and an ex vivo whole blood model under conditions of sepsis. J Pineal Res. 2014;56(4):427–38 [c].

[45] Wade AG, Farmer M, Harari G, et al. Add-on prolonged-release melatonin for cognitive function and sleep in mild to moderate Alzheimer's disease: a 6-month, randomized, placebo-controlled, multicenter trial. Clin Interv Aging. 2014;9:947–61 [C].

[46] Hansen MV, Andersen LT, Madsen MT, et al. Effect of melatonin on depressive symptoms and anxiety in patients undergoing breast cancer surgery: a randomized, double-blind, placebo-controlled trial. Breast Cancer Res Treat. 2014;145(3):683–95 [c].

[47] Pokharel K, Tripathi M, Gupta PK, et al. Premedication with oral alprazolam and melatonin combination: a comparison with either

alone—a randomized controlled factorial trial. Biomed Res Int. 2014;2014:356964 [C].

[48] Khezri MB, Oladi MR, Atlasbaf A. Effect of melatonin and gabapentin on anxiety and pain associated with retrobulbar eye block for cataract surgery: a randomized double-blind study. Indian J Pharmacol. 2013;45(6):581–6 [c].

[49] Fallah R, Shoroki FF, Ferdosian F. Safety and efficacy of melatonin in pediatric migraine prophylaxis. Curr Drug Saf. 2015;10(2):132–5 [c].

[50] Mostafavi A, Solhi M, Mohammadi MR, et al. Melatonin decreases olanzapine induced metabolic side-effects in adolescents with bipolar disorder: a randomized double-blind placebo-controlled trial. Acta Med Iran. 2014;52(10):734–9 [c].

[51] Bruni O, Alonso-Alconada D, Besag F, et al. Current role of melatonin in pediatric neurology: clinical recommendations. Eur J Paediatr Neurol. 2015;19(2):122–33 [M].

[52] Friedman JI, Soleimani L, McGonigle DP, et al. Pharmacological treatments of non-substance-withdrawal delirium: a systematic review of prospective trials. Am J Psychiatry. 2014;171(2):151–9 [M].

[53] Whitehouse AJ. Complementary and alternative medicine for autism spectrum disorders: rationale, safety and efficacy. J Paediatr Child Health. 2013;49(9):E438–42. quiz E442 [M].

[54] McCleery J, Cohen DA, Sharpley AL. Pharmacotherapies for sleep disturbances in Alzheimer's disease. Cochrane Database Syst Rev. 2014;3:CD009178 [M].

[55] Singer C, Tractenberg RE, Kaye J, et al. A multicenter, placebo-controlled trial of melatonin for sleep disturbance in Alzheimer's disease. Sleep. 2003;26(7):893–901 [M].

[56] Kuriyama A, Honda M, Hayashino Y. Ramelteon for the treatment of insomnia in adults: a systematic review and meta-analysis. Sleep Med. 2014;15(4):385–92 [M].

[57] Mukta M, Sahay PB. Role of misoprostol 600 mcg oral in active management of third stage of labor: a comparative study with oxytocin 10 IU i.m. J Obstet Gynaecol India. 2013;63(5):325–7 [C].

[58] Chaudhuri P, Mandi S, Mazumdar A. Rectally administered misoprostol as an alternative to intravenous oxytocin infusion for preventing post-partum hemorrhage after cesarean delivery. J Obstet Gynaecol Res. 2014;40(9):2023–30 [C].

[59] Tewatia R, Rani S, Srivastav U, et al. Sublingual misoprostol versus intravenous oxytocin in prevention of post-partum hemorrhage. Arch Gynecol Obstet. 2014;289(4):739–42 [c].

[60] Elgafor el Sharkwy IA. Carbetocin versus sublingual misoprostol plus oxytocin infusion for prevention of postpartum hemorrhage at cesarean section in patients with risk factors: a randomized, open trail study. Arch Gynecol Obstet. 2013;288(6):1231–6 [C].

[61] Wiberg-Itzel E, Pembe AB, Wray S, et al. Level of lactate in amniotic fluid and its relation to the use of oxytocin and adverse neonatal outcome. Acta Obstet Gynecol Scand. 2014;93(1):80–5 [c].

[62] Morikawa M, Cho K, Yamada T, et al. Do uterotonic drugs increase risk of abruptio placentae and eclampsia? Arch Gynecol Obstet. 2014;289(5):987–91 [c].

[63] Rosseland LA, Hauge TH, Grindheim G, et al. Changes in blood pressure and cardiac output during cesarean delivery: the effects of oxytocin and carbetocin compared with placebo. Anesthesiology. 2013;119(3):541–51 [c].

[64] Bruyere M, Ait Hamou N, Benhamou D, et al. QT interval prolongation following carbetocin in prevention of post-cesarean delivery hemorrhage. Int J Obstet Anesth. 2014;23(1):88–9 [c].

[65] Heuser CC, Knight S, Esplin MS, et al. Tachysystole in term labor: incidence, risk factors, outcomes, and effect on fetal heart tracings. Am J Obstet Gynecol. 2013;209(1). 32 e1–6 [C].

[66] Mameli S, Pisanu GM, Sardo S, et al. Oxytocin nasal spray in fibromyalgic patients. Rheumatol Int. 2014;34(8):1047–52 [c].

[67] Khan M, Balki M, Ahmed I, et al. Carbetocin at elective Cesarean delivery: a sequential allocation trial to determine the minimum effective dose. Can J Anaesth. 2014;61(3):242–8 [c].

[68] Anandakrishnan S, Balki M, Farine D, et al. Carbetocin at elective Cesarean delivery: a randomized controlled trial to determine the effective dose, part 2. Can J Anaesth. 2013;60(11):1054–60 [c].

[69] Gizzo S, Patrelli TS, Gangi SD, et al. Which uterotonic is better to prevent the postpartum hemorrhage? Latest news in terms of clinical efficacy, side effects, and contraindications: a systematic review. Reprod Sci. 2013;20(9):1011–9 [M].

[70] Vlachos DE, Pergialiotis V, Papantoniou N, et al. Oxytocin discontinuation after the active phase of labor is established. J Matern Fetal Neonatal Med. 2014;18:1–7 [M].

[71] Budden A, Chen LJ, Henry A. High-dose versus low-dose oxytocin infusion regimens for induction of labour at term. Cochrane Database Syst Rev. 2014;10:CD009701 [M].

[72] Kenyon S, Tokumasu H, Dowswell T, et al. High-dose versus low-dose oxytocin for augmentation of delayed labour. Cochrane Database Syst Rev. 2013;7:CD007201 [M].

[73] Preti A, Melis M, Siddi S, et al. Oxytocin and autism: a systematic review of randomized controlled trials. J Child Adolesc Psychopharmacol. 2014;24(2):54–68 [M].

[74] Nandhakumar A, Silverman GL. Acute hypoxemia in a parturient with primary ciliary dyskinesia following the administration of intravenous oxytocin: a case report. Can J Anaesth. 2013;60(12):1218–21 [A].

[75] Minowa Y, Hara K, Sata T. A case of myocardial ischemia inducedby oxytocin during cesarean section. Masui. 2013;62(8): 982–4 [A].

[76] Liu Y, Yang C, Li Z, et al. Safety, tolerability, pharmacokinetics, and pharmacodynamics of recombinant human parathyroid hormone (1-34) in healthy Chinese subjects. Clin Ther. 2014;36(6):940–52 [c].

[77] Fujita T, Fukunaga M, Itabashi A, et al. Once-weekly injection of low-dose teriparatide (28.2 mug) reduced the risk of vertebral fracture in patients with primary osteoporosis. Calcif Tissue Int. 2014;94(2):170–5 [C].

[78] Tsai JN, Uihlein AV, Lee H, et al. Teriparatide and denosumab, alone or combined, in women with postmenopausal osteoporosis: the DATA study randomised trial. Lancet. 2013;382(9886): 50–6 [C].

[79] Walker MD, Cusano NE, Sliney Jr J, et al. Combination therapy with risedronate and teriparatide in male osteoporosis. Endocrine. 2013;44(1):237–46 [c].

[80] Dominguez AR, Goldman SE. Nonuremic calciphylaxis in a patient with rheumatoid arthritis and osteoporosis treated with teriparatide. J Am Acad Dermatol. 2014;70(2):e41–2 [A].

[81] Delivanis DA, Bhargava A, Luthra P. Subungual exostosis in an osteoporotic patient treated with teriparatide. Endocr Pract. 2013;19(5):e115–7 [A].

[82] Caplin ME, Pavel M, Ruszniewski P. Lanreotide in metastatic enteropancreatic neuroendocrine tumors. N Engl J Med. 2014;371(16):1556–7 [C].

[83] Temmerman F, Gevers T, Ho TA, et al. Safety and efficacy of different lanreotide doses in the treatment of polycystic liver disease: pooled analysis of individual patient data. Aliment Pharmacol Ther. 2013;38(4):397–406 [C].

[84] Martin-Richard M, Massuti B, Pineda E, et al. Antiproliferative effects of lanreotide autogel in patients with progressive, well-differentiated neuroendocrine tumours: a Spanish, multicentre, open-label, single arm phase II study. BMC Cancer. 2013;13:427 [c].

[85] Myint TM, Rangan GK, Webster AC. Treatments to slow progression of autosomal dominant polycystic kidney disease: systematic review and meta-analysis of randomized trials. Nephrology. 2014;19(4):217–26 [M].

[86] Jayakrishnan TT, Groeschl RT, George B, et al. Review of the impact of antineoplastic therapies on the risk for cholelithiasis and acute cholecystitis. Ann Surg Oncol. 2014;21(1):240–7 [M].

[87] Chieffo C, Cook D, Xiang Q, et al. Efficacy and safety of an octreotide implant in the treatment of patients with acromegaly. J Clin Endocrinol Metab. 2013;98(10):4047–54 [C].

[88] Fukuhara N, Horiguchi K, Nishioka H, et al. Short-term preoperative octreotide treatment for TSH-secreting pituitary adenoma. Endocr J. 2015;62(1):21–7 [c].

[89] Nardone G, Compare D, Scarpignato C, et al. Long acting release-octreotide as "rescue" therapy to control angiodysplasia bleeding: a retrospective study of 98 cases. Dig Liver Dis. 2014;46(8):688–94 [c].

[90] Caroli A, Perico N, Perna A, et al. Effect of long acting somatostatin analogue on kidney and cyst growth in autosomal dominant polycystic kidney disease (ALADIN): a randomised, placebo-controlled, multicentre trial. Lancet. 2013;382(9903):1485–95 [c].

[91] Hoff PM, Saragiotto DF, Barrios CH, et al. Randomized phase III trial exploring the use of long-acting release octreotide in the prevention of chemotherapy-induced diarrhea in patients with colorectal cancer: the LARCID trial. J Clin Oncol. 2014;32(10):1006–11 [c].

[92] van Hulsteijn LT, van Duinen N, Verbist BM, et al. Effects of octreotide therapy in progressive head and neck paragangliomas: case series. Head Neck. 2013;35(12):E391–6 [A].

[93] Chen X, Shen G, Jiang J, et al. Pharmacokinetics and safety of subcutaneous pasireotide and intramuscular pasireotide long-acting release in Chinese male healthy volunteers: a phase I, single-center, open-label, randomized study. Clin Ther. 2014;36(8):1196–210 [c].

[94] Breitschaft A, Hu K, Hermosillo Resendiz K, et al. Management of hyperglycemia associated with pasireotide (SOM230): healthy volunteer study. Diabetes Res Clin Pract. 2014;103(3):458–65 [C].

[95] Petersenn S, Farrall AJ, De Block C, et al. Long-term efficacy and safety of subcutaneous pasireotide in acromegaly: results from an open-ended, multicenter, Phase II extension study. Pituitary. 2014;17(2):132–40 [c].

[96] Pivonello R, Petersenn S, Newell-Price J, et al. Pasireotide treatment significantly improves clinical signs and symptoms in patients with Cushing's disease: results from a Phase III study. Clin Endocrinol. 2014;81(3):408–17 [C].

[97] Shenouda M, Maldonado M, Wang Y, et al. An open-label dose-escalation study of once-daily and twice-daily pasireotide in healthy volunteers: safety, tolerability, and effects on glucose, insulin, and glucagon levels. Am J Ther. 2014;21(3):164–73 [C].

[98] Henry RR, Ciaraldi TP, Armstrong D, et al. Hyperglycemia associated with pasireotide: results from a mechanistic study in healthy volunteers. J Clin Endocrinol Metab. 2013;98(8):3446–53 [c].

[99] Deloose E, Bisschops R, Holvoet L, et al. A pilot study of the effects of the somatostatin analog pasireotide in postoperative dumping syndrome. Neurogastroenterol Motil. 2014;26(6):803–9 [c].

[100] Allen PJ. Pasireotide for postoperative pancreatic fistula. N Engl J Med. 2014;371(9):875–6 [C].

[101] Kinugawa K, Sato N, Inomata T, et al. Efficacy and safety of tolvaptan in heart failure patients with volume overload. Circ J. 2014;78(4):844–52 [C].

[102] Patra S, Kumar B, Harlalka KK, et al. Short term efficacy and safety of low dose tolvaptan in patients with acute decompensated heart failure with hyponatremia: a prospective observational pilot study from a single center in South India. Heart Views. 2014;15(1):1–5 [c].

[103] Nistor I, Bararu I, Apavaloaie MC, et al. Vasopressin receptor antagonists for the treatment of heart failure: a systematic review and meta-analysis of randomized controlled trials. Int Urol Nephrol. 2015;47(2):335–44 [M].

[104] Kalra A, Maharaj V, Goldsmith SR. Vasopressin receptor antagonists: from pivotal trials to current practice. Curr Heart Fail Rep. 2014;11(1):10–8 [R].

[105] Ahmed AF, Maarouf A, Shalaby E, et al. The impact of adding low-dose oral desmopressin therapy to tamsulosin therapy for treatment of nocturia owing to benign prostatic hyperplasia. World J Urol. 2015;33(5):649–57 [C].

[106] Goldberg H, Baniel J, Mano R, et al. Low-dose oral desmopressin for treatment of nocturia and nocturnal enuresis in patients after radical cystectomy and orthotopic urinary diversion. BJU Int. 2014;114(5):727–32 [c].

[107] Weiss JP, Herschorn S, Albei CD, et al. Efficacy and safety of low dose desmopressin orally disintegrating tablet in men with nocturia: results of a multicenter, randomized, double-blind, placebo controlled, parallel group study. J Urol. 2013;190(3):965–72 [C].

[108] Sharma R, Stein D. Hyponatremia after desmopressin (DDAVP) use in pediatric patients with bleeding disorders undergoing surgeries. J Pediatr Hematol Oncol. 2014;36(6):e371–5 [C].

[109] Ray S, Ray A. Non-surgical interventions for treating heavy menstrual bleeding (menorrhagia) in women with bleeding disorders. Cochrane Database Syst Rev. 2014;11: CD010338 [M].

[110] Ebell MH, Radke T, Gardner J. A systematic review of the efficacy and safety of desmopressin for nocturia in adults. J Urol. 2014;192(3):829–35 [M].

[111] Zachoval R, Krhut J, Sottner O, et al. Nocturnal polyuria, treatment with desmopressin. Ceska Gynekol. 2013;78(4):385–9 [M].

[112] Lucchini B, Simonetti GD, Ceschi A, et al. Severe signs of hyponatremia secondary to desmopressin treatment for enuresis: a systematic review. J Pediatr Urol. 2013;9(6 Pt B):1049–53 [M].

[113] Cetinel B, Tarcan T, Demirkesen O, et al. Management of lower urinary tract dysfunction in multiple sclerosis: a systematic review and Turkish consensus report. Neurourol Urodyn. 2013;32(8):1047–57 [M].

[114] Shah SN, Tran HA, Assal A, et al. In-stent thrombosis following DDAVP administration: case report and review of the literature. Blood Coagul Fibrinolysis. 2014;25(1):81–3 [A].

[115] Bhaskar P, John J, Bin Sallehuddin A. Polyuria after cessation of vasopressin in a child after cardiac surgery. J Cardiothorac Vasc Anesth. 2014;28(3):e24–5 [A].

[116] Ghosh S, Choudhary NS, Sharma AK, et al. Noradrenaline vs terlipressin in the treatment of type 2 hepatorenal syndrome: a randomized pilot study. Liver Int. 2013;33(8): 1187–93 [A].

[117] Wan S, Wan X, Zhu Q, et al. A comparative study of high-or low-dose terlipressin therapy in patients with cirrhosis and type 1 hepatorenal syndrome. Zhonghua Gan Zang Bing Za Zhi. 2014;22(5):349–53 [c].

[118] Sidhu SK, Das D. Terlipressin-induced QT prolongation. Intern Med J. 2013;43(9):1050–1 [A].

[119] Kim HR, Lee YS, Yim HJ, et al. Severe ischemic bowel necrosis caused by terlipressin during treatment of hepatorenal syndrome. Clin Mol Hepatol. 2013;19(4):417–20 [A].

[120] Wang YK, Hwang DY, Wang SS, et al. Terlipressin-induced hyponatremic encephalopathy in a noncirrhotic patient. Kaohsiung J Med Sci. 2013;29(12):691–4 [A].

[121] Zaki SA. Terlipressin-induced hyponatremic seizure in a child. Indian J Pharmacol. 2013;45(4):403–4 [A].

[122] Ozel Coskun BD, Karaman A, Gorkem H, et al. Terlipressin-induced ischemic skin necrosis: a rare association. Am J Case Rep. 2014;15:476–9 [A].

[123] Cho SY, Kim SJ, Jeong CW, et al. Under general anesthesia arginine vasopressin prevents hypotension but impairs cerebral oxygenation during arthroscopic shoulder surgery in the beach chair position. Anesth Analg. 2013;117(6):1436–43 [c].

[124] Van Haren RM, Thorson CM, Ogilvie MP, et al. Vasopressin for cerebral perfusion pressure management in patients with severe traumatic brain injury: preliminary results of a randomized controlled trial. J Trauma Acute Care Surg. 2013;75(6):1024–30 discussion 30 [c].

[125] Acker SN, Kinsella JP, Abman SH, et al. Vasopressin improves hemodynamic status in infants with congenital diaphragmatic hernia. J Pediatr. 2014;165(1). 53–8.e1 [c].

43

Drugs that Affect Lipid Metabolism

Robert D. Beckett*,1, *Andrea L. Wilhite*†

*Drug Information Center, Manchester University College of Pharmacy, Fort Wayne, IN, USA
†Manchester University College of Pharmacy, Fort Wayne, IN, USA
1Corresponding author: rdbeckett@manchester.edu

Bile Acid Sequestrants [SED-15, 1902; SEDA-36, 676]

Bile acid sequestrants are ion exchange polymers that bind to bile acids in the gastrointestinal tract, leading to decreased low density lipoprotein (LDL), cholesterol and total cholesterol. As a class, bile acid sequestrants are not substantially absorbed through the gastrointestinal tract. Common adverse drug effects include constipation, dyspepsia, and nausea; however, more serious events such as abdominal distention, dysphagia, fecal impaction, gastrointestinal obstruction, and pancreatitis have been reported.

Cholestyramine

No relevant publications from the review period were identified.

Colesevelam

A systematic review assessing colesevelam for treatment of heterozygous familial hypercholesterolemia identified two relevant studies through a search with Clinicaltrials.gov, PubMed, and Google Scholar [1M]. Unsurprisingly, most common colesevelam-related adverse effects were gastrointestinal events; however, unlike previous reports, there was similar risk for constipation relative to placebo (9% versus 5%) in adult patients and risk was minimal in pediatric (less than 2% of patients) population. The overall rate of adverse effects was low and rarely led to study discontinuation.

A randomized, double-blind, placebo-controlled trial assigned 140 patients with dyslipidemia and elevated fasting glucose to receive colesevelam 3750 mg orally once daily or placebo for 14–18 weeks [2c]. Each patient also received niacin 500 mg orally daily titrated to 2000 mg orally daily and aspirin 325 mg orally daily. The study

found minimal safety impact from addition of colesevelam. One serious adverse effect, a case of atrial fibrillation that ultimately resolved, occurred and was determined not to be treatment-related. Fourteen adverse drug effects led to early termination of therapy for 13 subjects (9%); of these, only five were considered to be totally or partially due to colesevelam. Of all adverse effects occurring in the combination therapy group, 40% were considered to be related to colesevelam (i.e., not niacin) while in the placebo group, 36% were similarly considered to be unrelated to niacin. The study provided limited information regarding specific adverse effects experienced by patients.

A retrospective, observational, cross-sectional study assessed 1239 patients who received colesevelam over a 7-year study period in order to assess clinical outcomes in patients with hypercholesterolemia, diabetes mellitus, or both [3c]. Unfortunately, adverse effects data were not gathered as part of this study.

Bile acid sequestrants, including colesevelam, are known to decrease systemic absorption of many medications. A report of three pharmacokinetic studies assessing impact of colesevelam on absorption of glimepiride, glipizide extended release (ER), and olmesartan found that area under the curve (AUC) was reduced by 19%, 13%, and 37%, respectively, during coadministration with colesevelam ($p < 0.05$ for each) [4c]. Results were not statistically significant when colesevelam administration was separated by 4 hours, with the exception of olmesartan (15% reduction, $p < 0.05$). The study was conducted in healthy patients; no adverse events occurred, but coadministration of colesevelam with each drug could result in decreased treatment effectiveness.

Colestipol

No relevant publications from the review period were identified.

© 2015 Elsevier B.V. All rights reserved.

Cholesteryl Ester Transfer Protein Inhibitors [SEDA-32, 723; SEDA-35, 810; SEDA-36, 677]

The only cholesteryl ester transfer protein inhibitor currently approved in the United States is ezetimibe. Ezetimibe decreases gastrointestinal absorption of cholesterol and other phytosterols, leading to decreases in LDL and total cholesterol, with minor increases in high density lipoprotein cholesterol (HDL). Ezetimibe is generally well tolerated with few patients experiencing adverse drug effects at greater rates than patients treated with placebo. Musculoskeletal effects, including myalgia and increased creatine kinase, have been reported but are more common in combination with other agents.

Ezetimibe

Results from recent studies of ezetimibe underscore previous studies, finding the drug to be well tolerated. A prospective, observational study assessed safety of ezetimibe 10 mg orally daily in combination with bezafibrate 400 mg orally daily in 659 Japanese patients [5c]. Incidence of adverse drug reaction was 6.2% of patients (95% confidence interval [CI] 4.6–8.4%) at 12 months. The most common adverse drug reactions were increased blood creatine phosphokinase (threshold not defined; 1.5%), myalgia (0.8%), gallstones (0.6%), and increased blood creatinine (threshold not defined; 0.6%). Aggregate changes in laboratory parameters (e.g., serum creatinine, liver injury tests, creatine phosphokinase) were not clinically significant.

In a randomized, open-label trial of patients with chronic kidney disease, 286 patients with LDL cholesterol greater than 120 mg/dL despite statin therapy received add-on ezetimibe 10 mg orally daily or statin titration (defined as doubling the dose) [6c]. Safety results underscored previous data: among patients with stage 3 to 5 chronic kidney disease, 38% in the statin titration group experienced muscle-related adverse effects compared to 10% of patients in the combination group. In this subgroup, 12% of patients in the statin titration group experienced liver-related toxicity compared to 3% of patients in the combination group. No patients developed a creatine kinase level greater than 5-times upper limit of normal.

A retrospective, observational study assessed the safety of ezetimibe in cardiac patients receiving calcineurin inhibitors [7c]. For 71 patients (61% receiving cyclosporine and 35% receiving tacrolimus), no difference was observed in terms of drug concentration (mean 101 ng/mL at baseline vs. 106 ng/mL at follow up; mean 9.1 ng/mL at baseline vs. 7.0 ng/mL at follow up) or calcineurin inhibitor dosing (mean 206 mg per day at baseline vs. 213 mg per day at follow up; mean 4.0 mg per day at baseline vs. 3.8 mg per day at follow up) for cyclosporine or tacrolimus, respectively. The most common adverse events were myalgia (5.6%), abdominal pain (2.8%), diarrhea (2.8%), and liver transaminases greater than 3-times upper limit of normal (2.8%).

A single-arm study placed 15 human immunodeficiency virus (HIV)-infected adults with stable, ritonavir-boosted antiretroviral therapy and LDL between 130 and 190 mg/dL on ezetimibe 10 mg orally for 8 weeks [8c]. No differences in CD-4 count, hematological parameters, plasma HIV-1 RNA, or routine biochemistry, were observed from baseline to end of study.

Nicotinic Acid Derivatives [SED-15, 2512; SEDA-34, 728; SEDA-35, 815; SEDA-36, 679]

Niacin (nicotinic acid) is a B-complex vitamin metabolized to coenzymes necessary for lipid metabolism; it is not precisely clear how niacin reduces LDL. Niacin is also known to reduce total cholesterol and triglycerides, and to increase HDL. The most common adverse drug effect associated with niacin is peripheral vasodilation that can manifest as flushing, pruritus, warmth, tingling, and orthostatic events. Incidence of this effect is substantially reduced in sustained release or controlled release formulations, but these formulations have been associated with hepatotoxicity. Laropiprant is a prostaglandin antagonist used in combination with niacin to reduce vasodilation. Niacin has also been associated with gastrointestinal adverse effects including abdominal pain, diarrhea, dyspepsia, nausea, and vomiting. A meta-analysis of five prospective, randomized, controlled trials of adults on hemodialysis or peritoneal dialysis who received niacin or placebo was conducted [9M]. The study underscored previous information, finding increased risk for flushing with niacin compared to placebo (relative risk [RR] 33; 95% CI 4.7–231) and increased risk for thrombocytopenia with niacinamide compared to placebo (RR 2.82; 95% CI 1.14–6.94).

A double-blind, clinical trial randomized 25 673 patients age 50–80 years with history of cardiovascular disease or diabetes mellitus to treatment with niacin/laropiprant 2 g/40 mg total daily dose or placebo for a mean duration of 3.9 years [10C]. Rates of death (6.2% vs. 5.7%, $p = 0.08$) and cancer diagnosis (4.8% vs. 4.7%, $p = 0.67$) were similar between niacin/laropiprant and placebo; however, incidence of serious adverse events was higher with niacin/laropiprant (55.6% vs. 52.7%, $p < 0.001$). Serious adverse events more common with niacin–laropiprant included infections (8.0% vs. 6.6%, $p < 0.001$), gastrointestinal events (including bleeding and peptic ulceration; 4.8% vs. 3.8%, $p < 0.001$), musculoskeletal events (including myopathy; 3.7% vs. 3.0%, $p < 0.001$), and bleeding events (2.5% vs. 1.9%, $p < 0.001$).

Additionally, new-onset diabetes (5.7% vs. 4.3%, $p < 0.001$) and serious disruptions in diabetes control (11.1% vs. 7.5%, $p < 0.001$) were more common with niacin/laropiprant.

A randomized, controlled trial compared extended release niacin 1500–2000 mg per day to placebo, containing 50 mg niacin to maintain blinding [11C]. Mean treatment duration was 36 months. All patients were at least 45 years of age with established cardiovascular disease and low HDL (less than 40 mg/dL for men and less than 50 mg/dL for women) and receiving concomitant simvastatin. A final analysis found increased risk for ischemic stroke (1.86% vs. 1.06%, hazard ratio [HR] 1.78; 95% CI 1.00–3.17) and a composite of ischemic and hemorrhagic stroke (2.10% vs. 1.24%; HR 1.73; 95% CI 1.01–2.96) with niacin compared to placebo. In a multivariate analysis, niacin was not associated with increased risk for ischemic stroke (HR 1.74; 95% CI 0.97–3.11), but age of at least 65 years (HR 3.58; 95% CI 1.82–7.05) and history of stroke, transient ischemic attack, or carotid disease (HR 2.18; 95% CI 1.82–7.05) were statistically significant.

A randomized, double-blind clinical trial enrolled patients age ranged 18–80 years with mixed hyperlipidemia (LDL 130–190 mg/dL and triglycerides 150–500 mg/dL) not at LDL goal [12c]. Patients were randomized to the following treatment groups: extended release niacin/laropiprant 2 g/40 mg plus simvastatin 20 mg orally daily, extended release niacin/laropiprant 2 g/40 mg plus simvastatin 40 mg orally daily, atorvastatin 10 mg orally daily, atorvastatin 20 mg orally daily, atorvastatin 40 mg orally daily, or atorvastatin 80 mg orally daily. In a pooled analysis comparing niacin/laropiprant groups to atorvastatin groups, incidence of clinical adverse experiences (59.6% vs. 45.9%) and treatment-related clinical adverse experiences (40.7% vs. 15.8%) was higher with niacin/laropiprant. Differences were primarily due to flushing (21.7% vs. 3.0%) and pruritus (6.0% vs. 0.6%) symptoms. There was no difference in terms of serious adverse events.

Psychiatric

A 52-year-old man with no psychiatric history, previously on niacin 500 mg orally daily, was increased to 1000 mg orally daily despite previous complain of hot flashes [13A]. Within 1 week, the patient experienced a manic-like psychotic episode consisting of elevated mood, labile affect, psychomotor agitation, flight of ideas, delusions of grandeur, and delusions of thought broadcasting. He was acutely treated with haloperidol 10 mg intramuscular and diazepam 10 mg intramuscular, and subsequently discharged on risperidone 1 mg orally daily and ordered not to take niacin. The patient subsequently self-discontinued risperidone with no further psychiatric symptoms.

Skin

A study of 201 Chinese patients with dyslipidemia taking extended release niacin/laropiprant 1000 mg/20 mg orally daily for 12 weeks identified 28 (14%) who experienced pruritic cutaneous eruption within a median of 4 or 5 days after increasing the dose to 2000 mg/40 mg or starting treatment, respectively [14A]. Patients who experienced the rash were older (mean 61 vs. 56 years, $p = 0.011$), had lower body mass index (mean 25 vs. 27.5 kg/m², $p = 0.002$), were more likely to be on other lipid-lowering therapy (82% vs. 61%, $p = 0.032$), and had lower baseline LDL (mean 102 mg/dL vs. 124 mg/dL). The addition of laropiprant, a genetic factor specific to the southern Chinese population, and a pharmacokinetic effect related to lower BMI were proposed as possible reasons for this new adverse effect.

A descriptive, cross-sectional study of 306 patients newly prescribed extended release niacin conducted routine assessments of flushing severity and impact on patient satisfaction [15c]. Following 1 week of treatment, 16%, 12%, and 3% of patients reported moderate, severe, and extreme flushing, respectively. Flushing was associated with substantial increases in irritation and frustration with decreases in patient satisfaction. Forty-four percent of patients discontinued treatment by the end of the 13-month study. Of these patients, 55% discontinued due to flushing symptoms. While risk for flushing with niacin is well described in the literature, this study provides additional information describing impact on patient treatment outcomes specifically with extended release niacin.

Fibric Acid Derivatives [SED-15, 1358; SEDA-32, 804; SEDA-333, 922; SEDA-34, 724; SEDA-35, 812]

Fibrates primarily exert their effects through the lowering of triglycerides. These medications are generally considered first line agents in patients with elevated triglycerides. Literature has not shown cardiovascular reduction benefits with the use of fibrates; however, these agents are often used in patients who are at risk for pancreatitis due to high triglyceride levels. Common adverse effects of this class include gastrointestinal disturbances, elevated liver enzymes, and myalgias and myopathy. In particular, gemfibrozil should not be used in combination with statins due to a drug interaction leading to an increased risk of myalgia, myopathy and rhabdomyolysis.

Gemfibrozil

No relevant publications from the review period were identified.

Fenofibrate

URINARY TRACT

A case report of a 53-year-old man diagnosed with familial juvenile hyperuricemic nephropathy and chronic renal disease was initiated on fenofibrate 160 mg orally daily [16c]. His baseline labs included creatinine 3.2 mg/dL, LDL 99 mg/dL (controlled with atorvastatin 40 mg orally daily), and triglycerides (TG) 275 mg/dL. One month after initiating fenofibrate, his serum creatinine increased to 4.2 mg/dL. The patient did not have any symptoms associated with rhabdomyolysis. Fenofibrate was discontinued and 3 months later serum creatinine decreased to baseline levels of 3.2 mg/dL, suggesting fenofibrate administration may be associated with further renal function impairment without a cause of rhabdomyolysis.

HMG-CoA Reductase Inhibitors [SED-15, 1632; SEDA-32, 807; SEDA-33, 924; SEDA-34, 725; SEDA-35, 812]

HMG-CoA reductase inhibitors, also known as "statins," are a widely used class of medications used to treat dyslipidemia and reduce cardiovascular risk. These agents have been well studied and are considered first line therapy in patients at risk for cardiovascular disease. It has been widely documented and seen in clinical practice that all statins pose a risk for myopathy, myalgia and very rarely, rhabdomyolysis. Other adverse effects have caused more controversy in the literature and are described below.

Cataracts

The relationship between statins and cataracts remains controversial in the current literature. Randomized clinical trials have not identified an association between statins and cataracts, while observational studies have had variable results regarding statin use and association with cataracts, including association, no association, protective effects, or variable effects depending on age and duration of statin use [17c,18c,19c,20c,21M]. Current studies have many confounding factors impacting the interpretation of the data to date.

A retrospective cohort study evaluated the association between statin use and risk of cataract surgery in 50165 elderly, Chinese patients; of these, 17670 required surgical intervention for cataracts over the 11-year study period review [18c]. The adjusted hazard ratio for cataract surgery was 1.20 (95% CI 1.14–1.27, $p < 0.001$) in statin users compared with control group suggesting an increased risk of cataract surgery in those using statins. A nested case–control study done in two different populations assessed the regular use of any statin on the risk of cataract and need for surgical intervention

[19c]. Statin use was associated with a greater risk for cataract formation and surgery (adjusted RR, 1.27; 95% CI 1.24–1.30). In a retrospective, propensity score-matched cohort analysis, risk for development of cataracts among 13,626 statin users and 32,623 non-statin users were evaluated [20c]. Statin use was found to be associated with a higher risk for cataract (OR 1.09; 95% CI 1.02–1.17). Further, the group was evaluated to determine if duration of statin use impacted risk of cataract. It was found that cumulative simvastatin years were related to increased risk (OR 1.001; $p < 0.001$). A meta-analysis evaluated studies related to cataract formation and the use of statins and found a decrease in cataracts with statins (OR 0.81; 95% CI 0.71–0.93, $p = 0.0022$), suggesting a protective effect against cataracts of statins [21M].

Diabetes

Previous observational studies and meta-analyses have suggested that statins are associated with an increased risk of developing diabetes mellitus. These studies also have suggested that more potent statins, particularly simvastatin and atorvastatin, have a slight increase in diabetes compared to pravastatin. Evidence has not demonstrated a clear, causal relationship between statins and diabetes, and benefits of statins should also be considered when making clinical decisions regarding treatment in patients [22c,23M,24c,25C,26c,27c,28c].

A population-based retrospective cohort study examined the risk of new-onset diabetes mellitus (NODM) among patients treated with different statins [27c]. Over the 14-year study period, 471,250 patients were identified for evaluation. Various statins were used among the study population, with atorvastatin accounting for the majority (56.9%). The crude event rate for incident diabetes was highest for atorvastatin (30.7 outcomes per 1000 person years) and rosuvastatin (34.21 outcomes per 1000 person years) compared with pravastatin (22.64 outcomes per 1000 person years). Simvastatin, fluvastatin, and lovastatin had crude events similar to pravastatin. Atorvastatin (HR 1.22; 95% CI 1.15–1.29), rosuvastatin (HR 1.18; 95% CI 1.10–1.26) and simvastatin (HR 1.10; 95% CI 1.04–1.17) showed increased rates of a diabetes diagnosis compared to pravastatin, the reference drug used in all analyses. This demonstrates that higher potency statins may have a higher risk of causing new-onset diabetes compared to lower potency statins.

A retrospective analysis assessed the risk of NODM compared to the reduction of cardiovascular events and death after statin therapy in 9055 pre-diabetic patients, 3288 of whom were receiving statins [28c]. Statin therapy was associated with an increased occurrence of NODM (HR 1.20; 95% CI 1.08–1.32) and a reduction in cardiovascular events and death (HR 0.70; 95% CI 0.61–0.80) compared with nonusers. This study suggests that while there may be an increased risk of NODM in patients treated with statins, benefits of cardiovascular events and reduction in death should be considered when determining treatment of statins in patients.

Pancreatitis

Original observational studies and case reports previously provided evidence that statins may cause pancreatitis [29c,30c,31c]. Further studies have not established a causal relationship between statins and pancreatitis; with some evidence pointing towards protective effects and others suggesting causation of pancreatitis [32M,33c,34c]. The evidence remains controversial. The evidence to date does not demonstrate a clear association with pancreatitis.

A retrospective cohort study assessed effects of simvastatin in relationship to risk of new onset, acute pancreatitis over a 7-year study period [35c]. Among 707 236 patients receiving simvastatin, risk of acute pancreatitis was significantly reduced compared to the reference population (crude incidence rate ratio 0.63; 95% CI 0.59–0.67, $p < 0.0001$).

In a case report, a 58-year-old male had a TG level of 317 mg/dL, no history of alcohol use, and was taking valproic acid, omeprazole, and simvastatin for 10 years [36c]. Venlafaxine had been initiated 6 weeks prior to hospital admission. The patient had a computed tomography (CT) scan of the abdomen confirming pancreatitis. Venlafaxine and simvastatin are both metabolized extensively by CYP3A4, suggesting the drug interaction as a possible cause of the acute pancreatitis episode. Simvastatin was discontinued, prompt resolution of the episode was noted, and lab values returned to normal. This case report affirms that drug interactions should be taken into account with statins. Patients should be monitored closely for potential toxicities of statins when used in combination with other drugs that alter pharmacokinetic properties.

Exercise

Myopathy and myalgias are well documented in the literature and are clinically common with the use of statins. Evidence suggests that exercise may exacerbate these statin-related side effects [37c,38c,39c,40c].

In a randomized, controlled trial, patients were assigned to a 12-week aerobic exercise training program ($n = 21$) or to an exercise program in combination with simvastatin 40 mg by mouth daily ($n = 20$). The study showed that simvastatin attenuated increases in cardiorespiratory fitness in response to the exercise training program ($p < 0.005$). Simvastatin also prevented exercise training induced increases in skeletal muscle citrate synthase activity, a marker of mitochondrial content ($p < 0.05$) [41c].

Cancer

The literature remains inconclusive on cancer risks associated with the use of statins. There are ongoing studies regarding the impact of statin use on various cancers such as gastric, breast, colon, pancreatic, lung and liver [42S]. Studies to date have found conflicting evidence.

An inception cohort study used populated-based Danish registries to evaluate the use of statins on survival in patients with glioblastoma multiforme (GBM) [43c]. A total of 113 statin-exposed patients were included in the study and matched to 226 patients who had not used statins prior to diagnosis of GBM. Use of a statin prior to GBM diagnosis did not significantly demonstrate reduced all-cause death (HR 0.79; 95% CI 0.63–1.00) compared to non-statin use. Longer duration of statin use (at least 5 years) also showed no significance in reducing all-cause death (HR 0.75; 95% CI 0.47–1.20).

A cross-sectional study evaluated the association between statin use and abnormal prostate-specific antigen (PSA) levels [44c]. The study found that statin use is associated with a reduction in the probability that an older male will have an abnormal PSA value. It is important to recognize that PSA is often elevated in males without prostate cancer and while statins may lower this value, this finding cannot be correlated to reduced cancer risks.

A meta-analysis evaluating statin effect on gastric cancer incidence suggested that statins have favorable results in this specific cancer. It was found that statins were inversely related to risk of gastric cancer (RR 0.56; 95% CI 0.35–0.90) [45M].

Psychiatric

Previously, there were observational studies suggesting a potential risk of statin use and depression. Many other studies have shown improvements in depression when lipid levels are high and treated with statins. Recently, three additional studies have been published that associate statins with a reduction in risk of depression [46c,47c,48c]. One study demonstrated patients with untreated high cholesterol levels have more depression than those appropriately treated with a statin [48c]. These results in conjunction with other previous studies, confirm that no causal relationship has been established between depression and statin use.

References

[1] Davidson M. The efficacy of colesevelam HCl in the treatment of heterozygous familial hypercholesterolemia in pediatric and adult patients. Clin Ther. 2013;35(8):1247–52 [M].

[2] Davidson MH, Rooney M, Pollock E, et al. Effect of colesevelam and niacin on low-density lipoprotein cholesterol and glycemic control in subjects with dyslipidemia and impaired fasting glucose. J Clin Lipidol. 2013;7(5):423–32 [c].

[3] Romanelli RJ, Leahy A, Jukes T, et al. Colesevelam in the treatment of hypercholesterolemia and hyperglycemia: a retrospective analysis from an ambulatory care medical network. Curr Med Res Opin. 2013;29(12):1747–56 [c].

[4] He L, Wickremasingha P, Lee J, et al. The effects of colesevelam HCl on the single-dose pharmacokinetics of glimepiride, extended-release glipizide, and olmesartan medoxomil. J Clin Pharmacol. 2013;54(1):61–9 [c].

[5] Teramoto T, Abe K, Taneyama T. Safety and efficacy of long-term combination therapy with bezafibrate and ezetimibe in patients with dyslipidemia in the prospective, observational J-COMPATIBLE study. Cardiovasc Diabetol. 2012;12:163 [c].

[6] Suzuki H, Watanabe Y, Kumagai H, et al. Comparative efficacy and adverse effects of the addition of ezetimibe to statin versus statin titration in chronic kidney disease patients. Ther Adv Cardiovasc Dis. 2013;7(6):306–15 [c].

[7] Makkar KM, Sanoski CA, Goldberg LR, et al. An observational study of ezetimibe in cardiac transplant recipients receiving calcineurin inhibitors. Ann Pharmacother. 2013;47(11):1457–62 [c].

[8] Leyes P, Martinez E, Larrousse M, et al. Effects of ezetimibe on cholesterol metabolism in HIV-infected patients with protease inhibitor-associated dyslipidemia: a single-arm intervention trial. BMC Infect Dis. 2014;14:497 [c].

[9] He Y-M, Feng L, Huo D-M, et al. Benefits and harm of niacin and its analog for renal dialysis patients: a systematic review and meta-analysis. Int Urol Nephrol. 2014;46:433–42 [M].

[10] Landray MJ, Haynes R, Hopewell JC, et al. Effects of extended-release niacin with laropiprant in high-risk patients. N Engl J Med. 2014;371(3):203–12 [C].

[11] Teo KK, Goldstein LB, Chaitman BR, et al. Extended-release niacin therapy and risk of ischemic stroke in patients with cardiovascular disease. Stroke. 2013;44:2688–93 [C].

[12] Chen F, Maccubbin D, Yan L, et al. Lipid-altering efficacy and safety profile of co-administered extended release niacin/laropiprant and simvastatin versus atorvastatin in patients with mixed hyperlipidemia. Int J Cardiol. 2013;167:225–31 [c].

[13] Loebl T, Raskin S. A novel case report: acute manic psychotic episode after treatment with niacin. J Neuropsychiatry Clin Neurosci. 2013;25(4):E14 [A].

[14] Yang Y-L, Hu M, Chang M, et al. A high incidence of exanthematous eruption associated with niacin/laropiprant combination in Hong Kong Chinese patients. J Clin Pharm Ther. 2013;38:528–32 [A].

[15] Rhodes T, Norquist JM, Sisk CM, et al. The association of flushing bother, impact, treatment satisfaction and discontinuation of niacin therapy. Int J Clin Pract. 2013;67(12):1238–46 [c].

[16] Salguerio G, Beltran LM, Torres RJ, et al. Fenofibrate increase serum creatinine in a patient with familial nephropathy associated to hyperuricemia. Nucleosides Nucleotides Nucleic Acids. 2014;33(4–6):181–4 [c].

[17] Fong DS, Poon KT. Recent statin use and cataract surgery. Am J Ophthalmol. 2012;153:222–8 [c].

[18] Lai CL, Shau WY, Chang CH, et al. Statin use and cataract surgery: a nationwide retrospective cohort study in elderly ethnic Chinese patients. Drug Saf. 2013;36:1017–24 [c].

[19] Wise SJ, Nathoo NA, Etminan M, et al. Statin use and risk for cataract: a nested case–control study of 2 populations in Canada and the United States. Can J Cardiol. 2014;30(12):1613–9 [c].

[20] Leuschen J, Mortensen EM, Frei CR, et al. Association of statin use with cataracts: a propensity score-matched analysis. JAMA Ophthalmol. 2013;131(11):1427–34 [c].

[21] Kostis JB, Dobrzynski JM. Prevention of cataracts by statins: a meta-analysis. J Cardiovasc Pharmacol Ther. 2014;19(2):191–200 [M].

[22] Freeman DJ, Norrie J, Sattar N, et al. Pravastatin and the development of diabetes mellitus: evidence for a protective treatment effect in the West of Scotland Coronary Prevention Study. Circulation. 2001;103:357–62 [c].

[23] Preiss D, Seshasai SR, Welsh P, et al. Risk of incident diabetes with intensive-dose compared with moderate-dose statin therapy: a meta-analysis. JAMA. 2011;305:2556–64 [M].

[24] Culver AL, Ockene IS, Balasubramanian R, et al. Statin use and risk of diabetes mellitus in postmenopausal women in the women's health initiative. Arch Intern Med. 2012;172:144–52 [c].

[25] Ridker PM, Pradhan A, MacFadyen JG, et al. Cardiovascular benefits and diabetes risks of statin therapy in primary prevention: an analysis from the JUPITER trial. Lancet. 2012;380:565–71 [C].

[26] Axsom K, Berger JS. Statins and diabetes: the good, the bad, and the unknown. Curr Atheroscler Rep. 2013;15:1–7 [c].

[27] Carter AA, Gomes T, Camacho X, et al. Risk of incident diabetes among patients treated with statins: population based study. BMJ. 2013;365:1–11 [c].

[28] Wang KL, Liu CJ, Chao TF, et al. Risk of new-onset diabetes mellitus versus reduction in cardiovascular events with statin therapy. Am J Cardiol. 2014;113:631–6 [c].

[29] Anagnostopoulos GK, Tsiakos S, Margantinis G, et al. Acute pancreatitis due to pravastatin therapy. JOP. 2003;4:129–32 [c].

[30] McDonald KB, Garber BG, Perreault MM. Pancreatitis associated with simvastatin plus fenofibrate. Ann Pharmacother. 2002;36:275–9 [c].

[31] Tysk C, Al-Eryani AY, Shawabkeh AA. Acute pancreatitis induced by fluvastatin therapy. J Clin Gastroenterol. 2002;35:406–8 [c].

[32] Preiss D, Tikkanen MJ, Welsh P, et al. Lipid-modifying therapies and risk of pancreatitis: a meta-analysis. JAMA. 2012;308:804–11 [M].

[33] Gornik I, Gasparovic V, Gubarev V, et al. Prior statin therapy is associated with milder course and better outcome in acute pancreatitis—a cohort study. Pancreatology. 2013;13:196–200 [c].

[34] Pulkkinen J, Kastarinen H, Kiviniemi V, et al. Statin use in patients with acute pancreatitis and symptomatic gallstone disease. Pancreas. 2014;43(4):638–41 [c].

[35] Bechien WU, Pandol SJ, Liu AI. Simvastatin in associated with reduced risk of acute pancreatitis: findings from a regional integrated healthcare system. Gut. 2015;64:133–8 [c].

[36] Etienne D, Reda Y. Statins and their role in acute pancreatitis: case report and literature review. World J Gastrointest Pharmacol Ther. 2014;5(3):191–5 [c].

[37] Semple SJ. Statin therapy, myopathy and exercise—a case report. Lipids Health Dis. 2012;11:40 [c].

[38] Farmer JA. The effect of statins on skeletal muscle function: the STOMP trial. Curr Atheroscler Rep. 2013;15:347 [c].

[39] Murlasits Z, Radak Z. The effects of statin medications on aerobic exercise capacity and training adaptations. Sports Med. 2014;44(11):1519–30 [c].

[40] Mikus CR, Boyle LJ, Borengasser SJ, et al. Simvastatin impairs exercise training adaptations. J Am Coll Cardiol. 2013;62(8):709–14 [c].

[41] Panayiotou G, Paschalis V, Nikolaidis MG, et al. No adverse effects of statins on muscle function and health-related parameters in the elderly: an exercise study. Scand J Med Sci Sports. 2013;23(5):556–67 [c].

[42] U.S. National Institutes of Health. Clinical trials, www.clinicaltrials.gov [S].

[43] Gaist D, Hallas J, Friis S, et al. Statin use and survival following glioblastoma multiforme. Cancer Epidemiol. 2014;38(6):722–7 [c].

[44] Shi Y, Fung KZ, Feedland SJ, et al. Statin medications are associated with a lower probability of having an abnormal screening prostate-specific antigen result. Urology. 2014;84(5):1058–65 [c].

[45] Ma Z, Wang W, Jin G, et al. Effect of statins on gastric cancer incidence: a meta-analysis of case control studies. J Cancer Res Ther. 2014;10(4):859–65 [M].

[46] Redlich C, Berk M, Williams LJ, et al. Statin use and risk of depression: a Swedish national cohort study. BMC Psychiatry. 2014;14:348–56 [c].

[47] Haghighi M, Khodakarami S, Jahangard L, et al. In a randomized, double-blind clinical trial, adjuvant atorvastatin improved symptoms of depression and blood lipid values in patients suffering from severe major depressive disorder. J Psychiatr Res. 2014;58:109–14 [c].

[48] Chuang C, Tse-Yen Y, Chih-Hsin M, et al. Hyperlipidemia, statin use and the risk of developing depression: a nationwide retrospective cohort study. Gen Hosp Psychiatry. 2014;36(5):497–501 [c].

44

Cytostatic Agents

Sipan Keshishyan*, Vikas Sehdev†, David Reeves‡, Sidhartha D. Ray*,1

*Department of Pharmaceutical Sciences, Manchester University College of Pharmacy, Fort Wayne, IN, USA
†Division of Pharmaceutical Sciences, Arnold & Marie Schwartz College of Pharmacy and Health Sciences, Long Island University, Brooklyn, NY, USA
‡Department of Pharmacy Practice, College of Pharmacy and Health Sciences, Butler University, Indianapolis, IN, USA
1Corresponding author: sdray@manchester.edu

INTRODUCTION

The class of antimetabolite chemotherapeutic agents can be broken down into the pyrimidine analogues, purine analogues, and the antifolate analogues. Given the size of this class of medications and the diversity in their actions and tolerability, this chapter will focus on adverse effects of the pyrimidine analogues. Though there are overlapping toxicities among the agents, each one has a unique toxicity profile. Recent additions to our understanding of these toxicity profiles are summarized in this chapter.

PYRIMIDINE ANALOGUES

Pyrimidine analogues are a sub-class of the anti-cancer antimetabolite agents. They possess potent activity against various malignancies (both solid tumors and hematologic malignancies, depending on the agent) and have been widely studied and utilized in cancer treatment protocols. Adverse effects are common in this class of medications and largely depend on the drug dose and schedule utilized.

AZACITIDINE (5-AZACITIDINE)

Azacitidine is frequently used for the treatment of myelodysplastic syndrome (MDS), chronic myelomonocytic leukemia (CMML), and acute myeloid leukemia (AML) [1]. It is an antimetabolite and a demethylating agent that exhibits anticancer activity by interfering with DNA, RNA, and protein synthesis and also by restoring expression of tumor suppressor genes via inhibition of DNA methylation in malignant cells.

The recommended therapeutic dose of azacitidine for treatment of various hematologic abnormalities is 75 mg/m^2 via subcutaneous or i.v. route daily for 7 days every 28 days [1]. Azacitidine is an effective anticancer agent but causes considerable adverse effects even when administered at recommended doses. Hematologic toxicities are the most common adverse events associated with azacitidine treatment and tend to be the most severe. Non-hematologic toxicities such as cardiovascular, fatigue, gastrointestinal, pain, and injection site reactions tend to be less severe in nature.

Cardiovascular

The multicenter Austrian Azacitidine Registry gathered clinical data on 302 AML patients and 48 CMML patients treated with recommended doses of azacitidine. The study reported development of cardiovascular abnormalities in 33 AML patients and 10 CMML patients. Severe grade 3–4 cardiovascular events were observed in 29/33 AML patients and 8/10 CMML patients [2c,3c]. Cardiac events included left ventricular output failure (AML: 23 events; CMML: 12 events in 6 patients), arrhythmia (AML: 7 events; CMML: 12 events), cardiac ischemia (CMML: 3 events), myocardial infarction (AML: 3 events), hypertension (AML: 5 events), angina pectoris (AML: 1 event), valvular insufficiency (CMML: 1 event), and sudden cardiac death (CMML: 1event) [2c,3c]. However, out of the group of patients experiencing a cardiovascular event, 61% of those with AML and 70% of those with CMML had a preexisting cardiovascular condition and worsening was not attributed to azacitidine therapy.

© 2015 Elsevier B.V. All rights reserved.

In addition, a rare case of acute myocarditis was reported in a 50-year-old patient who was diagnosed with and treated for MDS (refractory anemia with excess blasts or RAEB II) [4A]. The patient received azacitidine ($75 \, mg/m^2$ for 7 days every 28 days) along with ondansetron (8 mg b.i.d) to suppress emesis. The patient reported localized chest pains during the 2nd day of the second cycle and 4th day of the third cycle with azacitidine and ondansetron combination. Abnormal ECG profile and elevated levels of troponin were observed during both instances. Cardiac magnetic resonance imaging (MRI) was completed to confirm myocarditis. Moreover, serologic testing ruled out myocarditis due to viral infection and coronary catheterization ruled out ondansetron induced coronary vasoconstriction. Based on the work up, the patient was determined to have a rare case of azacitidine induced myocarditis.

Infection

In a retrospective clinical study, 300 MDS patients, receiving either azacitidine (203 patients) or decitabine (97 patients) as first line therapy, were analyzed and compared for therapy associated adverse effects [5c]. The patients received subcutaneous treatment with azacitidine at the recommended dose of $75 \, mg/m^2$ for 7 consecutive days at 4-week intervals. The rate of infectious episodes requiring IV antimicrobial agents was 11.8 per 100 cycles of azacitidine. In another study, 130 patients older than 50 years of age with relapsed or refractory AML were analyzed for adverse effects caused by azacitidine therapy [6c]. Documented infections or febrile neutropenia were reported in 74 patients during the first 4 cycles of the treatment and 53 out of the aforementioned 74 patients suffered a severe infectious episode resulting in hospitalization.

As highlighted above, like most cytotoxic agents, azacitidine treatment is associated with myelosuppression which increases the risk of infection and is often managed via dose reduction. The dose dependent nature of myelosuppression was demonstrated in a retrospective clinical study of 173 patients diagnosed with high risk MDS or AML, where it was observed that patients who received azacitidine doses of $75 \, mg/m^2$ for 7 days reported more than twice (34% patients) the number of infectious episodes than patients who received $75 \, mg/m^2$ for 5 days only (14.9% patients) [7c]. Bacteria were identified as the major causative pathogens as they were detected in 25 cases. Viral or fungal infections of the upper respiratory tract were also identified in 2 cases each.

In addition to the study above, others have described fungal and viral infections during azacitidine treatment. In the Austrian report of 48 CMML patients described earlier, the majority of infectious events were pulmonary infections, herpes simplex virus (HSV) and cytomegalovirus (CMV) reactivation [3c]. In the Austrian study of 302

AML patients described earlier, 22% of those requiring hospital admissions for an infectious event received antifungals while 14% received virostatics [2c]. In one additional case report, azacitidine therapy related reactivation of latent viral infection was reported in a 79-year-old Caucasian male who developed febrile neutropenia 1 week following his first cycle of azacitidine therapy [8A]. The patient developed diffuse papular erythematous rashes over various parts of his body. A subsequent biopsy of the skin revealed presence of varicella-zoster virus (VZV). This case demonstrated, for the first time, that azacitidine could mediate dissemination of primary VZV infection in patients suffering from MDS. This case, along with prior evidence of viral and fungal infections in patients receiving azacitidine, requires consideration when presented with a patient experiencing infectious symptoms.

Gastrointestinal

Mild gastrointestinal (GI) adverse events including constipation, diarrhea, nausea, and vomiting commonly occur in patients after treatment with azacitidine. The Austrian Azacitidine Registry data for adverse events observed in both AML and CMML patients showed that treatment with azacitidine primarily caused grade 1–2 nausea (AML: 10.9%; CMML: 8.3%), vomiting (AML: 3.0%; CMML: 2.1%), constipation (AML: 7.0%; CMML: 6.3%), diarrhea (AML: 8.6%; CMML: 12.5%), and other GI events (AML: 7.9%; CMML: 10.4%) [2c,3c]. In a recent study azacitidine was used as a frontline therapy for unfit acute myeloid leukemia patients [9c]. This study provided further evidence of gastrointestinal adverse effects in patients undergoing azacitidine therapy. A total of 117 gastrointestinal adverse effects were reported of which 91 events were of grade 1–2 severity and 26 events were of grade 3–5 severity [9c].

Hematologic

Bone marrow suppression is one of the most frequently observed adverse effects associated with azacitidine therapy. A comprehensive meta-analysis of 692 MDS patients from two phase II and two phase III clinical trials reported grade 3–4 neutropenia, anemia, thrombocytopenia, and febrile neutropenia in 76% (58–94%), 66% (50–82%), 56% (19–94%), and 29% (19–39%) of patients, respectively, receiving multiple cycles of the recommended dose ($75 \, mg/m^2$) of azacitidine [10M]. The observed hematologic toxicities were transient and most of the patients recovered before the next cycle. The Austrian Azacitidine Registry for AML and CMML patients also reported grade 3–4 hematologic toxicities as the most frequent form of adverse effects associated with azacitidine therapy. Severe neutropenia, thrombocytopenia, and anemia occurred in 35%, 30%, and 28% of the patients diagnosed with AML, respectively [2c]. A similar trend was observed in CMML patients where thrombocytopenia, neutropenia, and anemia occurred in 43.8%, 20.8%, and 39.6% patients, respectively [3c]. In a recent open-label phase II clinical trial, 74 patients diagnosed with MDS, AML or CMML were treated with 50 mg/m^2 of azacitidine for 10 consecutive days with or without entinostat. The treatment associated adverse event data indicated grade 3–4 anemia (53%), neutropenia (73%), and thrombocytopenia (72%) as the major form of drug induced toxicity [11c]. Bleeding, possibly a complication of thrombocytopenia, has also been described in azacitidine investigations with a frequency of 12–18%, of which 5% require hospitalization [2c,6c].

Respiratory

Respiratory adverse events are relatively mild and are likely a consequence of neutropenia associated with azacitidine therapy. In a retrospective study, 196 patients receiving azacitidine for treatment of MDS or AML were analyzed for disease progression and febrile events following therapy. Out of 146 febrile events reported, 59 events (40%) were pneumonia and 13 events (8.9%) were upper respiratory tract infections, respectively [12c]. In another retrospective study with 110 AML patients azacitidine treatment caused only 6 adverse events (0.9%) associated with the respiratory tract [9c].

Non-hematologic toxicities are typically relatively mild; however, one MDS patient was reported to develop fatal acute interstitial pneumonitis (AIP) due to treatment with azacitidine [13A]. A 72-year-old male diagnosed with MDS (RAEB-1) was treated with the standard dose of azacitidine. The patient developed pyrexia during the very first course of azacitidine treatment while exhibiting normal vital signs, good blood oxygen saturation levels, and no signs of infection. By the 7th day the patient manifested symptoms associated with difficulty in breathing. A subsequent X-ray and CT scan revealed interstitial opacity and bilateral pleural effusion. The patient was diagnosed with azacitidine induced AIP and was treated with corticosteroids, antibiotics, and antifungal agents. The patient showed improvement for the next 2 days but a subsequent round of azacitidine treatment worsened his respiratory condition. Pneumonitis has also been described in 6.7% of the elderly and frail population receiving azacitidine for the treatment of AML [14c].

Skin

Mild injection site reaction due to subcutaneous route of administration was one of the most common skin related adverse effects observed with azacitidine. Multiple clinical studies with MDS and AML patients reported injection site skin reactions that were mild (< grade 2) and not life threatening [2c,3c,9c,15c]. The injection site reactions mostly involved erythema of the site of injection. More serious dermatologic complications reported to be associated with azacitidine include Sweet's syndrome [16A], neutrophilic panniculitis [17A], necrotizing fasciitis [18A], and pyoderma gangrenosum. [19A].

Sweet's syndrome (acute febrile neutrophilic dermatosis) is characterized by an acute increase in body temperature, leukocytosis, and tender red skin lesions infiltrated with neutrophils. Trickett et al. described two clinical case studies where a 64-year-old male diagnosed with MDS and a 67-year-old male diagnosed with CMML were treated with the recommended dose of azacitidine [16A]. Both patients developed fever and severe skin rashes following treatment with azacitidine. Biopsy of the skin nodules was performed which revealed infiltration with neutrophils. The aforementioned symptoms improved after discontinuation of azacitidine and treatment with corticosteroids. In another case report, a 66-year-old female with MDS receiving azacitidine developed skin lesions on her lips, inner nose, and upper arms on day 3 of her second cycle [19A]. The lesions were unresponsive to antibiotics and progressed to 3–4 cm in diameter. A biopsy of the lesion was consistent with pyoderma gangrenosum. Azacitidine was withheld for two cycles along with prednisone and colchicine, the lesions healed, only to return upon rechallenge with azacitidine. The recurrence again responded to prednisone and the patient received a total of five cycles of azacitidine. Concomitant colchicine and prednisone were administered to control the skin lesions while receiving azacitidine.

Fatigue

In a phase II randomized trial evaluating the efficacy of azacitidine with or without entinostat, many patients experienced various degrees of fatigue. In the group treated with azacitidine alone, 9 patients (12%) developed grade 2 fatigue [11c]. In another study, fatigue was reported in as many as 39% of the patients [2c].

CYTARABINE

Cytarabine or cytosine arabinose is a nucleoside analogue that is approved by the FDA for the treatment of AML, chronic myeloid leukemia (CML), and meningeal leukemia (ML). In addition, it is used for the treatment of Hodgkin's lymphoma, malignant meningitis, mantle cell lymphoma, myelodysplastic syndrome, and non-Hodgkin's lymphoma. It is an antimetabolite that requires phosphorylation by deoxycytidine kinase (DCK) within the cells to form the active derivative ara-CTP (ara-Cytidine-5'-triphosphate) [20R]. The anti-cancer activity of cytarabine is attributed to ara-CTP mediated direct inhibition of DNA polymerase and replacement of deoxycytidine triphosphate (dCTP) by ara-CTP within the DNA during replication [20R]. Together, these mechanisms interfere with DNA synthesis during the S-phase of the cell cycle resulting in cancer cell death.

Cytarabine is mainly used for treatment of AML in combination with an anthracycline. In adults cytarabine is approved for use at low/intermediate dose ($100 \, mg/m^2$/day continuous i.v. infusion for 7 days or $100 \, mg/m^2$ i.v. every 12 hours for 7 days) as well as high dose ($3000 \, mg/m^2$ i.v. infusion over 1–3 hours every 12 hours for 2–6 days) for induction therapy in combination with other approved chemotherapeutic agents [21]. Bone marrow suppression with leukopenia, anemia, and thrombocytopenia are the most common serious adverse effects associated with cytarabine therapy [21]. Anaphylaxis, neuropathy, kidney disease, and infections have also been reported following treatment with cytarabine.

Respiratory

In a multicenter, randomized phase III study, 326 patients with refractory acute myeloid leukemia were treated with high-dose cytarabine+idarubicin or cytarabine+idarubicin+fludarabine. Pulmonary toxicities were reported in 8% of patients receiving cytarabine+idarubicin and 17% of patients receiving cytarabine+idarubicin+fludarabine. Patients were exposed to a high dose of cytarabine, $1000 \, mg/m^2$ as a 3-hour infusion every 12 hours. Pulmonary edema and dyspnea were the most reported pulmonary toxicities associated with the treatment [22C]. Reported toxicities were classified as grade 3 and 4 on the National Cancer Institute Common Terminology Criteria for Adverse Events (CTCAE) scale. A recent retrospective analysis of 15 patients receiving cytarabine monotherapy ($3000 \, mg/m^2$ every 12 hours) for relapsed/refractory AML demonstrated similar pulmonary outcomes in 4 patients (26%). Pulmonary toxicity in these four patients included dyspnea and oxygen desaturation as well as development of new pulmonary infiltrates. Unfortunately, an infectious etiology could not be ruled out in all cases [23c].

Cardiovascular

Cardiovascular events have rarely been reported with cytarabine; however, a recent case report described a serious cardiovascular adverse effect attributed to cytarabine treatment. The patient was a 58-year-old male receiving high dose cytarabine consolidation for AML. Six weeks after starting therapy, he developed severe dyspnea and cardiogenic shock. Echocardiogram demonstrated a reduced left ventricular function which returned to normal 5 months later. Electrocardiography did not show any lasting abnormalities. It was determined that the patient likely experienced Takotsubo cardiomyopathy which is an abrupt yet transient decline in cardiac function. It is also characterized by midventricular hypokinesia and compensatory hypercontractility which was demonstrated in this patient's echocardiogram [24A].

Hematologic

Myelosuppression is the main side effect of cytarabine and the majority of the patients treated with cytarabine eventually develop grade 3–4 hematologic toxicity. In a large clinical study conducted by the Cancer and Leukemia Group B (CALGB), 1088 adults patients newly diagnosed with AML were treated with a combination of cytarabine and daunorubicin to achieve complete remission followed by four courses of monthly maintenance treatment to prevent relapse [25C]. The maintenance treatment included low ($100 \, mg/m^2$/day for 5 days by continuous infusion), intermediate ($400 \, mg/m^2$/day for 5 days by continuous infusion), and high dose ($3000 \, mg/m^2$ as a 3-hour infusion every 12 hours two times a day on days 1, 3 and 5) cytarabine therapy and was administered to 203, 206, and 187 patients, respectively. The data for toxic side effects associated with cytarabine post-remission therapy clearly demonstrated an increase in neutropenia (NP) and thrombocytopenia (TCP) related hospitalization events with increasing doses of cytarabine (*Low dose*: NP—16% and TCP—28%; *Intermediate dose*: NP—59% and TCP—80%; *High dose*: NP—71% and TCP—86%) [25C]. In another retrospective study a total of 137 high dose ($2000 \, mg/m^2$ as a 3-hour infusion every 12 hours on days 1, 2, and 3) cytarabine treatment cycles were administered to 37 AML patients as post-remission consolidation therapy. High dose cytarabine resulted in severe life threatening events of anemia (79.6%), neutropenia (95.6%), and thrombocytopenia (96.4%) in these patients [26c].

Sensory

Neurotoxicity resulting in serious CNS abnormalities was reported in 12% of patients receiving high dose cytarabine as post-remission therapy in the CALGB study [25C]. Neurotoxicity was reversible in 60% of the patients; however, 40% developed permanent disability after treatment. It was also reported that patients aged 60 years or above were more susceptible to neurotoxic side effects of high dose cytarabine. In another study, 38 children and adolescents treated with liposomal cytarabine intrathecally for the treatment of malignant brain tumors and leptomeningeal dissemination developed visual and auditory disturbances. One patient with pre-existing hearing impairment developed hearing loss after 13 doses of liposomal cytarabine 50 mg. Hearing was regained with corticosteroid treatment. Visual disturbances were developed by 8 patients; furthermore, 6 of those patients developed double vision and papilledema. One patient developed decreasing visual sensitivity in one eye after the 5th dose of liposomal cytarabine 50 mg; the condition improved upon discontinuation of liposomal cytarabine [27c]. Given the irreversibility of the neurotoxicity in some patients, careful monitoring and early detection are key to preventing severe disability.

Skin

Dermatologic adverse events are mostly associated with high-dose cytarabine treatment regimens. The majority of the skin related adverse effects are mild and fade away within a few days. However, life-threatening severe skin reactions may occur predisposing a patient to infection and death. In one such clinical case a 13-year-old girl diagnosed with AML was treated with high dose cytarabine ($2000\ mg/m^2$ i.v. every 12 hours) [28A]. After 1 day of treatment the patient developed maculopapular rash all over the body that transformed into bullous lesions by day 2. Approximately 60% of the patient's body was covered with vesiculobullous lesions. Subsequent skin biopsy and histopathologic examination confirmed toxic epidermal necrolysis (TEN). The patient lost large areas of skin and developed septicemia resulting in her death on the 22nd day.

Gastrointestinal

High dose treatment with cytarabine has been correlated with relatively mild to moderate gastrointestinal adverse effects. In a clinical study toxic side effects of high dose cytarabine therapy were studied in 23 children diagnosed with different types of leukemia [29c]. Patients received high dose cytarabine (2000 or $3000\ mg/m^2$ every 12 hours) for a varying number of cycles as part of induction or consolidation therapy. Mild to severe nausea and vomiting were observed in all patients despite co-administration of antiemetics. Nausea and vomiting subsided once cytarabine treatment was stopped. Other gastrointestinal effects involved development of buccal mucositis (five patients), diarrhea (four patients), epigastric pain (two patients), pharyngitis (two patients), stomatitis (one patient), and esophagitis (one patient).

DECITABINE

Decitabine is an analogue of 2′-deoxycytidine that is approved by the FDA for treatment of MDS [30]. It has also been used for treatment of AML [30]. It is an antimetabolite that is phosphorylated after cellular uptake and replaces cytosine in DNA [31E]. This substitution results in inhibition of DNA methyltranferase (DNMT) and further DNA methylation is inhibited [32E]. Reduced methylation aids in activation of tumor suppressor and cell death mediating genes that further aid in cancer cell death and re-sensitization to other chemotherapeutic agents.

In adults diagnosed with MDS, decitabine treatment can be given as a 3-day regimen ($15\ mg/m^2$ i.v. as a 3-hour infusion every 8 hours for 3 days repeated every 6 weeks for at least 4 cycles) or a 5-day regimen ($20\ mg/m^2$/day i.v. as a 1-hour infusion for 5 days repeated every 4 weeks for at least 4 cycles) [30]. For AML, the 5-day regimen of decitabine has been used clinically [30].

Serious hematologic toxicities including anemia, neutropenia, myelosuppression, and thrombocytopenia are the major serious side effects associated with decitabine therapy. In addition, dermatologic, immunologic, and gastrointestinal adverse events have also been reported.

Cardiovascular

Decitabine mediated cardiovascular adverse events are relatively rare and mild. In one such case, a 75-year-old male diagnosed with AML and a past medical history of Diabetes mellitus type 2 presented to the emergency department with exertional dyspnea and chest tightness [33A]. A week prior to this emergency visit the patient had completed a second round of therapy with decitabine ($20\ mg/m^2$ for 10 days). Subsequent blood work, electrocardiogram, and left heart catheterization revealed that the patient's cardiac enzymes (troponin I and creatinine kinase MB) were elevated, he suffered from sinus tachycardia, and had developed nonobstructive coronary artery disease, respectively. The patient developed hypotension and required vasopressors. Development of these symptoms after treatment with decitabine indicated towards drug induced acute myocarditis. The aforementioned cardiomyopathy was transient and possibly related to decitabine as the patient's cardiac enzyme levels and echocardiogram normalized after discontinuation of decitabine. The patient received two additional cycles of decitabine reduced to 5 subsequent days of decitabine $20\ mg/m^2$ without any further cardiovascular issues.

Hematologic

Consistent with prior decitabine trials, a retrospective analysis of pooled data from two multicenter decitabine studies showed that the most common decitabine treatment related adverse events are hematologic and include thrombocytopenia, neutropenia and anemia [34M]. In a phase I/II study of safety and efficacy of decitabine and temozolomide, neutropenia was the most common grade 3–4 adverse event. Neutropenia occurred during the 4th or 5th week of the treatment and lasted for 7 days. Patients usually recovered within a couple of weeks after a dose modification [35C,36C].

Infection

In an open-label, prospective, observational study, 52 patients (age: 65–82 years) received decitabine treatment. Severe, grade 3–4 infection developed in 11 (21.2%) patients related to the decitabine treatment. Some of the infections resulted in death [37c]. In a review of decitabine usage in older patients with acute myeloid leukemia two studies were analyzed. Mild, grade 1–2, and severe, grade 3–4, infections that were associated with the decitabine treatment were pneumonia and urinary tract infection. Other rare, but severe grade 3–4 decitabine related infections were sepsis, septic shock and sinusitis [38R]. A study of younger patients (children and young adults) receiving low dose decitabine for acute myeloid leukemia was conducted in 8 patients. One patient developed Klebsiella bacteremia and another patient had febrile neutropenia with pseudomonal pneumonia and sepsis [39c]. These reports highlight that patients of all ages are at risk for infectious issues while receiving decitabine, likely due to its immunosuppressive properties.

Skin

In a phase I/II combination of decitabine and panitumumab in patients with colorectal cancer, 74% of 20 patients treated developed mild (grade 1–2), rash and 11% developed severe (grade 3–4), rash. Another skin related adverse effect was dry skin which developed in 16% of patients [40c]. Panitumumab is commonly associated with dermatologic adverse effects and is likely the agent driving the adverse effect rates in this report.

Neutrophilic eccrine hidradenitis (NEH) has been reported in patients suffering from leukemia and is characterized by edematous papules or plaques of skin that are sometimes associated with pustules. NEH could be a result of the cytotoxic effect of chemotherapeutic drugs or due to neutrophilic infiltration of the skin. Decitabine therapy has been reported to cause NEH [41A]. In one such case a 30-year-old women diagnosed with MDS (RAEB II) received a 5-day regimen of decitabine. Two weeks subsequent to the first course of therapy the patient developed neutropenic fever. Three days later the patient developed erythematous nodules on the right shin and an erythematous plaque over the left elbow.

These lesions further worsened over the next 5 days. Histopathologic examination was negative for any microbial infection; however, it did reveal neutrophil infiltration in the eccrine glands and dermal blood vessels. Together, these findings led to the diagnosis of NEH. After treatment with prednisolone the patient's fever and skin lesions improved. However, during the second round of decitabine therapy the aforementioned symptoms resumed once again. Increasing the prednisolone dose and discontinuation of decitabine resolved the skin lesions.

Gastrointestinal

Adverse effects associated with the gastrointestinal track related to the decitabine are usually mild (grade 1–2). In a multicenter, open-label, randomized phase II study, patients receiving decitabine + carboplatin developed nausea, vomiting and constipation. All of the gastrointestinal adverse effects were mild (grade 2) [42c]. In a phase I study of decitabine and rapamycin, reported gastrointestinal side effects were mild and included constipation, weight loss, decreased appetite, diarrhea, and nausea. More severe side effects included mucositis (grade 1–3) and GI bleeding (grade 4) [43c].

GEMCITABINE

Gemcitabine is an antimetabolite that requires phosphorylation to its active metabolite in order to inhibit DNA synthesis. It has activity in both hematologic and solid malignancies; however, the majority of its use is in solid malignancies including tumors of the gastrointestinal tract (pancreatic, biliary, etc.), bladder, and breast. Common adverse effects associated with gemcitabine include gastrointestinal effects (nausea/vomiting), hematologic effects (neutropenia, thrombocytopenia, anemia), and a flu-like syndrome.

Cardiovascular

In a randomized, placebo-controlled, double-blind, parallel-group phase III study, 275 patients assigned to receive gemcitabine developed several cardiovascular adverse events. In total 95 (35%) patients developed proteinuria with only 3 (1%) of the cases being severe (grade 3–4). Severe arterial and venous thromboembolic events were reported in 5 and 27 patients, respectively. Bleeding was reported in 20 (7%) patients and only 4 (1%) cases were grade 3–4. Hypertension was another adverse effect that was reported, with 17 patients (6%) experiencing high blood pressure. Only one patient (0.4%) in the gemcitabine treatment arm developed cardiac dysfunction [44C].

In addition to the above adverse events, multiple case reports have been recently published highlighting the cardiac and vascular effects of gemcitabine. Cardiomyopathy was described in one case of a 56-year-old male with pancreatic cancer after 2 cycles of gemcitabine $1000 \, mg/m^2$ IV on days 1, 8, and 15 of a 28-day cycle [45A]. The patient developed dyspnea on exertion, orthopnea and fatigue. His ejection fraction was 15–20% with global hypokinesia. Myocardial perfusion studies did not detect any ischemia. The patient was treated pharmacologically with a conventional heart failure regimen. The patient did not receive any further gemcitabine and his ejection fraction increased to 40% upon repeat examination a few months later. In another case report, a 40-year-old patient developed cutaneous vasculitis during cycle 1 of a regimen containing gemcitabine $1360 \, mg/m^2$ and cisplatin $100 \, mg/m^2$ [46A]. The patient presented with erythematous subcutaneous nodules in both the upper and lower extremities which were painful. Tests for infectious and autoimmune etiologies were negative and a biopsy showed perivascular inflammatory cell infiltrate without vessel wall necrosis along with transmural inflammation of the wall of medium sized arteries. Gemcitabine was discontinued and the patient was treated conservatively with non-steroidal anti-inflammatory drugs until resolution of the episode. Another patient developed large vessel vasculitis after receiving two cycles of gemcitabine $1000 \, mg/m^2$ of a 28 day cycle [47A]. Incidentally, she was found to have developed mid thoracic, aortic, and thoracoabdominal aortic and left femoral wall thickening consistent with arteritis on CT which was confirmed via a positron emission tomography (PET) scan. Gemcitabine was discontinued and the patient was started on prednisolone for 4 weeks. A repeat PET scan showed resolution of vasculitis. Monitoring for signs and symptoms of cardiovascular adverse effects in patients receiving gemcitabine is recommended as the adverse effects described above appear to be reversible with appropriate management.

Hematologic

The main dose limiting adverse event of gemcitabine therapy is myelosuppression, neutropenia being the most common [48c]. In a meta-analysis of 10 randomized controlled trials of gemcitabine monotherapy in pancreatic cancer. Hematologic adverse events were extracted; myelosuppression was reported to be the most common adverse event of gemcitabine. Neutropenia was the most reported form of myelosuppression with 388/1788 (21.7%) patients developing neutropenia while on gemcitabine monotherapy. Thrombocytopenia was reported in 155/1711 (9.1%) patients on gemcitabine monotherapy.

Anemia was reported in 123/1508 (1.5%) of the patients [49M]. Interestingly, in a retrospective study of 494 patients receiving gemcitabine based regimens, there was no difference in those ≥70 years of age and those <70 in terms of relative dose intensity and incidence of severe hematologic toxicity [50C]. However, grade 3/4 leucopenia was more common in the older age group (45% vs 9%, $p < 0.05$).

Thrombotic Microangiopathy

In a single center retrospective series, 264 patients previously treated with gemcitabine were evaluated for development of thrombotic microangiopathy. Three patients displaying signs of thrombotic microangiopathy were identified [51C].

A 63-year-old male with pancreatic adenocarcinoma received five cycles of gemcitabine $1000 \, mg/m^2$ weekly for 3 weeks followed by 1 week of rest. In total $15\,000 \, mg/m^2$ of gemcitabine was delivered. At the completion of the fifth cycle of gemcitabine treatment, the patient developed signs of thrombotic microangiopathy: acute renal impairment (serum creatinine $2.22 \, mg/dl$), thrombocytopenia (platelet count 43000) and hemolytic anemia (hemoglobin $6.8 \, g/dl$; LDH $3867 \, U/l$; schistocytes and elliptocytes in peripheral blood smear) [42c].

The second patient, a 30-year-old male with a high-risk non-seminomatous germ cell neoplasm, received gemcitabine $1000 \, mg/m^2$ on days 1, 8, and 15 of a 28-day cycle plus paclitaxel $100 \, mg/m^2$ on day 1. After completing five cycles of gemcitabine treatment, the patient presented with signs of thrombotic microangiopathy: acute renal injury (serum creatinine $5.15 \, mg/dl$), severe hemolytic anemia (hemoglobin $6.6 \, g/dl$, bilirubin $3.87 \, mg/dl$), thrombocytopenia (platelet count $70\,000/mm^3$), and altered mental status. Thrombotic microangiopathy was confirmed with peripheral blood smear [42c].

Lastly, a 39-year-old male with an undifferentiated nasopharyngeal neoplasm received gemcitabine $1250 \, mg/m^2$ on day 1, 8, and 15, every 28 days. After the second infusion, the patient presented with severe hemolytic anemia (hemoglobin $6.6 \, g/dl$), acute renal impairment, and shock [42c].

In addition to the above retrospective series, thrombotic microangiopathy has been recently described in numerous case reports [52A,53A,54A, 55A]. In 5 of these recent case reports the patients developed thrombotic microangiopathy after receiving gemcitabine for five cycles or more. All cases described similar signs to the above cases (anemia, thrombocytopenia, acute kidney injury and hypertension) and some required dialysis and plasma exchange. One patient failed to have a return of her renal function and required dialysis until her death due to cancer progression [52A].

Liver

In a randomized double-blinded, placebo-controlled phase II trial of simvastatin+gemcitabine compared with gemcitabine+placebo. Patients in the gemcitabine +placebo arm had an increase in liver enzyme levels. Creatine kinase was elevated in 1/10 (10%) of the patients, total bilirubin was elevated in 7 (12.5%), aspartate aminotransferase was elevated in 17 (30.4%), alanine transaminase was elevated in 18 (32.1%) and alkaline phosphatase was elevated in 23 (41.1%). Elevations in liver enzymes were common adverse events; however, the elevations were transient in nature and highly manageable with supportive care. Patients treated with simvastatin+gemcitabine had an increase in the liver enzyme levels as well, however there was no statistically significant difference between the groups [56c].

Infection

Infections are rare with gemcitabine treatment and can be severe (grade 3–4). The most common infection is febrile neutropenia [57c]. In a randomized controlled study of gemcitabine for unresectable pancreatic cancer, out of 46 patients treated with gemcitabine monotherapy, 7 (15.2%) developed an infection and 1 (2.2%) developed febrile neutropenia. All of the infections reported were grade 3–4; however they did not cause further complications [58c]. Due to the possible severity, monitoring for infections during treatment is important.

Gastrointestinal

Common gastrointestinal adverse events include nausea, vomiting and diarrhea [59c]. In a prospective, randomized, phase II trial of gemcitabine in advanced pancreatic cancer, 54 patients were treated with gemcitabine monotherapy. The most common gastrointestinal adverse event experienced by patients was nausea; with 20 (37%) of the patients experiencing nausea and 3 (5.6%) experiencing severe, grade 3–4, nausea. Vomiting was reported in 13 (14.1%) of patients with only 4 (7.6%) being considered severe. Diarrhea was only of mild severity and presented in 8 (14.8%) of the patients [60c].

A serious gastrointestinal adverse effect was recently published as a case report in which a 71-year-old male experienced severe ischemic colitis after his first dose of gemcitabine 1000 mg/m^2 and cisplatin 25 mg/m^2 [61A]. The patient presented with abdominal pain and was found to have intestinal necrosis via colonoscopy and received a colectomy and ileoceccal resection with ileostomy. Histologic examination of the tissue revealed inflammation and patchy ischemia throughout the entire colon and small intestine without arterial or venous thrombosis. The patient died due to renal failure 3 months after the episode. Due to the timing, this severe complication was believed to be related to the chemotherapy exposure.

Pain

Pain is very uncommon and usually mild (grade 1–2). In a 44 patient retrospective single center study of those with recurrent epithelial ovarian cancer treated with gemcitabine, grade 1 neuropathy was reported by 2 (4.7%) patients and grade 2 neuropathy was reported by 1 (2.3%) patient [62c]. In a randomized, open-label, non-comparative phase II trail, 144 patients with advanced biliary cancer were treated with the combination of gemcitabine+oxaliplatin with or without cetuximab. In the gemcitabine+oxaliplatin+cetuximab group, 48 (63%) patients developed grade 1–2 peripheral neuropathy and 18 (24%) patients developed grade 3 peripheral neuropathy. In the gemcitabine+oxaliplatin without cetuximab group, results were similar, 43 (63%) patients developed grade 1–2 peripheral neuropathy and 10 (15%) patients developed grade 3 peripheral neuropathy [63c].

Immunologic

In addition to the typical immune suppression caused by gemcitabine, it has also been associated with autoimmune adverse effects. A case report documented the occurrence of subacute cutaneous lupus erythematosus in a 71-year-old woman with breast cancer after her second weekly dose of gemcitabine [64A]. The patient developed erythematous annular patches with scale on her arms and pink papules on her chest along with fever and fatigue. Serology was positive for anti-Ro (SS-A), anti-La (SS-B), and anti nuclear antibodies. Gemcitabine was discontinued and the patient was treated with a topical steroid without resolution. Ultimately, a 20-day prednisone taper resulted in resolution.

Skin

Dermatologic toxicities secondary to gemcitabine are relatively rare and include generalized rash, radiation recall dermatitis and Stevens–Johnson syndrome. In addition to these, a recent case report described the occurrence of acute generalized exanthematous pustulosis 4 days after the first dose of gemcitabine in a 40-year-old male [65A]. The patient presented with a generalized erythematous eruption with pustules on the neck trunk and extremities. Skin biopsy revealed subcorneal pustule, exocytosis of neutrophils in the epidermis, and dermal edema. Gemcitabine was discontinued and symptoms resolved within 7 days after starting oral steroids and antihistamines.

Occular

A 64-year-old patient was reported to develop diffuse ischemic retinal vasculopathy after receiving gemcitabine 1000 mg/m² + oxaliplatin 100 mg/m² followed 6 weeks later by another dose of gemcitabine + cisplatin 25 mg/m² [66A]. The patient complained of painless bilateral vision loss. Treatment with panretinal photocoagulation in both eyes along with one intravitreal injection of bevacizumab was without success as the patients visual acuity was 20/400 in the right eye and count fingers in the left eye 2 months after presentation. It is unclear whether the vision impairment was due to gemcitabine or cisplatin; nonetheless, monitoring for vision impairment and prompt discontinuation may limit this adverse effect should it occur.

Musculoskeletal

Gemcitabine induced myopathy was recently described in a case of a 69-year-old patient with pancreatic cancer. The patient developed symptoms 1 day after the third dose of the second cycle of gemcitabine 1000 mg/m² days 1, 8, and 15 every 28 days [67A]. The patient developed erythema on both thighs with pain upon palpation. They had a motor deficiency at the level of the quadriceps and difficulty rising from a squat. Creatine kinase was 1858 IU/l and C reactive protein was 13.8 mg/dl. A muscle biopsy demonstrated post-necrotic generation and vascular proliferation. Gemcitabine was discontinued and the myopathy resolved. In another case report, a 44 years old experienced myositis; however, it was due to a radiation recall reaction [68A]. The patient presented 2 months after beginning therapy (gemcitabine + carboplatin) with pelvic pain along with erythema and swelling of the buttocks and groin. Creatine kinase was 1261 IU/l with a C-reactive protein of 140 mg/dl. Notably, the patient had a history of dermatomyositis. MRI revealed myositis within the area of prior radiation and gemcitabine was discontinued. The patient improved upon treatment with prednisolone.

FLUOROPYRIMIDINES

Fluorouracil and its prodrug, capecitabine, have been utilized in multiple malignancies including breast cancer and multiple gastrointestinal tumors. Capecitabine is metabolized via the liver and within tumor tissue to fluorouracil. Fluorouracil requires multiple conversions to form active metabolites with the main cytotoxic activity being via inhibition of thymidylate synthase. Common toxicities with both agents include gastrointestinal effects (mucositis, nausea, vomiting, etc.), as well as hand foot syndrome in those receiving continuous infusion fluorouracil and capecitabine. Patients receiving bolus fluorouracil infusions are at higher risk for myelosuppressive effects. Metabolism to inactive metabolites occurs via dihydropyrimidine dehydrogenase (DPD) and those with deficiency of DPD are at increased risk for toxicity with both medications.

FLUOROURACIL

Hematologic

In a multicenter, randomized, open-label, parallel group, phase II trial, 133 patients with esophageal cancer were treated with fluorouracil + cisplatin or fluorouracil + leucovorin + oxaliplatin (FOLFOX regimen). The most common grade 3–4 adverse effect in the fluorouracil + cisplatin treatment group was myelosuppression: Neutropenia in 38 (29%) patients, lymphopenia in 21 (16%) patients, anemia in 7 (6%) patients, thrombocytopenia in 9 (7%) patients [69c]. A phase III multicenter trial of 6 cycles of 5-fluorouracil + epirubicin + cyclophosphamide included 426 patients with breast cancer. As expected, 337 patients (79%) developed neutropenia, 29 patients (6.8%) developed leukopenia, 88 patients (21%) developed thrombocytopenia. All of the hematologic adverse effects were grade 3–4 [70C]. Complicating this further, patients with DPD deficiency are at an increased risk for more pronounced and prolonged myelosuppression due to delayed fluorouracil metabolism. A case report of a 71-year-old female receiving irinotecan, oxaliplatin, and fluorouracil for pancreatic cancer was recently published in which the woman developed prolonged neutropenia and neutropenic sepsis after her first cycle [71A]. Upon investigation, the patient was found to be heterozygous for a DPD mutation.

Neurologic

A 61-year-old male with esophageal cancer was treated with nedaplatin 90 mg/m² on day 1 followed by a continuous intravenous infusion of 5-fluorouracil 800 mg/m² for the next 5 days. After the final dose, the patient developed difficulty speaking, followed by left sided weakness. Physical examination that was performed on the patient showed that he was in a somnolent state and had left hemispatial neglect, a rightward gaze preference, left hemiplegia involving the face, and dysarthria. The patient was diagnosed with 5-fluorouracil-induced leukoencephalopathy with acute stroke-like presentation. A computed tomographic (CT) scan of the brain was performed 4 hours after symptom onset which revealed no abnormalities. The patient underwent intravenous recombinant tissue plasminogen activator (rtPA) therapy (0.6 mg/kg). Two days later, his neurologic complications were resolved with an exception of disturbed consciousness [72A].

Skin

Topical 5% 5-fluorouracil is known to cause toxicity, such as erythema, pain, and crusting/erosions. In an effort to develop a scale to measure this toxicity a trial enrolled and followed 954 US veterans at high risk for squamous or basal cell carcinomas. Grade 3–4 erythema occurred 344 times (27% of all erythema occurrences during the trial). Grade 1–2 crusting/erosions occurred 705 times; no grade 3–4 crusting/erosions were identified during the trial [73C]. In addition to the erythematous reactions to topical fluorouracil described in this trial, a case report has described an angioedema-like reaction in a patient receiving topical fluorouracil [74A]. The 77-year-old male with actinic keratosis was prescribed 0.5% fluorouracil cream. He admitted to applying the medication more frequently than prescribed and after 9 days, developed swelling in his hands. The patient then developed swelling of his lower lip and dysphonia. He was given a dose of IV corticosteroid followed by oral prednisone and his symptoms resolved over 2–3 days. The fluorouracil was discontinued along with lisinopril which he had been taking for approximately 2 years without incident. Hypersensitivity reactions such as this have been reported with IV fluorouracil administration; however, this was the first known case reported due to topical fluorouracil.

Gastrointestinal

Mucositis is one of the most common adverse effects of fluorouracil, it can be both severe (grade 3–4) and mild (grade 1–2). In a trial, 140 patients with locally advanced squamous cell carcinoma of the head and neck were given docetaxel + cisplatin + 5-fluorouracil. Dosing was as follows: docetaxel 50 mg/m^2 on day 1, cisplatin 60 mg/m^2 on day 4 and continuous 5-fluorouracil 600 mg/m^2/day on days 1–5. Grade 1–2 mucositis developed in 56 patients (40.0%). Other gastrointestinal adverse effects reported were: Grade 1–2 nausea/vomiting in 104 patients (74.3%) and grade 3 nausea/vomiting in 18 patients (12.9%), grade 1–2 diarrhea in 68 patients (48.6%) and grade 3 diarrhea in 11 patients (7.9%). No grade 4 gastrointestinal adverse effects were reported during this trial [75c,76c].

Cardiovascular

Cardiotoxicity is relatively uncommon but a serious and potentially life threatening adverse event of fluorouracil [77c,78c,79A]. In a retrospective study 42 patients, who previously have been given fluorouracil or capecitabine were identified. Types of cardiac toxicity developed by the patients included angina, acute arrhythmia, and myocardial infarction. The median number of cycles to the first cardiac event was one. Four patients had cardiac toxicity recognized and anti-anginal therapy initiated with nitrates and calcium antagonists. Despite the interventions they continued to experience further cardiac toxicity with subsequent chemotherapy cycles. Myocardial infraction was reported in 5 patients (12%) and ischemic pain was reported in 20 patients (48%) [77c]. A recent case report also described the development of Takotsubo syndrome in a patient receiving infusional fluorouracil (along with irinotecan and leucovorin; FOLFIRI regimen) [80A]. The 48-year-old male with gastric cancer developed tachycardia and dyspnea at the 34th hour of his 46-hour fluorouracil infusion. He was shown to have hypokinesis of the mid-apical segments and hyperkinesis of the basal segments on echocardiogram and his left ventricular ejection fraction was 15%. The patient then developed ventricular fibrillation and required intubation and intensive care for 36 hours. Subsequently, the patient recovered and after 27 days his ejection fraction rebounded to 50%.

A possible alternative for patients developing cardiac toxicity while receiving infusional fluorouracil is to rechallenge with a bolus fluorouracil regimen. In a case series of six patients, administration of bolus fluorouracil, after experiencing cardiotoxicity with infusional fluorouracil or capecitabine, was well tolerated without recurrence of cardiotoxicity [81c].

Fatigue

In an open-label, multicenter, phase II, randomized trial, patients with stage II rectal cancer were given adjuvant oxaliplatin + fluorouracil + leucovorin or fluorouracil + leucovorin. Both groups developed grade 1–2 fatigue as an adverse effect. In the fluorouracil + leucovorin group, 26 patients (17%) developed grade 1–2 fatigue. In the oxaliplatin + fluorouracil + leucovorin group 41 patients (28%) developed grade 1–2 fatigue [82C].

CAPECITABINE

Skin

Hand-foot syndrome (palmar-plantar erythrodysesthesia) is a common adverse effect of capecitabine [83C,84c,87c]. In a phase III, open-label, parallel, two-arm, multicenter trial of eribulin or capecitabine for the treatment of breast cancer, 546 patients were assigned to the capecitabine treatment group. All grades of hand-foot syndrome were reported in 246 (45.1%) patients in the capecitabine treatment group. Severe (grade 3) hand-foot syndrome was reported in 79 (14.5%) patients. Hand-foot syndrome was one of the leading causes of capecitabine discontinuation [83C].

In a randomized phase II trial, capecitabine was given to patients with advanced breast cancer. Mild (grade 1–2) skin fissures developed in 3 (21%) patients [84c]. In a phase II trial of fulvestrant with metronomic capecitabine for postmenopausal women with hormone receptor positive, HER2-negative metastatic breast cancer, 8 (19.5%) patients developed mild (grade 1–2) skin hyperpigmentation [85c]. In an interesting case published recently, a patient receiving capecitabine+bevacizumab for the treatment of breast cancer developed severe hand foot syndrome after the third cycle of chemotherapy [86A]. The symptoms resolved with a delay in therapy and dose reduction; however, the patient's finger prints were no longer present and did not return. Monitoring and prophylactic measures (regular application of moisturizers, etc.) should be undertaken when starting therapy with capecitabine.

Photosensitive lichenoid developed in a 75-year-old Caucasian woman receiving capecitabine for metastatic breast cancer. She presented in the dermatology clinic with pruritic eruption in the sun-exposed areas of her body starting 2 months after the initiation of capecitabine. The patient reported being exposed to the sun for a prolonged period of time during the treatment period. Furthermore, fingernail changes were present. Examination of the patient revealed numerous flat topped papules on extensor forearms, dorsal hands and anterior legs. Scaling and erythema were observed in the periungual areas with marked subungual hyperkeratosis. Diffuse erythema was also noted of the palmar and plantar surfaces. The patient was prescribed topical clobetasol propionate 0.05% ointment and systemic hydroxyzine as well as adherence to sun protection strategies. She noted an improvement in her eruption without any changes in her chemotherapeutic regimen [87A]. Prolonged sun exposure should be avoided while taking capecitabine.

Dermatomyositis developed in a 76-year-old man with metastatic gastric adenocarcinoma. The patient presented with diffuse rash and muscle weakness 2 weeks after receiving carboplatin+capecitabine 1 g orally twice daily. The patient previously received carboplatin monotherapy without any adverse events. Examination was performed revealing poikilodermatous plaques with shallow erosions scattered in a V-distribution on the upper chest and upper back. His hands contained erythematous, scaly papules symmetrically distributed over the metacarpophalangeal and interphalangeal joints as well as periungual erythema. The patient's creatine kinase was 2630 U/l and a punch biopsy of the shoulder revealed interface dermatitis with mild spongiosis, epidermal necrosis, and subepidermal vesicle formation [88A]. Symptoms resolved after a course of steroids and discontinuation of capecitabine; however, they flared upon reinitiation, requiring treatment with steroids and intravenous immune globulin. Again symptoms resolved.

Hematologic

In a phase I study of postoperative radiotherapy +capecitabine in patients with gastric cancer, 18 patients were analyzed. Neutropenia was a dose limiting adverse event at a capecitabine dose of 800 mg/m^2 twice daily [89c]. Myelosuppression was a common side effect and included: grade 1–2 leukopenia in 14 (77.8%) patients, grade 3–4 leukopenia in 2 (11.1%) patients, grade 1–2 neutropenia in 3 (16.7%) patients, grade 3–4 neutropenia in 1 (5.6%) patient, grade 1–2 anemia in 3 (16.7%) patients, and grade 1–2 thrombocytopenia in 5 (27.8%) patients [89c,90c].

Hemolytic anemia has also been described to occur with capecitabine. In a case report of a 61-year-old female receiving capecitabine for breast cancer, the patient developed hemolytic anemia which was determined to be autoimmune in nature based on a positive direct Coombs test [91A]. Another patient (70-year-old female with breast cancer) developed hemolytic anemia 4 days after starting capecitabine [92A]. Upon discontinuation of the medication, the hemolytic anemia resolved. It was determined that this patient had non-immune hemolytic anemia.

Gastrointestinal

In a multicenter, phase II study of trastuzumab +capecitabine+oxaliplatin in patients with advanced gastric cancer, 64 patients were screened and 55 patients were analyzed. Gastrointestinal adverse events were common and included: grade 1–2 nausea in 29 (50%) patients, grade 3–4 nausea in 1 (2%) patient, grade 1–2 constipation in 17 (30%) patients, grade 1–2 stomatitis in 11 (20%) patients, grade 3–4 stomatitis in 1 (3%) patient, grade 1–2 diarrhea in 20 (36%) patients and grade 3–4 diarrhea in 1 (2%) patient. There was one treatment related death due to severe diarrhea and complicated sepsis [93c,94c].

Colitis is an uncommon adverse effect of capecitabine treatment. A 45-year-old man with a history of gastroesophageal reflux disease presented with fatigue, nausea, vomiting, progressive dysphagia, and 20 pound weight loss. A CT scan revealed a large tumor at the gastroesophageal junction. Chemotherapy consisted of cisplatin 160 mg IV for 1 day, trastuzumab 638 mg IV for 1 day and capecitabine 200 mg twice a day for 14 days. On the second day of the third chemotherapy cycle, the patient presented with a new onset of lower abdominal pain, diarrhea and bright red blood per rectum. Abdominal exam noted tenderness to palpation and there was no evidence of neutropenia. Stool cultures were negative for bacterial infections and *Clostridium difficile*. Colonoscopy showed severe segmental colitis with erythema, edema, granularity and friability from 20 to 80 cm from the anal verge with sharp endoscopic definitions of the involved mucosa. A diagnosis of chemotherapy-induced colitis was made and capecitabine was discontinued. The patient's symptoms resolved and his condition improved during his hospital stay [95A].

Cardiovascular

In a 19 patient phase I trial, metastatic colorectal cancer was treated with radioimmunotherapy (131I-huA33) + capecitabine. One patient developed grade 3 cardiotoxicity which presented as chest pain associated with ST elevation secondary to capecitabine. This case resolved with treatment, but led to an early withdrawal from the study. Another patient developed episodes of retrosternal discomfort on exertion which may have represented pain of cardiac origin. No electrocardiogram abnormalities were found and a stress test suggested ischemia. The maximum tolerated dose of the combination was found to be $1.48 \, GBq/m^2$ 131I-huA33 combined with a capecitabine dose of $1250 \, mg/m^2/day$ [96c].

Cardiotoxicity is likely to be less common with capecitabine than fluorouracil due to the increased activity of its activating enzyme within tumor cells. Nonetheless, recent case reports are available describing coronary artery thrombosis and vasospasm as well as Takotsubo cardiomyopathy with capecitabine. Similar to the cardiac complications associated with fluorouracil, a patient receiving capecitabine + oxaliplatin for colon cancer developed acute coronary syndrome due to thrombotic coronary occlusion [97A]. Moreover, two case reports describe Takotsubo cardiomyopathy, which has also been described with fluorouracil (see Section Fluorouracil). The first case was an 81-year-old woman presenting with acute chest pain and dyspnea approximately 7 hours after her first dose of capecitabine. She was found to have apical dyskinesia with apical ballooning and a decline in ejection fraction (0.53) upon ventriculography. Moreover, on cardiovascular MRI, 5 days later, the patient had an ejection fraction of 44% with hypokinesia in the apical and mid-ventricular segments. Repeat MRI 4 weeks later showed resolution of wall motion abnormalities and normalized ventricular function [98A]. In the second, recently reported case report, a 55-year-old male with adenocarcinoma of the caecum presented with fatigue and chest pain 28 hours after starting capecitabine. He was found to have a low blood pressure (40 mmHg systolic) and echocardiogram demonstrated hypokinesia of the left ventricle and an ejection fraction of 15–20%. Capecitabine was discontinued and the patient began improving on hospital day 2. One week later, the patient had complete normalization of the ejection fraction to >55% [99A]. These two case reports describing Takotsubo cardiomyopathy demonstrate how quickly cardiotoxicity can manifest with capecitabine.

Neurologic

In a meta-analysis, capecitabine based treatment regimens were analyzed in patients with gastrointestinal cancer. Anorexia was the most common adverse event, with 202/340 (59%) patients developing anorexia in the capecitabine based treatment group [100M].

In a phase 2 study, 48 patients with metastatic breast cancer were treated with paclitaxel polyglumex + capecitabine. Treatment consisted of paclitaxel polyglumex $135 \, mg/m^2$ by intravenous infusion on day 1 + capecitabine $825 \, mg/m^2$ orally twice daily on days 1–14, repeated on a 3-week cycle. Peripheral sensory neuropathy was developed by 8% of patients in the trial [101c].

In addition to the above neurologic effects, capecitabine has also been associated with toxic encephalopathy. A 69-year-old male presented with recurrent generalized seizures 2.5 months after starting preoperative chemoradiotherapy with capecitabine for locally advanced rectal cancer. The patient received capecitabine $825 \, mg/m^2$ by mouth from day 1 to day 30 and pelvic radiation therapy totaling 45 Gy, 1.8 Gy/day from day 1 to day 30. Brain MRI revealed a diffuse, subcortical white matter alteration and the diagnosis of toxic encephalopathy was made after elimination of alternative causes of the neurological dysfunction. Chemotherapy was discontinued and complete resolution was achieved 3 months after discontinuation [102A].

Immunologic

Two case reports of subacute cutaneous lupus erythematosus have been reported in the literature recently. The first case was a 72-year-old woman with gastric cancer receiving capecitabine + oxaliplatin. One month after starting therapy, she developed multiple erythematous, indurated papules and plaques on the head, face, neck, trunk, forearms, and hands [103A]. Skin biopsy demonstrated interface dermatitis with perivascular lymphocytic infiltration. The patients antinuclear antibodies were >1:2560 and the anti-Ro antibodies were >1:240. Capecitabine was discontinued and the patient improved on oral and topical steroids. Capecitabine was reintroduced upon resolution and she developed extensive erythematous, violaceous, papulosquamous eruptions. Intravenous steroids and discontinuation of capecitabine once again led to resolution. In the second case, a 78-year-old woman with breast cancer developed erythematosquamous plaques on the face, neckline, upper back and forearms 10 days after starting therapy with capecitabine. A biopsy demonstrated epidermal atrophy with necrotic keratinocytes, vacuolar degeneration, perifollicular and perivascular lymphohistiocytic infiltrate. Antinuclear antibodies were 1/640 and anti-Ro antibodies were 0.83 IU/ml. Capecitabine was discontinued and the patient had resolution of plaques after 3 weeks [104A].

Acknowledgement

Authors gratefully acknowledge the assistance provided by Mr. Chance Dansforth, PharmD candidate and Dr. Robert Beckett during the preparation of this manuscript.

References

[1] Azacitidine. DrugPoint Summary. Micromedex 2.0. Truven Health Analytics, Inc. Greenwood Village, CO. Available at: http://www.micromedexsolutions.com. Accessed 2015 July 09. Last Modified 2015 June 11.

[2] Pleyer L, Burgstaller S, Girschikofsky M, et al. Azacitidine in 302 patients with WHO-defined acute myeloid leukemia: results from the Austrian Azacitidine Registry of the AGMT-Study Group. Ann Hematol. 2014;93(11):1825–38 [c].

[3] Pleyer L, Germing U, Sperr WR, et al. Azacitidine in CMML: matched-pair analyses of daily-life patients reveal modest effects on clinical course and survival. Leuk Res. 2014;38(4):475–83 [c].

[4] Bibault JE, Cambier N, Lemahieu JM, et al. Acute myocarditis induced by hypomethylating agents. J Clin Oncol. 2011;29(14):e411–2 [A].

[5] Lee YG, Kim I, Yoon SS, et al. Comparative analysis between azacitidine and decitabine for the treatment of myelodysplastic syndromes. Br J Haematol. 2013;161(3):339–47 [c].

[6] Itzykson R, Thepot S, Berthon C, et al. Azacitidine for the treatment of relapsed and refractory AML in older patients. Leuk Res. 2015;39(2):124–30 [c].

[7] Ofran Y, Filanovsky K, Gafter-Gvili A, et al. Higher infection rate after 7- compared with 5-day cycle of azacitidine in patients with higher-risk myelodysplastic syndrome. Clin Lymphoma Myeloma Leuk. 2015;15(6):e95–9 [c].

[8] Zhou G, Houldin AD. Disseminated varicella-zoster virus infection following azacitidine in a patient with myelodysplastic syndrome. Clin J Oncol Nurs. 2009;13(3):280–4 [A].

[9] Ramos F, Thepot S, Pleyer L, et al. Azacitidine frontline therapy for unfit acute myeloid leukemia patients: clinical use and outcome prediction. Leuk Res. 2015;39(3):296–306 [c].

[10] Xie M, Jiang Q, Xie Y. Comparison between decitabine and azacitidine for the treatment of myelodysplastic syndrome: a meta-analysis with 1,392 participants. Clin Lymphoma Myeloma Leuk. 2015;15(1):22–8 [M].

[11] Prebet T, Sun Z, Figueroa ME, et al. Prolonged administration of azacitidine with or without entinostat for myelodysplastic syndrome and acute myeloid leukemia with myelodysplasia-related changes: results of the US Leukemia Intergroup trial E1905. J Clin Oncol. 2014;32(12):1242–8 [c].

[12] Voso MT, Niscola P, Piciocchi A, et al. Standard dose and prolonged administration of azacitidine are associated with improved efficacy in a real-world group of patients with myelodysplastic syndrome or low blast count acute myeloid leukemia. Eur J Haematol. 2015; http://dx.doi.org/10.1111/ejh.12595. Epub ahead of print. [c].

[13] Kuroda J, Shimura Y, Mizutani S, et al. Azacitidine-associated acute interstitial pneumonitis. Intern Med. 2014;53(11):1165–9 [A].

[14] Passweg JR, Pabst T, Blum S, et al. Azacytidine for acute myeloid leukemia in elderly or frail patients: a phase II trial (SAKK 30/07). Leuk Lymphoma. 2014;55(1):87–91 [c].

[15] Falantes J, Delgado RG, Calderon-Cabrera C, et al. Multivariable time-dependent analysis of the impact of azacitidine in patients with lower-risk myelodysplastic syndrome and unfavorable specific lower-risk score. Leuk Res. 2015;39(1):52–7 [c].

[16] Trickett HB, Cumpston A, Craig M. Azacitidine-associated Sweet's syndrome. Am J Health Syst Pharm. 2012;69(10):869–71 [A].

[17] Kim IH, Youn JH, Shin SH, et al. Neutrophilic panniculitis following azacitidine treatment for myelodysplastic syndromes. Leuk Res. 2012;36(7):e146–8 [A].

[18] Niscola P, Tendas A, Cupelli L, et al. Necrotizing fasciitis in myelodysplastic syndrome: an exceptionally rare occurrence. Support Care Cancer. 2013;21(2):365–6 [A].

[19] Tseng E, Alhusayen R, Sade S, et al. Pyoderma gangrenosum secondary to azacitidine in myelodysplastic syndrome. Br J Haematol. 2015;169:461 [A].

[20] Galmarini CM, Mackey JR, Dumontet C. Nucleoside analogues: mechanisms of drug resistance and reversal strategies. Leukemia. 2001;15(6):875–90 [R].

[21] Cytarabine. DrugPoint Summary. Micromedex 2.0. Truven Health Analytics, Inc. Greenwood Village, CO. Available at: http://www.micromedexsolutions.com. Accessed 2015 July 07. Last Modified 2015 June 16.

[22] Fiegl M, Unterhalt M, Kern W, et al. Chemomodulation of sequential high-dose cytarabine by fludarabine in relapsed or refractory acute myeloid leukemia: a randomized trial of the AMLCG. Leukemia. 2013;28(5):1001–7. http://dx.doi.org/10.1038/leu.2013.297 [C].

[23] Wolach O, Itchaki G, Bar-Natan M, et al. High-dose cytarabine as salvage therapy for relapsed or refractory acute myeloid leukemia—is more better or more of the same. Hematol Oncol. 2015; http://dx.doi.org/10.1002/hon.2191. Epub ahead of print. [c].

[24] Bauman S, Huseynov A, Goranova D, et al. Takotsubo cardiomyopathy after severe consolidation therapy with high-dose intravenous cytarabine in a patient with acute myeloid leukemia. Oncol Res Treat. 2014;37:487–90 [A].

[25] Mayer RJ, Davis RB, Schiffer CA, et al. Intensive postremission chemotherapy in adults with acute myeloid leukemia. Cancer and Leukemia Group B. N Engl J Med. 1994;331(14):896–903 [C].

[26] Zhang W, Ding Y, Wu H, et al. Retrospective comparison of fludarabine in combination with intermediate-dose cytarabine versus high-dose cytarabine as consolidation therapies for acute myeloid leukemia. Medicine (Baltimore). 2014;93(27):e134 [c].

[27] Peyrl A, Sauermann R, Chocholous M, et al. Pharmacokinetics and toxicity of intrathecal liposomal cytarabine in children and adolescents following age-adapted dosing. Clin Pharmacokinet. 2014;53(2):165–73 [c].

[28] Ozkan A, Apak H, Celkan T, et al. Toxic epidermal necrolysis after the use of high-dose cytosine arabinoside. Pediatr Dermatol. 2001;18(1):38–40 [A].

[29] Andersson BS, Cogan BM, Keating MJ, et al. Subacute pulmonary failure complicating therapy with high-dose Ara-C in acute leukemia. Cancer. 1985;56(9):2181–4 [c].

[30] Decitabine. DrugPoint Summary. Micromedex 2.0. Truven Health Analytics, Inc. Greenwood Village, CO. Available at: http://www.micromedexsolutions.com. Accessed 2015 July 09. Last Modified 2015 June 11.

[31] Gore SD, Jones C, Kirkpatrick P. Decitabine. Nat Rev Drug Discov. 2006;5(11):891–2 [E].

[32] Baylin SB. DNA methylation and gene silencing in cancer. Nat Clin Pract Oncol. 2005;2(Suppl 1):S4–S11 [E].

[33] De C, Phookan J, Parikh V, et al. Decitabine induced transient cardiomyopathy: a case report. Clin Med Insights Oncol. 2012;6:325–9 [A].

[34] Jabbour E, Kantarjian H, O'Brien S, et al. Retrospective analysis of prognostic factors associated with response and overall survival by baseline marrow blast percentage in patients with myelodysplastic syndromes treated with decitabine. Clin Lymphoma Myeloma Leuk. 2013;13(5):592–6 [M].

[35] Tawbi HA, Beumer JH, Tarhini AA, et al. Safety and efficacy of decitabine in combination with temozolomide in metastatic melanoma: a phase I/II study and pharmacokinetic analysis. Ann Oncol. 2013;24(4):1112–9 [C].

[36] Garcia-Manero G, Jabbour E, Borthakur G, et al. Randomized open-label phase II study of decitabine in patients with low- or intermediate-risk myelodysplastic syndromes. J Clin Oncol. 2013;31(20):2548–53 [C].

[37] Zhao WH, Zeng QC, Huang BT, et al. Decitabine plus thalidomide yields more sustained survival rates than decitabine monotherapy for risk-tailored elderly patients with myelodysplastic syndrome. Leuk Res. 2015;39(4):424–8 [c].

[38] Curran MP. Decitabine: a review of its use in older patients with acute myeloid leukaemia. Drugs Aging. 2013;30(6):447–58 [R].

[39] Phillips CL, Davies SM, McMasters R, et al. Low dose decitabine in very high risk relapsed or refractory acute myeloid leukaemia in children and young adults. Br J Haematol. 2013;161(3):406–10 [c].

[40] Garrido-Laguna I, McGregor KA, et al. A phase I/II study of decitabine in combination with panitumumab in patients with wild-type (wt) KRAS metastatic colorectal cancer. Invest New Drugs. 2013;31(5):1257–64 [c].

[41] Ng ES, Aw DC, Tan KB, et al. Neutrophilic eccrine hidradenitis associated with decitabine. Leuk Res. 2009;34(5):e130–2 [A].

[42] Glasspool RM, Brown R, Gore ME, et al. A randomised, phase II trial of the DNA-hypomethylating agent 5-aza-2'-deoxycytidine (decitabine) in combination with carboplatin vs carboplatin alone in patients with recurrent, partially platinum-sensitive ovarian cancer. Br J Cancer. 2014;110(8):1923–9 [c].

[43] Liesveld JL, O'Dwyer K, Walker A, et al. A phase I study of decitabine and rapamycin in relapsed/refractory AML. Leuk Res. 2013;37(12):1622–7 [c].

[44] Rougier P, Riess H, Manges R, et al. Randomised, placebo-controlled, double-blind, parallel-group phase III study evaluating aflibercept in patients receiving first-line treatment with gemcitabine for metastatic pancreatic cancer. Eur J Cancer. 2013;49(12):2633–42 [C].

[45] Khan MF, Gottesman S, Boyella R, et al. Gemcitabine-induced cardiomyopathy: a case report and review of the literature. J Med Case Reports. 2014;8:220 [A].

[46] Contreras-Steyls M, Lopez-Navarro N, Gallego E, et al. Gemcitabine therapy-associated cutaneous vasculitis with a polyarteritis nodosa-like pattern. Int J Dermatol. 2013;52:1019–32 [A].

[47] Eyre TA, Gooding S, Patel I, et al. Gemcitabine-induced large vessel vasculitis demonstrated by PET CT: a rare, important side effect. Int J Hematol. 2014;99:798–800.

[48] Trouilloud I, Dupont-Gossard AC, Malka D, et al. Fixed-dose rate gemcitabine alone or alternating with FOLFIRI.3 (irinotecan, leucovorin and fluorouracil) in the first-line treatment of patients with metastatic pancreatic adenocarcinoma: an AGEO randomised phase II study (FIRGEM). Eur J Cancer. 2014;50(18):3116–24 [c].

[49] Li Q, Yuan Z, Yan H, et al. Comparison of gemcitabine combined with targeted agent therapy versus gemcitabine monotherapy in the management of advanced pancreatic cancer. Clin Ther. 2014;36(7):1054–63 [M].

[50] Crombag MR, DeVries Schultink AHM, et al. Incidence of hematologic toxicity in older adults treated with gemcitabine or a gemcitabine-containing regimen in routine clinical practice: a multicenter retrospective cohort study. Drugs Aging. 2014;31:737–47 [C].

[51] Leal F, Macedo LT, Carvalheira JB. Gemcitabine-related thrombotic microangiopathy: a single-centre retrospective series. J Chemother. 2014;26(3):169–72 [C].

[52] Richmond J, Gilbar P, Abro E. Gemcitabine-induced thrombotic microangiopathy. Intern Med J. 2013;43:1240–2 [A].

[53] Lee HW, Chung MJ, Kang H, et al. Gemcitabine-induced hemolytic uremic syndrome in pancreatic cancer: a case report and review of the literature. Gut Liver. 2014;8:109–12 [A].

[54] Held-Warmkessel J. Gemcitabine-associated thrombotic thrombocytopenic purpura and hemolytic uremic syndrome. Oncol Nurs Forum. 2014;41:551–3 [A].

[55] Yamada Y, Suzuki K, Nobata H, et al. Gemcitabine-induced hemolytic uremic syndrome mimicking scleroderma renal crisis presenting with Raynaud's phenomenon, positive antinuclear antibodies and hypertensive emergency. Intern Med. 2014;53:445–8 [A].

[56] Hong JY, Nam EM, Lee J, et al. Randomized double-blinded, placebo-controlled phase II trial of simvastatin and gemcitabine in advanced pancreatic cancer patients. Cancer Chemother Pharmacol. 2014;73(1):125–30 [c].

[57] Yang F, Li X, Chen KZ, et al. Tolerability and toxicity of adjuvant cisplatin and gemcitabine for treating non-small cell lung cancer. Chin Med J (Engl). 2013;126(11):2087–91 [c].

[58] Sudo K, Ishihara T, Hirata N, et al. Randomized controlled study of gemcitabine plus S-1 combination chemotherapy versus gemcitabine for unresectable pancreatic cancer. Cancer Chemother Pharmacol. 2014;73(2):389–96 [c].

[59] Shukuya T, Takahashi T, Imai H, et al. Comparison of cisplatin plus pemetrexed and cisplatin plus gemcitabine for the treatment of malignant pleural mesothelioma in Japanese patients. Respir Investig. 2014;52(2):101–6 [c].

[60] Bergmann L, Maute L, Heil G, et al. A prospective randomised phase-II trial with gemcitabine versus gemcitabine plus sunitinib in advanced pancreatic cancer: a study of the CESAR Central European Society for Anticancer Drug Research-EWIV. Eur J Cancer. 2015;51(1):27–36 [c].

[61] Osumi H, Ozaka M, Ishii H, et al. Severe ischemic colitis after treatment of bile-duct cancer using gemcitabine and cisplatin. Jpn J Clin Oncol. 2015;45(4):402–3 [A].

[62] Chanpanitkitchot S, Tangjitgamol S, Khunnarong J, et al. Treatment outcomes of gemcitabine in refractory or recurrent epithelial ovarian cancer patients. Asian Pac J Cancer Prev. 2014;15(13):5215–21 [c].

[63] Malka D, Cervera P, Foulon S, et al. Gemcitabine and oxaliplatin with or without cetuximab in advanced biliary-tract cancer (BINGO): a randomised, open-label, non-comparative phase 2 trial. Lancet Oncol. 2014;15(8):819–28 [c].

[64] Wiznia LE, Subtil A, Choi JN. Subacute cutaneous lupus erythematosus induced by chemotherapy. JAMA Dermatol. 2013;149:1071–5 [A].

[65] George J, De D, Mahajan R. Acute generalized exanthematous pustulosis caused by gemcitabine. Int J Dermatol. 2014;53:e158–239 [A].

[66] Sheyman AT, Wald KJ, Pahk P, et al. Gemcitabine associated retinopathy and nephropathy. Retin Cases Brief Rep. 2014;8:107–9 [A].

[67] Spielmann L, Messer L, Moreau P, et al. Gemcitabine-induced myopathy. Semin Arthritis Rheum. 2014;43:784–91 [A].

[68] Graf SW, Limaye VS, Cleland LG. Gemcitabine-induced radiation recall myositis in a patient with dermatomyositis. Int J Rheum Dis. 2014;17:696–7 [A].

[69] Conroy T, Galais MP, Raoul JL, et al. Definitive chemoradiotherapy with FOLFOX versus fluorouracil and cisplatin in patients with oesophageal cancer (PRODIGE5/ACCORD17): final results of a randomised, phase 2/3 trial. Lancet Oncol. 2014;15(3):305–14 [c].

[70] Delbaldo C, Serin D, Mousseau M, et al. A phase III adjuvant randomised trial of 6 cycles of 5-fluorouracil-epirubicine-cyclophosphamide (FEC100) versus 4 FEC 100 followed by 4 Taxol (FEC-T) in node positive breast cancer patients (Trial B2000). Eur J Cancer. 2014;50(1):23–30 [C].

[71] Suarez Martinez-Falero B, Gillmore R. A rare cause of susceptibility to neutropenic sepsis in a patient with metastatic pancreas cancer. BMJ Case Rep. 2014; http://dx.doi.org/10.1136/bcr-2013-202040. pii: bcr2013202040 [A].

[72] Kinno R, Kii Y, Uchiyama M, et al. 5-fluorouracil-induced leukoencephalopathy with acute stroke-like presentation fulfilling criteria for recombinant tissue plasminogen activator therapy. J Stroke Cerebrovasc Dis. 2014;23(2):387–9 [A].

[73] Korgavkar K, Firoz EF, Xiong M, et al. Measuring the severity of topical 5-fluorouracil toxicity. J Cutan Med Surg. 2014;18(4):229–35 [C].

[74] Maughan C, Lear W. Acute angioedema response to topical 5-fluorouracil therapy. Dermatol Online J. 2013;19:13 [A].

[75] Komatsu M, Shiono O, Taguchi T, et al. Concurrent chemoradiotherapy with docetaxel, cisplatin and 5-fluorouracil (TPF) in patients with locally advanced squamous cell carcinoma of the head and neck. Jpn J Clin Oncol. 2014;44(5):416–21 [c].

[76] Yoney A, Isikli L. Preoperative chemoradiation in locally advanced rectal cancer: a comparison of bolus 5-fluorouracil/leucovorin and capecitabine. Saudi J Gastroenterol. 2014;20(2):102–7.

[77] Ransom D, Wilson K, Fournier M, et al. Final results of Australasian Gastrointestinal Trials Group ARCTIC study: an audit of raltitrexed for patients with cardiac toxicity induced by fluoropyrimidines. Ann Oncol. 2014;25(1):117–21 [c].

[78] Rateesh S, Luis SA, Luis CR, et al. Myocardial infarction secondary to 5-fluorouracil: not an absolute contraindication to rechallenge? Int J Cardiol. 2014;172(2):e331–3 [c].

[79] Lestuzzi C, Vaccher E, Talamini R, et al. Effort myocardial ischemia during chemotherapy with 5-fluorouracil: an underestimated risk. Ann Oncol. 2014;25(5):1059–64 [A].

[80] Ozturk MA, Ozveren O, Cinar V, et al. Takotsubo syndrome: an underdiagnosed complication of 5-fluorouracil mimicking acute myocardial infarction. Blood Coagul Fibrinolysis. 2012;24:90–4 [A].

[81] Saif MW, Garcon MC, Rodriguez G, et al. Bolus 5-fluorouracil as an alternative in patients with cardiotoxicity associated with infusional 5-fluorouracil and capecitabine: a case series. In Vivo. 2013;27:531–4 [c].

[82] Hong YS, Nam BH, Kim KP, et al. Oxaliplatin, fluorouracil, and leucovorin versus fluorouracil and leucovorin as adjuvant chemotherapy for locally advanced rectal cancer after preoperative chemoradiotherapy (ADORE): an open-label, multicentre, phase 2, randomised controlled trial. Lancet Oncol. 2014;15(11):1245–53 [C].

[83] Kaufman PA, Awada A, Twelves C, et al. Phase III open-label randomized study of eribulin mesylate versus capecitabine in patients with locally advanced or metastatic breast cancer previously treated with an anthracycline and a taxane. J Clin Oncol. 2015;33(6):594–601 [C].

[84] Mita MM, Joy AA, Mita A, et al. Randomized phase II trial of the cyclin-dependent kinase inhibitor dinaciclib (MK-7965) versus capecitabine in patients with advanced breast cancer. Clin Breast Cancer. 2014;14(3):169–76 [c].

[85] Schwartzberg LS, Wang G, Somer BG, et al. Phase II trial of fulvestrant with metronomic capecitabine for postmenopausal women with hormone receptor-positive, HER2-negative metastatic breast cancer. Clin Breast Cancer. 2014;14(1):13–9 [c].

[86] Baden LR. Loss of fingerprints. N Engl J Med. 2015;372:16 [A].

[87] Walker G, Lane N, Parekh P. Photosensitive lichenoid drug eruption to capecitabine. J Am Acad Dermatol. 2014;71(2):e52–3 [A].

[88] Chen FW, Zhou X, Egbert BM, et al. Dermatomyositis associated with capecitabine in the setting of malignancy. J Am Acad Dermatol. 2014;70(2):e47–8 [A].

[89] Wang X, Jin J, Li YX, et al. Phase I study of postoperative radiotherapy combined with capecitabine for gastric cancer. World J Gastroenterol. 2014;20(4):1067–73 [A].

[90] Chao Y, Hsieh JS, Yeh HT, et al. A multicenter phase II study of biweekly capecitabine in combination with oxaliplatin as first-line chemotherapy in patients with locally advanced or metastatic gastric cancer. Cancer Chemother Pharmacol. 2014;73(4):799–806 [c].

[91] Sideris S, Loizidou A, Georgala A, et al. Autoimmune haemolytic anaema in a patient treated with capecitabine. Acta Clin Belg. 2013;68:135–7 [A].

[92] Shaaban H, Downs E, Shakouri P, et al. A rare case of non-immune hemolytic anemia in a patient with metastatic breast cancer treated with capecitabine. Med Oncol. 2013;30:321 [A].

[93] Ryu MH, Yoo C, Kim JG, et al. Multicenter phase II study of trastuzumab in combination with capecitabine and oxaliplatin for advanced gastric cancer. Eur J Cancer. 2015;51(4):482–8 [c].

[94] Smorenburg CH, de Groot SM, van Leeuwen-Stok AE, et al. A randomized phase III study comparing pegylated liposomal doxorubicin with capecitabine as first-line chemotherapy in elderly patients with metastatic breast cancer: results of the OMEGA study of the Dutch Breast Cancer Research Group BOOG. Ann Oncol. 2014;25(3):599–605 [c].

[95] Maggo G, Grover SC, Grin A. Capecitabine induced colitis. Pathol Res Pract. 2014;210(9):606–8 [A].

[96] Herbertson RA, Tebbutt NC, Lee FT, et al. Targeted chemoradiation in metastatic colorectal cancer: a phase I trial of 131I-huA33 with concurrent capecitabine. J Nucl Med. 2014;55(4):534–9 [c].

[97] a Dzaye OD, Cleator S, Nihoyannopoulos P. Acute coronary artery thrombosis and vasospasm following capecitabine in conjunction with oxaliplatin treatment for cancer. BMJ Case Rep. 2014; http://dx.doi.org/10.1136/bcr-2014-205567. pii: bcr2014205567 [A].

[98] Klag T, Cantara G, Ong P, et al. Epicardial coronary artery spasm as cause of capecitabine-induced takotsuo cardiomyopathy. Clin Res Cardiol. 2014;103:247–50 [A].

[99] Y-Hassan S, Tornvall P, Tornerud M, et al. Capecitabine caused cardiogenic shock through induction of global takotsubo syndrome. Cardiovasc Revasc Med. 2013;14:57–61 [A].

[100] Zhang X, Cao C, Zhang Q, et al. Comparison of the efficacy and safety of S-1-based and capecitabine-based regimens in gastrointestinal cancer: a meta-analysis. PLoS One. 2014;9(1):e84230 [M].

[101] Northfelt DW, Allred JB, Liu H, et al. Phase 2 trial of paclitaxel polyglumex with capecitabine for metastatic breast cancer. Am J Clin Oncol. 2014;37(2):167–71 [c].

[102] Lyros E, Walter S, Keller I, et al. Subacute reversible toxic encephalopathy related to treatment with capecitabine: a case report with literature review and discussion of pathophysiology. Neurotoxicology. 2014;42:8–11 [A].

[103] Ko JH, Hseih CI, Chou CY, et al. Capecitabine-induced subacute cutaneous lupus erythematosus: report of a case with positive rechallenge test. J Dermatol. 2013;40:939–40 [A].

[104] Kindem S, LLombart B, Requena C, et al. Subacute cutaneous lupus erythematosus after treatment with capecitabine. J Dermatol. 2013;40:75–6 [A].

45

Radiological Contrast Agents and Radiopharmaceuticals

Makoto Hasegawa, Tatsuya Gomi[1]

Department of Radiology, Ohashi Medical Center, Toho University, Tokyo, Japan
[1]Corresponding author: gomi@oha.toho-u.ac.jp

Introduction

Contrast agents are widely used in clinical practice to improve diagnostic performance of medical imaging. Various types of contrast agents exist; iodinated contrast agents which absorb more X-rays than human tissue are used for radiographic examinations such as computed tomography (CT), gadolinium based agents which have T1 relaxation time shortening effects are used for magnetic resonance imaging (MRI), and microbubbles which have a higher echogenicity compared to human tissue are used for ultrasound (US). Although these agents are indispensable in medical imaging, they are not risk free.

Adverse reactions to contrast agents can be classified as acute, late and very late by the timing of the reaction after administration of the agent. Acute reactions can be categorized as allergic-like or physiological by the type of reaction, and mild, moderate, or severe by the severity. Adverse reactions may affect various organ systems. Recent publications which cover various aspects of adverse reactions to contrast agents will be discussed in this chapter, including contrast induced nephropathy (CIN) and gadolinium accumulation.

Water-Soluble Intravascular Iodinated Contrast Agents [SEDA-33, 963; SEDA-34, 749; SEDA-35, 863; SEDA-36, 695]

There are four types of iodinated water-soluble contrast media, classified according to their physicochemical properties (Table 1). They are mainly used intravascularly, but can also be injected into body cavities, particularly the low-osmolar contrast agents. Some are also used for oral or rectal administration, and the high-osmolar water-soluble contrast agent diatrizoate is suitable only

for these purposes. Non-ionic agents can be used intrathecally for myelograms. Low osmolar and iso-osmolar iodinated contrast media have almost completely replaced high osmolar agents for intravascular use and administration into body cavities.

DRUG INTERACTIONS

Metformin, a biguanide oral antihyperglycaemic agent, is used to treat patients with noninsulin dependent diabetes mellitus. Metformin is thought to act by decreasing hepatic glucose production and enhancing peripheral glucose uptake as a result of increased sensitivity of peripheral tissues to insulin.

The most significant adverse effect of metformin therapy is the potential for the development of metformin-associated lactic acidosis in the susceptible patient. In the presence of certain comorbidities, which lead to decreased metabolism of lactate or increased anaerobic metabolism, *metformin should be discontinued at the time of an examination or procedure using IV iodinated contrast media.* Ideally, it should be withheld for 48 hours and administration can resume after reassessment of renal function [1M].

Types of Reactions

Adverse reactions that occur after contrast media injection typically occur within 20 minutes of the injection. An acute adverse reaction is an adverse reaction that occurs within 1 hour of injection. Acute reactions are classified as being of mild, moderate, and severe intensity. Types of reactions include mild symptoms such as nausea and itching and severe reactions such as hypotensive shock

© 2015 Elsevier B.V. All rights reserved.

TABLE 1 List of Few Iodinated Water-Soluble Contrast Media

Properties	Examples (INNs)	Brand names
High-osmolar ionic monomers	Diatrizoate	Angiografin, Hypaque, Gastrografin, Renografin, Urografin
	Iotalamic acid	Conray
	Ioxitalamic acid	Telebrix
	Metrizoate	Isopaque, Triosil
Low-osmolar ionic dimers	Ioxaglic acid	Hexabrix
Low-osmolar non-ionic monomers	Iobitridol	Xenetrix
	Iohexol	Omnipaque
	Iomeprol	Iomeron
	Iopamidol	Isovue, Niopam, Solutrast
	Iopentol	Imagopaque
	Iopromide	Ultravist
	Ioversol	Optiray
	Metrizamide	Amipaque
Iso-osmolar non-ionic dimers	Iodixanol	Visipaque
	Iosimenol	Iosmin
	Iotrolan	Isovist

and convulsions. A late adverse reaction to contrast medium is defined as a reaction that occurs at 1 hour to 1 week after injection. Maculopapular rashes, erythema, and pruritus are the commonest types of late reactions. A very late adverse reaction is a reaction that occurs at more than 1 week after contrast injection; this includes reactions such as thyrotoxicosis [2M]. The overall incidence of acute adverse reactions to low osmolar iodinated contrast media has been reported to be very low [1M].

The incidence of adverse reactions has previously been reported to be different among various low osmolar non-ionic contrast agents [3C]. A review of 59 915 individual case safety reports found 415 (0.7%) suspected adverse reactions to contrast media which included 44 serious cases. Hypersensitivity reactions were reported in the majority of cases. The contrast media with the highest number of reports were iohexol (40.7%), iomeprol (17.8%), iopamidol (12%) and diatrizoate (12%) [4C]. A study comparing iopromide and iomeprol found that iomeprol had a higher incidence in adverse reactions. The study included 62 539 CT scans and 10 348 urography scans using iopromide, and 34 308 CT scans and 2846 urography scans using iomeprol. 154 cases of reactions were reported for iopromide and 86 for iomeprol, being severe in 10 (6.5%) patients for iopromide vs 17 (19.8%) patients for iomeprol. A statistically significant difference was seen between the agents ($p < 0.003$), with adverse reactions being more severe for iomeprol [5C]. A study

comparing the safety profile of seven types of iodinated contrast media (iopromide, iohexol, iopamidol, iomeprol, ioversol, iobitridol, iodixanol) evaluated 6524 reports submitted to 15 Regional Pharmacovigilance Centers in Korea related to adverse events of contrast media. The study found that iopromide (45.5%), iohexol (16.9%), iopamidol (14.3%) and iomeprol (10.3%) were frequently reported contrast media. In the analysis of adverse reactions by organ class, platelet, bleeding and clotting disorders and urinary system disorders were more frequently reported for iodixanol than the other contrast media. The authors of this study suggest that the safety profiles of iodinated contrast media are significantly different [6C]. A meta-analysis investigating the difference of risk of cardiovascular events for iso-osmolar contrast agent (iodixanol) compared to low osmolar contrast agents found no statistical difference in the incidence of cardiovascular events [7M].

Salivary Glands

Iodide mumps is a rare adverse reaction after administration of iodinated contrast agents. Painless bilateral enlargements of the salivary glands are seen after administration of contrast agents. It is speculated to be due to accumulation of high concentration of iodine in the ductal system, which induces inflammation. Prognosis is reported to be good with conservative treatment alone

[8A,9A]. A case of iodide parotitis in a 51-year-old male patient has been reported after administration of iopamidol-370 during carotid artery stenting [10A]. Another case report suggested a 78-year-old male patient with a medical history of hypertension, chronic renal insufficiency, diabetes mellitus and hypothyroidism, who underwent contrast enhanced CT with iopromide experienced symptoms of iodide mumps and simultaneous neutrophilic dermatosis [11A].

Endocrine

Thyrotoxicosis is a type of very late adverse reaction seen after iodine-based contrast media exposure. Untreated Graves' disease and multinodular goiter and thyroid autonomy are risks for this adverse reaction. Patients with hyperthyroidism are usually advised not to have iodinated contrast media injection. Patients with normal thyroid function are thought to be at low risk for this condition [2M,12R,13R]. Yet, the iodine content in a usual dose of contrast media is very high compared to the recommended daily intake of iodine [14R], and hyperthyroidism from Wolf–Chaikoff effect as well as hypothyroidism from Jod-Basedow phenomenon may occur. A nested case–control study found an association between contrast media exposure and incident hyperthyroidism (thyrotropin level, at follow-up, below the normal range), incident overt hyperthyroidism (follow-up thyrotropin level ≤ 0.1 mIU/l), and incident hypothyroidism (thyrotropin level above the normal range). No association was found for incident overt hypothyroidism (follow-up thyrotropin level >10 mIU/l). The investigators of this study suggest that physicians should be aware of potential thyroidal complications associated with contrast medium administration [15C]. A prospective study investigating the effect of iodinated contrast media in 101 euthyroid patients undergoing coronary angiography compared free triiodothyronine (free T3), free thyroxine (free T4), and thyrotropin (TSH) before, 4 and 8 weeks after administration of iopromide. The study found that TSH levels showed significant decrease at 4 and 8 weeks compared to baseline level. Seven (6.9%) patients had subclinical hyperthyroidism at 4 weeks, and six (5.9%) patients had subclinical hyperthyroidism at 8 weeks. No patients developed overt or subclinical hypothyroidism [16c].

Cardiovascular

Cardiovascular adverse reactions from contrast agents such as angioedema, various types of arrhythmias, and hypotension have been reported. A case of a type 1 Brugada ECG unmasked by intracoronary contrast media administration has been reported in a 48-year-old patient who complained chest discomfort was found with ST segment elevation at his ambulance electrocardiograph. ST segment deviation was noted after injection of contrast medium (Omnipaque) [17A]. The exact cause is not known, but other substances are known to unmask Brugada ECG changes as well [18R,19r].

Skin

The most frequent delayed adverse reaction after contrast media administration is allergic-like and cutaneous [1M].

Iododerma is a type of halogenoderma in which cutaneous reactions occur after exposure to iodides. Some causes include iodine-131 treatment for hyperthyroidism and topical povidone–iodine [20c,21A]. These conditions have also been previously reported after administration of iodinated contrast agents [22A,23A]. Cases of iododerma have typically been reported in patients with renal insufficiency, such as a case of iododerma in a 60-year-old male patient after administration of ioversol, iohexol, and iodixanol [24A]. Yet, iododerma may occur in patients with relatively unimpaired renal function such as a case of iododerma in a 81-year-old female after administration of iodixanol [25A].

Allergic reactions to drugs usually do not occur on exposure to a single drug dose, and requires multiple doses during a sensitization phase. However, hypersensitivity reactions have been known to occur after the first exposure to contrast agents. A report described five patients who developed maculopapular exanthemas within 5–10 days after administration of a contrast agent for the first time. Monosensitization was found in 3 patients, and cross sensitization in 2 patients as evidenced by positive skin tests [26r].

Hematologic

Effects of contrast media on hemolysis have previously been reported to be low [27E,28E,29E]. A recent report suggests that some contrast media may alter erythrocyte morphology, and induce hemolysis *in vitro* [30E].

Immunologic

Anaphylactic reactions to contrast media in most cases are not IgE-mediated (in other words they are what used to be called "anaphylactoid", now called non-IgE-mediated anaphylactic reactions), and they may occur without previous sensitization. Nor do they occur consistently in patients who have had previous reactions to contrast media.

Radiation

Radiation dose increase in iodine-charged tissue has been previously reported in *in vitro* and *in vivo* experiments [31E,32E,33E]. This may result in induction of DNA double-strand break induction [34E]. An investigation evaluating this effect in contrast enhanced CT has calculated that radiation dose may increase in some organs compared to non-contrast enhanced CT [35c]. This effect was also demonstrated in a study of 62 patients who underwent CT cardiac examinations [36c].

Radiation recall is a rare clinical syndrome characterized by an acute inflammatory reaction at the site of prior radiation exposure. It is precipitated by the use of triggering agents, most commonly chemotherapeutic agents [37R,38A,39A,40R]. A case suspected of radiation recall precipitated by iodinated nonionic contrast media has been reported. The case was a 63-year-old woman with a previous history of adverse reaction to iodinated contrast media, penicillins and sulfa drugs who was diagnosed with breast cancer. The patient received neoadjuvant chemotherapy and mastectomy, and completed postmastectomy radiation, and also underwent contrast enhanced CT 7 weeks, 18 weeks and 2 years after radiation therapy for various reasons. The patient developed well demarcated erythema in the distribution of radiated areas after these scans which were suspected to be radiation recall dermatitis precipitated by the contrast media injections [41A].

Iodinated Radiocontrast-Induced Nephropathy

Contrast-induced nephropathy (CIN) is defined as renal hypofunction with an increase in the serum creatinine (SCr) concentration of 25% or more, or by 44 μmol/l (0.5 mg/dl) or more, and developing within 3 days after injection of an intravascular contrast medium in the absence of other causes.

Prevalence

The prevalence of CIN has been found to be as high as the third most common cause of acute kidney injury (AKI) in hospital acquired AKI [42c].

A study of 998 contrast enhanced CT in patients investigated the association of low osmolality iodinated contrast media. 58 patients were found to be at risk for CIN. Of the 58 patients at risk, two patients had CIN. The number of patients at risk, as well as the incidence of CIN was low [43]. Five hundred thirty-six patients underwent contrast enhanced CT with intravenous contrast media (Iohexol for patients with serum creatinine (SCr) less than 1.5 mg/dl and Iodixanol for those with SCr 1.5–2.0 mg/dl). The overall incidence of CIN was 15.3% (17 out of 111 patients). The results demonstrated that risk factors such as advanced age, diabetes mellitus (DM) and hypertension seems to predispose patients to CIN rather than abnormal baseline SCr [44C]. A study of 323 patients who underwent primary percutaneous coronary intervention investigated the incidence of CIN. All patients received iso-osmolar, nonionic contrast agent iodixanol. CIN occurred in 23 female and 26 male patients (25.0% vs 11.2%, p = 0.003). At multivariable analysis, reduced left ventricular ejection fraction (LVEF) (odds ratio [OR] 7.32 95% confidence interval [CI]: 2.60–21, p < 0.001) and female gender (OR 2.49 95% CI 1.22–5.07, p = 0.01) predicted CIN, whereas the occurrence of CIN (hazard ratio [HR] 3.65 95% CI 1.55–8.59, p = 0.003) and a Mehran risk score (MRS) ≥6 (HR 1.76 95% CI 1.13–2.74, p = 0.01) independently predicted long-term mortality [45c]. 423 contrast enhanced CT patients were included in a study to evaluate the role of inflammation in CIN. The patients were injected with intravenous contrast media (non-ionic iso-osmolar 350 mg/ml contrast media). Of these, 215 patients had elevated CRP and 208 normal CRP values. The incidence of CIN was 9.92%. Of the patients with inflammation, 29 (13.5%; CI, 8.90–18.07) developed CIN, while 13 (6.25%; CI, 2.96–9.54) of those without inflammation developed CIN [46c]. A study of 100 consecutive patients with stable CKD stages 2–4 who underwent coronary angiography found that the frequency of CIN was 11% (11 of 100), and 1 patient required dialysis. Serum NGAL increased ≥25% from baseline at 24 hours in 7 patients with CIN (p = 0.04). Serum CysC increased ≥25% from baseline at 24 hours in 4 patients with CIN (p = 0.008). Changes in serum NGAL and serum CysC from baseline at 24 hours (D values) could diagnose CIN 24 hours earlier than with serum NGAL showing a superior performance [47c]. A study evaluating the risk of CIN of patients undergoing TACE included, one hundred forty-one patients treated undergoing 305 consecutive sessions of TACE. They received a total of 2000 ml of the electrolyte solutions on the day of the procedure. An additional 500 ml of the initial electrolyte solution was administered on the following day. CIN by the present definition was observed after 2.6% of the TACE sessions. TACE is a relatively safe procedure in terms of the risk of CIN under vigorous periprocedural hydration and that the incidence of CIN is comparable to that of AKI associated with intravenous CM administration [48c]. A total of 79 cases received a contrast media dose of 250 ml or greater while undergoing a neuroendovascular procedure. For the control group, 79 cases in patients who received a CM dose of 75–249 ml while undergoing a neuroendovascular procedure during the same time period were selected at random for comparison. No cases of CIN occurred in the control group. In the high-dose cohort, there were four cases (5%) of CIN. Risk of developing CIN is relatively low in patients who undergo neuroendovascular procedures with CM doses of 250 ml or greater [49C]. In a study which included 90 patients who were hospitalized with a diagnosis of cancer and underwent contrast-enhanced CT, CIN was detected in 18 (20%) of these patients. The incidence of CIN after CT in hospitalized oncological patients was 20%. CIN developed 4.5 times more frequently in patients with cancer who had *undergone recent chemotherapy. Hypertension and the combination of bevacizumab/irinotecan may be additional risk factors for CIN development [50c].*

Prevention

A total of 4297 patient records were included in a study to evaluate hydration protocols in patients at risk for CIN. The mean percentage of high-risk patients for CIN was 14.6%. The mean percentage high-risk patients hydrated before contrast administration was 68.5% and was constant over time. Large variation between individual hospitals confirmed the difference in hospitals in correctly applying the guideline for preventing CIN [51C]. A large number of papers described that high-dose rosuvastatin loading before percutaneous coronary intervention was associated with a significantly lower incidence of CIN in patients with acute coronary syndrome [52c,53c,54C].

Management of Adverse Reactions

In patients who are at risk for an adverse reaction (patients who previously had moderate or severe acute reaction to an iodine-based contrast agent, patients with asthma or any allergy requiring medical treatment), premedication should be considered.

In patients who have previously reacted to iodinated contrast media, European Society of Urogenital Radiology guidelines on contrast media suggest the use of a different agent. Although clinical evidence of premedication is limited, the use of prednisolone 30 mg or methylprednisolone 32 mg orally 2 and 12 hours before the contrast agent should be considered for patients at risk [2M].

Breakthrough reactions are adverse reactions that occur in spite of premedications such as oral steroids in patients at risk. A study investigating the efficacy of premedications included 198 contrast enhanced CTs in patients who underwent an oral steroid premedication protocol because of risk factors such as previous adverse reactions to contrast media, and bronchial asthma. The study found nine breakthrough reactions. Most reactions were mild, and no severe reactions were reported [55c]. Although the number of cases is small, the incidence of breakthrough reactions after premedications seems to be low.

Susceptibility Factors

Known risk factors for adverse reactions to contrast agents include causes such as previous allergy like reactions to contrast media, bronchial asthma, renal insufficiency, patients with thyroid disorders.

A study which included 13 565 CT scans performed in cancer patients found that the incidence of acute allergy-like adverse reactions was higher in cancer patients undergoing concomitant antineoplastic treatment using taxanes. Estimated odds ratio was 2.06, and 95% confidence interval was 1.02–4.16 for patients receiving taxanes compare to patients not receiving treatment [56C].

Another study investigated the time dependence between adverse reactions to contrast agents and chemotherapy administration. The study included 3945 contrast enhanced studies in 1878 patients. Patients were classified into 4 groups by the type of antineoplastic treatment: platinum based, taxane based, platinum plus taxane, and other group. The time elapsed from the date of CT to the date of last chemotherapy was analyzed. 40 acute adverse reactions (1.01%) were reported, but no time dependency was found for the risk of acute adverse reactions [57C].

Repeated administration of contrast agents may increase the incidence of adverse reactions as well as severity. A report investigated the effect of repeated administrations in 23 684 exposures administrations to contrast media in 1861 patients with hepatocellular carcinoma. Adverse reactions occurred in 196 (0.83%) of patients. Cumulative probabilities for overall immediate reactions at the 10th, 20th, and 30th contrast enhanced CT examinations were 7.9%, 15.2%, and 24.1%, respectively, showing an increase incidence with cumulative exposures. The study also found that estimated hazard for overall adverse reactions decrease until around the 10th exposure, and rose with subsequent exposures. In addition, renal impairment was found to be a risk factor for adverse reactions [58C]. Another report investigating clinical characteristics related with development of anaphylactic shock after administration of contrast agents, which included 104 cases of anaphylaxis, found that patients who developed anaphylactic shock had a more frequent exposure to contrast agents compared to those who did not develop hypotension ($p = 0.004$) [59c].

There have been few case reports of myasthenic crisis development after intravenous contrast media injection, mostly from high-osmolality iodinated contrast agents. A previous investigation found that a statistically significant increase in disease related symptoms was seen within 1 day of injection, but no difference after 2 days [60c]. A 79-year-old man who was admitted to a hospital for progressive dysphagia and weight loss received an injection of low osmolality iodinated contrast agent (Iohexol) at contrast enhanced CT. The patient developed acute respiratory failure 2 hours later. The patient was diagnosed with myasthenia gravis after the scan [61A]. The course of the patient was consistent with the previous report. Caution is needed in patients with myasthenia gravis receiving contrast agents, and premedication for these patients may be necessary.

Multiple myeloma has been reported to be a risk factor for renal failure after administration of high osmolar ionic contrast media. Yet, in nonionic low and iso-osmolar contrast media, patients with multiple myeloma with a normal creatinine level have a low risk for developing CIN. β2-Microglobulin levels were associated with CIN in a previous report [62c], but assessment of Bence Jones proteinuria seems to be unnecessary for the evaluation of risk of kidney failure [62c,63R].

Diagnosis

Currently, there is no good clinical mechanism to predict the occurrence of adverse reaction to iodinated contrast agents. Skin tests are known to have a limited sensitivity and high specificity for patients with hypersensitivity. Preliminary intradermal skin testing with contrast agents is not predictive of adverse reactions, may itself be dangerous, and is not recommended [64C,65C]. They may have a modest utility in retrospectively evaluating severe adverse reactions. *In vitro* tests, such as basophil activation test, lymphocyte transformation test, and lymphocyte activation test, have been reported to be useful in previous reactors. However, the sensitivity and specificity of these tests have not been firmly established.

In a study to identify clinical characteristic related with anaphylactic shock, skin tests were performed in 51 patients after development of contrast media induced anaphylaxis. Overall skin test positivity was 64.7% and 81.8% in patients with anaphylactic shock [59c].

A study which included 106 patients with history of previous immediate hypersensitivity reactions to contrast media (ioversol 33.9%, iopamidol 31.1%, iomeprol 3.8%, iohexol 2.8%, ioxaglate 0.9%, iobitridol 0.9%, and unknown 26.4%), found 11 patients to be positive for intradermal test with the agent which caused the reaction. One patient showed cross reactivity in skin test to other agents.

Of the 11 patients with positive intradermal tests, 5 patients underwent controlled challenge test, 2 patients underwent computed tomography with an alternative skin test negative agent with no adverse reactions [66].

An investigation using leukocyte migration test to evaluate patients suspected with contrast media allergies found that the positive rate was 44% which was lower than that of other type of drugs (74%), which suggests that the involvement allergic reactions is quite low. In leukocyte migration test positive patients, 76% of the reactions were skin reactions, and 18% was anaphylactic reactions [67c].

MRI CONTRAST MEDIA

Gadolinium Salts [SEDA-33, 968; SEDA-34, 754; SEDA-35, 866; SEDA-36, 701]

Contrast enhancement is obtained by the T1 relaxation time shortening characteristics of gadolinium (Gd). From the type of use, these agents can be categorized into extracellular fluid agents, blood pool agents, and organ specific agents. Extracellular gadolinium-based contrast agents can be categorized as non-ionic and ionic from their charge, and linear or macrocyclic structure. Blood pool agents can be categorized into albumin binding gadolinium complexes such as gadofosveset and gadocoletic acid, and polymeric gadolinium complexes such as gadomelitol. The gadolinium salts that are used as contrast media in magnetic resonance imaging (MRI) and that have been assigned International Non-proprietary Names (INNs) by the WHO are listed in Table 2.

TABLE 2 Gadolinium Salts that Have Been Used as Contrast Media in Magnetic Resonance Imaging

Name (INN)	Brand name	Charge	Structure
Gadobenic acid	Multihance	Ionic	Linear
Gadobutrol	Gadovist	Non-ionic	Macrocyclic
Gadocoletic acid			
Gadodenterate			
Gadodiamide	Omniscan	Non-ionic	Linear
Gadofosveset	Ablavar	Ionic	Linear
Gadomelitol	Vistarem		
Gadopenamide			
Gadopentetic acid	Magnevist	Ionic	Linear
Gadoteric acid	Dotarem	Ionic	Macrocyclic
Gadoteridol	Prohance	Non-ionic	Macrocyclic
Gadoversetamide	OptiMARK	Ionic	Linear
Gadoxetic acid	Eovist, Primovist	Ionic	Ionic

Gadolinium agents are considered to have no nephrotoxicity at approved dosages for MRI. Therefore, MR with gadolinium has been used instead of contrast-enhanced CT in those at risk for developing worse renal failure if exposed to iodinated contrast media.

Multiorgan Damage

Nephrogenic systemic fibrosis (NSF) is a multisystemic disease in patients with renal insufficiency. Administration of gadolinium based contrast agents, especially linear-structured agents, has been associated with the development of NSF (Table 3). After the restriction of gadolinium based agents in high risk patients in guidelines, the number of new cases has decreased sharply. *Yet, clinicians should continue to be cautious when administering gadolinium based contrast agents; patients should be screened for renal insufficiency prior to administration* [68R,69M,70C,71A].

There is no specific treatment for NSF. Improvement of skin lesions after recovery of renal function [72A] and response to therapeutic plasma exchange have previously been reported [73A].

Gadolinium Accumulation

In vitro investigations have found that the chemical stability of gadolinium contrast agents are different according to their structure, with macrocyclic chelates being the most stable, and non-ionic linear chelates the least stable. Ionic agents are more stable than non-ionic agents. Evidence of stability has been demonstrated in *in vivo* experiments which found evidence that more gadolinium retention is seen in animals administered with non-ionic linear agent gadodiamide than ionic linear agent gadopentetate dimeglumine. Very small amounts of gadolinium were retained after macrocyclic agent administration [74M].

Free gadolinium is toxic to tissues, and acts as an inorganic blocker of voltage-gated calcium channels [75M,76R,77E]. The retention of gadolinium has been previously reported in a rat model [78E], and in human bone tissue [79c]. A recent study of comparing 19 patients who underwent contrast enhanced MRI and 16 patients who underwent unenhanced MRI has found that high signal intensity is seen in the dentate nucleus and globus pallidus on unenhanced T1-weighted MRI, with relation to cumulative dose, which may suggest gadolinium accumulation in these areas [80c]. Another study assessed the association between the serial number of gadolinium enhanced MRI and signal hyperintensity of the dentate nucleus. The study included 38 patients with multiple sclerosis and 37 patients with brain metastases. The study found that the hyperintensity of the dentate nucleus on unenhanced T1 weighted images progressively increased [81c]. The accumulation of gadolinium in the dentate nucleus may vary between structures of the agent used. A study comparing the hyperintensity of the dentate nucleus on unenhanced T1 weighted images between linear and macrocyclic agents found that high intensity of the dentate nucleus had a strong association with previous administration of linear agents, while no association was found with macrocyclic agents [82c]. There is lack of information on the long-term effects of gadolinium retention in these areas. Yet, clinician should be aware of the accumulation, and caution may be necessary when using linear agents.

TABLE 3 Risks of Systemic Fibrosis from Gadolinium-Containing Salts

Name (INN)	Chelate	Charge	Structure	Risk
Gadodiamide	DTPA-BMA	Non-ionic	Linear	High (3–7%)
Gadopentetic acid	DTPA	Ionic	Linear	High (0.1–1%)
Gadoversetamide	DTPA-BMEA	Non-ionic	Linear	High
Gadobenic acid	BOPTA	Ionic	Linear	Intermediate
Gadofosveset	DTPA-DPCP	Ionic	Linear	Intermediate
Gadoxetic acid	EOB-DTPA	Ionic	Linear	Intermediate
Gadobutrol	BT-DO3A	Non-ionic	Cyclic	Low
Gadoteric acid	DOTA	Ionic	Cyclic	Low
Gadoteridol	HP-DO3A	Non-ionic	Cyclic	Low

DPTA, diethylene triamine penta-acetic acid; BMA, 5,8-bis(carboxymethyl)-11-[2-(methylamino)-2-oxoethyl]-3-oxo-2,5,8,11-tetra-azatridecan-13-oic acid; BMEA, N,N'-bis[methoxyethylamide]; BOPTA, benzyloxypropionic tetra-acetic-acid; DPCP, N,N'-bis[pyridoxal-5-phosphate]-*trans*-1,2-cyclohexyldiamine-N,N'-diacetic acid; EOB-DTPA, ethoxybenzyldiethylene triamine penta-acetic acid; BT-DO3A, 10-[2,3-dihydroxy-1-hydroxymethylpropyl]-1,4,7,10-tetra-azacyclododecane-1,4,7-triacetic acid; HP-DO3A, 10-[2-hydroxypropyl]-1,4,7-tetra-azacyclododecane-1,4,7-triacetic acid; DOTA, 1,4,7,10-tetra-azacyclododecane-N,N',N'',N'''-tetra-acetic acid

Observational Studies

A phase 3 efficacy and safety trial of gadobutrol confirmed the safety of profile of the agent. The study included 343 patients, out of which 14 patients (4.1%) experienced at least one adverse event that was considered to be drug-related and was consistent previously published literature. All treatment-related adverse events were not serious. The most common drug-related adverse event was nausea ($n = 6$ [1.7%]) [83S].

The incidence and severity was compared between 4 different gadolinium based contrast agents (gadopentetate dimeglumine, gadoteridol, gadoterate meglumine, and gadoxetate disodium). The study retrospectively reviewed 10595 consecutive patients (4343 female; 6252 male; mean age, 63.8 ± 14.0 years) who underwent contrast-enhanced MRI. The study found that the overall incidence of adverse reactions was 0.45% (48/10595); 45 reactions were mild and three were moderate. No severe reactions were found. The incidence of acute adverse reactions was not significantly different between the 4 agents, but somewhat higher with gadoxetate disodium (0.82%) [84C].The renal safety of meglumine gadoterate (Gd-DOTA) was assessed 114 patients with known stage 3 or 4 chronic kidney disease according to the Kidney Disease Improving Global Outcomes (KDIGO) definition.

114 patients consisted of 70 patients who underwent Gd-DOTA enhanced MRI and 44 who underwent unenhanced MRI. The study showed a very similar low rate of CIN after Gd-DOTA-enhanced MRI (1.4%) and unenhanced MRI (0%) in patients with stage 3 or 4 CKD. One patient from the Gd-DOTA enhanced MRI group had a baseline serum creatinine level increase from 2.0 to 2.6 mg/dl after MRI, which returned to baseline within 2 weeks. No statistically significant difference was seen for adverse events between the groups ($p = 0.08$), and no signs suggestive of NSF were observed at 3 months follow-up [85c].

The safety of gadopentetate dimeglumine was assessed in a prospective case–control study of two age- and sex-matched groups ($n = 72$ for each group) of hospitalized patients high risk for AKI. Serum creatinine, albumin, uric acid, serum electrolytes, total cholesterol, low-density lipoprotein, triglyceride, liver enzymes, fasting blood glucose, hemoglobin A1C, and C-reactive protein (CRP) levels were measured before the procedures in all subjects. Serum creatinine, CRP, eGFR, serum cystatin C, NAG, and NGAL levels were measured at baseline, and at 6, 24, 72, and 168 hours after the procedures and albumin/creatinine ratio was measured in morning spot urine at baseline and 168 hours after the procedure. No cases of adverse effects, AKI, NSF were reported even in patients with chronic renal failure in both groups. The authors suggest that nephrotoxicity of gadopentetate dimeglumine is low even in patients at risk for AKI [86c].

A prospective comparison between 13 patients who received single dose (0.1 mmol/kg bodyweight) gadobenate dimeglumine and 15 patients who received double dose (0.2 mmol/kg bodyweight) gadopentetate dimeglumine for contrast-enhanced magnetic resonance angiography found no adverse events in both groups [87c]. The number of cases is small; therefore, it may be difficult assess the real incidence adverse reactions between the groups, but the incidence itself seems to be low.

Cardiovascular

Kounis syndrome is concurrence of acute coronary syndromes with conditions associated with mast cell activation, such as allergies or hypersensitivity and anaphylactic or anaphylactoid insults [88R,89R]. Type I occurs in patients without risk factors and normal coronary arteries, hence acute release of inflammatory cytokines causes coronary spasm and possible organ damage; type II occurs in patients with existing coronary artery disease (70% of all cases); and type III occurs in patients suffering from coronary artery thrombosis, including stent thrombosis where the aspirated thrombus contains a significant amount of mastocytes and eosinophils [90R]. A case of type I Kounis syndrome in a 46-year-old woman with multiple drug allergies after administration of gadoterate meglumine for brain MRI has been reported [91A].

Prevention

Breakthrough reactions, such as those seen with iodinated contrast media for CT, are adverse reactions that occur in spite of premedications in patients at risk. A study investigating the efficacy of premedications included 54 contrast enhanced MRIs in patients who underwent an oral steroid premedication protocol. The study found only 1 mild breakthrough reaction. The number of cases included in the study was small, yet the incidence of breakthrough reactions after premedications seems to be low. The authors suggest that, when the prior adverse reactions are mild, or when there is a history of asthma, following a premedication protocol may make it possible to safely perform contrast-enhanced examinations. Yet, in previous moderate or severe reactors, contrast should only be used with extreme caution even with premedication [55c].

Superparamagnetic Iron Oxide (SPIO) MRI Contrast Agents [SEDA-33, 970; SEDA-34, 757]

Iron oxide-containing contrast agents consist of suspended colloids of iron oxide nanoparticles, which reduce T2 MRI signals. They are taken up by the reticuloendothelial system. Superparamagnetic iron oxide

(SPIO) contrast agents are taken up by the liver and spleen. The ultrasmall superparamagnetic iron oxide (USPIO) contrast agents have a longer plasma circulation time and have greater uptake into marrow and lymph nodes. They also have a greater T1 shortening effect than SPIO contrast agents. For these characteristics, they have been investigated for liver imaging, macrophage imaging or blood pool agents.

Ferumoxytol is an intravenously injected superparamagnetic iron oxide coated with polyglucose sorbitol carboxymethylether, which is used for the treatment of anemia caused by low levels of iron in patients with chronic kidney disease. It has previously been used in the magnetic resonance imaging (MRI) of the central nervous system and lower extremities [92c,93c,94c,95c,96c]. A report investigated the efficacy of ferumoxytol for vascular assessment of lower extremity arterial disease in patients. The study included 10 patients suspected with arterial occlusive disease. Five patients with renal insufficiency were scanned with ferumoxytol, and 5 with gadolinium. No adverse reactions were found in both groups [97c].

ULTRASOUND CONTRAST AGENTS
[SEDA-32, 855; SEDA-33, 971; SEDA-34, 758; SEDA-35, 869; SEDA-36, 703]

A study investigating the safety of intravesical administration of a second-generation ultrasound contrast agent (SonoVue) included 1010 patients (563 girls, 447 boys; mean age: 2.9 years, range: 15 days to 17.6 years) with 2043 pelvi-ureter-units who underwent contrast-enhanced voiding urosonography. No cases of serious adverse events were recorded, and only 37 minor events were reported [98C].

A case report of a 60-year-old male patient who underwent contrast enhanced dobutamine stress echocardiography developed ST-segment elevation after administration of SonoVue. One minute after administration of a 1 ml bolus of SonoVue, the patient started complaining of nausea with profuse sweating and hypotension (100/45 mmHg). Two minutes later, sudden severe chest pain occurred and the ECG showed ST-segment elevation in leads II, III, aVF and V2–V4, with ST-segment depression in V2–V4, I, and aVL, and total AV-nodal block. Coronary angiography demonstrated spasm in the right coronary artery [99A].

References

[1] ACR Manual on Contrast Media, Version 9: American College of Radiology; 2013 [M].
[2] ESUR guidelines on contrasts media 8.1 European Society of Urogenital Radiology; 2013. Available from: http://www.esur.org/guidelines/ [M].
[3] Gomi T, Nagamoto M, Hasegawa M, et al. Are there any differences in acute adverse reactions among five low-osmolar non-ionic iodinated contrast media? Eur Radiol. 2010;20(7):1631–5 [C].
[4] Kalaiselvan V, Sharma S, Singh GN. Adverse reactions to contrast media: an analysis of spontaneous reports in the database of the pharmacovigilance programme of India. Drug Saf. 2014;37(9):703–10 [C].
[5] Garcia M, Aguirre U, Martinez A, et al. Acute adverse reactions to iopromide vs iomeprol: a retrospective analysis of spontaneous reporting from a radiology department. Br J Radiol. 2014;87(1033):20130511 [C].
[6] Seong JM, Choi NK, Lee J, et al. Comparison of the safety of seven iodinated contrast media. J Korean Med Sci. 2013;28(12):1703–10 [C].
[7] Zhang BC, Wu Q, Wang C, et al. A meta-analysis of the risk of total cardiovascular events of isosmolar iodixanol compared with low-osmolar contrast media. J Cardiol. 2014;63(4):260–8 [M].
[8] Kohri K, Miyoshi S, Nagahara A, et al. Bilateral parotid enlargement ("iodide mumps") following excretory urography. Radiology. 1977;122(3):654 [A].
[9] Bohora S, Harikrishnan S, Tharakan J. Iodide mumps. Int J Cardiol. 2008;130(1):82–3 [A].
[10] Kohat AK, Jayantee K, Phadke RV, et al. Beware of parotitis induced by iodine-containing contrast media. J Postgrad Med. 2014;60(1):75–6 [A].
[11] Fok JS, Ramachandran T, Berce M, et al. Radiocontrast-induced iodide sialadenopathy and neutrophilic dermatosis. Ann Allergy Asthma Immunol. 2014;112(3):267–8 [A].
[12] Lee SY, Rhee CM, Leung AM, et al. A review: radiographic iodinated contrast media-induced thyroid dysfunction. J Clin Endocrinol Metab. 2014;100(2):376–83. jc20143292 [R].
[13] Hudzik B, Zubelewicz-Szkodzinska B. Radiocontrast-induced thyroid dysfunction: is it common and what should we do about it? Clin Endocrinol (Oxf). 2014;80(3):322–7 [R].
[14] Trumbo P, Yates AA, Schlicker S, et al. Dietary reference intakes: vitamin A, vitamin K, arsenic, boron, chromium, copper, iodine, iron, manganese, molybdenum, nickel, silicon, vanadium, and zinc. J Am Diet Assoc. 2001;101(3):294–301 [R].
[15] Rhee CM, Bhan I, Alexander EK, et al. Association between iodinated contrast media exposure and incident hyperthyroidism and hypothyroidism. Arch Intern Med. 2012;172(2):153–9 [C].
[16] Ozkan S, Oysu AS, Kayatas K, et al. Thyroid functions after contrast agent administration for coronary angiography: a prospective observational study in euthyroid patients. Anadolu Kardiyol Derg. 2013;13(4):363–9 [c].
[17] Bowers RW, O'Kane P, Balasubramaniam RN. Type 1 Brugada ECG unmasked by intracoronary contrast media. Heart. 2013;99(2):147–8 [A].
[18] Sheikh AS, Ranjan K. Brugada syndrome: a review of the literature. Clin Med. 2014;14(5):482–9 [R].
[19] Rutledge M, Witthed A, Khouzam RN. It took a RedBull to unmask Brugada syndrome. Int J Cardiol. 2012;161(1):e14–5 [r].
[20] Paul AK, Al-Nahhas A, Ansari SM, et al. Skin eruptions following treatment with iodine-131 for hyperthyroidism: a rare and un-reported early/intermediate side effect. Nucl Med Rev Cent East Eur. 2005;8(2):125–7 [c].
[21] Aliagaoglu C, Turan H, Uslu E, et al. Iododerma following topical povidone-iodine application. Cutan Ocul Toxicol. 2013;32(4):339–40 [A].
[22] Sparrow GP. Iododerma due to radiographic contrast medium. J R Soc Med. 1979;72(1):60–1 [A].
[23] Sanda E, Rezac M. Toxic reactions to contrast substances. (Iododerma following sialography). Cesk Rentgenol. 1962;16:210–3 [A].
[24] Young AL, Grossman ME. Acute iododerma secondary to iodinated contrast media. Br J Dermatol. 2014;170(6):1377–9 [A].

[25] Rothman LR, Levender MM, Scharf MD, et al. Iododerma following serial computed tomography scans in a lung cancer patient. J Drugs Dermatol. 2013;12(5):574–6 [A].

[26] Bircher AJ, Brockow K, Grosber M, et al. Late elicitation of maculopapular exanthemas to iodinated contrast media after first exposure. Ann Allergy Asthma Immunol. 2013;111(6):576–7 [r].

[27] Tasaki T, Miura Y, Yamada Y, et al. The hematological and clinical effects of X-ray contrast medium contaminating autologous blood for transfusion purposes. Transfus Apher Sci. 2012;47(2):139–43 [E].

[28] Hayakawa K, Nakamura T, Shimizu Y. Role of hemolysis in potassium release by iodinated contrast medium. Eur Radiol. 1999;9(7):1357–61 [E].

[29] Hayakawa K, Nakamura T, Shimizu Y. Effect of hyperosmolality and cations on iodinated contrast medium-induced potassium release from human blood cells. Radiat Med. 2007;25(9):467–73 [E].

[30] Gerk U, Kruger A, Franke RP, et al. Effect of radiographic contrast media (Iodixanol, Iopromide) on hemolysis. Clin Hemorheol Microcirc. 2014;58(1):171–4 [E].

[31] Santos Mello R, Callisen H, Winter J, et al. Radiation dose enhancement in tumors with iodine. Med Phys. 1983;10(1):75–8 [E].

[32] Iwamoto KS, Cochran ST, Winter J, et al. Radiation dose enhancement therapy with iodine in rabbit VX-2 brain tumors. Radiother Oncol. 1987;8(2):161–70 [E].

[33] Mesa AV, Norman A, Solberg TD, et al. Dose distributions using kilovoltage x-rays and dose enhancement from iodine contrast agents. Phys Med Biol. 1999;44(8):1955–68 [E].

[34] Deinzer CK, Danova D, Kleb B, et al. Influence of different iodinated contrast media on the induction of DNA double-strand breaks after in vitro X-ray irradiation. Contrast Media Mol Imaging. 2014;9(4):259–67 [E].

[35] Amato E, Salamone I, Naso S, et al. Can contrast media increase organ doses in CT examinations? A clinical study. AJR Am J Roentgenol. 2013;200(6):1288–93 [c].

[36] Paul J, Jacobi V, Bazrafshan B, et al. Effect of contrast material on radiation dose in an adult cardiac dual-energy CT using retrospective ECG-gating. Health Phys. 2013;105(2):156–64 [c].

[37] Burris 3rd HA, Hurtig J. Radiation recall with anticancer agents. Oncologist. 2010;15(11):1227–37 [R].

[38] Guarneri C, Guarneri B. Radiation recall dermatitis. CMAJ. 2010;182(3):E150 [A].

[39] Heirwegh G, Bruyeer E, Renard M, et al. Radiation-recall myositis presenting as low-back pain (2010: 4b). Eur Radiol. 2010;20(7):1799–801 [A].

[40] Wernicke AG, Swistel AJ, Parashar B, et al. Levofloxacin-induced radiation recall dermatitis: a case report and a review of the literature. Clin Breast Cancer. 2010;10(5):404–6 [R].

[41] Lau SK, Rahimi A. Radiation recall precipitated by iodinated nonionic contrast. Pract Radiat Oncol. 2014;5(4):263–6 [A].

[42] Nash K, Hafeez A, Hou S. Hospital-acquired renal insufficiency. Am J Kidney Dis. 2002;39(5):930–6 [C].

[43] Moos SI, Nagan G, de Weijert RS, et al. Patients at risk for contrast-induced nephropathy and mid-term effects after contrast administration: a prospective cohort study. Neth J Med. 2014;72(7):363–71 [C].

[44] Hassen GW, Hwang A, Liu LL, et al. Follow up for emergency department patients after intravenous contrast and risk of nephropathy. West J Emerg Med. 2014;15(3):276–81 [C].

[45] Lucreziotti S, Centola M, Salerno-Uriarte D, et al. Female gender and contrast-induced nephropathy in primary percutaneous intervention for ST-segment elevation myocardial infarction. Int J Cardiol. 2014;174(1):37–42 [c].

[46] Kwasa EA, Vinayak S, Armstrong R. The role of inflammation in contrast-induced nephropathy. Br J Radiol. 2014;87(1041):20130738 [c].

[47] Alharazy SM, Kong N, Saidin R, et al. Serum neutrophil gelatinase-associated lipocalin and cystatin C are early biomarkers of contrast-induced nephropathy after coronary angiography in patients with chronic kidney disease. Angiology. 2014;65(5):436–42 [c].

[48] .Hayakawa K, Tanikake M, Kirishima T, et al. The incidence of contrast-induced nephropathy (CIN) following transarterial chemoembolisation (TACE) in patients with hepatocellular carcinoma (HCC). Eur Radiol. 2014;24(5):1105–11 [c].

[49] Prasad V, Gandhi D, Stokum C, et al. Incidence of contrast material-induced nephropathy after neuroendovascular procedures. Radiology. 2014;273(3):853–8 [C].

[50] Cicin I, Erdogan B, Gulsen E, et al. Incidence of contrast-induced nephropathy in hospitalised patients with cancer. Eur Radiol. 2014;24(1):184–90 [c].

[51] Schilp J, de Blok C, Langelaan M, et al. Guideline adherence for identification and hydration of high-risk hospital patients for contrast-induced nephropathy. BMC Nephrol. 2014;15:2 [C].

[52] Leoncini M, Toso A, Maioli M, et al. Early high-dose rosuvastatin for contrast-induced nephropathy prevention in acute coronary syndrome: results from the PRATO-ACS Study (protective effect of rosuvastatin and antiplatelet therapy on contrast-induced acute kidney injury and myocardial damage in patients with acute coronary syndrome). J Am Coll Cardiol. 2014;63(1):71–9 [c].

[53] Yun KH, Lim JH, Hwang KB, et al. Effect of high dose rosuvastatin loading before percutaneous coronary intervention on contrast-induced nephropathy. Korean Circ J. 2014;44(5):301–6 [c].

[54] Liu Y, Liu YH, Tan N, et al. Comparison of the efficacy of rosuvastatin versus atorvastatin in preventing contrast induced nephropathy in patient with chronic kidney disease undergoing percutaneous coronary intervention. PLoS One. 2014;9(10):e111124 [C].

[55] Jingu A, Fukuda J, Taketomi-Takahashi A, et al. Breakthrough reactions of iodinated and gadolinium contrast media after oral steroid premedication protocol. BMC Med Imaging. 2014;14:34 [c].

[56] Farolfi A, Della Luna C, Ragazzini A, et al. Taxanes as a risk factor for acute adverse reactions to iodinated contrast media in cancer patients. Oncologist. 2014;19(8):823–8 [C].

[57] Farolfi A, Carretta E, Luna CD, et al. Does the time between CT scan and chemotherapy increase the risk of acute adverse reactions to iodinated contrast media in cancer patients? BMC Cancer. 2014;14:792 [C].

[58] Fujiwara N, Tateishi R, Akahane M, et al. Changes in risk of immediate adverse reactions to iodinated contrast media by repeated administrations in patients with hepatocellular carcinoma. PLoS One. 2013;8(10):e76018 [C].

[59] Kim MH, Lee SY, Lee SE, et al. Anaphylaxis to iodinated contrast media: clinical characteristics related with development of anaphylactic shock. PLoS One. 2014;9(6):e100154 [c].

[60] Somashekar DK, Davenport MS, Cohan RH, et al. Effect of intravenous low-osmolality iodinated contrast media on patients with myasthenia gravis. Radiology. 2013;267(3):727–34 [c].

[61] Bonanni L, Dalla Vestra M, Zancanaro A, et al. Myasthenia gravis following low-osmolality iodinated contrast media. Case Rep Radiol. 2014;2014:963461 [A].

[62] Pahade JK, LeBedis CA, Raptopoulos VD, et al. Incidence of contrast-induced nephropathy in patients with multiple myeloma undergoing contrast-enhanced CT. AJR Am J Roentgenol. 2011;196(5):1094–101 [c].

[63] Mussap M, Merlini G. Pathogenesis of renal failure in multiple myeloma: any role of contrast media? Biomed Res Int. 2014;2014:167125 [R].

[64] Yamaguchi K, Katayama H, Takashima T, et al. Prediction of severe adverse reactions to ionic and nonionic contrast media in Japan: evaluation of pretesting. A report from the Japanese Committee on the Safety of Contrast Media. Radiology. 1991;178(2):363–7 [C].

[65] Kim SH, Jo EJ, Kim MY, et al. Clinical value of radiocontrast media skin tests as a prescreening and diagnostic tool in hypersensitivity reactions. Ann Allergy Asthma Immunol. 2013;110(4):258–62 [C].

[66] Prieto-Garcia A, Tomas M, Pineda R, et al. Skin test-positive immediate hypersensitivity reaction to iodinated contrast media: the role of controlled challenge testing. J Investig Allergol Clin Immunol. 2013;23(3):183–9 [c].

[67] Saito M, Abe M, Furukawa T, et al. Examination of patients suspected as having hypersensitivity to iodinated contrast media with leukocyte migration test. Biol Pharm Bull. 2014;37(11):1750–7 [c].

[68] Weller A, Barber JL, Olsen OE. Gadolinium and nephrogenic systemic fibrosis: an update. Pediatr Nephrol. 2014;29(10):1927–37 [R].

[69] Thomsen HS, Morcos SK, Almen T, et al. Nephrogenic systemic fibrosis and gadolinium-based contrast media: updated ESUR Contrast Medium Safety Committee guidelines. Eur Radiol. 2013;23(2):307–18 [M].

[70] Edwards BJ, Laumann AE, Nardone B, et al. Advancing pharmacovigilance through academic-legal collaboration: the case of gadolinium-based contrast agents and nephrogenic systemic fibrosis–a research on adverse drug events and reports (RADAR) report. Br J Radiol. 2014;87(1042):20140307 [C].

[71] Canga A, Kislikova M, Martinez-Galvez M, et al. Renal function, nephrogenic systemic fibrosis and other adverse reactions associated with gadolinium-based contrast media. Nefrologia. 2014;34(4):428–38 [R].

[72] Schad SG, Heitland P, Kuhn-Velten WN, et al. Time-dependent decrement of dermal gadolinium deposits and significant improvement of skin symptoms in a patient with nephrogenic systemic fibrosis after temporary renal failure. J Cutan Pathol. 2013;40(11):935–44 [A].

[73] Poisson JL, Low A, Park YA. The treatment of nephrogenic systemic fibrosis with therapeutic plasma exchange. J Clin Apher. 2013;28(4):317–20 [A].

[74] Thomsen HS, Morcos SK, Almen T. et. al, committee ECMS. Nephrogenic systemic fibrosis and gadolinium-based contrast media: updated ESUR Contrast Medium Safety Committee guidelines. Eur Radiol. 2013;23(2):307–18 [M].

[75] Idee JM, Fretellier N, Robic C, et al. The role of gadolinium chelates in the mechanism of nephrogenic systemic fibrosis: a critical update. Crit Rev Toxicol. 2014;44(10):895–913 [R].

[76] Idee JM, Port M, Dencausse A, et al. Involvement of gadolinium chelates in the mechanism of nephrogenic systemic fibrosis: an update. Radiol Clin North Am. 2009;47(5):855–69. vii [R].

[77] Okada E, Yamanaka M, Ishikawa O. New insights into the mechanism of abnormal calcification in nephrogenic systemic fibrosis—gadolinium promotes calcium deposition of mesenchymal stem cells and dermal fibroblasts. J Dermatol Sci. 2011;62(1):58–63 [E].

[78] Hope TA, Doherty A, Fu Y, et al. Gadolinium accumulation and fibrosis in the liver after administration of gadoxetate disodium in a rat model of active hepatic fibrosis. Radiology. 2012;264(2):423–7 [E].

[79] White GW, Gibby WA, Tweedle MF. Comparison of Gd(DTPA-BMA) (Omniscan) versus Gd(HP-DO3A) (ProHance) relative to gadolinium retention in human bone tissue by inductively coupled plasma mass spectroscopy. Invest Radiol. 2006;41(3):272–8 [c].

[80] Kanda T, Ishii K, Kawaguchi H, et al. High signal intensity in the dentate nucleus and globus pallidus on unenhanced T1-weighted MR images: relationship with increasing cumulative dose of a gadolinium-based contrast material. Radiology. 2014;270(3):834–41 [c].

[81] Errante Y, Cirimele V, Mallio CA, et al. Progressive increase of T1 signal intensity of the dentate nucleus on unenhanced magnetic resonance images is associated with cumulative doses of intravenously administered gadodiamide in patients with normal renal function, suggesting dechelation. Invest Radiol. 2014;49(10):685–90 [c].

[82] Kanda T, Osawa M, Oba H, et al. High signal intensity in dentate nucleus on unenhanced T1-weighted MR images: association with linear versus macrocyclic gadolinium chelate administration. Radiology. 2015;275(3):803–9. 140364 [c].

[83] Gutierrez JE, Rosenberg M, Duhaney M, et al. Phase 3 efficacy and safety trial of gadobutrol, a 1.0 molar macrocyclic MR imaging contrast agent, in patients referred for contrast-enhanced MR imaging of the central nervous system. J Magn Reson Imaging. 2015;41(3):788–96 [S].

[84] Okigawa T, Utsunomiya D, Tajiri S, et al. Incidence and severity of acute adverse reactions to four different gadolinium-based MR contrast agents. Magn Reson Med Sci. 2014;13(1):1–6 [C].

[85] Deray G, Rouviere O, Bacigalupo L, et al. Safety of meglumine gadoterate (Gd-DOTA)-enhanced MRI compared to unenhanced MRI in patients with chronic kidney disease (RESCUE study). Eur Radiol. 2013;23(5):1250–9 [c].

[86] Gok Oguz E, Kiykim A, Turgutalp K, et al. Lack of nephrotoxicity of gadopentetate dimeglumine-enhanced non-vascular MRI and MRI without contrast agent in patients at high-risk for acute kidney injury. Med Sci Monit. 2013;19:942–8 [c].

[87] Xing X, Zeng X, Li X, et al. Contrast-enhanced MR angiography: does a higher relaxivity MR contrast agent permit a reduction of the dose administered for routine vascular imaging applications? Radiol Med. 2015;120(2):239–50 [c].

[88] Kounis NG, Mazarakis A, Tsigkas G, et al. Kounis syndrome: a new twist on an old disease. Future Cardiol. 2011;7(6):805–24 [R].

[89] Kounis NG. Kounis syndrome (allergic angina and allergic myocardial infarction): a natural paradigm? Int J Cardiol. 2006;110(1):7–14 [R].

[90] Biteker M. A new classification of Kounis syndrome. Int J Cardiol. 2010;145(3):553 [R].

[91] Zlojtro M, Roginic S, Nikolic-Heitzler V, et al. Kounis syndrome: simultaneous occurrence of an allergic reaction and myocardial ischemia in a 46 year old patient after administration of contrast agent. Isr Med Assoc J. 2013;15(11):725–6 [A].

[92] Li W, Tutton S, Vu AT, et al. First-pass contrast-enhanced magnetic resonance angiography in humans using ferumoxytol, a novel ultrasmall superparamagnetic iron oxide (USPIO)-based blood pool agent. J Magn Reson Imaging. 2005;21(1):46–52 [c].

[93] Neuwelt EA, Varallyay CG, Manninger S, et al. The potential of ferumoxytol nanoparticle magnetic resonance imaging, perfusion, and angiography in central nervous system malignancy: a pilot study. Neurosurgery. 2007;60(4):601–11. discussion 11–2 [c].

[94] Stabi KL, Bendz LM. Ferumoxytol use as an intravenous contrast agent for magnetic resonance angiography. Ann Pharmacother. 2011;45(12):1571–5 [R].

[95] Ruangwattanapaisarn N, Hsiao A, Vasanawala SS. Ferumoxytol as an off-label contrast agent in body 3T MR angiography: a pilot study in children. Pediatr Radiol. 2015;45(6):831–9 [c].

[96] Bashir MR, Jaffe TA, Brennan TV, et al. Renal transplant imaging using magnetic resonance angiography with a nonnephrotoxic contrast agent. Transplantation. 2013;96(1):91–6 [c].

[97] Walker JP, Nosova E, Sigovan M, et al. Ferumoxytol-enhanced magnetic resonance angiography is a feasible method for the clinical evaluation of lower extremity arterial disease. Ann Vasc Surg. 2015;29(1):63–8 [c].

[98] Papadopoulou F, Ntoulia A, Siomou E, et al. Contrast-enhanced voiding urosonography with intravesical administration of a second-generation ultrasound contrast agent for diagnosis of vesicoureteral reflux: prospective evaluation of contrast safety in 1,010 children. Pediatr Radiol. 2014;44(6):719–28 [C].

[99] van Ginkel A, Sorgdrager B, de Graaf MA, et al. ST-segment elevation associated with allergic reaction to echocardiographic contrast agent administration. Neth Heart J. 2014;22(2):77–9 [A].

46

Treatments Used in Complementary and Alternative Medicine

H.W. Zhang*, Z.X. Lin*, K. Chan[†,1]

*School of Chinese Medicine, Faculty of Medicine, The Chinese University of Hong Kong, Shatin, N.T., Hong Kong SAR, PR China

[†]The National Institute of Complementary Medicine, University of Western Sydney, Penrith, NSW, Australia

[1]Corresponding author: Profkchan@gmail.com

INTRODUCTION

With an increasing use of complementary and alternative medicine by the general public worldwide, the safety issues of possible interactions between complementary and alternative medicine (CAM) and other medicines have attracted much more attention in recent years, especially in high-risk populations like cancer and preoperative patients. For example, a questionnaire survey of 100 consecutive gynecological outpatients in a cancer center in Germany reported that 64% of patients used CAM and 48% used at least one substance-based CAM. A third of all patients were in danger of interactions of CAM with cancer therapy, and more than half of all CAM users and three quarters of users of substance-based CAM are at risk of interactions [1c]. An analysis on the prescription data from 4975 patients in U.S. has found that 40% of 302 cancer patients and 43% of 908 non-cancer respondents had at least one potential drug interaction, and 12% were at risk for fatal or permanently debilitating effects [2C]. A survey conducted in Italy on 478 preoperative patients has found that 49.8% of these patients used at least one herbal remedy. Among them, 23.1% were actually exposed to at least one potential interaction [3C].

The general lack of compositional and toxicological information of a particular herbal product presents a challenge for clinical safety. A survey on 200 patients in a Hungarian hospital reported that of the 85.5% of patients who took supplementary products in the previous 2 weeks, 45.2% of them were detected with potentially severe drug–supplement interactions [4c].

An overview of 26 systematic reviews reported that many herbal medicinal products were adulterated or contaminated with dust, pollen, insects, rodent debris, parasites, microbes, fungi, mold, toxins, pesticides, toxic heavy metals and/or prescription drugs. The most severe adverse effects were agranulocytosis, meningitis, multi-organ failure, perinatal stroke, arsenic, lead or mercury poisoning, malignancies or carcinomas, hepatic encephalopathy, hepatorenal syndrome, nephrotoxicity, rhabdomyolysis, metabolic acidosis, renal or liver failure, cerebral edema, coma, intracerebral hemorrhage, and death. Adulteration and contamination were most commonly noted for traditional Indian and Chinese remedies, respectively [5M]. The needs for natural health product regulations, guidance on safety and toxicity testing of herbal medicinal products, and more stringent quality control measures have been proposed [6H].

TRADITIONAL CHINESE HERBAL MEDICINE PREPARATIONS

Traditional Chinese medicine (TCM) has a well-established theoretical system to understand, analyze, and use herbal medicines for the treatment of various diseases. Adverse effects associated with Chinese herbal medicines are greater if they are used under the guidance of modern medicine principles rather than TCM. Xiaochaihu Decoction is a popular traditional herbal formula which contains Bupleuri radix (Chaihu). "Xiaochaihu Decoction event (XCHDE)" occurred in late 1980s

© 2015 Elsevier B.V. All rights reserved.

in Japan, which involved some related adverse drug reaction (ADR), including interstitial pneumonitis, drug induced liver injury (DILI) and even death. A retrospective analysis on XCHD-related ADRs reported in China and Japan reported that XCHDE in Japan probably resulted from multiple factors, including combinatory use with interferon, application under the guidance of modern medicine theory and based on disease diagnosis instead of TCM syndrome differentiation. Few ADE cases, mostly manifesting with hypersensitivity responses of skin and perfuse perspiration, were reported for XCHD in China when compared to that in Japan [7H].

According to TCM theory, a herbal formula composed of a mixture of different herbal ingredients is designed to work synergistically to reduce possible toxicity of the product; however, clinical safety issues should not be overlooked. An observational study conducted in Taiwan found an association between the consumption of Chinese formulae composed of aristolochic acid-containing herbs such as Mutong (*Aristolochia manshuriensis* Caulis) and an increased risk of chronic kidney disease and urinary tract cancer. Dizziness, headache, stomachache, and diarrhea were believed to be probably related to a traditional formula named Suan Zao Ren Tang (Ziziphi Spinosae Semen Decoction) [8C]. A literature review of papers published since 2011 on TCM products and hepatotoxicity has identified some TCM herbal mixtures and individual herbs with potential health hazards. The herbal mixture products include Ban Tu Wan (Pill for Treating Alopecia), Jia Wei Xia Yao San (Augmented Rambling Powder), Kamishoyosan (a traditional Japanese herbal drug similar to Jia Wei Xia Yao San), Long Dan Xie Gan Tang (Decoction of Gentian to Purge the Liver), 'White flood' (a nutritional supplement) and Xiao Chai Hu Decoction (XCHD). The single herbs include Chinese green tea (*Camellia sinensis*, or Lucha in Chinese), Polygoni Multiflori Radix (Heshouwu), *Hovenia dulcis* (Jiguja), Notoginseng Radix Et Rhizoma (Sanqi), Angelicae Pubescentis Radix (Duhuo), Scutellariae Radix (Huangqin) [9R]. Among 1100 Hong Kong Chinese adults interviewed via telephone, 789 (71.7%) respondents reported the use of over-the-counter TCM products, and 25 (2.3%) of them reported at least one related adverse event (AE) in the past year. The most common AEs were allergic reactions, dizziness, and gastro-intestinal problems [10C]. The result of a survey conducted in Europe and China suggested the use of Chinese materia medica (CMM) appeared to be largely safe in both areas, except potential AEs with Pinelliae Rhizoma (Banxia), Persicae Semen (Taoren), Tripterygium Wilfordii Herba (Leigongteng), and Aconiti Radix (Chuanwu). In China, only a few toxic CMMs are commonly used, and some of them are used mainly for serious disorders and only be prescribed after proper preparation [11C].

Chushizhiyang Paste

Chushizhiyang paste (or Expel dampness to stop itching paste in English) is a topical Chinese herbal paste for the treatment of eczema, which is largely due to invasion of damp pathogen according to the TCM theory. Chushizhiyang paste is composed of Cnidii Fructus (Shechuangzi), Coptidis Rhizoma (huanglian), Phellodendri Chinensis Cortex (huangbo), Dictamni Cortex (Baixianpi), Sophorae Flavescentis Radix (Kushen), Polygoni Cuspidati Rhizoma (Huzhang), Violae Herba (Zihuadiding), Kochiae Fructus (Difuzi), Polygoni Avicularis Herba (Bianxu), Artemisiae Scopariae Herba (Yinchen), Atractylodis Rhizoma (Cangzhu), Zanthoxyli Pericarpium (Huajiao) and Borneolum Syntheticum (Bingpian). A case of contact dermatitis caused by this topical product has been reported [12A].

An 18-year-old man with chronic scrotum eczema developed strong itchiness and sting locally 1 hour after topical application of chushizhiyang paste. He subsequently developed swollen scrotum which extended to the right groin with increasing pain and itchiness after the second topical application. The paste was removed immediately, and the symptoms gradually subsided 24 hours after receiving injection of chlorphenamine maleate, dexamethasone sodium phosphate, and vitamin D_2 with calcium colloid.

Qizhengxiaotong Paste

Qizhengxiaotong paste (or Qizheng pain relieving paste), commonly used to relieve various musculoskeletal pain, is consisted of several traditional Tibetan medicines, including Lamiophlomis Herba (Duyiwei), Bubali Cornu (Shuiniujiao), Curcumae Longae Rhizoma (Jianghuang), Oxytropis Falcata (Jidou), and Myricaria bracteata (shuibaizhi). It was reported to cause skin allergic reactions, including acute or tardive rashes, 5–24 hours after topical application [13A,14A]. It has also been reported to cause nausea and vomiting [14A].

A 48-year-old man developed flushed face, staggering, and nausea and vomiting about 30 minutes after applying qizhengxiaotong paste to treat his frozen shoulder. The paste was removed immediately, and the symptoms gradually resolved after resting for 1 hour.

Shenqifuzheng Injection

Shenqifuzheng injection (or Codonopsis and Astragalus Injection of Restoring Energy) is made from Codonopsis Radix (Dangshen) and Astragali Radix (Huangqi), and has the function of strengthening the immune system and nourishing vitality. A post-marketing safety monitoring study reported that the incidence of an ADR was 1.85‰ among 20 100 cases, with 27 slight and 10 moderate cases, while no severe case was found. The adverse reaction symptoms included thrombocytopenia, rash, chills, palpitation, dyspnea, edema of a lower extremities, palpebral edema, and superficial vein inflammation [15C].

HERBAL MEDICINE

An overview of 50 systematic reviews on the adverse effects of herbal medicines (HMs) has found serious adverse effects from a number of herbs or herb parts from the following plants: *Pulvis standardisatus*, *Larrea tridentate*, *Piper methysticum* and *Cassia senna*. The most severe adverse effects were liver or kidney damage, colon perforation, carcinoma, coma and death [16M].

The safety of topical preparations containing botanical extracts needs more attention. A recent survey conducted in Italy reported that of the 1274 users of natural topical products, 139 (11%) reported cutaneous adverse reactions after botanical product application. The reactions were a worsening of the previous dermatitis or the development of new, different cutaneous symptoms and/or signs such as itching, burning, erythema, swelling, and vesiculation. The commonest botanically derived allergens were propolis, Compositae extracts, and *Melaleuca alternifolia* (tea tree) oil [17C].

GREEN TEA NUTRITIONAL SUPPLEMENTS

Green Tea Extract

Green tea, made from steaming of the leaves of tea plant *Camellia sinensis*, is a popular beverage consumed worldwide and generally considered safe. However, there has been increasing concern regarding the potential hepatotoxicity following the consumption of green tea extract [18M,19R]. A case of acute liver failure has been reported to be associated with green tea extract [20A].

A 16-year-old Hispanic boy presented with newly onset jaundice after taking several dietary supplements for weight loss which included Applied Nutrition® Green Tea Fat Burner for 60 days. His peak international normalised ratio (INR) and conjugated bilirubin (CB) increased dramatically. He gradually recovered 2 months after medical treatment.

As several possible causes were ruled out, and his liver histology was found to be consistent with previous cases of hepatotoxicity associated with green tea extract, it was believed that his liver injury could most likely be attributed to the weight loss supplement containing green tea extract.

SPECIFIC PLANTS

Astragali Radix (Huangqi)

The root of *Astragalus membranaceus* is one of the most often used qi tonifying herbs in TCM to treat various diseases. Adverse effects associated with the use of Astragalus Radix have been reported [21A].

A 70-year-old man developed dizziness, limb numbness, red face, chest tightness and scattered blisters and subsequent desquamation on both hands and feet after orally taking one decoction of a TCM formula named Huangqiguizhiwuwu tang (Decoction Made of Five Herbs Including Astragalus and Cinnamon Twigs) on the first treatment. The symptoms gradually subsided without any medical treatment. The similar symptoms reappeared after taking Huangqi with Xiangshaliujunzi tang (Six Gentlemen Decoction with Aucklandia and Amomum) on the second occasion. He was then diagnosed as exfoliative keratolysis, and recovered after topical application of fluocinonide and tretinoin ointment. Similar symptoms reoccurred twice subsequently after taking TCM formulae containing huangqi.

Luffa echinata (Bristly luffa)

Bristly luffa, a member of the Cucurbitaceae family, is found in East Asia and some parts of Africa. Its dried fruit is used in Ayurvedic medicine for various illnesses such as chronic bronchitis, dropsy, nephritis, intestinal and biliary colic, fever and jaundice. A case report indicates that excessive consumption of the fruit may be toxic to human [22A].

A 50-year-old man presented with acute onset of abdominal pain, vomiting, and bleeding per rectum 20 hours after consumption of 100–150 g of dried fruits of Bristly luffa soaked in water. He was found to have antral gastritis and duodenal erosions through upper gastrointestinal endoscopy examination and deranged liver function. He gradually recovered over a period of 7–10 days after receiving intravenous fluids, one unit of whole blood infusion and administrations of fresh frozen plasma, vitamin K, vasopressors and proton pump inhibitors.

Cade Oil

Cade oil is a kind of dark, faintly aromatic oil which is distilled from the branches and wood of *Juniperus oxycedrus*. It is used in some cosmetics preparations and incense. It is also used in Moroccan folk medicine for the treatment of bronchitis, abdominal pain and diarrhea, psychiatric disorders, cancer, fever, cephalgia, angina, weight loss, common cold, and hypotonia. The oil contains phenols, which are believed to be the most toxic components. An analysis of a Moroccan pharmacovigilance of herbal products database from January 1, 2004 to December 31, 2012 found that 30 (2.4%) of 1251 reported adverse events associated with herbal products were related to cade oil. Reported cases were mainly due to topical application (60%), oral ingestion (36.7%) or nasal application (3.3%). The reported adverse effects involved many organs but renal disorders were the most common. After hospitalization and with supportive and symptomatic treatment, 23 (76.7%) patients recovered and were discharged. However, three deaths (10%) were reported in relation to the use of cade oil. The results of WHO-UMC causality assessment demonstrated the adverse effects were rated as "probable" in 4 cases, "possible" in 24 cases, "unlikely" in 1 case and "unassessable" in 1 case [23R].

Cannabis sativa (Marijuana)

A survey of 313 patients with inflammatory bowel disease reported that 17.6% of respondents use Cannabis to relieve symptoms, with the majority by inhalational route (96.4%). Although Cannabis could subjectively improve pain and diarrheal symptoms, it was associated with higher risk of surgical treatment in patients with Crohn's disease. It was suspected that Cannabis use may mask the clinical symptoms related to the ongoing inflammation [24C].

Tribulus terrestris (Bulgarian tribulus)

Tribulus terrestris is an herb belonging to the Zygophyllaceae family which is indigenous to the Southern Europe, Southern Asia, Australia, and Africa. It is often used in the treatment of infertility, low sex drive, and erectile dysfunction. It is also used by athletes to increase muscle strength and improve performance in sports [25M,26C]. Bulgarian tribulus has been reported to increase transaminases via rhabdomyolysis [27A].

A 44-year-old man, with a history of Hodgkin's lymphoma, was referred to a gastroenterology/hepatology department for elevated transaminases. He was asymptomatic but admitted consuming alcohol every 2 weeks. Laboratory tests showed elevated liver function indexes that are higher than normal. He had recently taken Bulgarian tribulus for 2 weeks [route, dosage, indication and time to reaction onset not stated]. The herb was stopped, and transaminase measurement and creatine kinase were normalized within 10 days.

Mistletoe Extracts (Viscum album L.)

The commercially available mistletoe extracts are prepared from the semi-parasitic plant Viscum album (Loranthaceae). It is the most frequently used complementary medicine in the treatment of cancer patients in German-speaking countries [28M]. A multi-center, observational study has found that of 1923 cancer patients treated with subcutaneous injection of mistletoe extracts, 162 (8.4%) patients reported a total of 264 ADRs, with mild in 50.8%, moderate in 45.1%, and severe in 4.2% of the patients. The adverse reactions appeared to be dose-related and could be explained by the immune-stimulating, pharmacological activity of mistletoe [29C]. Intravenous mistletoe therapy seems to be safer than subcutaneous application. An observational study on 475 cancer patients who received intravenous infusions of Helixor, Abnoba viscum, or Iscador mistletoe preparations, 22 patients (4.6%) reported 32 ADRs of mild (59.4%) or moderate severity (40.6%) [30C].

Polygoni Multiflori Radix (Chinese Fleeceflower Root, Heshouwu)

A warning has been issued by China Food and Drug Administration for the potential risk of liver damage caused by raw and processed Polygoni Multiflori Radix. Generally, the cases of liver damage were mild or moderate, and mostly reversible. The main manifestations of the DILI associated with Heshouwu were weakness, poor digestion and anorexia, and jaundice. The risk of DILI may be increased by the following situations: (1) large dosage and long-term administration, (2) patients with history of liver damage caused by Polygoni Multiflori Radix, and (3) combined use with other medicines of potential liver toxicity. Raw Polygoni Multiflori Radix is more likely to cause liver damage than the processed plant [31S].

Smilacis Glabrae Rhizoma (Tufuling)

Smilacis Glabrae Rhizome, a traditional Chinese herb, is commonly used to expel dampness in the treatment of eczema, rheumatoid arthritis, urinary tract infection and other diseases. It has been reported to cause one case of allergic shock [32A].

A 45-year-old man with eczema suddenly developed nausea, palpitation, purple mouth and lip, respiratory distress, profuse sweating, and cold extremities when he manually smashed Smilacis Glabrae Rhizome for his prescribed topical paste. He gradually recovered 30 minutes after receiving inhalation of salbutamol and muscular injection of dexamethasone and adrenaline.

ACUPUNCTURE

Acupuncture seems generally safe to pregnant women. A systematic review has identified a total of 429 (incidence rate 1.9%) AEs in the 27 reports involving approximately 22 283 sessions of acupuncture in 2460 pregnant women. Among these AEs, 291 of them (incidence rate 1.3%) were evaluated as causally (certain, probably or possibly) related to acupuncture, and were rated as mild to moderate in severity, with needling pain being the most frequent. Severe AEs or deaths were few and all considered unlikely to have been caused by acupuncture [33M].

Acupuncture was reported to induce transient paralysis in one patient with history of idiopathic complex partial seizures (CPS) [34A].

A 38-year-old man had a history of CPS which was regarded as being well controlled by lamotrigine 150 mg and sodium valproate 2000 mg daily. Four hours after receiving the first session of mild acupuncture treatment for a painful musculoskeletal condition, he reported to have one of his vague staring episodes. During the second acupuncture treatment 3 weeks later, he developed heaviness, a tingling ice-cold sensation, loss of muscle power, and became unable to move his eyes and speak. He subsequently fell asleep for a few seconds, and gradually came around to normal after 50 minutes. He later experienced an increased frequency of CPS. Follow-up analysis suggested that the patient probably had comorbidities in the form of rapid eye movement sleep behaviour disorder and dysfunctional somatosensory/vestibular processing. Acupuncture may have triggered the adverse event via shared neurosubstrates.

Skin pigmentation changes have been reported to be associated with silver needle implantation, electroacupuncture and repeated strong manual stimulation of the needles [35A,36A]. A case of skin pigmentation and textural changes following repeated needling of Yintang (EX-HN3) has been reported [37A].

A 43-year-old Caucasian woman received intermittent acupuncture treatment on a weekly or biweekly basis over 6 years for heavy menstrual bleeding and clots. Yintang was used 95 times out of 98 treatments and GV20 (Baihui) in all the treatments along with other acupoints such as SP6 (Sanyinjiao), ST36 (Zusanli), LV3 (Taichong) and LI4 (Hegu). She reported a dark, beige, dry, scaly spot at the point of Yintang. The discoloration remained unresolved 10 months after cessation of all treatment.

CUPPING

A case report of cupping treatment administered on a patient undergoing concomitant therapy with bevacizumab, an angiogenesis inhibitor, suggested further research is needed on the safety issue of cupping during anticancer therapy, and raised awareness of the need to improve communication between CAM practitioners and oncologists when it comes to the care of patients with cancer [38A].

A 62-year-old Taiwanese man with advanced non-small-cell lung cancer (NSCLC) received four cycles of carboplatin AUC 6, paclitaxel 200 mg/m^2, and bevacizumab 15 mg/kg, and the maintenance dose of bevacizumab 15 mg/kg was continued once every 3 weeks. The patient underwent 3 sessions of glass dry cupping lasting 15 minutes on an every-other-day schedule for 18 days after receiving maintenance bevacizumab. He developed usual characteristic rounded skin ecchymoses at sites of cupping, which completely resolved 24 days after initial cupping. No overt cutaneous adverse events or bleeding was found.

MOXIBUSTION

The smoke of burned moxa during moxibustion treatment may cause adverse reaction. A case of allergic reaction has been reported to be associated with moxibustion treatment [39A].

A 50-year-old woman developed red and swollen eyes with tears, runny nose, sneezing, and flushed face with itching 3 days after receiving tui na and moxibustion treatment for recurrent low back pain. The moxibustion was stopped immediately, and her symptoms gradually resolved 3 days after topical application of cold pad and oral administration of cetirizine and prednisone.

OSTEOPATHY

Osteopathic treatment seems to be associated with vascular and neurological complications. The most frequent complication is stroke, spinal disc herniation with spinal cord compression, radiculopathy and cauda equina syndrome [40M]. A case of cervical disc herniation was reported to be associated with spinal manipulative therapy [41A].

A 33-year-old woman reported numbness and tingling feeling in her right posterior arm, together with marked weakness of the right upper extremity the following day after receiving an osteopathic treatment including cervical spine manipulation. The MRI revealed an interruption of the subarachnoid spaces (due to a right posterolateral disc herniation pushing back the spinal cord) in the spine at the C6–C7 location and a protrusion of the C4–C5 and C5–C6 discs. The condition was alleviated by surgical operation and subsequent physiotherapy.

TAI CHI

A systematic review on the safety of tai chi identified 153 eligible randomised controlled trials, of which only 50 trials (33%) included reported AEs. Reported

AEs were typically minor musculoskeletal aches and pains, and no intervention-related serious AEs were found [42M].

TUI NA

Tui na, also called Chinese medical massage, is a traditional hands-on manipulation treatment method guided by TCM theory. Through manual manipulations, tui na is used widely to treat various diseases, including not only musculoskeletal disorders, but also diseases of internal organs. Like acupuncture that may cause faint, tui na has been also reported to induce faint. Proper stimulation strength (non-excessive) of manipulation was suggested to avoid such events [43A].

A 38-year-old woman with neck pain developed minor faint after receiving the first tui na treatment intended to treat common cold. The symptom was relieved after 5-minute rest. Two weeks later, she suddenly developed dizziness, palpitation, nausea, pale face and lips, cold limbs with sweating after receiving another session of tui na treatment. She gradually recovered after drinking warm honey water and resting for about 30 minutes.

YOGA

Yoga, rooted in Indian philosophy, has become a worldwide popular way to promote physical and mental well-being through controlling the body and mind. A systematic review on 35 case reports and 2 case series of 76 subjects reported 27 AEs (35.5%) affecting the musculoskeletal system, 14 (18.4%) the nervous system, and 9 (11.8%) the eyes. Of these cases, 15 subjects (19.7%) fully recovered, 9 (11.3%) partially recovered, 1 (1.3%) did not recover, and 1 subject (1.3%) died. It is advisable for Yoga beginners to avoid extreme movements/stretching and be instructed by qualified instructors [44M].

References

[1] Zeller T, Muenstedt K, Stoll C, et al. Potential interactions of complementary and alternative medicine with cancer therapy in outpatients with gynecological cancer in a comprehensive cancer center. J Cancer Res Clin Oncol. 2013;139(3):357–65 [c].

[2] Chen L, Cheung WY. Potential drug interactions in patients with a history of cancer. Curr Oncol. 2014;21(2):e212–20 [C].

[3] Gallo E, Pugi A, Lucenteforte E, et al. Pharmacovigilance of herb-drug interactions among preoperative patients. Altern Ther Health Med. 2014;20(2):13–7 [C].

[4] Vegh A, Lanko E, Fittler A, et al. Identification and evaluation of drug-supplement interactions in Hungarian hospital patients. Int J Clin Pharm. 2014;36(2):451–9 [c].

[5] Posadzki P, Watson L, Ernst E. Contamination and adulteration of herbal medicinal products (HMPs): an overview of systematic reviews. Eur J Clin Pharmacol. 2013;69(3):295–307 [M].

[6] Neergheen-Bhujun VS. Underestimating the toxicological challenges associated with the use of herbal medicinal products in developing countries. Biomed Res Int. 2013;2013:804086 [H].

[7] Wu S, Sun H, Yang X, et al. Re-evaluation upon suspected event" is an approach for post-marketing clinical study: lessons from adverse drug events related to *Bupleuri Radix* preparations. Zhongguo Zhong Yao Za Zhi. 2014;39(15):2983–8 [Chinese] [H].

[8] Lai JN, Tang JL, Wang JD. Observational studies on evaluating the safety and adverse effects of traditional Chinese medicine. Evid Based Complement Alternat Med. 2013;2013:697893 [C].

[9] Teschke R, Wolff A, Frenzel C. Review article: herbal hepatotoxicity—an update on traditional Chinese medicine preparations. Aliment Pharmacol Ther. 2014;40(1):32–50 [R].

[10] Kim JH, Kwong EM, Chung VC, et al. Acute adverse events from over-the-counter Chinese herbal medicines: a population-based survey of Hong Kong Chinese. BMC Complement Altern Med. 2013;13:336 [C].

[11] Williamson E, Lorenc A, Booker A, et al. The rise of traditional Chinese medicine and its materia medica: a comparison of the frequency and safety of materials and species used in Europe and China. J Ethnopharmacol. 2013;149(2):453–62 [C].

[12] Liang YH. One case analysis of adverse effects caused by chushizhiyang paste. Chin J Hosp Pharm. 2013;33(12):1019–20 [Chinese] [A].

[13] Zhang W, Wu XQ, Wang Q. Eight cases of contact dermatitis caused by Qizhengxiaotong paste. Adverse Drug React J. 2009;5(6):57 [Chinese] [A].

[14] Zhang X, Bi LZ. Analysis on four cases of adverse effects caused by Qizhengxiaotong paste. J Pharm Res. 2013;32(11):680 [Chinese] [A].

[15] Ai Q, Zhang W, Xie Y. Post-marketing safety monitoring of shenqifuzheng injection: a solution made of dangshen (Radix Codonopsis) and huangqi (Radix Astragali Mongolici). J Tradit Chin Med. 2014;34(4):498–503 [C].

[16] Posadzki P, Watson LK, Ernst E. Adverse effects of herbal medicines: an overview of systematic reviews. Clin Med. 2013;13(1):7–12 [M].

[17] Corazza M, Borghi A, Gallo R, et al. Topical botanically derived products: use, skin reactions, and usefulness of patch tests. A multicentre Italian study. Contact Dermatitis. 2014;70(2):90–7 [C].

[18] Sarma D, Barrett M, Chavez M, et al. Safety of green tea extracts: a systematic review by the US Pharmacopeia. Drug Saf. 2008;31(6):469–84 [M].

[19] Mazzanti G, Menniti-Ippolito F, Moro P, et al. Hepatotoxicity from green tea: a review of the literature and two unpublished cases. Eur J Clin Pharmacol. 2009;65(4):331–41 [R].

[20] Beer S, Kearney DL, Phillips G, et al. Green tea extract: a potential cause of acute liver failure. World J Gastroenterol. 2013;19(31):5174–7 [A].

[21] Liu Y. One case of exfoliative keratolysis caused by oral Huangqi. J Emerg Tradit Chin Med. 2013;22(7):1251 [Chinese] [A].

[22] Giri S, Lokesh C, Sahu S, et al. Luffa echinata: healer plant or potential killer? J Postgrad Med. 2014;60(1):72–4 [A].

[23] Skalli S, Chebat A, Badrane N, et al. Side effects of cade oil in Morocco: an analysis of reports in the Moroccan herbal products database from 2004 to 2012. Food Chem Toxicol. 2014;64:81–5 [R].

[24] Devlin S, Kaplan GG, Panaccione R, et al. Cannabis use provides symptom relief in patients with inflammatory bowel disease but is associated with worse disease prognosis in patients with Crohn's disease. Inflamm Bowel Dis. 2014;20(3):472–80 [C].

[25] Qureshi A, Naughton DP, Petroczi A. A systematic review on the herbal extract *Tribulus terrestris* and the roots of its putative aphrodisiac and performance enhancing effect. J Diet Suppl. 2014;11(1):64–79 [M].

[26] Akhtari E, Raisi F, Keshavarz M, et al. *Tribulus terrestris* for treatment of sexual dysfunction in women: randomized double-blind placebo-controlled study. Daru. 2014;22:40 [C].

[27] Chen A, Lim B, Chaya C. Bulgarian tribulus side effect mimicking liver disease. Am J Gastroenterol. 2013;S353(108):1201 [A].

[28] Horneber MA, Bueschel G, Huber R, et al. Mistletoe therapy in oncology. Cochrane Database Syst Rev. 2008;2:CD003297 [M].

[29] Steele M, Axtner J, Happe A, et al. Adverse drug reactions and expected effects to therapy with subcutaneous mistletoe extracts (*Viscum album L.*) in cancer patients. Evid Based Complement Alternat Med. 2014;2014:724258 [C].

[30] Steele M, Axtner J, Happe A, et al. Safety of intravenous application of mistletoe (Viscum album L.) preparations in oncology: an observational study. Evid Based Complement Alternat Med. 2014;2014:236310 [C].

[31] China Food and Drug Administration Agency. Notice on the risk of liver injury caused by Heshouwu and its formulae. Chin Adv Drug React Inf Bull. 2014; (61). [Chinese] [S].

[32] Chen L, Zhou YZ, Li Ma. Once case of allergy caused by Tufuling. Pract J Med Pharm. 2013;30(7):666 [Chinese] [A].

[33] Park J, Sohn Y, White AR, et al. The safety of acupuncture during pregnancy: a systematic review. Acupunct Med. 2014;32(3):257–66 [M].

[34] Beable A. Transient paralysis during acupuncture therapy: a case report of an adverse event. Acupunct Med. 2013;31(3):319–24 [A].

[35] Tanita Y, Kato T, Hanada K, et al. Blue macules of localized argyria caused by implanted acupuncture needles. Electron microscopy and roentgenographic microanalysis of deposited metal. Arch Dermatol. 1985;121(12):1550–2 [A].

[36] Miao E. Skin changes after manual or electrical acupuncture. Acupunct Med. 2011;29(2):143–6 [A].

[37] Cooper F. A case study of pigmentation and textural changes associated with needling Yin Tang. J Acupunct Meridian Stud. 2014;7(2):95–7 [A].

[38] Klempner S, Costa D, Wu P, et al. Safety of cupping during bevacizumab therapy. J Altern Complement Med. 2013;19(8):729–31 [A].

[39] Zhao ZY, Ge M. Clinical analysis on three cases of allergy caused by moxibustion stick treatment. J External Ther Tradit Chin Med. 2013;22(6):39 [Chinese] [A].

[40] Ernst E. Manipulation of the cervical spine: a systematic review of case reports of serious adverse events, 1995-2001. Med J Aust. 2002;176(8):376–80 [M].

[41] Cicconi M, Mangiulli T, Bolino G. Onset of complications following cervical manipulation due to malpractice in osteopathic treatment: a case report. Med Sci Law. 2014;54(4):230–3 [A].

[42] Wayne P, Berkowitz D, Litrownik D, et al. What do we really know about the safety of tai chi? A systematic review of adverse event reports in randomized trials. Arch Phys Med Rehabil. 2014;95(12):2470–83 [M].

[43] Wang A, Yang LQ, Zeng KX, et al. Analysis of one case of faint caused by tuina. Chin Manipulation Rehabil Med. 2014;5(7):219–20 [A].

[44] Krucoff C, Dobos G. Adverse events associated with yoga: a systematic review of published case reports and case series. PLoS One. 2013;8(10):e75515 [M].

47

Miscellaneous Drugs, Materials, Medical Devices and Techniques

Anjan Nan[1]

Department of Pharmaceutical Sciences, University of Maryland Eastern Shore School of Pharmacy,
Princess Anne, MD, USA
[1]Corresponding author: anan@umes.edu

Aluminum (SEDA-36, 726)

Aluminum (Al) is a trivalent cation found in most animal and plant tissues and natural waters. Human beings are naturally exposed to Al in varying quantities in their daily lives from food, water and air. Even though there exists no formal characterization of health hazards, use of Al in numerous cosmetics such as antiperspirants, sunscreens and lipsticks, over the counter pharmaceuticals, injected vaccines that contain adjuvant Al as well as exposure in industrial settings may be a potential source of toxicity. The health risks due to aluminum exposure from antiperspirants has been reviewed by Guillard et al., who support the French safety agency recommendation to lower the concentration of Al in these products from 5% to 0.6% [1r]. Recent reports have also suggested the involvement of dietary Al in carcinogenic processes while long-term intake or exposure of Al-based compounds as food additives can account for neurodegenerative disorders like Alzheimer's disease (AD).

Nervous System

Walton and coworkers performed causality analysis [2r] to evaluate the extent to which the routine, life-long intake, and metabolism of aluminum compounds can account for Alzheimer's disease (AD), using Austin Bradford Hill's epidemiological and experimental causality criteria, including strength of the relationship, consistency, specificity, temporality, dose-dependent response, and biological rationale, coherence with existing knowledge, experimental evidence, and analogy. The casuality analysis suggested that routine ingestion of dietary aluminum (0.5–1.6 mg/kg bw/day) for an average adult results in low concentrations of Al being progressively taken up into the brain over a long prodromal phase. Being similar in ionic size as iron, Al can enter iron-dependent cells responsible for memory processing and reach toxic levels, deregulating iron homeostasis and causing microtubule depletion, eventually producing changes that result in disconnection of neuronal afferents and efferents, loss of function and regional atrophy. These reports were consistent with MRI findings in brains of patients with AD demonstrating the role of chronic Al uptake. Bhattacharjee et al. investigated the mechanism of selective transport of Al into the hippocampus of AD patients compared to age matched controls [3c]. They showed that the posterior cerebral artery had maximum Al deposition in AD patients compared to controls which is significant since this is the major artery that supplies blood to the hippocampus where AD appears to initiate.

LONG-TERM EFFECTS

Tumorigenicity

Al salts mainly Al-chlorhydrate (ACH) is an excipient widely used in underarm deodorant/antiperspirants that block sweat ducts upon application when it converts to insoluble Al-hydroxide. Recent *in vitro* studies using the MCF-7 breast cancer cell line by Iskakova for the first time alludes to the possible role of Al in breast cancer [4E]. Their studies show that Al-chlorhydrate can increase the migratory and invasive properties of breast cancer cells following long-term exposure (32 weeks). Although additional research is needed to investigate the translation of *in vitro* results to *in vivo*, such studies inject a sense of

© 2015 Elsevier B.V. All rights reserved.

urgency to reducing metal concentration in antiperspirant and related cosmetic products.

Artificial Sweeteners (SED-15, 348; SEDA-32, 892; SEDA-33, 1011; SEDA-35, 786)

Non-caloric artificial sweeteners (NAS) such as aspartame, sucralose and saccharin are widely consumed as they are generally considered to be safe and because of their projected beneficial health impact as opposed to sugar-sweetened products. In the US, 30% of adults and 15% of children aged 2–17 years consume low-calorie sweeteners [5R]. The Food and Drug Administration (FDA) has set acceptable daily intake (ADI) rate for aspartame of 50 mg/kg/day in the US. The estimated intake of aspartame as sweetener is about 1/10 of the ADI, and even exposure by heavy aspartame consumers does not exceed 30% of the ADI [6R]. However in recent years an increasing number of studies suggest that frequent consumption of these sugar substitutes may be counterintuitive leading to the risk of excessive weight gain, metabolic syndrome, type 2 diabetes and cardiovascular disease (reviewed in [5R]).

Metabolic Disorder

In a recent clinical study by Elinav et al. artificial sweeteners were shown to cause changes in glucose tolerance which is considered a marker of metabolic diseases like diabetes mellitus [5R]. A group of 7 healthy (non-diabetic) volunteers who do not normally consume artificial sweeteners were fed saccharin daily for 1 week. Four of these subjects were responders who developed poorer glycemic responses and had altered intestinal microbiota within 1 week, compared to other 3 subjects who were non-responders. Bacteria from the responders, sampled at the end of the trial, were introduced into mice who subsequently developed glucose intolerance whereas baseline samples (prior to consuming saccharin) or samples from non-responders did not show this effect. These findings provide evidence that NAS-induced dysbiosis has a role in inducing glucose intolerance seen in these patients. However, specific microbial compositions can predispose human patients to NAS-induced metabolic effects. Hence, the factors that contribute to such susceptibility warrants further investigation.

Long-Term Adverse Health Outcomes
CANCER

Although no large scale clinical studies have been reported to date, several animal studies investigated chronic exposure of aspartame starting from fetal period to development of cancer later in life [7R]. These studies demonstrated that aspartame induced carcinogenic lesions in rats when administered at 4–100 mg/kg body weight/day. Additionally, when rat fetuses were exposed to similar levels of aspartame from the 12th day of fetal life, an increased incidence of lymphomas, leukemias and breast tumors were observed later in life. The incidence of lymphomas and leukemias occurred earlier in life in female offspring when aspartame exposure started prenatally compared with adult life. It is believed that carcinogenic effects seen in these studies may be related to the metabolites (methanol) of aspartame rather than aspartame itself.

ALTERATION OF INTESTINAL MICROBIOTA

A potential mechanism that explains the relationship between artificial sweetener consumption and adverse metabolic outcomes is through the modulation of the intestinal microbiota that colonize the intestinal tract. The bacterial flora in the intestine impacts important physiological functions particularly innate and adaptive immunity and metabolism of dietary nutrients and xenobiotics. A decrease in the proportion of Firmicutes and Bacteroides in fecal samples has been found in individuals with type 2 diabetes and obesity, respectively. Intake of a mixture of sucralose and nutritive sweeteners for 12 weeks reduced the number of commensal bacteria such as Bifidobacterium, Lactobacillus and Bacteroides in rat. These alterations have been correlated with the development of insulin resistance, hyperlipidemia, increased adiposity and inflammation.

GLUCOSE INTOLERANCE

Elinav and coworkers showed that chronic consumption of artificial sweeteners leads to the development of glucose intolerance in mice through induction of compositional and functional alterations to the intestinal microbiota [8E]. These harmful metabolic effects are cured by antibiotic treatment and are fully transferrable to germ-free mice upon faecal transplantation from sweetener consuming mice. The authors also found significant positive correlations between sweetener consumption and metabolic syndrome related clinical parameters in data collected from 381 non-diabetic individuals. These parameters include increased weight and waist to hip ratio, higher fasting blood glucose, glycosylated hemoglobin and glucose tolerance test. In seven healthy volunteers who normally do not consume sweeteners, a 7-day study of saccharin consumption at FDA's acceptable daily intake rate (5 mg/kg body weight) resulted in significantly poorer glycemic response for 4 subjects after 5 days. The microbiome configurations of these subjects were different from the 3 non-responders. Stool transfer from these responders to germ free mice induced significant glucose intolerance.

APOPTOSIS

A recent study investigated the effects of chronic aspartame administration on rat brain [9E]. Aspartame exposure resulted in a significant increase in the enzymatic activity in protein carbonyl, lipid peroxidation levels, superoxide dismutase, glutathione-S-transferase, glutathione peroxidase and catalase activity in treated animals and a significant decrease in reduced glutathione, glutathione reductase and protein thiol, pointing out the generation of free radicals. The gene and protein expression of pro apoptotic marker Bax showed a marked increase whereas the anti-apoptotic marker Bcl-2 decreased markedly indicating that aspartame is harmful at cellular level. It is clear from this study that long-term aspartame exposure could alter the brain antioxidant status, and can induce apoptotic changes. Genotoxic and carcinogenic effects of aspartame has been recently reviewed providing useful guidance to consumers [10R].

NEUROBEHAVIORAL EFFECTS

There is also a growing body of mixed evidence on neurobehavioral effects of artificial sweeteners. Lindseth et al. recently conducted a trial to test the safe limits of aspartame over a short period of time [11c]. Healthy adults who consumed a high-aspartame diet (25 mg/kg bw/day) for a week and then a low-aspartame diet (10 mg/kg bw/day) for a week, with a 2-week washout between the diets, were examined for within-subject differences in cognition, depression, mood, and headache. Measures included weight of foods consumed containing aspartame, mood and depression scales, and cognitive tests for working memory and spatial orientation. When consuming high-aspartame diets, participants had more irritable mood, exhibited more depression, and performed significantly worse on spatial orientation tests. Aspartame consumption did not have an effect on working memory. The levels of aspartame used in this study were only one half of FDA's "safe" acceptable daily intake of 40–50 mg/kg bw/day. Such studies therefore warrant careful consideration when consuming food products with artificial sweeteners that may affect neurobehavioral health.

INSULIN RESISTANCE

Klein et al. evaluated the acute effects of another artificial sweetener sucralose commonly branded as Splenda, upon ingestion by obese subjects [12c]. Seventeen subjects (BMI $42.3 \pm 1.6 \, kg/m^2$) who did not use NAS and were insulin sensitive (insulin resistance score ≤ 2.6) were administered a 5 hour modified oral glucose tolerance test on two separate occasions preceded by consuming either sucralose or water (control) 10 min before the glucose load in a randomized cross-over trial. Compared to controls, sucralose ingestion caused a greater increase in peak plasma glucose concentrations (4.8 vs. 4.2 mmol/L; P = 0.03), a 20% greater increase in insulin area under the curve (AUC) (P < 0.03), 22% greater peak insulin secretion rate (P < 0.02), and a 7% decrease in insulin clearance (P = 0.04). Further after sucralose ingestion, a 23% decrease in insulin sensitivity index (P = 0.01) was observed, suggesting that sucralose may cause insulin resistance. Such data demonstrates that sucralose ingestion is not physiologically inert but affects the glycemic responses to an oral glucose load and potentiates glucose-induced insulin secretion in obese people who normally do not consume NAS.

BENZYL ALCOHOL (PRESERVATIVE)

Nervous System

Benzyl alcohol is an aqueous soluble preservative widely used in injectable pharmaceutical preparations as well as in cosmetic products. Although toxic in neonates and infants, it is generally recognized as safe by the FDA at concentrations up to 5% in adults. The effect of benzyl alcohol present as preservative in bacteriostatic normal saline has recently come under investigation when administered via intraarticular injection. Patients who undergo MRI-based arthrography for standard clinical indications are commonly administered a contrast agent like gadolinium diluted in bacteriostatic saline. Clifford et al. recently performed a clinical study to prospectively evaluate the effect of benzyl alcohol present in saline, on post-procedural pain in patients following direct shoulder arthrography [13c].

In this study 138 patients underwent MR arthrography. Using the Wong-Baker Faces Pain Scale, patients were asked to report their shoulder pain level before and after the procedure and also followed up for 2 days after the procedure. A control group of 62 patients received preservative-free saline solution as contrast agent diluent while a test group of 62 patients received saline containing 0.9% benzyl alcohol. The patients were randomized for this study and the effect of preservative vs. control on pain level was estimated with multiple regression.

The observed pain scale scores were significantly higher (0.79 units, $P = 0.0382$) with benzyl alcohol preservative compared with control (saline). In both study groups, the pain scale scores decreased slightly after the procedure, increased by roughly 1 unit over baseline for the test group and 0.3 unit over baseline for the control group by 6 hours after the procedure, were 0.50 unit over baseline for the test group and 0.12 unit over baseline for the control group at 24 hours, then fell to be slightly greater than baseline at 48 hours with benzyl alcohol and slightly less than baseline without benzyl alcohol. These trends over time were highly significant ($P < 0.0001$).

This report provides evidence of significantly increased patient discomfort when using normal saline preserved with benzyl alcohol as a diluent. This new study is consistent with similar findings reported in the literature [14c, 15c]. Therefore it warrants further investigation and caution while choosing the appropriate diluent for systemic administration of drugs or diagnostic agents.

Calcium (SEDA-36, 727)

Mouth and Teeth

Caphosol® (CP) is a commercially available electrolyte solution containing supersaturated calcium phosphate that is used as a mouth rinse to lubricate the oral mucosa and to maintain the integrity of the oral cavity by minimizing friction and dissolution of hardened mucous.

The CP mouth rinse has a similar composition as saliva, which is primarily water and salts. CP is marketed as an adjunct to standard oral care for treating mucositis that may be caused by radiation or high dose chemotherapy. Several clinical studies have shown positive effects of CP mouth rinses on the frequency, intensity and duration of oral mucositis in patients undergoing hematopoietic stem cell transplantation (HSCT). Nuyts et al. recently reported the first randomized clinical trial, evaluating the effect of adding a CP mouth rinse on the severity and evolution of oral mucositis in patients with head and neck cancer (HNC) treated with chemo-radiotherapy [16c].

Fifty-eight patients with malignant neoplasms of the head and neck receiving chemo-radiation were included in this study. The patients were randomized into a control group receiving standard of care ($n=31$) and a study group receiving standard of care plus daily CP mouth rinses ($n=27$) starting on the first day of chemo-radiation. Oral mucositis and dysphagia were assessed twice a week using the National Cancer Institute common toxicity criteria scale version 3, while oral pain was scored with a visual analog scale.

The study did not reveal any significant difference in grade III mucositis (59% vs. 71%; $P=0.25$) or dysphagia (33% vs. 42%, $P=0.39$) between the study group and the control group. Also no significant differences were found in time until development of peak mucositis (28.6 vs. 28.7 days; $P=0.48$), duration of peak mucositis (22.7 vs. 24.6 days; $P=0.31$), recuperation of peak dysphagia (20.5 vs. 24.2 days; $P=0.13$) and occurrence of severe pain (56 vs. 52%, $P=0.5$). Thus, this first randomized clinical study did not find any evidence supporting the addition of CP mouth rinse to standard of care use in daily practice. Similar findings were reported in two additional trials, one a Phase II multicenter trial [17C] and a prospective randomized study in pediatric cancer patients [18c] suggesting no added benefits of Caphosol use.

Catheter (SEDA-36, 728)

Urinary Tract

Urinary tract infections (UTI) associated with urinary catheters are a leading cause of secondary bacterial infections and account for approximately 20% of all hospital acquired bacteremias. Long-term indwelling bladder catheterization often results in bacterial colonization in the catheter forming an extensive biofilm on their surfaces. These biofilms are resistant to antibacterial agents and therefore must be removed to prevent the infection from spreading.

In a recent study, Nandkumar and coworkers investigated the prevalence of bacterial biofilms on vascular and Foley (bladder) catheters from patients who underwent neurosurgery in order to understand the nature of antibiotic resistant strains present associated with biofilms [19c]. 141 vascular catheter and 86 Foley catheter were retrieved for this study. Patients with any pre-existing infections were excluded. Skin swabs were collected from these patients after catheter retrieval. It was found that Staphylococcus was the most prevalent strain in vascular catheters some of which were Methicillin or Vancomycin resistant. Among the Foley catheter isolates, Enterococcus faecalis was the major isolate followed by E. coli, Staphylococcus, Klebsiella, Pseudomonas and Citrobacter. Most of the strains were resistant to multiple antibiotics. Although the patients selected did not show any clinical symptoms of infection, the presence of multi-drug resistant biofilms could potentially be of concern for hospital acquired infections. Biofilms form rapidly, within 1 to 3 days, on the intraluminal and extraluminal catheter surface. Therefore, the duration of catheterization is the strongest risk factor for bacteriuria development. Approximately 10–25% patients with bacteriuria progress to symptomatic UTI and 1–4% develop urosepsis. Going forward, development of a novel early warning sensor [20c] that can continually monitor for early stages of biofilm formation has gathered a lot of interest. It is currently under clinical evaluation and has the potential to improve the life of indwelling catheter users.

Choline (SEDA-36, 728)

Cardiovascular

Ongoing research in animal models as well as clinical investigations has now confirmed the association between acute egg yolk ingestion and formation of trimethylamine-N-oxide (TMAO) in the gut by the intestinal microbiota. Choline is particularly abundant in egg yolk and is converted to TMAO which is purported to be a risk factor for developing cardiovascular diseases. A recent study by Zeisel et al. specifically looked at possible relationship between egg consumption and increase in markers of inflammation or increased oxidation of LDL [21c]. The results of this study involving six volunteers, was that egg consumption of two or more increased plasma and urine TMAO concentrations significantly with 14% of total choline in eggs converted to TMAO. Future studies are warranted to confirm the association of TMAO and atherosclerosis.

Sexual Function

Choline is a water-soluble essential nutrient, grouped within the B-complex vitamins. It is found in foods such as fish, eggs, muscle meats and is also used as a dietary supplement in various diseases including liver, psychiatric and neurological disorders. While choline is generally safe, doses over the recommended daily intake levels

(550 mg–3.5 g/day for adults) are likely to cause side effects such as sweating, gastrointestinal distress, diarrhea and vomiting. Increasing dietary choline also is shown to increase the risk of colorectal cancer.

In a recent study, Bramanti and coworkers reported that choline could be a possible cause of hypersexuality [22A]. In this study, a 79-year-old man who was affected by memory loss was diagnosed with mild cognitive impairment and subsequently treated with oral choline supplementation of 1200 mg/day. After 6 weeks of regular choline consumption, the patient showed a pathological increase in libido with sexual urges. Interestingly while on choline the patient also reported significant improvement in erectile function. However after choline was withdrawn, the hypersexuality receded in about 5 days. Hypersexuality involves persistent uninhibited sexual behavior and may be a relatively unexplored new adverse effect of choline and related drugs and dietary supplements that act on the cholinergic pathway. Although hypersexuality is a common side effect of dopamine agonists, no exist on role of choline (a precursor of the parasympathetic neurotransmitter acetylcholine) in sexual function. Such report is the first of its kind and while it warrants further investigation, it emphasizes the need to be considered when treating and counselling patients with inappropriate sexual behavior.

Collagen (SEDA-36, 730)

Cardiovascular

Collagen-based vascular closure devices (VCD) are commonly used after catheterization with femoral access. However, data about complication rates due to the utilization of VCDs in patients with known peripheral artery disease (PAD) of the lower limbs are inconsistent and patients with significant PAD are excluded in most VCD trials. Erbel and coworkers reported a prospective clinical study to compare the efficacy and safety of a collagen-based VCD after coronary or lower limb intervention in patients with vs. without PAD [23c].

A total of 382 patients (268 men; mean age 65 years) undergoing either an endovascular procedure of the lower limb (PAD group, $n = 132$) or a percutaneous coronary intervention (PCI group, $n = 250$) via a common femoral artery access were enrolled in this study if hemostasis was achieved using the collagen-based commercial product namely Angio-Seal. Exclusion criteria were: treatment with Angio-Seal within the last 90 days; known allergy to bovine products; and a puncture adjacent to the femoral bifurcation. The study showed no significant differences (1.5% PAD vs. 1.2% PCI, $P = 1.0$) in the rate of major complications after utilization of a collagen-based VCD for femoral artery access site closure in patients with severe lower limb PAD compared to those without. The major complications recorded were bleeding, large hematoma, pseudoaneurysm, vessel occlusion, and dissection. However, complications in the PAD group tended to be more severe, with the need for surgical repair. After utilization of Angio-Seal, 2 patients developed major complications such as stenosis of the puncture site or a total occlusion of the femoral artery. This was caused by the anchor and collagen plug located intravasally, triggering a thrombogenic occlusion of the vessel. There was a trend toward higher prevalence of complications with increasing size of closure device and with the stage of PAD. Therefore, Angio-Seal safety in patients with significant PAD needs further evaluation in larger trials.

Cremophor

Cardiovascular

Cremophor EL (CrEL) is a formulation vehicle used to improve solubility of various poorly-water soluble drugs, including the anticancer agent paclitaxel (Taxol). In contrast to earlier reports, CrEL is not an inert vehicle, but exerts a range of biological effects, some of which have important clinical implications. Its use has been associated with severe anaphylactoid hypersensitivity reactions, hyperlipidemia, abnormal lipoprotein patterns, aggregation of erythrocytes and peripheral neuropathy. The pharmacokinetic behavior of CrEL is dose-independent, although its clearance is highly influenced by duration of the infusion. This is particularly important since CrEL can affect the disposition of various drugs by changing the unbound drug concentration through micellar encapsulation.

Schiffelers and coworkers report a study that investigated the effects of CrEL-PTX on red blood cells (RBCs) and compared these with the effects observed after exposure to a novel nanoparticle albumin-bound PTX formulation, marketed as Abraxane® [24E]. The study results showed that CrEL caused RBC lysis and induction of phosphatidylserine exposure which in turn had an increased association with endothelial cells. CrEL was also responsible for vesiculation of RBCs. Abraxane formulated in albumin (no CrEL) did not induce any of these effects on RBCs, indicating that the choice of excipients can have a pronounced influence on the efficacy and side effects of anticancer drugs. This is the first time new insights are provided into the side effect of CrEL which is likely to have implications for patients with erythrocyte disorders.

Vitamin D Supplement

Vitamin D is a fat-soluble vitamin that is naturally present in very few foods and is widely available as dietary additive or supplement. It is biologically inert and undergoes hydroxylation in the liver (to 25-hydroxy Vitamin D) and the kidney (to 1, 25-dihydroxy Vitamin D) for activation. Vitamin D promotes calcium absorption in the gut and maintains adequate serum calcium and phosphate concentrations to enable normal mineralization of bone. It is also needed for bone growth and bone remodeling by osteoblasts and osteoclasts Vitamin D sufficiency prevents rickets in children and osteomalacia in adults.

Although Vitamin D toxicity is rare in children, increased use of Vitamin D formulations can increase the potential for toxicity. Vitamin D intoxication is known to cause hypercalcemia in children and has renal, cardiac and neurological consequences. Fede et al. recently presented two cases of hypervitaminosis due to self-medication of over the counter Vitamin D supplements [25A]. A 12-year-old boy was hospitalized for abdominal pain, constipation and vomiting. Upon routine biochemistry, it was determined that he had severe hypocalcaemia and renal failure. Plasma 25-OH Vitamin D level was very high while parathyroid hormone was suppressed. Renal ultrasound showed nephrolithiasis. Hydration, diuretics and prednisone induced a progressive reduction of calcium levels. His brother, who was receiving the same treatment, was hospitalized although asymptomatic. Normal serum calcium and renal function were revealed, while 25-OH Vitamin D was high and parathyroid hormone was suppressed. Upon examination of the Vitamin D content of the over-the-counter supplement a higher amount was found than declared. Vitamin D administration therefore implies several risks and must be prescribed only when needed and under strict medical control.

Vitamin D is available in two mono-hydroxy forms: Ergocalciferol (Vitamin D2) and Cholecalciferol (Vitamin D3). Both are found as dietary supplements and in various food items naturally or after fortification. Additionally, the active di-hydroxy form is also available commercially for treatment of hypocalcemia.

In light of a growing body of research, recent reports of Vitamin D intoxication and increased use of Vitamin D supplements, the Drugs and Therapeutics committee of the Pediatric Endocrine Society (PES) performed a systematic review of the safety of currently recommended high Vitamin D doses as well as reported cases of intoxications in pediatrics (reviewed in [26R]). Based on their findings, the recent cases of intoxication were related to manufacturing or formulation errors, or high total intake in the range of 240 000–4 500 000 IU (total dose). The current safety guidelines limit the upper level intake in children in the range of 1000–5000 IU/day for 2–4 weeks.

In adult patients with primary hyperparathyroidism (PHPT) Vitamin D insufficiency is commonly observed. However, Vitamin D supplementation is not prescribed in these patients because of the possible risk of hypercalcemia or hypercalciuria. There is limited data on effects of Vitamin D supplementation in PHPT patients.

Case report [27A]:

- Two women (A: 53 years/BMI 28 and B: 63 years/BMI 24) with diagnosed PHPT and Vitamin D deficiency were erroneously prescribed 2 400 000 IU (300 000 IU/day for 8 days) and 4 500 000 U (300 000 U/day for 15 days) of Vitamin D3, respectively. They were supposed to take only a single oral dose of 300 000 IU. The patients were followed for 4 months and ionized calcium, creatinine, PTH, 25-hydroxy Vitamin D, 1, 25-dihydroxy Vitamin D and urinary calcium/creatinine levels were measured. During the observational period 25-hydroxy-Vitamin D levels rose quickly and attained values higher than 150 ng/mL during the first month in patient B and during the second month in patient A, reaching ≤70 ng/mL by the end of the observation period. PTH levels, in turn, quickly declined after the Vitamin D load and began to rise again from the second month. The patients were asked to increase their daily water intake (more than 3 L/day). They did not develop any symptom or clinical sign of hypercalcemia. After 4 months the patients were operated on, because of osteoporosis, and a parathyroid adenoma was removed in both. Even 1 year after surgery the patients did not developed any complications. The unintentional over-supplementation of Vitamin D caused a moderate increase of hypercalcemia and hypercalciuria and was not associated with clinical signs of toxicity. However, the negative correlation initially found between 25OHD and PTH levels strongly suggests that PTH secretion may be modulated by Vitamin D even in patients with PHPT.

Dapsone Gel

Systemic Toxicity

Aczone® is a FDA approved topical 5% gel formulation of dapsone which is used to treat inflammatory and non-inflammatory acne. Dapsone is an antibacterial antibiotic that blocks myeloperoxidase during inflammation. The most common side effects of ACZONE® Gel are dryness, redness, oiliness, and peeling of the skin being treated. Dapsone is also available as oral pill which has been related to cause hemolytic anemia. However, it is believed that topical absorption of dapsone does not result in large enough systemic drug concentration to cause clinical symptoms. Interestingly, a rare instance of adverse effect was recently reported [28A] after topical dapsone gel use for facial acne. A 19-year-old woman (51 kg) who used Aczone for a week developed headache, shortness of breath and blue lips and fingers. Upon examination she showed a methemoglobin level of 20.3% compared to a normal value of <0.1%. She had perioral and acral cyanosis which were resolved upon subsequent treatment with intravenous methylene blue. After 2 hours of treatment, her methemoglobin level came down below 2%. Urinary drug screening revealed presence of dapsone. There is no established explanation for this rare side-effect as the patient had no open wounds that would promote greater drug absorption. This case report therefore highlights the potential for systemic drug absorption and toxicity with therapeutic use of topical drug formulations.

Disulfiram (SED-15, 1148; SEDA-31, 760; SEDA-32, 895; SEDA-33, 1016; SEDA-34, 791; SEDA-36, 731)

Neurological

Disulfiram (tetraethylthiuram disulfide) is a quaternary ammonium compound used for treating alcohol dependency for over 60 years. It is an inhibitor of dopamine-β-hydroxylase causing an increase in the concentration of dopamine in the brain. Initially, when disulfiram was being used, the doses were much higher (1000–3000 mg) than today (250–500 mg) due to reports of neurotoxicity, delirium, and psychosis.

Alves et al. reports a case of a rare complication when using disulfiram for alcoholism treatment in a patient in alcoholic abstinence [29A]. A 42-year-old male developed psychotic symptoms 3 weeks after initiating treatment with disulfiram for alcohol dependency. The patient had a history of chronic alcoholism for 12 years and was under disulfiram treatment (250 mg/day) for 1 month, with no other past history of psychiatric illness. The symptoms worsened after he initiated alcohol consumption, while taking disulfiram. When he was admitted at the emergency room he presented symptoms of alcohol disulfiram reaction with tachycardia, sweating, and vomiting. Serological examination showed hepatic alterations (GGT-124, ALT-92); alcohol was positive—0.07. After the patient was hospitalized disulfiram was suspended the patient became asymptomatic in 4 days remained asymptomatic after 6 weeks. Treatment with disulfiram can lead to the appearance of psychosis, which can be related to alcohol-induced psychotic disorder based on symptoms, such as delusions and auditory and visual hallucinations. In clinical practice, psychosis in the context of alcoholism with disulfiram therapy is often neglected and should be taken into account. Patients with a family history of psychosis are more vulnerable to precipitants of psychosis than others due to genetic predisposition. The patient's father was previously diagnosed with chronic alcoholism when he presented with psychotic symptoms. Because of this family history, this patient may have low levels of dopamine-β-hydroxylase; so, when disulfiram blocks it, there is a greater predisposition to the development of psychosis. Other recent studies reported have alluded to side-effects of disulfiram ingestion including hepatic failure [30A] and risks of myocardial infarction [31A].

Fluoride (SED-15, 1395; SEDA-32, 892; SEDA-33, 1017; SEDA-34, 791; SEDA-36, 733)

Fluoride is ingested primarily through consuming drinking water. Although safe and even healthy at low concentrations, sustained consumption of large amounts of soluble fluoride salts is dangerous. Referring to a common salt of fluoride, sodium fluoride (NaF), the lethal dose for most adult humans is estimated at 5–10 g (which is equivalent to 32–64 mg/kg elemental fluoride/kg body weight). Ingestion of fluoride can produce gastrointestinal discomfort at doses at least 15–20 times lower (0.2–0.3 mg/kg or 100–150 mg for a 50 kg person) than lethal doses. Although helpful for dental health in low dosage, chronic exposure to fluoride in large amounts interferes with bone formation. In this way, the most widespread examples of fluoride poisoning arise from consumption of ground water that is abnormally fluoride-rich.

Recent review of the literature points to several reports of Fluoride related side-effects that may not be neglected. In one study, children of Kalmar County Sweden were evaluated who ingest water from wells enriched with Fluorine [32c]. The levels of Fluorine in these wells were above the US EPA limit of 0.06 mg/kg-day. As much as 48% of these children were assessed to be at risk after exposure from drinking water and when taking into account other possible exposure pathways such as beverages and food, ingestion of toothpaste, dust inhalation, the number increased to 77%. Thus, total exposure should consider all possible pathways.

Another study looked at interaction of fluoride and gene expression in apoptosis or inflammatory processes in 72 children (6–12 years old) with chronic exposure to Fluoride (5.3 mg/L) in drinking water and in food cooked with the same water [33c]. CD25 gene expression levels and urine concentrations of F were negatively correlated. Age and height influenced the expression of cIAP-1, whereas XIAP expression was correlated only with age. Additionally, there was a lower percentage of CD25- and CD40-positive cells in the group of 6- to 8-year-old children exposed to the highest concentrations of F when compared to the 9- to 12-year-old group. These changes could potentially decrease immune responses in children exposed to F.

Another study conducted in Gaya district of Bihar, India analyzed groundwater used for drinking and cooking for fluoride, and conducted health surveys [34c]. Survey data showed that more than 50% of adults and more than 55% of children had complaints of gastrointestinal (GI) disturbances in the fluoride-rich areas (2.36±0.23 mg/L) while less than 20% of adults and less than 10% of children complained of GI problems in the control areas (0.59±0.03 mg/L). Hematological analyses showed occurrence of anemia with lowered hemoglobin, hematocrit, mean corpuscular volume, mean corpuscular hemoglobin and mean corpuscular hemoglobin concentration in the fluorotic subjects.

Gelatin (SED-15, 885; SEDA-34, 792; SEDA-36, 734)

Cardiovascular

FloSeal and SurgiFlo hemostatic matrices are commonly used in surgical procedures (other than ophthalmic) to as adjunct to hemostasis to promote coagulation and minimize blood loss. They are composed of bovine and porcine gelatin matrix, respectively, that can be injected into pedicles to stop osseous bleeding during pedicle screw insertion. The gelatin matrix is made of cross-linked gelatin spheres and is mixed with thrombin immediately prior to application.

Woerz reports 2 pediatric spinal deformity reconstructive surgery patients who experienced intraoperative cardiovascular issues after the intraosseous administration of FloSeal [35A].

Case #1: An 11-year-old female with adolescent idiopathic scoliosis was undergoing routine posterior spinal instrumentation and fusion. During placement of the fourth pedicle screw, the patient developed profound hypotension, tachycardia, and elevated airway pressures requiring intravenous epinephrine and phenylephrine for hemodynamic support. Postoperative work-up demonstrated a positive immunoassay for bovine gelatin. When surgery was performed 1 week later, without the use of FloSeal, no episodes of hemodynamic instability were reported.
Case #2: A 9-year-old female with juvenile idiopathic scoliosis who was undergoing a growing spine construct was administered SurgiFlo into 2 pedicle tracts after which there was profound hypotension, tachycardia, and elevated airway pressures. When surgery was repeated 2 weeks later, without the use of SurgiFlo, no episodes of hemodynamic instability were reported.

Both patients showed symptoms for anaphylaxis immediately following the administration of gelatin-based matrices. A similar incident was recently reported [36A] for a 9-year-old boy who also had an episode of anaphylaxis after measles, mumps, and rubella vaccines were administered which are known to contain gelatin. Although gelatin allergy has been well described in type 1 hypersensitivity reactions to vaccines, these are the first known reported cases of intraoperative anaphylaxis associated with hemostatic agents. Patients who are atopic, asthmatic, and allergic are more likely to develop hypersensitivity than individuals who are not allergic. Gelatin in FloSeal or SurgiFlo is derived from bovine sources, and there is high cross reactivity between mammalian gelatin antigens. The results also emphasize the need for determining preoperative history of allergy and immunotesting for animal derived gelatin products.

Glycine

Cardiovascular

WATER FOR IRRIGATION

1.5% Glycine irrigation USP is a sterile non-pyrogenic aqueous solution typically used during transurethral prostatic or bladder surgery. Typically with glycine there is no risk of allergy as it is an endogenous amino acid. Hahn et al. recently argued that Glycine for irrigation use should be avoided completely [37R], based on a systematic review of literature on preclinical and clinical studies. Overall he looked at 11 animal studies, 3 in healthy subjects and 6 patients where Glycine solution was used during transurethral resection of the prostate. These studies showed adverse effects after administration or absorption of glycine solution. It also indicated that higher concentrations of glycine such as 2.2% were more toxic than 1.5% glycine. The side effects included tissue damage or higher mortality (in animals) or increased symptoms (volunteers and patients).

In the mouse models, earlier studies have indicated myocardial hypoxia and inflammation upon glycine infusion [38E]. In another study glycine 1.5% caused hypo-osmotic pressure and rupturing of the histoskeleton in pigs [39E]. In healthy volunteers, glycine infusion generally caused symptoms like prickling sensation of the skin, flushing, blurred vision, discomfort, slight nausea and exhaustion. These effects correlated with a corresponding increase of blood ammonia to 354 μM which was 10 folds higher than the normal level. In clinical studies with patients undergoing transurethral resection of prostate, one study showed statistically significant circulatory symptoms like increased fluid absorption (>1 L). Additionally, neurological symptoms like nausea, headache and visual impairment were also seen to a greater magnitude compared to when mannitol was used instead. Rise in blood ammonia was also reported in some patients. Potential mechanism for high ammonia levels are not clear while the inhibitory neurotransmitter properties are believed to account for impaired vision. Overall these studies diminish the enthusiasm for use of glycine as a superior irrigation fluid compared to other alternatives.

DIETARY GLYCINE

Elliott and coworkers reported a study to assess the role of dietary glycine on blood pressure [40C]. Animal protein intake through red meat consumption is believed to have a direct relationship to elevated blood pressure. Animal protein is abundant in several amino acids like glycine, alanine, arginine, histidine, lysine etc. In the reported cross-sectional epidemiological study 4680 subjects (age 40–60 years) from 17 random population samples in China, Japan, United Kingdom and United States were monitored for blood pressure and dietary records and urine samples were analyzed.

The percentage of dietary glycine in total protein intake was directly related to blood pressure. It was estimated that for each additional 0.71 g/day of glycine, there was an increase in systolic blood pressure of 2–3 mmHg. BP differences associated with higher glycine intake higher in Western subjects than in East Asians. Interestingly in Westerners, meat was the main dietary source of glycine but not in East Asians who got it more from vegetable and fish. However, further studies are needed to demonstrate reproducibility of this effect. In related preclinical studies in sugar-fed rats, an inverse effect was observed instead of a direct effect. Biological mechanisms for the direct association observed in this study needs to be investigated.

Glycols (SED-15, 1516; SEDA-30, 567; SEDA-34, 792; SEDA-33, 1017)

Ethylene Glycol

URINARY TRACT

Ethylene glycol found in antifreeze fluids/car coolants, air-conditioning systems is a relatively common cause of acute renal toxicity in humans. This is frequently caused by accidental ingestion of this sweet tasting colorless, odorless liquid but also intentional abuse as a cheap alcohol substitute. Mortality rate from such acute poisoning is high ($\sim$30%) second only to methanol intoxication. Recently, a case was reported [41A] of a 52-year-old farmer who was admitted to the emergency department due to feeling unwell and anuria and edema for 2 days and subsequently diagnosed with advanced renal failure. He had aspirated antifreeze into his mouth several time a week ago. When feeling headache and nausea he drank alcohol as well.

This case was interesting as there were no neurodepression right away but only nausea initially. However, prolonged renal failure was seen in a week when he developed acute kidney injury which was believed to be due to ethylene glycol ingestion as was evidenced by appearance of calcium oxalate crystals in renal biopsy. Oxalic acid is the metabolic end-product of ethylene glycol metabolism.

Propylene Glycol

Propylene glycol (PG) is a synthetic co-solvent used as a solubility enhancing additive in many drug formulations. The FDA has classified propylene glycol as "generally recognized as safe" (GRAS) for use in food. The potential for systemic toxicity secondary to propylene glycol has traditionally been considered to be low in adult patients; however, several case reports associating PG with hyperosmolality, elevated anion gap metabolic acidosis, hemolysis, neurotoxicity, and acute renal insufficiency have challenged this assumption. Most of the time the drugs products containing propylene glycol as an excipient, are administered to critically ill patients with co-medications. Thus, it is difficult to identify the effects specifically due to PG. Bhat et al. recently reported a case of PG toxicity related to infusion of antiepileptic drugs phenobarbital and phenytoin in patients with refractory status epilepticus [42A]. PG toxicity include lactic acidosis, renal failure, and multiorgan failure mimicking sepsis. Prior renal disease is an important precipitating factor for toxicity.

In another study [43A], continuous IV infusion of pentobarbital was associated with PG intoxication with severe acidosis that was resolved upon withdrawal of the formulation.

TOXICITY IN CHILDREN

A recent review by Pageler et al., comprehensively presents adverse effects of propylene glycol use in pediatric population providing safe prescribing guidelines [44M]. The study covers medical literature from 1970 to 2010. Key summary of their findings provides evidence of CNS and cardiotoxicity associated with PG administration as excipients of medications. PG tends to accumulate with chronic use in pediatric patients particularly those in the intensive care units undergoing continuous drug infusions. Commonly used drugs that contained PG include lorazepam, phenobarbital, and digoxin. PG is not significantly serum protein bound and can be cleared by hemodialysis.

Electronic Cigarettes

Use of electronic nicotine delivery devices like e-cigarettes is rapidly gaining in popularity in the USA. In e-cigarettes nicotine along with other components are aerosolized prior to inhalation. Scientific evidence regarding the human health effects of e-cigarettes are however limited and confusing due to lack of standardized testing methods. While e-cigarette aerosol may contain fewer toxic ingredients than cigarette smoke, studies evaluating whether e-cigarettes are less harmful than cigarettes are largely inconclusive.

Besides nicotine, hazards can arise from other constituents of liquids, such as solvents, flavors, additives and contaminants. Glycol and glycerol vapor are common components of most e-cigarette refill solutions [45E]. Analysis of various vaping solutions has revealed concentrations of PG ranging from 60 percent to 90%, and up to 15% glycerin although some vendors have reported mixtures of equal parts and others substitute glycerin and water for PG completely. PG is a known upper airway irritant when administered in aerosolized form. This could be of potential concern to people with chronic lung disease such as asthma, emphysema or chronic bronchitis. PG mist may also dry out mucous membranes and eyes. Although PG does not cause cytotoxic effects long-term inhalation of vapor associated with e-cigarette use could lead to different behavior because of the reduction of particle size and increase in surface area of exposure. Of the limited studies reported there was evidence of decrease in exhaled nitric oxide (FeNO) and increase in respiratory impedance and respiratory flow resistance similar to cigarette use [46c].

Another ingredient commonly found in analyzed e-cigarette liquids is formaldehyde which is a carcinogen and a known degradation products of propylene glycol. In one study Goniewicz and colleagues detected 3 carbonyls namely formaldehyde, acetaldehyde and acroleinfrom 12 brands of e-cigarettes [47E] although the levels were 9–450 times lower compared to emissions form tobacco cigarettes. In another study, looking at several samples of e-cigarette vapors (produced by thermal degradation of propylene glycol in presence of oxygen during vaping process), more than 2% of the total solvent were shown to convert to formaldehyde reaching concentrations higher than that of nicotine [48E]. Others studies have shown that vapors generated from various commercial e-cigarette solutions expose users to toxic carbonyls, including the carcinogens formaldehyde and acetaldehyde [49E, 50E]. In fact, the highest levels of carbonyls were observed in vapors generated from PG-based solutions. The amount of formaldehyde exposure from e-cigs is particularly high when they are vaped at high voltage using a variable-voltage battery.

To date limited clinical studies evaluating the effects of short-term e-cigarette use on cardiovascular and respiratory functional outcomes have shown that even if some harmful effects of vaping are reported, these are considerably milder compared with smoking conventional cigarettes. However, it is difficult to assess the prognostic implications of these studies; longer-term data are needed before any definite conclusions are made. There are limited data on the chronic inhalation of these chemicals by humans, although and none of them specifically investigated the role of glycols. The readers are encouraged to read a recent comprehensive review of safety evaluation and risk assessment of electronic cigarettes by Polosa and coworkers [51R].

Hyaluronidase

Sensory Systems: Eye

Hyaluronidase (Hylase Dessau®) is a hyaluronic acid-metabolizing enzyme, which has been shown to enhance drug diffusion and thereby increasing the efficacy of local anesthetics. It is used in management of lower eyelid edema associated with cosmetic procedure. Hyaluronic acid-based dermal fillers are often employed as safe operative procedures although rare complications involve development of eyelid edema which could be an indication of systemic or periorbital diseases. Gerber et al. conducted a study to evaluate the efficacy of hyaluronidase in the management of lower eyelid edema with the hypothesis that it loosens the extracellular matrix [52c]. In this retrospective analysis, 20 patients with lower eyelid edema were treated with 0.2–0.5 mL Hylase (20–75 IU) per eyelid. Although hyaluronidase rapidly and effectively resolved eyelid edema after single injection, it was noted that for two cases, it also partly or completely dissolved the injected hyaluronic acid fillers possibly due to injection of a large volume. This negatively impacts tear-trough augmentations such as bruising, color changes, and swelling and warrants additional diagnostic measures. It is important to note some related *in vitro* studies like those by Marazzi and coworkers evaluated the role of hyaluronidase on skin and soft tissue viability [53E]. It was reported that high concentrations of this enzyme can inhibit skin viability. Also concentration-dependent hyaluronidase toxicity was mentioned to be a cause of postoperative periorbital inflammation after cataract surgery following regional anesthesia [54A, 55A].

Hydroxyethyl Starch (SEDA-36, 734)

Renal Toxicity

Hydroxyethyl starch (HES) solutions like Voluven, Hespan or Hextend (6% solution) are widely used for the treatment of hypovolemia (low blood volume) when plasma volume expansion is desired. Low-molecular-weight HES like Voluven (MW 130 000) have shown increased risk of AKI and mortality in recent large randomized trials (reviewed in [56R]). However, these studies focused on critically ill patients (i.e., sepsis and major trauma) who were given large volumes of HES. But unlike critical care patients who are often given high-dose HES over prolonged periods, surgical patients are typically given smaller amounts over just a few hours. It remains unknown whether the adverse effects of HES observed in critically ill patients apply to routine surgical patients.

Kurz et al. recently evaluated the association between intraoperative HES administration and postoperative kidney function after noncardiac surgery [57C]. For this purpose, Hextend was chosen (high molecular weight, 670 000). The authors reviewed 14 680 patients receiving colloids with 14 680 patients receiving noncolloidal balanced salt solutions aka crystalloids. Data suggested that the odds of developing a more serious level of AKI with Hextend were 21% (6–38%) greater than with crystalloid only ($P = 0.001$). AKI risk increased as a function of colloid volume ($P < 0.001$). In contrast, the relationship between colloid use and AKI did not differ on baseline AKI risk ($P = 0.84$). There was no association between colloid use and risk of in-hospital ($P = 0.81$) or 90-day ($P = 0.02$) mortality. Thus, dose-dependent renal toxicity associated with Hextend in patients having noncardiac surgery is consistent with randomized trials in critical care patients.

Although the exact mechanism remains unclear, the potential for colloids to cause kidney injury is well known. HES with MW smaller than the renal threshold (60–70 kDa) are excreted in urine. Larger molecules are broken down by α-amylase before being excreted by the kidneys. Larger MW HES circulate in the blood stream longer. Subsequently, HES induces tubular swelling and osmotic necrosis due to cytoplasmic vacuole formation which is believed to cause renal toxicity. Such effects are clearly molecular weight related. Thus, Voluven with lower molecular weight and lower degree of substitution is expected to be better tolerated than Hextend.

Latex (SED-15, 2005; SEDA-31, 761; SEDA-33, 1018; SEDA-34, 792; SEDA-36, 736)

Immunologic

In the 1990s powdered, natural rubber latex glove related allergy was widespread in healthcare workers. Subsequent use of powder-free, low protein latex gloves significantly reduced the incidences. However, small number of reports of occupational latex allergy still emerge. A review of literature was performed by Ahmed et al. to determine the optimal management of workers with type 1 latex allergy [58R]. The review suggests a strong evidence that symptoms and markers of sensitization in latex-allergic individuals were related to using natural rubber latex gloves at workplace. Even if sensitized individuals wear powder-free latex gloves they are at risk of exposure from co-workers who use the powdered latex gloves.

Powdered latex gloves continue to be widely used in hospitals in developing countries due to the low cost. A cross-sectional study in female nurses in Thai hospitals [59c] reported not only dermal but also respiratory symptoms like sneezing, rhinitis and even asthma associated with wearing more than 15 pairs of latex gloves in a day. Rui et al. reported on a 10-year follow-up of 9660 healthcare workers in-between 2000 and 2009, where many subjects were found with allergic symptoms related to common allergens are at higher risk [60c].

An interesting pilot study was reported on prenatal latex sensitization in patients with congenital disorder like spinabifida [61c]. These patients are believed to be particularly at risk of IgE-mediated latex sensitization and hypersensitivity reactions. The prevalence among these patients are much higher (25–65%) compared to healthy children (0.7%). Latex specific and total IgE levels in these patients were significantly higher than healthy individuals ($P = 0.001$). There is now increasing evidence suggesting that prenatal exposure to allergens plays an important role in the development of allergy. The presence of allergen-specific T cells at the time of birth may imply that specific immune responses can develop in the womb. Also contact of latex allergens with cerebrospinal fluid or the meningeal layer induces localized allergic reactions. This pilot study thus gives novel insights in the immunological reactions related to spina bifida. The increased latex-specific IgE levels could possibly be associated with the occurrence of a latex allergy in the future.

Liposome

Dose-Limiting Toxicity

Nanomedicines like Pegylated liposomes are novel drug delivery systems that provide increased tumor delivery of anticancer chemotherapeutics while concurrently reduced non-selective toxicity. These nanocarriers are approximately 100 nm in diameter and have a lipid bilayer shell with anticancer drugs encapsulated in its aqueous core. Liposomes are unique in that they can improve drug solubility and alter the biodistribution and pharmacokinetics of the small molecule drug payload in favor of the target site i.e. tumor. Pegylation i.e. modification of the surface of these liposomes with a water-soluble polymer polyethylene glycol provides stealth properties to these liposomes allowing them circulate longer in the body and evade uptake by the reticuloendothelial system (liver and spleen). Pegylated liposome formulation of doxorubicin (Doxil®) is FDA approved for treatment of patients with refractory ovarian cancer. Although the safety of Doxil is well characterized limited information exists regarding the clinical risk factors for ovarian cancer patients who develop palmar plantar erythrodysesthesia (PPE, also known as hand-foot syndrome). This is a complication that occurs in 30% of ovarian cancer patients treated with Doxil and is characterized by redness and tenderness of palms and soles and sometimes blistering leading to severe impairment of daily functions. Gehrig et al. conducted a retrospective analysis of recurrent ovarian cancer patients who underwent treatment with Doxil from 2005–2009[62c]. Results show that 23% of the 133 patients studied, developed PPE. Unlike previous reports 75% of these patients developed PPE within the first 3 cycles of infusion which suggests early onset of PPE. The PPE development was non-dose limiting and not associated with receiving prior chemotherapy. The magnitude of PPE toxicity was believed to be less possibly due to preventive measure that were taken such as use of corticosteroids (dexamethasone) prior to each infusion. Doxil appeared to be metabolized by a different biological system than typical small molecule cytotoxic drugs. Because of Doxil's ability to evade the RES system, it shows poorer clearance, decreased monocyte count and consequently increased risk of PPE toxicity. Another reason for increased PPE toxicity could be related to the size of Doxil. Because of it macromolecular nature Doxil preferentially localizes in areas of high vascular permeability like palms and soles due to the well characterized "Enhanced Permeability and Retention" (EPR) effect.

Overall from this single center study, several observations were made that warrants further investigation of the mechanism of metabolism of Doxil. Recent advances in the design and development of nanoscale drug carriers like liposomes, dendrimers, gold nanoparticles, etc. are promising to improve the conventional chemotherapy regimens and outcomes, however, further understanding of their mechanism of action and biological fate will be necessary for clinical success of these novel nanomedicines.

Magnesium (SEDA-36, 736)

Drug Overdose

Magnesium (Mg) is commonly found in over-the-counter medications. It is often used as a laxative, so diarrhea after taking a Mg-based laxative can be a mild symptom of magnesium overdose. Antacids also contain magnesium. In the absence of renal impairment, excess Mg is removed by the kidneys. Mg is an essential mineral that helps muscles function and maintain energy. Mg overdose hypermagnesemia, generally occurs when magnesium is ingested in large quantities in the form of a supplement, either as a pill or a liquid. It is very rare to experience a magnesium overdose by consuming foods that have naturally occurring magnesium in them, such as fruits and vegetables or nuts and whole grains.

People with impaired kidney function are at the greatest risk for magnesium overdose. Even a moderate magnesium overdose may cause a drop in blood pressure in those with kidney disease. Nagao et al. recently reported a fatal case of hypermagnesemia caused by oral ingestion of milk containing $MgCl_2$ [63A]. Upon autopsy no other injury or illness was observed while the serum Mg

concentration was 10.2 mg/dL. Reports like this alludes to the potential risks of Mg containing food and supplements.

Drug–Drug Interactions

Mg over the past 20 years have been used to inhibit preterm labor. Antenatal exposure to Mg-sulfate has shown to reduce the risk of intraventricular hemorrhage, cerebral palsy, and neonatal mortality associated with preterm birth. The proposed mechanism of action is that Mg dilates blood vessels in the brain, attenuates hypoxia and prevents brain damage. It is also believed to decrease calcium entry to the brain. However, one cause of concern reported by Sherwin et al. is the possibility of cardiopulmonary drug-drug interactions with Mg-sulfate ($MgSO_4$) [64c]. In this report, pregnant women admitted to a hospital during 2009–2011 were studied if they received one or more doses of $MgSO_4$ concomitantly with other medications like aminoglycoside antibiotics, antacids, laxatives, calcium channel blockers, corticosteroids, diuretics, Vitamin D analogs, which were all contraindicated in patients receiving $MgSO_4$. The most commonly identified potentially interacting drugs were calcium channel blockers, diuretics and antacids/laxatives. Most of these interactions resulted in longer hospital stays for these women. Three women who received the diuretic drug furosemide experienced cardiac arrest. This report can be put in context of an older but alarming report of correlation between $MgSO_4$ therapy and pediatric mortality in premature newborns [65c]. $MgSO_4$ should be used with caution for management of fetal distress when there is clear evidence of increased uterine activity.

Treatment of Migraine

Magnesium oxide is frequently used as pills to prevent migraine at doses of 400–500 mg/day. Acutely, it can also be given intravenously as $MgSO_4$ at 1–2 g. Dose-responsive diarrhea and cramping is often seen as a side effect. It is believed that Mg may prevent the wave of brain signaling which produces the visual and sensory changes that are the common forms of aura. Mg also has improved platelet function and decreased release or blocking of pain transmitting chemicals in the brain such as Substance P and glutamate. Mg may also prevent narrowing of brain blood vessels caused by the neurotransmitter serotonin. Parmar et al. recently reported a double-blind, randomized controlled trial to assess the efficacy and tolerability of intravenous Mg for treatment of acute migraine in adults [66M]. Meta-analysis of 295 patients failed to show the beneficial effects of IV Mg in reducing acute migraine or pain in adults. On the other hand, patients treated with Mg experienced more side-effects such as dizziness, irregular heartbeat, and sweating. Thus, results of Mg are therapy of migraine is less convincing than what reports on the internet or social media claim.

Miltefosine

Pancreas

Visceral leishmaniasis (VL) or kala-azar is recognized by the WHO as one of the top 10 most important infectious disease which is very common in developing countries including India, Brazil and Sudan. Miltefosine is an alkylphosphocholine drug which was recently introduced as the first oral drug in treatment of VL and in countries like India is prescribed as first line treatment. Although side effects of this drug include GI toxicity like diarrhea, vomiting, association of acute pancreatitis was not reported previously as was the case with its predecessor sodium stibogluconate that is now discontinued due to drug resistance. Das and coworkers recently reported a case of fatal acute pancreatitis is a VL patient during treatment with Miltefosine [67A]. A 41-year-old male with prolonged fever and hepatomegaly but normal hepatic and renal function was tested positive for VL. He was initially put on Miltefosine capsules (50 mg twice daily for 28 days). On day 13 of treatment he showed diffuse abdominal pain, paleness, vomiting and abdominal tenderness. This was diagnosed as acute pancreatitis concurrently with VL. Blood test showed higher TLC, lower hemoglobin, and higher serum enzymes, blood urea nitrogen and serum creatinine. CT scan of the abdomen revealed features of acute necrotizing pancreatitis. The patient was put on antibiotics and IV fluids but died 3 days later because of renal failure and septicemia. Based on the Naranjo Casualty score the development of acute pancreatitis was believed to be related to Miltefosine. This case is also interesting as pancreatitis is typically associated with patients who are coinfected with VL and HIV. In this case, the patient was immunocompetent. Thus, this study warrants further investigation of adverse drug reaction of Miltefosine using hematological and biochemical markers.

Parabens

Parabens are para hydroxybenzoic acid esters commonly referred to a group of compounds used as preservatives in pharmaceuticals, food and cosmetic products. Methyl- and propyl-parabens are the most prevalent of these esters. At low concentrations, they have a broad spectrum of activity against yeasts, molds and bacteria. They are chemically stable under physiological conditions and generally have low degree of systemic toxicity. Around the turn of the millennium there were several reports of estrogenic activity and carcinogenic potential of parabens and the FDA has regulated the allowable content of parabens in cosmetic products to 0.4% for a single ester and 0.8% for mixtures of all parabens.

The average daily total personal paraben exposure is estimated to be 76 mg, with cosmetics and personal care products accounting for 50 mg, 25 mg from pharmaceutical products, and 1 mg from food. In recent human studies repeat application of methyl parabens containing topical formulations have shown increase in compound accumulation in the stratum corneum (outermost layer) of the skin. Oral or intravenous parabens are typically metabolized by esterases within the intestine and liver.

Parabens have been detected in urine, serum, breast milk and seminal fluid. Koeppe et al. observed an inverse association between urinary levels of parabens and serum thyroid hormone concentration in adult females [68c]. Parabens are frequently detected in the urine, also among pregnant women and children. Parabens are also found in the human placental tissue and a strong correlation between urinary paraben concentrations of pregnant women and their matching newborn infants indicate the transfer of the compound from the mother to the fetus. In a few studies, parabens levels were correlated with biomarkers of oxidative DNA damage in pregnant women. Although the correlations might be coincidental, it is still a possibility that parabens, even at very low concentrations, influence organism homeostasis.

Tumorigenicity

Another worrisome observation has been the detection of parabens in breast tissue from patients with breast cancer [69R]. One hypothesis relates to use of underarm deodorant and an increased incidence of breast cancer in the upper lateral breast area. Further research involving humans are therefore necessary to assess possible adverse effects of parabens. Additionally, the influence of parabens on tissues of the immune and the central nervous system should be tested.

Phenol/Phthalate

Mutagenicity

Overexposure of children and neonates to endocrine disruptive compounds (EDC) like phthalates and phenols can potentially impact their structural and functional development and can influence disease manifestation later in life. Phthalates are diesters of phthalic acid widely used in a variety of consumer products like varnishes, lotions as well as in medical devices. Bisphenol-A (BPA) is widely used in plastic containers. Exposure to these harmful chemicals can occur via dietary ingestion, skin absorption or parenterally through injections.

A growing body of evidence suggests that epigenetic mechanisms can alter gene–environment interactions. Imprinted genes like IGF2 and H19 play a major role in fetal and placental growth and thus may be the developmental origins of disease. To date few studies examined whether epigenetic profiles in tissues were altered following exposure to phenols and phthalates. Michels and coworkers analyzed placental tissue of 196 women to investigate how first trimester individual and phthalate and phenol biomarker exposure correlates with H19 and IGF2 methylation and allele-specific expression in placenta samples [70c]. Overall, greater correlation was found among the urinary concentrations of phthalate biomarkers than of phenols. Epigenetic modifications in the placenta following EDC exposure were found to be sexually dimorphic. Statistically, significant sex interactions were observed for phenols and phthalates. For IFG2, male placenta samples were more susceptible to altered DNA methylation following phenol exposures, while female placenta samples were more susceptible following phthalate exposures. Neither methylation nor expression of these imprinted regions had a significant impact on birth length or birth weight. The mechanisms of how phthalates and phenols exert epigenetic effects are currently under investigation; however, this study provides new insight into the epigenetic mechanisms that occur following exposure to EDCs. For a review of current human and animal studies examining the effects of BPA exposure on reproduction, behavior and carcinogenesis focusing on epigenetic mechanisms please consult the paper reported by Bielajew et al. [71R].

Sclerotherapy (SED-15, 3107; SEDA-33, 1021; SEDA-34, 795)

Cardiovascular

Sclerotherapy is a medical procedure used to eliminate varicose veins and spider veins. The procedure involves an injection of a solution (generally a salt solution of 1% polidocanol or sodium tetradecyl sulfate) directly into the vein. The solution irritates the lining of the blood vessel, causing it to swell and stick together, and the blood to clot. Over time, the vessel turns into scar tissue that fades from view. Ultrasound-guided foam sclerotherapy is widely used alternatives to surgery for the treatment of varicose veins. Randomized trials and meta-analyses have shown these treatments to be effective in the short term but the safety and quality of life was not assessed previously as a primary outcome of foam sclerotherapy.

A recent clinical trial entitled "Comparison of Laser, Surgery, and Foam Sclerotherapy (CLASS) was conducted to assess quality of life and other outcomes of varicose vein treatment [72C]. Seven hundred ninety-eight participants with primary varicose veins at 11 centers in the United Kingdom were evaluated and primary outcomes at 6 months of disease-specific quality of life and generic quality of life were recorded. Secondary outcomes of complication and clinical success were also measured. It was observed that the mean disease-specific quality of life was worse after treatment with foam than after surgery ($P=0.006$). The frequency of procedural complications like deep vein thrombosis in the foam group (6%) was higher compared to laser treatment (1%). Interestingly, the frequency of serious adverse events was approximately 3% for foam sclerotherapy. Clinical success based on successful ablation of the main trunks of the saphenous vein was less for foam treatment than surgery ($P<0.001$).

The foam sclerosant, which is made of a mixture of air and a sclerosant such as polidocanol or sodium tetradecyl sulfate, is considered advantageous over the traditional liquid sclerosants as they are compact solutions and displace the blood column rather than being dissolved in the circulating blood. Also foam adheres to the walls of the vein better and has a higher contact surface area for the endothelium. Chang et al. reported a comparative study to look at efficacy and adverse effects of treatment of varicose tributaries using foam versus liquid sclerotherapy [73c]. Patients were enrolled during 2007–2009. The foam or liquid sclerosant was injected through a microcatheter followed by endovenous laser ablation (EVLA).

Varicose tributaries demonstrated complete sclerosis in greater fraction of foam treated patients (92.7%) compared to liquid treatment (71.8%) ($P=0.014$). However, adverse effects monitored such as bruising, pain or tenderness and hyperpigmentation were also associated more with foam treated groups. This study indicated that foam sclerotherapy is more effective but also carries more complications than liquid sclerotherapy.

Sevelamer (SEDA-36, 743)

Renal Toxicity

Phosphorus retention is considered to be one of the main cardiovascular risk factors for patients with chronic kidney disease (CKD). Increased phosphate levels have been attributed to the development of vascular calcification in CKD patients. Higher serum phosphorus levels are correlated with aortic valve sclerosis and aortic and mitral annular calcification in the elderly population. The National Kidney Foundation recommends that serum levels of phosphate should be maintained between 3.5 and 5.5 mg/dL, because above this level patient survival significantly decline. Dietary phosphate restriction together with the use of phosphate binders are proposed to control phosphate levels.

Phosphate binders can be divided into calcium-containing (e.g. calcium carbonate/acetate) or non-calcium containing (e.g. Sevelamer). Calcium-containing compounds have reported risk of hypercalcemia and parathyroid suppression. Sevelamer hydrochloride

(Renagel) is a synthetic FDA approved compound that can be used as an efficient medication for phosphate control, with a lower risk of side effects. However, several clinical trials have compared the risk of vascular calcification between Sevelamer and calcium salts with inconsistent results.

A number of adverse effects have been associated with Sevelamer [74c], especially metabolic acidosis. Treatment of hemodialysis patients for 6 weeks with Sevelamer resulted in decrease of serum bicarbonate level. Sevelamer is a non-absorbable polymer, which contains 17% chloride by weight, as amine hydrochloride. Upon phosphate binding or sequestration of bile acids or binding to bicarbonates in the small intestine, HCl is thought to be released resulting in metabolic acidosis. The other side effect of Sevelamer is increased risk of gastrointestinal upset, including bloating, diarrhea, and constipation.

Silicone oil (Heavy) (SED-15, 3137; SEDA-31, 766; SEDA-33, 1022; SEDA-34, 796; SEDA-36, 743)

Sensory Systems

Silicone oil (polydimethylsiloxane, PDMS) is used as a tamponade agent in retinal detachment surgery to displace the retina towards the eye wall by surface tension and close retinal breaks due to lower specific gravity (than the vitreous humor). Tamponade agents are known to prevent proliferative vitreoretinopathy (PVR). Silicone oils are chemically stable and non-immunogenic. However, PDMS provides good support only for superior retina. They are less useful for closing inferior retinal breaks for which more ideal are tamponades that are heavier than water such as heavy silicone oil (HSO). HSOs are mixtures of PDMS and semifluorinated alkanes (SFAs) that have high viscosity. A recent review by Semeraro et al. describes the physicochemical properties of various HSOs and their efficacy and safety profiles in the context of intraocular inflammation induced by these compounds [75R]. Specifically discussed are four mechanisms involved in the inflammatory response: (1) toxicity due to impurities or the instability of the agent, (2) direct toxicity and immunogenicity, (3) oil emulsification, and (4) mechanical injury due to gravity. Four different types of commercially available HSOs were reviewed. The side effects such an inflammatory reaction, macular epiretinal membranes, increased intraocular pressure, cataract and emulsification of HSOs were however comparable to PDMS. A related review by Gastaud and Bailif reviewed the short- and long-term complications associated with HSO use in management of complicated retinal detachment surgery [76R].

Roessler and coworkers reported a retrospective clinical study to determine the short-term and long-term complications associated with HSO use in 100 patient eyes following primary vitreoretinal surgery [77c]. Complete ophthalmological examination was performed before and after treatment. The mean intraocular pressure (IOP) increased from 13.3 ± 5.6 to 23.3 ± 8.5 mmHg after surgery but decreased to 13.7 ± 7.2 mmHg after HSO removal. Secondary IOP raise due to emulsification of the silicone oil was seen in 29 eyes after 7.8 ± 4.5 weeks. Other complications observed with HSO installation were persistent corneal erosion ($n = 3$) and prolonged anterior chamber inflammation ($n = 29$). In 13 eyes recurrent retinal detachments occurred during follow-up. The authors concluded that potential complications associated with HSO use should be taken into account when making the decision if to use and when to remove HSO in complicated retinal surgery. Other recent reports suggest neurotrophic corneal ulceration following retinal detachment surgery that maybe associated with HSO use [78A].

Talc (SED-15, 3592; SEDA-32, 898; SEDA-34, 797; SEDA-36, 744)

Tumorigenicity

Talcum powder is made from talc, a mineral made up mainly of magnesium, silicon, and oxygen. As a powder, it is an excellent moisture absorber, and helps cut down on friction, making it useful for keeping skin dry and helping to prevent rashes. It is widely used in cosmetic products such as baby powder and adult body and facial powders. Talc products available in the US are asbestos free. Several recent studies have looked at the possible link between talcum powder and cancer of the ovary. So far most findings yielded mixed results with no strong correlations. These types of studies not free of bias because they often rely on a person's memory of past history of talc use. A recent prospective cohort study was reported that assessed perineal powder use and risk of ovarian cancer in women [79c]. The primary outcome assessed was self-reported ovarian cancer centrally adjudicated by physicians. Unfortunately, this study concluded that perineal powder use did not contribute to the risk of ovarian cancer. It is possible that even if an individual woman has an increased risk, the overall potential is likely very small. Still, talc continues to be widely used in many products, so continued research is warranted to determine if the perceived increased risk is real.

References

[1] Pineau A, Fauconneau B, Sappino AP, et al. If exposure to aluminium in antiperspirants presents health risks, its content should be reduced. J Trace Elem Med Biol. 2014;28(2):147–50 [r].

[2] Walton JR. Chronic aluminum intake causes Alzheimer's disease: applying Sir Austin Bradford Hill's causality criteria. J Alzheimer's Dis. 2014;40(4):765–838 [r].

[3] Bhattacharjee S, Zhao Y, Hill JM, et al. Selective accumulation of aluminum in cerebral arteries in Alzheimer's disease (AD). J Inorg Biochem. 2013;126:35–7 [c].

[4] Darbre PD, Bakir A, Iskakova E. Effect of aluminium on migratory and invasive properties of MCF-7 human breast cancer cells in culture. J Inorg Biochem. 2013;128:245–9 [E].

[5] Swithers SE. Artificial sweeteners produce the counterintuitive effect of inducing metabolic derangements. Trends Endocrinol Metab. 2013;24(9):431–41 [R].

[6] Marinovich M, Galli CL, Bosetti C, et al. Aspartame, low-calorie sweeteners and disease: regulatory safety and epidemiological issues. Food Chem Toxicol. 2013;60:109–15 [R].

[7] Araujo JR, Martel F, Keating E. Exposure to non-nutritive sweeteners during pregnancy and lactation: impact in programming of metabolic diseases in the progeny later in life. Reprod Toxicol. 2014;49C:196–201 [R].

[8] Suez J, Korem T, Zeevi D, et al. Artificial sweeteners induce glucose intolerance by altering the gut microbiota. Nature. 2014;514(7521):181–6 [E].

[9] Ashok I, Sheeladevi R. Biochemical responses and mitochondrial mediated activation of apoptosis on long-term effect of aspartame in rat brain. Redox Biol. 2014;2:820–31 [E].

[10] Yilmaz S, Ucar A. A review of the genotoxic and carcinogenic effects of aspartame: does it safe or not? Cytotechnology. 2014;66(6):875–81 [R].

[11] Lindseth GN, Coolahan SE, Petros TV, et al. Neurobehavioral effects of aspartame consumption. Res Nurs Health. 2014;37(3):185–93 [c].

[12] Pepino MY, Tiemann CD, Patterson BW, et al. Sucralose affects glycemic and hormonal responses to an oral glucose load. Diabetes Care. 2013;36(9):2530–5 [c].

[13] Storey TF, Gilbride G, Clifford K. Postprocedural pain in shoulder arthrography: differences between using preservative-free normal saline and normal saline with benzyl alcohol as an intraarticular contrast diluent. AJR Am J Roentgenol. 2014;203(5):1059–62 [c].

[14] Deguzman ZC, O'Mara SK, Sulo S, et al. Bacteriostatic normal saline compared with buffered 1% lidocaine when injected intradermally as a local anesthetic to reduce pain during intravenous catheter insertion. J Perianesth Nurs. 2012;27(6):399–407 [c].

[15] Minogue SC, Sun DA. Bacteriostatic saline containing benzyl alcohol decreases the pain associated with the injection of propofol. Anesth Analg. 2005;100(3):683–6 [c].

[16] Lambrecht M, Mercier C, Geussens Y, et al. The effect of a supersaturated calcium phosphate mouth rinse on the development of oral mucositis in head and neck cancer patients treated with (chemo) radiation: a single-center, randomized, prospective study of a calcium phosphate mouth rinse + standard of care versus standard of care. Support Care Cancer. 2013;21(10):2663–70 [c].

[17] Rao NG, Trotti A, Kim J, et al. Phase II multicenter trial of Caphosol for the reduction of mucositis in patients receiving radiation therapy for head and neck cancer. Oral Oncol. 2014;50(8):765–9 [C].

[18] Raphael MF, den Boer AM, Kollen WJ, et al. Caphosol, a therapeutic option in case of cancer therapy-induced oral mucositis in children? Results from a prospective multicenter double blind randomized controlled trial. Support Care Cancer. 2014;22(1):3–6 [c].

[19] Pradeep Kumar SS, Easwer HV, Maya Nandkumar A. Multiple drug resistant bacterial biofilms on implanted catheters— a reservoir of infection. J Assoc Physicians India. 2013;61(10):702–7 [c].

[20] Long A, Edwards J, Thompson R, et al. A clinical evaluation of a sensor to detect blockage due to crystalline biofilm formation on indwelling urinary catheters. BJU Int. 2014;114(2):278–85 [c].

[21] Miller CA, Corbin KD, da Costa KA, et al. Effect of egg ingestion on trimethylamine-N-oxide production in humans: a randomized, controlled, dose-response study. Am J Clin Nutr. 2014;100(3):778–86 [c].

[22] Calabro RS, Cordici F, Genovese C, et al. Choline associated hypersexuality in a 79-year-old man. Arch Sex Behav. 2014;43(1):187–9 [A].

[23] Kara K, Kahlert P, Mahabadi AA, et al. Comparison of collagen-based vascular closure devices in patients with vs. without severe peripheral artery disease. J Endovasc Ther. 2014;21(1):79–84 [c].

[24] Vader P, Fens MH, Sachini N, et al. Taxol((R))-induced phosphatidylserine exposure and microvesicle formation in red blood cells is mediated by its vehicle Cremophor((R)) EL. Nanomedicine. 2013;8(7):1127–35 [E].

[25] Conti G, Chirico V, Lacquaniti A, et al. Vitamin D intoxication in two brothers: be careful with dietary supplements. J Pediatr Endocrinol Metab. 2014;27(7-8):763–7 [A].

[26] Vogiatzi MG, Jacobson-Dickman E, DeBoer MD, et al. Vitamin D supplementation and risk of toxicity in pediatrics: a review of current literature. J Clin Endocrinol Metab. 2014;99(4):1132–41 [R].

[27] Battista C, Viti R, Minisola S, et al. Over-supplementation of vitamin D in two patients with primary hyperparathyroidism. Hormones. 2013;12(4):598–601 [A].

[28] Swartzentruber GS, Yanta JH, Pizon AF. Methemoglobinemia as a complication of topical dapsone. N Engl J Med. 2015;372(5):491–2 [A].

[29] de Melo RC, Lopes R, Alves JC. A case of psychosis in disulfiram treatment for alcoholism. Case Rep Psychiatry. 2014;2014:561092 [A].

[30] Watts TE, Pandey RA, Vancil TJ. Fatal fulminant hepatic failure related to the use of disulfiram. J Ark Med Soc. 2014;110(13):280–3 [A].

[31] Amuchastegui T, Amuchastegui M, Donohue T. Disulfiram–alcohol reaction mimicking an acute coronary syndrome. Conn Med. 2014;78(2):81–4 [A].

[32] Augustsson A, Berger T. Assessing the risk of an excess fluoride intake among Swedish children in households with private wells— expanding static single-source methods to a probabilistic multi-exposure-pathway approach. Environ Int. 2014;68:192–9 [c].

[33] Estrada-Capetillo BL, Ortiz-Perez MD, Salgado-Bustamante M, et al. Arsenic and fluoride co-exposure affects the expression of apoptotic and inflammatory genes and proteins in mononuclear cells from children. Mutat Res Genet Toxicol Environ Mutagen. 2014;761:27–34 [c].

[34] Yasmin S, Ranjan S, D'Souza D. Haematological changes in fluorotic adults and children in fluoride endemic regions of Gaya district, Bihar, India. Environ Geochem Health. 2014;36(3):421–5 [c].

[35] Luhmann SJ, Sucato DJ, Bacharier L, et al. Intraoperative anaphylaxis secondary to intraosseous gelatin administration. J Pediatr Orthop. 2013;33(5):e58–60 [A].

[36] Agarwal NS, Spalding C, Nassef M. Life-threatening intraoperative anaphylaxis to gelatin in Floseal during pediatric spinal surgery. J Allergy Clin Immunol Pract. 2015;3(1):110–1 [A].

[37] Hahn RG. Glycine 1.5% for irrigation should be abandoned. Urol Int. 2013;91(3):249–55 [R].

[38] Hahn RG, Zhang W, Rajs J. Pathology of the heart after overhydration with glycine solution in the mouse. APMIS. 1996;104(12):915–20 [E].

[39] Sandfeldt L, Riddez L, Rajs J, et al. High-dose intravenous infusion of irrigating fluids containing glycine and mannitol in the pig. J Surg Res. 2001;95(2):114–25 [E].

[40] Stamler J, Brown IJ, Daviglus ML, et al. Dietary glycine and blood pressure: the International Study on macro/micronutrients and blood pressure. Am J Clin Nutr. 2013;98(1):136–45 [C].

[41] Liberek T, Sliwarska J, Czurak K, et al. Prolonged renal failure in the course of atypical ethylene glycol intoxication. Acta Biochim Pol. 2013;60(4):661–3 [A].

[42] Pillai U, Hothi JC, Bhat ZY. Severe propylene glycol toxicity secondary to use of anti-epileptics. Am J Ther. 2014;21(4):e106–9 [A].

[43] Pugin D, Foreman B, De Marchis GM, et al. Is pentobarbital safe and efficacious in the treatment of super-refractory status epilepticus: a cohort study. Crit Care. 2014;18(3):R103 [A].

[44] Lim TY, Poole RL, Pageler NM. Propylene glycol toxicity in children. J Pediatr Pharmacol Ther. 2014;19(4):277–82 [M].

[45] Hutzler C, Paschke M, Kruschinski S, et al. Chemical hazards present in liquids and vapors of electronic cigarettes. Arch Toxicol. 2014;88(7):1295–308 [E].

[46] Callahan-Lyon P. Electronic cigarettes: human health effects. Tob Control. 2014;23(Suppl 2):ii36–40 [c].

[47] Goniewicz ML, Knysak J, Gawron M, et al. Levels of selected carcinogens and toxicants in vapour from electronic cigarettes. Tob Control. 2014;23(2):133–9 [E].

[48] Jensen RP, Luo W, Pankow JF, et al. Hidden formaldehyde in e-cigarette aerosols. N Engl J Med. 2015;372(4):392–4 [E].

[49] Kosmider L, Sobczak A, Fik M, et al. Carbonyl compounds in electronic cigarette vapors: effects of nicotine solvent and battery output voltage. Nicotine Tob Res. 2014;16(10):1319–26 [E].

[50] Burstyn I. Peering through the mist: systematic review of what the chemistry of contaminants in electronic cigarettes tells us about health risks. BMC Public Health. 2014;14:18 [R].

[51] Farsalinos KE, Polosa R. Safety evaluation and risk assessment of electronic cigarettes as tobacco cigarette substitutes: a systematic review. Ther Adv Drug Saf. 2014;5(2):67–86 [R].

[52] Hilton S, Schrumpf H, Buhren BA, et al. Hyaluronidase injection for the treatment of eyelid edema: a retrospective analysis of 20 patients. Eur J Med Res. 2014;19:30 [c].

[53] Cavallini M, Antonioli B, Gazzola R, et al. Hyaluronidases for treating complications by hyaluronic acid dermal fillers: evaluation of the effects on cell cultures and human skin. Eur J Plast Surg. 2013;36(8):477–84 [E].

[54] Park S, Lim LT. Orbital inflammation secondary to a delayed hypersensitivity reaction to sub-Tenon's hyaluronidase. Semin Ophthalmol. 2014;29(2):57–8 [A].

[55] Zamora-Alejo K, Moore S, Leatherbarrow B, et al. Hyaluronidase toxicity: a possible cause of postoperative periorbital inflammation. Clin Exp Ophthalmol. 2013;41(2):122–6 [A].

[56] Patel A, Waheed U, Brett SJ. Randomised trials of 6% tetrastarch (hydroxyethyl starch 130/0.4 or 0.42) for severe sepsis reporting mortality: systematic review and meta-analysis. Intensive Care Med. 2013;39(5):811–22 [A].

[57] Kashy BK, Podolyak A, Makarova N, et al. Effect of hydroxyethyl starch on postoperative kidney function in patients having noncardiac surgery. Anesthesiology. 2014;121(4):730–9 [C].

[58] Madan I, Cullinan P, Ahmed SM. Occupational management of type I latex allergy. Occup Med. 2013;63(6):395–404 [R].

[59] Supapvanich C, Povey AC, de Vocht F. Respiratory and dermal symptoms in Thai nurses using latex products. Occup Med. 2013;63(6):425–8 [c].

[60] Larese Filon F, Bochdanovits L, Capuzzo C, et al. Ten years incidence of natural rubber latex sensitization and symptoms in a prospective cohort of health care workers using non-powdered latex gloves 2000-2009. Int Arch Occup Environ Health. 2014;87(5):463–9 [c].

[61] Boettcher M, Goettler S, Eschenburg G, et al. Prenatal latex sensitization in patients with spina bifida: a pilot study. J Neurosurg Pediatr. 2014;13:291–4 [c].

[62] Ko EM, Lippmann Q, Caron WP, et al. Clinical risk factors of PEGylated liposomal doxorubicin induced palmar plantar erythrodysesthesia in recurrent ovarian cancer patients. Gynecol Oncol. 2013;131(3):683–8 [c].

[63] Torikoshi-Hatano A, Namera A, Shiraishi H, et al. A fatal case of hypermagnesemia caused by ingesting magnesium chloride as a folk remedy. J Forensic Sci. 2013;58(6):1673–5 [A].

[64] Campbell SC, Stockmann C, Balch A, et al. Intrapartum magnesium sulfate and the potential for cardiopulmonary drug-drug interactions. Ther Drug Monit. 2014;36(4):544–8 [c].

[65] Mittendorf R, Covert R, Boman J, et al. Is tocolytic magnesium sulphate associated with increased total paediatric mortality? Lancet. 1997;350(9090):1517–8 [c].

[66] Choi H, Parmar N. The use of intravenous magnesium sulphate for acute migraine: meta-analysis of randomized controlled trials. Eur J Emerg Med. 2014;21(1):2–9 [M].

[67] Pandey K, Singh D, Lal CS, et al. Fatal acute pancreatitis in a patient with visceral leishmaniasis during miltefosine treatment. J Postgrad Med. 2013;59(4):306–8 [A].

[68] Bledzka D, Gromadzinska J, Wasowicz W. Parabens. From environmental studies to human health. Environ Int. 2014;67:27–42 [c].

[69] Kirchhof MG, de Gannes GC. The health controversies of parabens. Skin Therapy Lett. 2013;18(2):5–7 [R].

[70] LaRocca J, Binder AM, McElrath TF, et al. The impact of first trimester phthalate and phenol exposure on IGF2/H19 genomic imprinting and birth outcomes. Environ Res. 2014;133:396–406 [c].

[71] Mileva G, Baker SL, Konkle AT, et al. Bisphenol-A: epigenetic reprogramming and effects on reproduction and behavior. Int J Environ Res Public Health. 2014;11(7):7537–61 [R].

[72] Brittenden J, Cotton SC, Elders A, et al. A randomized trial comparing treatments for varicose veins. N Engl J Med. 2014;371(13):1218–27 [C].

[73] Park SW, Yun IJ, Hwang JJ, et al. Fluoroscopy-guided endovenous sclerotherapy using a microcatheter prior to endovenous laser ablation: comparison between liquid and foam sclerotherapy for varicose tributaries. Korean J Radiol. 2014;15(4):481–7 [c].

[74] Ossareh S. Clinical and economic aspects of sevelamer therapy in end-stage renal disease patients. Int J Nephrol Renov Dis. 2014;7:161–8.

[75] Morescalchi F, Costagliola C, Duse S, et al. Heavy silicone oil and intraocular inflammation. BioMed Res Int. 2014;574825:1–16 [R].

[76] Baillif S, Gastaud P. Complications of silicone oil tamponade. J Fr Ophtalmol. 2014;37(3):259–65 [R].

[77] Schwarzer H, Mazinani B, Plange N, et al. Clinical observations and occurrence of complications following heavy silicone oil surgery. BioMed Res Int. 2014;706809:1–5 [c].

[78] Banerjee PJ, Chandra A, Sullivan PM, et al. Neurotrophic corneal ulceration after retinal detachment surgery with retinectomy and endolaser: a case series. JAMA Ophthalmol. 2014;132(6):750–2 [A].

[79] Houghton SC, Reeves KW, Hankinson SE, et al. Perineal powder use and risk of ovarian cancer. J Natl Cancer Inst. 2014;106(9):dju208 1–6 [c].

Reviewer List

Name	Surname	Affiliation
Robert	Beckett	Drug Information Center, Manchester University College of Pharmacy, Fort Wayne, IN, USA
Nick	Bello, PhD	Department of Animal Sciences School of Environmental and Biological Sciences Rutgers, The State University of New Jersey 84 Lipman Drive New Brunswick, NJ 08901
Gary M.	Besinque, PharmD, FCSHP	Adjunct Assistant Professor of Pharmacy Practice - USC School of Pharmacy, Pharmacist Evidence Analyst and Strategist, Formulary Group - Cardiovascular Health, Drug Information Services, Kaiser Permanente - California Regions, Kaiser Permanente Independence Park - 1st Floor, 12254 Bellflower Blvd, Downey, CA 90242-4894, USA
Chance	Densford, BS, PharmD Candidate	Manchester University College of Pharmacy, Fort wayne, IN 46845
Carol R.	Gardner, PhD	Associate Professor, Rutgers University, Ernest Mario School of Pharmacy, Department of Pharmacology and Toxicology, Piscataway, NJ 08854-8020, USA
Joshua P.	Gray, PhD	Department of Science, United States Coast Guard Academy, New London, CT, USA
Kristopher	Hall, BS, PharmD candidate	Manchester University College of Pharmacy, Fort wayne, IN 46845.
Herb J.	Halley, PharmD	Assoc. Professor, BCPS, Director of Experiential Education, Manchester University College of Pharmacy, Fort wayne, IN 46845.

Name	Surname	Affiliation
Mary E.	Kiersma, PharmD, PhD	Department of Pharmaceutical Sciences Manchester University College of Pharmacy Fort Wayne, IN 46845
Kathryn	Loeser, PharmD candidate	Manchester University College of Pharmacy, Fort wayne, IN 46845.
Risha	Patel, PharmD candidate	Manchester University College of Pharmacy, Fort wayne, IN 46845.
Alan	Polnariev	College of Pharmacy, University of Florida, Gainesville, FL, USA
Hana	Raber, PharmD	Saint Joseph Regional Medical Center, Mishawaka, IN, USA
Sidhartha D.	Ray, PhD, FACN	Department of Pharmaceutical Sciences, Manchester University College of Pharmacy, Fort Wayne, IN, USA
David M.	Ribnicky, PhD	Department of Plant Biology & Pathology, Rutgers University, New Brunswick, NJ 08901
Brian	Spoelhoeff, PharmD, BCPS	Department of Pharmacy, Johns Hopkins Bayview Medical Center, Baltimore, MD, USA
Sidney J.	Stohs, PhD, FACN, ATS, FAATS	Dean Emeritus, Creighton University school of pharmacy, Omaha, NE 68178, USA
Andrew J.	Wiemer, PhD	Assistant Professor of Medicinal Chemistry, Department of Pharmaceutical Sciences, University of Connecticut, USA

Index of Drugs

For drug–drug interactions see the separate index. In pages 633–634.

Note: Page numbers followed by "*f*" indicate figures and "*t*" indicate tables.

Index of Drug-Drug Interactions

Index of Adverse Effects and Adverse Reactions

CPI Antony Rowe
Chippenham, UK
2015-11-05 15:46